Health Promotion Points

Home Care Considerations

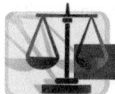

Legal & Ethical Considerations

NURSING CARE PLANS

Patient Teaching

Continued

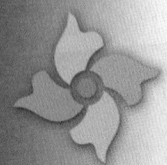

SPECIAL FEATURES—cont'd

Safety Alert

Skills

Steps

Continued

COMPANION CD-ROM RESOURCES

ADDITIONAL NURSING CARE PLANS, SKILLS, STEPS, AND PROCESS RECORDING

Nursing Care Plan 8-1: Care of the Patient with Impaired Communication
Nursing Care Plan 16-2: Care of the Patient with a Foot Wound
Nursing Care Plan 17-2: Care of the Patient Under Droplet Precautions
Sample of Process Recording 8-1: Communicating with the Patient Who Is Withdrawn
Skill 37-2: Performing a Surgical Prep
Steps 36-4: Changing the IV Tube

ANIMATIONS

Auscultation of Heart Valves
Cardiac Cycle During Systole and Diastole
Changes in Body Proportion
Classification of Joints: Condyloid Joint (Hand)
Classification of Joints: Gliding Joint (Hand)
Classification of Joints: Hinge Joint
Classification of Joints: Saddle Joint (Hand)
Comparison of Drug Absorption by Route of Administration
Digestion, Entire Process
Distribution: Fat-Soluble vs. Water-Soluble Drugs
Drug Movement Through the Body
Drug Receptors: Agonists
Functions of the Respiratory System
Insertion of Foley Catheter (male and female)
The Kidneys
Main Organ: Large Intestine
Menstrual Cycle
Metabolic Rates
Motor Pathways and Clinical Evaluation
Nasogastric Tube Placement (procedure)
Opening an Airway (emergency)
Oxygen Administration
Patterns of Respirations
Percussion Tones
Pulse Oximeter
Pulse Quality
Pulse Variations
Receptor Interaction
Reflex Arc
Respirations
Sensory Pathways and Clinical Evaluation of Central Nervous System

AUDIO CLIPS

Aortic Ejection Sound Related to S1
Bronchial Breath Sounds
Bronchovesicular Breath Sounds
Diastolic Murmur
Fourth Heart Sound (S4)
Fourth Heart Sound (S4) with Bell Held Lightly then Applied Firmly
High-Pitched Crackles
High-Pitched Wheeze
Low-Pitched Crackles
Low-Pitched Wheeze
Midsystolic Click Sound Related to S1
Murmurs: Blowing, Harsh or Rough, and Rumble
Murmurs: High, Medium, and Low
Paradoxical Split Sound Related to S2
Pericardial Friction Rub
Pleural Friction Rub
Pulmonic Ejection Sound Related to S1
S1 at Various Locations
S2 at Various Locations
Single S1
Single S2
Stridor
Systolic Murmur
Third Heart Sound (S3)
Vesicular Breath Sounds
Wide Split Sound Related to S2

CRITICAL THINKING REVIEW

DORLAND'S AUDIO PRONUNCIATIONS

FLUIDS AND ELECTROLYTES MODULE

FORMS

Admission Record for Skilled Nursing
Medication Administration Record
Patient Admission Assessment Form

HELPFUL PHRASES FOR COMMUNICATING IN SPANISH

MATHEMATICS REVIEW

Roman Numerals
Fractions
Decimals
Percentage
Proportion
Fahrenheit and Celsius
Systems of Measurement

PERFORMANCE CHECKLISTS FOR SKILLS AND STEPS

VIDEO CLIPS

Auscultation: Abdomen, Bowel Sounds (Adult Male)
Auscultation: Carotid Artery (adult male)
Dressing Changes: Wet to Dry
Enteral Feedings
Evaluation: Central Vision and Visual Acuity (adult male)
Evaluation: Pupil Responses, Direct and Accomodation, Cranial Nerves III, IV, and VI—Oculomotor, Trochlear and Abducens Nerves (adult male)
Evaluation: Pupil Responses, Direct and Consensual (older adult female)
Evaluation: Sensory, Light Touch; Face, Upper and Lower Extremities, Cranial Nerve V—Trigeminal Nerve (older adult female)
Evaluation: Smell, Cranial Nerve I—Olfactory Nerve (adult male)
Inspection and Palpation: Breathing and Respiratory Excursion, Anterior Chest (adult male)
Inspection and Palpation: Cardiac Auscultory Landmarks (adult male)
Inspection and Palpation: Cardiac, Anterior Chest (adult female)
Inspection and Palpation: External Ear (adult male)
Inspection and Palpation: External Eye (adult male)
Inspection and Palpation: Muscular Development (adult male)
Inspection and Palpation: Pulses, Lower Extremities (adult female)
Inspection and Palpation: Respiration, Respiratory Excursion and Tactile Fremitus, Posterior Chest (adult male)
Inspection and Palpation: Standing Position (younger adult male)
Inspection and Percussion: Diaphragmatic Excursion (adult male)
Inspection: Ear Canal (adult male)
Inspection: Female Breasts (sitting position) (adult female)
Inspection: Fine Motor Coordination, Lower Extremities (older adult female)
Inspection: Fine Motor Coordination, Upper Extremities (older adult male)
Inspection: Gait (older adult female)
Inspection: General Muscular Strength (adult male)
Inspection: Nose (adult female)
Intake and Output
Intradermal Medications
Intramuscular Injections
Midstream Urine Collection
Palpation: Abdomen Superficial and Deep (adult male)
Palpation: Female Breasts (supine position) (adult female)
Percussion: Abdomen (adult male)
Percussion: Anterior Thorax (adult male)
Percussion: Liver (adult male)
Percussion: Spleen (adult male)
Positioning and Transfers
Pulse: Measuring an Apical Pulse
Respirations: How to Measure Respirations
Sputum Specimen
Sterile Gloving
Subcutaneous Injections
Urinary Catheter Care
Wound VAC

FUNDAMENTAL CONCEPTS AND SKILLS FOR NURSING

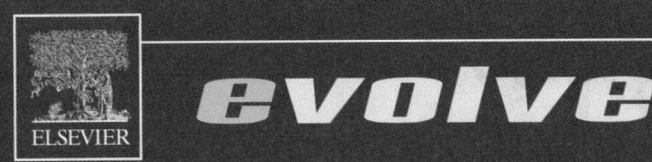

To access your Student Resources, visit the web address below:

http://evolve.elsevier.com/deWit/fundamental/

Evolve® Student Resources for *Fundamental Concepts and Skills for Nursing,* **3rd Edition,** offer the following features:

Student Resources

- **NCLEX-PN® Examination–Style Interactive Review Questions**
  Test your knowledge with interactive questions and rationales for correct and incorrect responses.

- **Animations**
  Learn through vivid visualizations of anatomy and physiology and physiologic processes.

- **Audio and Video Clips**
  Content comes alive with authentic heart and lung sounds and assessment skill videos.

- **Mathematics Review**
  Build a solid foundation for medication administration with this review of basic arithmetic skills.

- **Dorland's Audio Pronunciations**
  Learn to pronounce difficult medical terms with this helpful tool.

- **Forms, Additional Care Plans, Skills and Steps, Performance Checklists, Useful Resources**

- **Additional Resources**
  Electronic Anatomy and Physiology Body Spectrum book, Concept Map Creator, Helpful Phrases for Communicating in Spanish, and more!

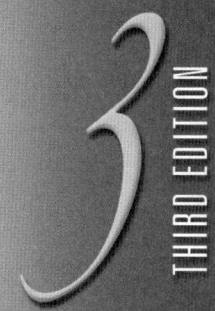

THIRD EDITION

FUNDAMENTAL CONCEPTS AND SKILLS FOR NURSING

Susan C. deWit, MSN, RN, CNS, PHN

Formerly, Instructor of Nursing
El Centro College
Dallas, Texas

Photographs by Jack Sanders, Portland, Oregon

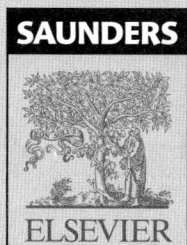

SAUNDERS

ELSEVIER

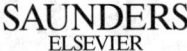

11830 Westline Industrial Drive
St. Louis, Missouri 63146

Notice

Knowledge and best practice in this field are constantly changing. As new research and experience broaden our knowledge, changes in practice, treatment and drug therapy may become necessary or appropriate. Readers are advised to check the most current information provided (i) on procedures featured or (ii) by the manufacturer of each product to be administered, to verify the recommended dose or formula, the method and duration of administration, and contraindications. It is the responsibility of the practitioner, relying on their own experience and knowledge of the patient, to make diagnoses, to determine dosages and the best treatment for each individual patient, and to take all appropriate safety precautions. To the fullest extent of the law, neither the Publisher nor the Author assumes any liability for any injury and/or damage to persons or property arising out of or related to any use of the material contained in this book.

The Publisher

Previous editions copyrighted 2001, 2005

Library of Congress Cataloging-in-Publication Data

DeWit, Susan C.
  Fundamental concepts and skills for nursing / Susan C. DeWit ; photographs by Jack Sanders. — 3rd ed.
    p. ; cm.
  Includes bibliographical references and index.
  ISBN-13: 978-1-4160-5228-9 (pbk. : alk. paper)
  ISBN-10: 1-4160-5228-3 (pbk. : alk. paper)   1.   Nursing.   I. Title.
  [DNLM: 1.   Nursing Process. 2.   Nursing Care.   WY 100 D521f 2009]
  RT41.D443 2009
  610.73—dc22   2008032018

Vice President, Publishing Director: Sally Schrefer
Executive Publisher: Tom Wilhelm
Managing Editor: Robin Levin Richman
Developmental Editor: Mayoor Jaiswal
Publishing Services Manager: Jeffrey Patterson
Senior Project Manager: Mary G. Stueck
Book Designer: Teresa McBryan
Marketing Project Manager: Jamie Kitsis

Printed in Canada

Last digit is the print number: 9 8 7 6 5 4 3 2 1

To my lovely daughter and great son-in-law,
Kristen and Scott Webster, who I wish lived closer to me

To my extended family and young cousins
who bring support, love, and fun

To my contributors, colleagues, and editors who lend
insight and depth to my research and writing

To the nursing students who work so hard to gain knowledge
and to excellently apply it in their chosen profession

and

To the memory of my aunt, "Bogie,"
who will always be in my heart.

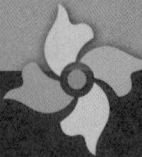

Contributors/Reviewers

CONTRIBUTORS

CAROL DALLRED, MSN, RNC, WHCNP
Advanced Practice Nurse
University of Texas
M.D. Anderson Cancer Center
Houston, Texas

CANDICE K. KUMAGAI, MSN, RN
Instructor in Clinical Nursing
University of Texas at Austin
Austin, Texas

PATRICIA A. O'NEILL, MSN, RN, CCRN
Nursing Instructor
DeAnza College
Cupertino, California

FRANCES M. WARRICK, RN, MS
Program Coordinator, Vocational Nursing
El Centro College
Dallas, Texas

BARBARA WRAY WAYLAND, ASN, RN
Consultant and Writer
San Luis Obispo, California
Formerly, Nurse Educator
Marian Hospital
Santa Maria, California;
Former Director of Nursing
San Luis Obispo General Hospital
San Luis Obispo, California

REVIEWERS

JEAN BURDEN, BSN, RN
Instructor
Ohio Hi-Point Career Center
Bellefontaine, Ohio

BRIGITTE L. CASTEEL, MSN, RN
Associate Professor; Program Director
Practical Nursing Program
Mountain Empire Community College
Big Stone Gap, Virginia

MICHELE CISLO, RN, MA, CPN
Assistant Professor, Practical Nursing
Union County College
Plainfield, New Jersey

BRENDA INGRAHAM CUCUKOV, BSN, RN, BS
Instructor
Vineland Adult School of LPN
Vineland, New Jersey

JEANNE HATELY, PhD, MSN, RN, PLNC
Regional Nursing Director
Corinthian Colleges, Inc.
Santa Ana, California

MARY ANN KENNEDY, BSN, RNC, MAT
Instructor
J.M. Wright Technical School
Stamford, Connecticut

CAROLYN H. LANGER, MSN, RN
Instructor
State of Connecticut Practical Nurse Program
Middletown, Connecticut

KAY B. O'NEAL, MSN, RN
Instructor
El Centro Community College
Dallas, Texas

ELAINE POLAN, PhD, RNC, MS
Instructor
Vocational Education & Extension Board
Practical Nurse Program
Uniondale, New York

CARLOTTA SOUTH, RN, AAS, ADN
Instructor
San Jacinot College North
Houston, Texas

COLLENE THAXTON, MS, BS
Instructor
Mount Wachusett Community College
Devens, Massachusetts

ANN LEIPHART UNHOLZ, BSN, RN, MS
Adjunct Instructor (retired)
J.S. Reynolds Community College;
Director Health and Medical Sciences
Henrico County Public Schools
Richmond, Virginia

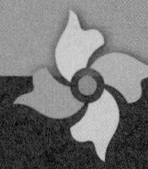

To the Instructor

Fundamental Concepts and Skills for Nursing, third edition, written especially for LPN/LVN students, incorporates aspects of nursing in all of the major settings in which LPN/LVNs are employed: hospitals, long-term care facilities, clinics, physicians' offices, and home care agencies.

This text teaches all the basic concepts and fundamental skills that an LPN/LVN needs in current practice. The material is presented from simple to complex, with clarity and conciseness of language, making the fundamental concepts and skills content readily comprehended by beginning nursing students. Because there are so many students with English as their second language entering nursing, this book has been reviewed and edited by an English-as-a-Second-Language specialist to make the language as clear as possible.

As the role of the LPN/LVN expands, there is an even greater need for a thorough knowledge of the nursing process and problem solving. **Nursing process** is the underlying theme of the text and is interwoven with these six threads: (1) focus on the patient as a consumer of health care with psychosocial as well as physical needs; (2) critical thinking as a tool for learning, problem solving, and developing clinical judgment; (3) communication as an essential tool for the art and practice of nursing; (4) collaboration with other health care workers and the use of management and supervision to provide coordinated, cost-effective patient care; (5) teaching for the maintenance of wellness and promotion of self-care; and (6) integration of cultural sensitivity and cultural competence into patient care.

It is important to remember that because of the difference in state laws, LPN/LVNs in some states may be certified to perform a variety of tasks related to IV fluid therapy, but in other states IV therapy is not within the scope of practice. We do include skills on IV therapy since so many schools teach a separate short course on it for IV certification for their students. Consult your state nurse practice act for more information.

ORGANIZATION OF THE TEXT

CONTENT

The text is divided into the following nine units: *One,* Introduction to Nursing and the Health Care System; *Two,* The Nursing Process; *Three,* Communication in Nursing; *Four,* Developmental, Psychosocial, and Cultural Considerations; *Five,* Basic Nursing Skills; *Six,* Meeting Basic Physiologic Needs; *Seven,* Medication Administration; *Eight,* Care of the Surgical and Immobile Patient; *Nine,* Caring for the Elderly.

In this third edition, we are pleased to include the following new content:
- The most current CPR guidelines from the American Heart Association are included along with the latest information for families on the new guidelines on bystander CPR
- The new MyPyramid is presented and dietary guidelines have been updated
- Evidence-based nursing and best practices
- Updated isolation information from the CDC
- Current immunization guidelines
- Ethnopharmacy (how patients from different ethnicities metabolize drugs)

The following key content areas and major concepts are covered:
- Health care delivery, collaborative care, and changing role of the LPN/LVN
- Concepts of the nursing process and their application to clinical situations
- Nurse-patient and family communication
- Professional communication
- Management, supervision, and delegation
- Health promotion and patient education
- *Healthy People 2010* Objectives and National Patient Safety Goals
- Growth and development from infancy through adulthood, with special attention to the aging population
- Cultural sensitivity in nursing care, with an additional perspective provided by an English-as-a-Second-Language specialist
- Full chapter on loss, grief, end-of-life care, and palliative care
- Basic nursing skills, including current information about infection control in the health care setting and home, dangers of drug-resistant infections, prevention of pressure ulcers, patient safety, and assessment of health status
- Concepts and skills needed to meet basic physiologic needs, including the latest in pain control interventions
- Complete unit on medication knowledge and administration, with a section on blood product administration
- A chapter on the administration of intravenous fluids and medications
- Care of surgical patients, care of immobile patients, including those needing care of wounds and pressure ulcers; promotion of musculoskeletal function
- Physiologic and psychosocial care of the aging patient

STANDARD LPN THREADS FEATURES

The following LPN Threads features are found in *Fundamental Concepts and Skills for Nursing*, third edition:

- **Full-color design, cover, photos,** and **illustrations** are visually appealing and pedagogically useful.
- **ESL (English as a Second Language)** considerations figure prominently in both the textbook and its Student Learning Guide. An ESL specialist has reviewed all chapters during development to make sure they will be clearly understood by ESL students and students with limited proficiency in English.
- **Key Terms with phonetic pronunciations and text page references** help improve and supplement terminology and language skills of ESL students and students with limited proficiency in English before they enter clinical practice. Key Terms are in color at first mention in the text (all Key Terms are in the Glossary).
- **Objectives** (numbered) in the chapter opener and divided into Theory and Clinical categories provide a framework for content and are especially important to the TEACH Lesson Plans for the book, which is structured around chapter objectives.
- **Critical Thinking Activities** at the end of chapters include a realistic clinical case scenario and a clinical situation, both of which provide ample opportunity for students to hone their critical thinking skills. *Answers are provided in the TEACH Instructor Resources on the Evolve website.*
- **Key Points** are located at the end of chapters and summarize chapter highlights.

SPECIAL FEATURES

The following pedagogic features help students understand and apply the chapter content:

- **Overview of Structure and Function:** In chapters where an understanding of anatomy and physiology is necessary to comprehend the chapter content, a brief **review of the body system** directly precedes the main text of the chapter.
- **Application of the Nursing Process:** Once the basic concepts of nursing and the nursing process are introduced in Unit Two, the **nursing process** is integrated in succeeding chapters.
- **Assignment Considerations** provide suggestions for assigning or delegating tasks or work to other health team members.
- **Clinical Cues** contain pointers for practical application in the clinical setting.
- **Communication Cues** address **therapeutic communication** and developing facility in interacting with patients and other health professionals,

which are major components of nursing education. This feature presents typical dialogue and ways to handle different situations.

- **Complementary & Alternative Therapies** provide information on different therapies for specific problems.
- **Concept Maps** are visualizations of processes that help students make sense of information that is typically more difficult to learn.
- **Cultural Cues** provide specific information to consider when working with a patient from a particular culture.
- **Elder Care Points** highlight points of care for the older population and appear throughout the chapters to emphasize the changes that occur with age and the adjustments needed for delivery of nursing care to older adults. **Elder Care Points** are also presented within the Skills, where appropriate, in various chapters. Together with Chapters 13, 40, and 41 on nursing care specific to the older adult, this content covers the major areas of gerontology in the LPN/LVN curriculum.
- **Focused Assessment** provides a guide to assess a particular body system.
- **Health Promotion Points** highlight patient teaching for wellness and disease prevention.
- **Home Care Considerations** highlight the changes necessary to adapt nursing care skills and techniques to the needs of the patient in the home setting. These are also presented within the Skills, where appropriate, in various chapters.
- **Legal & Ethical Considerations** focus on specific legal or ethical concerns.
- **Patient Teaching** highlights special teaching points and teaching plans for promoting wellness, preventing illness, and encouraging self care.
- **NCLEX-PN® Examination–Style Review Questions** at the end of each chapter include multiple-choice and alternate-format questions to help students familiarize themselves with the format and prepare for the examination. *Answers are provided at the end of the book.*
- **Nursing Care Plans:** These illustrate each step of the nursing process. Each nursing diagnosis is supported by the accompanying assessment data, and Critical Thinking Questions are provided at the end of each care plan. The nursing care plan has been chosen as the focus for care planning since it is such an integral part of teaching the **nursing process**. A sample critical pathway is included in Chapter 6 to illustrate how collaborative care is planned and implemented. *Answers to Critical Thinking Questions in the Nursing Care Plans are provided in the TEACH Instructor Resources on the Evolve website.*
- **Safety Alerts** point out specific concerns for patient safety and ways to prevent harm to patients.

- **Skills:** Seventy-five of the major skills that require mastery in most LPN/LVN programs are presented with full-color photographs in a step-by-step format that emphasizes use of the nursing process and includes rationales for each step, as well as Critical Thinking Questions at the end of each skill. Performance Checklists for all skills are located in the Student Learning Guide. Additional Performance Checklists can be found on the Companion CD-ROM and on the Evolve website. *Answers to Critical Thinking Questions in these Skills are provided in the TEACH Instructor Resources on the Evolve website.*

- **Steps:** Steps are shorter versions of skills. These 37 other procedures that nurses are expected to perform are presented step-by-step with rationales. Performance Checklists for all steps are found on the Companion CD-ROM and on the Evolve website.

- **Think Critically About . . .** boxes ask students to think critically about the chapter content or to **apply concepts** outside the context of the chapter.

- **Appendixes:** *Appendix 1* provides the ANA Standards of Practice. *Appendix 2* presents the ANA Code of Ethics. *Appendix 3* represents the Standard Steps protocol for the performance of each Skill and Step. *Appendix 4* provides the NFLPN Code for Nurses. *Appendix 5* lists the CDC Standard Precautions for the care of all patients. *Appendix 6* contains a table of the basic common laboratory test values. A detailed version of most common laboratory test values can be found on the Evolve website. *Appendix 7* offers some basic therapeutic diets for various types of patients. *Appendix 8* presents the basic principles, prefixes, suffixes, and abbreviations needed to learn medical terminology. *Appendix 9* provides the Answer Key for the NCLEX-PN® Examination–Style Review Questions at the end of each chapter.

- **Bolded text** throughout the narrative emphasizes key concepts and practice.

TEACHING AND LEARNING PACKAGE

We provide a rich, abundant collection of supplemental resources for both instructors and students.

FOR THE INSTRUCTOR
TEACH Instructor Resources

The new, comprehensive TEACH Instructor Resources on the Evolve website provide a wealth of material to meet your teaching needs, in addition to everything in the Student Resources, including NCLEX-PN® Examination–Style Interactive Review Questions:

- **ExamView Test Bank** contains over 1000 NCLEX-PN® Examination–Style Questions, multiple-choice as well as alternate-format questions.

- **TEACH Lesson Plans with PowerPoint Lecture Outlines,** based on textbook chapter learning objectives, provide a roadmap to link and integrate all parts of the educational package. These concise and straightforward lesson plans can be modified or combined to meet scheduling and teaching needs.

- **PowerPoint Presentation** provides over 2000 text and image slides.

- **Open-Book Quizzes** for each chapter in the textbook vary instructor testing options.

- **Image Collection** includes all the illustrations and photographs from the book plus supplemental images from other Elsevier titles that can be easily incorporated into the PowerPoint presentations.

- **iClicker (Audience Response) Questions** promote interactive learning and feedback for instructors in the classroom.

- **Answer Keys** to the Critical Thinking Activities and Critical Thinking Questions in the textbook, and Student Learning Guide activities and exercises.

FOR THE STUDENT

- **Companion CD-ROM** (bound with text) includes Audio and Video Clips; Animations, including ARCHIE-MD® animations of Anatomy and Physiology; Dorland's Audio Pronunciations; Helpful Phrases for Communicating in Spanish; Critical Thinking Review; Mathematics Review; Fluids and Electrolytes Module; selected forms used in health care settings; additional Nursing Care Plans; additional Skills and Steps; and Performance Checklists for all Skills and Steps.

- **Student Learning Guide** contains various types of questions and activities including the following sections: **Terminology; Short Answer; Completion; Multiple Choice NCLEX-PN® Examination Review Questions; Application of the Nursing Process; Priority Setting; Identification; Review of Structure and Function; Critical Thinking Activities; Clinical Activities; and Steps Toward Better Communication Activities.** The activities are designed to (1) reinforce material in the text chapter; (2) provide practice in priority setting; (3) guide practice in application of the nursing process; and (4) stimulate synthesis, analysis, and application necessary for the development of critical thinking skills and clinical judgment. **Performance Checklists** for Skills are included for each chapter, beginning with Chapter 15.

- **Application of the Nursing Process** helps students make the connection between the conceptual nursing process, often very difficult to comprehend, and real-life patient care.

- The special section, **Steps Toward Better Communication,** is written by an English-as-a-Second-

Language specialist to assist students with limited proficiency in English to gain a greater command of English pronunciation and medical language, while reinforcing chapter content. This section is subdivided into Vocabulary Building Glossary, Completion Exercise, Vocabulary Exercise, Word Attack Skills, Communication Exercise, and Cultural Points. There are examples and practice in appropriate dialogue needed for patient interaction and delegation of tasks.

- *Answers to questions in the Student Learning Guide appear in the TEACH Instructor Resources on Evolve.*
- **Evolve Learning System Student Resources** include everything on the Companion CD as well as the Anatomy and Physiology Body Spectrum Coloring Book, a Concept Map Creator, forms used in health care settings; most common laboratory test values; and useful resources. NCLEX-PN® Examination–Style Interactive Review Questions test your students' knowledge and help in preparation for licensure.
- **Virtual Clinical Excursion (VCE)** is an interactive workbook CD-ROM that guides the student through a multifloor virtual hospital in a hands-on clinical experience. With limited clinical space for LPN/LVN students, the VCE is an excellent opportunity for "hands-on" practice.

● ● ●

Teaching nursing has been one of the most exciting and gratifying phases of my life. I hope this textbook and its ancillaries make your job as an instructor easier and class preparation more time-efficient. May your students find excitement and joy in learning and applying the information you impart in the clinical setting.

SUSAN C. deWIT, MSN, RN, CNS, PHN

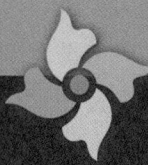

LPN Threads

Fundamental Concepts and Skills for Nursing, third edition, shares some features and design elements with other LPN titles on the Elsevier list. The purpose of these LPN Threads is to make it easier for students and instructors to use the variety of books required by the relatively brief and demanding LPN curriculum.

The shared features in *Fundamental Concepts and Skills for Nursing*, third edition, include the following:

- A **reading level evaluation** is performed on every manuscript chapter during the book's development. The purpose is to increase the consistency among chapters and to make the text easy to understand.
- Cover and internal **design similarities**. The colorful, student-friendly design encourages the reading and learning of the core content.
- Numbered lists of **Objectives** that begin each chapter.
- **Key Terms** with phonetic pronunciations and page number references at the beginning of each chapter. The key terms are in color the first time they appear in the chapter.
- **Critical Thinking Questions** at the end of every Nursing Care Plan.
- Bulleted lists of **Key Points** at the end of each chapter.
- A **Bibliography** at the end of the text.
- A **Glossary** at the end of the text.
- A wide variety of Special Features related to critical thinking, clinical practice, care of the older adult, health promotion, safety, patient teaching, complementary and alternative therapies, communication, home health care, legal and ethical considerations, delegation and assignment, and more!

And for instructors . . .

- An **ExamView Test Bank** with the following categories of information: Topic, Step of the Nursing Process, Objective, Cognitive Level, NCLEX-PN® Category of Client Need, Correct Answer, Rationale, and Text Page Reference.
- A **PowerPoint slide presentation** in the TEACH Instructors Resources on Evolve.
- **Lesson Plans** in the TEACH Instructor Resources on Evolve.
- A **PowerPoint Lecture Outline** in the TEACH Instructor Resources on Evolve.
- **Open-Book Quizzes** in the TEACH Instructor Resources on Evolve.
- **Student Learning Guide answer key** in the TEACH Instructor Resources on Evolve.
- **Tips for teaching English as a Second Language (ESL) students** in the TEACH Instructor Resources on Evolve.

In addition to content and design threads, these LPN textbooks benefit from the advice and input of the Elsevier LPN Advisory Board.

LPN Advisory Board

SHIRLEY ANDERSON, MSN
Kirkwood Community College
Cedar Rapids, Iowa

M. GIE ARCHER, MS, RN, C, WHCNP
Dean of Health Sciences
LVN Program Coordinator
North Central Texas College
Gainesville, Texas

MARY BROTHERS, MEd, RN
Coordinator, Garnet Career Center School of
   Practical Nursing
Charleston, West Virginia

PATRICIA A. CASTALDI, RN, BSN, MSN
Union County College
Plainfield, New Jersey

MARY ANN COSGAREA, RN, BSN
PN Coordinator/Health Coordinator
Portage Lakes Career Center
Green, Ohio

DOLORES ANN COTTON, RN, BSN, MS
Meridian Technology Center
Stillwater, Oklahoma

LORA LEE CRAWFORD, RN, BSN
Emanuel Turlock Vocational Nursing
   Program
Turlock, California

RUTH ANN ECKENSTEIN, RN, BS, MED
Oklahoma Department of Career and
   Technology Education
Stillwater, Oklahoma

GAIL ANN HAMILTON FINNEY, RN, MSN
Nursing Education Specialist
Concorde Career Colleges, INC
Mission, Kansas

PAM HINCKLEY, RN, MSN
Redlands Adult School
Redlands, California

DEBORAH W. KELLER, RN, BSN, MSN
Erie Huron Ottawa Vocational Education
   School of Practical Nursing
Milan, Ohio

PATTY KNECHT, MSN, RN
Nursing Program Director
Center for Arts & Technology
Brandywine Campus
Coatesville, Pennsylvania

**LIEUTENANT COLONEL (RET) TERESA Y. McPHER-
SON, RN, BSN, MSN**
LVN Program Director
Nursing Education
St. Philip's College
San Antonio, Texas

FRANCES NEU, MS, BSN, RN
Supervisor, Adult Ed Health
Butler Technology and Career Development
   Schools
Fairfield Township, Ohio

DIANNA DANCED SCHERLIN, MS, RN
National Director of Nursing
Lincoln Educational Services
West Orange, New Jersey

BEVERLEY TURNER, MA, RN
Director, Vocational Nursing Department
Maric College, San Diego Campus
San Diego, California

C. SUE WEIDMAN, RN, BSN
Brown Mackie College Nurse Specialist
Forest, Ohio

SISTER ANN WIESEN, RN, MRA
Erwin Technical Center
Tampa, Florida

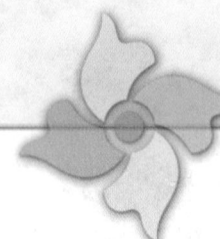

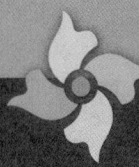

Acknowledgments

Fundamental Concepts and Skills for Nursing is the result of the creative efforts of many people. I am especially grateful to the contributors, consultants, and reviewers for their expertise, suggestions, and finished work. Their perspectives from the various geographical areas of the United States and Canada have lent a broader viewpoint of current nursing practice.

Thanks to the following people for their hard work and dedication to prepare a great ancillary package with the textbook: Patricia Delmoe for the ExamView test bank; Daniel Matusiak for the Open Book Quizzes; Mary E. Lewis for the NCLEX-PN® Examination–Style Interactive Review Questions; Amanda Swisher for iClicker Questions; Charla Hollin and Suzy Harrington for the PowerPoint presentation; and Jennifer Ponto for the TEACH Lesson Plans. The dedicated staff at Elsevier has provided tireless support and expertise from the initial concept of the book to the cohesive finished product. Special thanks to Terri Wood, former Senior Acquisitions Editor for the first edition, whose vision, attention to detail, and excellent managerial skills were key to the project's success. I am very grateful to Robin Levin Richman, Managing Editor, who attended to every detail throughout each phase of the book's creation for both the first and second editions. Her friendship, wonderful sense of humor, constant support, patience, and commitment to excellence assisted with maintaining the quality of the text for this third edition. Thanks to Mayoor Jaiswal, my Developmental Editor, who oversaw every detail throughout this revision, and is skilled, patient, and very helpful. Marie Thomas, Editorial Assistant, has been, as usual, extremely efficient and helpful and has attended to every request very quickly. Mary Stueck, our production manager, made certain that problems were solved and skillfully attended to all aspects of production and printing of the text. Megan Westerfeld's copyediting skills and phenomenal attention to the details of the text enhanced the continuity and readability of the text. Jamie Kitsis, Marketing Manager, applied her creative ideas to promote the book and announce its presence to students and instructors. The design of the book, following the Threads design of other Elsevier LPN/LVN texts, was provided by Teresa McBryan. Thanks for all the efforts of these diligent, creative, professional people.

Thanks to Gail Boehme, our English-as-a-Second-Language specialist, who reviewed manuscript and made suggestions that make this text more understandable for the student with limited proficiency in English. Thanks to Kathleen Stilling, RN, MS, who provided help with clinical questions, review of page proof, and checking URLS, statistics, and countless other details. I could not do this book without her. The artistry, many hours, and creative eye of Jack Sanders, our photographer, lent the visual appeal and clinical detail needed to illustrate the concepts and skills of all three editions. Ginger Navarro, RN, did a wonderful job coordinating the photography shoots, facilities, and models for the third edition. The fine artwork in the first edition was provided by Observatory Group, Inc of Cincinnati, Ohio, and continues to enhance the colorful presentation and provide clinical detail for the skills in the book. New art work was rendered by Graphic World, and has added pleasing visuals to this edition.

Many thanks also to Southwest Washington Medical Center and in-patient surgery units, and particularly the beautiful new orthopedic unit where photos were taken for this third edition. Thanks to the employees who contributed their time and talents to the first and second editions—Michael Burdick, RN; George Vaughan, Respiratory Therapist; George Hess; Vanessa Givands; Michele Reeves, RN; Rebecca Juan, RN; Dale T. Vaughn; George Ellis; James A. Jones; Lani Ching; Nancy Sloan, RN; Patricia Madsen; Pamela Hess; Melvin F. Warren; Norbu Moenbook, CNA; Jan Rezac, CNA; Rena Rataczak, LPN; Terry Moreno; Scott Reistar, RN; Matt Haven, RN; Debra McQueen. Gratitude to Susan Hastings, Jennifer Clark, Ginger Navarro, Francisco Navarro, Elyssa Morris, Rossana Gratrix, Ryan Parker, Jerry Hooper, Darrell Coffey, Oyelena Mitibjeck, Deborah Werst, Lettie Tadeo, Yony Russell, Olga Perez, Carrie Lujan, and Joel Gilinsky who were models in this third edition. staff and residents of Rose Vista Nursing Center; staff and students of Clark County Skills Center; staff and residents of Better Options Adult Family Home of Vancouver, Solvang Lutheran Home, Solvang, California; Marian Medical Center of Santa Maria, California; and models for the first edition Patricia Madsen, Seth, Micah, and Becca Wilkerson, Savannah and Scott Thacker, Chitra Prentice, Royce Wallace, and Janie Boxer.

Appreciation to all my nursing colleagues who comprise my e-mail network across the country and who contributed expertise and encouragement throughout the project.

SUSAN C. deWIT, MSN, RN, CNS, PHN

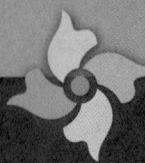

To the Student

Designed specifically with the LPN/LVN student in mind, *Fundamental Concepts and Skills for Nursing,* third edition, will help you learn basic nursing care with its visually appealing and easy-to-use format.

COMPANION CD-ROM

Packaged with the textbook, this includes audio pronunciations from *Dorland's Medical Dictionary;* health assessment videos and audio clips; animations; Mathematics Review; Fluids and Electrolytes Tutorial; selected complete medical record forms; additional Nursing Care Plans, Skills, and Steps; and much more. Using these resources as you study can help you master the material.

Following are some of the numerous special features that will help you understand and apply the material.

Theory and Clinical Objectives highlight the chapter's main learning goals

Key Terms with phonetic pronunciations and text page references are identified in bold color and defined when they first appear in the chapter

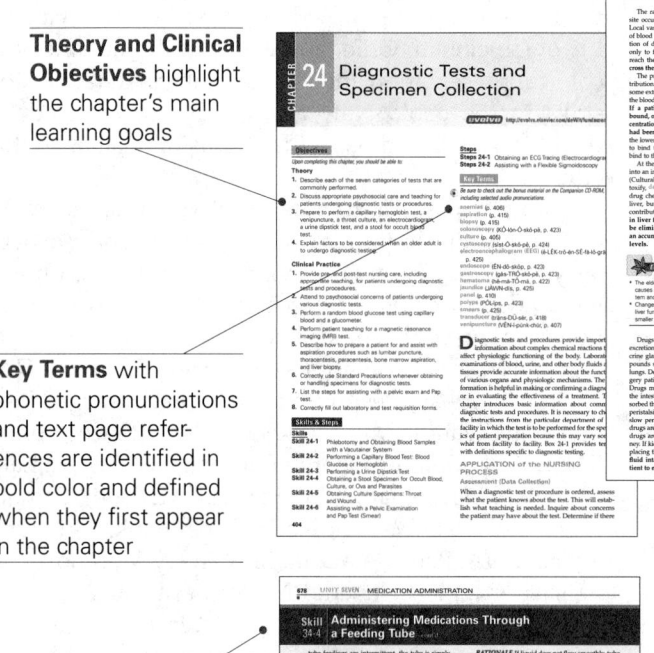

Cultural Cues provide information and strategies to help the nurse give culturally sensitive care

Assignment Considerations address the responsibility of the LPN/LVN for assigning tasks and, if permitted, delegating tasks to unlicensed assistive personnel

Skills provide illustrated, step-by-step instructions for performing key nursing procedures, and include clear actions and rationales, and Critical Thinking Questions

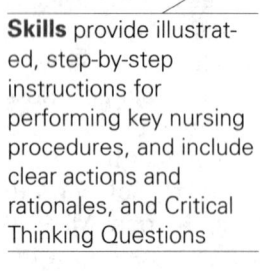

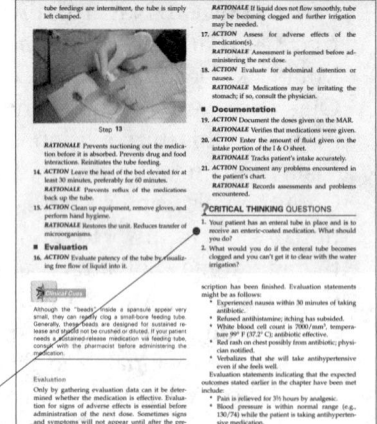

Critically Thinking Questions appear at the end of every Skill

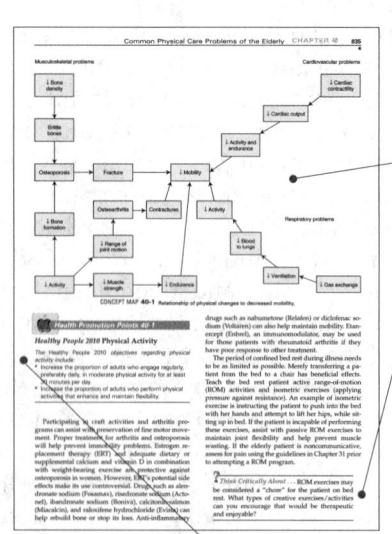

Concept Maps help visualize difficult content

Think Critically About . . . boxes encourage students to synthesize information and apply concepts beyond the scope of the chapter

Health Promotion Points address supporting wellness and preventing disease, including content on diet, infection control, and more

Overview of Structure and Function provides a basic review of anatomy and physiology with a special section on changes due to aging

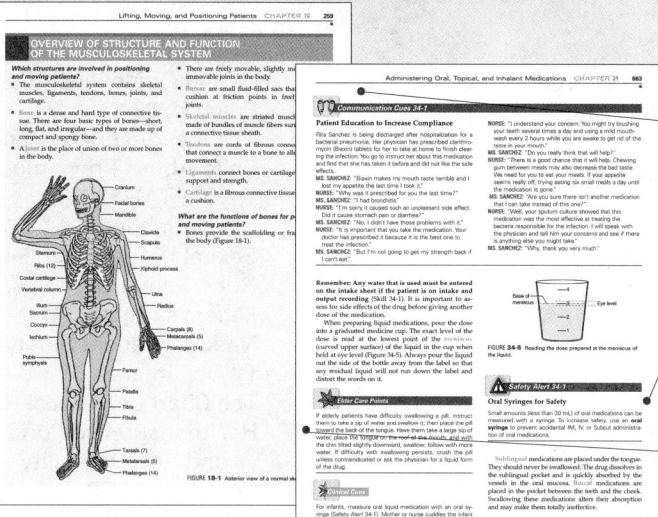

Communication Cues present sample nurse-patient dialogues and instructive therapeutic communication techniques

Safety Alerts highlight potentially dangerous situations as well as common clinical mistakes, to help students recognize and prevent errors

Elder Care Points introduce students to the unique care issues that affect older adults

Application of the Nursing Process and **Nursing Care Plans** help you to apply the nursing process to real-life situations

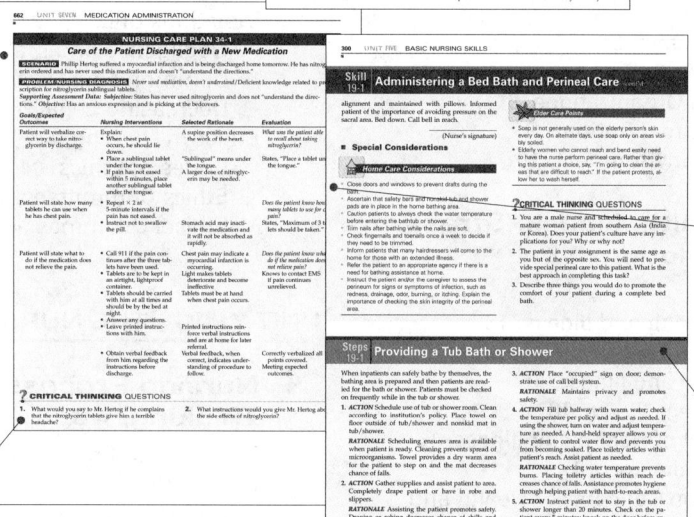

Home Care Considerations focus on how to adapt nursing skills and techniques to the home care setting

Critical Thinking Questions appear at the end of Nursing Care Plans and Skills

Steps are short, non-illustrated Skills with Actions and Rationales

Patient Teaching boxes offer step-by-step instructions to help nurses educate patients and their families about proper post-hospital care

Key Points summarize main chapter concepts

NCLEX-PN® Examination–Style Review Questions at the end of each chapter include multiple-choice and alternate-format questions to prepare students for the exam

Legal & Ethical Considerations cover a wide range of issues and dilemmas that nurses face every day in providing care in a variety of settings

Critical Thinking Activities are short scenarios with related questions to help develop problem-solving skills

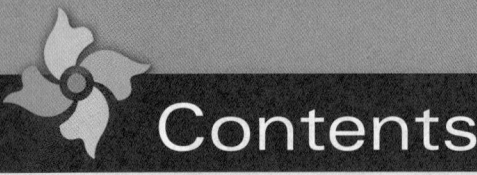
Contents

UNIT **FIVE**   BASIC NURSING SKILLS

16 Infection Prevention and Control: Protective Mechanisms and Asepsis, 209

17 Infection Prevention and Control in the Hospital and Home, 234

18 Lifting, Moving, and Positioning Patients, 258

19 Assisting with Hygiene, Personal Care, Skin Care, and the Prevention of Pressure Ulcers, 288

20 Patient Environment and Safety, 315

APPENDIXES

CHAPTER 1

Nursing and the Health Care System

evolve http://evolve.elsevier.com/deWit/fundamental/

Objectives

Upon completing this chapter, you should be able to:

Theory

1. Describe Florence Nightingale's influence on nurses' training.
2. Explain why nursing is both an art and a science.
3. Indicate how evidence-based practice is helpful in nursing.
4. Trace the growth of nursing in the United States from the Civil War to the present.
5. Discuss the ways in which the desirable attributes of the nurse might be demonstrated.
6. Identify the educational ladder that is available to nurses.
7. Describe educational pathways open to the LPN upon graduation.
8. Compare methods of delivery of nursing care.
9. List four practice settings in which LPNs may find employment.
10. Identify segments within the various levels of health care.
11. Explain how a health maintenance organization and a preferred provider organization differ.
12. Relate how the managed care system has affected your own health care.

Clinical Practice

1. Write your own definition of nursing.
2. Discuss how the standards of practice for the LPN/LVN are applied in the clinical setting.
3. List the practice areas in the community in which you could be employed as a vocational nurse.

Key Terms

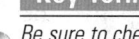
Be sure to check the bonus material on the Companion CD-ROM, including selected audio pronunciations.

apprenticeship (ă-PRĔN-tĭ-shĭp, p. 2)
aseptically (ā-SĔP-tĭk-ăl-lē, p. 4)
capitated cost (p. 9)
diagnosis-related groups (DRGs) (dī-ăg-NŌS-ĭs, p. 9)
evidence-based nursing (p. 4)
health maintenance organizations (HMOs) (āch-ĕm-ō, p. 9)
implement (ĬM-plĕ-mĕnt, p. 6)
integrated delivery network (p. 9)
interventions (p. 3)
invasive procedures (ĭn-VĀ-sĭv, p. 3)

nursing process (p. 6)
nursing theory (p. 4)
practice acts (p. 6)
preferred provider organizations (PPOs) (p. 9)

HISTORICAL OVERVIEW

The art of nursing arose in primitive times when one person simply cared for another who was sick. As family groups banded together into communities, certain individuals extended themselves to care for the ill, the helpless, and the elderly. During this period, nursing consisted of comforting, caring for basic needs, and using herbal remedies.

NURSING IN ENGLAND AND EUROPE

As civilizations appeared, nurses were under the direction of the priest-physicians because illness was often believed to be caused by sin or the gods' displeasure. With the growth of Christianity, caring for the sick became a function of religious orders. The Christian St. Paul introduced a deaconess named Phoebe, a practical nurse, to Rome. She was the first visiting nurse. Both men and women tended the sick during this period. Nursing became a recognized vocation during the Crusades (1100 to 1200 AD) as hospitals were built to care for the large number of pilgrims needing health care.

The service provided by the religious orders in England changed with the break between King Henry VIII of England and the Catholic Church in the 1500s. The nuns and priests were sent out of the country. The patients in their hospitals were abandoned; the hospitals became the responsibility of the government. Criminals, widows, and orphans were recruited, and in exchange for housing and food, they tended the sick. The drunken nurse-midwives Sairey Gamp and Betsy Prig, as portrayed in Charles Dickens' 1849 novel *Martin Chuzzlewit*, were typical of hospital nurses at the time. Health care conditions became very bad.

Florence Nightingale

In the mid-1800s Florence Nightingale, an Englishwoman, felt a calling by God to become a nurse. Nightingale studied in Germany with a Protestant order of women who cared for the sick. She went on to reform and manage a charity hospital for ill governesses. During the Crimean War, Florence Nightingale asked the Secretary of War to allow her to train women to care for the sick and wounded. By cleaning up the wards and improving ventilation, sanitation, and nutrition, her group of 38 nurses lowered the death rate from 60% to 1%. The Nightingale nurses made their rounds after dark with the aid of a lighted oil lamp. The lamp became the official symbol of nursing. Florence Nightingale kept records and statistics that reinforced her theories of care, many of which are still valid today.

Funds were given out of gratitude by the servicemen and their families. These funds were used to begin the first Nightingale training school for nurses, located in England at St. Thomas Hospital. Nightingale based her curriculum on the following beliefs:

- Nutrition is an important part of nursing care.
- Fresh, clean air is beneficial to the sick.
- Sick people need occupational and recreational therapy.
- Nurses should help identify and meet patients' personal needs, including providing emotional support.
- There are two conditions to which nursing should be directed: health and illness.
- Nursing is distinct and separate from the practice of medicine and should be taught by nurses.
- Continuing education is needed for nurses.

These beliefs are still the foundation of nursing today.

Think Critically About ... How is the tradition of combining religion and medical care still evident today?

NURSING IN NORTH AMERICA

Nursing care was sadly lacking during the Civil War in America. The Union government finally appointed Dorothea Dix, a social worker, to organize women volunteers to provide nursing care for the soldiers. These workers were like the nursing assistants of today. Clara Barton took volunteers into the field hospitals to care for soldiers of both armies. She later founded the American Red Cross. Lillian Wald took nursing out into the community, and in 1893 she established the Henry Street Settlement Service in New York City. In the period following the Civil War, nurses' training was essentially an apprenticeship (learning by doing). Over time, the schooling became more formal and the hospital-based training period lengthened from 6 months to 3 years. Graduates of the training program received a diploma. **In an era when women were expected to remain at home and be subservient to men, nurses' training became a way to obtain further education and employment that could provide independence for women.**

In 1892 the New York Young Women's Christian Association (YWCA) started the Ballard School, which

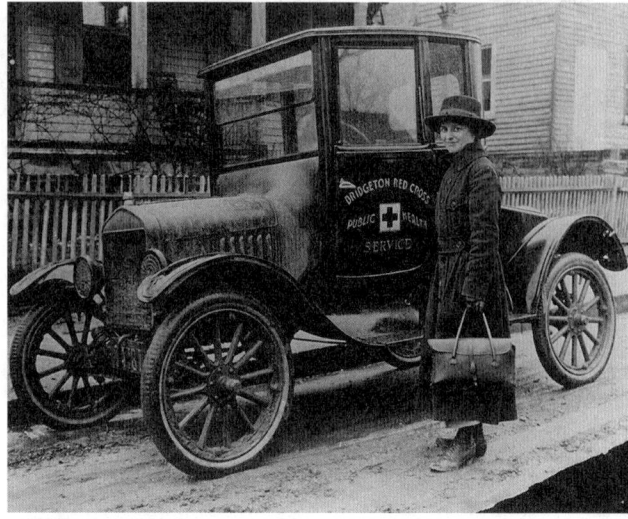

FIGURE **1-1** A Red Cross public health nurse poses with her Model T Ford before setting out on her rounds. (Photo courtesy of The American National Red Cross.)

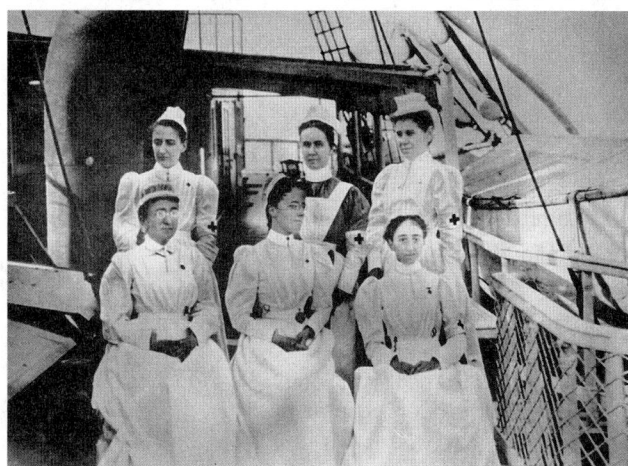

FIGURE **1-2** During the Spanish-American War in 1898, nurses traveled by sea to care for soldiers in need. (Photo courtesy of The American National Red Cross.)

offered a 3-month course in practical nursing. Students were trained to care for infants, children, and the elderly in the home. A legacy left by Thomas Thompson allowed Richard Bradley, the executor of the will, to open a practical nursing school in Brattleboro, Vermont, in 1907. In 1918 a group of women opened the Household Nursing School in Boston to train nurses to care for the sick at home. Later this school was called the Shepard Gill School of Practical Nursing.

The training in the Nightingale schools varied considerably from that of the U.S. nursing schools. The Nightingale program was well organized, with classes held separately from practical experience on the wards. The core curriculum was the same in all schools. Instruction was provided by a trained nurse and was focused on nursing care.

In the United States, the students staffed the hospital and worked without pay. There were no formal classes; education was achieved through work. There

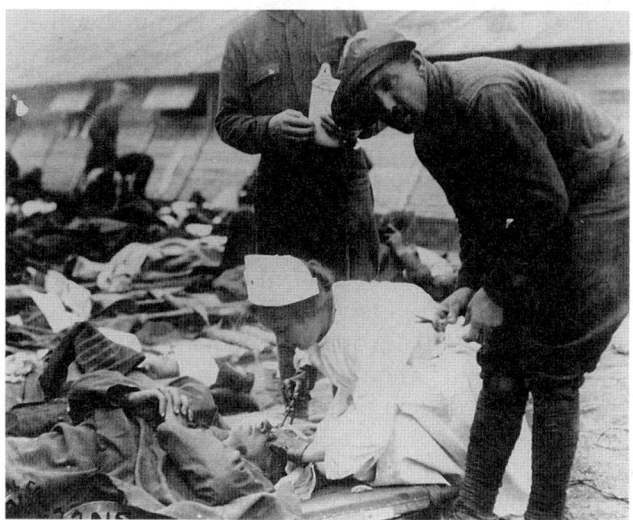

FIGURE **1-3** During World War I, a Red Cross nurse at a field hospital in France bathes the eyes of a gassed patient from the U.S. Army. (Photo courtesy of The American National Red Cross.)

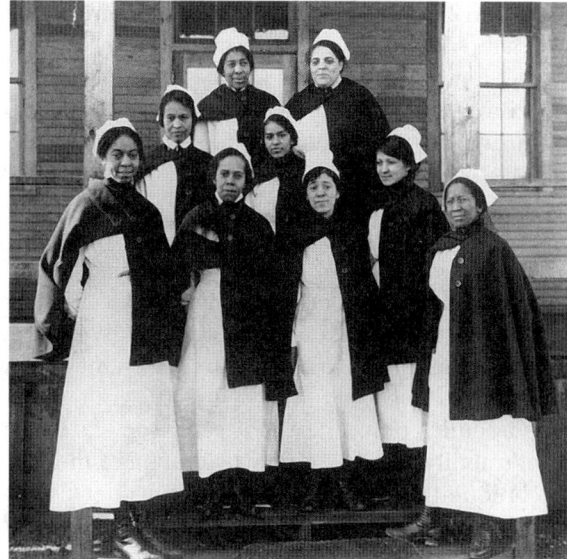

FIGURE **1-4** Some of the first African American nurses to serve with the U.S. Army standing outside their quarters at Camp Sherman in Chillicothe, Ohio. (Photo courtesy of The American National Red Cross.)

was no set curriculum, and content varied depending on the type of cases present in the hospital. Instruction was done at the bedside by the physician and therefore came from a medical viewpoint.

In the 20th century nurses moved out into the community. They worked with the poor in the cities, provided midwifery services, and taught prenatal, obstetric, and child care (Figure 1-1). Nurses were present during wartime, providing essential care on all fronts (Figure 1-2). During World War I, nurses worked behind the lines to care for sick and wounded soldiers (Figure 1-3). Also, the first African American nurses to serve in the U.S. Army paved the way for others to follow (Figure 1-4). World War II created a great demand for nurses in military hospitals, and training programs had to be increased (Figure 1-5). Congress passed a bill to draft nurses, but the declaration of peace occurred before it was enacted. Nurses continue to serve in times of military crisis, as they have for Operation Iraqi Freedom.

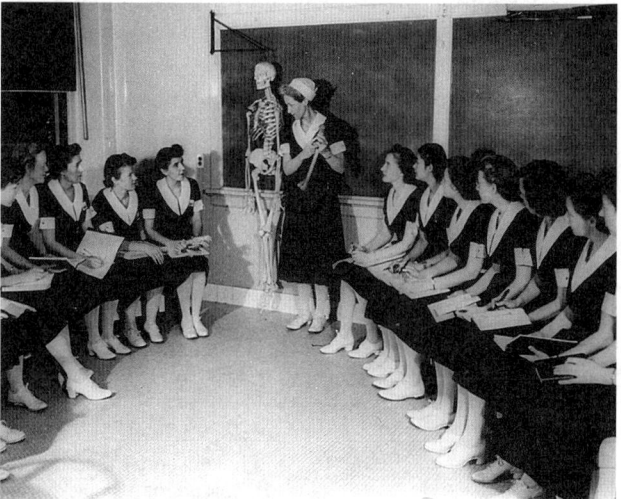

FIGURE **1-5** A group of nursing students during the 1930s or 1940s in an anatomy class at Walter Reed General Hospital, Washington, DC.

THE ART AND SCIENCE OF NURSING

There are many definitions of nursing, and as you progress through your nursing career, ideas about what nursing is will grow and change. Among the various definitions, the following four common goals appear:

- To promote wellness
- To prevent illness
- To facilitate coping
- To restore health

To accomplish these goals, the practical nurse takes on the role of caregiver, educator, collaborator, and manager. Caregiving skills are interventions aimed at restoring and maintaining a person's health. Interventions are actions taken to improve, maintain, or restore health or prevent illness. An example would be assist-

ing a patient with hygiene tasks such as bathing and brushing the teeth. Today caregiving skills extend to using highly technical equipment for medical therapies and protecting the safety of the patient undergoing invasive procedures (procedures that require entry into the body). Nurses provide both physical and emotional care to patients. By performing various tasks and working closely with the patient, nurses develop a concern for the patient's well-being. **The nurse's goal is to encourage growth toward wellness so that the patient can once again be self-reliant.**

Health teaching and counseling are functions of the practical nurse and are directed toward promoting wellness and preventing illness. Teaching about medications and how to **aseptically** (without introducing infectious material) change dressings are examples of this role. Emotional support and comfort are incorporated in care, and the nurse is an advocate for the patient during times of health-related stress.

The licensed practical nurse (LPN) or licensed vocational nurse (LVN) collaborates with the registered nurse (RN) and other members of the health care team to provide continuity of care. Care for the patient is planned jointly by all members of the health care team. Minor tasks such as taking vital signs or giving a bed bath may be assigned to the nursing assistant or other ancillary personnel.

Therapeutic communication techniques facilitate a patient's ability to cope. Active listening is a therapeutic technique that helps the patient consider possible solutions when a problem occurs. Establishing a good nurse-patient relationship is necessary to gain the patient's trust so that teaching and other communications are well received.

Initially nursing was an art—it consisted of performing certain acts of care skillfully, with intuition and creativity. Over time, a scientific base was combined with the art of nursing. From this body of knowledge, the nurse can choose interventions that are most likely to produce desired outcomes for the patient.

As this scientific base for nursing has developed, various scholars have proposed theories concerning the process of nursing. A **nursing theory** is a statement about relationships among concepts or facts, based on existing information. Nursing theorists generally base their beliefs on the relationships among humans, environment, health, and nursing. Table 1-1 provides a

brief explanation of some of the major nursing theories. A particular theory may be the basis of a nursing school's curriculum structure and part of its philosophy of how nursing care is delivered. Nursing strives to maintain recognition as a profession. For this reason, ongoing research is essential to add to the scientific knowledge base.

EVIDENCE-BASED PRACTICE

The promotion of **evidence-based nursing** has become stronger around the world over the last decade. It involves the "integration of best research evidence with clinical expertise and patient values to facilitate clinical decision making" (DiCenso et al., 2005). Students are being taught the skills to discriminate between high-quality and flawed research and to interpret the study results. Nurses are being strongly encouraged to seek evidence for their practice throughout their careers. Evidence-based practice is using the best scientific evidence from research to guide decision making (Benefield, 2002). Evidence-based nursing is used to help determine "best practices." Best practices are optimal techniques, procedures, or programs identified by one or more organizations that improve care effectiveness or efficiency while providing positive patient outcomes (Huffman, 2005). Clinical field experience and evidence-based research are used to establish the best practices for patient care.

Think Critically About . . . Which role of the nurse appeals to you the most?

Table 1-1 *Selected Nursing Theories*

THEORIST	GOAL OF NURSING	PRACTICE FRAMEWORK
Virginia Henderson (1955)	To help clients gain independence in meeting their needs as quickly as possible	14 fundamental needs
Dorothy Johnson (1968)	To reduce stress, allowing the client to recover as quickly as possible	Seven behavioral subsystems in an adaptation model
Martha Rogers (1970)	To achieve maximum level of wellness	Concept of "unitary man" evolving along the life process
Dorothea Orem (1971)	To care for and help clients with various needs attain self-care	Self-care deficits
Betty Neumann (1972)	To assist individuals, families, and groups to attain and maintain maximum levels of total wellness through purposeful interventions	Systems model with stress reduction as its goal. Nursing care occurs on various levels: primary prevention, secondary prevention, or tertiary prevention
Sister Callista Roy (1976)	To identify types of demands placed on client and client's adaptation to them	Four adaptive modes: physiologic, psychological, sociologic, and independence
Jean Watson (1979)	To promote health, restore clients to health, and prevent illness	"Carative" factors with caring as an interpersonal process used to meet human needs
Rosemarie Parse (1987)	To assist client in interaction with the environment and in co-creating health. To sustain a safe and protective environment	Human Becoming: patients are open, mutual, and constantly interacting with the environment. Health is constantly changing
Patricia Benner and Judith Wrubel (1989)	To care about the client as an individual	Primacy of caring: caring is central and allows for the giving and receiving of help. Caring extends to all aspects of care of the client

CURRENT NURSING PRACTICE

As nursing has grown and changed to meet the needs of society, laws have been made and standards set that govern the practice of the profession. In 2004 the American Nurses Association (ANA) revised the Standards of Nursing Practice (see Appendix 1). These standards for the professional registered nurse protect the nurse, the patient, and the health care agency where nursing care is given. The practical nurse follows standards as written by the National Federation of Licensed Practical Nurses to deliver safe, knowledgeable, nursing care (Box 1-1, Appendix 4). The National Association for Practical Nurse Education and Service (NAPNES) has formulated an additional set of standards for practical nurses (see Chapter 3). In Canada, another set of similar standards guides the practice of nursing (Box 1-2).

Box 1-1 | *Nursing Practice Standards for the Licensed Practical/Vocational Nurse*

EDUCATION

The Licensed Practical/Vocational Nurse

1. Shall complete a formal education program in practical nursing approved by the appropriate nursing authority in a state.
2. Shall successfully pass the National Council Licensure Examination for Practical Nurses.
3. Shall participate in initial orientation within the employing institution.

LEGAL/ETHICAL STATUS

The Licensed Practical/Vocational Nurse

1. Shall hold a current license to practice nursing as an LP/VN in accordance with the law of the state wherein employed.
2. Shall know the scope of nursing practice authorized by the Nursing Practice Act in the state wherein employed.
3. Shall have a personal commitment to fulfill the legal responsibilities inherent in good nursing practice.
4. Shall take responsible actions in situations wherein there is unprofessional conduct by a peer or other health care provider.
5. Shall recognize and have a commitment to meet the ethical and moral obligations of the practice of nursing.
6. Shall not accept or perform professional responsibilities which the individual knows (s)he is not competent to perform.

PRACTICE

The Licensed Practical/Vocational Nurse

1. Shall accept assigned responsibilities as an accountable member of the health care team.
2. Shall function within the limits of educational preparation and experience as related to the assigned duties.
3. Shall function with other members of the health care team in promoting and maintaining health, preventing disease and disability, caring for and rehabilitating individuals who are experiencing an altered health state, and contributing to the ultimate quality of life until death.
4. Shall know and utilize the nursing process in planning, implementing, and evaluating health services and nursing care for the individual patient or group.
   a. Planning: the planning of nursing includes:
      (1) Assessment/data collection of health status of the individual patient, the family and community groups
      (2) Reporting information gained from assessment/data collection
      (3) The identification of health goals

   b. Implementation: the plan for nursing care is put into practice to achieve the stated goals and includes:
      (1) Observing, recording, and reporting significant changes which require intervention or different goals
      (2) Applying nursing knowledge and skills to promote and maintain health, to prevent disease and disability and to optimize functional capabilities of an individual patient
      (3) Assisting the patient and family with activities of daily living and encouraging self-care as appropriate
      (4) Carrying out therapeutic regimens and protocols prescribed by personnel pursuant to authorized state law
   c. Evaluations: the plan for nursing care and its implementations are evaluated to measure the progress toward the stated goals and will include appropriate person and/or groups to determine:
      (1) The relevancy of current goals in relation to the progress of the individual patient
      (2) The involvement of the recipients of care in the evaluation process
      (3) The quality of the nursing action in the implementation of the plan
      (4) A re-ordering of priorities or new goal setting in the care plan
5. Shall participate in peer review and other evaluation processes.
6. Shall participate in the development of policies concerning the health and nursing needs of society and in the roles and functions of the LP/VN.

CONTINUING EDUCATION

The Licensed Practical/Vocational Nurse

1. Shall be responsible for maintaining the highest possible level of professional competence at all times.
2. Shall periodically reassess career goals and select continuing education activities which will help to achieve these goals.
3. Shall take advantage of continuing education and certification opportunities which will lead to personal growth and professional development.
4. Shall seek and participate in continuing education activities which are approved for credit by appropriate organizations, such as the NFLPN.

SPECIALIZED NURSING PRACTICE

The Licensed Practical/Vocational Nurse

1. Shall have had at least 1 year's experience in nursing at the staff level.

Continued

Box 1-1 *Nursing Practice Standards for the Licensed Practical/Vocational Nurse—cont'd*

2. Shall present personal qualifications that are indicative of potential abilities for practice in the chosen specialized nursing area.
3. Shall present evidence of completion of a program or course that is approved by an appropriate agency to provide the knowledge and skills necessary for effective nursing services in the specialized field.
4. Shall meet all of the standards of practice as set forth in this document.

GLOSSARY

Authorized (Acts of Nursing)
Those nursing activities made legal through state nurse practice acts.

Lateral Expansion of Knowledge
An extension of the basic core of information learned in the school of practical nursing.

Peer Review
A formal evaluation of performance on the job by other LP/VNs.

Specialized Nursing Practice
A restricted field of nursing in which a person is particularly skilled and has specific knowledge.

Therapeutic Regimens
Regulated plans designed to bring about effective treatment of disease.

Career Advancement
A change of career goal.

LP/VN
A combined abbreviation for Licensed Practical Nurse and Licensed Vocational Nurse. The LVN is the title used in California and Texas for the nurses who are called LPNs in other states.

Milieu
One's environment and surroundings.

Protocols
Courses of treatment which include specific steps to be performed in a stated order.

Box 1-2 *Canadian Nurses Association Standards for Nursing Practice*

These four standards are necessarily interdependent and interrelated.

Standard I. Nursing practice requires that a conceptual model(s) for nursing be the basis for that practice.

Nurses are required to have a clear idea, conception, or understanding of (1) goal, (2) client, (3) role of the nurse, (4) source of difficulty, (5) focus and modes of intervention, and (6) consequences.

Standard II. Nursing practice requires the effective use of the nursing process.

Nurses are required in any practice setting to do the following: (1) collection of data, (2) analysis of data, (3) planning of the intervention, (4) implementation of the intervention, and (5) evaluation.

Standard III. Nursing practice requires that the helping relationship be the nature of the client-nurse interaction.

Nurses are required to perform the following parts of the helping relationship: (1) initiation, (2) maintenance, and (3) termination.

Standard IV. Nursing practice requires nurses to fulfill professional responsibilities.

Nurses are expected to respect or comply with the following: (1) legislation, (2) ethics, and (3) collaboration.

Adapted from Canadian Nurses Association. (1987). *Standards for Nursing Practice.* Prepared and revised by a Task Group to Develop a Definition of Nursing Practice and Standards for Nursing Practice. Ottawa: Canadian Nurses Association.

Nurse practice acts have been established in each of the states of the United States and in the provinces of Canada to regulate the practice of nursing. Each state has a regulatory body that makes and enforces rules and regulations for the nursing profession. The practice acts generally define activities in which nurses may engage, state the legal requirements and titles for nursing licensure, and establish the education needed for licensure. **The practice acts are designed to protect the public, and they define the legal scope of practice.** Policy and procedure books are established by each facility that hires nurses. These books define which procedures each professional can perform in that facility as well as specify step-by-step guidelines for the way that facility wants a procedure performed.

The nursing process emerged during the 1970s and 1980s as an organized, deliberate, systematic way to deliver nursing care. The nursing process provides a way to implement (to put into action) caregiving, and it combines the science and the art of nursing. The nurse focuses on the patient as an individual, identifies health care needs and strengths of the patient, establishes and implements a plan of action to meet those needs, and evaluates the outcomes of the plan. It is a circular process involving ongoing assessment. The nursing process is presented in depth in Unit Two: The Nursing Process.

NURSING EDUCATION PATHWAYS

Formal education has been another way to build a professional image for nursing. Nursing education has been mostly moved from hospital training schools into institutions of higher learning. There are two levels of entry into nursing: practical (or vocational) nursing and professional (registered) nursing. Often a student studies to become a certified nursing assistant before going up the "ladder" to practical/vocational training. Each educational program produces graduates with skills for a particular level of entry into practice. A nursing assistant program is short, averaging 6 to

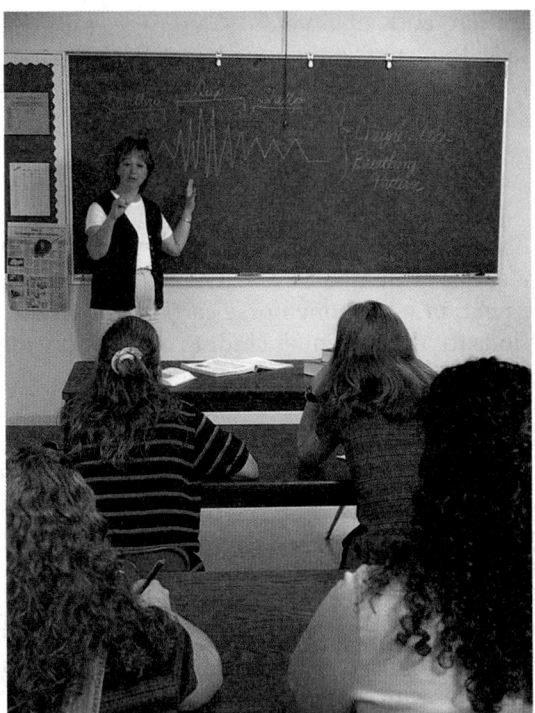

FIGURE **1-6** Present-day nursing students.

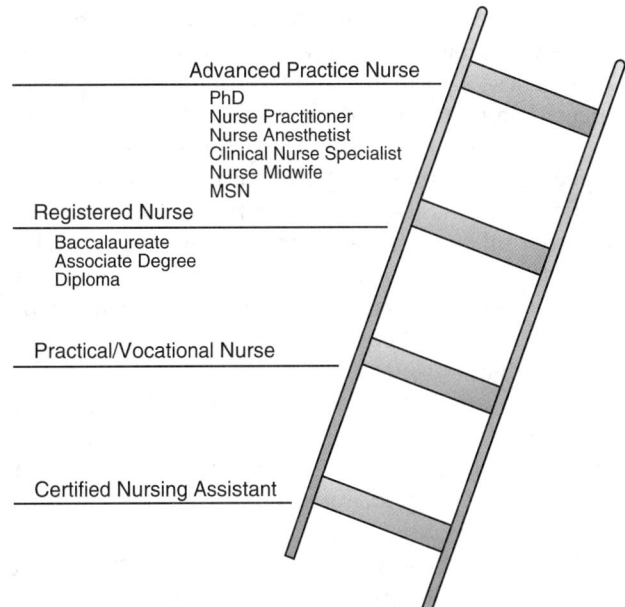

FIGURE **1-7** Nursing education ladder.

8 weeks. Basic personal care and basic nursing skills are taught. The practical nursing program generally takes 12 to 18 months to complete. The professional nursing program (RN) requires 2 to 5 years of education, depending on the type of degree sought (Figure 1-6). If the student has already obtained a practical/ vocational nursing license, the program may require only one more year to become an RN.

PRACTICAL NURSING

Practical nursing was created to fill a gap left by nurses who enlisted in the military services during World War II. Programs were developed to train practical nurses to care for well people and those who were mildly or chronically ill or past the acute stage of illness. Registered nurses could then concentrate on the acutely ill. A need for practical nurses continued after the war, and the National Association for Practical Nurse Education and Service (NAPNES) was formed to standardize practical nurse education and to establish licensure criteria for graduates. Practical nursing programs are offered in vocational schools, hospitals, proprietary schools, and community colleges. Graduates take the National Council Licensure Examination for Practical Nurses (NCLEX-PN®) after program completion. Successfully passing the exam and obtaining licensure allows the use of the initials LVN or LPN after one's name. **Practical nurses provide direct patient care under the supervision of a registered nurse, physician, or dentist.** Many community colleges have structured the practical nurse curriculum so that graduates can easily enter the second year of the registered nursing program. This type of curriculum is consid-

ered a "ladder program." Many LPN/LVN programs require that the entering student be a certified nursing assistant (Figure 1-7).

After completion of an LPN/LVN curriculum and/ or licensure, the graduate can seek certification by NAPNES in pharmacology and long-term care. The pharmacology examination can be taken online. Pharmacology certification is for 5 years and can then be renewed.

REGISTERED NURSING

Graduates of three different educational programs are qualified to take the registered nurse licensure exam (NCLEX-RN®): a hospital-based diploma program, a 2-year associate degree program at a community college, or a 4-year baccalaureate nursing program at a college or university. Registered nurses may provide bedside care or care in the community, or supervise others in managing care of multiple patients.

Diploma schools decreased as the desire to improve the professional image of nursing through more formal education occurred. Hospitals could no longer afford to provide the expensive diploma programs. Diploma nurses are very well trained in skills compared with the students of other programs. They spend a far greater number of clinical hours working directly with patients, but they do not get as broad a base of scientific knowledge as college-educated nurses receive.

Associate degree programs attract the majority of registered nurse students. The associate degree nurse is considered a *technical* nurse and is not specifically prepared to work in a management position, although many do. Graduates of these programs have 2 years of clinical experience along with their academic classes.

Baccalaureate nursing programs prepare nurses who have managerial skills as well as bedside nursing skills. These graduates are considered *professional* nurses. The push toward professionalism for nursing has caused the ANA to propose that the baccalaureate degree be necessary for entry into professional nursing practice. There has been considerable controversy over this proposal because the many registered nurses who graduated from diploma or associate degree programs feel that their jobs may be threatened by such a proposal. To date, most employers do not distinguish between the various educational programs of the registered nurse, and view graduates of all three programs as the same. Another concern is that, if the more expensive and longer program is required to become a professional registered nurse, employers would have to pay higher salaries. The nursing shortage has also tempered the thrust for all nurses to be baccalaureate prepared since the program is twice as long.

ADVANCED PRACTICE NURSING

Graduate programs are available in nursing for both master's and doctorate degrees. Nurses who pursue higher education are prepared as specialists in the various clinical branches of nursing, in research, or in administration. Another form of advanced education is the nurse practitioner program. Registered nurses continue their training in a specialty such as family practice, pediatrics, maternity, psychiatry, adult health nursing, or geriatrics, and once licensed can practice more independently than as a registered nurse. Nurse practitioners usually provide care in an outpatient, ambulatory care, or community-based setting. In many states they can treat patients on their own and write prescriptions under the direction of a physician. A certified nurse-midwife (CNM) is a registered nurse with further training in midwifery. Certification is by examination through the American College of Nurse-Midwives.

The ANA set up a separate American Nurses Credentialing Center to enhance the professional image of nursing. Registered nurses who have experience in a particular specialty may take a comprehensive examination. Passing the exam provides the nurse with certification of expertise in that specialty. Certification is also available for the practical nurse under a program developed by NAPNES.

DELIVERY OF NURSING CARE

Various systems of delivering nursing care have been tried through the years. Today various adaptations are devised to meet the specific needs of the patients and nurses. *Functional nursing care* was the first care delivery system for the practical nurse. Practical nurses performed a series of tasks such as administration of medication and treatments. Care was rather fragmented. *Team nursing* evolved in the 1950s and extended into the mid-1970s. A registered nurse was the team leader who coordinated care for a group of patients. Work tasks were assigned to the other members of the team, the practical nurses and the nurses' aides. This system worked fairly well as long as there was excellent communication among the members and the team leader evaluated care delivered. *Total patient care* came next, in which one nurse carried out all nursing functions for the patient, including medication administration. This was an effort to provide less fragmented care for the patient.

Primary nursing appeared in the late 1960s and 1970s. In this system, one nurse plans and directs care for a patient over a 24-hour period. This method eliminated fragmentation of care between shifts. When the primary nurse is off duty, an associate nurse takes over the care and planning. Today, primary nursing is often modified with the use of cross-trained personnel assigned to help with duties. To increase the level of productivity, ancillary workers supervised by the RN are trained in multiple functions, such as clerical and housekeeping tasks and vital sign measurement and phlebotomy. This system has not been entirely satisfactory. Presently, because research is showing better patient outcomes with more of the care being delivered by nurses, there is a trend back to *total patient care.*

PRACTICE SETTINGS

Practical nurses work in areas where there is supervision by a registered nurse, physician, or dentist. Community nursing, school nursing, and public health nursing presently are primarily the arena of the professional registered nurse. Practice settings for the LPN/LVN include the following:

- *Hospitals:* Restorative care is provided to ill or injured patients
- *Extended care facilities:* Facilities for intermediate or long-term care where personal care and skilled care is provided for those requiring rehabilitation or custodial care
- *Physicians' offices:* Ambulatory patients receive preventive care or treatment of an illness or injury
- *Ambulatory clinics:* Ambulatory patients come for preventive care or treatment of an illness or injury; often treatment by specialty groups is available on site
- *Renal dialysis centers:* Patients with kidney failure receive renal dialysis treatments
- *Hospices:* Supportive treatment is provided for patients who are terminally ill
- *Home health agencies:* In-home care is provided to patients by nurses who visit the home

- *Neighborhood emergency centers:* Minor emergency care is provided to patients within the community setting

As the role of the practical nurse expands, employment in other practice settings is possible.

TODAY'S HEALTH CARE SYSTEM

In times past, most medical care was provided by physicians in private practice. With the technological advances in medicine and the flood of new drugs on the market, health care costs have risen dramatically. Although the use of magnetic resonance imaging (MRI) and computed tomography (CT) provides much more data than a standard radiograph, both cost much more. Microsurgical techniques allow procedures that would not have been possible 20 years ago. The elderly are living longer and needing more years of medical care and many prescription drugs.

Diagnosis-related groups (DRGs) were created by Medicare in 1983 as an attempt to contain health care costs. **The DRG system means that a hospital receives a set amount of money for a patient who is hospitalized with a certain diagnosis.** If a patient is admitted with pneumonia, only a certain number of days of hospitalization are allowed and will be paid for by Medicare. If the patient has other known problems, they are mentioned when he is admitted. It is to the advantage of the hospital and physician to indicate all possible diagnoses when the patient enters the hospital. If the patient with pneumonia also has diabetes, the length of stay is likely to be longer. Adding this diagnosis at admission provides an extra measure of money for the patient's care. Private insurance companies have adjusted their payments in many instances to be more in line with what Medicare will pay for the same problem. This system has created a large amount of paperwork for all health care agencies and caregivers. In 2008 Medicare will stop paying hospitals for care related to preventable hospital-acquired conditions. This means that if a patient contracts an infection as a result of poor catheter care or poor aseptic techniques while in the hospital, the hospital will not be paid for the care and extra days the patient is there to clear the infection. **To clearly prove patient needs and proper care, nursing documentation of patient assessment and identified need become very important.**

In December of 2003, Congress passed the controversial Medicare Prescription Drug Modernization and Improvement Act, which is meant to supply financial relief to seniors who take multiple prescription drugs. The way the law is written and the intricacies of the program have caused many problems. About 6 million low-income and disabled persons found their drug coverage reduced from former levels. Many retirees have been forced to go from private insurance–funded prescription coverage to this new government program. Although beneficial to low-income participants, it provides only modest relief for middle-income seniors. Medicare recipients have the option to forego traditional Medicare coverage and receive vouchers for private insurance coverage, mainly from health maintenance organizations, that will provide some prescription drug coverage. There will be very high deductibles for the drug coverage. Legislative work is underway to correct problems with the Medicare Prescription Drug Program.

LEVELS OF HEALTH CARE

An emphasis on managing health care rather than on managing illness is coming to the forefront. There is more focus on maintaining wellness and on providing preventive care. The integrated delivery network is a set of providers and services organized to deliver coordinated care to promote wellness, care for illness, and promote rehabilitation. This type of network performs these services for a set or capitated cost, meaning that they are paid a set fee for every patient enrolled in the network each year.

There are six levels of care within the health care system: preventive, primary, secondary, tertiary, restorative, and continuing care (Figure 1-8). The levels of care show the scope of services and settings where patients receive care across the spectrum of health and illness. Box 1-3 depicts the types of specific services available within the various levels of care.

HEALTH MAINTENANCE ORGANIZATIONS

The need to decrease the high cost of medical care has caused health care providers to group together to provide services. Health maintenance organizations (HMOs), a type of group practice, enroll patients for a set fee per month. They provide a limited network of physicians, hospitals, and other health care providers from which to choose. Two national HMOs are Kaiser Permanente and Family Health Plan (FHP). The patient or employer pays a monthly fee for the insurance, and a small copayment may be required from the patient for each visit. Patients must be referred by their primary physician for diagnostic tests, hospitalization (including emergency room visits), and consultation with a specialist. Part of the philosophy of the HMO is that because the patient does not pay the full cost for each visit, earlier treatment will be sought and serious illness can be avoided. **One goal of the HMO is to keep patients healthy and out of the hospital.**

PREFERRED PROVIDER ORGANIZATIONS

Large businesses and insured groups may contract with preferred provider organizations (PPOs). PPOs offer a discount on fees in return for a large pool of

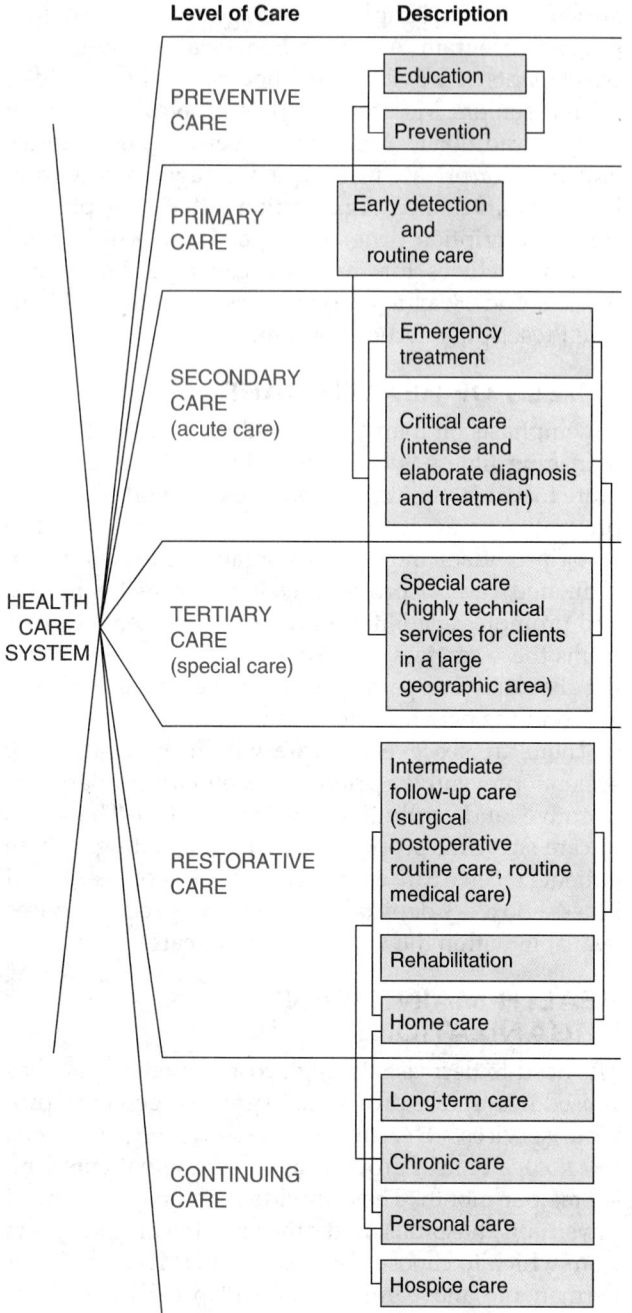

FIGURE **1-8** Levels of health care.

PREVENTIVE CARE AND PRIMARY CARE
- Health Promotion
  - Prenatal care
  - Well-baby care
  - Nutrition counseling
  - Exercise classes
  - Family planning
  - Meditation classes
  - Emergency preparedness classes
  - Fire prevention classes
  - Mature driver courses
  - Smoking cessation classes
  - School physical exams
- Illness Prevention
  - Immunization clinic
  - Blood pressure screening
  - Health fairs and screenings
  - Mental health counseling and crisis intervention
  - Child safety classes
  - Annual physical checkups
  - Vision screenings

SECONDARY CARE (ACUTE CARE)
- Radiologic procedures
- Laboratory and diagnostic procedures
- Surgical procedures
- Inpatient services
- Emergency care
- Restorative care
- Rehabilitation services
  - Physical therapy
  - Speech therapy
  - Occupational therapy
- Home health care
- Cardiovascular and pulmonary outpatient rehabilitation

TERTIARY CARE (CONTINUING CARE)
- Extended (long-term) care
- Chronic disease management
- In-home personal care
- Hospice care

potential patients. Using PPOs allows insurance companies to keep their premium rates lower and in turn makes insurance coverage of employees less expensive for employers. Patients then choose a physician from the list of those associated with the PPO. There are usually a larger number of physicians to choose from in a PPO than in an HMO.

THE MANAGED CARE ENVIRONMENT

There is considerable controversy about the effectiveness of this managed care approach to health care. Patients find that they cannot establish a long-term relationship with a physician because employers' con-

tracts with PPOs change frequently, and HMOs find that physicians frequently leave for employment elsewhere. Patients resent having to see their primary physician before seeing other specialists.

Nurses must constantly think critically about cost containment while trying to give optimal care to patients. **Vigilant assessment with documentation is more important than ever in order to catch beginning complications before they become serious.** Budgeting issues for every department and unit in a health care agency concern each employee. The nurse who forgets to discontinue a heating pad the patient is no longer using, or forgets to charge for an item taken from the supply cart, is costing the nursing unit and the health care agency money. Documentation is exacting because every treatment and each use of equipment must be documented **with evidence showing it is needed.**

In an effort to cut costs, many hospitals are cross-training personnel to fulfill more than one function. Unit secretaries may be training to be electrocardiography (ECG) monitor technicians or housekeeping staff may be trained to perform tasks usually done by nursing assistants, such as taking vital signs. Fewer nurses are found on nursing units than before, and they care for a larger number of patients. Nurses must learn to be good managers and to maximize use of ancillary personnel in order to accomplish their work.

Health care agencies are beginning to find that nurses are very necessary to the agency and can provide a much better quality of care than ancillary workers. With time, a balanced ratio of qualified, licensed personnel to patients will again occur.

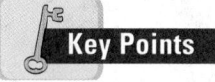
Key Points

- Providing comfort, tending to basic needs, and using herbal remedies were the functions of nurses in early civilizations.
- Florence Nightingale trained to become a nurse in the mid-1800s and started the first school of nursing in England.
- Nightingale's beliefs about nursing hold true today.
- Dorothea Dix organized volunteer "nurses" during the Civil War.
- Nurses' training became a way for women to obtain further education and a means of employment that could provide independence.
- In the early 1900s, U.S. training school nurses staffed the hospitals, learned on the job, and worked without pay.
- Nurses moved from hospitals out into the community in the 20th century and provided midwifery services as well as teaching regarding prenatal, obstetric, and child care.
- Nursing expanded during World War II.
- Nursing is an art and a science.
- Evidence-based practice is used to help establish "best practices" to employ for positive patient outcomes.
- The educational ladder in nursing progresses from the nursing assistant to the advanced practice nurse.
- The goals of nursing are to promote wellness, prevent illness, facilitate coping, and restore health.
- The roles of the practical nurse are caregiver, educator, collaborator, and manager.
- Various nursing scholars have developed theories of nursing.
- Standards of Nursing Practice protect the nurse, the patient, and the health care agency where the nurse practices.
- The nurse practice acts define activities in which nurses may engage and state the legal requirements and titles for organizations that enroll patients and supply all of their medical care. These organizations contract with physicians and facilities to provide medical care.
- There are six levels of care within the health care system.
- Health care costs have risen dramatically, and every effort is being made to cut costs.

 Go to your **Companion CD-ROM** for an Audio Glossary, animations, video clips, and more.

evolve Be sure to visit the companion Evolve site at http://evolve.elsevier.com/deWit/fundamental/ for additional online resources.

NCLEX-PN® EXAMINATION-STYLE REVIEW QUESTIONS

*Choose the **best** answer(s) for each question.*

1. When nursing was taken out into the community, nursing education was essentially:
   1. an apprenticeship.
   2. a 3-month course.
   3. a short hospital course.
   4. a 1-year program.

2. The American Red Cross was founded by _____ _____, as an outgrowth of service during the _____ war. *(Fill in the blanks.)*
   1. Dorothea Dix, First World
   2. Clara Barton, Civil
   3. Lillian Wald, Second World
   4. Florence Nightingale, Crimean

3. In setting up her nurses' training, Florence Nightingale carried out her belief that: *(Select all that apply.)*
   1. recreational therapy is essential to recovery.
   2. large classes are detrimental to learning.
   3. nursing should be taught by nurses.
   4. proper nutrition is essential to recovery from illness.
   5. any woman could be trained to be a nurse.
   6. sick people need occupational and recreational therapy.
   7. fresh, clean air is beneficial to the sick.

4. Inherent in any definition or philosophy of nursing are several core concepts. The core concepts include: *(Select all that apply.)*
   1. promoting wellness.
   2. providing direction.
   3. facilitating coping.
   4. sacrificing self for others.
   5. preventing illness.
   6. restoring health.
   7. working with diligence.

5. A nursing theory is:

   1. scientifically based.
   2. devised by graduate students.
   3. based on skills.
   4. based on existing information.

6. One main difference between a licensed practical nurse and a registered nurse is that the licensed practical nurse:

   1. usually is responsible for giving medications.
   2. performs only noninvasive procedures.
   3. cares for fewer patients than the registered nurse.
   4. is required to work in a supervised setting.

7. Which of the following nursing education programs prepares a nurse for a management role?

   1. Nurse practitioner program
   2. Associate degree nursing program
   3. Baccalaureate nursing program
   4. Practical nursing program

8. Which one of the following would be an example of collaborative practice?

   1. Showing the patient how to cleanse a wound
   2. Speaking with the social worker about the patient's insurance problems

3. Administering each of a patient's prescribed medications
4. Asking the nursing assistant to take the vital signs on three patients

9. An advantage to the patient of a managed health care system is:

   1. always receiving care from the same physician.
   2. paying lower health insurance costs and small copayments.
   3. the ease of quickly seeing a specialist.
   4. being able to walk into the clinic without an appointment.

10. An example of illness prevention activities would be:

    1. applying a dressing to a wound.
    2. performing vision screenings.
    3. referring a patient to a physician.
    4. promoting prenatal care.

CRITICAL THINKING ACTIVITIES *Read each clinical scenario and discuss the questions with your classmates.*

Scenario A
What type of employment do you think would appeal to you after graduation?

Scenario B
If you wish to continue your education after graduation from the practical nursing program, what path do you think would be best for you?

Scenario C
What are some ways that could be used to contain the high cost of medical care?

CHAPTER 2

Concepts of Health, Illness, Stress, and Health Promotion

Objectives

Upon completing this chapter, you should be able to:

Theory

1. Compare traditional and current views of the meanings of health and illness.
2. Describe what the word "health" means to you.
3. Define what "sickness" means to you.
4. Discuss why nurses need to be aware of any cultural, educational, and social differences that might exist between themselves and their patients.
5. Compare cultural/racial differences in disease predisposition and communication between the main cultures and different races.
6. List the components of holistic health care.
7. Identify the four areas of human needs and give an example within each level of need.
8. Identify ways in which the body adapts to maintain homeostasis.
9. Explain why a particular stressor may be experienced differently by two people.
10. List the common signs and symptoms of stress.
11. Identify four ways in which a nurse can help decrease stress and anxiety for patients.

Clinical Practice

1. Observe patients during the data-gathering process and interview process and determine their views on health and illness.
2. Recognize cultural differences in health care concepts and behaviors in the clinical setting and be able to share those observations with fellow students.
3. Determine a patient's status on Maslow's hierarchy during a clinical experience.
4. Describe alterations in homeostasis as observed in the clinical setting.
5. Document observations about stress-reduction techniques used by staff or patients during a clinical experience.

Key Terms

Be sure to check the bonus material on the Companion CD-ROM, including selected audio pronunciations.

acute illness (p. 14)
adaptation (p. 14)
asymptomatic (ā-sĭmp-tō-MĂ-tĭk, p. 16)
autonomic (p. 21)
chronic illness (p. 14)

convalescence (kŏn-vă-LĔ-sĕns, p. 14)
coping (p. 16)
defense mechanisms (p. 25)
disease (p. 13)
etiology (ē-tē-Ŏ-lō-jē, p. 14)
health (p. 13)
hierarchy (HĪ-ĕr-ăr-kē, p. 18)
holistic (hō-LĬS-tĭc, p. 18)
homeostasis (hō-mĕ-ō-STĀ-sĭs, p. 21)
idiopathic (ĭd-ē-ō-PĂTH-ĭk, p. 14)
illness (p. 13)
maladaptation (măl-ă-dăp-TĀ-shŭn, p. 14)
primary illness (p. 14)
secondary illness (p. 14)
self-actualization (SĔLF ăk-tū-ăl-ĭ-ZĀ-shŭn, p. 21)
stress (p. 18)
stressor (p. 21)
terminal illness (p. 14)
wellness (p. 14)

HEALTH AND ILLNESS

The word "health" means many different things to people. For some health is the absence of disease (pathologic process that causes illness); for others it means optimum functioning on every level. "Health" comes from a word that means "wholeness." According to the Miller-Keane dictionary, health is "a relative state in which one is able to function well physically, mentally, socially, and spiritually in order to express the full range of one's unique potentialities within the environment in which one is living."

It is important to define what you believe *health* and *illness* (disease of body or mind) to mean, because your perception of these terms influences what you say and do when caring for patients. Because of cultural, educational, and social differences, you and the patient could have totally different ideas about health and illness and what constitutes "good" health and effective health practices. Before working with patients to accomplish health care goals, try to discover their beliefs about health and illness.

TRADITIONAL VIEWS OF HEALTH AND ILLNESS

The traditional view of health in Western culture was influenced by Plato, Aristotle, and other philosophers who were concerned only with biologic well-being.

For many years an acceptable definition of health was simply "the absence of disease."

In 1946 the World Health Organization redefined health as "the state of complete physical, mental, and social well-being and not merely the absence of disease or infirmity."

In 1974 a change was finally made in the Federal Employees Compensation Act to reimburse federal employees for treatment by psychologists and psychiatrists. Treatment of mental illness became recognized as a legitimate medical cost. Following the lead of the federal government, other third-party payers (such as insurance companies) made similar changes in the 1970s. This willingness to pay for medical care for illnesses other than clearly defined physical diseases reflected a new and expanded understanding of the nature of health.

From birth to death, the health status of an individual can vary from day to day or even hour to hour. People who are partially or completely paralyzed, suffering from a chronic (persisting for a long time) illness, deaf or blind, or living with an anatomic defect may think of themselves as fairly healthy and lead full and productive lives. None of these people can be labeled as "sick," nor can any one of them be called completely healthy. There are others who have no identifiable organic disease who nevertheless do not feel well and are not able to live their lives to the fullest.

Illness is a pronounced deviation from normal health (sickness). Illness is an unavoidable, common part of life. We all occasionally have a cold or the flu. Illness is a personal thing; it is subjective. **Only the person can tell you if she feels ill.** Illness may have a detectable basis in disease or trauma or it may not. Disease is a pathologic process with a definite set of signs and symptoms; disease causes illness.

An acute illness is one that develops suddenly and resolves in a short time. Intestinal flu is an example of an acute illness. *Chronic illness,* such as hypertension, tends to develop slowly over a long period and last throughout life. A terminal illness is one for which there is no cure available; it ends in death. In the terminal phase of illness, death usually occurs within a short period, such as a few months, weeks, or days.

A primary illness is one that develops without being caused by another health problem. A secondary illness results from or is caused by a primary illness. Peripheral vascular disease resulting from diabetes is an example of a secondary illness and occurs because of the effect diabetes has on blood vessels.

Some diseases are inherited (genetic) or congenital (present at birth). Sickle cell anemia is an inherited disease. Fetal alcohol syndrome (FAS) is a congenital disorder caused by the intake of alcohol during pregnancy. An idiopathic illness is one for which there is no known etiology (cause).

?
• *Think Critically About* . . . How is depression looked at? Is it considered an illness, a character weakness, or something else among your family and friends? You may find many examples of differences in how people view health as you explore the answer to this question.

STAGES OF ILLNESS

Illness occurs in stages; there is a transition stage (onset), an acceptance stage (sick role), and a convalescence stage (recovery). When experiencing illness, people act in ways called *illness behaviors.* These behaviors include how people monitor the body, define and interpret symptoms, seek health care, and follow advice and self-care measures to regain wellness (physical and mental well-being). Illness behavior varies according to the stage of illness and the beliefs of the individual.

Transition Stage

The onset of illness may consist of vague, nonspecific symptoms. During this period one may deny feeling ill, but recognize that symptoms of an illness are present. Acknowledgment of a health problem occurs. As symptoms continue or worsen, self-medication may be used or medical assistance may be sought.

Acceptance Stage

Acceptance occurs as denial of illness stops and a "sick role" is assumed. This involves acknowledging illness and engaging in measures to become well. There is withdrawal from usual responsibilities and roles. Remedies from the pharmacy or home medicine cabinet may be used, or the person may go home and go to bed. If symptoms continue to worsen, medical treatment may be sought. Some people will put off going to a physician as long as possible. Fear of what the problem may be and of undergoing examination and diagnostic procedures often causes anxiety.

Convalescence Stage

Convalescence is the process of recovering after the illness and regaining health. If the illness or disease is chronic, a total recovery phase is replaced by adaptation (adjustment in structure or habits) to limitations and positive use of remaining capabilities, or by maladaptation (lack of adjustment).

?
• *Think Critically About* . . . What are the behaviors that different members of your family display when they assume the sick role?

CURRENT VIEWS OF HEALTH AND ILLNESS

Contemporary definitions of health and illness are more abstract and philosophical, and therefore more vague, than the precise definitions based on measurable criteria. **In general, being healthy means being able to function well physically and mentally and to express the full range of one's potentialities within the environment in which one is living.**

This concept takes health beyond the level of meeting basic physiologic needs and recognizes people's need to accept themselves as worthwhile, to live in harmony with others, and to express their personalities fully, thereby becoming more *self-actualized* (reaching one's full potential) and fulfilled. In the words of René Dubos, "Health is primarily a measure of each person's ability to do (what he wants to do) and become what he wants to become."

Current views of health and illness are based on the thoughts and ideas of men such as René Dubos and Halbert Dunn, who urged people to look at these concepts in a new and different way. Realizing that people are dynamic beings whose state of health changes daily and even hourly, they suggest that it is better to think of each person as being located somewhere on a graduated scale or continuous spectrum (continuum) ranging from obvious disease through the absence of detectable disease to a state of optimum functioning in every aspect of life. Figure 2-1 shows a model for the current view of health and illness as dynamic states of being. The phrase *high-level wellness* was first used by Dunn to signify the ideal state of health in every dimension of the human personality. Dunn does not consider high-level wellness to be the same as good health. He thinks of health as being a relatively passive state, one that a person enjoys because of hereditary and environmental factors that are essentially beyond the control of the person. High-level wellness, on the other hand, is described as a dynamic and active movement toward fulfillment of one's potential.

In Dunn's view, each person accepts responsibility for and takes an active part in improving and maintaining her own state of wellness. A person with a high level of wellness does so by virtue of her own efforts. A person who works at achieving high-level wellness improves her self-esteem, is able to accept and give love and concern for others, and lives each day of her life to its fullest insofar as possible.

In the contemporary view, health and illness are relative, rather than absolute, terms. This means that each person's state of health depends on many different things beyond biologic fitness. Figure 2-2 shows the variables that influence health and illness. Among the personal, psychosocial, and spiritual factors that influence a person's state of health at any given moment are the values and beliefs about what it means to be healthy and what it means to be sick, the image of oneself, and the ability to reach out and relate to others and to search for and find meaning and purpose in life. From this point of view, health is never a static state.

Think Critically About . . . Where do you place yourself on Dunn's continuum?

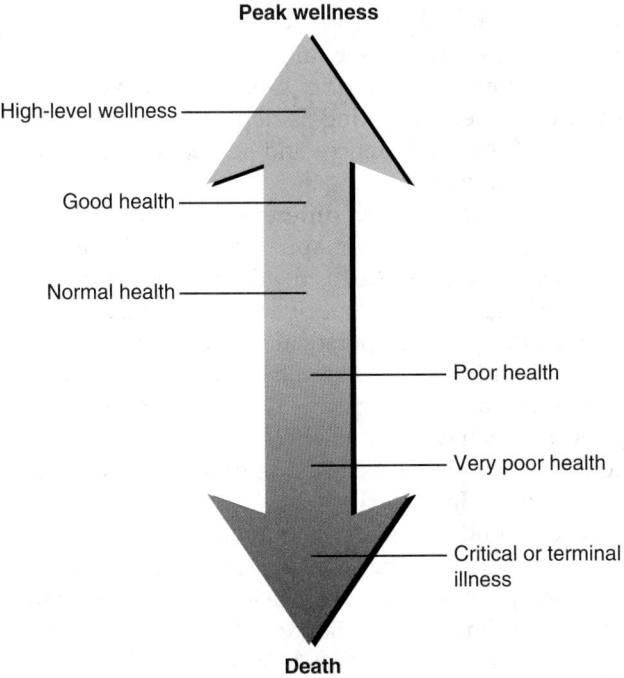

FIGURE **2-1** Health-illness continuum.

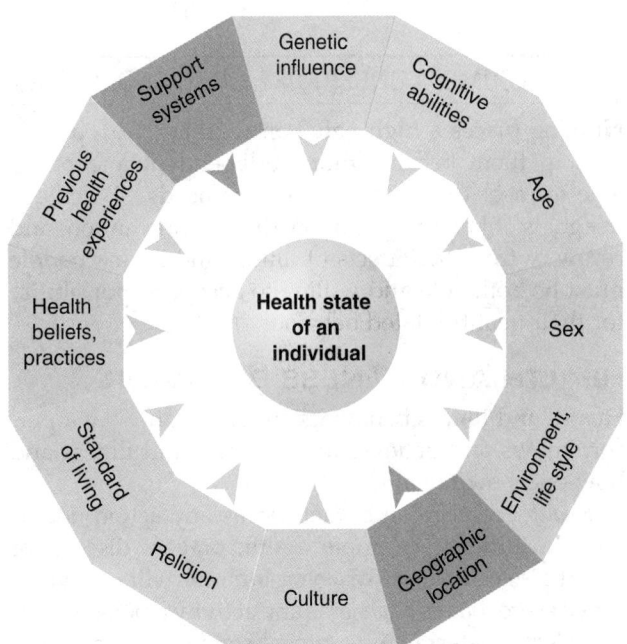

FIGURE **2-2** Multiple variables influence health and illness.

IMPLICATIONS OF CURRENT VIEWS

These views of the nature of health and illness have greatly added to the complexity of health care. They challenge the traditional single-minded goal of curing disease. In the delivery of nursing care, current concepts of health and illness reinforce the value of nursing as primarily a caring profession.

A common theme in all of nursing theory is that nursing is concerned with helping people cope with adverse physiologic, psychosocial, and spiritual responses to illness, rather than with treating the illness itself. Although the nurse is involved in the curing of those who are ill or injured, this goal is primarily under the control of the physician. Nurses have traditionally been concerned with promoting good health habits in their patients and giving them the support they need to cope with illness. Since Florence Nightingale, nurses have encouraged a wholesome environment in the home, hospital or other health care agency, and community.

The nurse knows that it is ultimately the inner resources of the individual that determine whether she will be able to function at an optimum level.

Nurses seek to help patients utilize their coping (adjusting to or accepting challenges) abilities to best advantage and to adapt to conditions that cannot be changed. The patient with a chronic and incurable illness can be helped to minimize its harmful effects and can be encouraged to continue to set and attain goals in other dimensions of life. A patient who is permanently disabled because of traumatic injury is not necessarily limited in every other aspect of life, and it is possible for terminally ill patients to live their final days more fully and perhaps with greater meaning and purpose than during any other stage of life.

THE CONSUMER CONCEPT OF HEALTH AND ILLNESS

Nursing places a high value on working with people to help them become more independent and better able to meet their own health care needs. To achieve the goals of health promotion, disease prevention, and recovery from the effects of illness and injury, people must be both able and willing to accept responsibility for their health-related behavior.

HEALTH AND ILLNESS BEHAVIOR

Health and illness behaviors are based on what a person knows and believes about health and illness and how one's own health is assessed.

Health behavior can be defined as any action undertaken in order to promote health, prevent disease, or detect disease in an early, asymptomatic (without symptoms) stage. *Illness behavior* is any activity a person takes in order to determine her actual state of health and to seek a suitable remedy for a health problem.

Some examples of health behavior might include watching dietary intake to avoid becoming overweight, engaging in a regular program of exercise, taking care to obtain available immunizations against communicable diseases, and monthly self-examination of the breasts or testes. These behaviors are encouraged by health care providers because they are perceived by them as valuable. **If a patient does not undertake these behaviors when they have been recommended, then the nurse must consider whether there is a conflict in values between health care personnel and the patient.** Because of cultural and personal differences, not everyone views certain health practices and behaviors in the same way. What one eats or refuses to eat can be influenced by religious and cultural beliefs. Whether one allows oneself or one's children to be immunized can be dictated by religious convictions and restrictions. Early detection of disease can depend on a person's knowledge about normal physiology and psychology, and signs of abnormal conditions of the body and mind.

Illness behavior is equally complex. Because it involves actions undertaken by an ill person, the underlying question to be answered by the person is "What does it mean to be ill?" or "How do I know I am ill?" The nurse must consider what the person knows about health and deviations from health, and what is believed to be an appropriate remedy for the health problems. Examples of illness behavior include consulting a physician or nurse, consulting the pharmacist, visiting a neighborhood health care clinic, and taking prescribed medications.

CULTURAL INFLUENCES ON CONCEPTS OF HEALTH AND ILLNESS

Great cultural diversity in the United States brings many differences between the values and practices of various ethnic and minority groups. Effective nursing care, whatever the setting, is dependent on an appreciation of these differences and adjustments in care to accommodate them.

Some areas in which differences among racial and ethnic groups are most apparent are attitudes and practices related to birth, death, and general health care; susceptibility to specific diseases; responses to pain and suffering; personal hygiene and sense of privacy; and adjustment to life changes. Additionally, the words and concepts used to communicate feelings and behaviors related to health practices and remedies for sickness are quite different in each cultural group (Table 2-1).

The attitudes, beliefs, and practices of a cultural group may or may not conform to the nurse's idea of what is a productive and beneficial action of health promotion or illness prevention (Cultural Cues 2-1). Typically, health care professionals in the United States and other countries influenced by Western medical science

Table 2-1 | *Cross-Cultural Examples of Cultural Phenomena Affecting Nursing Care*

NATIONS OF ORIGIN	COMMUNICATION	SPACE	TIME ORIENTATION	SOCIAL ORGANIZATION	ENVIRONMENTAL CONTROL	BIOLOGIC VARIATIONS
Asian China Hawaii Philippines Korea Japan Southeast Asia (Laos, Cambodia, Vietnam)	National language preference Dialects, written characters Use of silence Nonverbal and contextual cuing	Noncontact people	Present	Family: hierarchical structure, loyalty Devotion to tradition Many religions, including Taoism, Buddhism, Islam, and Christianity Community social organizations	Traditional health and illness beliefs Use of traditional medicines Traditional practitioners: Chinese physicians and herbalists	Liver cancer Stomach cancer Coccidioidomycosis Hypertension Lactose intolerance
African West coast (as slaves) Many African countries West Indian islands Dominican Republic Haiti Jamaica	National languages Dialect: pidgin, creole, Spanish, and French	Close personal space	Present over future	Family: many female, single parent Large, extended family networks Strong church affiliation within community Community social organizations	Traditional health and illness beliefs Folk medicine tradition Traditional healer: rootworker	Sickle cell anemia Hypertension Esophageal cancer Stomach cancer Coccidioidomycosis Lactose intolerance
Europe Germany England Italy Ireland Other European countries	National languages Many learn English immediately	Noncontact people Aloof Distant Southern countries: closer contact and touch	Future over present	Nuclear families Extended families Judeo-Christian religions Community social organizations	Primary reliance on modern health care system Traditional health and illness beliefs Some remaining folk medicine traditions	Breast cancer Heart disease Diabetes mellitus Thalassemia
American Indian 500 American Indian tribes Aleuts Eskimos	Tribal languages Use of silence and body language	Space very important and has no boundaries	Present	Extremely family oriented Biologic and extended families Children taught to respect traditions Community social organizations	Traditional health and illness beliefs Folk medicine tradition Traditional healer: medicine man	Accidents Heart disease Cirrhosis of the liver Diabetes mellitus
Hispanic countries Spain Cuba Mexico Central and South America	Spanish or Portuguese primary language	Tactile relationships Touch Handshakes Embracing Value physical presence	Present	Nuclear family Extended families *Compadragos;* godparents Community social organizations	Traditional health and illness beliefs Folk medicine tradition Traditional healers: *curandero, esperitista, partera, señora*	Diabetes mellitus Parasites Coccidioidomycosis Lactose intolerance

From Potter, P.A., & Perry, A.G. (2005). *Fundamentals of Nursing* (6th ed.). St. Louis: Elsevier Mosby. Compiled by Rachel Spector, RN, PhD.

have been taught according to the values and beliefs of a white, middle-class society. At the same time, the cultural groups that they care for may not necessarily share these values and beliefs. Unless this conflict is resolved in some way, there may be a problem in communication and in meeting the goals of health care. The problem for the nurse will occur because of unrealistic expectations

of what the patient can be convinced to do or of what can be done for her. The patient may experience problems because the quality and type of care desired may not be delivered.

Many cultural health beliefs are based on folk medicine passed down through the generations within a culture. Many cultures have their own healers—for

Touching

It is important to know the cultural beliefs of your patient with respect to touching before beginning a hands-on examination. You may need to ask permission to touch, or you may need a relative in the room. The patient may insist that someone of the same sex perform the examination.

example, a *medicine man, shaman,* or *curandero.* Those within the culture often seek the advice of this person before going to a licensed health professional. Beliefs in the various cures that the cultural healer suggests are very powerful. Respect for the person's cultural beliefs in all areas is necessary on the part of the nurse in order to gain the trust of the patient and for advice and teaching to be effective.

Assessment must be done without criticism, with an open mind, and with active listening. Judgmental terms such as *noncompliant, uncooperative, ignorant, lazy,* or *unmotivated* should not be used to describe another person's health behavior.

There should be no conditions or strings attached to the unspoken contract between the nurse and the patient. The nurse need not condone what a patient is doing or not doing to maintain or restore health. The nursing point of view may be respectfully conveyed to the patient. Each patient must be dealt with as a unique individual whose concepts of health and illness and health care might be different from one's own.

? *Think Critically About . . .* Are there health practices within your family that differ from those of your friends or classmates?

THE HOLISTIC APPROACH

Nurses take a holistic approach to caring for the sick and promoting wellness. A holistic approach is one that considers the biologic, psychological, sociologic, and spiritual aspects and needs of the person. The current focus on holism was stimulated by Jan Smuts, a noted South African who formulated a philosophical theory of holism. The value we place on human life, our ability to deal with sickness and death, and our decisions about how to behave toward other people are all profoundly influenced by our basic beliefs about other humans and our relationships with them. Some basic beliefs central to the holistic approach are as follows:

- Each person is a unique integration of body, mind, and spirit, and the unified whole is more than the sum of the body parts. A change in one

aspect of a person's life brings about change in every aspect of her being and alters the quality of the whole.
- Each person has potential for growth in knowledge and skills and in becoming more loving toward herself and others.
- Humans are naturally inclined to be healthy; each of us has responsibility for our own well-being, self-healing, and self-care.
- The "person" of an individual belongs to herself; therefore, decisions about what happens to that person rightfully belong to the owner.
- The focal point of healing efforts is the person, not the disease or injury.
- The relationship between health care professionals and their patients should be one of mutual cooperation. Health care providers intervene on behalf of the adult patient only when their help is sought by the patient or when health needs cannot be met.

In holistic health care, traditional methods of surgical intervention and drug prescription are being combined with or replaced by acupuncture, acupressure, biofeedback, meditation to reduce tension and stress (biologic reactions to an adverse stimulus), and various relaxation techniques for the management of pain, to name but a few of the less traditional approaches. Chiropractic care, once looked upon as questionable, is now covered by many insurance companies. Insurance companies are becoming more inclined to pay for acupressure for treatment of pain.

MASLOW'S THEORY OF BASIC NEEDS

Nurses attempt to assist patients to meet their needs and thereby achieve a higher level of health. People respond to needs as "whole" and integrated beings. Abraham Maslow, a psychologist, identified basic needs necessary for existence and higher level needs for healthy integration of the whole being. He proposed a hierarchy of human needs as an explanation for the forces that motivate human behavior. A hierarchy is defined as the arrangement of objects, elements, or values in order of their importance. Many nursing programs are built on Maslow's basic needs. Figure 2-3 shows Maslow's original hierarchy of needs and an adaptation of the hierarchy used to determine priorities of nursing care. Theoretically, the basic physical needs such as food, air, water, and rest must be satisfied before the higher emotional-level needs emerge. This is true in general, **but the order in which needs are felt and become important to an individual is different from person to person and from situation to situation.**

Once a human need is met, it does not remain satisfied forever. This is obviously true in regard to food, water, air, and other basic first-level physiologic needs. As well as continually needing food, people need continued assurance that they are important, held in es-

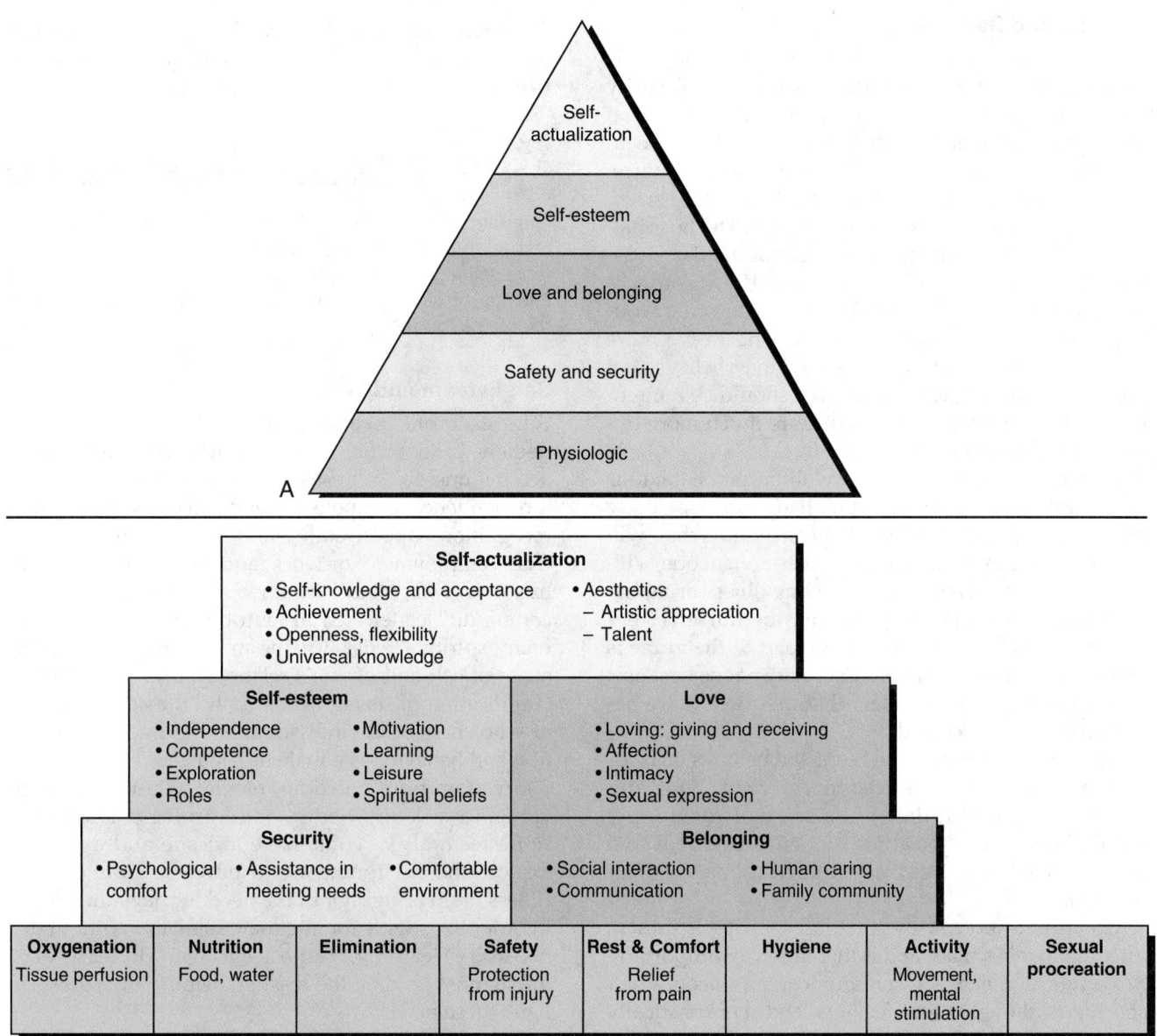

FIGURE **2-3 A,** Maslow's hierarchy of needs. **B,** Evolving hierarchy of needs adapted by nursing to help to determine priorities of care.

teem, safe, and secure from harm. The patient who is receiving medications and treatments for her illness also needs personal contact with loving and caring people.

Physiologic Needs

Fundamental physical needs are essential to maintaining life. The first physiologic need is for oxygen and is immediately followed by the need for adequate cardiovascular function to supply the tissues with blood. The needs for adequate nutrition and for elimination come next.

Basic safety needs are almost as important as physiologic needs. If the patient cannot be protected from the dangers of a being burned or a severe fall, attending to her physiologic needs is useless. **Protection from physical harm, from a nursing standpoint, is often equivalent in importance to physical needs.**

The need for rest comes next and includes freedom from pain, which can greatly interfere with rest. Hygiene needs follow the need for rest because good hygiene is a part of providing comfort and adds a measure of safety and protection against the invasion of bacteria.

Musculoskeletal activity is also a basic physiologic need, because without activity of the muscles and joints, atrophy and deformity will occur, preventing normal function of the muscles and joints. Nurses therefore attend to assisting the patient with movement and ambulation or perform passive range-of-motion exercises for immobile patients.

Sexual expression is a physiologic and psychological need. Survival of a group in society clearly depends on sexual intercourse as a means of procreation to extend the existence of the group. Gratification of sexual needs fits best in the areas of self-esteem and love.

Security and Belonging

Once basic physiologic needs are satisfied, the needs for security and belonging demand attention. Security for patients mainly depends on the reassurance that their physiologic and safety needs will be met. Security also includes protection from psychological harm; freedom from anxiety and fear; and the need for structure, order, and a peaceful environment. The hospitalized child and the elderly person are particularly susceptible to stress created by an unfamiliar, disorderly, or hazardous environment. People value order, routine, and rhythm in their daily lives and thrive more readily in an environment in which they believe that these things are present, although it should be remembered that orderliness and routine are much more important to some people than to others.

Adults who suddenly become ill might be anxious about finances, loss of control, change in their body image, continuation of employment, and what will happen to them in the future if they must cope with the effects of a permanently disabling illness or injury. Therefore, emotional support from the nurse is very important. **Active listening on the part of the nurse is essential in meeting patients' security needs because, to feel secure, they must feel that their needs are being accurately perceived.**

Each person needs to feel that she belongs or is attached to others. People need to feel cared about, and they function best if they feel a sense of community with others. Some social interaction is essential to a sense of well-being and psychological balance (Figure 2-4).

Communication is the method by which human interaction takes place and is therefore very important. Providing a means of communication, encouraging sharing of thoughts and feelings, and therapeutically interacting with the patient is the core of good nursing practice. One can perhaps meet the basic physiologic needs of a patient without communication, but it is impossible to meet other needs if good communication is not present. **Adequate feedback and clarification and validation of communication are essential.**

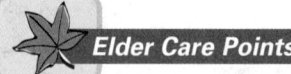

Elder Care Points

Familiarity helps establish secure feelings. If someone comes into an elderly patient's room or house and rearranges that person's belongings, it threatens the person's feelings of security because she no longer knows where things are located.

Self-Esteem and Love

Self-esteem and love are interrelated, since it is apparent that one cannot truly love others until one first loves or accepts oneself. Self-esteem develops from feelings of independence, competence, and self-respect and from recognition, appreciation, and respect from others. One's employment, or work, and various roles (e.g., as husband/wife, father/mother, brother/sister, child, community leader, etc.) all contribute to self-esteem. For many, spiritual belief systems are an integral part of the sense of self and of one's relationship to the universe. Gratification of sexual needs contributes to the feeling of wholeness of the individual and to one's identification and behavior as a male or a female.

Freedom from boredom, mental stimulation, motivation to seek knowledge, and learning play a role in self-esteem also. People have a desire and a need to explore the environment and universe around them. Illness often brings about the need for new knowledge in order to provide for adequate self-care. Without this necessary learning, self-esteem will decrease. The nurse must become the teacher, helping the patient to meet these needs.

Balance in a person's life is brought about by the ability to enjoy leisure activity, to play, and to seek things that bring a measure of happiness.

Illness and adversity, particularly physical adversity, often damage the patient's self-esteem. Nurses can be instrumental in helping to rebuild feelings of competence, independence, and self-respect.

Love consists of both giving and receiving. Without love and attention, an infant will withdraw and gradually die despite having its physiologic needs met. Extreme, prolonged deprivation of love and esteem can bring about neurotic behavior and organic illness.

Intimacy—the greater degree of connectedness, of feeling that one understands and is understood by another—is one of the fibers of love. The achievement of intimacy is the developmental task of the teenager and young adult. However, illness can greatly interfere with intimacy for all adults. Nurses need to assist patients to find ways for intimacy needs to be fulfilled, especially in patients with long-term or chronic illnesses.

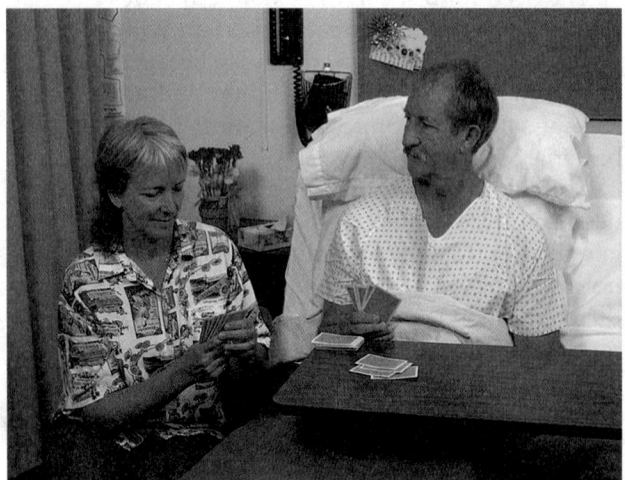

FIGURE **2-4** Spouse sharing leisure time with patient.

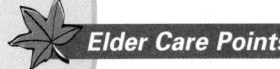
Elder Care Points

An elderly person who no longer has a mate or family, and whose close friends have all died, may become discouraged and depressed. Depression may progress to the degree that the person feels there is nothing left for which to live. This person needs psychological support and social integration so that new friends can be made who will provide a measure of caring and attachment.

Self-Actualization

Self-actualization (reaching one's full potential) is an area to which people do not advance until the physiologic, security and belonging, self-esteem, and love needs have been met. Self-actualization occurs when individuals are very comfortable with themselves and are certain of their beliefs and values. These people are self-reliant, flexible, and open to new ideas; have sought knowledge and truth; and function close to their full potential. Creative expression, whether in an area of performance or appreciation, is part of the self-actualization process. Self-actualization is an ongoing process, not something reached at a particular point in time. Nursing actions that facilitate self-actualization are pertinent mainly during rehabilitation periods, when the nurse assists the patient to strive to achieve full potential.

Humans are rational, decision-making beings. A person is believed to want to have control over her life, even when choosing dependence over independence. Although a person is free to choose, there is no guarantee that every choice will be a wise one. Patients can and do decide not to take physician-prescribed medications, to continue drinking to excess, or to ignore advice of any kind offered by health care professionals. Nurses must understand that behavior is based on what a person perceives to be a need and how highly that person values satisfaction of that need.

? *Think Critically About . . .* If you were ill and hospitalized, how would you prioritize the basic needs for yourself? Which areas would be most important to you in that situation?

HOMEOSTASIS

Homeostasis is a term first coined by W.B. Cannon in 1939 to describe a tendency of biologic systems to maintain stability of the internal environment by continually adjusting to changes necessary for survival. The suffix *-stasis* indicates a static, or balanced state, involving continual adaptation, movement, and change. The term implies a steady state or equilibrium in which there are variations within set limits. These variations take place in a predictable manner—for example, variations in body temperature, changes in the acidity and alkalinity of body fluids, hormonal production and release, and other changes that occur during every 24-hour period. In health, continuous adaptation and change must take place in the internal environment in order to maintain its steady state (equilibrium). Another word for homeostasis is "equilibrium."

In order to enjoy some degree of health and sense of well-being, one must adapt to factors in the *external* environment. In other words, one needs to be in harmony with elements outside oneself by interacting with and integrating various elements into one's life. These elements include the physical, biologic, and psychosocial factors in the world in which one lives and works.

To live in harmony with external environmental factors requires both adaptability and stability.

Wellness is maintained or regained, at least in part, when one is able to keep a sense of balance while adapting to factors that can upset that balance. These factors include such life experiences as socialization, education, mental and physical stress, satisfactions, and rewards. Perhaps one of the most crucial of factors in today's world is change. When change is required, additional stress is put on a person's inner resources, and this in turn can increase susceptibility to illness. Health and illness are dynamic states; therefore, adaptability to a changing external environment is essential to stability and health. Adaptation that results in illness is considered maladaptation.

When the equilibrium of the body is disturbed, *stress* occurs. Stress is the sum of biologic reactions that take place in response to any stressor (adverse stimulus). The stressor may be physical, mental, or emotional and can come from within the body or from the environment. **Stress disturbs the homeostasis of the organism and causes the body to attempt to adapt.** Physical or psychological illness may result from excessive stress or ineffective coping mechanisms.

ADAPTATION

To adapt is to respond to change. The systems of the body have self-regulatory mechanisms to maintain homeostasis. These mechanisms require pathways of communication between the brain and the various body systems. Coordination of the central nervous system, the autonomic (not subject to voluntary control) nervous system, and the endocrine system is required for the body to adjust, adapt, and maintain equilibrium.

The central nervous system, consisting of the brain and spinal cord, coordinates adaptation within the body. The cortex, the thinking part of the brain, communicates with the midbrain and brainstem, which contain many of the structures involved in adaptation and maintenance of physiologic functions. Along with

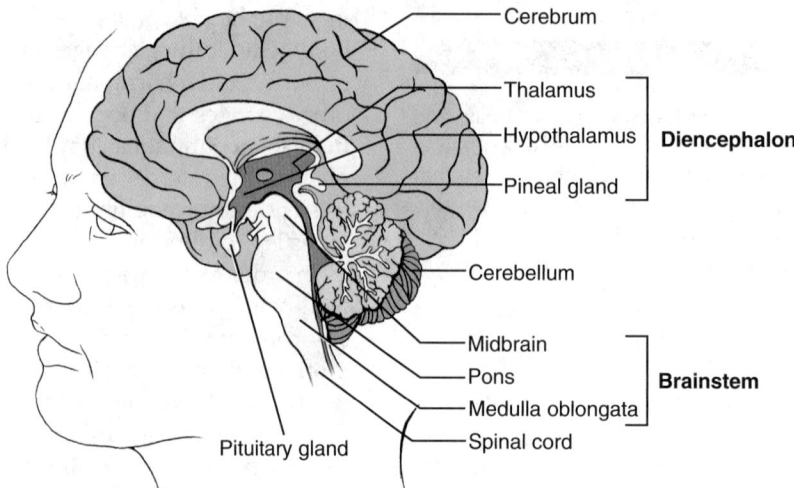

FIGURE **2-5** Central nervous system structures.

the action of the endocrine glands, these structures regulate breathing, heart action, blood pressure, body temperature, hunger, and sleepiness (Figure 2-5).

The reticular activating system (RAS), a bundle of nerve fibers in the brainstem, transmits messages to the cortex from the sensory receptors of the body and carries messages back to the hypothalamus in the midbrain to regulate physiologic functions. The hypothalamus helps regulate the autonomic nervous system and the secretion of hormones by the endocrine system.

The autonomic nervous system regulates physiologic functions that are essentially automatic and beyond voluntary control. It is divided into the sympathetic and parasympathetic nervous systems. These two divisions act like the gas and the brake pedals of a car as they increase or decrease physiologic response of the systems and organs of the body. For example, during vigorous exercise, the sympathetic nervous system sends messages to the bronchi of the lungs to dilate so that more oxygen can be delivered. In contrast, when stepping out into bright sunlight, the parasympathetic system relays messages to the muscles controlling the iris of the eye to constrict the pupil so that less light is allowed to hit the retina.

When the brain perceives a situation as threatening, the sympathetic nervous system stimulates the physiologic functions needed for *fight or flight*. This is the type of reaction that occurs when you are suddenly confronted by a very large, snarling dog on a walking path. The alarmed individual becomes more alert, breathes more deeply, and has muscles poised for fight or flight, and the heart pumps harder. Once the threatening situation is over, the parasympathetic nervous system works to restore equilibrium. In certain situations, the parasympathetic system may be stimulated to slow systems down as a protective measure against a perceived threat.

Although the autonomic nervous system reacts immediately to a perceived threat, the endocrine system must become involved to sustain the fight-or-flight

state. The glands of the endocrine system produce hormones that act on other organs or systems of the body (Figure 2-6). Initiation of a stimulus for hormone production comes from the cortex of the brain and travels to the hypothalamus. The hypothalamus activates the pituitary gland, which in turn secretes hormones that stimulate the other endocrine glands. As long as the body's capacity is not overtaxed, the central nervous system, autonomic nervous system, and endocrine system regulate body systems to maintain

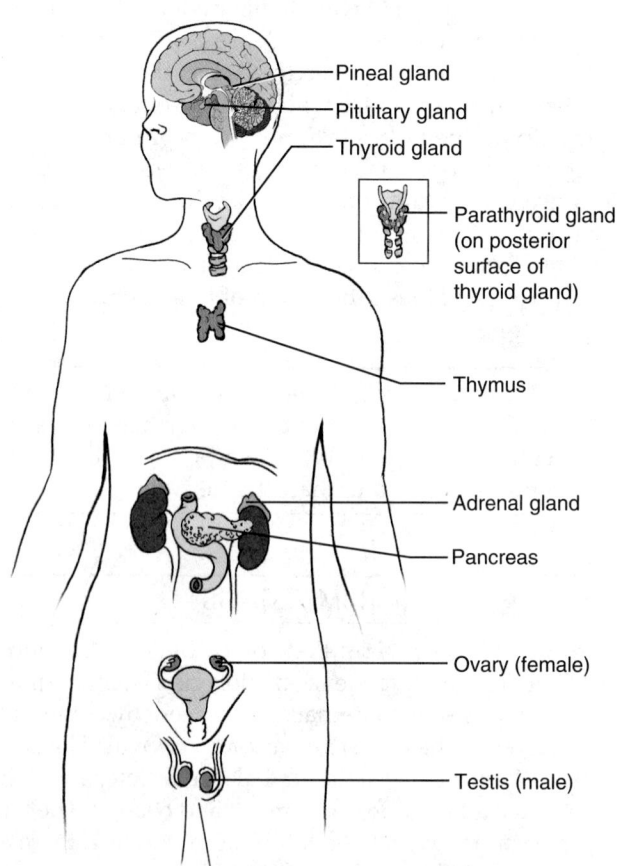

FIGURE **2-6** Major endocrine glands.

Table 2-2 | *Alarm Reaction: Comparison of Sympathetic and Parasympathetic Actions*

ORGAN	SYMPATHETIC ACTION	PARASYMPATHETIC ACTION
Iris of eye	Dilates—pupil becomes larger	Constricts—pupil becomes smaller
Bronchial tubes	Dilate—provide greater air flow	Constrict
Salivary glands	Stimulate thick secretions—dry mouth	Stimulate profuse, watery secretions
Heart	Increases rate and strength of contraction	Decreases rate; no effect on strength of contraction
Blood vessels	Generally constrict—increased blood pressure	No effect for many
Sweat glands	Stimulate sweat production	No effect
Intestines	Inhibit mobility—possible constipation	Stimulate motility and secretion
Liver	Stimulates glycogen breakdown for energy	No effect
Adrenal medulla	Stimulates secretion of epinephrine and norepinephrine	No effect

Adapted from Herlihy, B., & Maebius, N.K. (2007). *The Human Body in Health and Illness* (3rd ed., p. 205). Philadelphia: Elsevier Science.

Box 2-1 | *Common Signs and Symptoms of Stress*

PHYSICAL EFFECTS
- Dry mouth
- Rapid pulse
- Rapid, shallow breathing
- Sweaty palms or generally increased perspiration
- Shakiness and tremors
- Increased blood pressure
- Frequent urination
- Muscle tenseness
- Inability to sit still; tapping fingers on table, pumping leg up and down
- Talking rapidly; stammering
- "Butterflies" in stomach
- Dizziness or feeling light-headed
- Inability to control tears

PSYCHOLOGICAL EFFECTS
- Confusion and forgetfulness
- Anxiety
- Irritability
- Labile moods
- Quick to anger
- Depression

Box 2-2 | *Stress-Related Diseases and Disorders*

- Headaches
- Gastritis
- Asthma
- Low back pain
- Connective tissue disease
- Ulcerative colitis
- Irritable bowel syndrome
- Allergies
- Hypertension
- Cancer
- Sexual dysfunction
- Crohn's disease
- Eating disorders
- Infection*

*Excessive stress weakens the immune system, making the person more vulnerable to invasion by pathogens.

---

homeostasis. Table 2-2 presents body responses when a fight-or-flight reaction occurs. Common signs and symptoms of stress are listed in Box 2-1.

Think Critically About . . . What signs and symptoms does the threat of a major lecture examination cause in you?

The General Adaptation Syndrome

In 1950 Hans Selye, a Canadian physician, published his research-based theories on stress. He found that no matter what the nature of the stressor was, the same nonspecific physical response occurred. The body attempted to deal with stressors by secretion of hormones that caused adaptive responses. Selye concluded that stress plays a role in every disease process because of faulty adaptation (maladaptation) by the body. If the body overreacts in defending itself, there is a surplus of hormones that are favorable to the development of inflammation, and problems such as allergy, arthritis, and asthma may develop. When the body underreacts, too many anti-inflammatory hormones are circulating and serious infection or peptic ulcers may result.

Selye stated that a general adaptation syndrome (GAS) occurs in response to *long-term* exposure to stress. The stages are the *alarm stage,* the *stage of resistance,* and the *stage of exhaustion.* Brief stress responses result in adjustment by homeostatic mechanisms, and equilibrium is restored. During the alarm stage, hormone release mobilizes the body's defenses. Nonspecific signs of illness such as a slight rise in temperature, a loss of energy, decreased appetite, and a general feeling of malaise occur. During the second stage, the stage of resistance, the body is battling for equilibrium. If this stage is excessive or prolonged, the response becomes maladaptive and a pathologic condition occurs, which may be in the form of a stress-related disorder. Box 2-2 lists diseases and disorders considered to be stress related.

The stage of exhaustion occurs if the stressor is severe enough or is present over a long enough period of time to deplete the body's resources for adaptation. Critical illness or death results (Figure 2-7). Examples

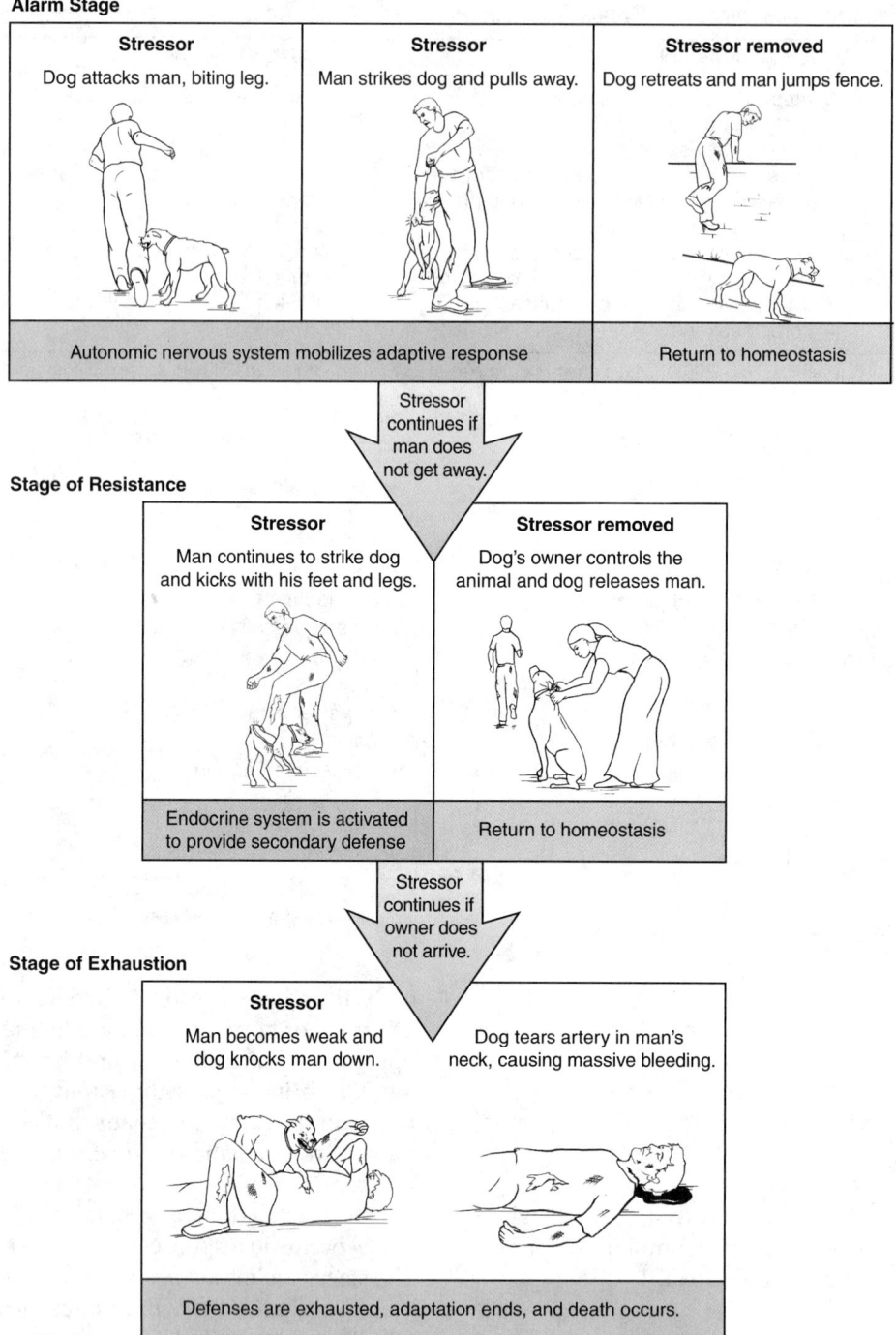

Alarm Stage

Stressor	Stressor	Stressor removed
Dog attacks man, biting leg.	Man strikes dog and pulls away.	Dog retreats and man jumps fence.

Autonomic nervous system mobilizes adaptive response	Return to homeostasis

Stressor continues if man does not get away.

Stage of Resistance

Stressor	Stressor removed
Man continues to strike dog and kicks with his feet and legs.	Dog's owner controls the animal and dog releases man.

Endocrine system is activated to provide secondary defense	Return to homeostasis

Stressor continues if owner does not arrive.

Stage of Exhaustion

Stressor	
Man becomes weak and dog knocks man down.	Dog tears artery in man's neck, causing massive bleeding.

Defenses are exhausted, adaptation ends, and death occurs.

FIGURE **2-7** Stages of the general adaptation syndrome.

of stressors that cause the GAS include trauma, burns, infection, severe cold, and emotional upsets.

Selye believed the body adapts to local stressors in similar ways. The local response is called the *local adaptation syndrome* (LAS). This takes place within a single organ or area of the body, such as when a cut finger becomes inflamed.

THE EFFECTS OF STRESS

We all react or adapt to stress in our own way. What may cause a very mild reaction in one person may cause a much stronger reaction in someone else. A stressor can be helpful or harmful depending on the person's

- Perception of the stressor
- Degree of health and fitness
- Previous life experiences and personality
- Available social support system
- Personal coping mechanisms

When there is a total absence of stress, we may become bored and cease to achieve personal growth. Common patient stressors are found in Box 2-3.

Box 2-3 | **Common Patient Stressors**

- Having to wear an ill-fitting gown that opens down the back
- Sharing a room with a stranger
- Being dependent on others for toileting or bathing
- Sleeping in a different bed with a different pillow
- Eating meals at different times than usual
- Being awakened at odd hours and many times
- Too many or too few visitors
- Worrying about medical costs, home bills, family needs
- Being uncertain of the diagnosis and what will happen
- Not understanding medical terms
- Having to deal with many health care workers who are strangers
- Not being able to obtain desired foods, drinks, or objects
- Being left on a stretcher in a hall without sufficient warm covers
- Having to wait for tests to be done or for the physician to come
- Being stuck with a needle repeatedly for laboratory specimens or intravenous (IV) therapy
- Having other health care workers barge in during toileting or cleansing
- Having different personnel providing care each day

Think Critically About . . . Can you make a list of the stressors in your life at this time?

Coping with Stress

The body has several types of physiologic defenses. Unbroken skin and an intact immune system that protect us against invasion of viral and bacterial stressors are two examples. Psychological defenses include the personality trait of toughness. Tough people believe that life has meaning and that people can influence the environment, and they see change as a challenge. Hardy people cope well. *Coping* means adjusting to or solving challenges. Coping mechanisms help us to resist and master stressors. Coping mechanisms are learned and, once used successfully, they become part of our psychological defense armor. There are three types of coping responses:

- Actions or thoughts that change the situation so it is no longer stressful
- Alteration of thoughts to control the meaning of the situation before it triggers a stress response
- Control of thoughts and actions to stop a stress reaction

Ways to achieve these responses are:

- Seeking information (eliminates fear of the unknown)
- Taking direct action (taking yourself away from a dangerous situation)
- Stopping an unhelpful reaction (refraining from shouting or throwing things when angered)
- Discussing the situation with someone from your social support system
- Using defense mechanisms to perceive the situation differently

Defense Mechanisms. Defense mechanisms are strategies that protect us from increasing anxiety. Defense mechanisms reduce both anxiety and the secretion of stress hormones. Defense mechanisms are used to maintain and improve our self-esteem. Unconsciously using defense mechanisms gives us time to solve the problem and adapt in a positive manner. Using defense mechanisms relieves tension and lessens anxiety. However, they can be overused in a maladaptive way as well. Table 2-3 describes commonly used defense mechanisms and gives examples.

Think Critically About . . . What coping mechanisms do you use the most?

Stress Reduction Techniques. Box 2-4 lists measures that help reduce stress and anxiety in patients. Other measures that help to control the degree of anxiety and reaction to stressors include progressive relaxation, imagery, massage, biofeedback, yoga, and meditation. An additional method of stress reduction is regular physical exercise. Exercise causes endorphin release, which promotes a feeling of well-being and tranquility. More information on these techniques can be found in Chapter 31.

HEALTH PROMOTION AND ILLNESS PREVENTION

A national initiative toward better health was begun in the 1970s. The latest update of direction, goals, and objectives is *Healthy People 2010: With Understanding and Improving Health and Objectives for Improving Health* (U.S. Department of Health and Human Services, 2000). It is a comprehensive set of objectives for disease prevention and health promotion for the nation and was created by scientists. The overall goals are to (1) increase the quality and years of healthy life, and (2) eliminate health disparities. There are 28 focus areas and more than 400 objectives with a target for improvements to be achieved by the year 2010. Every nurse has a responsibility to patients to promote better health through teaching about illness prevention, periodic diagnostic testing for cancer and diabetes, and safe health practices. Encouraging achievement of appropriate weight, regular exercise, adequate sleep, proper nutrition, quitting use of tobacco products, refraining from recreational drug use, and moderation of alcohol intake should be a standard part of nursing care. Practices to prevent back injury, latex allergy, spread of infectious agents, and needlestick injury help safeguard the health of the nurse.

Table 2-3 *Common Defense Mechanisms*

DEFENSE MECHANISMS	CHARACTERISTICS	EXAMPLE
Repression	Blocking a wish or desire from conscious expression.	You forget the name of someone for whom you have intense negative feelings.
Denial	A more serious form of repression. Person lives as though an unwanted piece of information or reality does not exist. There is a persistent refusal to be swayed by evidence.	An alcoholic states, "I do not have a problem with alcohol. I never drink before 5:00 P.M. My stomach problems and liver problems are caused by something else."
Projection	Attributing an unconscious impulse, attitude, or behavior to someone else (blaming or scape-goating).	A man who is attracted to his friend's wife on an unconscious level accuses his own wife of flirting with his friend.
Reaction-formation	An intense feeling regarding an object, person, or feeling is out of awareness and is unknowingly acted out consciously in an opposite manner.	You treat someone whom you unconsciously dislike intensely in an overly friendly manner.
Regression	Returning to an earlier level of adaptation when severely threatened.	A child resumes bedwetting, after having long since stopped, when her baby brother is born and fussed over at home.
Rationalization	Unconsciously falsifying an experience by giving a contrived, socially acceptable, and logical explanation to justify an unpleasant experience or questionable behavior.	A student who did not study for an examination blames his failure on the teacher's poor lecture material and the unfairness of the examination.
Identification	Modeling behavior after someone else.	A 6-year-old girl dresses up in her mother's dress and high-heeled shoes.
Introjection	A more primitive form of identification. More closely relates to unconscious imitation.	A child who becomes irritable after angry interactions with a parent, taking in ("swallowing whole") the image of the angry parent, which grows into himself.
Displacement	Discharging intense feelings for one person onto another object or person who is less threatening, thereby satisfying an impulse with a substitute object.	A child who has been scolded by her mother hits her doll with a hairbrush.
Sublimation	Rechanneling an impulse into a more socially desirable object. You forget the name of someone for whom you have intense negative feelings.	A student satisfies sexual curiosity by conducting sophisticated research into sexual behaviors.

Adapted from Varcarolis, E.M. (2002). *Foundations of Psychiatric Mental Health Nursing* (4th ed., p. 26). Philadelphia: Saunders.

Box 2-4 *Measures to Help Reduce Stress and Anxiety in Patients*

- Explain everything—hospital routine; how the TV, lights, curtains, etc., work; procedures; and diagnostic tests.
- Listen carefully to the patient; answer questions.
- Provide privacy.
- Treat the patient with respect.
- Answer call lights promptly.
- Protect confidentiality.
- Check on the patient frequently.
- Make certain that dietary needs and wants are satisfied as much as possible.
- Return to the patient's bedside when you say you will.
- Bring requested as-needed (PRN) medication promptly; do not allow pain to go untreated.
- Provide uninterrupted rest and sleep periods; coordinate care and treatments.
- Keep visitors within acceptable numbers and time limits per patient's desire.
- Keep noise to a minimum.
- Insist that roommates respect each other's rights.
- Try to keep patient advised as to when to expect diagnostic tests to be performed and when the physician usually makes rounds.
- Allow the patient some control; give choices for time of bathing, ambulating, etc.
- Keep the room temperature adjusted to patient's comfort.

Illness prevention practices are related to health promotion. They consist of voluntary actions that an individual takes to decrease the potential or actual threat of illness. Such actions are divided into primary, secondary, and tertiary prevention. *Primary prevention* avoids or delays occurrence of a specific disease or disorder.

Secondary prevention consists of following guidelines for screening for diseases that are easily treated if found early or for detecting return of a disease. *Tertiary prevention* consists of rehabilitation measures after the disease or disorder has stabilized. Health Promotion Points 2-1 lists such behaviors. Following such health practices

Health Promotion Points 2-1

Health Promotion Behaviors

PRIMARY PREVENTION
- Wearing seat belts, helmets
- Eating well-balanced meals
- Not smoking
- Consuming no or minimal alcohol
- Being immunized
- Maintaining ideal body weight

SECONDARY PREVENTION
- Having yearly Papanicolaou (Pap) smear tests
- Performing a monthly breast or testicular self-examination
- Having mammograms as recommended
- Getting skin tests for tuberculosis screening
- Having routine tonometry tests to detect glaucoma

TERTIARY PREVENTION
- Following a cardiac rehabilitation program
- Pursuing rehabilitation programs for stroke, head injury, or arthritis

Modified from Ignatavicius, D.D., & Workman, M.L. (2006). *Medical-Surgical Nursing: Critical Thinking for Collaborative Care* (5th ed., p. 6). Philadelphia: Elsevier Saunders.

has been associated with a greater degree of health for persons of any age, sex, or economic status. The United States and Canada have published goals for essential health care services. The priorities in *Healthy People 2010* involve teaching for disease and accident prevention, health promotion, and self-care behaviors (see Chapter 9). While caring for patients in different settings, you should always assist patients to mobilize and maintain appropriate coping mechanisms and teach practices that promote good health. Specific *Healthy People 2010* objectives are included in the appropriate sections throughout this text.

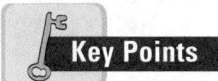

Key Points

- The word "health" comes from a word meaning "wholeness" and means many different things to people.
- Cultural, educational, and social factors affect how people view health and illness.
- The World Health Organization states that health is "the state of complete physical, mental, and social well-being and not merely the absence of disease or infirmity."
- Illness occurs in stages; there is a transition stage (onset), an acceptance stage (sick role), and convalescence stage (recovery).
- A contemporary definition of being healthy means being able to function well physically and mentally and to express the full range of one's potentialities within the environment in which one is living.
- Dubos and Dunn promoted the philosophy that health and illness are dynamic states of being, constantly altering, and that each person moves up and down within a spectrum ranging from obvious disease through the absence of detectable disease and on to a state of optimum functioning in all aspects of life.
- Nursing is concerned with helping people cope with adverse physiologic, psychosocial, and spiritual responses to illness, rather than treating the illness itself.
- The essential task of nursing is to enhance and support a patient's healing strengths by helping her to utilize coping abilities to best advantage and to adapt to conditions that cannot be changed.
- A major goal of nursing is to get people to take charge of their own health and to take positive steps to preserve or enhance it through positive health promotion or illness prevention actions.
- Different cultures have different values and beliefs about health and illness. Cultural practices must be understood and respected by the nurse.
- A holistic approach considers the physiologic, psychological, sociologic, and spiritual aspects and needs of the individual.
- Maslow described a hierarchy of needs that nursing has adopted for prioritizing patient problems and care. The five areas of need established by Maslow are physiologic, safety and security, love and belonging, self-esteem, and self-actualization.
- Homeostasis is the tendency of the body's biologic systems to constantly adjust to maintain constant conditions that are optimal to maintaining life and health. It involves continual adaptation (response to change).
- Stress disturbs homeostasis and causes the body to attempt to adapt.
- When the body receives a threat, the sympathetic nervous system stimulates the physiologic functions needed for fight or flight. Once the threat is over, the parasympathetic nervous system mediates to return the physiologic functions to normal.
- As long as the body's capacity is not overtaxed, the central nervous system, autonomic nervous system, and endocrine system regulate the body to maintain homeostasis. If the body is overtaxed, critical illness or death occurs.
- Hans Selye developed the theory of the general adaptation syndrome, which occurs in three stages: the alarm stage, the stage of resistance, and the stage of exhaustion.
- Coping mechanisms are learned to help in the defense against stress. Defense mechanisms are unconscious strategies that protect us from increasing anxiety.
- Measures that help control stress and anxiety are progressive relaxation, imagery, massage, biofeedback, yoga, meditation, and regular exercise.
- Health can be promoted by personal practices regarding diet, exercise, rest, and refraining from health risk behaviors.

- Illness may be prevented by voluntary actions regarding health care practices, screening tests, and participation in treatment regimens.
- *Healthy People 2010* is a set of national goals to promote better health by increasing the quality and years of healthy life and by eliminating health disparities.

 Go to your **Companion CD-ROM** for an Audio Glossary, animations, video clips, and more.

evolve Be sure to visit the companion Evolve site at http://evolve.elsevier.com/deWit/fundamental/ for additional online resources.

NCLEX-PN® EXAMINATION-STYLE REVIEW QUESTIONS

*Choose the **best** answer(s) for each question.*

1. Which one of the following statements **best** describes health? Health is:
   1. a relative state of being.
   2. the total state of physical and psychological well-being.
   3. the state of functioning well physically, mentally, and socially.
   4. being free of sickness or infirmity.

2. Taking on the sick role occurs when a patient:
   1. recognizes that vague aches and pains are present.
   2. states that she might be getting a cold.
   3. refuses to see a physician even though her cough is constant.
   4. buying and taking a couple of aspirin.

3. Current views of health include the concept of:
   1. rarely allowing oneself to become ill.
   2. allowing others to take responsibility for one's health.
   3. personal endeavor to better oneself.
   4. expressing the full range of one's potentialities.

4. The ability of a person to function at an optimum level is primarily dependent on:
   1. inner resources of the person.
   2. considerate, expert nursing care.
   3. high-quality medical treatment.
   4. a solid support system.

5. It is important to assess a patient's *actual* cultural beliefs because:
   1. a patient may not adhere to the usual health beliefs of her culture.
   2. cultural beliefs play a major role in how the patient perceives herself.
   3. the family's beliefs are inherent in the patient.
   4. cultural diversity is present in all parts of the United States.

6. When nurses set priorities of patient needs according to Maslow's hierarchy, they should: *(Select all that apply.)*
   1. only consider physiologic needs.
   2. consider airway status first.
   3. consider safety a high priority.
   4. place self-esteem needs before security needs.
   5. place activity needs before belonging needs.
   6. consider elimination needs before rest and comfort needs.

7. A patient had major surgery and says she's worried about what is happening at home, is worried about not being there to coach the soccer team tomorrow, is feeling pain, and wants to see her husband. Which one of the following actions would you take **first?**
   1. Tell her not to worry about things at home.
   2. Allow her to call the children at home.
   3. Administer pain medication.
   4. Check to see who might be able to coach the soccer team.
   5. Put in a call to her husband so she can obtain information and have him arrange for someone to coach the soccer team.

8. Which one of the following is the **best** description of homeostasis?
   1. It is the tendency of the body to constantly adjust to changing conditions.
   2. It occurs when the equilibrium of the body is disturbed.
   3. It is the biologic reaction that takes place in response to a stressor.
   4. It is a static condition of the body during health.

9. The effects of stress on a person partially depend on:
   1. the presence of prior illness.
   2. the time of day it occurs.
   3. the surrounding environment.
   4. the perception of the stressor.

10. Selye's theory of general adaptation states that homeostasis will be regained:
    1. by the actions of the endocrine system.
    2. in spite of the person's state of health.
    3. unless adaptive mechanisms are overwhelmed.
    4. when the stressor is relieved.

CRITICAL THINKING ACTIVITIES *Read each clinical scenario and discuss the questions with your classmates.*

1. Share some of your family values and beliefs that contribute to your own definition of health.

2. What does illness mean to you?

3. How can you increase your ability to effectively cope with stress?

4. How would you go about helping a patient mobilize her coping mechanisms?

Legal and Ethical Aspects of Nursing

Objectives

Upon completing this chapter, you should be able to:

Theory

1. Explain the legal requirements for the practice of nursing, and how they relate to a student nurse.
2. Identify the consequences of violating the nurse practice act.
3. Examine the issue of professional accountability, professional discipline, and continuing education for licensed nurses.
4. Compare and contrast the terms *negligence* and *malpractice.*
5. Discuss what you can do to protect yourself from lawsuits or the damages of lawsuits.
6. Differentiate a code of ethics from laws or regulations governing nursing, and compare the similarities of the codes of ethics from the NFLPN, NAPNES, and ANA.
7. Describe the NAPNES standards of practice.

Clinical Practice

1. Reflect on how laws relating to discrimination, workplace safety, child abuse, and sexual harassment affect your nursing practice.
2. Discuss the National Patient Safety Goals and identify where these can be found.
3. Interpret rights that a patient has in a hospital, nursing home, community setting, or psychiatric facility.
4. Describe three factors necessary for informed consent.
5. Explain advance directives and the advantage of having them written out.

Key Terms

Be sure to check the bonus material on the Companion CD-ROM, including selected audio pronunciations.

accountability (ă-kŏwn-tă-BĬ-lĭ-tē, p. 31)
advance directive (p. 38)
assault (ă-SĂLT, p. 40)
assignment (p. 31)
battery (p. 40)
competent (p. 38)
confidential (cŏn-fĭ-DĔN-shŭl, p. 35)
consent (p. 37)
defamation (dĕ-fă-MĀ-shŭn, p. 40)
delegation (p. 31)
discrimination (p. 34)

do not resuscitate (DNR) (rē-SŬ-sĭ-tāt, p. 39)
ethical codes, ethical principles, ethics committee (p. 29)
ethics (p. 44)
euthanasia (yū-thă-NĀ-zhē-ă, p. 45)
false imprisonment (p. 41)
health care agent (p. 39)
incident report (p. 42)
invasion of privacy (p. 40)
laws (p. 30)
liability (lī-ă-BĬL-ĭ-tē, p. 38)
libel (LĪ-bŭl, p. 40)
living will (p. 38)
malpractice (măl-PRĂK-tĭs, p. 39)
negligence (p. 39)
nurse practice act (p. 31)
Occupational Safety and Health Act (OSHA) (ŏ-kŭ-PĀ-shŭn-ŭl, p. 32)
patient advocate (ĂD-vō-kăt, p. 39)
privilege (PRĬ-vĭ-lĕj, p. 29)
protective devices (p. 41)
prudent (p. 39)
reciprocity (rĕ-cĭ-PRŎ-cĭ-tē, p. 31)
release (p. 38)
sentinel event (p. 35)
sexual harassment (hă-RĂS-mĭnt, p. 34)
slander (p. 40)
standards of care (p. 32)
statutes (p. 30)
tort (p. 30)
whistle-blowing (p. 45)

An understanding of legal and ethical codes is essential for nurses to practice safely and to protect the rights of patients and co-workers. Nurses work in situations that give them privilege (permission to do what is usually not permitted in other circumstances) to a patient's body and emotions. Laws define the boundaries of that privilege and make clear the nurse's rights and responsibilities. Ethical codes (actions and beliefs approved of by a particular group of people) are different from laws, and are important because not all situations are covered by a law, and there may not be one *right* action. In these situations, ethical principles (rules of right and wrong from an ethical point of view) are applied, often by an ethics committee (a committee formed to consider ethical problems).

SOURCE OF LAW

Laws are rules of conduct that are established by our government (the specialized vocabulary used in reference to legal terms is defined in Box 3-1). In the United States, law comes from three sources: the Constitution and Bill of Rights; laws made by elected officials; and regulations made by agencies created by these elected officials. Constitutional laws, both federal and state, provide for basic rights and create the legislative bodies (senate and assembly) that write laws governing our lives.

Judicial law results when a law or court decision is challenged in the courts and the judge affirms or reverses the decision. This is called "establishing a precedent," because in the future other judges will base their decisions on the preceding or earlier decision. Our federal Supreme Court is the highest court to which an appeal of a court decision can be brought. A well-known health care issue that has been ruled on by the Supreme Court was *Roe v. Wade* (1972), which established a woman's right to obtain an elective abortion. More recently, state courts are hearing cases challenging laws that deal with abortion, euthanasia, and assisted suicide.

Administrative law comes from agencies created by the legislature. In health care, agencies such as the Department of Health and Human Services or Office of Professional Licensing oversee nursing and the other health care professions. These agencies write regulations or rules that control the profession and its practice. Administrative law governs schools of nursing, licensure, hospitals, nursing homes, and home health agencies, as well as health care insurance such as Medicare, Medicaid, and private insurance company policies.

CIVIL AND CRIMINAL LAW

Statutes (laws) may be either civil or criminal. Civil law guarantees individual rights, and a tort is a violation of civil law. You may be guilty of a tort if you harm a patient, for example, by administering the wrong dose or type of medication. A lawsuit may result, and, if the **defendant** is found guilty, a monetary award may be given to the **plaintiff.**

A **crime** is a wrong against society, and imprisonment and/or fines may result if one is convicted of a

---

Box 3-1 | *Legal Terms and Definitions*

Advance directive: Written statement expressing wishes of the patient regarding future consent for or refusal of treatment if the patient is incapable of participating in decision making.

Appeal: Challenge to a court decision; a higher court will judge whether the original decision is affirmed or reversed.

Civil rights, civil law: Personal or individual conditions (e.g., life, liberty, privacy) guaranteed by the Constitution, Bill of Rights, and federal or regulatory law.

Competent: Mentally and emotionally able to understand and act (make choices). Able to appreciate consequences of actions.

Controlled substance: Specific drugs with a potential for abuse, such as narcotics, tranquilizers, stimulants, and sedatives. Laws regulate how these are prescribed, dispensed, and stored.

Crime: Violation of public law.

Defendant: Person accused of violation of public law (crime) or civil law (tort).

Damages: The monetary award to an injured plaintiff when the defendant is found responsible for the injury.

Emancipated minor: Person under 18 years of age who is legally considered an adult, usually because of marriage, parenthood, or enlistment in the armed services.

Felony: A serious crime that may result in a prison term of more than 1 year.

Health care agent: Person designated by the patient to make health care decisions when the patient is incapacitated (not able to make those decisions). Usually part of an advance directive.

Liability: Responsibility to pay or compensate for a loss or injury that results from one's negligence.

Litigation: Lawsuit; legal process to prove facts of a dispute.

Malpractice: Failure to do, or doing, what a prudent (reasonable) professional would or would not do; results in harm or injury to a patient who is in the professional's care.

Malpractice insurance: Policy that protects nurse from expense of defending self from lawsuit; will pay the amount awarded up to policy limits if nurse is found guilty of malpractice.

Medical power of attorney: Legal assignment of ability to make health care decisions for another person. Similar to a health care agent.

Misdemeanor: Less serious crime than felony; may result in fines, imprisonment of 1 year or less, or both.

Negligence: Failure to do what a prudent (reasonable) person would do, or doing what a reasonable person would not do; results in harm or injury to another person.

Plaintiff: Person who believes he or she has been injured by the actions of another, and seeks to prove it in a court of law.

Power of attorney: Legal action to allow a person to conduct business matters for another.

Precedent: A judicial decision that is used as a guide to interpreting the law and deciding cases afterward.

Privileged relationship: One that requires confidentiality; trust that information gained in the relationship will not be made public.

Statute: Legal term for a law.

Tort: Violation of a civil law, a wrong against an individual.

crime. Criminal action charges in nursing could come about if a nurse was involved in drug diversion, patient abuse, intentional death, or mercy killing. Serious crimes are called **felonies** and are punished with long prison terms of a year of more, or even the death penalty; less serious crimes are **misdemeanors,** and may result in prison terms of less than a year, monetary fines, or both.

LAWS RELATED TO NURSING PRACTICE AND LICENSURE

NURSE PRACTICE ACT

State licensure is required to practice nursing in the United States, and each state writes its own laws and regulations regarding licensure, in what is called a nurse practice act. This law defines the scope of nursing practice, and provides for the regulation of the profession by a state board of nursing.

SCOPE OF PRACTICE

The nurse practice act in each state sets forth the scope of practice in that state. This includes the definition of nursing for the registered professional nurse (RN) and the licensed practical or vocational nurse (LPN or LVN) and may include definitions for advanced practice nurses such as nurse practitioners or nurse anesthetists. Nurse practice acts regulate the degree of dependence or independence of a licensed nurse with regard to other nurses, physicians, and health care providers. For example, an LPN/LVN practices under the direction of an RN, physician, or dentist. Nurses must follow the lawful order of a physician unless it is harmful to the patient, and must have a physician order to perform certain functions, such as administering prescription drugs or placing a patient in a protective device.

LICENSURE

Eligibility for licensure is determined by each state's board of nursing, usually involving completion of an approved educational program. The National Council of State Boards of Nursing, which develops the National Council Licensure Examination (NCLEX), has a representative from each of the state boards of nursing in the United States who has input on the exam. A passing score on this computer-adapted test is accepted by the states for initial licensure when all other state requirements for eligibility are met. A current issue regarding licensure involves national licensure, or automatic reciprocity (recognition of one state's nursing license by another state). Although a growing number of states have developed reciprocity agreements, nurses who wish to practice in more than one state may need to apply for the nursing license in each state in which they practice. National licensure would recognize a state license in all other states.

Student Nurses

Student nurses, although they are not yet licensed, are held to the same standards as a licensed nurse. This means that although a student nurse may not perform a task as quickly or as smoothly as the licensed nurse, the student will achieve the same outcome without harm to the patient. The student is legally responsible for her own actions or inaction, and many schools require the student to carry **malpractice insurance.** The instructor who supervises a student is responsible for proper instruction and adequate supervision and evaluation of a student. Instructors are responsible for assigning students to patients of an appropriate level of complexity so that they do not jeopardize patient safety. A student's responsibility is to consult with the instructor when she is unsure in a situation, or when a patient's condition is changing rapidly. **Student nurses need to know the nurse practice act and its definition of nursing in the state in which they are practicing, and not exceed the scope of practice for their state. It is not legal to do something beyond the scope of nursing practice just because you were told to do so.** Hospitals or health care agencies may impose limitations on student practice, but they may not add duties or responsibilities beyond the scope of practice in that state.

PROFESSIONAL ACCOUNTABILITY

Accountability is taking responsibility for one's actions. Professional accountability is a nurse's responsibility to meet the health care needs of the patient in a safe and caring way. In order to do so, students must prepare themselves in the classroom with **theory**—the textbook description of patient needs and nursing interventions—and then apply that information in the clinical setting. Accountability means asking for assistance when unsure, performing nursing tasks in the safe and prescribed manner, reporting and documenting assessments and interventions, and evaluating the care given and the patient's response to that care. As a licensed nurse, accountability means all of the above, plus a commitment to continuing education to stay current and knowledgeable.

Delegation

Delegation is the assignment of duties to another person. Some states differentiate between delegation (only to another licensed person) and assignment, which can be done to an unlicensed person, such as a nursing assistant. An LPN may supervise nursing assistants, technicians, or other LPNs (Assignment Considerations 3-1). The nurse is responsible for ensuring patient safety and the observation of patient rights. It is the delegating nurse's duty to supervise and evaluate the care a licensed or unlicensed person provides.

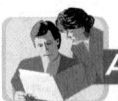

Assignment Considerations 3-1

Nurse's Responsibilities

When a licensed nurse gives an assignment to another person, the nurse is responsible for ensuring that the person has the skills and abilities to safely perform the assignment, and that an unlicensed person is not performing acts restricted to nursing under the law.

Standards of Care

Legally, you are responsible for your actions under the nurse practice act and according to the standards of care that are approved by the profession. These standards are defined in nursing procedure books, institutional manuals of policies and procedures or protocols, and nursing journals that outline current skills or techniques. On a national level, standards of care have been identified and published for clinical practice and specialty areas by professional nursing organizations. These standards provide a way of judging the quality and effectiveness of patient care, and in legal cases determine whether a nurse acted correctly (see Boxes 1-1 and 1-2). Standards of care are continually being revised as better treatments and techniques are continually being updated and revised with nursing research. What is the standard today may not be the standard of care next year; therefore, it is crucial that the LPN/LVN keep abreast of current standards with continuing education.

PROFESSIONAL DISCIPLINE

State boards of nursing are also responsible for discipline within the profession. When a licensed nurse is charged with a violation of the nurse practice act, there will be a hearing to determine if the charges are true. The most common charges brought against nurses include substance abuse (drug and alcohol related), incompetence (doing something that can or did harm a patient, such as medication errors), and negligence (discussed later). **It is considered negligence not to report another professional's misconduct.** When a nurse is found guilty of professional misconduct, the penalties may result in a temporary suspension or loss of licensure.

CONTINUING EDUCATION

Many states have adopted laws that require evidence of continuing education after a nurse has passed the licensing exam. Once licensed, it is expected that the nurse will function safely in any nursing situation. Therefore, it is necessary for nurses to continue their education about changes in health care practice, pharmacology, and technology in order to practice safely. Nurses may stay current by attending programs provided by their employer; through participation in their professional organization; by attending workshops, seminars, or presentations on health care topics; by reading professional nursing journals; by formal continuing education in colleges; or by correspondence courses.

LAWS AND GUIDELINES AFFECTING NURSING PRACTICE

When a licensed nurse accepts employment with an agency or individual, the nurse is bound to work within the law and regulations governing nursing in that state. There are also federal laws that regulate safety and health in the workplace, and forbid discrimination and sexual harassment. Although not law, the "Patient Care Partnership: Understanding Expectations, Rights, and Responsibilities" provides ethical guidelines for nursing practice (Box 3-2).

OCCUPATIONAL SAFETY AND HEALTH ACT (OSHA)

The Occupational Safety and Health Act (OSHA) was passed in 1970 to improve the work environment in areas that affect workers' health or safety. It includes regulations for handling infectious or toxic materials, radiation safeguards, and the use of electrical equipment. Health care agencies, as a result of OSHA requirements, provide mandatory orientation and continuing education regarding a wide range of topics from isolation procedures and blood-borne pathogen (disease-producing organism) exposure, to fire or bomb threats and lifting and evacuation procedures.

Safe storage and handling of toxic chemicals and drugs are important parts of OSHA. Each facility is required to keep a record of hazardous substances, which includes seemingly harmless liquids such as bleach and disinfectants, as well as obviously dangerous chemicals. The facility must store them properly in designated areas, and maintain material safety data sheets (MSDS), which outline the hazard the substance can pose. Employees must be updated on these workplace hazards and know the location of the MSDS collection.

CHILD ABUSE PREVENTION AND TREATMENT ACT (CAPTA)

The Child Abuse Prevention and Treatment Act (CAPTA) is a federal law. It was passed in 1973 and was rewritten in October 1996. This law defines child abuse and neglect as "any recent act, or failure to act, that results in imminent risk of serious harm, death, serious physical or emotional harm, sexual abuse, or exploitation of a child by a parent or caretaker who is responsible for the child's welfare." A child is a person under the age of 18 unless state law specifies a younger age. Many children who are victims of abuse are too young to speak for themselves. CAPTA states that licensed health care personnel are required to report

Box 3-2 *Patient Care Partnership: Understanding Expectations, Rights, and Responsibilities*

When you need hospital care, your doctor and the nurses and other professionals at our hospital are committed to working with you and your family to meet your health care needs. Our dedicated doctors and staff serve the community in all its ethnic, religious, and economic diversity. Our goal is for you and your family to have the same care and attention we would want for our families and ourselves.

The sections below explain some of the basics about how you can expect to be treated during your hospital stay. They also cover what we will need from you to care for you better. If you have questions at any time, please ask them. Unasked or unanswered questions can add to the stress of being in the hospital. Your comfort and confidence in your care are very important to us.

WHAT TO EXPECT DURING YOUR HOSPITAL STAY

- **High quality hospital care.** Our first priority is to provide you the care you need, when you need it, with skill, compassion, and respect. Tell your caregivers if you have concerns about your care or if you have pain. You have the right to know the identity of doctors, nurses, and others involved in your care, as well as when they are students, residents, or other trainees.
- **A clean and safe environment.** Our hospital works hard to keep you safe. We use special policies and procedures to avoid mistakes in your care and keep you free from abuse or neglect. If anything unexpected and significant happens during your hospital stay, you will be told what happened and any resulting changes in your care will be discussed with you.
- **Involvement in your care.** You and your doctor often make decisions about your care before you go to the hospital. Other times, especially in emergencies, those decisions are made during your hospital stay. When they take place, making decisions should include:
  - Discussing your medical condition and information about medically appropriate treatment choices. To make informed decisions with your doctor, you need to understand several things:
    — The benefits and risks of each treatment.
    — Whether it is experimental or part of a research study.
    — What you can reasonably expect from your treatment and any long-term effects it might have on your quality of life.
    — What you and your family will need to do after you leave the hospital.
    — The financial consequences of using uncovered services or out-of-network providers.
    Please tell your caregivers if you need more information about treatment choices.
  - Discussing your treatment plan. When you enter the hospital, you sign a general consent to treatment. In some cases, such as surgery or experimental treatment, you may be asked to confirm in writing that you understand what is planned and agree to it. This process protects your right to consent to or refuse a treatment. Your doctor will explain the medical consequences of refusing recommended treatment. It also protects your right to decide if you want to participate in a research study.
  - Getting information from you. Your caregivers need complete and correct information about your health and coverage so that they can make good decisions about your care. That includes:
    — Past illnesses, surgeries, or hospital stays.
    — Past allergic reactions.
    — Any medicines or diet supplements (such as vitamins and herbs) that you are taking.
    — Any network or admission requirements under your health plan.
  - Understanding your health care goals and values. You may have health care goals and values or spiritual beliefs that are important to your well-being. They will be taken into account as much as possible throughout your hospital stay. Make sure your doctor, your family, and your care team know your wishes.
  - Understanding who should make decisions when you cannot. If you have signed a health care power of attorney stating who should speak for you if you become unable to make health care decisions for yourself, or a "living will" or "advance directive" that states your wishes about end-of-life care, give copies to your doctor, your family, and your care team. If you or your family need help making difficult decisions, counselors, chaplains, and others are available to help.
- **Protection of your privacy.** We respect the confidentiality of your relationship with your doctor and other caregivers, and the sensitive information about your health and health care that are part of that relationship. State and federal laws and hospital operating policies protect the privacy of your medical information. You will receive a Notice of Privacy Practices that describes the ways that we use, disclose, and safeguard patient information and that explains how you can obtain a copy of information from our records about your care.
- **Help preparing you and your family for when you leave the hospital.** Your doctor works with hospital staff and professionals in your community. You and your family also play an important role. The success of your treatment often depends on your efforts to follow medication, diet, and therapy plans. Your family may need to help care for you at home. You can expect us to help you identify sources of follow-up care and to let you know if our hospital has a financial interest in any referrals. As long as you agree we can share information about your care with them, we will coordinate our activities with your caregivers outside the hospital. You can also expect to receive information and, where possible, training about the self-care you will need when you go home.

From American Hospital Association. (2003). *Patient Care Partnership: Understanding Expectations, Rights, and Responsibilities*. Chicago: American Hospital Association. © 2003 by the American Hospital Association.

Continued

Box 3-2 *Patient Care Partnership: Understanding Expectations, Rights, and Responsibilities—cont'd*

- **Help with your bill and filing insurance claims.** Our staff will file claims for you with health care insurers or other programs such as Medicare and Medicaid. They will also help your doctor with needed documentation. Hospital bills and insurance coverage are often confusing. If you have questions about your bill, contact our business office. If you need help understanding your insurance coverage or health plan, start with your insurance company or health benefits manager. If you do not have health coverage, we will try to help you and

your family find financial help or make other arrangements. We need your help with collecting needed information and other requirements to obtain coverage or assistance.

While you are here, you will receive more detailed notices about some of the rights you have as a hospital patient and how to exercise them. We are always interested in improving. If you have questions, comments, or concerns, please contact _____.

---

child abuse. Each facility usually has guidelines on how to report child abuse.

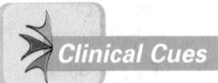

In the case of child abuse, the account of the injury or accident given by the caregiver is often inconsistent with the physical signs and symptoms. A student should bring any suspicions of child abuse to the attention of the instructor.

DISCRIMINATION

Discrimination is making a decision or treating a person based on a class or group to which he belongs, such as race, religion, or sex, rather than on his individual qualities. In 1964, federal legislation made it illegal for employers to *discriminate* (to hire, promote, or fire employees on the basis of race, color, religion, sex, or national origin). The law has been amended to include protection for people with disabilities, as well as discrimination based on age. Disability has been broadly interpreted to include physical or mental impairment that seriously interferes with a person's ability to carry on one or more life activities. It particularly protects people with human immunodeficiency virus (HIV) infection or acquired immunodeficiency syndrome (AIDS), or those who are recovering from drug or alcohol addiction. It is not legal for employers to ask questions on an employment application that would indicate race or other protected categories, or health status. It also requires employers to make reasonable accommodations for persons with a disability.

SEXUAL HARASSMENT

Sexual harassment is defined by the Equal Employment Opportunity Commission (EEOC) as "unwelcome sexual advances, requests for sexual favors, and other verbal or physical conduct of a sexual nature." Sexual harassment is illegal when it is used as a condition of employment or promotion or when it interferes with job performance. Sexual harassment prohibition has been further applied in schools and in the clinical setting. Student nurses and their instructors need to recognize what sexual harassment is; to refrain from conversation or actions that create a hostile, intimidat-

ing, or offensive atmosphere; and to report actions that are sexually harassing in the classroom or clinical setting. In our society, in which sexual comments and activities are commonplace on television or in movies, we must be aware of the right time and place for sexually suggestive or explicit words or touch. It is appropriate to state, "I am offended by your language (conversation, inappropriate touch)." If the sexually explicit or harassing behavior continues, it should be reported to your supervisor.

GOOD SAMARITAN LAWS

Good Samaritan laws are those that protect a health care professional from liability if she stops to provide aid in an emergency. In most states there is no legal requirement for a nurse to provide aid in an emergency, but if a nurse does provide care in an emergency, liability is limited unless there is evidence of gross negligence or intentional misconduct. These laws do not apply to employed emergency response workers.

PATIENT'S RIGHTS

In 1972, with revision in 1992, the American Hospital Association (AHA) developed the "Patient's Bill of Rights," a list of rights the patient could expect and responsibilities that the hospital may not violate. In 2003, this document was revised into "The Patient Care Partnership: Understanding Expectations, Rights, and Responsibilities" (see Box 3-2). Although this is an ethical, not a legal, document, state legislators have written laws that prohibit certain actions or guarantee particular rights. Since the first patient bill of rights, which was hospital oriented, many others have been published, particularly for residents of nursing homes and those in psychiatric units. These documents emphasize that patients continue to have rights even if they are helpless and sick. They seek to preserve the dignity, privacy, freedom of movement, and information needs of the patient.

Under some legally specified conditions, certain rights may be temporarily suspended, such as in an emergency when the patient is unconscious or unable to communicate. Other conditions would include the patient who is in danger of injury and cannot protect himself from harm, or to protect the public from harm. However, patients with psychiatric disorders in most

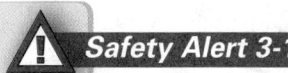

Safety Alert 3-1

Communication and Safety

Safe and effective patient care depends on complete communication between caregivers. *"Handoff" communication* describes times when information is passed from one caregiver to another, such as a change-of-shift report, patient transfer to another unit or facility, or contacting the physician. Patient safety during these times depends on effective, complete communication.

---

states cannot be held against their will for more than 2 or 3 days, unless they are a distinct danger to self or others, or are gravely disabled, which means unable to provide for their basic needs of food, shelter, or clothing. The current principle is to protect the rights of harmless individuals to be different, to disagree with the majority, to live their own lives, and to seek their own solutions to private difficulties.

NATIONAL PATIENT SAFETY GOALS

The International Center for Safety of The Joint Commission (formerly known as the Joint Commission on Accreditation of Healthcare Organizations [JCAHO]) has developed goals to promote specific improvements in patient safety. The goals attempt to provide evidence-based and expert-based solutions to areas that have been problematic in terms of patient safety. The Joint Commission's National Patient Safety Goals are updated every year, and are available on their website (www.jcipatientsafety.org). It is in the best interest of patient safety and quality nursing care for all nurses to review these goals on an annual basis.

A sentinel event is an unexpected patient care event that results in death or serious injury (or risk thereof) to the patient. One of the National Patient Safety Goals is to improve the effectiveness of communication among caregivers, since the most frequently cited cause of a sentinel event by The Joint Commission is communication (Safety Alert 3-1). During "handoff" communication, there is a risk that critical patient care information might be lost due to lack of communication. One form of communication, termed the *SBAR method of communication,* is a strategy that reduces the likelihood of critical patient details being lost. SBAR is an acronym that stands for situation, background, assessment, and recommendation (Communication Cues 3-1).

SBAR is also useful when communicating with physicians, because nurses and physicians are taught different ways to communicate patient information in their educational processes. Nurses are taught to communicate in narrative form, and to include every possible detail, whereas physicians are taught to communicate using brief "bullet" points. This SBAR format encourages caregivers to communicate in a way that is concise, yet complete.

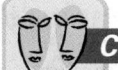

Communication Cues 3-1

Example of SBAR Communication

SITUATION: You are communicating the 3:00 P.M. change-of-shift report for a 65-year-old patient who was admitted 3 days ago with pneumonia.

BACKGROUND: Mrs. Smith is a 65-year-old patient who was admitted 3 days ago with pneumonia and shortness of breath. She has completed 3 days of antibiotic therapy, nebulizer treatments every 4 hours, and continuous supplemental oxygen therapy.

ASSESSMENT: Mrs. Smith has clear lung sounds, and her pulse oximeter reads 98% on 2 L of oxygen. Vital signs: T 98.8°, P 86, R 22, BP 128/72. She ambulated twice this shift down the length of the hall and denies shortness of breath. She has an occasional cough, productive of yellow sputum.

RECOMMENDATION: Monitor pulse oximeter readings with vital signs once a shift; administer antibiotics and nebulizer treatments on time, ambulate one more time this evening; consider administering PRN cough medicine at bedtime.

Key: *BP*, blood pressure; *P*, pulse; *PRN*, as needed; *R*, respirations; *T*, temperature.

The National Patient Safety Goals and requirements apply to nearly 15,000 hospitals and health care organizations that are accredited by The Joint Commission. There are specific goals for numerous types of patient care areas, such as ambulatory care, assisted living, behavioral health, home care, long-term care, and others. The goals for hospitals are listed in Box 3-3.

LEGAL DOCUMENTS

THE CHART OR MEDICAL RECORD

When a person enters the health care system to visit a physician, clinic, hospital, or emergency room, or to receive home health care, a record is begun (or continued) that documents that person's health status or problem and the care given. That record is a legal document that includes records of all assessments, tests, and care provided. The chart, or medical record, is confidential (kept private), meaning that only people directly associated with the care of that patient have legal access to the information in the chart. **The chart is the property of the hospital or agency or physician, not the patient.** However, the patient does have the right of access to the chart, and copies of information in the chart may be authorized by the patient to be provided to other agencies—for example, if a patient transfers from one physician or health care facility to another. Health care researchers and insurance companies may also gain access to chart information with the patient's permission.

Student nurses must protect the confidentiality of their patients. Charts may not be copied by students to use for report purposes. Reports or notes on patients

---

Box 3-3 | *2009 Critical Access Hospital National Patient Safety Goals*

Goal **Improve the accuracy of patient identification.**
- Use at least two patient identifiers when providing care, treatment, or services.
- Eliminate transfusion errors related to (patient) misidentification.

Goal **Improve the effectiveness of communication among caregivers.**
- For verbal or telephone orders or for telephonic reporting of critical test results, verify the complete order or test result by having the person receiving the information record and "read back" the complete order or test result.
- Standardize a list of abbreviations, acronyms, symbols, and dose designations that are not to be used throughout the organization.
- Measure, assess, and, if appropriate, take action to improve the timeliness of reporting, and the timeliness of receipt by the responsible licensed caregiver, of critical test results and values.
- Implement a standardized approach to "hand-off" communications, including an opportunity to ask and respond to questions.
- Implement a standardized approach to "hand-off" communications, including an opportunity to ask and respond to questions.

Goal **Improve the safety of using medications.**
- Identify and, at a minimum, annually review a list of look-alike/sound-alike drugs used by the organization, and take action to prevent errors involving the interchange of these drugs.
- Label all medications, medication containers (e.g., syringes, medicine cups, basins), or other solutions on and off the sterile field.
- Reduce the likelihood of patient harm associated with the use of anticoagulation therapy.

Goal **Reduce the risk of health care–associated infections.**
- Comply with current World Health Organization (WHO) Hand Hygiene Guidelines or Centers for Disease Control and Prevention (CDC) hand hygiene guidelines.
- Manage as sentinel events all identified cases of unanticipated death or major permanent loss of function associated with a health care–associated infection.
- Implement evidence-based practices to prevent health care–associated infections due to multiple drug-resistant organisms in critical access hospitals.
- Implement best practices or evidence-based guidelines to prevent central line-associated bloodstream infections.
- Implement best practices for preventing surgical site infections.

Goal **Accurately and completely reconcile medications across the continuum of care.**
- There is a process for comparing the patient's current medications with those ordered for the patient while under the care of the organization.
- A complete list of the patient's medications is communicated to the next provider of service when a patient is referred or transferred to another setting, service, practitioner, or level of care within or outside the organization. The complete list of medications is also provided to the patient on discharge from the facility.
- A reconciled medication list is provided to the patient.

Goal **Reduce the risk of patient harm resulting from falls.**
- Implement a fall reduction program, including an evaluation of the effectiveness of the program.

Goal **Encourage patients' active involvement in their own care as a patient safety strategy.**
- Define and communicate the means for patients and their families to report concerns about safety and encourage them to do so.

Goal **Improve recognition and response to changes in a patient's condition.**
- The organization selects a suitable method that enables health care staff members to directly request additional assistance from a specially trained individual(s) when the patient's condition appears to be worsening.

Adapted from The Joint Commission. (2007). National Patient Safety Goals. Available at www.jointcommission.org/PatientSafety/NationalPatientSafetyGoals/08_cah_npsgs.htm.

---

used for school purposes (case studies, nursing care plans, student task or skills lists) should not identify the patient by name. Case discussion should indicate "a 67-year-old man" rather than "Mr. Joe Morales."

As a legal document, the chart is used to determine the truth of what happened—what was done or not done—to a patient during a period of time. Therefore, its contents always need to be accurate, pertinent, and timely. Erasures or changes to a patient's chart may suggest covering up or dishonesty. Charting should be focused on the patient, and the nursing care provided. Remember that the chart may be introduced as evidence in a court case, and do not make inappropriate chart notations. Charting guidelines are covered in Chapter 7.

HEALTH INSURANCE PORTABILITY AND ACCOUNTABILITY ACT (HIPAA)

The Health Insurance Portability and Accountability Act of 1996 (HIPAA) called for the creation of regulations regarding patient privacy and electronic medical records. Failure to comply with the rules may lead to civil penalties. Intentional violation of the regulations can lead to sizable fines and time in jail. Box 3-4 presents the six patient rights covered in these regulations.

A considerable amount of information about patients is shared among health care professionals within an agency each day. The new federal privacy regulations took effect in April 2003. The privacy rules, which are part of HIPAA, protect the way patient in-

Box 3-4 *Rights Provided by HIPAA (Health Insurance Portability and Accountability Act)*

HIPAA covers six patient rights and provider responsibilities:

Consent: Written consents must contain a clause that says the patient agrees to allow the provider to use and disclose his information for treatment, payment, and health care operations. A notice must be attached to the consent form.

Notice: The provider's obligations are outlined regarding the privacy of the patient's health care information. It includes the six patient rights and responsibilities of the provider. It details how the patient information will be protected and a process for filing a complaint if the patient believes privacy rights have been violated.

Access: The patient has the right to inspect and copy his medical record.

Amendment: A patient has the right to amend his record for the purpose of accuracy.

Accounting for disclosures: Providers are held accountable for how patients' medical information is handled. Tracking of any disclosures of information not related to treatment, payment, or health care operations, or that were not authorized by the patient, must occur.

Restriction of disclosure: The patient can request that the provider restrict the use and disclosure of his information. The provider does not, however, have to grant the request.

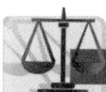

Legal & Ethical Considerations 3-1

Protecting Patient Privacy

- Keep interactions with patients as private as possible. If your patient is not in a private room, take care to lower your voice to restrict others from hearing what is said.
- Remember that any discussions about patients in clinical postconference are for educational purposes only and not for gossip. These discussions should never contain identifying information, and should not be discussed outside the clinical conference or classroom setting, such as in a hospital elevator or cafeteria.
- Do not leave patient information on display. If you use a clipboard, place a cover sheet to shield patient data from wandering eyes.
- Prior to providing any information about your patient to anyone not directly involved in the patient's care (such as patient's friends or family), check for authorization to release health-related information.
- Never photocopy the patient's medical record for any purpose.
- Never blog about your clinical day. Even without providing identifying patient information, it is too easy to breach patient confidentiality, and you may be punished and/or fined!
- Remove all identifying information from personal notes or assignments. Maintain such notes in a secure and confidential manner, even if they contain no identifying patient information. They must not be left unattended at school, at home, in your car, or on your computer. Shred or destroy all such documents once the purpose has been fulfilled (e.g., once your assignment has been graded and recorded).

formation is conveyed and stored. HIPAA also dictates to whom information may be revealed. Many nurses are now afraid to share *any* patient information with family members for fear of violating the HIPAA privacy rule. The rule states that disclosing medical information to family members, close personal friends, or other individuals identified by the patient for involvement in the patient's care *is* permitted if *the patient does not object*. It is important, then, to make certain you have the patient's consent to relay information about his health care to family members. It is also important to know and follow the hospital's policies as well.

The HIPAA rules also give patients the right to the information in their medical records as well as the right to emend an erroneous record. Privacy and confidentiality of patient information have always been part of the ethical code of nurses, physicians, and health care facilities; the new rules have simply increased awareness of the need for confidentiality and imposed new guidelines. Charts and flow sheets must be secured and not left where they may be viewed by others. Public displays of patient information (on a white board in the nurse's station for example) are not acceptable. Nurses need to be careful with printouts, such as the Kardex sheet or Care Plan, and be certain that they are shredded or disposed of properly when the shift is over. When working with a patient in a double room or multiple-bed ward, voices need to be lowered to prevent others from hearing what is said. Patients must sign a specific release

form if they desire information be sent to another agency, physician, or insurance company (Legal & Ethical Considerations 3-1).

CONSENTS AND RELEASES

A consent is permission given by the patient or his legal representative. Consents or *releases* are legal documents that record the patient's permission to perform a treatment or surgery, or to give information to insurance companies or other health care providers (Box 3-5).

Informed consent indicates the patient's participation in the decision-making process. The person signing must have knowledge of what the consent allows and be able to make a knowledgeable decision. In a consent for surgery or treatment, the patient must be told, in terms he can understand, the risks and benefits of the proposed treatment, what the consequences may be of not having the procedure done, and the name of the health care professional who will perform the procedure. This information is usually provided by the professional performing the procedure. **If the patient has any questions, they should be satisfactorily answered before the patient signs the consent. It is important to determine that proper consent has been obtained, both legally *and ethically*. Failure to obtain a valid informed consent may lead to charges of as-**

Box 3-5 | *Types of Consents*

Admission agreement: Commonly obtained at the time of admission to a hospital, this form spells out the hospital's or facility's responsibility to the patient. The hospital agrees to provide room, meals, basic nursing care, and medical care prescribed by the physician. The patient consents to diagnostic services, such as radiographs, medication administration, and nursing treatments. The patient acknowledges responsibility to pay for the services. Consent to bill insurance companies and provide medical information about the patient to receive payment are usually part of the admission agreement.

Operative consent: All surgical or invasive procedures, such as repair of a hernia or removal of the appendix, **biopsies** (taking a piece of tissue to examine), and many diagnostic tests that are **invasive** (involve an incision or cutting of the patient's body, or the introduction of an instrument into a body cavity) require an operative consent. It may be called a surgical consent, or permission for surgery or anesthesia. **The physician, surgeon, or anesthesiologist who performs the procedure is responsible for explaining the procedure, its risks and benefits, and possible alternative options.**

Consent to receive blood: A consent to receive a blood transfusion would indicate that the patient was informed of the benefits and risks of transfusion, as is done for surgical or invasive procedures. Some patients hold religious beliefs that would prohibit transfusions, even in life-threatening situations.

Research consent: Clinical research is carried out only with the patient's informed consent about the possible risks, consequences, and benefits of the research. A patient always has the right to refuse to participate in a research study, and no patient may be given a research drug or treatment without his informed consent.

Consent to release information: A specific consent to release confidential patient information to other agencies or people is required before the information may be released. An exception is that information may be shared between consulting or referring physicians without a specific consent.

Other consents: Special consents are required to perform an autopsy, donate organs after death, or be photographed, and for the disposal of body parts during surgery.

---

sault and battery, or invasion of privacy. (These charges are fully explained later in this chapter.)

In order to be valid, a consent must be signed by the person or the legal agent for that person. Consents must be freely signed without threat or pressure, and must be witnessed by another adult. *Consent can be withdrawn at any time before the procedure or treatment is started.* When a person is older than 18 years and competent, he must sign the consent for treatment. A competent person is one who is legally fit (mentally and emotionally). A person is considered incompetent if he is unconscious, under the influence of mind-altering drugs (including

alcohol or narcotics, such as "premedication" for the procedure), or declared legally incompetent, such as in cases of chronic dementia or mental deficiency. In these situations, a next of kin, appointed guardian, or one who holds a durable power of attorney (discussed later) has legal authority to give consent. Minors (younger than 18 years) may not give legal consent; their parents or guardians have this right. If a child's parents are divorced, the custodial parent is the legal representative. Stepparents usually cannot give consent unless they have legally adopted the child. **An emancipated minor, or one who has established independence by moving away from parents or through service in the armed forces, marriage, or pregnancy, is considered legally capable of signing a consent.**

Implied consent is assumed when, in a life-threatening emergency, consent cannot be obtained from the patient or family. The law agrees with this. Consent may be obtained by telephone if it is witnessed by two persons who hear the consent of the family member.

A release is a legal form used to excuse one party from liability (responsibility). A commonly used release is a *Leave Against Medical Advice* (or *Leave AMA*). This form is used by a hospital or facility when a patient does not accept the physician's recommendation for hospitalization, and leaves the agency. The form documents that the reasons for continuing hospitalization or treatment, and risks of leaving without treatment, have been explained to the patient. If the patient refuses to sign the release, that is noted and witnessed. The term *release* may also refer to forms used to authorize an agency to send confidential health care information to another agency, school, or insurance company.

WITNESSING WILLS OR OTHER LEGAL DOCUMENTS

Occasionally, nurses may be asked to witness a will or other legal document. Although there is no legal reason not to do so, most hospitals and health care agencies have policies against this. The reason is that wills or legal documents may be contested, and the nurse who witnessed the document can be called to court to testify regarding the patient's health or mental condition, or relationship to visitors. To avoid this conflict, hospitals often provide business office personnel or a notary public to witness the signature. To witness the signing of a legal document, you need not know the content of the document. Legally, it is necessary only that the witness confirms that the signature or mark is made under no influence (drug or otherwise) and that the person knows what he is signing.

ADVANCE DIRECTIVES

An advance directive, sometimes called a "living will," is a consent that has been constructed before the need for it arises. It spells out a patient's wishes regarding surgery as well as diagnostic and therapeutic treatments. Clear direction for making decisions is then present if the patient suffers an accident or illness that results in the patient being unresponsive or incompetent, and unable to make the decision. This has become very important because technology in health care allows the prolonging and maintaining of life with sophisticated treatments that may cause conflict among family members or between the health care professionals and the family as to how the patient would want to live (or die) in this situation. When a person puts in writing his wishes regarding life support and the use of medical technology, both the medical community and the family have clear direction. A *durable power of attorney* is a document that gives legal power *to* a health care agent (surrogate decision maker), who is a person chosen by the patient to follow the patient's advance directives and make medical decisions on his behalf.

All 50 states recognize advance directives, but each state regulates advance directives differently, and an advance directive from one state may not be recognized in another, depending on the similarities or differences in their laws. Advance directives do not expire; it is a good idea for the patient to review his advance directive periodically, to be certain it still reflects his wishes. Historically, emergency medical technicians (EMTs) have not been able to honor advance directives. Therefore, if a patient had an advance directive limiting the types of care he wanted, and a loved one called 9-1-1, the EMTs had to perform any and all procedures to stabilize the patient and bring him to the hospital. Many states have enacted laws to allow EMTs to honor DNR orders and/or advance directives, provided documentation is available at the scene.

Do not resuscitate (DNR) orders are written by a physician when the patient has indicated a desire to be allowed to die if he stops breathing or his heart stops. In this situation, no cardiac compressions or assisted breathing (cardiopulmonary resuscitation [CPR]) would be started. **It is very important for nursing personnel to know who is to be resuscitated and who is NOT.** A nurse who attempts to resuscitate a patient who has a physician's DNR order would be acting without the patient's consent, and committing battery.

It is also illegal to call for or participate in a "slow code." In a slow code, there is no DNR order but staff do not respond quickly to a patient who has stopped breathing or whose heart has stopped, so that the CPR will not be effective. This is usually done because the patient has a terminal condition.

VIOLATIONS OF LAW

There are a number of civil laws that nurses need to know about in order to practice safely and within the legal system. A nurse needs to know not only the law

---

Box 3-6 *Elements of Malpractice*

Duty: The obligation to use due care (e.g., a nurse has a duty to monitor the condition of the patient for whom she is caring).

Breach of duty: Failure to use due care (e.g., a nurse fails to check the vital signs or condition of the patient after surgery; or a nurse begins CPR on a patient who has a DNR order).

Causation: The action or inaction by the nurse causes the injury, or harm to the patient. There must be a direct link between the breach of duty and the injury. The nurse's failure to check the patient's condition could lead to an undetected loss of blood that causes the patient's death.

Injury or damages: The actual harm or disorder that results from the negligence. Injury or damages may be physical, emotional, or financial. Pain and suffering, loss of ability to continue in a job, physical or emotional disability, extended hospitalization, or death would all be considered injury or damage in a negligence action.

---

in regard to her own practice but also how to act as a patient advocate, one who speaks for and protects the rights of the patient.

NEGLIGENCE AND MALPRACTICE

Negligence is simply defined as failing to do something a reasonably prudent (sensible and careful) person would do, or doing something a reasonably prudent person would **NOT** do.

Malpractice is negligence by a professional person. The person does not act according to professional standards of care as a reasonably prudent professional would. **In nursing malpractice, a reasonably prudent person is a similarly educated, licensed, and experienced nurse.** An example of nursing malpractice would be if a nurse did not check the patient's vital signs and condition after surgery, there was hemorrhage, and the patient went into shock and died.

In order to prove malpractice, there are four elements that must be present: duty, a breach of duty, causation, and injury (Box 3-6). If even one of these four elements is not present, the nurse was not guilty of malpractice. For example, if a nurse made a clinical error that did not result in harm to the patient, the event would not be considered to be malpractice; however, it would be a deviation from the standard of care, and as such could be grounds for discipline by the employer, the licensing board, or both.

COMMON LEGAL ISSUES

Nurses have access to private information and personal contact that is permitted by their professional caregiver role. With that right to information and touch come legal responsibilities to respect the patient's privacy, to protect the patient's safety, and to ensure the patient's right to make decisions. When legal boundaries are violated, and injury occurs, nurses may be subject to **litigation** (a lawsuit).

Assault and Battery

Assault is the threat to harm another, or even to threaten to touch another without that person's permission. The person being threatened must believe that the nurse has the ability to carry out the threat. Battery is the actual physical contact that has been refused or that is carried out against the person's will. An example of assault would be the nurse who says "If you don't let me give you this injection, two other nurses will hold you down so I can give it to you." Battery would occur when a patient is held down to receive an injection he has refused. It would also include the rough physical handling of an excited, confused, or psychotic patient in ways that would be described as angry, violent, or negligent.

Adults who are alert and oriented have the right to refuse medications, baths, treatments, dressing changes, irrigations, insertion of a catheter, and diagnostic tests as well as surgery. Even if the test or procedure is necessary for the well-being or comfort of the patient, the patient has the legal right to refuse. **It is the nurse's responsibility to explain the reason why a particular drug or treatment is important. However, if the patient still refuses, the nurse should obtain a release from liability because the treatment is not done or the drug is not taken.** Performing a procedure without the proper consent is battery (except in emergency situations when the patient is unable to give consent).

Elder Care Points

Although an elderly person may be forgetful and require supervision of activities of daily living, he still has rights of privacy and self-determination (the right to consent to or refuse treatments). Nurses need to document carefully any explanations given and the patient's ability to understand the benefits, risks, and consequences of decisions.

Defamation

Defamation is when one person makes remarks about another person that are untrue, and the remarks damage that other person's reputation. There are two forms of defamation: slander (oral) and libel (written). Two nurses may be overheard talking about a physician in a way that holds the physician up to ridicule or contempt. If another person decides never to use that physician because of the derogatory comments, the physician's reputation is damaged and the nurses may be guilty of slander. An example of libel is a letter or newspaper article quotation that states that a person is incompetent or dishonest. The loss of respect for and trust of the person may result in damage to his reputation and loss of business. A person sued for slander or libel may be found innocent if the statements made were true, or were said or written with no intent to harm the person, but for a justified purpose.

Invasion of Privacy

Invasion of privacy occurs when there has been a violation of the confidential and privileged nature of a professional relationship. When patients entrust themselves to our care, it is with the expectation of confidentiality—that what is told to the health care professional and what is learned about the patient's health and personal history is private information to which no one else should have access.

Invasion of privacy occurs when unauthorized persons learn of the patient's history, condition, or treatment from the professional caregiver. It might include the nurse's giving information over the telephone to a caller who asks about the patient's condition. It occurs when health care workers are overheard carelessly discussing their patients in the elevator or cafeteria. It occurs when a next-door neighbor asks about another neighbor who is in the hospital and the nurse tells him about the patient's condition. It occurs when a nurse, out of curiosity, reads the chart of a public figure who has been admitted to her unit, but to whom the nurse is not assigned or responsible. Releasing information to a newspaper, another health care agency, an insurance company, or a person without the patient's valid consent is invasion of privacy. However, **nurses are required by law in most states to report information regarding child or elder abuse, sexual abuse, or violent acts that may be crimes (stab or gunshot wounds).** When such reporting is done in good faith, the nurse cannot be held liable for invasion of privacy. Nurses must be aware of the required reporting procedures for abuse or crime where they work.

Invasion of privacy extends to leaving the curtains or door open while a treatment or procedure is being done, or to leaving patients in a position that might cause them loss of dignity or embarrassment. Exposing the patient's body more than necessary, or leaving a confused and agitated patient in a hallway where he might behave in ways that would be embarrassing if he were not confused and agitated, are also examples of invasion of privacy. Interviewing a patient or family member in a room with only a curtain between the patients, or where conversation can be overheard, allows confidential information to be heard by unauthorized persons. **The reasonable and prudent nurse does for the patient what the patient cannot do for himself—covers the patient's body, protects him from public exposure, and preserves his dignity.**

A growing area of concern regarding privacy has to do with computerized data banks and the Internet. Many health care agencies are computerizing their records, and nurses (as well as physicians, laboratory technicians, pharmacists, dietitians, and unit clerks) can enter information about patients in that facility as well as retrieve it. Nurses must be careful to ensure the patient's privacy when entering or using data in a computer network. HIPAA, discussed earlier in the chapter, sets rules governing transmission of patient data (electronic, telephone, fax), such as the requirement that the sending facility must have reasonable safeguards in place to ensure the data are sent where they were intended to be sent and are treated in a confidential manner. A national data bank is envisioned in the future that could allow health care practitioners to access a patient's medical record wherever that patient sought care—from California to New York, from a clinic to a major medical center, from a private practice physician to a pharmacist at the local drugstore—but the need for safeguards to prevent unauthorized access, as well as the reluctance of many people to have confidential health information so readily accessible, may delay this from becoming a reality very soon.

False Imprisonment

Just as a patient has the right to refuse medications or tests or treatments, a patient has the right to leave a hospital or health care facility or to move about in it. Preventing such a person from leaving, or restricting his movements in the facility, is false imprisonment. When a person wants to leave the hospital against the advice of the physician, a release to leave "against medical advice" (AMA) is used. The patient, by signing the form, releases the hospital and staff of any consequences that occur as a result of the patient's leaving. It is also important to follow your facility's policies regarding a competent adult who wishes to leave AMA. The policy may include finding out the reason why the patient wishes to leave, informing the physician, informing the patient of the risks of refusing treatments, and carefully documenting all aspects of the situation.

Persons who have psychiatric disorders may be admitted to a psychiatric unit on a voluntary or involuntary basis. A person who is admitted voluntarily agrees to the admission and can refuse or accept any treatment, and can leave the facility as a regular discharge. If the physician believes the patient should not be discharged, the patient can sign an AMA release.

An involuntary admission is made against the patient's wishes, to protect him from self-harm or from harming others. There is a limit to the time (usually 72 hours) a person can be detained without consent. During that time, if the patient does not agree to a voluntary admission, and there remains the belief that the person is a threat to self or others, two psychiatrists can petition a judge to issue a court order for the patient to be held in the psychiatric facility for a specific period of time.

Protective Devices. The inappropriate use of devices that limit a person's mobility is a nursing action that can result in charges of false imprisonment. Protective devices may be mechanical, such as locks, rails, belts, or garments that prevent a person from getting out of a room, bed, or chair, or they may be chemical: drugs such as sedatives or tranquilizers that so sedate the patient that he is unable to move about. **A physician order is necessary for any protective device, mechanical or chemical.** Creative nurses and health care facilities have developed ways of allowing for mobility while protecting the confused or agitated person from danger. Nurses must be alert to the abuse of protective devices when other less restrictive techniques may be effective. Clearly a reasonable and prudent nurse will carefully assess a patient's potential for falls or other harm, and document the need for and proper application of physician-ordered protective devices to ensure the patient's safety. Nurses should consult with their supervisor about using protective devices in an emergency situation when no physician order is available. Documentation of the need to protect the patient from harm and securing the physician order as soon as possible protect the nurse from liability for charges of false imprisonment or malpractice.

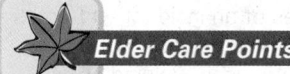
Elder Care Points

Careful assessment of an elderly patient's mental status, medications, potential for orthostatic hypotension, balance, and mobility can identify the patient with a risk for falls and injury. Specific nursing interventions can then be identified and used to protect the patient from injury.

DECREASING LEGAL RISK
Nursing Competence

Although nurses cannot prevent a lawsuit from being filed, several nursing actions can reduce the likelihood of a suit (Box 3-7). **First and most important is competent and well-documented nursing care.** Nursing *competence* is defined as possessing the suitable skill, knowledge, and experience necessary to provide adequate nursing care. Establishing rapport and effective communication skills can create a relationship in which patient anger or misunderstanding can be resolved rather than grow to lawsuit proportions. Competence in nursing also includes following the proper policies and procedures and upholding the standards of care. Sometimes in nursing you may observe another nurse "bending the rules" in an unsafe way to save time; as a novice in the field, you may feel peer pressure to do things in a way that is "the way things are done on this unit." Rule bending might appear to be the only solution on a unit that is chronically understaffed, but it only provides a temporary solution. What is more likely needed is a permanent change in the situation that will make rule bending unnecessary. If there are hospital rules that are out-of-date or unrealistic, it is important to get involved (e.g., on the hospital's policy committee) to change these rules, rather than work around them.

Box 3-7 *Guidelines to Reduce Legal Risk*

1. **Maintain competence**
   - Learn skills thoroughly.
   - Know the state law for nursing practice.
   - Know and follow your employer's institutional policies.
   - Develop the ability to evaluate your knowledge and performance; identify areas in which you are weak and work to improve these.
   - Attend continuing education programs and keep abreast of changes in health care.
   - Keep records of workshops or seminars you attend.
   - Identify experienced nurses whose competence you respect, and seek their assistance when you are unfamiliar with equipment or a technique.
2. **Document fully**—there is an expression in nursing that says "If you didn't chart it, it didn't get done."
   - Accurate, factual, and timely charting of nursing assessments, plans, interventions, and evaluations are essential to prove that nursing care that meets standards of care was carried out.
   - Anecdotal records are a tool for nurses to use in assisting their memory. Anecdotal records are the nurse's recollection or notes of an incident written as close to the time of the incident as possible, and kept by the nurse in a secure place. Relying on memory is a poor way to prove what a nurse did or did not do. Lawsuits often take years from the date of occurrence of an event to the filing and notice of a lawsuit.
3. **Establish rapport**
   - Develop rapport and treat each patient with respect: identify yourself, smile, listen attentively, address patients by their preferred name.
   - Be careful of damaging the relationship between the patient and his physician or other staff by engaging in critical or negative conversation with the patient.
   - Listen to patient complaints and communicate professionally to attempt to resolve problems.
4. **Communicate effectively**
   - Therapeutic communication techniques can allow the patient to express feelings without the nurse agreeing or supporting charges of incompetence or negligence.
   - Notify your supervisor of any situation in which a patient or family members are dissatisfied with the nursing care received, or with another health care professional.
   - Follow the procedure for communication with the risk management team.
5. **Take care of yourself**
   - Be at your best for every clinical day.
   - Follow the principles of proper nutrition and regular exercise; obtain adequate, restful sleep.
   - Recognize that fatigue is a significant factor in making clinical errors: refrain from working hours in excess of what you can safely do, even though the money may be tempting.

Situations sometimes occur in which a patient believes he has suffered an injury or loss. Documentation is the key element in proving that nursing actions used were appropriate, thus protecting the nurse from liability.

Potential lawsuits may be avoided by early identification of dissatisfied patients. Many facilities have risk management teams composed of people specially trained to deal with situations that may put the facility at risk for a lawsuit. Part of a comprehensive risk management program would include in-service programs to promote safety, preventive maintenance for equipment and the physical plant, and counseling and interventions in situations that pose potential for lawsuits.

? *Think Critically About . . .* How would you respond to a patient who complains to you that the nurse on the night shift ignored his call for assistance for 45 minutes, that the nurse said that the unit was short staffed, and the patient should not bother them unless it was absolutely necessary?

Incident or Occurrence Reports

If there is an occurrence that is out of the ordinary, an incident (occurrence) report is often used to document what happened, the facts about the incident, and who was involved or witnessed it. The incident report is a tool used by the risk management department (see Chapter 10). This report is useful for several reasons. It allows the facility to note dangerous patterns—for example, if several visitors or staff have tripped and fallen in the same location, or if a change in the appearance of a medication might have been a factor in several recent similar medication errors. The incident report also serves as an immediate recall of an occurrence that may result in injury or damages and future lawsuit. Some examples of when an incident report might be written include when a medication error is made, a patient falls out of bed, or a visitor faints in the hall (Figure 3-1). **Incident reports are generally not filed as part of the patient's chart; no reference to the incident report is made in the patient's chart,** although the medically relevant details about the incident, if they relate to patient care, should be included in the progress notes. Incident reports should be timely, factual, and concise, and should not contain unnecessary details, such as explanations about why the event might have occurred.

Liability Insurance

Liability insurance does not provide protection from being sued. It can, however, protect the livelihood and assets of a nurse should the nurse get sued. If a nurse is sued, liability insurance pays for the expenses of a law-

BASSETT HEALTHCARE
INCIDENT/VARIANCE REPORT
#1001 4/88 rev. 8/94; 4/98; 6/98; 7/98 (f:\riskmgt\.doc)

COMPUTER LOG # _____

Instructions: Complete form immediately after an incident occurs. Send original to Quality/Risk Management Department within 24 hours of incident and keep copy for department use.

INCIDENT DATE: _____   TIME: _____

IDENTIFICATION ☐ EMPLOYEE; DEPT: _____   ☐ PATIENT ☐ VISITOR ☐ VOLUNTEER ☐ OTHER

LAST NAME: _____   FIRST NAME: _____

CHART #: _____   AGE: _____   SEX: ☐ MALE ☐ FEMALE

Incident Location

☐ MIBH   ☐ O'CONNOR
☐ Emergency Services
☐ Health Center: _____
☐ Inpatient Services   Unit/Room: _____
☐ Food Services
☐ Laboratory: Section: _____
☐ Operative Services; Unit: _____

☐ Other
☐ Outpatient Services
       Clinic: _____
☐ Outside Property
       Clinic: _____
☐ Pharmacy
☐ Radiology
☐ Rehabilitative Services

Category:

☐ Fall (Describe injury/no injury below)
☐ Fracture/Dislocation
☐ Burn
☐ Chemical burn
☐ Contusion/laceration
☐ Back/muscle strain
☐ Blood/Body Fluid Exposure
       ☐ Blood   ☐ Other body fluid _____
       ☐ Clean needle   ☐ Contaminated needle
       Source patient chart #: _____
☐ Patient Care Equipment
       Equipment type/tag #: _____
       ☐ Equipment not available
       ☐ Electrical problem/shock
       ☐ Mechanical problem
☐ Procedural Variance
       ☐ Laboratory specimen/testing error
       ☐ Improper prep of a patient for a procedure
       ☐ Improper sharps disposal
       ☐ Other
☐ Security Variance
       ☐ Hospital property loss
       ☐ Personal property loss
       ☐ Suspected crime/assault
☐ Other

☐ Medication   Which med? _____
       ☐ Adverse reaction
       ☐ Drug omitted
       ☐ Extra dose given
       ☐ Patient with history of allergy
       ☐ Transcription error
       ☐ Incorrect dose
       ☐ Incorrect time
       ☐ Incorrect route
       ☐ Incorrect patient
       ☐ Incorrect medication
       ☐ Other: _____
☐ IV Variance
       ☐ Allergic/adverse reaction
       ☐ Contaminated/outdated
       ☐ Drug omitted
       ☐ Extra dose given
       ☐ Mislabeled drug/solution
       ☐ Incorrect rate of flow
       ☐ Incorrect dose
       ☐ Incorrect IV solution
       ☐ Incorrect patient
       ☐ Incorrect time
       ☐ Transcription error
       ☐ Other: _____
☐ Patient left AMA without signing AMA form

Brief Description:
(Required for employee incidents) _____
_____
_____

Seen by provider?
☐ No ☐ Yes Date: _____
       Outcome: _____
       _____
       _____

_____
SIGNATURE AND TITLE OF PERSON COMPLETING THIS FORM   DATE

_____
SIGNATURE OF MANAGER/SUPERVISOR   DATE

FIGURE 3-1 Sample incident report.

yer to defend the nurse and pays any award won by the plaintiff up to the limits of the policy. It may also pay for attorney costs and related costs if the nurse is subjected to review by the state board of nursing. Having liability insurance does not increase the nurse's chances of being sued, and most authors agree that it is unwise to rely on your employer's liability insurance policy to protect you, because there may be situations in which the interests of the institution are at odds with your legal interests. Nursing liability insurance is relatively inexpensive, and is available through nursing organizations as well as private insurance companies.

ETHICS IN NURSING

Ethics or *ethical principles* are rules of conduct that have been agreed to by a particular group. They are based on the consensus (agreement) of the group that these rules are believed to be morally right or proper for that group. Professional groups such as physicians, nurses, and lawyers have developed codes of ethics that guide the person in that profession to act in ways approved by the group. Ethics are different from laws, in that they are voluntary. There are no prescribed legal penalties for violating a code of ethics, although in many instances, violation of a professional code of ethics may result in disciplinary action by a licensing or regulating agency. In some cases, ethics and the law overlap—for example, in dealing with issues of confidentiality. But in many cases, ethics deal with ideals or situations in which there is no right or wrong solution to a problem and about which thoughtful, caring people may hold opposing views. Areas of debate continue about life-and-death issues such as abortion, life support, and euthanasia.

Ethics are closely linked with **values,** the worth or importance of an action or belief to an individual. An ethical **dilemma** (problem or conflict) may result when people hold differing values. Codes of ethics attempt to provide a framework for making professional decisions.

Think Critically About . . . How would you react to a patient who refuses surgery that might prolong and perhaps enhance the patient's life? What values do you hold regarding quality of life, right to die, and self-determination? Is there a difference if the patient is 23 years old or 87 years old?

CODES OF ETHICS

The International Council of Nurses (ICN), the American Nurses Association (ANA), the National Association for Practical Nurse Education and Service (NAPNES), and the National Federation of Licensed

---

Box 3-8 | *NAPNES Code of Ethics*

The Licensed Practical/Vocational Nurse Shall:
1. Consider as a basic obligation the conservation of life and the prevention of disease.
2. Promote and protect the physical, mental, emotional, and spiritual health of the patient and his family.
3. Fulfill all duties faithfully and efficiently.
4. Function within established legal guidelines.
5. Accept personal responsibility (for his/her acts) and seek to merit the respect and confidence of all members of the health team.
6. Hold in confidence all matters coming to his/her knowledge, in the practice of his/her profession, and in no way and at no time violate this confidence.
7. Give conscientious service and charge just remuneration.
8. Learn and respect the religious and cultural beliefs of his/her patient and of all people.
9. Meet his/her obligation to the patient by keeping abreast of current trends in health care through reading and continuing education.
10. As a citizen of the United States of America, uphold the laws of the land and seek to promote legislation that will meet the health needs of its people.

NAPNES (2004). *Standards of Practice for Licensed Practical/Vocational Nurses.* Available at www.napnes.org/standards.pdf.

Practical Nurses (NFLPN) have developed codes of ethics for nurses (Box 3-8). Although the codes are worded differently, they have many commonalities. They all indicate the following:
- A respect for human dignity, the individual, and provision of nursing care that is not affected by race, religion, lifestyle, or culture.
- A commitment to continuing education, to maintaining competence, and to contributing to improved practice.
- The confidential nature of the nurse-patient relationship, outlining behaviors that bring credit to the profession and protect the public.

In addition, NAPNES has set standards for nursing practice since 1941 (Box 3-9). The standards represent the foundation for the provision of safe and competent nursing practice. Competency implies knowledge, understanding, and skills that transcend specific tasks and is guided by a commitment to ethical/legal principles. Box 3-10 refers to the NFLPN Code for Licensed Practical/Vocational Nurses (see also Appendix 4).

ETHICS COMMITTEES

Many health care facilities have ethics committees that are composed of people from various departments such as nursing, medicine, surgery, psychiatry, pharmacy, legal, economics, spiritual, and social work. Together they develop policies, address issues in their facility, and come to a better understanding of ethical dilemmas from different viewpoints.

Box 3-9 **NAPNES Standards of Practice for Licensed Practical/Vocational Nurses**

The LPN/LVN Student on program completion will display the following standards and competencies:

- **Professional Behaviors:** Demonstrate accountability and professionalism according to legal and ethical standards.
- **Communication:** Effectively communicate with patients, significant others, and health care team members.
- **Assessment:** Collect holistic assessment data, communicate that data to health care providers and evaluate patient responses to interventions.
- **Caring:** Demonstrate a caring and empathic approach to patient care.
- **Planning and Interventions:** Collaborate with the healthcare team to utilize assessment data to plan, revise, implement and evaluate patient care.
- **Managing:** Under supervision, implement patient care and assign care to unlicensed assistive personnel.

Adapted from NAPNES Standards of Practice and Educational Competencies of Graduates of Practical/Vocational Nursing Programs. National Association for Practical Nurse Education and Service, Inc. 2007. (Full text available on Companion CD-ROM.)

Box 3-10 **NFLPN Code for Licensed Practical/Vocational Nurses**

1. Know the scope of maximum utilization of the LP/VN as specified by the nurse practice act and function within this scope.
2. Safeguard the confidential information acquired from any source about the patient.
3. Provide health care to all patients regardless of race, creed, cultural background, disease, or lifestyle.
4. Uphold the highest standards in personal appearance, language, dress, and demeanor.
5. Stay informed about issues affecting the practice of nursing and delivery of healthcare and, where appropriate, participate in government and policy decisions.
6. Accept the responsibility for safe nursing by keeping oneself mentally and physically fit and educationally prepared to practice.
7. Accept responsibility for membership in NFLPN and participate in its efforts to maintain the established standards of nursing practice and employment policies which lead to quality patient care.

ETHICAL DILEMMAS

Many ethical dilemmas may face the nurse today. A current issue revolves around life-and-death decisions. When a patient is diagnosed with a terminal illness, there are often conflicting opinions among family members and even the health care team about seeking life-prolonging treatment versus refusing such treatment. Patients have the right to information about alternative as well as conventional treatment options, with their risks, consequences, and benefits. Nurses must honor the right of the patient to choose or refuse any treatment or procedure, even if it would not be the nurse's choice.

Perhaps even more difficult is the choice to initiate or terminate life support or treatment. Questions of whether to allow a patient to stop artificial feedings, or not to treat an infection with antibiotics in a terminally ill person, often raise uncomfortable feelings in nurses. Respecting and supporting a patient's informed choice regarding treatment is respecting the patient's right to self-determination. Providing compassionate care at the end of life honors the person's decision to live his remaining time in the way he chooses.

Another ethical issue involves **assisted suicide,** which is aiding a person (providing the means) to end his life. The Supreme Court in June 1997 held that there was no constitutional right to physician-assisted suicide. Legally, at this time assisted suicide is a crime except in Oregon, which has enacted an assisted suicide law. Assisted suicide is often confused with euthanasia, or mercy killing. Euthanasia is the act of ending another person's life, with or without the person's consent, to end actual or potential suffering. It is not legal in any state.

Yet nurses may have to deal with a patient who asks for help to die. Participation in assisted suicide is a violation of the ANA *Code for Nurses,* as well as the ethical tradition of "do no harm." The issue remains very controversial, with caring people holding different values.

On a daily basis, nurses face personal ethical decisions involving honesty, whistle-blowing (reporting illegal or unethical actions), and provision of care. Our professional code of ethics dictates that we act as patient advocates and safeguard our patients from harm. Who will know if a nurse gives a wrong medication, or fails to assess an unconscious patient? Should a nurse report suspected incompetence or impairment of a fellow nurse or physician? What care can be omitted in a short-staffed unit where all the needs are urgent? How does a nurse treat difficult patients—those who are abusive or who arouse feelings of anger or hatred, such as a person convicted of brutal crimes?

Nursing codes of ethics provide guidelines for behavior that promote excellence in patient care and the profession. They promote values such as dignity, honesty, integrity, and compassion.

On an institutional level, the question of "which of many patients is chosen for the liver transplant?" may occupy an ethics committee. On a state and national level, legislators choose where to spend money, and write laws that affect health care. Those decisions are influenced by ethics and values, and nurses can have an impact by sharing their ethical concern for patients and speaking up for patients' rights.

Nurses can consciously consider what is right or wrong for them, in light of personal values. When a nurse feels confused or conflicted about the right course of action in a situation, talking with other nurses, the unit supervisor, or the ethics committee in the agency can assist the nurse to solve the problem from an ethical viewpoint.

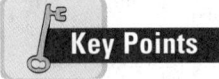

Key Points

- Legislators, agencies, and courts create laws; codes of ethics are written by professional organizations. Laws are civil (private) or criminal (public). A civil wrong is a tort; a public wrong is a crime.
- Nursing is governed by state nurse practice acts, which define the scope of practice. State boards of nursing administer the law. Standards of care are developed by professional organizations. Students are held to the same standards and laws as the professional.
- Professional accountability means taking responsibility for one's own actions. Nurses may delegate patient care to unlicensed personnel, but they remain responsible for the safe, effective delivery of patient care.
- Continuing education is an ethical responsibility to keep knowledge and skills current and safe. In many states it is a legal requirement for continuing licensure.
- The Occupational Safety and Health Act (OSHA) monitors the workplace for the health and safety of its employees.
- The Child Abuse Prevention and Treatment Act (CAPTA) requires licensed nurses and other health care professionals to report child abuse.
- The "Patient Care Partnership" recognizes that patients do not lose their civil rights when they are hospitalized.
- Consent is necessary to perform invasive procedures, to divulge confidential information, or to conduct research. Consent must be legally obtained to show the patient's permission.

- Types of advance directives include living wills and a medical power of attorney. A living will allows a patient to express his wishes about medical treatment; a medical power of attorney gives legal power to a person to make decisions when the patient is unable.
- HIPAA regulations strictly guard the privacy of patient information. They require a specific signed consent for release of information.
- Negligence and malpractice are common torts in health care; assault, battery, defamation, invasion of privacy, or false imprisonment may result in malpractice torts.
- A successful lawsuit requires the following four elements to be proven: duty, breach of duty, causation, and injury.
- Competent nursing practice, careful documentation, development of a caring relationship with patients, and communicating professionally can reduce one's likelihood of being named in a lawsuit. Patient safety, medication/treatment errors, and failure to assess are frequent areas of suits for nurses.
- Malpractice insurance protects nurses from financial damages in the event of a lawsuit, and provides legal assistance.
- Codes of ethics have been developed by nursing organizations and provide principles to guide behavior in situations in which there may be no "right" answer.
- Ethical dilemmas result when people hold differing views on issues. Ethics committees can provide an interdisciplinary approach to solving ethical dilemmas.

 Go to your **Companion CD-ROM** for an Audio Glossary, animations, video clips, and more.

evolve Be sure to visit the companion Evolve site at http://evolve.elsevier.com/deWit/fundamental/ for additional online resources.

NCLEX-PN® EXAMINATION-STYLE REVIEW QUESTIONS

*Choose the **best** answer(s) for each of the following questions.*

1. The practice of nursing is regulated by:
   1. state boards of nursing.
   2. the National Council of State Boards of Nursing.
   3. the American Nurses Association.
   4. the American Hospital Association.

2. Which of the following actions would be considered an invasion of a patient's privacy? *(Select all that apply.)*
   1. Discussing the comatose patient's condition with his father-in-law.
   2. Discussing the outcome of a patient's test with another nurse from the unit while in an elevator with other people.
   3. Relaying information about the patient's concerns to the nurse who will care for him on the next shift.
   4. Relaying a complaint by the patient's wife to the charge nurse.

5. Posting a blog on your personal website about a difficult clinical day, including information about the hospital and patient's diagnosis but NOT stating the patient's name.

3. Which of the following actions would be classed as assault? *(Select all that apply.)*
   1. Telling the patient for the second time that you will bring the pain medication as soon as it is time for it.
   2. Restraining the patient's feet because he is kicking the nurse when an injection is to be administered.
   3. Threatening not to bring a meal tray if the patient won't behave.
   4. Grasping the patient's upper arm snugly when administering a subcutaneous insulin injection.
   5. Informing the patient that if he attempts to get out of bed one more time, he will be restrained.

4. For a nurse to be found guilty of malpractice when a patient has been injured, it would have to be shown that she did not:

   1. take responsibility for a medication error.
   2. do what a reasonably prudent nurse would have done in a similar patient care situation.
   3. remember to put up the side rails on the bed to prevent the patient from falling out of bed.
   4. keep the details of a patient's diagnosis and care private.

5. An advance directive is a consent that:

   1. gives a relative the power of attorney over financial affairs.
   2. spells out the incapacitated patient's wishes regarding tests and treatments.
   3. provides consent for specific organs to be donated in the event of death.
   4. puts the burden of medical decisions on a close relative or friend.

6. The visitor of one of your patients, stops you in the hall and says, "I hope you will not try to revive my neighbor if her heart stops." The correct response is:

   1. "That decision is up to the physician."
   2. "We are all trained in CPR."
   3. "I understand your concern, but I can't discuss your neighbor's care with you."
   4. "There is a 'do not resuscitate' order on her chart."

7. A physician advises a patient to accept intravenous fluids, which she refuses. The nurse says to the patient, "You must have the fluids if you want to stay in the hospital and have us take care of you." The nurse is:

   1. correct in insisting on fluid replacement.
   2. violating the patient's right to refuse treatment.
   3. not providing specific enough information about the options available for fluid replacement.
   4. giving information so the patient can make an informed refusal of fluids.
   5. wrong in speaking to the patient; the daughter should make the decision for or against fluid replacement.

8. Your newly admitted patient is found wandering in the hall. An aide helps her back to bed, and asks you if the patient should be placed in a protective device to keep her from wandering. You tell the aide to use a protective device. By providing this instruction, you are:

   1. liable for charges of false imprisonment.
   2. acting in the patient's best interests.
   3. guilty of a crime.
   4. not responsible for what the nursing assistant does.

9. Your patient asks you, "What do you think of my physician?" You mention that the physician doesn't seem to care about her patients, or how well their symptoms are managed. As a result, the patient switches to another physician. The physician may have grounds to sue you for:

   1. malpractice.
   2. slander.
   3. libel.
   4. invasion of privacy.

10. For a patient to successfully win a malpractice claim, which of the following elements must be proven? *(Select all that apply.)*

    1. Duty
    2. Breach of duty
    3. Lack of caring
    4. Harm or damage
    5. Cause-and-effect relationship
    6. Intent
    7. Fraud

CRITICAL THINKING ACTIVITIES *Read each clinical scenario and discuss the questions with your classmates.*

Scenario A
Jose Morales is a 46-year-old husband and father of two grown children. He has painful metastatic bone cancer. He is being discharged with a pain management program that still does not completely ease his pain. He tells you that he plans to "end it all" once he is at home, and asks you to help him with information about what kind and how much medication it would take so his death did not look like suicide. He also warns you not to tell anyone of his plans, because of "confidentiality."

1. Describe how you would answer his questions about assisted suicide.
2. Discuss the issue of confidentiality among the health care team versus invasion of privacy. How would you handle his request not to tell anyone?

Scenario B
You are a staff nurse at a skilled nursing facility on the evening shift. One 66-year-old woman who is very confused and agitated is pacing in the halls, entering other residents' rooms, and attempting to leave the building. Another nurse grabs the patient roughly and shouts at her, "If you don't stay in your room, I'm going to tie you in that bed." The nurse escorts the patient to her room, pushes her into a chair, and ties a sheet across the patient's lap to prevent her from getting out of the chair.

1. Identify the legal and ethical violations the nurse has committed.
2. What is your legal and ethical responsibility in this situation?

Scenario C
How would you respond to a physician at the clinic where you work who asks you embarrassing questions about your sexual experience, and suggests that you would benefit in your job if you entertained him at your home?

4 Nursing Process and Critical Thinking

evolve http://evolve.elsevier.com/deWit/fundamental/

Objectives

Upon completing this chapter, you should be able to:

Theory

1. Explain the use of the nursing process.
2. Identify the components of the nursing process.
3. State what "critical thinking" means.
4. Identify the steps of the problem-solving process.
5. List the steps used in making decisions.
6. Discuss the use of critical thinking in nursing.
7. Identify ways to improve critical thinking skills.
8. Explain the basic principles of setting priorities for nursing care.
9. List factors to be considered when setting priorities.
10. Apply the critical thinking process to a real-life problem.

Clinical Practice

1. Apply nursing process to a patient care assignment.
2. Use critical thinking to prioritize care for a patient assignment.

Key Terms

 Be sure to check the bonus material on the Companion CD-ROM, including selected audio pronunciations.

assessment (data collection) (p. 49)
critical thinking (p. 49)
decision making (pp. 49, 50)
evaluation (p. 49)
implementation (p. 49)
nursing diagnosis (p. 49)
nursing process (p. 48)
outcomes (p. 48)
planning (p. 49)
priority (prī-ŌR-ĭ-tē, p. 52)
scientific method (sī-ĕn-TĬ-fĭk, p. 48)

THE NURSING PROCESS

The nursing process is a way of thinking and acting based on the scientific method (a step-by-step process with observable results used by scientists to solve problems). The nursing process is a tool for identifying patients' problems and an organized method for meeting patients' needs. It was developed in the 1950s to describe the independent role of the nurse in providing patient care. Nurses are taught to use this framework consistently and methodically (Figure 4-1).

The five components of the nursing process are assessment (data collection), nursing diagnosis, planning, implementation, and evaluation. Box 4-1 provides a brief explanation of each component. The goals of the systematic, dynamic process are to explore patients' health status, identify actual or potential health care problems, determine desired outcomes (results of actions), deliver specific nursing interventions to solve the problems and promote health, and evaluate care given to determine whether outcomes have been achieved. The components often overlap as the nurse continually assesses and evaluates effects of actions. The role of the LPN/LVN is shown in Table 4-1 on p. 50 as set by the LPN/LVN Standards described by the National Federation of Licensed Practical/Vocational Nurses (NFLPN). The LPN role is explained more fully in Chapters 5 and 6.

The construction of a plan of care for the patient is a collaborative process among the nurse, the patient, and other health team members. **Patient input during the planning stage results in more success with the plan of care.** Registered nurses are officially responsible for the initiation of nursing care plans for each patient, but the LPN/LVN assists with each part of the care plan. The LPN is often responsible for data collection to assist the RN with the assessment phase. The nursing process allows for constant alterations in the plan of care as patients' conditions change.

The nursing process is similar to other methods used to organize tasks in daily life. In planning a week's meals at home, the goal is to supply each family member with good nutrition. The assessment or data collection phase involves deciding what might be served and surveying the supplies on hand needed for the food preparation. These data are analyzed to determine what must be purchased at the store, to plan specific menus, and to plan for deviation from normal meals, such as school lunches or quick dinners before a child's basketball game. Implementation includes shopping, preparing and serving the meals, and cleaning up afterward. Evaluation is performed to determine whether the plan was successful: Did the family members eat what was served? Was there too much

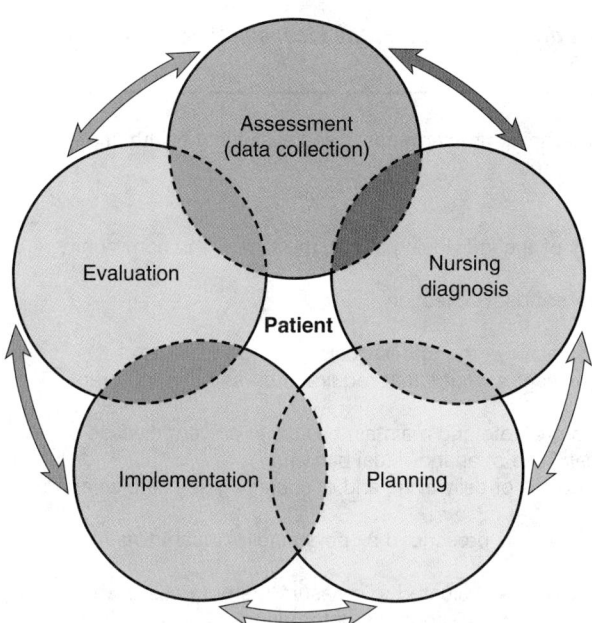

FIGURE **4-1** The nursing process—a dynamic, overlapping, continuous process centering on the patient.

Box 4-1 *Components of the Nursing Process*

Assessment (data collection): Collecting, organizing, documenting, and validating data about a patient's health status. Assessment data are obtained from the patient, the family, the physician, diagnostic tests, and information about the patient from other health professionals.

Nursing diagnosis: The process by which the assessment data are sorted and analyzed so that specific actual and potential health problems are identified. The factors contributing to the problems are considered and specific nursing diagnoses are chosen for the patient's care plan.

Planning: A series of steps by which the nurse and the patient set priorities and goals to eliminate or diminish the identified problems. The goals are stated as specific expected outcomes. The nurse and the patient collaborate and choose specific interventions for each nursing diagnosis. The interventions assist the patient to meet the expected outcomes. The expected outcomes and nursing interventions are listed on the patient's nursing care plan.

Implementation: Carrying out the nursing interventions in a systematic way. The nurse carries out the interventions or delegates some of them to an appropriate person. The patient's response to the care given is documented on the patient's chart.

Evaluation: Assessing the patient's response to the nursing interventions. The responses are compared with the expected outcomes to see to what extent the outcomes have been achieved. The entire care plan is reassessed in this phase, and any changes needed are made.

---

left over? Should something have been prepared differently? Was the expected outcome of balanced nutrition for each family member met? If not, how could the plan be altered for next week? This is not a new way of thinking and doing; the process is just being applied in a nursing context.

? *Think Critically About . . .* Can you think of something you do frequently in which you use this type of process for thinking and accomplishing things?

CRITICAL THINKING

It is necessary to think critically to use the nursing process successfully and to develop good clinical judgment. What does this mean? **Critical** means requiring careful judgment. **Thinking,** in this context, means to reason. Critical thinking **is directed, purposeful, mental activity by which ideas are evaluated, plans are constructed, and desired outcomes are decided.** Critical thinking is necessary to make reliable observations regarding health status and to draw sound conclusions from the data obtained. Critical thinking is needed for creative problem solving and for the production of new ideas and solutions. It is essential for the evaluation of information received from others as well. Critical thinking is the keystone of good clinical decision making and the development of clinical judgment.

PROBLEM SOLVING AND DECISION MAKING

Nursing is a discipline that incorporates scientific knowledge and methods of research. Scientists use a consistent, logical method to solve problems. In the scientific method, the scientist first defines the problem, then gathers information, analyzes the information, and develops solutions. The scientist makes a decision about which solution to use, implements the decision, and then evaluates the outcome of the decision. The nursing process has many similar characteristics. Table 4-2 compares the scientific method with the nursing process.

The *problem-solving* process has the following several steps:

- First, define the problem clearly.
- Second, consider all possible alternatives as solutions to the problem.
- Third, consider the possible outcomes for each alternative.
- Fourth, predict the likelihood of each outcome occurring.
- Finally, choose the alternative with the best chance of success that has the fewest undesirable outcomes.

Table 4-1 *Correlation of Nursing Process and the NFLPN Nursing Practice Standards for the Licensed Practical/Vocational Nurse*

	STANDARD Shall know and utilize the nursing process in planning, implementing, and evaluating health services and nursing care for the individual patient or group.
1. *Assessment*	*RN Function*
2. *Nursing Diagnosis*	*RN Function*
3. Planning	1. Assessment/data collection of health status of the individual patient, the family, and community groups 2. Reporting information gained from assessment/data collection 3. The identification of health goals
4. Implementation	The plan for nursing care is put into practice to achieve the stated goals and includes: 1. Observing, recording, and reporting significant changes that require intervention or different goals. 2. Applying nursing knowledge and skills to promote and maintain health, to prevent disease and disability and to optimize functional capabilities of an individual patient. 3. Assisting the patient and family with activities of daily living and encouraging self-care as appropriate. 4. Carrying out therapeutic regimens and protocols prescribed by personnel pursuant to authorized state law.
5. Evaluation	The plan for nursing care and its implementations are evaluated to measure the progress toward the stated goals and will include appropriate person and/or groups to determine: 1. The relevancy of current goals in relation to the progress of the individual patient. 2. The involvement of the recipients of care in the evaluation process. 3. The quality of the nursing action in the implementation of the plan. 4. A re-ordering of priorities or new goal setting in the care plan.

Copyright © 2003 National Federation of Licensed Practical Nurses, Inc. From National Federation of Licensed Practical Nurses, Inc., 605 Poole Drive, Garner, NC 27529. Phone: 919/779-0046. Fax: 919/779-5642. www.nflpn.org/practice_standards4web.pdf.

Table 4-2 *Comparison of Scientific Method and the Nursing Process*

SCIENTIFIC METHOD STEP	NURSING PROCESS STEP
Define the problem Gather information	**Assessment (Data Collection)** History taking, physical assessment, results of diagnostic tests
Analyze the information (data)	**Nursing Diagnosis** Consider assessment database and identify problems; choose nursing diagnoses
Develop solutions Make a decision	**Planning** Determine desired outcomes Choose interventions to achieve those outcomes
Implement the decision	**Implementation** Carry out the interventions
Evaluate the decision	**Evaluation** Assess the result of the interventions; determine if outcomes have been achieved; revise the plan if outcomes are not being met; terminate interventions no longer needed

Decisions are necessary to solve problems. Nurses make decisions in each step of the nursing process. Good decision making is choosing the best actions to meet a desired goal and is part of the critical thinking process. Nurses often have to make quick decisions in moments of crisis; they also assist patients to make decisions. Nurses must problem-solve continually. Critical thinking improves the outcomes of the problem-solving process.

SKILLS FOR CRITICAL THINKING

Critical thinking involves a variety of skills. Foundation skills are effective reading, effective writing, attentive listening, and effective communicating. Effective reading involves reading material in a way that helps you pick out the main ideas and relevant data. Reading a paragraph and then restating the main ideas to yourself is one way to read critically.

Effective writing concerns writing thoughts coherently and concisely, yet clearly. Writing clearly, logically, and concisely is a learned skill. Evaluating what you write helps improve this skill.

Attentive listening is consciously focusing on the topic of discussion. Attentive listening takes a lot of practice. With our busy lives, we tend to rush ahead to form an answer or ask a question rather than wait until the speaker has finished. Pay attention to each word and the meaning the speaker is trying to convey (Figure 4-2). To practice attentive listening, work with a partner. Have your partner tell you about something that interests her. When she is finished, repeat back the main ideas of what was stated. Confirm with the speaker that you heard correctly.

Effective communicating requires speaking in a disciplined manner. The disciplined speaker thinks about

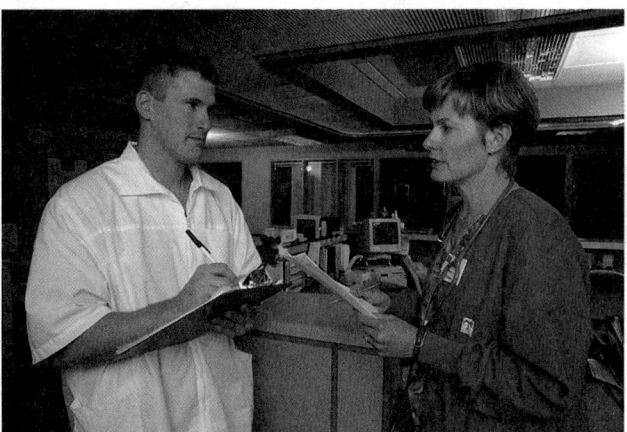

FIGURE **4-2** Student listening attentively to staff nurse.

what to say and how to state it clearly and concisely in a logical way before beginning to speak. Effective speaking follows attentive listening. Much communication in our fast-paced society results in spontaneous response without conscious thought, and misunderstanding often occurs. Taking time to consider your response before beginning to speak is another good way to improve this skill. Group interactions that provide feedback will help you assess and improve your speaking skill. Other skills and attributes found in the critical thinker are listed in Box 4-2. Practicing careful consideration of problems and purposeful thinking, rather than random thinking, will help you develop these skills and attributes.

A technique that nursing students have found helpful is *concept mapping*. Concept mapping promotes critical thinking. It helps students learn to synthesize pertinent assessment data, develop care plans that are comprehensive and holistic, link nursing interventions with health problems and nursing diagnoses, and effectively implement the plan of care. It can help you see relationships within a concept or relationships between concepts. Concept mapping will help you gather data in a logical manner and then group those data in a meaningful way. Concept Map 4-1 shows the possible demands on a student nurse's life and related responsibilities. This map does not show the interrelationships between the items depicted. Looking at it, try to visualize how one area may be affected by another. For example, study hours and work hours will probably affect the time available for sleep. Multiple lines could be drawn to show the interrelationships. Once you are familiar with the nursing process and begin to take care of patients, you will see how effective concept mapping can be in helping you to devise and carry out patient care. Concept mapping is helpful in learning about the pathophysiology of a disease and how it affects the body. It can be used to show relationships between ideas. You will find various concept maps throughout this text.

Think Critically About . . . What critical thinking skills do you already use? Give some examples. Which critical thinking skill do you think is most important?

CRITICAL THINKING IN NURSING

Critical thinking in nursing requires skills and experience as well as knowledge. Professional standards and codes of ethics influence a nurse's critical thinking.

Critical thinking is applied to the nursing process in many ways. **Assessment (data collection)** is carried out in an organized, systematic way. Data are gathered to determine and eliminate or manage actual or potential health problems. The data are accurately recorded. Ways of helping patients obtain optimum wellness and independence are identified.

Nursing diagnosis requires analysis of data gathered during assessment, clustering related information, identifying problem areas, and choosing appropriate nursing diagnoses.

Planning involves determining specific desired outcomes for each nursing diagnosis. While planning interventions to achieve those outcomes, one considers ways to promote optimum wellness and independence. How to achieve the desired outcomes in the most timely, cost-effective way is decided.

Implementation is begun by preparing to perform the interventions. Equipment and supplies are gathered and procedures are thought through before beginning them. Interventions are performed and responses to them are assessed. Changes in interventions

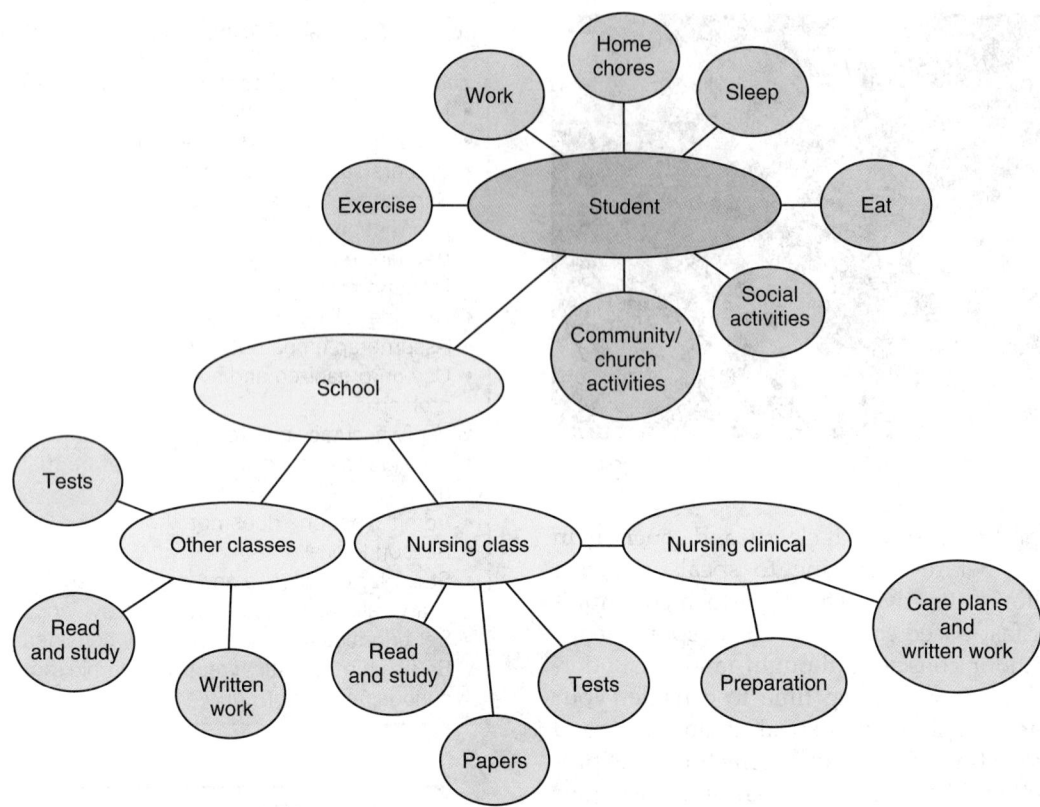

CONCEPT MAP **4-1** Demands on a student nurse's life and associated responsibilities.

are instituted as needed. Accurate documentation of interventions and patient response occurs.

Evaluation is carried out by gathering data to determine if expected outcomes have been achieved. When interventions are not achieving expected outcomes, reconsideration of what needs to be done occurs. Aspects of the plan of care are modified or terminated as appropriate.

PRIORITY SETTING AND WORK ORGANIZATION

Critical thinking is applied to setting priorities for patient care. Nurses must also be able to prioritize the tasks assigned to them. A priority is more important than something else at that time. **Priority setting (prioritizing) involves placing nursing diagnoses or nursing interventions in order of importance.** Life-threatening problems are of a *high priority*. Problems that threaten health or coping ability are of a *medium priority*. *Low-priority* problems are ones that do not have a major effect on the person if not attended to that day or even that week. Prioritizing patient problems is usually based on the adaptation of Maslow's hierarchy of needs (see Figure 2-3). Setting these priorities will be discussed in Chapter 5.

Priority setting for work organization requires consideration of several factors. As a student, you begin by prioritizing care for one patient. After graduation, you will need to prioritize care for many patients.

When beginning your shift (or clinical day), go over your patient assignment worksheet, the Kardex, or the computer patient care plan and determine what needs to be done in the next hour. These items are of a high priority. Some tasks that may need to be done are vital signs, daily weights before breakfast, blood sugar readings before eating, morning insulin injections, preoperative assessments, and administration of medication for pain control.

When looking at prioritizing such tasks, you must consider what will happen if the task is not done on time. The recovering patient whose vital signs have been stable for the past 24 hours probably will not suffer a bad consequence if you do not take her vital signs right at 8 A.M. The diabetic who is hospitalized to control her disease really needs to have her blood sugar checked and her insulin given and may suffer an alteration in her health status if these tasks are not completed on time.

Other factors to be considered are the surgery schedule, degree of stability of each patient in your care, amount of time it will take to perform each task for each patient, availability of help, medication orders, unforeseen problems that occur, and physicians making rounds who ask you to do a task on a patient who isn't yours. Knowledge, critical thinking, and clinical judgment will help you prioritize the tasks of your workload.

When all tasks have a rather high priority and there is no way you can do them all alone, you must assign some tasks to others. After prioritizing your tasks for

ASSIGNMENT/WORK ORGANIZATION SHEET

Patient/Room #	7:30	8:00	9:00	10:00	11:00	12:00	1:00	2:00	3:00
J. G. 526	V.S. Quick Assess	Shower Δ dressing	Meds chart	Full Assess chart		V.S.	Pre-op Teaching chart	I+O Tape report	Close Chart
G. H. 528A	V.S. ✓Feed Pump	Quick Assess	Meds Full Assess	chart	Teaching ✓Feed Pump	V.S.	meds	I+O	Close chart ✓Feed Pump
S. S. 528B	V.S. ✓IV Quick Assess	med ✓IV	Full Assess chart	✓IV	✓IV	V.S. Teaching	✓IV Δ dressing	I+O	Close Chart

FIGURE **4-3** One example of a work organization sheet for a shift.

the first hour, consider priorities for the rest of the shift. Figure 4-3 shows one type of work organization sheet.

? *Think Critically About . . .* How would you respond if you are about to go to check a patient's blood sugar and administer her insulin, and a physician asks you to put on a wound dressing for a patient who is not assigned to you?

Priorities constantly change because patient needs and conditions change frequently. To maintain organization with your workload, you must be flexible and you must frequently reorder your tasks. You should reconsider your work organization plan at least every 2 hours during your shift, reprioritizing as needed.

APPLICATION OF PROBLEM SOLVING AND CRITICAL THINKING

The emergency room is a good place to observe how nurses prioritize care and solve problems. When the emergency room nurse is faced with three patients seeking help, the problem of how to deal with all three patients and quickly make a decision about who is treated first must be solved. The first patient complains of severe chest pain; the second has a fever and a very bad cough; the third has a laceration on her chin and is bleeding. The problem: Which patient to treat first?

There are six possibilities for the order of treatment. When considering the possible outcome of choosing each alternative, the nurse looks at the consequences of placing each patient first, second, or third. If the woman with the laceration is chosen to be first, the outcomes might be (1) she will stop bleeding; (2) the man with chest pain may be having a heart attack and may die, or he may be diagnosed with severe indigestion; and (3) the woman with the fever and cough may become angry and cause a commotion. If the man with the chest pain is chosen to be first to be treated, the outcomes might be (1) his life may be saved, or it may be determined he has severe indigestion; (2) the woman with the laceration may lose more blood, or the bleeding may stop by applying pressure while she is waiting to be treated; and (3) the woman with the cough and fever may cause a commotion or may be courteous about waiting.

Considering the likelihood of each outcome occurring is the next step. The nurse looks at the three patients and estimates that the man with chest pain has at least a 65% chance of it being a life-threatening heart attack and a 35% chance that he has indigestion; the chance of the woman with the fever and sore throat causing a commotion is about 5%, and the chance of this woman courteously waiting about 95%. If you choose the man with the chest pain to be treated first, the chance of the woman with the laceration losing a serious amount of blood is about 20% while the chance of stopping the blood with pressure while awaiting treatment is about 80% or better. Since the chance of a bad outcome is highest for the man with the chest pain, you choose to have him treated first. **The goal is to avoid having your decision cause injury to anyone.**

Besides ordering treatment for emergency room patients, you must decide many things each day, such as what size needle is best to use for an injection, what to tell the patient or her family about her prognosis, which tasks to assign and which to do yourself, which staff to assign to which patients, and which nursing diagnosis has the highest priority for a patient on a particular day. **With critical thinking skills, you can weigh many factors and skillfully solve problems, making good decisions a majority of the time.** No one makes perfect decisions all the time. Learning to apply the nursing process well will assist you to gain clinical judgment and to follow logical processes automatically when solving problems and making decisions. **Operating in a critical thinking mode while pursuing your nursing studies will help you develop the clinical judgment necessary for safe nursing practice.**

The nursing process is a way of thinking as well as organizing. In this dynamic process, the nurse is constantly gathering data and evaluating. The next two chapters explain the components of the nursing process more thoroughly. The bibliography for this chapter identifies resources for the student who wishes to enhance learning by improving critical thinking skills.

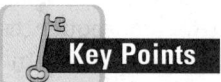

Key Points

- The nursing process is a way of thinking and acting based on the scientific method. It is a framework for planning, implementing, and evaluating nursing care.
- RNs are officially responsible for the initiation of nursing care plans, but LPN/LVNs assist with the care plan, evaluate care, and help revise through collaboration with other health team members (see Table 4-1).

- The components of the nursing process are assessment, nursing diagnosis, planning, implementation, and evaluation (see Box 4-1).
- Formulating a plan of care is a collaborative process among the nurse, the patient, and other health team members.
- The nursing process has many characteristics that are similar to the scientific method (see Table 4-2).
- The steps to problem solving are (1) define the problem clearly; (2) consider all possible alternatives; (3) consider the possible outcomes for each alternative; (4) predict the likelihood of each outcome occurring; and (5) choose the alternative with the best chance of success and the least undesirable outcomes.
- Critical thinking improves the outcomes of the problem-solving process.
- Critical thinking is directed, purposeful, mental activity by which ideas are created and evaluated, plans are constructed, and desired outcomes are decided.
- Critical thinking is necessary to make reliable observations regarding health status and to draw sound conclusions from the data obtained.
- Critical thinking involves a variety of skills; effective reading, effective writing, attentive listening, and effective communicating are the foundation skills.
- Practicing careful consideration of problems and purposeful thinking increases critical thinking skills (see Box 4-2).
- Critical thinking is applied within each component of the nursing process.
- Priority setting involves placing tasks, nursing diagnoses, or nursing interventions in order of importance.
- Nurses use priority setting for work organization. Priorities constantly change as patient needs change.
- With critical thinking, factors can be weighed, problems skillfully solved, and good decisions made a majority of the time.

 Go to your **Companion CD-ROM** for an Audio Glossary, animations, video clips, and more.

evolve Be sure to visit the companion Evolve site at http://evolve.elsevier.com/deWit/fundamental/ for additional online resources.

NCLEX-PN® EXAMINATION-STYLE REVIEW QUESTIONS

*Choose the **best** answer for each question.*

1. _____ during the planning stage of the nursing process results in more success. *(Fill in the blank.)*

2. The planning phase of the nursing process correlates with which step of the scientific method?
   1. Brainstorming
   2. Data analysis
   3. Developing solutions
   4. Implementing the decision

3. Priorities of care change constantly because: *(Select all that apply.)*
   1. the nurse's workload may change as patients are admitted.
   2. physicians' orders may change throughout the shift.
   3. a patient's condition may deteriorate.
   4. tests or therapies may not be done on time.
   5. many visitors are in the rooms.

4. Critical thinking is necessary to:

1. plan nursing care.
2. organize care for several patients.
3. collaborate with others.
4. draw sound conclusions from assessment data.

5. Attributes of critical thinkers include: *(Select all that apply.)*

1. setting priorities.
2. consulting physicians.
3. verifying accuracy and reliability of data.
4. reasoning logically.
5. accepting others' decisions.
6. being flexible.
7. recognizing inconsistencies in data gathered.

6. The first step in problem solving involves:

1. setting priorities for tasks.
2. organizing the workload.
3. considering alternatives of action.
4. defining the problem clearly.

7. Critical thinking will help you in the clinical setting to:

1. delegate work efficiently.
2. make good decisions most of the time.
3. identify nursing diagnoses.
4. write care plans more effectively.

CRITICAL THINKING ACTIVITIES *Read each clinical scenario and discuss the questions with your classmates.*

Scenario A

As a student, you have several tasks to complete. There is an Anatomy and Physiology test 4 days away. A comprehensive paper is due in 1 week and you just collected the library materials you need for it. A 50-page reading assignment needs to be completed for lecture the day after tomorrow.

1. How would you organize to accomplish these tasks?
2. In what order of priority would you place each of these tasks? Explain why you place each task within the order you've chosen.

Scenario B

Your clinical area does not have sphygmomanometers (blood pressure cuffs) on the wall by each patient; portable ones are used. You need to take 8 A.M. vital signs (temperature, pulse, respiration rate, and blood pressure) quickly, and there is no portable unit available right now. How would you solve this problem?

Scenario C

Your clinical assignment is for:

  M.H., age 72; diagnosis: pneumonia
  F.S., age 52; diagnosis: leg ulcer
  J.P., age 78; diagnosis: abdominal hernia repair
  It is 9:45 A.M. If J.P. needs to be ambulated three times a day, M.H. needs his antibiotic given at 10 A.M., and F.S. needs her dressing changed this morning, in what order would you do these tasks? How did you make this decision?

Objectives

Upon completing this chapter, you should be able to:

Theory

1. Identify the purpose of assessment (data collection).
2. Differentiate objective data from subjective data.
3. Identify sources of data for the formulation of a patient database.
4. Discuss the three basic methods used to gather a patient database.
5. Correlate patient problems with nursing diagnoses from the accepted North American Nursing Diagnosis Association–International (NANDA-I) list.
6. Identify appropriate outcome criteria for selected nursing diagnoses.
7. Plan goals for each patient and write outcome criteria for the chosen nursing diagnoses.

Clinical Practice

1. Collect assessment data for a patient and document it.
2. Analyze the data collected to determine patient needs.
3. Identify appropriate nursing diagnoses from the NANDA list for each assigned patient.
4. Prioritize the nursing diagnoses.
5. Write specific goal/outcome statements.
6. Plan appropriate nursing interventions to assist the patient in attaining the goals/expected outcomes.

Key Terms

Be sure to check out the bonus material on the Companion CD-ROM, including selected audio pronunciations.

cues (KĔWS, p. 62)
data (p. 56)
database (p. 56)
defining characteristics (p. 65)
etiologic factors (ē-tē-ō-LŌ-jĭk, p. 65)
expected outcome (p. 67)
goal (p. 66)
inferences (ĬN-fĕr-ĕn-sĕs, p. 63)
interview (p. 57)
nursing diagnosis (p. 63)
objective data (p. 57)
signs (p. 65)
subjective data (p. 57)
symptoms (p. 65)

ASSESSMENT (DATA COLLECTION)

In this chapter we will discuss the first three steps in the nursing process: assessment and data collection, nursing diagnosis, and planning. **Assessment** consists of gathering information about patients and their needs using a variety of methods. During the assessment phase of the nursing process, data (pieces of information on a specific topic) are systematically obtained, organized into a logical database (all the information gathered about a patient), and documented. Although assessment is an RN function rather than an LPN/LVN function according to most state nurse practice acts, LPN/LVNs assist the RN in the gathering of data. Data collection is a large part of assessment. Assessment for the LPN/LVN is guided by the National Federation of Licensed Practical Nurses (NFLPN) Standard 4 under the Planning area of the nursing process: "The planning of nursing includes assessment/data collection of health status of the individual patient, the family and community groups" (see Box 1-1). An RN is designated as the staff member who must perform the initial admission assessment of each patient. However, the **LPN/LVN is often asked to assist with this task and participates in carrying out the plan by continuing to collect data** (Assignment Considerations 5-1).

There are various approaches to data collection. One is a structured format to obtain a comprehensive database based on the 11 functional health patterns as formulated by Mary Gordon (Box 5-1). After data in all 11 areas are collected, a review is performed to see if there are patterns indicating problems. The assessment data are then compared with the patient's baselines, such as usual blood pressure, heart rate, weight, and so forth. The functional patterns represent the interaction between the patient and the environment. The 11 patterns are each part of a whole, and any one pattern is understood only in conjunction with the other 10 patterns. The analysis and comparisons help the nurse identify patient strengths and patient weaknesses. Many nursing schools teach this approach.

A second method of data collection is to begin with areas in which problems are evident, such as pain. Factors causing or affecting the pain are explored. This is a *focused assessment* because it is concerned with one very specific problem. The assessment and data collec-

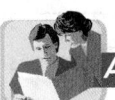

Assignment Considerations 5-1

Assigning Admission Tasks

If assistive personnel are available to help, you may assign the tasks of weighing, measuring, and obtaining a urine specimen for the newly admitted patient. The assistant could open the admission supplies and set up the patient's room. Be certain to alert the assistant of any safety measures needed for the patient.

Box 5-1 *Gordon's 11 Health Patterns*

- Health perception–health management pattern
- Nutritional-metabolic pattern
- Elimination pattern
- Activity-exercise pattern
- Cognitive-perceptual pattern
- Sleep-rest pattern
- Self-perception–self-concept pattern
- Role-relationship pattern
- Sexuality-reproductive pattern
- Coping-stress-tolerance pattern
- Value-belief pattern

For each pattern, the following are assessed:

FUNCTIONAL
- Present function
- Personal habits
- Lifestyle and cultural factors
- Age-related factors

DYSFUNCTIONAL
- History of dysfunction
- Diagnostic test abnormalities
- Risk factors related to medical treatment plan

   All problems identified within a pattern are considered according to their relationship to the other functional patterns. Nursing focus is aimed at improving the patient's functional status in each pattern area.

From Gordon, M. (1994). *Nursing Diagnosis: Process and Application* (3rd ed.). St. Louis: Mosby. Adapted from Harkreader, H., Hogan, M.A., & Thobaben, M. (2007). *Fundamentals of Nursing: Caring and Clinical Judgment* (2nd ed., p. 107). Philadelphia: Elsevier Saunders.

Table 5-1 | *Examples of Subjective and Objective Data*

SUBJECTIVE DATA EXAMPLES	OBJECTIVE DATA EXAMPLES
"I have a headache."	Temperature 101.4° F (38.6° C)
"I am nauseated."	135 mL emesis at 08:20
"The sharp pain is in my hip."	Bruise on right hip
"I've been feeling really blue lately."	Eyes downcast, flat affect
"I've been lonely since my husband died."	Only one visitor seen in room all day
"I'm tired all the time."	Hb 10.5 mg/dL, HCT 31%
"I'm afraid I have cancer."	Pathology report states tissue is adenosarcoma

Key: *Hb*, Hemoglobin; *HCT*, hematocrit.

views the patient to find out his major complaints, performs a physical examination, and determines the patient's overall health status. Information is also gathered by observing the patient, reading the chart or other sources of written information, and consulting with the family, significant others, and other health professionals. Data obtained from the patient verbally are called subjective data. A headache, tingling in the feet, or pain in the shoulder is only apparent to the patient, and only the patient can describe or verify such symptoms. These are examples of subjective data.

Information obtained through the senses and hands-on physical examination is objective data. The observed inabilities of a patient to grasp a glass in his left hand or to support his body when standing are examples of objective data. Vital signs, physical examination findings, and results of diagnostic tests are also objective data (Table 5-1).

Other sources of data are the physician's history and physical, ancillary staff notes, and the admission note. The data collection is guided by a printed form that is filled out and placed in each patient's chart. The nursing student may be assigned to interview patients using a more comprehensive form as part of a learning experience. Figure 5-1 shows a portion of a typical nursing admission assessment and data collection form used in the hospital setting. Other sections of the form include skin, nutrition, personal habits, pain, education, and psychological/spiritual assessments. The full form is located on the **CD-ROM** accompanying this text.

Think Critically About . . . Can you think of two other pieces of information that might be obtained during an assessment that would be subjective data?

THE INTERVIEW

The interview is focused on gathering data and is not a social interaction. Good communication is vital to adequate assessment. Communication may be verbal—

tion then progress to how the problem affects other areas of the patient's life. If the patient is in acute distress, a focused assessment may be performed before a total assessment and data collection are completed.

A third method is to assess every area in Maslow's hierarchy of basic needs (see Figure 2-3).

Whatever method is used, assessment and data collection must be comprehensive, covering all aspects of the patient: physical, psychosocial, and spiritual.

An admission assessment and data collection interview (conversation where facts are obtained) is usually performed when patients are assigned to the nursing unit, enter the care of a home health agency, or become residents in a long-term care facility. The nurse inter-

ADMISSION DATE & TIME:	PRIMARY LANGUAGE IF NOT ENGLISH	ADMITTED FROM: ☐ ED ☐ ECF ☒ HOME ☐ DIRECT _____ ☐ OTHER _____	HT. 5' 3" IN. ☐ STATED ☐ MEASURED	WT. 138# ☒ STANDING ☐ BED SCALE ☐ CHAIR SCALE	REASON FOR DEFERRED WT.
5/20/09 ROOM NUMBER: 427 B	☐ SIGN LANGUAGE	MODE OF TRANSFER. ☐ W/C ☐ BED ☐ GURNEY ☐ AMBULATED			

Patient Statement / Complaint:

C.V.A. Left-sided paresis. Cannot bear weight

VITAL SIGNS
T 97⁸ F. R 14 /min.
R   L
P 92 BP 148/94

Instruction of Routines and Services to Patient/Family

- ☑ Nurse call system / Intercom
- ☑ Bed controls
- ☑ Side Rails
- ☑ Telephone/TV
- ☑ Pastoral Care
- ☑ Visiting policy / Cellular Phone Use
- ☑ Smoking policy
- ☑ Identiband

SIGNATURE & TITLE

The valuables/personal effects policy has been explained, and, I understand that Marian Medical Center does not assume responsibility for valuables (money, jewelry, or other personal effects) not secured in the Marian Medical Center safe.

John C. Thompson Signature
Patient or Responsible Person
Husband

La poliza tocante objetos de valor ha sido explicada, y yo entiendo que Marian Medical Center no asume responsabilidad por estos objetos (alhajas, dinero, etc.) o cualquier otra prenda personal que no sea asegurada en la caja fuerte de Marian Medical Center.

_____ Firma
Paciente o persona responsable por el paciente

MEDICAL HISTORY

	YES	NO
Diabetes	☐	☑
Asthma	☐	☑
Epilepsy	☐	☑
Family Bleeding Tend.	☐	☑
Glaucoma	☐	☑
Cardiac	☐	☑

Any other Medical/Surgical Conditions:

PHARMACY

CURRENT MEDICATIONS: (Prescribed and non-prescribed)

DISPOSITION OF MEDICATIONS: ☐ Home ☐ To Pharmacy
Medications sent to Pharmacy noted on Administrative Data Screen.

Medication	Dosage	Frequency	Last Dose	Medication	Dosage	Frequency	Last Dose
Synthroid	0.05 mg.	qd	9 AM				
MOM	30cc	qhoc	10 pm				
Lo Dose ASA (81 mg)		qd	9 AM				

Do you take any vitamin or food supplements or herbal remedies? ☑ Yes ☐ No List: Multiple Vitamin, Vitamin E

ALLERGIES

		TYPE OF REACTION	MEDICATIONS/FOODS	TYPE OF REACTION
NO KNOWN ALLERGIES ☐				
ADHESIVE TAPE: YES ☐ NO ☑			Milk - Lactose Intol.	diarrhea/Bloating
IODINE SKIN PREP: YES ☐ NO ☑				
LATEX: YES ☐ NO ☑				
PCN		Skin rash		
SULFA		Hives		

PAGE 1

PATIENT ADDRESSOGRAPH

MARY THOMPSON
#0194628
ROOM 427 B
AL Johnson, M.D.

Marian Medical Center
✚ CHW
1400 East Church Street
Santa Maria, CA 93454

L.V.N. Signature: _S. Heartland LVN_
R.N. Signature: _J. Hoppe, RN_

PATIENT ADMISSION ASSESSMENT

S6010-8 (9/02)

FIGURE **5-1** Example of a patient admission assessment form. This is the first page of a four-page form; the entire form is included on your Companion CD-ROM.

NEUROLOGICAL STATUS

PUPIL SIZE CHART

| 1mm | 2mm | 3mm | 4mm | 5mm | 6mm | 7mm | 8mm | 9mm |

N Normal   S Sluggish   NR Non-Reactive

LEVEL OF CONSCIOUSNESS: ☐ ALERT   ☐ ORIENTED
☐ Confused   ☐ Slow to respond/Comprehend
☐ Disoriented   ☒ Lethargic   ☐ Vertigo
☒ Pupils: Size & reaction: Right *4mm*   Left: *4 mm*

SENSORY LIMITATIONS: ☐ WNL
☐ Taste   ☐ Speech   ☐ Sight
☒ Touch *Left*   ☐ Smell   ☐ Hearing

	If Pt. Uses	If with Patient
Glasses	☒	☒
Contact Lenses ☐ R ☐ L	☐	☐
Hearing Aid ☐ R ☐ L	☐	☐

FUNCTIONAL STATUS (LEVEL OF SELF CARE)

MOBILITY: ☐ WNL   ☐ Decreased mobility over last month
Limitations:

		If Pt Uses	If with Patient
☒ Walking	☒ Stairs		
☒ Transfer	☒ Standing Cane/Crutches/Walker	☐	☐
☒ Turning in bed	☐ Generalized Weakness Artificial Limbs ☐ R ☐ L	☐	☐
	Brace	☐	☐

☒ Request Rehab. Services consult
☒ Acute onset
☐ Changes in mobility in the last month
☐

WEAKNESS PARALYSIS/TRAUMA/SURGERY *Left sided weakness*
MOTOR FUNCTION
RUE→ ☐ WNL ☐ Weak ☐ Absent
RLE→ ☐ WNL ☐ Weak ☐ Absent
LUE→ ☐ WNL ☒ Weak ☐ Absent   ASSISTANCE REQUIRED:
LLE→ ☐ WNL ☒ Weak ☐ Absent   ☒ Hygiene/Grooming   ☒ Dressing   ☐ Meals   ☒ Other *Transfers*

SAFETY RISK

		Score			Score
1. History of falling	No 0		5. Gait		
	Yes 25	0	Normal/bedrest/wheelchair	0	
2. Secondary diagnosis	No 0		Weak	10	
More than 1 medical dx	Yes 15	0	Impaired	20	X
3. Ambulatory Aid:			6. Mental Status:		
None/Bedrest/Nurse assist	No 0		Oriented to own ability	0	0
Crutches/Cane/Walker	Yes 15		Overestimates/forgets		
Furniture	Yes 30	X	limitations	15	
4. IV therapy/Saline lock	No 0				
	Yes 20	X			

Total Score *70*

☒ > 51 Initiate Safety Risk Protocol Care Plan Identified at High Risk for Fall

RESPIRATORY

☐ WNL BREATH SOUNDS RATE
☐ Accessory Muscles   ☒ Secretions   ☐ Nasal Flaring
☐ Dyspnea   ☐ Tracheostomy   ☐ Orthopnea
☒ Abnormal Breath Sounds   ☐ Tachypnea   ☐ Cough
☐ Oxygen ☐ Type _____

Crackles @ lung base

CARDIO VASCULAR

☐ WNL REGULAR RHYTHM, RATE
☐ Abnormal Pulses   ☐ Abnormal Heart Sounds   ☐ Pedal Edema
Apical/Radial/Pedal   ☐ Jugular Vein Distension   ☐ Pacemaker

abnormal BP

GASTRO INTESTINAL

☐ WNL   ☐ INCONTINENT OF BOWEL
☐ NAUSEA/VOMITING   ☐ OCCASIONAL   ☐ FREQUENT
☐ TUBES   ☒ BOWEL SOUNDS
  ☐ N/G ☐ GT ☐ J/T   ☒ NORMAL ☐ HYPO ☐ HYPER ☐ ABSENT
☐ OTHER _____   ☐ CONSTIPATION   ☐ DIARRHEA
☒ BLOODY STOOL   ☐ ABDOMINAL DISTENSION
☒ LAST BOWEL MOVEMENT: *5/20/09*   ☐ ABDOMINAL TENDERNESS/PAIN
☐ OSTOMY/ELIMINATION AIDS   LOCATION _____
  ☒ OTHER *ON MOM* _____

Genitourinary / GYN

☐ Anuric   ☐ WNL
☐ Nocturia   ☐ Other: _____
☐ Burning   ☐ Catheter
☐ Urgency   Date Placed _____
☒ Urinary Incontinence
☐ Urinary Frequency
☐ Stress Incontinence

GYN
☐ Not Applicable
☐ Vaginal Discharge
☐ Unusual Bleeding
  Pad Count _____
☐ Pregnant
☐ LMP _____

☐ If pregnant and over 20 weeks, complete OB Assessment.

Obtain prenatal record from L&D or Obstetrician

PAGE 2

FIGURE **5-1, cont'd** Example of a patient admission assessment form. This is the second page of a four-page form; the entire form is included on your Companion CD-ROM.

Cultural Cues 5-1

Be Attentive to Cultural Needs

If your patient is of a different culture, recall the specifics of cultural differences in communication, personal space, and expected courtesies. Obtain an interpreter if there is a language barrier to good communication.

talking and listening—or nonverbal, which involves noting facial expressions, body posture, movement, and gestures (Cultural Cues 5-1). The course of the interaction is directed to elicit specific information concerning the patient's health status or feelings about her health.

The interview contains three basic stages: (1) the opening, when rapport is established with the patient; (2) the body of the interview, when the necessary questions are presented; and (3) the closing segment of the interview. After establishing rapport, discuss the purpose of the interview. While asking the necessary questions, examine the patient. Indicate the closing of the interview by stating, "Do you have any questions?" or, "I would be glad to answer any questions you have." Another way of closing the interview is to say something like, "Well, I guess that's all I need for now." Thank patients for their time, express some concern for their welfare, and tell them what will happen next. Summarize their problems and tell them when you will be back (see Chapter 8).

After the initial assessment, you will continue to gather data about the patient each time there is an encounter. **Assessment is an ongoing process.** If you are assigned to a patient in the days after the admission, a quick chart review can provide data needed to provide adequate care.

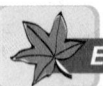

Elder Care Points

When interviewing an elderly person, allow more time because the person will probably have a more extensive history and may take a little longer to recall the needed information.

CHART REVIEW

A chart review is a data collection tool that assists in obtaining the information needed to intelligently interview the patient or to prepare adequately for the day's patient assignment. To perform a chart review, methodically look through the chart, checking the sections listed in Box 5-2. Of course, if the patient has just been admitted, you can seek information only from the face sheet and the physician's orders.

To do a review in preparation for your clinical assignment, look first at the face sheet and then at the most current physician's orders, as well as those of the

---

Box 5-2 | *Quick Chart Review*

Look for the following information:

Face sheet: Age, sex, marital status/significant other, religion, occupation, residence, next of kin and address, allergies, insurance status

Physician's orders: Admitting diagnosis, date of admission; current orders regarding diet, activity, frequency of vital signs measurement, daily weight, treatments, medications, diagnostic tests ordered, IV fluids, therapies ordered

Nurse's notes: Status during the last 24 hours

Physician's progress notes: Findings from last 2 days; status of problems

Medication administration record (MAR): Medications received, frequency of PRN medications, allergies

Physician's patient history and physical: Current complaint, chronic problems, physical finding abnormalities, allergies, impressions

Surgery operative report: Procedure done; organs removed; type of incision, drains or equipment in place, blood loss, problems during surgery

Pathology report: Presence of malignancy or infection

Current diagnostic tests: Check for any abnormal findings: CBC, UA, blood chemistries, x-ray films, culture and sensitivity, other tests

Nursing admission history and assessment: Reason for hospitalization, average number of cigarettes smoked per day, average amount of alcohol consumed per day, last bowel movement, special diet requirements, use of aids or prostheses (e.g., hearing aid or eyeglasses), medications taken regularly, identification of significant other, previous hospitalizations or surgeries, baseline vital signs, physical abnormalities

Fall risk assessment: Risk factors to consider; safety measures to provide

Skin assessment: Risk factors to consider; areas needing inspection and care

Nursing care plan or problem list

Key: *CBC,* Complete blood count; *IV,* intravenous; *PRN,* as necessary; *UA,* urinalysis.

previous 2 days. Check the medication profile (medication administration record, or MAR) to find out what medications the patient is receiving and whether the MAR contains current orders. This will provide information about concurrent chronic conditions that may not be initially evident. Read the physician's admitting history and physical assessment if they are included in the chart. Scan any surgical procedure reports and accompanying pathology reports, paying particular attention to the conclusions. Note the psychosocial data on the face sheet. Does the patient live with family or a significant other? This information gives some idea of available support systems. Next, check the nurse's notes from the previous 24 to 48 hours, and then scan the current diagnostic test results. Read the nursing care plan or care map. Finally, read the nurse's admission assessment for data concerning events leading up to this hospitalization, pre-

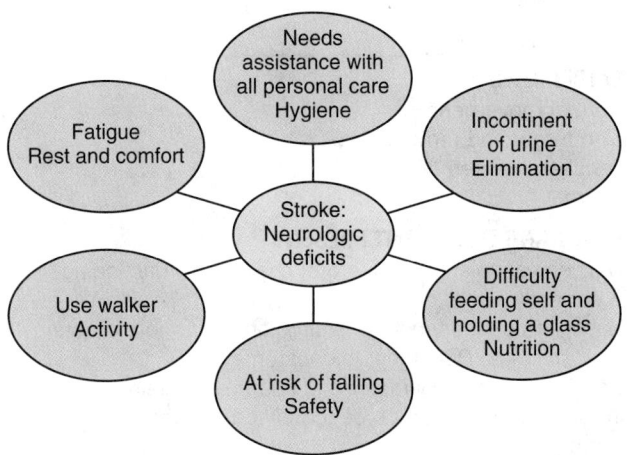

CONCEPT MAP **5-1** Health problems and needs of patient Victoria Torres from data given.

vious hospital and illness experiences, other chronic health problems, and a history of allergies.

To visualize the nursing process in action, consider the following scenario:

> Victoria Torres, age 76, room 728, bed A, suffered a stroke 3 days ago and has left-sided weakness (hemiparesis). She has difficulty with bladder control and urinary incontinence. She is left-handed, cannot firmly grasp objects, and therefore needs assistance with all personal care. She is receiving physical therapy to strengthen the muscles in her left arm and leg and is learning to walk with a walker, but she tires very easily.

This information alone can help you begin to plan care for the patient. Concept Map 5-1 shows the relationships between Mrs. Torres' identified health problems and Maslow's areas of basic need for which nursing assistance is indicated. However, you would need to systematically gather data to obtain a full picture of the patient's problems and needs.

PHYSICAL EXAMINATION

A physical examination is conducted by the registered nurse. However, parts of this examination may be delegated to the LPN/LVN. To conduct the examination, use techniques of inspection (looking), auscultation (listening), palpation (touching), and percussion (thumping). (These techniques are discussed in Chapter 22.) The examination is carried out in a systematic manner and begins with measuring height and weight and the vital signs. A history of what drugs the patient is taking and drug allergies is recorded. The list should include any over-the-counter medications the patient uses, including herbal preparations, as well as prescription drugs. A brief medical history is noted. Inquiries as to special assistive devices needed reveal whether the patient uses a hearing aid, glasses, cane, prosthesis, or dentures. Then a review of systems is required. Usually there is a section on the assessment and data collection form for a psychosocial history as well. Often there is a

section regarding needed assistance for self-care. A nutrition and skin assessment are performed and noted. A risk screening for falls may be required, and a determination of educational or discharge planning needs is performed so that appropriate planning can begin.

Listen to the heart and lungs of the patient and perform a physical examination, paying particular attention to any system in which the patient is expressing a problem. If he has abdominal pain, you would auscultate and palpate the abdomen. If he complains of a joint hurting, you would examine the joint and check the range of motion of the extremity. If a urinalysis has been ordered, you would obtain a urine specimen before leaving the patient.

After the admission assessment, each patient should be visited and assessed during the first hour of each shift. Perform a head-to-toe examination, which should take approximately 10 minutes. Box 5-3 presents areas to cover for this assessment and data collection procedure. Later in the shift, particular problem areas for each patient should be explored in greater depth. Listen to the heart and lungs of patients with respiratory or heart problems; examine the abdomen of the patient with gastrointestinal tract problems or abdominal pain; perform a neurologic examination on the patient with a neurologic disorder. At the time of the initial data collection and assessment, determine what supplies and equipment will be needed for the patient for the shift. Ongoing nursing data collection and examination focus on the body systems in which there is a problem or potential problem. Concept Map 5-1 linked the patient's reasons for needing care with the basic needs areas identified in the information about Mrs. Torres. Concept Map 5-2 on p. 63 shows how data should be gathered for every basic need and then must be analyzed in order to define Mrs. Torres' problems and attach the appropriate nursing diagnosis label. This map includes the next nursing process step, planning.

Think Critically About . . . From the information about Victoria Torres that has been given, which areas do you think would need in-depth assessment?

ASSESSMENT IN LONG-TERM CARE

An extensive initial assessment is performed when a patient enters a long-term care facility. Reassessment is done at fixed intervals and as the patient's condition changes. For Medicare patients, a reassessment by an RN is necessary every 90 days, and the care plan is reviewed and revised at that time. Besides the physical assessment, health history, and medication history, a functional assessment is performed. The functional assessment supplies a picture of the activities of daily living (ADLs) with which the patient will need assistance. An assessment of personal preferences regard-

Box 5-3 *Quick Head-to-Toe Assessment*

INITIAL OBSERVATION
Breathing
How patient is feeling
Appearance
Affect
Skin color

HEAD
Level of consciousness
Ability to communicate
Mentation status
Appearance of eyes

VITAL SIGNS
Temperature
Pulse: rate, rhythm
Respirations: rate, pattern and depth; oxygen saturation
Blood pressure: compare with previous readings

HEART AND LUNG ASSESSMENT, NEUROLOGIC CHECK
Auscultation of heart and lungs will be done to determine a baseline; neurologic check is done now if ordered or indicated.

ABDOMEN
Shape
Soft or hard
Bowel sounds
Appetite
Last bowel movement
Voiding status

EXTREMITIES
Normal movement
Skin turgor and temperature
Peripheral pulses
Edema

TUBES AND EQUIPMENT PRESENT
Oxygen cannula: liter flow rate; chest tube functioning correctly
Nasogastric tube: suction setting, amount and character of drainage; PEG tube; jejunostomy tube
Urinary catheter: character and quantity of drainage
Intravenous catheters: type; condition of site(s), fluid in progress, rate
Percutaneous endoscopic gastrostomy (PEG): intact, skin condition
Dressings: location, character and amount of drainage, wound suction device, drains
Pulse oximeter: intact probe; readings
Traction: correct weight, body alignment, weights hanging free
Sequential compression device: correct application, turned on
Continuous passive motion: machine set and applied correctly; turned on
Cardiac monitor: leads placed correctly; alarm parameters set

PAIN STATUS
Use a pain scale (e.g., 1 to 10)

ing routines for bathing, sleeping, daytime activities, food likes and dislikes, hobbies, and so forth is also completed. A fall risk assessment (see Figure 20-3) and a comprehensive skin assessment (see Figure 19-2) are part of the admission procedure. A mental status assessment completes the admission process. **Usually the LPN/LVN collects data for the RN, who will finalize the assessment.**

ASSESSMENT IN HOME HEALTH CARE

The initial patient assessment in the home is usually performed by the RN. The family is assessed regarding attitude and ability to help with care of the patient, their ability to provide emotional support for the patient, their ability to cope with the situation, and teaching that will need to be provided for them. The nurse must work within the patient and family's territory, and that requires a shift in attitude and perspective as compared to working in a health care facility. The LPN/LVN, when doing private duty in a home, will need to perform daily assessments and maintain the necessary documentation. Changes found on assessment should be reported to the RN supervisor.

ANALYSIS

Once the information has been gathered, the database is analyzed for **cues** that indicate deviations from the norm. **Cues** **are pieces of data or information that**

influence decisions. Problems are identified so that nursing diagnoses can be written by the RN as required by ANA Standard II: **Diagnosis** (see Appendix 1). The LPN/LVN may assist in this process.

The database is analyzed, pieces of data are sorted, related data are grouped (clustered), and missing data are identified. An example of a cluster of data would be a need to void frequently, occasional incontinence of urine, and some burning upon urination. These data are all related to a urinary system problem. This activity depends on the nurse's knowledge base and previous experience. The student uses texts to read about the underlying condition, signs and symptoms, and causes. The database is reviewed for signs and symptoms of abnormalities. Once cues are identified, they are grouped, and inferences can be made regarding the patient's problems. While clustering the data, you interpret the possible meaning of the cues.

From Mrs. Torres' situation, cues that suggest a problem exists include the following: she cannot firmly grasp objects with her left hand; she will need to use a walker to support herself when ambulating; and she is incontinent of urine. Factors contributing to the problem are also important. In Mrs. Torres' case, the fact that she has suffered a stroke (cerebrovascular accident) and has some neurologic impairment is pertinent. Nursing diagnosis statements are used to state the specific problems.

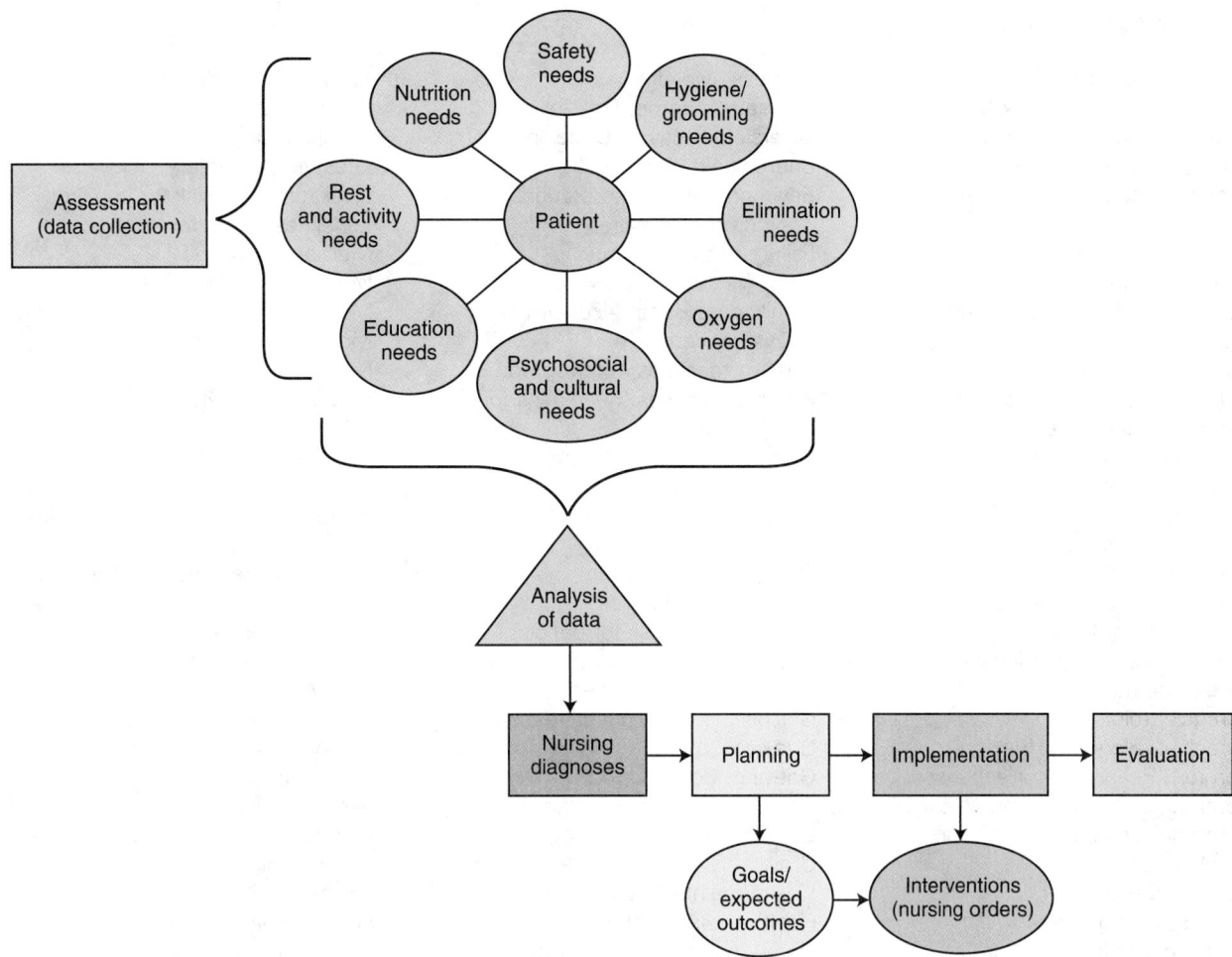

CONCEPT MAP **5-2** Basic needs and the nursing process.

Inferences (conclusions made based on observed data) made from the data include: Mrs. Torres' mobility is decreased; she cannot perform self-care unassisted; she has left-sided weakness and is at risk of injury from a fall; and she is incontinent of urine. She will need encouragement and reinforcement for her physical therapy program. Concept Map 5-2 shows how the assessment data collected by all techniques are analyzed. The map indicates the next steps to be completed in the nursing process: nursing diagnosis, planning with goals and expected outcomes, implementation with the selection of interventions to help the patient meet the expected outcomes, and evaluation to see if the outcomes have been met.

NURSING DIAGNOSIS

The second step of the nursing process results in the development of a diagnostic statement or a nursing diagnosis. **A nursing diagnosis statement indicates the patient's actual health status or the risk of a problem developing, the causative or related factors, and specific defining characteristics (signs and symptoms).** The medical diagnosis (i.e., stroke or cerebro-

vascular accident) is **never** included in the construction of the nursing diagnosis. Although registered nurses formulate nursing diagnoses, LPNs/LVNs are expected to be able to complete a plan of care after the nursing diagnoses have been designated.

The diagnostic labels have been formulated by the North American Nursing Diagnosis Association–International (NANDA-I) and are revised every 2 years. Ongoing research continues in order to validate the diagnostic labels and to support new nursing diagnoses, which are then added to the official NANDA list.

Once the nursing diagnoses are identified, the planning phase occurs. The NANDA list of diagnostic labels is used to form the first part (stem) of the nursing diagnoses used in nursing care plans. The nursing diagnosis describes a health problem amenable to nursing intervention. Box 5-4 shows the current list of approved NANDA nursing diagnoses. The stem label (the problem) is combined with the cause or causative factors. An example of a nursing diagnosis for Mrs. Torres might be Reflex urinary incontinence related to neurologic impairment, as evidenced by the inability to retain urine. "Reflex urinary incontinence" is the stem. Another nursing diagnosis appropriate for Victoria Torres is Impaired physical

Box 5-4 **NANDA-I Nursing Diagnoses**

Activity intolerance
Activity intolerance, Risk for
Airway clearance, Ineffective
Allergy response, Latex
Allergy response, Risk for latex
Anxiety
Anxiety, Death
Aspiration, Risk for
Attachment, Risk for impaired parent/child
Autonomic dysreflexia
Autonomic dysreflexia, Risk for
Behavior, Risk-prone health
Body image, Disturbed
Body temperature, Risk for imbalanced
Bowel incontinence
Breastfeeding, Effective
Breastfeeding, Ineffective
Breastfeeding, Interrupted
Breathing pattern, Ineffective
Cardiac output, Decreased
Caregiver role strain
Caregiver role strain, Risk for
Comfort, Readiness for enhanced
Communication, Impaired verbal
Communication, Readiness for enhanced
Conflict, Decisional
Conflict, Parental role
Confusion, Acute
Confusion, Chronic
Confusion, Risk for Acute
Constipation
Constipation, Perceived
Constipation, Risk for
Contamination
Contamination, Risk for
Coping, Compromised family
Coping, Defensive
Coping, Disabled family
Coping, Ineffective
Coping, Ineffective community
Coping, Readiness for enhanced
Coping, Readiness for enhanced community
Coping, Readiness for enhanced family
Death syndrome, Risk for sudden infant
Decision making, Readiness for enhanced
Denial, Ineffective
Dentition, Impaired
Development, Risk for delayed
Diarrhea
Dignity, Risk for compromised human

Distress, Moral
Disuse syndrome, Risk for
Diversional activity, Deficient
Energy field, Disturbed
Environmental interpretation syndrome, Impaired
Failure to thrive, Adult
Falls, Risk for
Family processes: Alcoholism, Dysfunctional
Family processes, Interrupted
Family processes, Readiness for enhanced
Fatigue
Fear
Fluid balance, Readiness for enhanced
Fluid volume, Deficient
Fluid volume, Excess
Fluid volume, Risk for deficient
Fluid volume, Risk for imbalanced
Gas exchange, Impaired
Glucose, Risk for unstable blood
Grieving
Grieving, Complicated
Grieving, Risk for complicated
Growth and development, Delayed
Growth, Risk for disproportionate
Health maintenance, Ineffective
Health-seeking behaviors
Home maintenance, Impaired
Hope, Readiness for enhanced
Hopelessness
Hyperthermia
Hypothermia
Identity, Disturbed personal
Immunization status, Readiness for enhanced
Incontinence, Functional urinary
Incontinence, Overflow urinary
Incontinence, Reflex urinary
Incontinence, Stress urinary
Incontinence, Total urinary
Incontinence, Urge urinary
Incontinence, Risk for urge urinary
Infant behavior, Disorganized
Infant behavior, Risk for disorganized
Infant behavior, Readiness for enhanced organized
Infant feeding pattern, Ineffective
Infection, Risk for
Injury, Risk for
Injury, Risk for perioperative positioning
Insomnia
Intracranial adaptive capacity, Decreased

Knowledge, Deficient
Knowledge, Readiness for enhanced
Lifestyle, Sedentary
Liver function, Risk for impaired
Loneliness, Risk for
Memory, Impaired
Mobility, Impaired bed
Mobility, Impaired physical
Mobility, Impaired wheelchair
Nausea
Neglect, Unilateral
Noncompliance
Nutrition: less than body requirements, Imbalanced
Nutrition: more than body requirements, Imbalanced
Nutrition, Readiness for enhanced
Nutrition: more than body requirements, Risk for imbalanced
Oral mucous membrane, Impaired
Pain, Acute
Pain, Chronic
Parenting, Readiness for enhanced
Parenting, Impaired
Parenting, Risk for impaired
Peripheral neurovascular dysfunction, Risk for
Poisoning, Risk for
Post-trauma syndrome
Post-trauma syndrome, Risk for
Power, Readiness for enhanced
Powerlessness
Powerlessness, Risk for
Protection, Ineffective
Rape-trauma syndrome
Rape-trauma syndrome: compound reaction
Rape-trauma syndrome: silent reaction
Religiosity, Impaired
Religiosity, Readiness for enhanced
Religiosity, Risk for impaired
Relocation stress syndrome
Relocation stress syndrome, Risk for
Role performance, Ineffective
Self-care, Readiness for enhanced
Self-care deficit, Bathing/hygiene
Self-care deficit, Dressing/grooming
Self-care deficit, Feeding
Self-care deficit, Toileting
Self-concept, Readiness for enhanced
Self-esteem, Chronic low
Self-esteem, Situational low
Self-esteem, Risk for situational low
Self-mutilation

From North American Nursing Diagnosis Association–International (NANDA-I). (2007). *NANDA Nursing Diagnoses: Definitions and Classifications 2006.* Philadelphia: Author. Copyright © 2006 by the North American Nursing Diagnosis Association–International.

Box 5-4 | *NANDA Nursing Diagnoses—cont'd*

Self-mutilation, Risk for	Suffocation, Risk for	Tissue integrity, Impaired
Sensory perception, Disturbed	Suicide, Risk for	Tissue perfusion, Ineffective
Sexual dysfunction	Surgical recovery, Delayed	Transfer ability, Impaired
Sexuality pattern, Ineffective	Swallowing, Impaired	Trauma, Risk for
Skin integrity, Impaired	Therapeutic regimen management,	Urinary elimination, Impaired
Skin integrity, Risk for impaired	Effective	Urinary elimination, Readiness for
Sleep deprivation	Therapeutic regimen management,	enhanced
Sleep, Readiness for enhanced	Ineffective	Urinary retention
Social interaction, Impaired	Therapeutic regimen management,	Ventilation, Impaired spontaneous
Social isolation	Ineffective community	Ventilatory weaning response,
Sorrow, Chronic	Therapeutic regimen management,	Dysfunctional
Spiritual distress	Ineffective family	Violence, Risk for other-directed
Spiritual distress, Risk for	Therapeutic regimen management,	Violence, Risk for self-directed
Spiritual well-being, Readiness for	Readiness for enhanced	Walking, Impaired
enhanced	Thermoregulation, Ineffective	Wandering
Stress overload	Thought processes, Disturbed	

mobility related to decreased motor function and left-sided muscular weakness, as evidenced by the inability to bear weight on the left leg. Because of her left-sided weakness, Mrs. Torres is at high risk for falling. This potential problem should be included on the care plan. The appropriate nursing diagnosis is Risk for injury related to neurologic impairment and muscular weakness as evidenced by inability to support body weight. Handbooks are available that present each of the approved nursing diagnosis labels, their defining characteristics, possible etiologic factors, and possible nursing interventions.

Think Critically About . . . Do the above nursing diagnoses with the problem related to a basic need apply to Concept Map 5-1?

ETIOLOGIC FACTORS

Etiologic factors are the causes of the problem. In Mrs. Torres' case, the etiologic factor for her decreased mobility is neurologic impairment. Signs are abnormalities that can be verified by repeat examination and are objective data. A bruise on the arm would be a sign. Symptoms are data the patient has said are occurring that cannot be verified by examination; symptoms are subjective data. A headache would be a symptom. You cannot see or verify that the patient actually has a headache; you must trust what the patient tells you.

DEFINING CHARACTERISTICS

Defining characteristics are those characteristics (signs and symptoms) that must be present for a particular nursing diagnosis to be appropriate for that patient. These supply the evidence that the nursing diagnosis is valid. Nursing diagnoses differ from medical diagnoses in that the nursing diagnosis *defines the patient's*

Table 5-2 | *Construction of a Nursing Diagnosis*

Nursing diagnosis = Problem + Etiology (cause) + Signs and symptoms	
Problem	Nursing diagnosis label (stem)
Etiology	Related to (etiologic or causative factors)
Signs and symptoms	As evidenced by (defining characteristics)

response to illness, whereas the medical diagnosis *labels the illness.* Table 5-2 shows the way in which a nursing diagnosis is constructed.

PRIORITIZATION OF PROBLEMS

Priorities of care are set so that the nurse will first attend to the most important interventions for the high-priority problems for each patient. Then, as time permits, the lower priority problems will be considered.

Once the nursing diagnoses have been designated, they are ranked according to their importance. This order can be guided by the hierarchy of needs adapted from Maslow (see Figure 2-3), by the patient's beliefs regarding the level of importance of each problem, and by what is most life threatening or problematic for the patient. **Physiologic needs for basic survival take precedence.** One of the first rules concerning priorities of care is that the **airway always comes first.** Without an adequate airway, the patient will die very quickly. Circulation usually is the next priority: Failure of the heart and loss of too much blood will also quickly cause death. Thereafter, the nurse must consult with and involve the patient in determining the priority of needs. A patient in considerable pain will usually give pain relief a higher priority than the need for food, at least on a short-term basis.

After physiologic needs are met, safety problems take priority. For a patient at risk for injury related to

Box 5-5 | *Selected Nursing Diagnoses Commonly Found for Long-Term Care Residents*

- Impaired swallowing r/t weakness or paralysis of the swallowing muscles.
- Risk for aspiration r/t impaired swallowing, depressed gag reflex, or decreased level of consciousness.
- Impaired verbal communication r/t changes in the cerebral hemispheres.
- Self-care deficit r/t impaired mobility, disturbed thought processes, or sensory impairment.
- Disturbed thought processes r/t damage to cerebral tissue.
- Impaired urinary elimination: incontinence r/t decreased ability to control elimination.
- Risk for injury r/t falls, weakness, or altered thought processes.
- Self-esteem, situational low r/t change in appearance, loss of self-control, role changes, or dependence on others to meet basic needs.
- Imbalanced nutrition: less than body requirements r/t decreased oral intake.
- Risk for imbalanced fluid volume r/t inadequate fluid intake or excessive fluid loss.
- Chronic pain r/t chronic disease process.
- Impaired skin integrity r/t damage to skin associated with friction, pressure, or shearing.
- Impaired physical mobility r/t loss of muscle mass, tone, or strength, or paralysis.
- Risk for constipation r/t medication side effects, decreased GI motility, loss of nervous control over defecation reflex, or decreased activity.
- Impaired social interaction r/t depressed mood, withdrawal, or impaired communication.
- Disturbed thought processes r/t inaccurate interpretation of environment.
- Ineffective coping r/t inability to function at previous level, poor problem solving, or poor cognitive function.
- Wandering.

Key: *GI,* Gastrointestinal; *r/t,* related to.

increased intracranial pressure as evidenced by decreased level of consciousness, safety is the priority need. Increasing intracranial pressure can be lethal. Nursing judgment is crucial to the setting of priorities. Nurses draw on their knowledge of the disease or disorder in question, the database, and their experience with similar patients. Critical thinking is used to make astute judgments regarding priorities.

After physiologic and safety needs have been met, the psychosocial needs of love and belonging, self-esteem, and self-actualization are given attention. **Every nurse must attempt to look at each patient holistically, keeping psychosocial needs in mind while working on physical problems.** Calling patients by their correct names, giving them opportunities to make some decisions about their care, protecting their privacy, and showing respect help meet psychosocial needs.

NURSING DIAGNOSIS IN LONG-TERM CARE

As an LPN/LVN employed in a long-term care facility, you will begin the care planning process when a patient is admitted. The supervising RN will review the care plan, modify it as needed, and finalize it for the chart. The same process is used to analyze data, identify problems and safety concerns, and to choose nursing diagnoses appropriate for the new resident. Box 5-5 shows some of the more common nursing diagnoses found for residents in long-term care facilities. Once the nursing diagnoses are chosen, the plan is individualized for the resident.

NURSING DIAGNOSIS IN HOME HEALTH CARE

In addition to the patient's problems, nursing diagnosis in this setting must include any problems identified in the family's ability to cope with the illness or situation and any teaching needs for care of the patient. The care plan encompasses the whole family rather than just the patient.

PLANNING

The third step of the nursing process is planning, and it correlates with the fourth NFLPN Standard, part 3, "the identification of health goals" (see Box 1-1).

EXPECTED OUTCOMES (GOALS)

A **goal** is a broad idea of what is to be achieved through nursing intervention. **Short-term goals** are those that are achievable within 7 to 10 days or before discharge, whereas long-term goals take many weeks or months to achieve. **Long-term goals** often relate to rehabilitation. When goals are written as expected outcomes, it is easier to evaluate whether interventions have helped the patient succeed in meeting them. Questions that the nurse considers in this part of the planning process are as follows:

- What are the goals for this patient? How can they be expressed as expected outcomes so that the success of nursing care can be easily evaluated?
- Should the goals for this patient be both short term and long term?
- What are the priorities of care?

A short-term goal regarding Mrs. Torres' incontinence might be that she stays dry for 2 hours at a time between toiletings. A long-term goal for this problem would be that she achieves total urinary continence.

Concept Map 5-3 shows how data for every basic need area have been collected and the data analyzed to identify problems and nursing diagnoses for Mrs. Torres. Goals have been formulated and converted into expected outcomes, and interventions have been chosen.

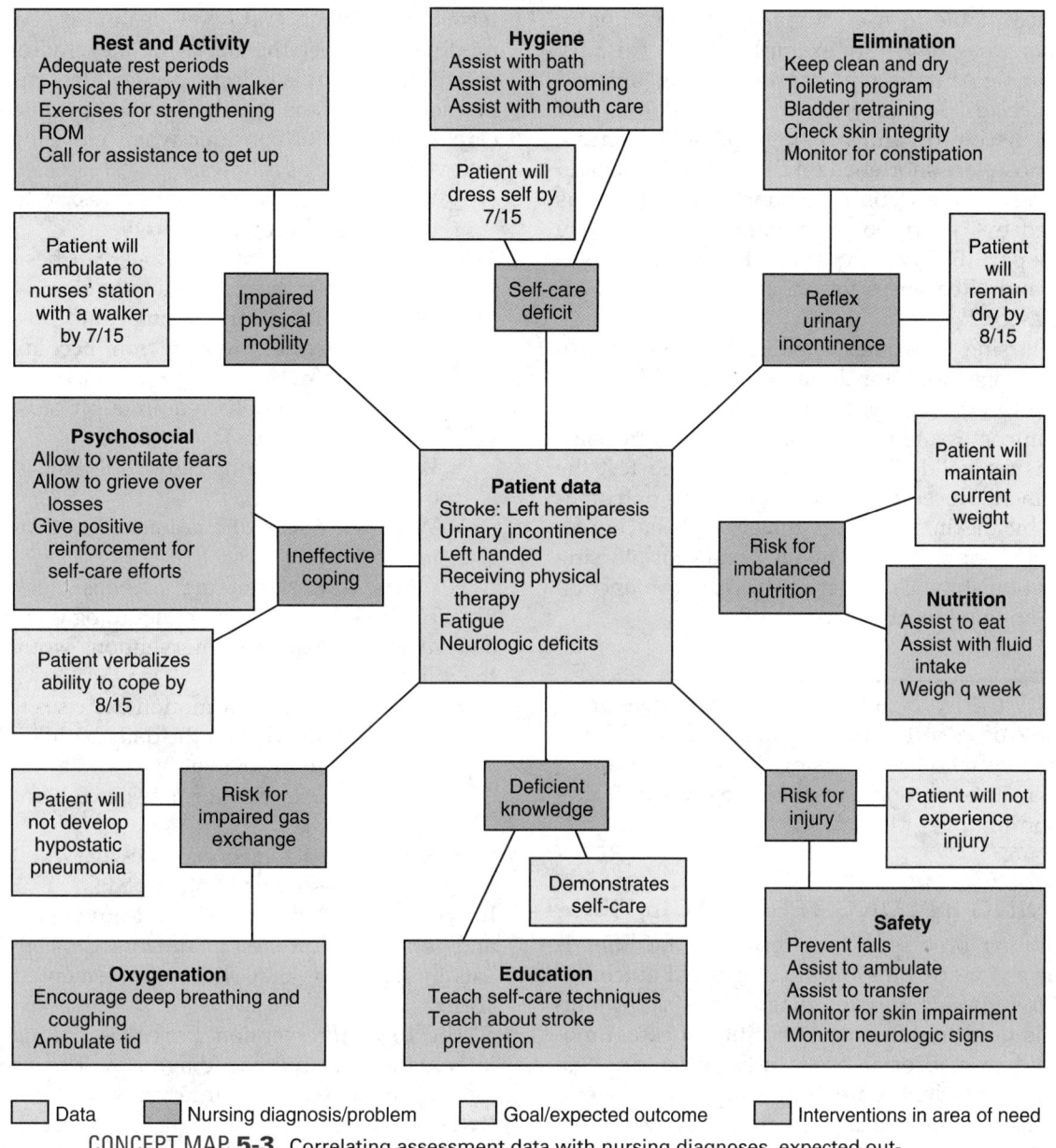

CONCEPT MAP **5-3**   Correlating assessment data with nursing diagnoses, expected outcomes, and interventions for all basic needs for Mrs. Torres.

Expected outcomes are derived from the goals. An expected outcome is a specific statement of the goal the patient is expected to achieve as a result of nursing intervention. An expected outcome for Mrs. Torres' nursing diagnosis of Impaired physical mobility related to left-sided muscular weakness, as evidenced by inability to bear weight on the left leg, might be "Patient uses a walker to ambulate to the nurses' station without assistance by July 10." The expected outcome should also contain measurable criteria that can be evaluated to see whether the outcome has been achieved. For example, for Mrs. Torres' nursing diagnosis of Reflex urinary incontinence related to neurologic impairment as evidenced by inability to retain urine, an appropriate expected outcome might be "Patient voids in bedpan every 2 hours while awake without intervening episodes of incontinence by July 10." If the nurse assists Mrs. Torres with the bedpan every 2 hours and she voids each time, the expected outcome would be met. If Mrs. Torres is wet between voidings, the goal of remaining dry during waking hours would not have been met. **An expected outcome should be realistic and attainable and should have a defined time line.** Collaboration with the patient regarding the expected outcomes is important. There must be agreement on the importance of the expected outcome with the patient and other health professionals involved in the patient's care. Some health facilities use the term *discharge criteria* in place of *expected outcome. Desired outcome* is another term often used for expected outcome.

It is acceptable to use standard abbreviations in the nursing diagnosis—for example, "Pain r/t injury to right ankle AEB discomfort and swelling" instead of "Pain *related to* injury to the right ankle *as evidenced by* discomfort and swelling." Sometimes nursing diagnoses are shortened on the hospital care plan by leaving off the defining characteristics (the "as evidenced by" part). Some nursing diagnoses only have one part. Examples include "Rape-trauma syndrome" and "Readiness for enhanced organized infant behavior."

The Nursing Outcomes Classification (NOC) provides language labels for desired outcomes. The purposes are to (1) identify, label, validate, and classify patient outcomes and indicators; (2) field test the classifications for validation; and (3) define and test the measurement procedures to determine if the outcomes are met by the interventions that have been implemented. This project is run by the Center for Nursing Classification at the University of Iowa, in conjunction with the ongoing work of NANDA-I.

? *Think Critically About* . . . Can you give an example of a short-term and a long-term goal for the patient who has a nursing diagnosis of Pain r/t skin interruption as evidenced by surgical incision?

PLANNING IN LONG-TERM FACILITIES

The planning process in long-term care facilities is the same as for any other facility. Expected outcomes are written for each nursing diagnosis. Maslow's hierarchy is used to determine priorities of care. Emotional and psychosocial needs must be addressed. Safety of the resident is a high priority. Family members are usually invited to the care planning session so that they have input into the care of their loved one. They are also invited to periodic reviews of the care plan.

PLANNING IN HOME HEALTH CARE

Family members concerned with care of the patient are collaborated with when choosing the expected outcomes. This helps the family to feel involved and gives a feeling of some control over what will be occurring in their home and for their loved one. Needs of the family are considered throughout the care planning process.

INTERVENTIONS (NURSING ORDERS)

The nurse selects appropriate nursing interventions to alleviate the problems and assist the patient in achieving the expected outcomes. Consider all possible interventions for relief of the problems, then select those most likely to be effective. Write them on the nursing care plan as nursing orders. Interventions for long-term care residents and home health care patients are modified to meet the needs of the environment in which the patient is living. Specific interventions may be included for the family members in home health care. Questions to consider when choosing nursing interventions are as follows:

- What nursing actions are necessary to monitor the status of a high-risk problem?
- Which nursing interventions can best help the patient reach the expected outcomes?
- What nursing interventions could possibly prevent a potential problem from becoming an actual problem?
- Which interventions require a physician's order (dependent actions)?
- Which interventions fall within the nurse's license to practice?
- What is the scientific rationale for using each intervention?

For Mrs. Torres' nursing diagnosis of Impaired physical mobility related to neurologic impairment and muscular weakness, interventions would include the following:

- Assist with range-of-motion exercises for her left arm and hand during the daily bath, in the afternoon, and in the evening.
- Instruct her to call for assistance before getting out of bed.
- Reinforce teaching of exercises that will strengthen her muscles while lying in bed.

Interventions listed should include giving medications and performing ordered treatments. Concept Map 5-3 lists interventions that will be implemented for Mrs. Torres.

The Iowa Intervention Project is linking nursing interventions to nursing diagnoses. The project has developed a Nursing Interventions Classification (NIC) taxonomy. The nurse must still individualize the interventions to the patient's needs. The nurse uses critical thinking to link the correct interventions to the nursing diagnosis for a specific patient. There are seven domains in the NIC taxonomy: Physiological: Basic; Physiological: Complex, Behavioral, Safety, Family, Health System, and Community. A thorough explanation of the taxonomy can be found in Bulechek and McCloskey (2000).

Concept Map 5-2 shows the nursing diagnoses, goals, and interventions appropriate for Mrs. Torres. The nursing care plan in Figure 5-2 shows further development of the concepts for four nursing diagnoses to meet Mrs. Torres' individual needs based on the assessment data.

? *Think Critically About* . . . Can you support each nursing diagnosis in Concept Map 5-2 with the corresponding assessment data?

DOCUMENTATION OF THE PLAN

The nursing care plan is supposed to be initiated by a registered nurse. In reality, LPNs/LVNs often construct a plan for the approval of the RN. The planning process is not finished until the nursing care plan is in the patient's chart or medical record. If the LPN/LVN has constructed the care plan, the RN reviews it before it is placed into the chart. Many health care facilities now use computerized programs to assist in constructing the nursing care plan. The nurse chooses the appropriate nursing diagnoses and then is presented with computer screens from which to choose the ex-

pected outcomes and the nursing interventions. The nurse can change or modify outcomes and interventions in order to individualize the plan. Once the entire plan is constructed, it is printed out, reviewed, and placed in the chart.

Some facilities use a standardized care plan and the nurse adds and deletes items in order to individualize the plan. The nursing care plan should be constructed right after the admission database is collected. It must be readily available to each nurse who is assigned to the patient. Once each 24 hours, the care plan is reviewed and updated. Necessary changes

---

NURSING CARE PLAN

Sample Nursing Care Plan

SCENARIO

Victoria Torres suffered a stroke (CVA) and has left-sided paresis (muscle weakness). She is unable to bear weight on her left leg and cannot grasp items with her left hand. She is incontinent of urine. The following is the nursing care plan written for her. Date of initiation: 6/16

PROBLEM/NURSING DIAGNOSIS Impaired physical mobility related to decreased motor function and muscular weakness, as evidenced by inability to bear weight on left leg.

Goals/Expected Outcomes	Nursing Intervention	Selected Rationale	Evaluation
Patient will ambulate to the nurse's station using walker, unassisted, by 7/1.	Encourage active ROM to right leg and arm q 4 hr while awake.	Active ROM works muscles and prevents atrophy as well as helping them maintain strength.	*Is patient ambulating unassisted?* Yes, but only for a short distance. Continue plan.
	Assist patient in walking with walker in room tid.	Using the walker promotes confidence and helps build stamina for walking.	
	Encourage patient to walk with walker in hall at least once daily; assist as needed.	Positive reinforcement encourages the desired behavior.	
	Reinforce instructions from physical therapist for exercises and walker use.	Reinforcing instructions helps patient remember them and to perform exercises and use walker correctly.	

PROBLEM/NURSING DIAGNOSIS Reflex incontinence related to neurologic impairment, as evidenced by inability to retain urine.

Goals/Expected Outcomes	Nursing Intervention	Selected Rationale	Evaluation
Voids in bedpan q 2 hr while awake without intervening episodes of urinary incontinence by 6/30.	Collaborate on voiding schedule times. Keep schedule at bedside.	Patient knows her usual pattern for voiding.	*Have there been episodes of incontinence?* No.
	Assist patient to use bedpan.	Conserves energy and prevents spilling.	Expected outcome met 6/18.
	Praise patient for each 2-hr period of continence.	Positive reinforcement encourages the desired behavior.	
	Discuss patient's feelings about bladder problem and progress with retraining.	Allows patient to ventilate feelings; reduces anxiety.	

Key: *ROM,* Range of motion; *tid,* three times a day.

FIGURE **5-2** Example of a hospital-style nursing care plan.   *Continued*

■

NURSING CARE PLAN—cont'd

PROBLEM/NURSING DIAGNOSIS Risk for injury related to neurologic impairment and muscular weakness, as evidenced by inability to bear weight on left leg.

Goals/Expected Outcomes	Nursing Intervention	Selected Rationale	Evaluation
Will not suffer injury from fall at any time. Will compensate for neurologic impairment with use of aids for ambulation by 7/1.	Keep walker positioned by bed for ease of use. Encourage to use walker whenever out of bed.	Object close at hand encourages use. Encouragement prompts desired action.	*Has patient suffered any injury?* No. *Is patient using a walker?* Yes.
	Ask to use call bell for assistance whenever she needs to get up.	Assistance helps prevent falls.	Continue plan.
	Assess muscular strength, balance, and ability to walk safely with walker daily.	Patient must have sufficient muscle strength to safely use walker.	

PROBLEM/NURSING DIAGNOSIS Self-care deficit, hygiene and grooming, related to muscular impairment, as evidenced by inability to grasp items with dominant left hand and inability to walk without assistance.

Goals/Expected Outcomes	Nursing Intervention	Selected Rationale	Evaluation
Will assist with bath by bathing left extremities by 6/26.	Assist with hygiene and grooming activities; encourage patient to participate.	Encouragement prompts desired action.	*Is patient performing some part of ADLs using the right extremities?* Not yet.
Will attempt to brush hair with right hand by 6/26.	Collaborate with patient regarding daily goals; praise all accomplishments and attempts at self-care.	Goals are more likely to be achieved if the patient helps set the goals.	*Is patient attempting to wash left arm?* Not yet.
Will brush teeth with right hand by 6/30.	Assist patient in attempts at brushing teeth and combing hair using right hand.	Undue fatigue prevents successful achievement of the activity.	Continue plan.
Will learn to put clothes on right extremities before discharge.	Reinforce occupational therapist's instructions for dressing self; supervise practice and give encouragement.	Positive reinforcement encourages the desired behavior.	
	Prevent patient from becoming overtired when attempting own hygiene activities; space activities.		

FIGURE 5-2, cont'd Example of a hospital-style nursing care plan.

can be made to it at any time. The new plan must be printed and placed in the patient's record. Implementation and evaluation of the care plan are discussed in Chapter 6. Many hospitals are using a collaborative "care map" or "clinical pathway" type of plan that incorporates all interventions by the various members of the health care team (see Chapter 6). The nursing care plan is incorporated into the total collaborative plan.

Interventions for the long-term care resident are chosen in the same manner and individualized. There are generally more long-term goals/expected outcomes than short-term ones on the care plan since the resident will most likely be in the facility for an extended period of time.

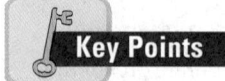 **Key Points**

- Assessment, the first step of the nursing process, begins at admission with the admission interview, history, and physical assessment.
- Subjective data are information that the patient that are apparent only to the patient and can be described or verified only by the patient.
- Objective data are facts that are obtained through using the senses and hands-on physical assessment.
- A database is compiled through the interview, physical assessment, talking with family and significant others, communication with other health professionals, and a chart review that includes surveying results of diagnostic tests. The database is all the information obtained.

- A concept map linked to basic needs can be constructed once patient problems are identified.
- Assessment is a continual, ongoing process.
- A chart review is useful for gathering information for the nursing database and for obtaining information for a student assignment.
- A nursing history and assessment are performed at admission (see Figure 5-1).
- The nurse should perform a quick head-to-toe assessment of each assigned patient at the beginning of each shift (see Box 5-3).
- A functional assessment is performed on patients being admitted to a long-term care facility.
- Emotional and psychosocial concerns are always considered when formulating a plan of care for the long-term care resident.
- Analysis is used to sort and group assessment data so that nursing diagnoses can be chosen and priorities can be set.
- A nursing diagnosis statement indicates the patient's actual health status or a potential problem, the causative or related factors, and specific defining characteristics (signs and symptoms).
- Nursing diagnoses should be chosen from the NANDA approved list (see Box 5-4).
- Expected outcomes are written based on the nursing diagnoses and problems.

- An expected outcome should be realistic, attainable, and measurable; have a defined time line; and be easily evaluated.
- Planning is the third step of the nursing process and involves choosing appropriate nursing interventions and documenting the plan.
- Nursing orders are the interventions chosen that will best assist the patient to achieve the expected outcomes.
- A concept map can be constructed showing the areas of need, nursing diagnoses, goals, and nursing interventions. A complete nursing care plan can be constructed from the assessment data and the concept map.
- A nursing care plan should be documented in the medical record soon after the admission assessment.
- The nursing care plan is reviewed and updated every 24 hours.

 Go to your **Companion CD-ROM** for an Audio Glossary, animations, video clips, and more.

evolve Be sure to visit the companion Evolve site at http://evolve.elsevier.com/deWit/fundamental/ for additional online resources.

NCLEX-PN® EXAMINATION-STYLE REVIEW QUESTIONS

*Choose the **best** answer for each question.*

1. Everyone has basic needs that must be satisfied in order to grow and develop. Your patient has pneumonia, is very weak, and has a headache from "coughing so hard." Which one of the following needs has the *highest* priority?

   1. The need for social interaction
   2. The need for physical activity
   3. The need for pain relief
   4. The need for oxygen

2. Which one of the following is the etiologic factor in the nursing diagnosis Impaired physical mobility r/t left-sided muscular weakness, as evidenced by the inability to use the left arm for activities of daily living?

   1. Impaired physical mobility
   2. Left-sided muscular weakness
   3. As evidenced by
   4. Inability to use the left arm

3. An example of an approved, correctly written NANDA nursing diagnosis for the patient is:

   1. Pain r/t abdominal surgery as evidenced by surgical report.
   2. Risk for injury r/t neurologic impairment as evidenced by paralysis of right leg.
   3. Risk for deficient fluid volume r/t nausea and vomiting.
   4. Constipation r/t complaint of no BM yesterday.

4. The patient's temperature is 100.4° F (38° C). The skin on her forehead is warm and dry. She has been incontinent and her bed is wet. She is complaining of being very tired. Which of the data are subjective? *(Select all that apply.)*

   1. Temperature is 100.4° F (38° C).
   2. States, "I'm very uncomfortable."
   3. Bed is wet.
   4. Complains of being very tired.
   5. Skin is warm and dry.
   6. States, "I have a headache."

5. Which one of the following nursing interventions for the patient in question 4 would you rank as the *highest* priority?

   1. Allow patient to rest.
   2. Change the bed linens and gown.
   3. Medicate for headache pain.
   4. Apply lotion to skin.

6. The role of the LPN/LVN in the patient admission procedure differs from that of the RN and might include: *(Select all that apply.)*

   1. writes nursing diagnoses for the patient's care plan.
   2. obtains an ordered urine specimen.
   3. takes the patient's history.
   4. assists with physical data collection.
   5. orients the patient to the unit.
   6. performs a thorough admission assessment.

7. When performing a chart review for data collection:
   1. always take the chart to a private place.
   2. read all of the nurse's notes since admission.
   3. remember to look at the medication administration record.
   4. commit what you read to memory.

8. A long-term goal/outcome would be:
   1. Will walk without assistance within 3 weeks.
   2. Pain will be controlled with medication within 24 hours.
   3. Nausea will be controlled before discharge.
   4. Will make correct diet choices by the end of the week.

9. Which one of the following is stated as a goal rather than an expected outcome?
   1. Patient will resume full job activities within 3 weeks.
   2. Patient will perform exercises three times a day.
   3. Patient will regain use of left arm and leg.
   4. Physical therapist will instruct patient in use of walker before discharge.

10. Which one of the following is a correctly stated expected outcome?
   1. Sit in the chair three times a day.
   2. Patient will walk to the end of the hall this week.
   3. Use the incentive spirometer every 2 hours.
   4. Patient will respond to pain medication.

CRITICAL THINKING ACTIVITIES *Read each clinical scenario and discuss the questions with your classmates.*

Scenario A
The physician's admitting diagnosis for Rachel Himmel is pneumonia. Her nursing diagnosis is Impaired gas exchange r/t excessive lung secretions AEB crackles in both lungs. Discuss the difference between nursing diagnoses and medical diagnoses.

Scenario B
From the NANDA-I list of approved nursing diagnoses, select the one that best fits the following patient assessment data: Patient unable to walk around house without becoming short of breath. Becomes fatigued after bathing and dressing in the morning. Had a severe case of the flu 2 weeks ago.

Scenario C
Develop a short-term and a long-term goal for Leora Chang, who fell, fractured her hip, and had a hip-pinning surgery 3 days ago.

Scenario D
Choose nursing interventions for the above patient for the nursing diagnosis Impaired skin integrity related to surgical procedure AEB incisional wound on left hip.

Implementation and Evaluation

Objectives

Upon completing this chapter, you should be able to:

Theory

1. Identify factors to consider in implementing the plan of care.
2. Set priorities for providing care to a group of patients.
3. List the Standard Steps commonly carried out for all nursing procedures.
4. Identify the steps a nurse uses to evaluate care given.
5. Discuss the evaluation process and how it correlates with expected outcomes.
6. Explain the term *continuous quality improvement* and how it relates to the improvement of health care.

Clinical Practice

1. Develop a useful method of organizing work for the day.
2. Use the Standard Steps for all nursing procedures.
3. Write a nursing care plan for an assigned patient.
4. Implement a nursing care plan and evaluate care provided.
5. Revise the nursing care plan as needed.

Key Terms

Be sure to check out the bonus material on the Companion CD-ROM, including selected audio pronunciations.

chart (p. 78)
clinical pathway/care map (p. 74)
continuous quality improvement (p. 80)
dependent nursing action (p. 74)
documentation (p. 77)
evaluation (p. 76)
implementation (p. 73)
independent nursing action (p. 74)
interdependent action (p. 74)
interventions (p. 73)
nursing audit (ĀW-dĭt, p. 79)
outcome-based quality improvement (OBQI) (p. 79)
time-fixed (p. 73)
time-flexible (p. 73)

IMPLEMENTATION

Implementation follows assessment, nursing diagnosis, and planning. The fourth step of the nursing process is derived from the National Federation of Licensed Practical Nurses (NFLPN) practice standards. The standards for the LPN/LVN concerning implementation are in Box 6-1. During the implementation (carrying out) phase, the nursing interventions or nursing orders (actions) listed on the nursing care plan are carried out. Implementing care for a group of patients requires good work organization. There are many ways of organizing the shift's work, but in all instances, priorities of tasks must first be set.

PRIORITY SETTING

Tasks for the shift must be determined and then prioritized. The change-of-shift report gives clues about high-priority tasks and imminent deadlines for certain tasks to be accomplished. Use a worksheet as discussed in Chapter 4 and write down important information from the change-of-shift report. Sequential, time-related tasks should be entered for each assigned patient. For example, write the intravenous (IV) flow rate and the fluid that will be used when the IV container is changed, and the expected time for changing the fluid (Safety Alert 6-1). Note the time of the last administered dose of pain medication. If a patient is to have preoperative medication at 8 A.M., the preoperative routine must be completed prior to that time. Time-flexible (can be done any time) tasks are entered onto the worksheet schedule between time-fixed (must be done at a set time) tasks. Critical thinking is essential to form a good work plan.

Note patient needs, such as tissues, on the worksheet so you can bring the items on the next visit to the patient. When planning time for uninterrupted care, consider the following:

- If visitors will be coming
- When diagnostic tests are scheduled
- What time the physician may come to see the patient
- Medication administration schedules

The work schedule may need to be revised after the initial shift assessment. Priorities of care for the patient may need to be altered if the patient's condition becomes more acute. Review the work organization sheet in Figure 4-3. It takes practice to correctly set priorities for multiple patients.

Box 6-1 | *NFLPN Nursing Practice Standards Regarding Implementation and Evaluation*

Standard 4 b states that:

"**Implementation:** The plan for nursing care is put into practice to achieve the stated goals and includes:

(1) Observing, recording and reporting significant changes which require intervention or different goals.

(2) Applying nursing knowledge and skills to promote and maintain health, to prevent disease and disability and to optimize functional capabilities of an individual patient.

(3) Assisting the patient and family with activities of daily living and encouraging self-care as appropriate.

(4) Carrying out therapeutic regimens and protocols prescribed by personnel pursuant to authorized state law."

Standard 4 c states that:

"**Evaluation:** The plan for nursing care and its implementations are evaluated to measure the progress toward the stated goals and will include appropriate person and/or groups to determine:

(1) The relevancy of current goals in relation to the progress of the individual patient.

(2) The involvement of the recipients of care in the evaluation process.

(3) The quality of the nursing action in the implementation of the plan.

(4) A re-ordering of priorities or new goal setting in the care plan."

Copyright © 2003 National Federation of Licensed Practical Nurses, Inc. From National Federation of Licensed Practical Nurses, Inc., 605 Poole Drive, Garner, NC 27529. Phone: 919/779-0046. Fax: 919/779-5642. www.nflpn.org.

 Safety Alert 6-1

IV Fluid Orders

Whether your state allows you to hang IV fluids or not, you should be aware of what fluid should be currently being administered and which fluid is to be started during your shift. Do not solely rely on the information from the change-of-shift report. Check the container in progress yourself and verify it with the health care provider's order. Check the order for the fluid that is to follow the present one as well.

CONSIDERATIONS FOR CARE DELIVERY

Before carrying out the specific interventions listed on the plan of care, identify the reason for the intervention, the rationale for the intervention, the usual standard of care, the expected outcome, and any potential dangers. A danger might be the possibility of introducing microorganisms during an invasive procedure.

Each intervention is either an independent nursing action or a dependent nursing action. An independent nursing action does not require a physician's order, but it does require critical thinking and nursing judgment.

Nursing judgment is derived from experience and knowledge. Each time you think critically about a patient problem, you build the knowledge base that will contribute to your ability to make accurate nursing judgments. The more experience you gain working with patients, the more reliable your nursing judgment will be. Teaching a patient about the side effects of a medication is an independent nursing action. The administration of a medication is a dependent nursing action because giving medication requires a physician's order. Giving a back massage would be an independent nursing action; ordering a heating pad and applying it to a patient is a dependent nursing action. Assisting the speech therapist by helping the patient practice speech exercises would be an interdependent action. Interdependent actions are those that come from collaborative care planning.

There is often controversy about whether a dressing change requires a physician's order. The general rule is that the initial dressing placed at the end of surgery is changed only by the surgeon unless there is a direct order to change it. If drainage is extensive, the dressing is reinforced with sterile materials. After the surgeon has changed the dressing, there is usually an order to change the dressing as needed or every day or two. Some hospitals have standard protocols for subsequent dressing changes. **Check the facility's policy.** Another topic that is often questioned is whether a hot pack or cold pack can be applied without a physician's order. The general practice seems to be that applying a warm, moist pack to an inflamed IV area without an order is accepted practice. Again, some hospitals have standard protocols for this situation. Usually cold packs will be applied to a sprain or strain in the emergency room even before the patient sees the physician when an injury has occurred. There should be a written standard protocol for this situation. Technically, no dressing should be changed, or any hot or cold pack applied, unless there is a standard protocol or physician's order in place.

Think Critically About . . . Can you think of other instances in which a question has arisen about whether a physician's order is needed? What about on night shift when a patient develops a high fever? Can the nurse use cold packs to bring the temperature down?

INTERDISCIPLINARY CARE

Many hospitals and health care agencies are using a collaborative type of plan of care referred to as an interdisciplinary care plan, a clinical pathway/care map, or a collaborative care plan. It is a step-by-step approach to the total care of the patient. This multidisciplinary approach to patient care is an outgrowth of managed care. All disciplines involved in the care of the patient provide input to the plan. Figure 6-1 presents a portion of a

ICD-9 Code **578.9**	ELOS **4 days**			
Nursing Diagnosis/ Collaborative Problem	**Expected Outcome (The patient is expected to . . .)**	**Met/Not Met**	**Reason**	**Date/Initials**
Fluid volume, deficient (hypovolemia)	Have stable vital signs (VS) and no evidence of active bleeding			
Electrolyte imbalance	Have electrolytes within normal limits and no signs or symptoms of electrolyte imbalance			
Risk for recurrent gastro-intestinal bleeding	Follow discharge instructions regarding medications, diet lifestyle changes, early detection			

Aspect of Care	Date_____ **Day 1**	Date_____ **Day 2**	Date_____ **Day 3**	Date_____ **Day 4**
Assessment	VS q1-4h, depending on stability Monitor vomitus and stool for gross and occult blood (OB) Systems assessment	VS q2-4h, depending on stability Monitor vomitus and stool System assessment Assess for weakness, postural hypotension	VS four times daily Monitor vomitus and stool Systems assessment Assess for weakness, postural hypotension	VS four times daily Systems assessment Monitor stools for occult blood
Teaching	Orient to hospital and unit Review clinical pathway/care plan with patient and family Reinforce importance of NPO, medications, IVs, and diagnostic studies	Teach pre- and post-test care for endoscopic examination	Begin discharge teaching, including • Medications • Diet • Lifestyle changes • When to call MD • Monitoring stools	Reinforce/review discharge instructions
Consults	Gastroenterology/ surgery Social worker	N/A	Dietitian	N/A
Lab Tests	CBC with diff, SMA-6 (6/60), INR(PT)/APTT, type and crossmatch, stools for OB	Hgb and Hct, stools for OB	Hgb and Hct, stools for OB	Hgb and Hct
Other Tests	Chest x-ray if >40 yr or if history of cardiac disease	Endoscopy	N/A	N/A
Medications	Ranitidine (H$_2$ antagonist), continuous IV or IVPB Blood transfusions until Hgb and Hct increase to baseline range Discontinue all other nonessential medications	Same as Day 1 (blood, if indicated, for low Hgb and Hct)	PO antacids, sucralfate, and/or H$_2$ antagonist Discontinue IV medications	PO antacids, sucralfate, and/or H$_2$ antagonist
Treatments/Interventions	I & O q8h Head of bed elevated at least 30 degrees, unless severely hypotensive If severely hypotensive, may need shock blocks	Same as Day 1	Discontinue I & O	N/A

FIGURE **6-1** Example of a clinical pathway.

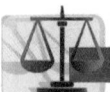

Legal & Ethical Considerations 6-1

Standards of Care

Legally, standards of care are set by the nurse practice act of your state, the professional association standards, and the agency's policies and procedures. Each agency has a policy and procedures manual. It is wise to look over the procedures you will be performing to make certain that nothing differs from the procedure you learned at school. Differences might be in the type of antiseptic solution used or in the steps to perform the procedure. If anything untoward happens to the patient as a result of the procedure, such as a nosocomial infection, you will be held accountable according to the procedure as described in the agency manual.

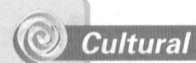

Cultural Cues 6-1

Honor Cultural Practices

Inquire about cultural practices related to bathing, touching, touching by the opposite sex, attitudes toward teaching, and so forth. In certain cultures it is not acceptable for persons other than relatives or very close friends to touch one another. This is particularly true for many people from the Middle East. Muslim women and those from Mexico and Central and South America are very modest, and there are often taboos about having someone of the opposite sex assist with intimate tasks. Older Japanese men may not listen to the instructions or teaching provided by a younger person or a female.

---

sample clinical pathway. **The nursing care plan is not part of the patient's chart when an interdisciplinary care plan is used; however, the nursing process is still utilized.** Evaluation is judgment of the effectiveness of the intervention or plan and is a collaborative process. Such pathways are standardized for particular medical diagnoses and then customized for the patient at the time of admission. A case manager, usually an RN, is in charge of reviewing the patient's progress along the path to see that actions are carried out and to determine whether the patient will achieve the expected outcomes in the predicted amount of time. These plans have been shown to be cost-effective in the delivery of health care.

IMPLEMENTING CARE

When a nursing intervention on the care plan calls for a procedure to be performed, review the hospital procedure manual regarding the particular steps involved. Each hospital has particular requirements for the way a procedure is to be carried out. Employees and students are expected to perform at the designated standard of care listed in the procedure manual (Legal & Ethical Considerations 6-1).

For efficient use of time, consider which interventions for a particular patient can be combined. Generally, baths and bed making are combined, and the time in the room is used to gather more assessment data or to begin implementing the teaching plan (Cultural Cues 6-1). Range-of-motion exercises may also be incorporated into the bath routine. Critical thinking helps with organization.

There are some Standard Steps that are always followed when performing a nursing procedure. These steps are introduced in Box 6-2 and are also included in Appendix 3. The steps are based on the standards of clinical practice, the rights of patients, and safe nursing practice.

Implementation in Long-Term Care

Most of the routine care of the residents in a long-term care facility is assigned to nursing assistants.

Baths and personal care are done by nursing assistants. Exercise interventions are provided by nursing assistants, physical therapy aides, or restorative aides. Medications are administered by licensed nurses or by nursing assistants with certification in medication administration. The licensed nurse on duty who is assigned to a group of patients is responsible for assigning and overseeing the work of the nursing assistants (Assignment Considerations 6-1). **The nurse performs any invasive procedure and any sterile procedure.** It is wise to spot-check the documentation of nursing assistants since the nurse is ultimately responsible for adequate documentation on care of the patient. Assignment guidelines are provided in Chapter 10.

Implementation in Home Health Care

Although the nurse makes periodic visits to the home, unless a private-duty LPN/LVN is required, the family and/or patient will be implementing the interventions on the care plan. The nurse does the teaching that enables the family member or patient to properly administer medications, change dressings, perform range-of-motion or help with other exercises, perform treatments, and so forth. Often the nurse performs any procedure for which strict sterility is mandatory or any procedure that is invasive and could cause serious harm to the patient. The nurse should ask the patient or family member to keep track of care given and to call if there is a change in condition. At each visit, the nurse reviews the documentation to see that the care plan is being carried out properly. The family should have a phone number at which the nurse can be reached and should be encouraged to call with questions or concerns.

DOCUMENTATION OF THE NURSING PROCESS

Each time a procedure is performed, a medication is administered, vital signs are measured, or something

Box 6-2 | Standard Steps for All Nursing Procedures

AT THE BEGINNING OF THE PROCEDURE

- **Step A: Perform the task according to protocol.**

  Mentally review the steps of the task beforehand. If you are uncertain how to do a task, ask your team leader, resource nurse, instructor, or charge nurse. Plan for efficiency of time and effort while delivering safe care.

- **Step B: Check the order, collect the equipment and supplies, and perform hand hygiene.**

  Verify that the procedure is to be done for the patient. Check the agency's policy and procedure manual for the accepted method of performing the procedure. Process equipment and supply charges. Take all equipment and supplies to the patient's room.

- **Step C: Identify and prepare the patient.**

  Greet the patient, introduce yourself, and check the patient's identification using two identifiers such as the armband and asking the birth date. Explain what you are going to do in terms the patient can understand. Elicit questions and answer clearly. Provide necessary teaching related to the procedure to be performed.

- **Step D: Provide privacy and institute safety precautions; arrange the supplies and equipment.**

  Close the door or curtains and drape the patient before beginning the procedure or discussing information the person might want kept confidential. Check equipment for breaks or wear and for safety. Set up the equipment and supplies in an orderly, methodical fashion. Raise the bed to an appropriate working height. Raise the side rail before turning the patient, and be certain that the wheels are locked. Perform hand hygiene to prevent contaminating the patient with organisms from the chart, the nurses' station, and the supply room.

DURING THE PROCEDURE

- **Step E: Use Standard Precautions and aseptic technique as appropriate.**

  Protect yourself from blood and body fluids by wearing gloves. If there is a danger of splashing blood or body fluids, wear protective glasses or goggles and an imperme-able cover gown or apron. Be very careful with sharp instruments and needles so as not to nick your skin. (See Appendix 5: Standard Precautions).

AT THE END OF THE PROCEDURE

- **Step X: Remove gloves and other protective equipment.**

  After making certain the patient is clean and dry, dispose of used supplies, remove goggles and other protective equipment and discard or store appropriately. To remove gloves without contaminating yourself, begin by pulling one glove off without touching your skin; hold the removed glove in the palm of the remaining gloved hand and then reach to the inside of the other glove and roll it down the hand. Dispose of the gloves in the trash. Perform hand hygiene immediately.

- **Step Y: Restore the unit. Collect the used equipment; dispose of, clean, or store items in the proper places.**

  Make the person comfortable, tidy the bed and unit, place the call light and personal items within reach, and provide for safety by lowering the bed. Remove used equipment. Soiled linens are placed in a soiled-linen hamper. Reusable items are cleaned and returned to the storage or processing area (central supply). Discontinue use of the equipment on the computer so no further charges will be made. Remove unsightly, odorous, or potentially infectious trash from the room. Inquire if anything else is needed. Perform hand hygiene before leaving the room.

- **Step Z: Record and report the procedure.**

  Document assessment findings and the details of the procedure performed, or care given, in the chart. Include any problems encountered and the patient's response to the care or treatment. The recording should be accurate, specific, concise, and appropriate and should include the specific time the procedure was performed and how it was done. Report abnormalities encountered to the charge nurse or physician.

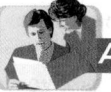

Assignment Considerations 6-1

Safely Assigning Tasks

It is the licensed nurse's responsibility to know the capability of the person to whom a task is assigned. Each assistive person should have documentation of the tasks that he can safely perform in his personnel file.

Be certain that the person to whom you assign a task for a particular resident or patient knows any safety requirements particular to that person and any precautions that must be taken while performing the task. For example, is the patient hard of hearing, and needs a hearing aid turned on? Does the patient have weakness on one side? (If so, state which side.)

is done that is a planned part of nursing care, a notation must be made in the chart. **Nurses' notes must indicate that the nursing care plan has been carried out.** If an intervention on the care plan is not mentioned in charting, it is considered not done. **It is wise to review the nursing care plan before beginning care to have a clear idea of all of the areas that need written** documentation (recording of pertinent data on the clinical record). Most hospitals require that some note be made about each problem or nursing diagnosis at least once every 24 hours. Long-term care facilities require a written note every 7 days or *when the patient's condition changes.* **Care is documented on flow sheets daily.**

After implementing care for the patient, document that care in the patient's medical record. Routine items such as bathing are recorded on the care flow sheet (see Figure 7-1). If a new problem is encountered, such as beginning skin breakdown, a nurse's note is required to document the assessment findings, the nursing diagnosis, and the plan to correct or alleviate the problem. The sooner care is documented after it is given the better. Many hospitals require that nurses chart (document) on each patient at least every 2 hours. Guidelines for charting are given in Chapter 7.

> **?**
> *Think Critically About . . .* Look at the sample hospital-style care plan in Chapter 5 (Figure 5-2). Can you identify which actions are independent, dependent, and interdependent?

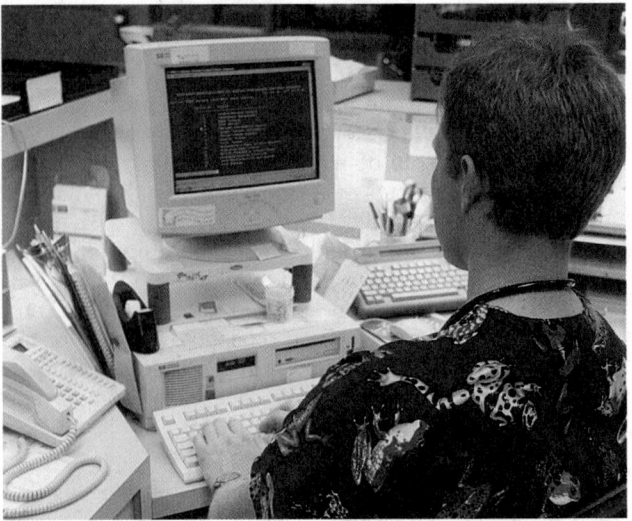

FIGURE **6-2** Nurse revising the nursing care plan.

EVALUATION

The fifth and final step of the nursing process is based on NFLPN Standard 4 c: **Evaluation** (see Box 6-1). Once the interventions have been carried out, you must determine whether they are effective in helping the patient reach the expected outcomes. If the expected outcomes have been reached, then goals have been met. Compare actual outcomes to the expected outcomes to determine whether progress has been made. For example, patient Victoria Torres (from Chapter 5) should be assessed throughout the day to see if she remains dry, uses the bedpan, and empties her bladder every 2 hours. If, for example, Mrs. Torres is assisted with the bedpan every 2 hours but at 11:30 P.M. she soiled the bed because she could not hold her urine any longer, then you should consider why this happened. Did she drink an excessive amount of fluid at dinner? Was there a considerable delay between the time Mrs. Torres called for assistance to urinate and the time someone entered her room to assist her? Progress has been made toward the expected outcome, but does the plan need to be changed by assisting her to urinate more frequently or to provide prompt assistance? **Evaluation is a continual process.** The patient should provide feedback, when possible, about whether the expected outcome is being met.

> **?**
> *Think Critically About . . .* How might you evaluate whether the medication you are giving a patient for pain is effective?

EVALUATION IN LONG-TERM CARE

Evaluation is based on data obtained from assessment, analysis of the data, and determination as to whether the specific expected outcomes are being met. The resident and family should be consulted to find out if the care plan is meeting needs adequately. The nurse considers whether the interventions on the plan are the best to meet the expected outcomes for those outcomes not yet met. If not, the plan is revised.

EVALUATION IN HOME HEALTH CARE

The nurse periodically assesses the results of the interventions and analyses to see if the expected outcomes are met. The patient and family are included in the process for input as to whether the care plan is meeting their needs. If expected outcomes are not being met, the interventions are revised.

REVISION OF THE NURSING CARE PLAN

Ineffective interventions must be revised. If the interventions have been so effective that the problem is resolved and the nursing diagnosis is no longer appropriate, it is marked "resolved" on the nursing care plan. **If the expected outcomes are considered met, the nurses' notes must contain data to support this.** Nursing care plans in the hospital are revised as often as every 24 hours, with resolved problems inactivated, new problems added, interventions revised, and progress toward outcomes evaluated. This is frequently done directly on the unit computer (Figure 6-2). The LPN/LVN collaborates with the RN during this process.

Each nurse determines whether there is a better, more efficient intervention to help the patient achieve the expected outcomes. Constant evaluation is an integral part of every aspect of nursing. Concept Map 6-1 includes the last step of the nursing process. It depicts how, if an expected outcome is not met, the plan must be revised with different interventions.

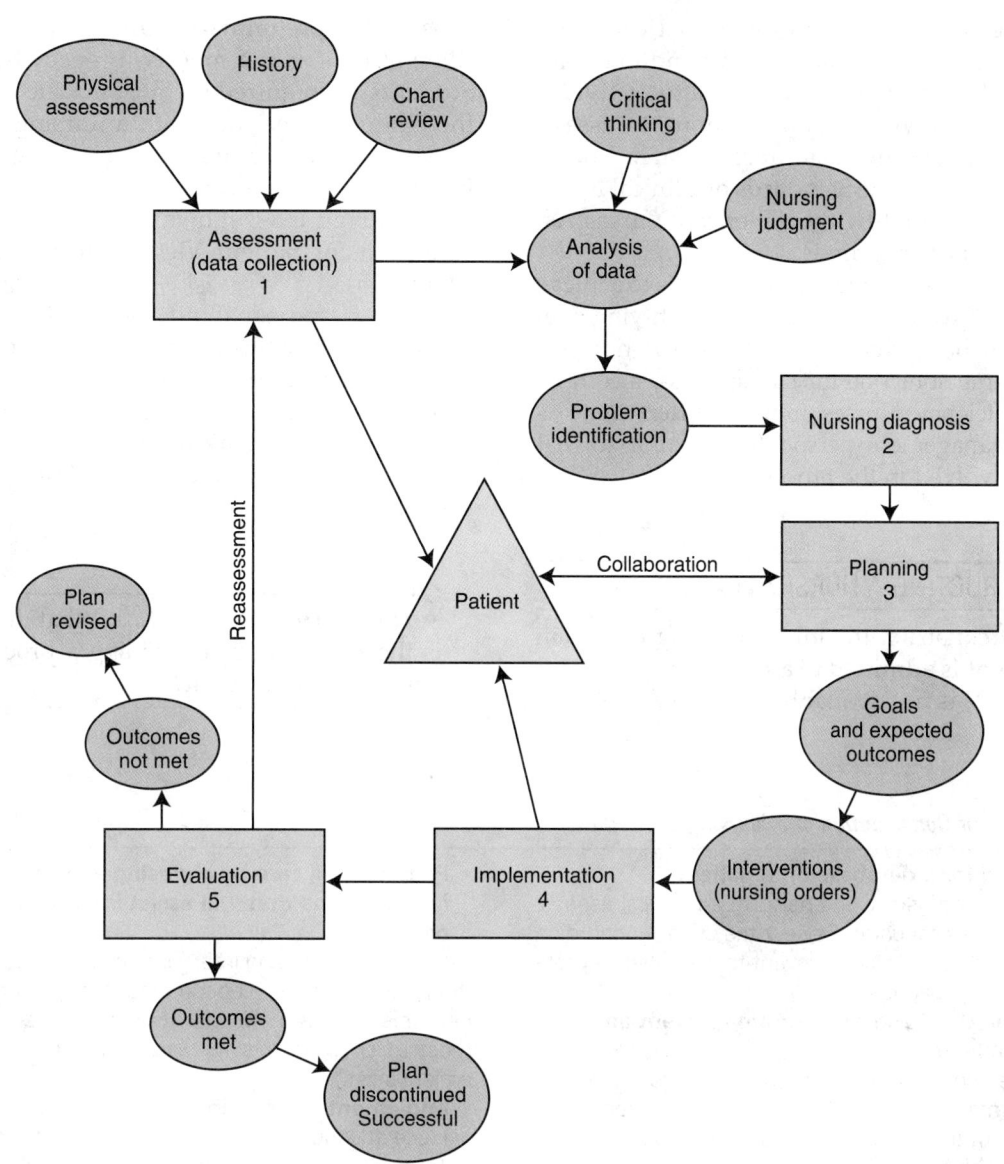

CONCEPT MAP **6-1**   The nursing process in action.

QUALITY IMPROVEMENT

Overall, evaluation of nursing practice includes determining whether the nurse's actions were carried out with regard to the safety of the patient. Safety for the nurse and other workers is evaluated. A determination is made as to whether nursing practice has been performed in a cost-effective, time-efficient manner.

Outcome-based quality improvement (OBQI) (improvement of the quality of performance) programs are used to evaluate nursing care delivered to patients. The goal of these programs is the improvement of nursing practice. The program is usually agency-wide, incorporating nursing audits and evaluation regarding compliance with standards for ev-

ery department. The audits are based on whether outcomes are being met. A nursing audit is the examination of a series of patient records to determine if nursing care for those patients met particular standards and particular outcomes. For example, if IV cannulas are to be changed every 72 hours, the charts are examined to see if there is a notation every 72 hours that the cannula was changed. The outcome is usually expressed as a percentage of compliance (e.g., 98% of IV cannulas were changed every 72 hours over a specific time period). If the standard of care is that each nursing diagnosis will be addressed in documentation every 24 hours, then a set number of charts might be audited to see if the nurses on that unit are meeting this standard. An audit is most often performed on medical records of patients who have been discharged. Every hospital must perform both medical and nursing audits to achieve and maintain accreditation. *Process* evaluations look at the activities of the nurses and what they have done to assess, plan, implement, and evaluate nursing care. Process evaluation criteria are the Standards of Clinical Nursing Practice developed by the American Nurses Association (ANA) (Appendix 1).

The purpose of evaluating nursing care is to achieve continuous quality improvement by identifying specific areas that need changes. Evaluation is not performed to blame someone for carelessness, incompetence, or inefficiency. Nurses on a unit often rotate as the quality management person for the unit so that everyone is involved in the process.

CONSTRUCTING A NURSING CARE PLAN

The RN may construct the initial nursing care plan or, if the patient is admitted to a long-term care facility when an RN is not available, the LPN/LVN may construct a preliminary nursing care plan that an RN will review and modify as needed the next day. Students are required by most instructors to come to the clinical experience with a nursing care plan, or concept map, in hand for their assigned patients. Box 6-3 provides guidelines for the care planning process. Figure 6-3 shows a sample student nursing care plan for patient Victoria Torres (discussed in Chapter 5).

Having studied about the parts of the nursing process and how the process as a whole is applied to care planning and to the practice of nursing, you should begin to incorporate the principles into your thinking. **The nursing process is inherent in every aspect of nursing and is a tool for success as a nurse.**

Think Critically About . . . What do you think is the rationale for explaining a procedure to a patient before doing it?

Box 6-3 | *Steps for Construction of a Nursing Care Plan*

- **Collect data for a database on a patient.**

  Obtain a patient history and perform a physical assessment (gather physical data). Review the chart, noting data and current laboratory values relevant to the patient's problems or admitting diagnosis.
- **Analyze the database to determine current and potential problems.**

  Group data according to body system and review for areas of abnormalities or problems. Identify problems and collaborate with the patient to see that she also considers each one a problem.
- **Choose appropriate nursing diagnoses based on defining characteristics of the patient's problems.**

  Collaborate with the RN in choosing nursing diagnoses from the NANDA accepted diagnoses list: terminology = problem + cause + signs and symptoms.
- **Rank the nursing diagnoses in order of priority.**

  Confer, if possible, with the patient about the priorities of the patient's problems and needs. Physiologic needs for oxygen and circulation must be met first. Number the diagnoses according to priority.
- **Plan the nursing care by defining goals and writing expected outcomes.**

  Define the overall goals and write specific expected outcomes that will be easy to determine through evaluation if they have been achieved. Include a time frame for each outcome to be achieved.
- **Plan nursing care by choosing appropriate nursing interventions that will assist in achieving the outcomes.**

  Consider all nursing interventions known to be useful for the type of problem; choose those that can be expected to help this patient meet the goals and expected outcomes most quickly. Do this for each nursing diagnosis on the patient's list.
- **Implement the nursing interventions.**

  Place the nursing care plan in the chart or Kardex, or enter it into the computer. Communicate the plan of care to staff members on other shifts. Carry out the nursing interventions using the standard steps for all nursing procedures.
- **Evaluate the actual outcomes of each nursing intervention; determine whether progress toward achieving the expected outcomes has been made.**

  Gather data via patient reassessment and document in the chart the result of the nursing interventions. Once every 24 hours, read over the nursing care plan and determine whether it is meeting the expected outcomes or needs to be revised. Determine whether there are nursing diagnoses that have been resolved and can be discontinued. Consider whether any data indicate that a new nursing diagnosis should be added. In collaboration with the RN, add new nursing diagnoses as indicated by the data. Continue to seek patient input on the care plan and goals.

NURSING CARE PLAN

Sample Student Nursing Care Plan Based on the Situation for Victoria Torres

PROBLEM/NURSING DIAGNOSIS Weak left extremities/Impaired physical mobility related to decreased motor function and left-sided muscular weakness, as evidenced by inability to bear weight on left leg.

Supporting assessment data *Objective:* CVA 6/16; left-sided weakness, unable to bear weight on left leg; cannot grasp with left hand; is left handed.

Planning/Goals/ Expected Outcomes	Implementation/ Nursing Interventions	Selected Rationale	Evaluation*
ST: Will walk to the nurses' station using walker, unassisted by 7/1.	Encourage active ROM to left leg and arm q 4 hr while awake.	ROM prevents atrophy of muscles and helps maintain strength.	*Is patient walking with walker unassisted? How far?* Attempts ROM by self when encouraged; performed ROM × 2 this shift.
LT: Will walk unassisted to the end of hall using walker by discharge.	Assist patient in walking with walker in room tid.	Assistance helps prevent falls and offers encouragement.	Used walker during physical therapy × 2.
	Encourage to walk with walker in hall at least once daily; assist as needed.	Encouragement provides some motivation.	Up with walker to bathroom × 1 this shift; needs assistance to get up from bed.
	Reinforce instructions from physical therapist for exercises and walker use.	Reinforcing instructions helps patient remember them.	Reviewed physical therapist's instructions for walker use. Progressing toward meeting expected outcomes; continue plan.

PROBLEM/NURSING DIAGNOSIS Left-sided weakness/Risk for injury from fall related to neurologic impairment and muscle weakness, as evidenced by inability to bear weight on left leg.

Supporting assessment data *Objective:* CVA 6/16; unable to support body weight on left leg; balance shaky, lists to side; cannot grasp with left hand; staggers when tries to walk unaided.

Planning/Goals/ Expected Outcomes	Implementation/ Nursing Interventions	Selected Rationale	Evaluation*
LT: Will not suffer injury from fall at any time.	Keep walker positioned by bed.	Object close at hand encourages use.	*Has patient suffered any injury from a fall? Is patient using aids to ambulation?* Walker is placed within reach toward foot of bed.
LT: Will compensate for neurologic impairment with use of aids to ambulation by 7/15.	Encourage to use walker whenever out of bed.	Encouragement prompts desired behavior.	States willingness to use walker at all times; is afraid of falling.
	Ask to use call bell for assistance whenever fatigued and needs to get up.	Assistance helps prevent falls.	Rang for assistance to get up this P.M.; states she is tired from all the visitors.
	Assess muscular strength, balance, and ability to walk safely with walker q 3 d.	Helps prevent falls should condition deteriorate.	Right arm and leg still weak; cannot fully support self without walker. Balance seems to be improving with walker use. Becoming more adept at moving walker and judging how to get around furniture; meeting expected outcomes; continue plan.

*Evaluation statements are examples of documentation indicating interventions have been carried out and the patient's response to them. The results of the actions reflect whether expected outcomes are being met.

Key: *CVA*, Cerebrovascular accident; *d*, day; *hr*, hours; *LT*, long term; *q*, every; *ROM*, range of motion; *ST*, short term; *tid*, three times a day; *UA*, urinalysis.

FIGURE **6-3** Sample student nursing care plan.   *Continued*

NURSING CARE PLAN—cont'd

PROBLEM/NURSING DIAGNOSIS Wetting the bed/Reflex incontinence related to neurologic impairment as evidenced by inability to retain urine.
Supporting assessment data: Objective: Unable to control bladder consistently since CVA; frequent urinary incontinence; UA normal; no foul odor to urine.

Planning/Goals/ Expected Outcomes	Implementation/ Nursing Interventions	Selected Rationale	Evaluation*
ST: Will void in bedpan q 2 hr while awake without intervening episodes of urinary incontinence by 6/30.	Collaborate on voiding schedule times. Keep schedule at bedside. Remind patient to ask for bedpan. Assist with bedpan.	Patient knows her usual pattern for voiding.	*Has patient had episodes of incontinence?* 2-hr schedule beginning after breakfast instituted.
LT: Will experience no episodes of incontinence by discharge.	Praise patient for each 2-hr period of continence.	Positive reinforcement encourages the desired behavior and helps self-esteem.	Used bedpan at designated times; praise given. One soiling of bed at 23:30 P.M. Patient upset about bed soiling; states does see some progress. Achieving expected outcomes; continue plan.

PROBLEM/NURSING DIAGNOSIS Unable to use left extremities/Self-care deficit, hygiene and grooming, related to muscular impairment, as evidenced by inability to grasp items with dominant left hand and inability to walk without assistance.
Supporting assessment data: Subjective: States, "I can't seem to do anything with this arm and leg." *Objective:* CVA 6/16. Left-sided weakness of both extremities.

Planning/Goals/ Expected Outcomes	Implementation/ Nursing Interventions	Selected Rationale	Evaluation*
ST: Will assist with bath by bathing left extremities by 6/26.	Assist with hygiene and grooming activities; encourage patient to participate.	Demonstrates caring.	*What hygiene and grooming activities has patient performed independently?* States she wishes to bathe herself without assistance; will attempt to do more of bath as fatigue decreases.
ST: Will attempt to brush hair with right hand by 6/26.	Collaborate with patient on daily goals; praise all accomplishments and attempts at self-care.	Participation in goal setting helps patient "own" the goal and desire to suceed in achieving it.	Attempted to brush hair; unable to do more than three strokes.
ST: Will brush teeth with right hand 6/30.	Assist patient in attempts at brushing teeth and combing hair using right hand.	Encouragement and praise help reinforce positive behaviors and increase self-esteem.	Occupational therapy scheduled for Friday. Willing to do more than wash face tomorrow.
LT: Will learn to put clothes on left extremities before discharge.	Reinforce occupational therapist's instructions for dressing self; supervise practice and give encouragement.	Reinforcement helps patient recall how to efficiently dress; supervision helps prevent frustration.	Praised for use of hairbrush. Will attempt to brush her own teeth tomorrow.
LT: Will perform her own hygiene and grooming within 3 mo.	Prevent patient from becoming overtired when attempting her own hygiene activities; space activities.	Neurologic damage to the brain causes easy fatigue. Fatigue will interfere with success and cause frustration.	Beginning to achieve expected outcomes; continue plan.

❓ CRITICAL THINKING QUESTIONS

1. While helping the patient with ROM excerises, she says to you, "Will I ever be able to walk normally again?" What would be the most therapeutic reply to this question?
2. How would you explain to the patient why it is important for her to use the call bell and ask for assistance when she desires to get up from the bed?
3. What is the rationale for praising the patient for each 2-hr period of continence?

FIGURE **6-3, cont'd** Sample student nursing care plan.

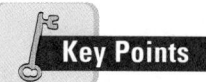

Key Points

- During the implementation step of the nursing process, the planned nursing interventions are carried out.
- Priorities of care are more easily determined if there is a well-organized work plan for the shift.
- Before carrying out interventions, the reason for the intervention, the usual standard of care, the expected outcome, and any potential danger should be understood.
- An independent nursing action is one that the nurse can perform without a physician's order.
- A dependent nursing action requires a physician's order before it can be legally carried out.
- An interdependent action is one derived from collaborative planning between two or more health care professionals.
- A clinical pathway or interdisciplinary care map contains the actions to be carried out by all of the health professionals involved in the patient's care. It is a managed care tool and is used to speed a patient to recovery as quickly and cost-effectively as possible.
- The family and resident are invited to the care planning conference in the long-term care facility.
- The care plan for the home health patient encompasses the needs and concerns of the family as well as the patient.

- Documentation of nursing care is essential and should be done soon after an action has been completed.
- Documentation must show the progress toward attainment of outcomes.
- Evaluation involves reassessment of data to determine whether the expected outcomes have been achieved.
- After evaluation, revision of the nursing care plan is performed.
- Quality improvement programs are used to evaluate nursing care provided to patients.
- The goal of a quality improvement program is improvement of nursing practice and patient care.
- Construction of a nursing care plan involves assessing the patient, analyzing the data, identifying nursing problems, prioritizing the problems, deciding on goals, writing expected outcomes, and choosing interventions. After the plan is implemented, the outcomes of the interventions are evaluated and the plan is revised as needed.

 Go to your **Companion CD-ROM** for an Audio Glossary, animations, video clips, and more.

evolve Be sure to visit the companion Evolve site at http://evolve.elsevier.com/deWit/fundamental/ for additional online resources.

NCLEX-PN® EXAMINATION-STYLE REVIEW QUESTIONS

*Choose the **best** answer(s) for each question.*

1. You assist a patient with her bath, change her dressing, rub her back, give her her medication, and ambulate her. Which of the following are examples of an independent nursing action? *(Select all that apply.)*

   1. Teaching the side effects of the medication
   2. Changing her dressing
   3. Ambulating her
   4. Giving her a back rub
   5. Giving a bath
   6. Administering medication

2. Before carrying out a dependent nursing action, the nurse: *(Select all that apply.)*

   1. makes certain the family is in agreement with the order.
   2. verifies that the physician's order is on the chart.
   3. considers whether there is any contraindication for the action.
   4. chooses an appropriate time to carry out the action.
   5. gathers all equipment and supplies needed for the action.

3. You evaluated the care provided to the patient by determining:

   1. if she is beginning to improve.
   2. whether all planned interventions were carried out.
   3. whether expected outcomes have been achieved.
   4. if she is well enough for discharge.

4. If evaluation determines that outcomes are not being achieved,

   1. a new nursing care plan must be written.
   2. the nursing care plan is revised.
   3. the interventions are continued.
   4. a change in physician's orders may need to occur.

5. Outcome-based quality improvement programs require nursing audits. The goal of such programs is the
   _____. *(Fill in the blank.)*

6. A difference in the assessment of the patient entering a long-term care facility versus that of a hospital patient is that the long-term care resident is assessed for:

   1. functional abilities.
   2. psychosocial concerns.
   3. emotional concerns.
   4. skin problems.

7. Nursing and medical audits:

   1. only evaluate overall agency performance.
   2. determine if a nursing unit is efficient.
   3. are for the purpose of improving profit.
   4. are essential for hospital accreditation.

8. An example of a dependent nursing action would be:
   1. starting the continuous passive motion (CPM) machine.
   2. providing a back massage.
   3. encouraging the consumption of more fluid.
   4. changing the patient's linens after an episode of incontinence.

9. To perform proper evaluation of care provided, you must:
   1. determine the effectiveness of the interventions.
   2. document the care that was provided.
   3. carry out all interventions on the care plan.
   4. plan when to carry out the interventions.

10. The patient's order reads: ampicillin 50 mg/kg/day, PO q 6 hr. The patient weighs 110 lb. How many milligrams (mg) per dose should you give? _____.
    (Fill in the blank.)

CRITICAL THINKING ACTIVITIES *Read each clinical scenario and discuss the questions with your classmates.*

Scenario A
Construct a nursing care plan from the following scenario: Mark Hansen, a 45-year-old, is admitted with a fractured femur. He is placed in skeletal traction. His nursing diagnoses are Impaired physical mobility r/t immobilization by traction and Self-care deficit, bathing, grooming, and toileting r/t immobilization.

Scenario B
Discuss and compare dependent and independent nursing actions that are on your care plan for Mr. Hansen.

Scenario C
What would you need to know about the order for traction in order to properly carry out care for this patient?

Documentation of Nursing Care

Objectives

Upon completing this chapter, you should be able to:

Theory

1. Identify three purposes of documentation.
2. Correlate the nursing process with the process of charting.
3. Discuss maintaining confidentiality of medical records.
4. Compare and contrast the five main methods of written documentation.
5. List the legal guidelines for recording on medical records.
6. Relate the approved way to correct entries in medical records that were made in error.

Clinical Practice

1. Correctly make entries on a daily care flow sheet.
2. Use a systematic way of charting to ensure that all pertinent information has been included.
3. Document the characterization of signs or symptoms in a sample charting situation.
4. Apply the general charting guidelines in the clinical setting.

Key Terms

Be sure to check out the bonus material on the Companion CD-ROM, including selected audio pronunciations.

case management system charting (p. 87)
charting (p. 85)
charting by exception (p. 87)
computer-assisted charting (p. 87)
computerized provider order entry (CPOE) (p. 93)
electronic health record (EHR) (p. 92)
focus charting (p. 87)
medical record (chart) (p. 85)
PIE charting (p. 89)
problem-oriented medical record (POMR) charting (p. 87)
protocols (PRŌ-tō-kŏls, p. 91)
source-oriented (narrative) charting (p. 87)

PURPOSES OF DOCUMENTATION

Documentation provides a written record of the history, treatment, care, and response of the patient while under the care of a health care provider. It acts as a guide for reimbursement of costs of care, may serve as evidence of care in a court of law, shows the use of the nursing process, and provides data for quality assurance studies. Each person who provides care for the patient adds written documentation to the medical record (chart). The medical record contains all orders, tests, treatments, and care that occurred during the time the person was under the care of the health care provider. The chart is a communication tool for the professionals involved in caring for the patient. By documenting, each care provider tells the other health team members what has been done, how the patient has responded, and the current plan for care. Many different forms are used for documentation, and the most common forms are shown in the chapters specific to their content; for example, an intravenous (IV) flow sheet is shown in Chapter 36 (Administering Intravenous Solutions and Medications). A sample list of common chart forms is provided in Table 7-1.

Insurance companies and Medicare rely on documentation in order to determine actual length of stay, procedures performed, and diagnoses established, and to calculate charges due for reimbursement. Each piece of equipment in service must be documented. Charts must display data that support the medical and nursing diagnoses listed. Evaluation data indicating that the treatment was successful or unsuccessful must be present to justify the duration of the hospital stay. Documentation of this type is also necessary for accreditation of the health care agency. Charts are also used for research data collection. For example, statistics may be compiled for the number of cases of pneumonia treated, the average age of the patients, and to see which treatments were the most effective.

The medical record is a legal record and can be used as evidence of events that occurred or treatment that was given. When documentation is thorough, the record provides a way to show that accepted standards of care have been met.

Documentation, also called charting, is used to track the application of the nursing process. The nurse writes down observations made about the patient's condition, notes the care and treatment that was delivered, and adds the patient's response. Documentation shows progress toward the expected outcomes listed on the nursing care plan.

Documentation is useful for supervisory purposes to determine how the staff are performing. Charting is audited as part of the health care agency's quality improvement program. Evidence that care adheres to accepted standards should be present in the nurse's notes. The results of chart audits tell nurse managers where improvement may be needed.

DOCUMENTATION AND THE NURSING PROCESS

The written nursing care plan or interdisciplinary care plan provides the framework for the nurse's documentation. Charting is organized by nursing diagnosis or

Table 7-1 *Forms Used for Hospital Documentation*

FORM	TYPE OF INFORMATION
GENERAL FORMS	
Face sheet	Patient data, including the patient's name, address, phone number, next of kin, hospital identification number, religious preference, place of employment, insurance company, occupation, name of admitting physician, and admitting diagnosis
Physician's orders	The physician's directives for patient care
Graphic sheet	Record of serial measurements and observations, such as temperature, pulse, respiration, blood pressure, weight
Nursing care plan	Plan of care for the patient, including nursing diagnoses, goals/expected outcomes, and nursing interventions
Nurse's notes	Written report of the nursing process (i.e., assessment, nursing diagnosis, planning, implementation, and evaluation); record of interventions implemented and the patient's response to them
Care flow sheet	Form on which checkmarks or short entries are made to indicate dietary intake, type of bath, wound dressing changes, oxygen in use, physician visits, equipment in use, level of activity, and so forth
Medication administration record (MAR)	Documentation of all medications ordered, doses given, and doses not taken by the patient
History and physical examination forms	Physician's record of the patient's medical history and findings of the current physical examination
Nurse's admission history and assessment	Nurse's current history, including usual habits, medications usually taken, and physical assessment findings at admission
Progress sheet	Physician's notes regarding the patient's progress
Laboratory reports	Results of laboratory tests
Radiology reports	Results of x-ray examinations
Admission forms	Information on patient identification, conditions for admission, and consent for general medical and nursing care
Intake and output (I&O) record	Serial record of 24-hour intake and output
SPECIAL FORMS	
Ancillary staff sheets	Records of treatments by physical therapists, occupational therapists, respiratory therapists, and so forth
Discharge planning sheet	Records by social services, home health agencies, case managers, and clinical nurse specialists regarding the discharge plans and needs of the patient
Consultation sheet	Record of another physician called in to consult by the attending physician
Surgical or treatment consent form	Patient authorization for surgery or treatment
MISCELLANEOUS FORMS	
Diabetic flow sheet	Record of blood sugar determinations and amounts of insulin administered
Preoperative checklist	List used to verify that the patient is ready to go to surgery
Frequent observations sheet	Used when very frequent measurements of vital signs or neurologic assessments are needed (e.g., after surgery or after head trauma)
Intravenous (IV) flow sheet	Record of IV fluids and additives infused, type of IV catheter in use, date tubing was changed, date dressing was applied
Transfer form	Information pertinent for the transfer of the patient to another unit or facility
Discharge form	Information about instructions given regarding wound care, medications, rest, activity restrictions, needed exercises, diet, and signs and symptoms to report to the physician; also includes when to next see the physician
Skin risk assessment	Data from thorough skin assessment upon admission; evaluation of risk factors for skin breakdown; diagrams showing areas of redness, breaks in the skin, or pressure ulcers
Fall risk assessment	Information regarding the potential fall risk of the patient; particularly used for frail, elderly, or neuromuscularly impaired patients
Pain assessment	Record of pain level, when assessed, measures to reduce it, effectiveness of treatment

problem. An initial assessment is charted for each shift. Standard areas of assessment are usually noted on flow sheets, and a written note is added if an abnormality exists. Nursing diagnoses or problems are entered on the plan of care, which is created soon after the admission assessment is complete. The plan is reviewed and updated every 24 hours. Implementation of each intervention is documented either on a flow sheet or within the nursing notes. The specifics of what was done and how, plus the patient response, are entered in the chart. Evaluation statements are placed in the nurse's notes and indicate progress toward the stated expected outcomes and goals. Evaluation data must be documented showing that expected outcomes have been achieved before a nursing diagnosis is marked "resolved" or deleted from the nursing care plan. When expected outcomes are not being met, the plan of care is altered.

> **?**
> • *Think Critically About* . . . If evaluation data are not showing progress toward expected outcomes, what part of the nursing care plan needs to be altered? Where in the chart would this be done?

THE MEDICAL RECORD

The **medical record,** or **chart,** contains data on a patient's stay in the health facility or while under the care of a health care provider. Each type of facility has a particular set of forms used to record information about the patient.

As a legal record, its contents must be kept **confidential** and can only be given out with the patient's written consent because it contains personal information regarding the patient. **Only those health professionals caring directly for the patient, or those involved in research or teaching, should have access to the chart.** Protecting the privacy of the patient is of prime importance. Patient information is not discussed with others who are not directly involved in the patient's care.

The chart is the property of the health facility or agency, not of the patient or physician. Patients do have a right to information contained in the chart under certain circumstances (see Chapter 3). Keeping the patient and the family informed in a clear and timely manner usually satisfies their need for such information. After the patient has been discharged, the chart is sent to the medical records or health information department for safekeeping. It can be retrieved if the patient is admitted to service again within a 10-year span.

> **?**
> • *Think Critically About* . . . What would you say to your neighbor, who sees you working on the unit on which her sister's husband is a patient, if she asks you to check and see what her brother-in-law's physician has charted about his condition?

METHODS OF DOCUMENTATION (CHARTING)

Different methods of charting are used in various health care agencies. The six main methods of charting are (1) source-oriented (narrative) charting, which focuses on the patient's disease; (2) problem-oriented medical record (POMR) charting, which focuses on the problems experienced by the patient as a result of being ill or on the defined nursing diagnoses reflecting those problems; (3) focus charting, which centers on the patient from a positive perspective; (4) charting by exception, which focuses on deviations from predefined norms, using preset protocols and standards of care; (5) computer-assisted charting, where data are input to the computer; and (6) case management system charting, which tracks variances from the clinical pathway.

Whatever method of documentation is used, you are required to chart the patient's progress periodically during the shift or at the time of a home health visit. The chart entries are either in your notes or on the various flow sheets (Figure 7-1). Flow sheets track routine assessments, treatments, and frequently given care. The specific time frame required for charting is found in the agency's policy and procedure manual. Some agencies require one note per patient contact, others require charting every 1 to 3 hours during the shift.

SOURCE-ORIENTED OR NARRATIVE CHARTING

These records are organized according to the source of information. There are separate forms for nurses, physicians, dietitians, and other health care professionals to document their assessment findings and plan the patient's care. Narrative notes are phrases and sentences written without any standardized structure, content, or form. Narrative charting used in source-oriented records requires documentation of patient care in chronologic order. Assessments usually follow a body systems format. The content is similar to a set of dated and timed journal entries (Figure 7-2).

Advantages of the source-oriented (narrative) method are as follows:

- It gives information on the patient's condition and care in chronologic order.
- It indicates the patient's baseline condition for each shift.
- It includes aspects of all steps of the nursing process.

Disadvantages of the source-oriented, or narrative, method are as follows:

- It encourages documentation of both normal and abnormal findings, making it difficult to separate pertinent from irrelevant information.
- It requires extensive charting time by the staff.
- It discourages physicians and other health team members from reading all parts of the chart because of the lengthy descriptive entries in it.

FLOWSHEET	10/10	10/11		Doe, John B.
ADLs—cont'd	11-7	7-3	3-11	Neverland Hospital From 10/10/09 to 10/11/09
Ambulate		done RN FR 10:00 done self FR 14:00		Room 645-1 ADM 10/09/09 Age 63Y Sex M MD Sawbucks, Jackson ID 4620958 MR 102756
Activity response		tolerated well FR 08:00 tolerated well FR 10:00 tolerated well FR 14:00	tolerated well FR 16:00 tolerated well RJK 20:00 tolerated well RJK 22:00	
Feeding		self assist FR 08:00 self assist FRI 12:00		
Diet		regular FR 08:00 regular FR 12:00		
Ate %		80% FR 08:00 80% FR 12:00		
Hygiene		assist bath perineal care skin care back rub linen change FR 10:00		
Standard prec		yes FR 08:00 yes FR 10:00	yes RJK 20:00 yes RJK 22:00	
SKIN	11-7	7-3	3-11	
Skin assmnt	WNL RJK 00:00	WNL FR 08:00	WNL RJK 20:00	
Braden sc	21 RJK 00:00	21 FR 08:00	21 RJK 22:00	
INC/WDS UPPER	11-7	7-3	3-11	
L shoulder				
Wound type	incision RJK 00:00	incision FR 08:00	incision RJK 20:00	
Wound appearance	dry clean RJK 00:00	dry clean FR 08:00	dry clean RJK 20:00	
L shoulder				
Wound dressing	dry intact checked RJK 00:00	dry intact checked FR 08:00	dry intact checked RJK 20:00	
IV LINES	11-7	7-3	3-11	
R subclavian				
Line type	triple RJK 00:00	triple FR 08:00	triple RJK 20:00	
Rutken, Frances (FR) RN		Kahn, Roland J. (RTK) LPN		

FIGURE **7-1** Computer activity flow sheet.

PROBLEM-ORIENTED MEDICAL RECORD (POMR) CHARTING

A system developed by Dr. Lawrence Weed has been used since the late 1960s. It focuses on patient status rather than on medical or nursing care. POMR charting emphasizes the problem-solving approach to patient care and provides a method for communicating what, when, and how things are to be done in order to meet the needs of the patient. The POMR contains five basic parts: the database, the problem list, the plan, the progress notes, and the discharge summary (Table 7-2). The precise form these records take varies greatly between agencies, but the essentials of charting are the same.

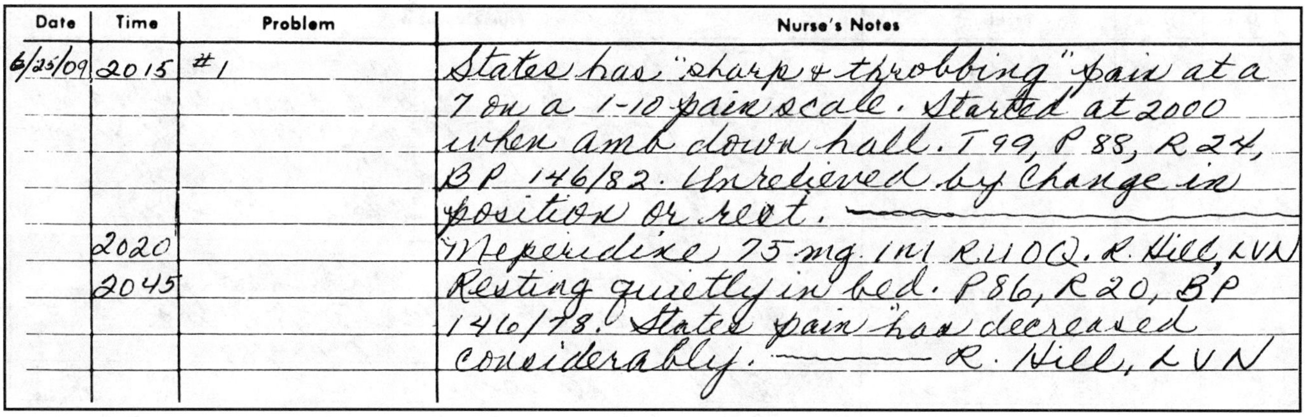

Date	Time	Problem	Nurse's Notes
6/23/09	2015	#1	States has "sharp & throbbing" pain at a 7 on a 1-10 pain scale. Started at 2000 when amb down hall. T 99, P 88, R 24, BP 146/82. Unrelieved by change in position or rest. ————
	2020		Meperidine 75 mg. IM RUOQ. R. Hill, LVN
	2045		Resting quietly in bed. P 86, R 20, BP 146/78. States pain has decreased considerably. ———— R. Hill, LVN

FIGURE **7-2** Example of source-oriented (narrative) charting.

Table **7-2** *Major Components of the Problem-Oriented Medical Record*

AREA	CONTENTS
Database	Initial assessment, general health history, findings of the physical examination, results of diagnostic and laboratory tests, psychosocial information, nursing assessment, patient's response to the illness or problem.
Problem list	A list of problems derived from the information in the database. The list is continually updated with resolved problems deleted and new problems added. Problems are listed in the chronologic order in which they were identified, not by priority. Both actual and potential problems are listed.
Plan	A three-part plan of care is devised based on the identified problems. For each problem there is a plan for diagnostic studies, a therapeutic plan, and a teaching plan. The physician orders therapies for medical problems and the nurse orders care for nursing problems.
Progress notes	Contain the assessments, plans, and orders of the physicians, nurses, and other therapists involved in the patient's care. Notes are organized by problem number from the problem list, and each problem is addressed in the SOAP format: S = subjective data that include symptoms and patient's description of the problem O = objective data based on health care team's observations, physical examination, and diagnostic tests A = assessment or analysis of the meaning of the data obtained P = plan to resolve the problem It is not essential to write a progress note on each problem every day.
Discharge summary	A summary of the problems the patient had, how they were resolved, and the plan for care after discharge.

As this documentation method evolved, the original *SOAP* format for progress notes (*S—subjective* information, *O—objective* data, *A—assessment* data, and *P—plan*) was modified to *SOAPIE* and *SOAPIER*. The additional letters stand for *I—implementation, E—evaluation,* and *R—revision.* It is not necessary to use each component of the SOAPIER format each time you make an entry. If there are no subjective data, the "S" can be omitted or labeled "none." If there is no revision, the "R" can be left out (Figure 7-3).

Advantages of the POMR method of documentation are as follows:

• It provides documentation of comprehensive care by focusing on patients and their problems.
• It promotes the problem-solving approach to care.
• It improves continuity of care and communication by keeping relevant data related to a problem all in one place so that it is more available to all who are providing care.
• It allows easy auditing of patient records in evaluating staff performance or quality of patient care.

• It requires continual evaluation and revision of the plan of care.
• It reinforces application of the nursing process.

Disadvantages of the POMR method of documentation are as follows:

• It results in loss of chronologic charting.
• It is more difficult to track trends in patient status.
• It fragments data because of the increased number of flow sheets required.

PIE Charting

Another offshoot of this method is PIE charting: *P—problem* identification, *I—interventions,* and *E—evaluation.* This type of charting follows the nursing process and uses nursing diagnoses while placing the plan of care within the nurses' progress notes. It differs from SOAP notes because it does not use a traditional nursing care plan or require narrative charting of the assessment data as long as they are normal. The problems, teaching, and discharge needs are listed under

Date	Time	Problem	Nurse's Notes
7/18/09	0800	#2 Pain, Abdominal	S. States having RUQ pain radiating to rt shoulder. Is "like a knife is poking me." States is a 6 on a scale of 1-10. "It started after I ate the bacon." States feels nauseous, but no vomiting.
			O. Pale, diaphoretic and shaky. Splinting abdomen c̄ hands. T 100°F, P 112, R 22, BP 134/88.
			A. Abdominal pain
			P. Institute NPO status; medicate when in order received; notify physician. ———— J. Sims, RN

A

Date	Time	Problem	Nurse's Notes
6/25/09	16²⁰	#1 Hyperthermia	S. States feeling "warm and restless".
			O. Face flushed; skin hot to touch. T 103°F, P 120, R 26, BP 160/90.
			A. Hyperthermia r/t wound infection.
			P. Medicate for ↑ temp.
	16²⁵		I. Acetaminophen 500 mg. P.O. with full glass of H₂O. Gown changed. Heat turned down; blanket removed.
	17⁰⁰		E. T 101.6°F, P 95, R 24; temp falling. States is feeling better. Skin cooler to touch. ———— M. Bailey LPN

B

FIGURE **7-3** **A,** Example of problem-oriented medical record (POMR) charting. **B,** Example of SOAPIE (subjective, objective, assessment, plan, implementation, evaluation) charting.

the *P* of the PIE format. Nursing diagnoses are kept on a problem list *(P)*, and each charting entry is marked with the problem number and title. With this method, the daily assessment information is placed on special flow sheets and duplication of the information is avoided. Interventions performed are documented under *I*. The outcomes of the interventions are evaluated and documented under *E* (Figure 7-4). When assessment data are abnormal, an *A* is added (APIE).

FOCUS CHARTING

Focus charting is similar to the POMR system but it substitutes *focus* for the *problem*, eliminating the negative connotation attached to "problem." Focus charting is directed at a nursing diagnosis (e.g., pain), a patient problem (pressure sore), a concern (decreased food intake), a sign (fever), a symptom (anxiety), or an event (return from surgery). The note has three components: D—data, A—action, and R—response (DAR) or D—data, A—action, and E—evaluation (DAE) (Figure 7-5). The data component contains subjective and objective information that describes or supports the focus of the note. The action component includes interventions performed or to be implemented. The response component describes the outcomes of the interventions and whether the goal has been met.

The advantages of focus charting are as follows:
- It is compatible with the use of the nursing process.
- It shortens charting time by using many flow sheets and checklists.
- The focus is not limited to patient problems or nursing diagnoses.

Date	Time	Problem	Nurse's Notes
7/18/09	14²⁰	Pain & IT ROM exercise of Rt. knee by CPM machine.	P. Reinstruct in use of PCA and measures for distraction. I. Instructions for use of PCA given; encouraged to watch a TV movie for distraction. Knee position on CPM machine ok; machine functioning at ordered settings. Repositioned upper body for comfort.
	14⁵⁰		E. Using PCA as needed. Pain decreased. States is tolerable at 3 on a scale of 1-10. Watching movie. ———— C. Harris, LPN

FIGURE **7-4** Example of PIE (problem, intervention, evaluation) charting.

DATE	HOUR	FOCUS	PATIENT PROGRESS
7/21/09	1300	Impaired skin integrity Rt. ankle	D. Slt serous drainage on dressing wound 1 x 2 cm. c̄ lt. red border; no odor; states hurts slightly ———— A. Cleansed c̄ sterile saline. DuoDerm thin applied. R. Wound clean; minimal drainage present. T. Harper RN

FIGURE **7-5** Example of focus charting.

The disadvantages of focus charting are as follows:
- If the database is not sufficient, patient problems may be missed.
- It does not adhere to charting with the focus on nursing diagnoses and expected outcomes.

CHARTING BY EXCEPTION

Charting by exception was developed in the early 1970s by a group of nurses at St. Luke's Medical Center in Milwaukee, Wisconsin. The goal was to decrease the lengthy narrative entries of traditional charting systems and reduce repetition of data. **Charting by exception is based on the assumption that all standards of practice are carried out and met with a normal or expected response *unless otherwise documented.*** Agency-wide and unit-specific protocols (standard procedures) and standards of nursing care are the heart of the system. The standards and protocols are integrated into flow sheets and forms, and the nurse needs only to document abnormal findings or responses correlated with the nursing diagnoses listed on the nursing care plan (Figure 7-6). **A longhand note is written only when the standardized statement on the form is not met** (Figure 7-7, p. 93). Otherwise only a signature is necessary.

Charting by exception is the direct opposite of the adage, "If it wasn't charted, it wasn't done." Charting by exception assumes that, unless documented to the contrary, all standards and protocols were followed and all assessment values were within accepted limits. This type of charting may present some problems with legalities when a chart is called into court because only abnormalities are documented in written words.

The advantages of charting by exception are as follows:
- It highlights abnormal data and patient trends.
- It decreases narrative charting time.
- It eliminates duplication of charting.

GUIDELINES FOR USE OF THE NURSING/PHYSICIAN ORDER FLOW SHEET

1. Indicate the Nursing Diagnosis that relates to the nursing order in the far left-hand column of the category boxes. If the order is a physician order, indicate "D.O." ("Doctor Order") instead of the nursing diagnosis number.
2. Indicate the nursing or physician order. If the nursing order includes an assessment to be completed, use the following protocol:
   a. *NEUROLOGIC ASSESSMENT* - will include orientation, pupil movement, sensation, quality of speech/swallowing, and memory.
   b. *CARDIOVASCULAR ASSESSMENT* - will include apical pulse, neck veins, CRT, peripheral pulses, edema, and calf tenderness.
   c. *RESPIRATORY ASSESSMENT* - will include respiratory characteristics, breath sounds, cough, sputum, color of nailbeds/mucous membranes, and CRT.
   d. *GASTROINTESTINAL ASSESSMENT* - will include abdominal appearance, bowel sounds, palpation, diet tolerance, and stools.
   e. *URINARY ASSESSMENT* - will include voiding patterns, bladder distention, and urine characteristics.
   f. *INTEGUMENTARY ASSESSMENT* - will include skin color, skin temperature, skin integrity, and condition of mucous membranes.
   g. *MUSCULOSKELETAL ASSESSMENT* - will include joint swelling, tenderness, limitations in ROM, muscle strength, and condition of surrounding tissue.
   h. *NEUROVASCULAR ASSESSMENT* - will include color, temperature, movement, CRT, peripheral pulses, edema, and patient description of sensation to affected extremity.
   i. *SURGICAL DRESSING/INCISIONAL ASSESSMENT* - will include condition of surgical dressing and/or color, temperature, tenderness of surrounding tissue, condition of sutures/staples/steri-strips, approximation of wound edges, and presence of any drainage.
   j. *PAIN ASSESSMENT* - will include patient description, location, duration, intensity, radiation, precipitating factors.
   k. *POST-MYELOGRAM COMPLICATION ASSESSMENT* - will include headache, nausea, and vomiting.
   l. *MYELOGRAM SITE ASSESSMENT* - will include presence of ecchymosis and drainage.

OR

Specify exactly which parts of assessment should be completed.
3. Top of sheet should be dated. Time should be indicated in the small box in upper right-hand corner of each category box.
4. Upon carrying out an order that has no significant findings. a "✓" in the appropriate category box is sufficient to indicate it was done. If the order includes an assessment, the following parameters will be considered a negative assessment and constitute the use of a "✓".
   a. *NEUROLOGIC ASSESSMENT* - Alert and oriented to person, place, and time. Behavior appropriate to situation. Pupils equal and reactive to light. Active ROM of all extremities with symmetry of strength. No paresthesia. Verbalization clear and understandable. Swallowing without coughing and choking on liquids and solids. Memory intact.
   b. *CARDIOVASCULAR ASSESSMENT* - Regular apical pulse, S_1 and S_2 audible. Neck veins flat at 45 degrees. CRT <3 sec. Peripheral pulses palpable. No edema. No calf tenderness.
   c. *RESPIRATORY ASSESSMENT* - Respirations 10-20/min at rest. Respirations quiet and regular. Breath sounds vesicular through both lung fields, bronchial over major airways, with no adventitious sounds. Sputum clear. Nailbeds and mucous membrane pink. CRT <3 sec.
   d. *GASTROINTESTINAL ASSESSMENT* - Abdomen soft. Bowel sounds active (5-34/min.) No pain with palpation. Tolerates prescribed diet without nausea and vomiting. Having BMs within own normal pattern and consistency.
   e. *URINARY ASSESSMENT* - Able to empty bladder without dysuria. Bladder not distended after voiding. Urine clear and yellow to amber.
   f. *INTEGUMENTARY ASSESSMENT* - Skin color within patient's norm. Skin warm and intact. Mucous membranes moist.
   g. *MUSCULOSKELETAL ASSESSMENT* - Absence of joint swelling and tenderness. Normal ROM of all joints. NO muscle weakness. Surrounding tissues show no evidence of inflammation, nodules, nail changes, ulcerations, or rashes.
   h. *NEUROVASCULAR ASSESSMENT* - Affected extremity is pink, warm and movable within patient's average ROM. CRT <3 sec. Peripheral pulses palpable. No edema. Sensation intact without numbness or paresthesia.
   i. *SURGICAL DRESSING/INCISIONAL ASSESSMENT* - Dressing dry and intact. No evidence of redness, increased temperature, or tenderness is surrounding tissue. Sutures/staples/steri-strips intact. Wound edges well-approximated. No drainage present.
   j. *PAIN ASSESSMENT* - If medication alone relieves pain and expected outcome is met, documentation on the Medication Profile is sufficient. No specific problem needs to be identified in the Nurses' Notes or Flow Sheet.
   k. *POST-MYELOGRAM COMPLICATION ASSESSMENT* - Absence of headache, nausea, and vomiting.
   l. *MYELOGRAM SITE ASSESSMENT* - Steri-strip dry and intact. No drainage present.
5. Upon carrying out an order that has significant findings, an asterisk is entered in the appropriate box. An asterisk (*) in the category box indicates to "See Significant Findings Section."
6. If status remains unchanged from previous asterisk entry, current entry may be indicated with an "→."
7. If an order no longer needs to be carried out, the next unused category box in that row indicate "order D/Ced," and a line should be drawn through the remaining boxes. Any unused rows can be left blank.
8. Each flow sheet is used for 24 hours.

FIGURE **7-6** Guidelines for the use of the nursing or physician order flow sheet. These guidelines appear on the reverse side of the first page of the flow sheet.

Disadvantages of charting by exception are as follows:

- It requires development of detailed protocols and standards.
- It requires retraining staff to use unfamiliar methods of record keeping and recording.
- Nurses become so used to *not* charting that important data are sometimes omitted.

COMPUTER-ASSISTED CHARTING

An electronic health record (EHR) is a computerized comprehensive record of a patient's history and care across all facilities and admissions. This type of record is a goal for the future for every patient. Systems are currently under design and study to accomplish this goal. Security and confidentiality of records are still major concerns (Legal & Ethical Considerations 7-1, on

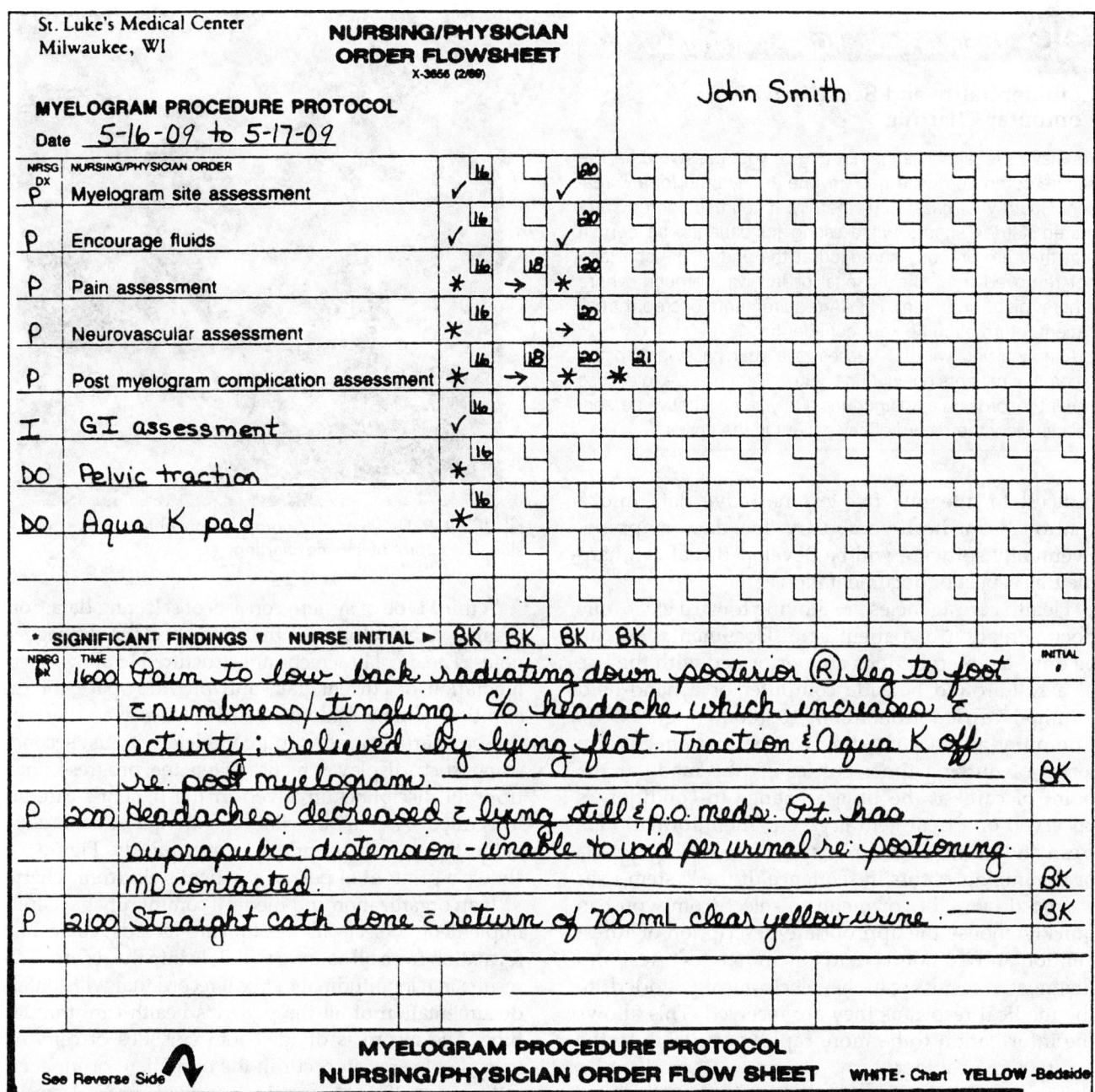

FIGURE **7-7** Physical assessment documentation on a nursing or physician order flow sheet, with significant findings noted.

p. 94). Within a hospital system, computer records are protected by passwords and a firewall. With the addition of wireless technology for ease of entry from any place in the hospital, the security issues have increased. Each user who has access to a patient record must have a secure password. Passwords must be changed regularly in order to maintain security of the records. Encryption as well as authentication software is used when reports are transmitted outside of the health care facility campus.

Computerized provider order entry (CPOE) provides for efficiency of work flow because when orders are entered into the computer, there is automatic routing to the appropriate clinical areas for action. For example, a physician order for a new medication is ordered on the computer. That order is automatically posted to the electronic medication administration record (eMAR) for that patient. The order is always legible and transcribing errors are eliminated.

There are problems with the vocabulary used for computer entries in that terminology that is appropriate for the entire interdisciplinary team is needed. The Systematized Nomenclature of Medicine Clinical Terms is a reference vocabulary developed for this purpose. This is important for evidence-based practice in order for researchers to understand the relationships in the data to predict trends and consequences of care (Lunney et al., 2005). At this time, it is

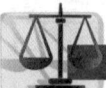

Legal & Ethical Considerations 7-1

Confidentiality and Security with Computer Charting

You have a legal obligation not to give your password for the secure computer system to anyone at any time for any reason. Guard your password carefully. If you use printed automated Kardex sheets while caring for patients, be certain that they are properly shredded at the end of the shift and not removed from the hospital or left lying around where others might find them. HIPAA requirements decree that all patient information be kept confidential.

Although you will have access via your password to the records of patients on your unit, you will not be able to access patient records on any other unit. Only administrative personnel can view the record of any patient in the hospital.

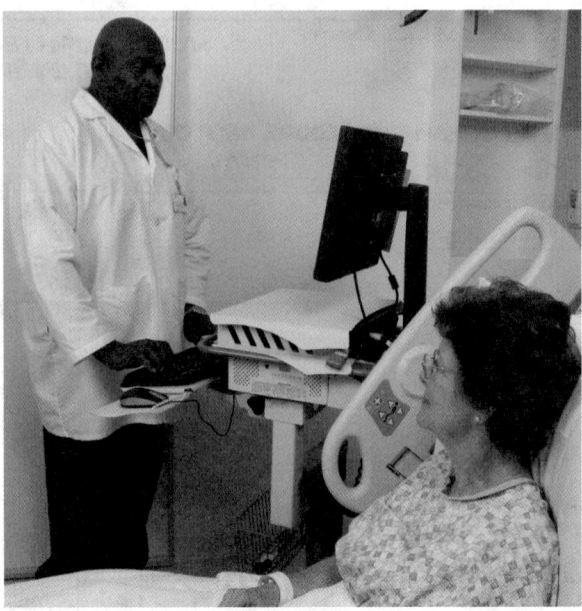

FIGURE **7-8** Nurse using a computer on wheels at the bedside to do point-of-service charting.

difficult to integrate free-text narrative data into a controlled medical vocabulary for data mapping. Eventually software will be developed that can handle this aspect of documentation.

Health care agencies are moving toward electronic documentation of patient care. Documentation can be done as interventions are performed with the use of a roll-around bedside computer or a hand-held terminal carried from room to room (Figure 7-8). Computer-assisted charting can be cost-effective in terms of nursing time. Entries can be made at the point of care, at the time a change in condition is observed or a treatment is given. The information is fresh and no time has to be spent in recalling details or organizing events in sequence. If the system uses a drop-down table or menu to select from, you can quickly choose the appropriate description or intervention and do not have to key in free text. Test and diagnostic results can be electronically added to the medical record as they are received. This allows the information to be more rapidly available to the health care provider.

There are variations of computerized systems for charting. Any documentation system can be supported using electronic documentation. Some organizations use a combination of manual and electronic documentation. For example, some produce a flow sheet with the expected patient outcomes and nursing interventions listed. The nurse initials those interventions that were implemented, writes a narrative note for other necessary information, and adds the printout page to the chart. This adds some limited electronic functions to a basically manual system.

Other systems use the POMR format and produce a prioritized problem list. A plan of care is constructed by selecting the diagnoses, expected outcomes, and nursing interventions from specific screens on the computer and keystroking in required information. A touch screen may be part of the system for choosing the items on the screen.

A third type of system consists of selecting data from display screens to build the flow sheets and progress notes. The display screens are structured to allow documentation of current data and provide space for the addition of new findings. Much of the everyday care can be charted rapidly and completely in just seconds using such display screens. Often the progress notes from all disciplines involved in the patient's care are integrated. A chart of vital sign trends or laboratory value trends can be printed very quickly. Figure 7-9 shows a printout of part of a patient's electronic chart.

If an organization and medical community have fully implemented electronic health care records, clinical information from all sources will flow into the record. This results in a longitudinal medical record that will contain documentation of all the patient's health care through time. The record is divided into episodes of care. An episode of care can occur in the outpatient or inpatient setting, any time the patient received medical assessment and/or medical intervention. As mentioned earlier, lab results, diagnostic imaging results, pathology reports, medication administration, and other information from all care delivery settings will be available via the electronic health care record. This provides virtually instant access to a complete medical history. Compare this to reviewing paper medical records from a variety of settings to assess a patient's medical history.

At this time in today's health care environment, a fully integrated electronic health care record is not common. There are multiple vendors for electronic health care record systems. Integration of these systems with an agency's current needs requires computer programming and interfaces. These activities are expensive and time-consuming. Organizations must be prepared for a significant investment of time and finances to develop a true longitudinal electronic health care record.

Doe, John
Charity Hospital
Assessments/Interventions
FROM; 10/8/09 07:00 TO: 10/8/09 23:30
ROOM 123-01 ADM: 10/8/09 05:21
AGE: 56Y   SEX: M   MD: J. Jones
ID: 000004444
Page 4

FLOWSHEET	10/07	10/08		
INC/WDS UPPER-cont'd	11-7	7-3	3-11	11-7
Wound dressing		dry intact checked CP 14:14	dry intact checked CP 16:11	stained stain marked checked CP 23:06 stained stain marked checked NI 23:30
L shoulder				
Closure type		tegaderm CP 14:14	tegaderm CP 16:11	
Closure condition		intact CP 14:14	intact CP 16:11	
Davol #1				
Location		L shoulder CP 14:14	L shoulder CP 16:11	L shoulder NI 23:30
Drains		patent draining suction emptied CP 14:14	patent draining suction emptied CP 16:11	patent draining NI 23:30
Drain drainage		moderate sero-sanguin CP 14:14	moderate sero-sanguin CP 16:11	sero-sanguin NI 23:30
Medicated incis		done CP 14:14	done CP 16:11	
Teaching inc/wnd		done SeeMultidisForm CP 14:14	done SeeMultidisForm CP 16:11	
Incis intv resp		tolerated CP 14:14	tolerated CP 16:11	

FIGURE **7-9** Example of part of a patient's electronic chart.

Most commonly, organizations with an electronic medical record have a system that collects the health care record while the patient is within that system. The medical information is collected while the patient receives services as an inpatient or outpatient of that specific health care system. Physicians may be able to access health care information from that system from their offices. However, the clinic medical record and the hospital systems medical record may still remain separate and require access to both systems to review.

There are some considerations when using an electronic documentation system. One is confidentiality. Every individual who accesses the medical record has a password that is necessary for access to the assigned patient's chart. Based on her position or job code, the person will be given a level of security that will allow access to only the specific information required for the job. When working on documentation at the computer, **you should never leave the terminal while part of a patient's chart is on the screen.** Terminals should be situated so that passersby cannot view the information displayed. Organizations will have very specific policies outlining access, security, and use of the electronic health care record.

Electronic records place vital information instantly at the tips of the health care provider's fingers because a review of previous problems, treatments, and responses can be viewed immediately. In 2006, The Joint Commission (formerly JCAHO) started requiring that a patient's medical record must document his language and communication needs. When cultural information about the patient is entered, all of the health care team has access to it (Cultural Cues 7-1).

Advantages of computer-assisted documentation include the following:

- The date and time of the notation are automatically recorded.
- Notes are always legible and easy to read.

- There is quick communication between departments about patient needs.
- It allows multiple health care providers to access the same patient's information at one time.
- If well designed, it can reduce documentation time.
- Electronic records can be retrieved very quickly (as long as the computer is up and running).
- If designed correctly, reimbursement for services rendered is faster and more complete because of complete and accurate documentation.
- A true electronic medical record can provide a complete longitudinal record of the patient's medical history at one point of access.
- Well-designed integrated systems can reduce errors, thus having a positive impact on patient safety.

Disadvantages include the following:
- A very sophisticated security system is necessary to prevent unauthorized personnel from accessing patient records.
- Initial costs are considerable because many more terminals and an appropriate networking system

must be purchased and interfaced for the system to work efficiently.
- Implementation of a full system can take a considerable length of time. This results in the need to use two systems, paper and electronic, during that transition.
- There is significant cost and time involved in training staff to use the system.
- Computer downtime can create problems of input, access, and transfer of information. Well-established backup plans (downtime procedures) must be developed.

CASE MANAGEMENT SYSTEM CHARTING

Case management is a method of organizing patient care through an episode of illness so that clinical outcomes are achieved within an expected time frame and at a predictable cost (see Chapters 1 and 2). A clinical pathway or interdisciplinary care plan takes the place of the nursing care plan (see Figure 6-1). Documentation of variances is placed on the back of the pathway sheets. For example, a patient is admitted for abdominal surgery. The wound is healing well, but the patient develops pneumonia. The variance would be documented as in Figure 7-10.

? *Think Critically About* . . . Which method of charting seems as if it would be the easiest for you? Can you explain why?

THE DOCUMENTATION PROCESS

When documenting patient care, the patient's needs, problems, and activities should be presented in terms of *behaviors*. The notes focus on the immediate past

Variation	Cause	Action Taken
Airway Clearance	Pneumonia 7/23	7/23 ↑ fluids to 2000 ml/day 7/24 Proventil inhaler for wheeze 7/24 Incentive spirometer use q 1° while awake 7/26 Instruct in home O₂ use 7/26 UnitAir contacted for oxygen delivery

FIGURE **7-10** Example of variance charting.

Table 7-3 *Abbreviations, Acronyms, and Symbols Not to Be Used in Documentation*

ABBREVIATION	POTENTIAL PROBLEM	PREFERRED TERM
U (for "unit")	Mistaken as zero, four, or "cc."	Write "unit"
IU (for "international unit")	Mistaken as "IV" (intravenous) or "10" (ten).	Write "international unit"
q A.M., q P.M.	Mistaken for "9" A.M. or "9" P.M.	Write, " morning, daily", "evening, daily" or "every morning" or "every evening"
Q.D. Q.O.D. (Latin abbreviations for "once daily" and "every other day")	Mistaken for each other. The period after the Q can be mistaken for an "I" and the "O" can be mistaken for "I."	Write "daily" and "every other day"
Trailing zero (*X*.0 mg) Lack of leading zero (.*X* mg)	Decimal point is missed.	Never write a zero by itself after a decimal point (*X* mg), and always use a zero before a decimal point (0.*X* mg)
MS (for "morphine sulfate") MSO_4, $MgSO_4$ (for "magnesium sulfate")	Confused for one another.	Write "morphine sulfate" or "magnesium sulfate"
μg (for "microgram")	Mistaken for mg (milligrams), resulting in 1000-fold dosing overdose.	Write "mcg"
H.S. (for "half-strength" or as Latin abbreviation for "bedtime")	Mistaken for either "half-strength" or "hour of sleep" (at bedtime). q. H.S. mistaken for "every hour." All can result in a dosing error.	Write out "half-strength" or "at bedtime"
T.I.W. (for "three times a week")	Mistaken for "three times a day" or "twice weekly," resulting in an overdose	Write "3 times weekly" or "three times weekly"
S.C. or S.Q. (for "subcutaneous")	Mistaken as SL for "sublingual," or "5 every."	Write "Sub-Q," "subQ," "subcut.," or "subcutaneously"
D/C (for "discharge")	Interpreted as "discontinue" whatever medications follow (typically discharge meds).	Write "discharge"
c.c. (for "cubic centimeter")	Mistaken for U ("units") when poorly written.	Write "ml" for milliliters
A.S., A.D., A.U. (Latin abbreviations for "left ear," "right ear," or "both ears") O.S., O.D., O.U. (Latin abbreviation for "left eye," "right eye," or "both eyes")	Mistaken for each other (e.g., AS for OS, AD for OD, AU for OU)	Write: "left ear," "right ear" or "both ears"; "left eye," "right eye," or "both eyes

and the present, never the future. For example, after assisting a patient to ambulate, you would chart something like "Ambulated 20 feet down the hall and back ×3 with minimal assistance."

Charting should be accurate, brief, and complete. When charting follows these guidelines, it presents a photographic view of the patient to anyone who reads the nursing notes.

ACCURACY IN CHARTING

Be specific and definite in using words or phrases that convey the meaning you wish expressed. Use of the words "appears to" or "seems" in phrases such as "appears to be resting" should be avoided. Chart the behavior; the patient either is or is not resting. Words that have ambiguous meanings and slang should not be used in charting. For example, how much is "a little," "a small amount," or a "large amount"? What do phrases such as "ate well," "taking fluids poorly," and "decubitus on sacrum" mean? Although such words give a general idea of what is meant, they are not specific. Someone else reading the notes will not know if

the patient who "ate well" had a half a piece of toast, juice, and a cup of coffee or ate a bowl of cereal, scrambled eggs, two slices of bacon, 4 oz of orange juice, and two cups of coffee. Instead of charting a conclusion such as "taking fluids poorly," chart the behavior and the specific amounts of liquid taken in a particular amount of time, such as "given fluids at frequent intervals, but takes only a few swallows; intake from 0700–1000: 30 mL of coffee, 60 mL of orange juice, and 50 mL of water." Although a chart entry of "decubitus on sacrum" points to a patient problem, a better description is "skin of back clear, except for 4-cm reddened area over sacrum." Specific data about size, amounts, and other measurements provide a means for determining whether the condition is getting better, getting worse, or staying the same. Rather than use the term "tolerated well," describe what happened, even if it is a statement such as "walked in hall without problems."

Table 7-3 provides a list of dangerous abbreviations, acronyms, and symbols that should not be used within a medical record.

HOME HEALTH SKILLED NURSING NOTE

PATIENT NAME Thompson, James	MEDICAL RECORDS # 56043	SERVICE DATE 12-4-09	DAY SA SU M TU W TH (F)	TIME IN 3:10p	TIME OUT 4:00p

VISIT CODE ○ADMISSION ✗SCHEDULED VISIT ○SUPERVISORY VISIT ○DISCHARGE ○UNSCHEDULED (EXPLAIN IN NOTES)	DISCIPLINE ○RN ✗LVN/LPN	MILEAGE FROM: Jones TO: Thompson TOTAL MILES DRIVEN: 21	PAYOR ✗MEDICARE ○MEDICAID ○INSURANCE ○CONTRACT ○PRIVATE ○OTHER:

EMPLOYEE NAME: Anders, Julia	EMPLOYEE NUMBER: 473	EMPLOYEE SIGNATURE/TITLE J. Anders LVN

PATIENT SIGNATURE James Thompson	I WAS SEEN BY THE NURSE TODAY, CARE WAS PERFORMED IN A SATISFACTORY MANNER, AND I AGREE TO THE TERMS AND CONDITIONS SET FORTH ON THIS FORM.	LAB SPECIMEN COLLECTED TYPE: Urine C+S DELIVERED TO: General Hosp

CLINICAL FINDINGS:
T 101 AP ___ RP 92 R 20 B/P 146/86 (○STAND ✗SIT ○LIE) WEIGHT ___

WOUND EVALUATION: L: ___ W ___ D ___ LOCATION: ___ COLOR: ___ DRAINAGE: ___ ODOR: ___

SUPPLIES USED: gloves, sterile urine cup

NURSING OBSERVATION AND ASSESSMENT Indicate areas of concern with an X and address in narrative.

CARDIOVASCULAR:		GASTROINTESTINAL		NUTRITION		NEUROLOGICAL	
Rate and Rhythm	X	Bowel Sounds		Appetite		Syncope/Vertigo	
Chest Pain		Nausea/Vomiting		Fluid Intake		Headache/LOC	
Neck Vein Distention		Constipation/Diarrhea		**SKIN**		Grasp	
Edema		Incontinence (Bowel)		Injury/Wound/Incision/Ulceration		Pupillary Reaction	
Ascites		Colostomy/Ileostomy		Jaundice/Pallor/Cyanosis		(Movement)Tremors s/p CVA	X
Dysrhythmia		Difficulty Swallowing		Turgor/Hydration		Vision	
Peripheral Pulses		**GENITO-URINARY**		Rash/Itching		Hearing	
RESPIRATORY		Burning/Pain	X	**MUSCULOSKELETAL**		Verbalization	
Lung Sounds		Distention/Retention		Balance/Endurance/Weakness	X	Tactile Sensation	
Cough/Sputum		Frequency/Urgency/Hesitation	X	Pain		**PSYCHOSOCIAL/EMOTIONAL**	
Dyspnea/SOB/Orthopnea COPD	X	Incontinence (Bladder)		**SAFETY**		(Anxious)Depressed.	X
Trach/Vent		Color/Odor	X	Falls	X	(Confused)Forgetful/Disoriented	X
Oxygen		Catheter/Ileoconduit		Other:		Affect/Thought Process/Coping	

ACTIVITY LEVEL ○INDEPENDENT ○MINIMAL ASSIST ✗MODERATE ASSIST ○DEPENDENT IN ALL ADLs   Reason Homebound (R) hemiparesis severe dyspnea on exertion

INTERVENTIONS

○CATHETER ○IMPACTION ○INJECTION ○TUBE FEEDING ○ACTIVITY RESTRICTIONS ○IV THERAPY ○OTHER (list)
○DRESSING CHANGE ○ENEMA ○DIABETIC CARE ○TRACH CARE ○NUTRITION ○TPN
○PRESSURE WOUND ✗BOWEL(BLADDER) ○INSULIN ○RESPIRATORY CARE ✗MEDICATIONS ○CHEMO
○VENIPUNCTURE ○C/P INSTRUCTION ✗DISEASE PHYSIOLOGY ○TERMINAL CARE ✗SAFETY ○CENTRAL LINE
○CHEST PT ○C/V INSTRUCTION ○OSTOMY CARE ○BEDRIDDEN CARE ○PAIN MANAGEMENT ✗UNIV PREC UTILIZED

ASSESSMENT NOTES, INTERVENTION SPECIFICS AND OUTCOME

Mr. Thompson's urine has developed foul odor + he c/o pain on urination. Also confused + febrile, agitated. More unsteady when ambulation. Wife states he fell 2 days ago but she did not call anyone. No injuries apparent, she states he did not hit his head. Fever + urine odor began yesterday.

SPECIFICS TAUGHT: Encourage clean fluids; begin antibiotics when they arrive from pharmacy - be sure to finish. disorientation

CONTACT WITH OTHERS: WHO: Dr Smith   REASON: Fever, urine odor, recent fall

ORDERS RECEIVED? ○NO ✗YES: Urine for C+S; antibiotics will be ordered.

CARE PLAN REVISED? ✗NO ○YES: Pt has hx of UTI, so already monitoring Wife does well managing antibiotics. Given written inst.

ASSESSMENT OF AIDE SERVICES: AIDE PRESENT? ○YES ✗NO   CARE PLAN FOLLOWED? ✗YES ○NO   PATIENT NEEDS MET? ✗YES ○NO
ASSIGNMENT SHEET UPDATED? ✗YES ○NO   AIDE USES GOOD CLINICAL SKILLS? ✗YES ○NO   PATIENT/CAREGIVER EXPRESSES SATISFACTION? ✗YES ○NO

Comments: Wife states P Jones CHHA very thorough and gentle.

FIGURE **7-11** Example of home care agency charting.

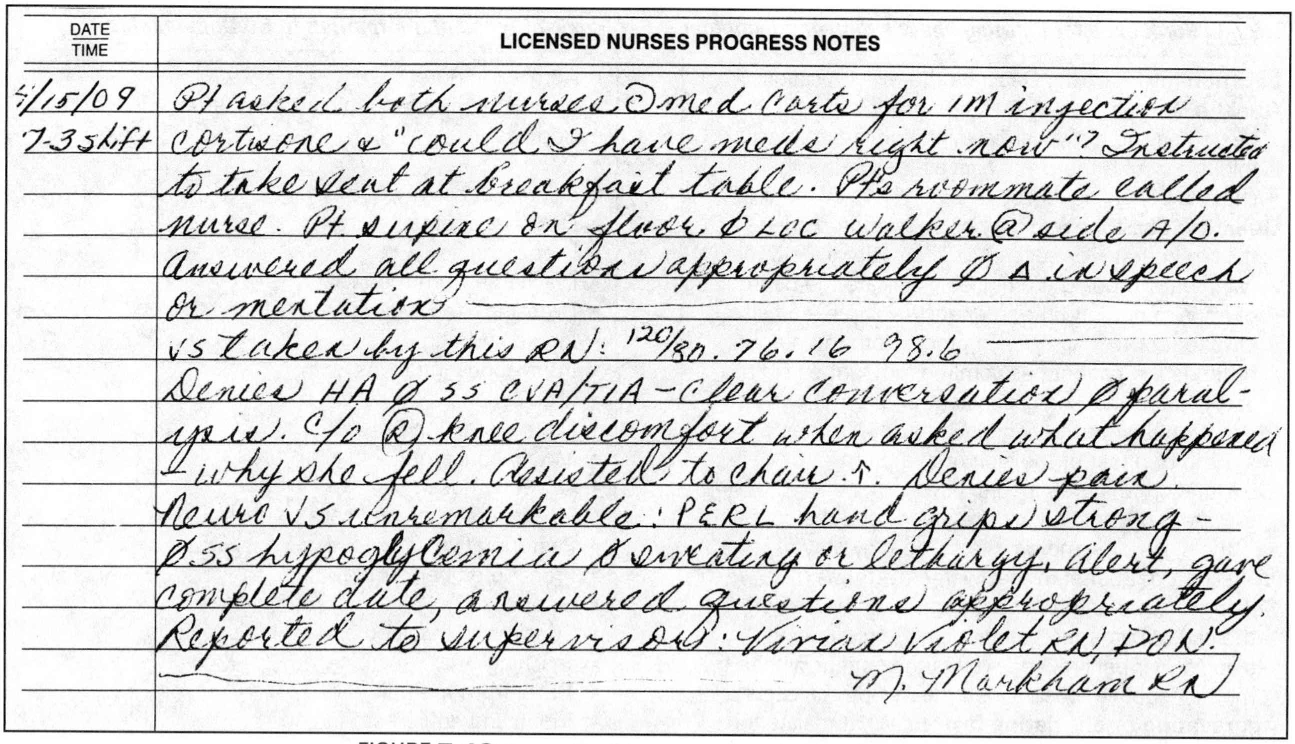

DATE TIME	LICENSED NURSES PROGRESS NOTES
4/15/09 7-3 shift	Pt asked both nurses @ med carts for IM injection cortisone & "could I have meds right now"? Instructed to take seat at breakfast table. Pt's roommate called nurse. Pt supine on floor @ LOC walker @ side A/O. Answered all questions appropriately $\emptyset$ Δ in speech or mentation — vs taken by this RN: $^{120}/_{80}$. 76. 16 98.6 — Denies HA $\emptyset$ ss CVA/TIA - clear conversation $\emptyset$ paralysis. C/o ® knee discomfort when asked what happened & why she fell. Assisted to chair ↑. Denies pain. Neuro vs unremarkable: PERL hand grips strong — $\emptyset$ ss hypoglycemia $\emptyset$ sweating or lethargy. Alert, gave complete date, answered questions appropriately. Reported to supervisor: Vivian Violet RN, DON. M. Markham RN

FIGURE 7-12 Example of long-term care facility charting.

BREVITY IN CHARTING

When charting, sentences are not necessary. Articles (*a, an, the*) may be omitted. Because the chart is about a particular patient, the word "patient" is left out whenever it is the subject of the sentence. Each statement should begin with a capital letter and end with a period. Rather than stating "Patient left for surgery via stretcher at 10:15," simply state "To surgery via stretcher at 10:15."

Abbreviations, acronyms, and symbols acceptable to the agency are used in charting to save time and space. Each agency has its own list of acceptable abbreviations and symbols. This list is usually found in the policy and procedures manual. A list of commonly used abbreviations and symbols is provided in Appendix 8.

You must choose which behaviors and observations are noteworthy or your nurse's notes will be lengthy and irrelevant. In most agencies, if data are recorded on a flow sheet, they need not be documented again in the nurse's notes. For example, the number of times the patient voids during the shift can simply be entered on the flow sheet under the proper section. No other notation is made in the nurse's notes unless there was a problem or some significant data related to urination. A good way to begin to learn what should and should not be charted is to read over the notes of experienced nurses who are known to chart accurately and well. **A rule of thumb is that if the behavior or finding is abnormal or a change from previous behavior or data, chart it.**

LEGIBILITY AND COMPLETENESS IN CHARTING

Legibility is extremely important when charting. The medical record may be called into court, and what you wrote may be scrutinized and evaluated. If the writing is not easily legible, misperceptions of what was written can occur.

However, completeness is more important than brevity. You should record information about the patient's needs and problems and also specify the nursing care given for those needs or problems. If you chart "Skin at IV site reddened and slightly swollen," you must include a note about what you did about the problem. The full note should read "Skin at right forearm IV site reddened and slightly swollen in 4-cm area. IV dc'd and warm moist pack applied for 20 minutes. Redness and swelling receding. IV restarted in left hand with 20-ga catheter."

What constitutes complete charting may vary among hospitals, extended-care facilities, and other health care agencies. Home care charting must particularly note safety factors in place and the need for continued care (Figure 7-11). Long-term care facilities may require only a monthly summary for patients in stable condition or a note when their condition changes (Figure 7-12), whereas hospitals caring for acutely ill patients require continual documentation of the patient's condition, with entries made every few hours. For completeness in charting about a sign or a symptom of the patient, note something about each of the seven factors listed in Box 7-1.

Box 7-1 | *Guidelines for Charting about a Sign or a Symptom*

Location in the body: Describe the exact location.

Quality: Describe in patient's terms; for example, a person having a myocardial infarction (heart attack) might describe the chest pain as feeling like the chest is being "squeezed in a vise."

Quantity: Chart the intensity of the symptoms (i.e., mild, moderate, or severe). Use a scale of 1–10 for pain, with 10 being the highest. Indicate the degree of impairment; and the frequency, volume, and size or extent of the sign or symptom. Note the number of times the patient has vomited, amount each time, and whether nausea is constant or intermittent.

Chronology: Note the sequence of development:
a. Time of onset of the sign or symptom
b. Duration (minutes, hours, days)
c. Pattern of variation and frequency and the course of the signs or symptoms (e.g., do they stay the same, get better, or get worse over time?).

Setting: Where is the patient (e.g., at home, in bed, in the car), what is the patient doing (e.g., running, sleeping, or eating), and who is the patient with (e.g., mother, spouse, boss) when the symptoms occur?

Aggravating or alleviating factors: What makes the signs or symptoms worse and what makes them better? Does a hot shower make a skin rash worse? Does eating cause more or less pain?

Associated manifestations: Signs and symptoms rarely occur singly. For instance, does the patient have nausea before vomiting? Has there been a weight change since the onset of vomiting?

Box 7-2 | *Types of Information to Be Documented*

- Admission note
- Assessment data for all body systems
- Body care
- Death
- Degree of activity
- Diagnostic tests
- Diet and fluids
- Discharge from the facility
- Dressings and wound care
- Intake and output
- Intravenous infusions
- Medications
- Mental state and mood
- Mood, concerns, or discomfort
- Oxygen in use
- Physician's visits and calls to physician
- Postoperative care
- Procedures performed
- Sleep
- Specimens obtained and their disposition
- Teaching
- Travel from the unit
- Tubes and equipment in use
- Visitors

WHAT TO DOCUMENT

In addition to assessment data related to signs and symptoms, information on the topics in Box 7-2 is to be documented either on flow sheets or in the nurse's notes. The charting examples included with the procedures throughout this book show how to describe different types of information.

General Charting Guidelines

In addition to those mentioned above, there are several other general rules to consider when charting. They are presented in Box 7-3. Figure 7-13 (p. 102) shows the use of regular versus military time for chart entries.

THE KARDEX

Many organizations have eliminated the use of the Kardex. If it is used, however, it needs to be up to date. Though it is not a part of the permanent medical record, the Kardex is a quick reference for current information about the patient and ordered treatments. When used, it is kept at the desk with the unit secretary. It usually consists of a folded card for each patient in a holder that can be quickly flipped from one patient to another. The unit secretary and the primary nurse assigned to

the patient update the information daily. Information kept on the Kardex includes the following:

- Room number, patient name, age, sex, admitting diagnosis, and physician's name
- Date of surgery
- Type of diet ordered
- Scheduled tests or procedures
- Level of activity permitted
- Notations regarding tubes, machines, and other equipment in use
- Nursing orders for assistive or comfort measures
- List of medications prescribed by name
- IV fluids ordered

Hospitals that have instituted a completely computerized patient care system may not have this type of Kardex anymore. In its place, worksheets or working care plans are printed out for each patient each shift. The nurse assigned to the patient receives the printed sheet or reviews an electronic plan of care before or during the report on patients from the previous shift. The unit secretary has a census sheet or an electronic census board listing the room numbers, patient names, and diagnoses. For the computerized system, these sheets are automatically updated as new orders are keyed into the computer.

The printed working care plans can be used to organize your work. They also serve well if you write pertinent information that will be needed for charting onto the form as you work. Noting the time at which PRN (as necessary) medications are given, the amounts of intake and output, vital signs, wound appearance,

Box 7-3 | *General Guidelines for Charting*

- Verify the name on the chart and the page *before* beginning to chart. Each page should have an imprint of the patient's name and hospital number on it.
- Chart the initial assessment at the beginning of the shift.
- Preferably use black ink; blue may be acceptable in your agency.
- Place date at beginning of day's entries and time each entry; use either a regular clock or a 24-hour clock (military time; see Figure 7-13).
- Charting is done only by the person who made the observation or performed the intervention and who is legally responsible for the accuracy and quality of care.
- Write legibly or print.
- After the note is complete, sign with one initial plus last name and title (e.g., J. Jones, LPN; M. White, SVN). Many agencies ask students to add "student" or their school initials behind their title.
- Chart objective data after completing each task. Nothing is ever charted before it is actually done.
- No blank lines are left in the charting. A horizontal line is drawn through the center of an empty line or part of a line. A line is drawn through a space or "N/A" (not applicable) is written if information asked for on forms does not apply to the patient.
- A late entry may be made if something has been forgotten. Write the time of the entry, circle it, and write "late entry" and your initials above the time.

Example of a late entry:

DATE	TIME	PROBLEM	NURSE'S NOTES
8/22/09	0900	#3	Voided 450 mL clear, straw-colored urine. States no "burning, urgency," or ↑ frequency of voiding.
	0930	#2	Amb to door of room & back c̄ assistance. States caused no pain.
	0945	Late entry for (0900)	Clean cath urine collected & sent to lab for UA. ——————— J. Biggs, LPN

- Clearly identify care given by another health care team member.
- When a patient refuses a medication, a circle is placed on the medication administration record around the time the medication was to be given, and an explanation for the refusal is recorded in the progress notes. Any refusals of treatments are also recorded in the chart. The exact words the patient uses when refusing to comply with the treatment regimen should be documented. Document any instructions given to the patient and any patient behaviors that are against the instructions.
- Spell chart entries correctly. Use a dictionary to check words you are unsure how to spell.
- Use only ink on the medical record. Entries should never be erased or obliterated with liquid correction fluid. Deleted entries may be questioned if the chart is used later in a court of law. If you suspect that a medical order or progress note is incorrect, seek clarification from the person who wrote the order or the note. If you make an error when charting, draw a line through the incorrect word or phrase and write the word "error" above it; add the date and your initials. Some agencies require the words "mistaken entry" or "incorrect entry" rather than "error."

Example of error correction:

DATE	HOUR	FOCUS	PATIENT PROGRESS
7/22/09	12⁴⁵	Impaired skin integrity Rt. ankle.	D. Slt. ~~sanguineous~~ *error J. Harper* serous drainage on dressing. Wound 1 x 2 cm c̄ lt. red border; no odor; states hurts "a bit." ———
			A. Cleansed c̄ sterile saline. Duoderm thin applied. ———
			R. Wound healing. J. Harper RN

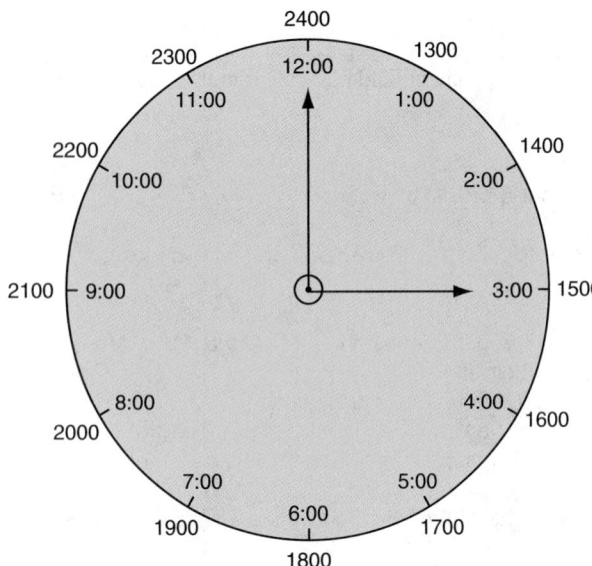

FIGURE **7-13** Military time versus civilian time.

and so on makes it easy to chart the information quickly once the chart is in hand or you are at the computer terminal. When using a printed care plan, it is important to remember that the printed sheet is only as current as the time it was printed. If orders have changed or been added, you must look at the electronic medical record. When an electronic system is used, staff should use the electronic system and not depend on printed reports.

If used, the Kardex can be a reference when giving a report on your patients. It also serves as a quick reference guide for the unit secretary in locating patients and when answering staff questions related to a particular patient. Although it takes time and practice to learn to chart efficiently and well, it is a major part of a nurse's job and should be viewed as an important skill.

Documentation of medication administration is covered in Chapter 34.

 **Key Points**

- Documentation provides a communication tool for the health care team; maintains a written record of the history, care, and treatment of the patient; is a legal record; is a quality assurance tool; and provides a basis for reimbursement of services rendered by Medicare/Medicaid, insurance companies, and third-party payers.
- The nursing care plan is the framework for nursing documentation.

- Charting is organized by nursing diagnosis or problem.
- Evaluation data that are documented must show progress toward expected outcomes.
- Information in the medical record must be kept confidential, and only those health professionals directly involved in the patient's care should have access to the record.
- There are six main methods of charting: (1) source-oriented (narrative) style; (2) problem-oriented medical record (POMR) style; (3) focus charting; (4) charting by exception; (5) computer charting; and (6) case management system charting.
- Besides nurses' and physicians' progress notes, there are many flow sheets that are used to document patient information.
- An advantage of the source-oriented method is that information on the patient's condition and care is listed in chronologic order.
- An advantage of the POMR system is that it improves continuity of care by keeping relevant data related to a problem all in one place.
- An advantage of focus charting is that it shortens charting time by using many flow sheets and checklists.
- Although charting by exception highlights abnormal data and patient trends, it presents problems if called into court because only abnormal findings are documented in written word.
- Computer charting is very expensive to institute but saves considerable nursing time.
- Case management system charting tracks variances from the care map.
- Documentation should show the application of the nursing process.
- Your charting should present a photographic view of the patient's condition and care.
- Charting must be objective, accurate, brief, and complete.
- Chart the patient's behaviors and statements, not the nurse's opinions.
- The list of activities and data that must be charted about the patient each day is extensive.
- Guidelines for charting tell the nurse when, what, and how to document patient assessments, activities, and interventions.
- The Kardex is a quick reference for current information about the patient and ordered treatments.

 Go to your **Companion CD-ROM** for an Audio Glossary, animations, video clips, and more.

evolve Be sure to visit the companion Evolve site at http://evolve.elsevier.com/deWit/fundamental/ for additional online resources.

NCLEX-PN® EXAMINATION-STYLE REVIEW QUESTIONS

*Choose the **best** answer(s) for each question.*

1. Which accreditation agency provides the guidelines for required documentation?
   1. American Nurses Association
   2. National League for Nursing
   3. The Joint Commission
   4. The American Hospital Association

2. When an error is made in charting, the nurse remedies it by:
   1. lining out the entry, dating it, and initializing it.
   2. recopying the sheet and destroying the original.
   3. using an eraser to remove the entry.
   4. painting over the entry with liquid correction fluid.

3. Patients frequently request copies of their medical records. You understand that:
   1. they have a right to a copy of their record after discharge.
   2. only health care staff have the right to read the record.
   3. the patient and family have a right to read the record.
   4. the physician must write an order for the release of the record.

4. One characteristic differentiating source-oriented (narrative) charting from POMR charting is:
   1. a specific order of forms in the chart.
   2. a focus on the patient's problems.
   3. the separation of notes on medical care and nursing care.
   4. patient identification stamped on each form.

5. When charting, it is wise to always:
   1. include the names of all visitors with the time of the visit.
   2. check that you are on the right chart or screen and on the right date.
   3. sign your full name, date, and time on each sheet.
   4. use acronyms you are familiar with to shorten notes.

6. When a patient's medical record is needed as evidence for a legal action, you are aware that the record is the property of:
   1. the patient.
   2. the patient's lawyer.
   3. the court.
   4. the health care agency.

7. The advantage of POMR charting when using an interdisciplinary care system is that:
   1. all charting is done on flow sheets.
   2. not as many flow sheets are used.
   3. all members of the team chart in a sequential order.
   4. nurses only have to chart on flow sheets.

8. The assumption in charting by exception is that:
   1. if it was not charted, it was not done.
   2. patient care is charted chronologically.
   3. unless otherwise documented, all standards have been met.
   4. a SOAPIER format note must be made each shift.

9. An advantage of computer charting is that:
   1. computers are always up, running, and available.
   2. security of information is guaranteed with the computer system.
   3. others can see what is being input as the nurse works with the charting screens.
   4. it is cost-effective because it saves nursing time compared to writing out notes.

10. When charting the patient's condition and nursing care, the nurse records: *(Select all that apply.)*
    1. activities planned for a later date.
    2. goals for the medical treatment and evaluation.
    3. the interventions performed and the patient's responses.
    4. patient statements and behaviors that are observed.
    5. clinical data measurements.

CRITICAL THINKING ACTIVITIES *Read each clinical scenario and discuss the questions with your classmates.*

Scenario A
Read the following scenario and then write out a POMR progress note and a focus charting note using the data given.

Marvin Barnes was admitted with impaired gas exchange r/t excessive pulmonary secretions. When you go to assess him, you discover that his temperature is 102.6° F (38.9° C), pulse 77, respirations 26 and shallow, and blood pressure 147/92 mm Hg. He is coughing and produces yellow-green sputum. He is having difficulty stopping the cough. He has

oxygen via nasal cannula running at 3 L/min. He has acetaminophen ordered for fever over 100.2° F (38° C). You tell him that you will be back with medicine for his fever and that you will call the physician for an order for some cough medicine to relieve the cough.

Scenario B
Discuss the guidelines that will help you chart so that you would be protected if there is a lawsuit involving a patient to whom you had given care.

evolve http://evolve.elsevier.com/deWit/fundamental/

Objectives

Upon completing this chapter, you should be able to:

Theory

1. Describe the components of the communication process.
2. List three factors that influence the way a person communicates.
3. Compare effective communication techniques with blocks to communication.
4. Describe the difference between a therapeutic nurse-patient relationship and a social relationship.
5. Discuss the importance of communication in the collaborative process.
6. List three guidelines for effective communication with a physician by telephone.
7. Identify four ways to delegate effectively.
8. Discuss five ways in which the computer is used for communication within the health care agency.

Clinical Practice

1. Use interviewing skills to obtain an admission history from a patient.
2. Interact therapeutically in a goal-directed situation with a patient.
3. Communicate effectively with a patient who has an impairment of communication.
4. Give an effective report on assigned patients to your team leader or charge nurse.

Key Terms

 Be sure to check out the bonus material on the Companion CD-ROM, including selected audio pronunciations

active listening (p. 105)
aphasia (ă-FĀ-zē-a, p. 113)
body language (p. 104)
communication (kō-myū-nĭ-KĀ-shŭn, p. 104)
confidentiality (kŏn-fĭ-dĕn-shē-ĂL-ĭ-tē, p. 112)
congruent (kŏn-GRŪ-ĕnt, p. 104)
delegate (DĔ-lĕ-gāt, p. 116)
empathy (ĔM-pă-thē, p. 112)
feedback (p. 105)
incongruent (ĭn-kŏn-GRŪ-ĕnt, p. 106)
input (p. 116)
nonverbal (NŎN-vĕr-bŭl, p. 104)
perception (pĕr-CĔP-shŭn, p. 105)
rapport (ră-PŌR, p. 111)

SBAR (p. 115)
shift report (p. 114)
therapeutic (thĕr-ă-PYŪ-tĭk, p. 108)
therapeutic communication (p. 107)
verbal (VĔR-bŭl, p. 104)

THE COMMUNICATION PROCESS

Communication occurs when one person sends a message to another person who receives it, processes it, and indicates that the message has been interpreted (Figure 8-1). The receiver must acknowledge that the message has been received and comprehended for the communication to be complete. By its nature, communication is a continuous, circular process and occurs in two ways, **verbal** (in words) and **nonverbal** (without words). Verbal communication consists of words either spoken or written. Nonverbal communication is conveyed without words by gesture, expression, body posture, intonation, and general appearance. Nonverbal communication is often referred to as **body language.** Nonverbal communication conveys more of what a person feels, thinks, and means than what is actually stated in words (Figure 8-2). Sometimes the person's nonverbal communication is not **congruent** (in agreement) with the verbal communication. If you state that you want to sit and talk for a while and then sit with legs crossed and a foot bouncing rapidly during the conversation, the message is one of impatience rather than attentive listening.

? *Think Critically About . . .* Look at Figure 8-2. Identify six or seven examples of nonverbal communication that the nurse is using in this nurse-patient depiction.

You can learn more about patients by observing nonverbal behavior. **Anxiety, fear, and pain are often expressed by nonverbal cues.** Wincing when turning, a pinched expression, or nervously picking at the bed covers may indicate what patients are really feeling, although they say they are fine. Experience will increase your ability to assess nonverbal communication. Rigid body posture or slow movements often in-

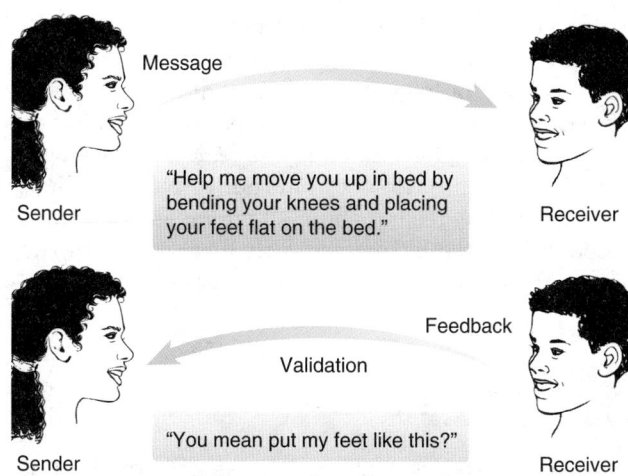

Message

Sender

"Help me move you up in bed by bending your knees and placing your feet flat on the bed."

Receiver

Feedback

Validation

"You mean put my feet like this?"

Sender

Receiver

FIGURE **8-1** The communication process.

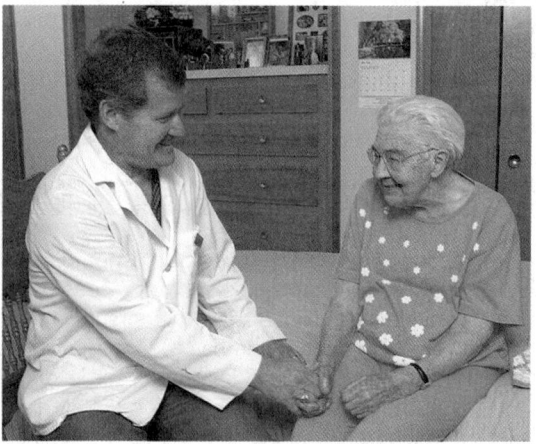

FIGURE **8-2** Nonverbal communication signals that the nurse is interested in the patient and what she is saying.

dicate pain. Restless movements may indicate anxiety. Validate perception (recognition and interpretation of sensory stimuli) of nonverbal communication with the patient. This can be done by asking about feelings and thoughts. For, example, "Mrs. Lopez, you seem a little restless [and anxious] today. Would you like to talk about something?"

Good communication requires active listening (mind and senses are focused on what is being said), timely feedback (responding), and validation of assumptions about nonverbal cues.

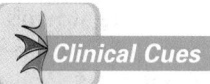

Giving positive feedback increases the likelihood that a desired behavior will be repeated. For example, you are trying to get Mrs. Panopoulous to independently perform activities of daily living. *"Mrs. Panopoulous, I saw you combing your own hair this morning. (State the observed behavior.) I really liked the way that you styled it. (Give praise.) Keep up the good work!"* (State the desired behavior.)

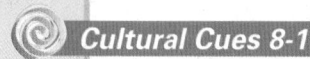 *Cultural Cues 8-1*

Eye Contact

Most Americans expect direct eye contact when interacting with someone; other cultures—for example, traditionally Japanese, Chinese, Vietnamese, and Laotians—believe that it is rude to look directly at someone. For Jamaicans, direct eye contact toward an authority figure or between strangers may indicate a challenge. In order to determine how eye contact is used in your patient's culture, observe how your patient interacts with others. Also, make opportunities to talk with colleagues from different cultures to learn about eye contact and other communication issues.

FACTORS AFFECTING COMMUNICATION

Culture, past experience, emotions, mood, attitude, perceptions of the individual, and self-concept all contribute to the way people communicate. Every culture has norms for appropriate communication. The norms include the distance between communicators, whether eye contact should be established, the tone of voice, and the amount of gestures used.

Cultural Differences

Individuals differ in the amount of personal space they need between them and the person with whom they are speaking. In the United States, 18 inches to 4 feet is the amount of distance that individuals place between themselves and a new acquaintance. This distance is called *personal space*. The distance lessens when people converse with someone with whom they are intimate. When people are not acquainted, they maintain a social distance of 4 to 12 feet if they have a choice. In general, American Indians, northern Europeans, and Asians maintain more distance from others than do Hispanic, southern European, or Middle Eastern people. Cultural Cues 8-1 presents cultural considerations of making eye contact during communication.

Past Experience

All of our experiences affect how we perceive what is communicated to us. Interpretation of messages is influenced by cultural values, level of education, familiarity with the topic, occupation, and type of previous life experiences.

Think Critically About . . . You are with Mrs. Ito and the doctor walks in and says, "A cardiac catheterization needs to be done to see if the coronary arteries are blocked." The patient has limited experience with hospitalization and medical terminology. She shyly looks down at her hands. It is unclear if she understands. What could you do?

Emotions and Mood

Emotions and mood can drastically affect the way messages are sent or interpreted. **A highly anxious person may not correctly hear what is said, or may interpret the message totally differently than the sender intended. A depressed person tends to use few words. A person who is upset or stressed may speak in a loud, harsh tone or be more abrupt than usual.**

Attitude

A person's attitude affects how a message is worded and the body language that accompanies it. When your attitude is one of acceptance of the patient, caring and concern are displayed by open, attentive body language. If you disapprove of the patient's behavior, you may use a closed body stance and stern expression and be somewhat distant during interactions. Someone with an accepting attitude will make an effort to understand what a person is trying to convey during the communication.

You should try to be open and attentive to patients' communications, to maintain a nonjudgmental attitude, and to remember not to take personally the unpleasant things a patient might say when upset or frightened.

COMMUNICATION SKILLS

Some people are more effective communicators than others. Effective communication can be learned by improving basic communication skills.

Active Listening

Active listening requires great concentration and focused energy. All the senses are used to interpret verbal and nonverbal messages, attention is on what the speaker is saying, and the mind is focused on the interaction. Listen for feelings as well as words. It takes practice to tune out other thoughts that try to intrude and not to start formulating a response until the speaker is finished. When you are an active listener, you demonstrate interest in the patient, and a trusting relationship can be built. An active listener maintains eye contact without staring, gives the patient full attention, and makes a conscious effort to block out other sounds and distractions. The active listener does not interrupt the speaker and waits for the full message before interpreting what is said. Responding to the content and feelings of the message by stating what you, as the listener, understand was said by the patient completes the process. Nonverbal cues that indicate active listening are leaning forward, focusing on the speaker's face, nodding slightly to indicate the message is being heard, and maintaining an open body posture.

Interpreting Nonverbal Messages

The speaker's posture, gestures, tone, facial expression, and eye movements should be observed. A smile or frown, hunched-down posture, or hand-wringing all express feelings. When taking in nonverbal messages, it is important to remember that they must be interpreted in the context of the *speaker's* culture, not the listener's. The listener must decide if the nonverbal messages are congruent with the spoken message. Mixed messages, in which the words do not fit the nonverbal indications, leave an uneasy feeling about an interaction. When the verbal and nonverbal messages are incongruent (do not agree), the listener should explore what the speaker really desires to communicate.

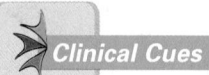

Clinical Cues

Laughing, smiling, and appropriate use of humor can decrease stress and anxiety and have a positive effect on the immune system (Christie & Moore, 2005). Encourage and support your patient's efforts to smile and be positive; however, be sensitive to incongruent behaviors. If you think your patient is smiling to cover her fears or anxieties, then provide openings for her to express her true feelings.

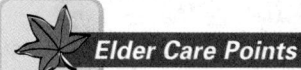

Elder Care Points

When interacting with an elderly person, try not to speak too quickly. Allow more time for the person to process your message and formulate a response. Face the person so that your lips can be seen and so that she has the optimal chance of hearing what you say. Many elderly have some degree of hearing loss. If the person wears a hearing aid, be certain it is in place and turned on before the interaction begins.

Obtaining Feedback

A vital part of communication is checking to see if you interpreted a message in the way the speaker meant it. This can be accomplished by rephrasing the meaning of the message or directly asking a feedback question, such as "Is your headache severe?" "Are you uncertain about having this surgery?" or "Does the idea of having anesthesia scare you?" The response received from the question should verify whether the original message sent was interpreted correctly.

Focusing

Keeping attention focused on the communication task at hand can save time. The effective communicator refocuses the other person gently to the issue at hand when the focus has wandered. Occasionally the approach, "We'll come back to that later, but right now I need to know..." will quickly refocus the communication. At other times, commenting "I think we were talking about..." is what is needed.

Adjusting Style

The patient's style and level of usual communication should be considered when interacting. If the person is a slow, calm communicator, adjust to that pace. If a response is slow in coming, allow plenty of time for consideration and a response; try not to display impatience. If it is comfortable for the patient to display feelings only in the context of telling a story about a related topic, allow enough time for full development of the topic so that the feelings can be adequately expressed (Cultural Cues 8-2).

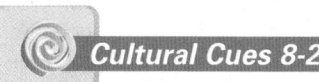

Cultural Cues 8-2

Conversational Pace and Flow

Long pauses are a natural part of conversation in some cultures. This is often found among Native Americans. Do not be too quick to assume the speaker is finished. Among some cultural groups, giving a direct "no" answer is considered rude, so maintaining silence means "no." This may be true of those raised in a Japanese family. Often it is necessary to "give permission" to ask questions. Certain groups regard asking questions as rude or disrespectful.

THERAPEUTIC COMMUNICATION TECHNIQUES

Therapeutic communication (communication that is focused on the needs of the patient) promotes understanding between the sender and the receiver. There are various phrases or cues that may be used to promote such understanding or facilitate an interaction between a patient and the nurse. These techniques should be used judiciously and in a varied manner or the interaction will feel stilted and uncomfortable. Common therapeutic communication techniques are presented in Table 8-1.

SILENCE

Appropriate use of silence is one of the hardest techniques for most students to develop. The new nurse is often uncomfortable with silence, and so tends to be too quick to end it. Silence gives the patient time to think and respond. When the nurse remains attentive and uses body language indicating patience and interest, the patient is encouraged to verbalize feelings or thoughts.

Table 8-1 | *Therapeutic Communication Techniques*

TECHNIQUE	EXAMPLE	RATIONALE
General leads	"Go on." "I see." "Uh huh." "Please continue."	Encourages patient to continue or elaborate.
Open-ended questions or statements	"Tell me more about that feeling." "I'd like to hear more about... ."	Encourages patient to elaborate rather than answer in one or two words.
Offering self	"I'm here to listen." "Can I help in some way?"	Shows caring, concern, and readiness to help.
Restatement	Patient says, "I tossed and turned last night." Nurse says, "You feel like you were awake all night."	Restates in different words what the patient said; encourages further communication on that topic.
Reflection	Patient says, "I'm so scared about the surgery; anesthesia terrifies me." Nurse says, "Something scares you about anesthesia?" Patient looks scared. Nurse says, "You look scared."	Reflects received message back to patient. It also encourages further verbalization of feelings. Reflects feelings. Can also be used if patient is unable to verbalize or if nonverbal information is incongruent with verbal.
Seeking clarification	Patient says, "Having my little girl come to visit me was so hard. I'm so upset." Nurse says, "Something about your daughter's visit upset you?"	Seeks clarification about the source of the upset feeling. Helps the patient clarify unclear thoughts or ideas.
Focusing	"Do you have any questions about your chemotherapy?"	Asking a goal-directed question helps the patient focus on key concerns.
Encouraging elaboration	"Tell me what that felt like." "I need more information about that." "Tell me more about that experience."	Helps the patient describe more fully the concern or problem under discussion.
Giving information	"The test results take at least 48 hours." "You will get a preoperative injection that will make you sleepy before you are taken to the operating room."	Informs the patient of information relevant to specific health care or situation.
Looking at alternatives	"Have you thought about...?" "You might want to think about... ." "Would this be an option?"	Helps patients see options and consider alternatives to make their own decisions about health care.
Silence	Patient says, "I don't know if I should have chemotherapy, radiation, or both." Nurse remains silent.	The nurse maintains silence, sitting attentively but quietly. This allows patients time to gather their thoughts and sort them out.
Summarizing	"You've identified your alternatives pretty clearly." "You are aware of the important signs and symptoms to report to your physician; you plan to call to make an appointment next week."	Sums up the important points of an interaction.

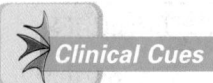

If you are having trouble with using silence, remember, you are not passively waiting for the patient to speak. You are observing and analyzing nonverbal behaviors during this silence. Note the patient's body position (i.e., relaxed, tense, shifting), expression on the face (i.e., thoughtful, sad, distant), conditions of the environment (i.e., organized, presence or lack of personal items), and indicators of emotional duress (i.e., picking at nails, pulling at hair, restless feet movements). These observations provide a significant amount of objective data.

OPEN-ENDED QUESTIONS

An open-ended question is broad, indicating only the topic, and it requires an answer of more than a word or two. Use of an open-ended question or statement allows the patient to elaborate on a subject or to choose aspects of the subject to be discussed. Open-ended questions or statements are helpful to open up the conversation or to proceed to a new topic. They usually cannot be answered with one word or just "yes" or "no." "Tell me about your day" versus "Did you have a good day?" or "How did you sleep?" versus "Did you sleep well?" are examples of open-ended versus closed questions. The closed question forces the listener to stick directly to the topic and to be concise. **Open-ended questions create an inviting atmosphere for sharing thoughts, feelings, and concerns.**

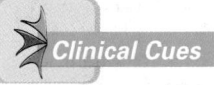

Closed questions are usually not considered part of the therapeutic communication process; however, there are times when closed questions are appropriate: when you are gathering information ("Have you ever had a blood transfusion?"), if the patient is highly anxious ("Are you hurt?") or confused ("Do you need to go to the toilet?"), or if the patient is at a very young developmental age ("Would you like the red one or the blue one?").

RESTATING

You listen for the basic message the patient is conveying and then rephrase the heart of the message. If the patient states, "My son hasn't been to see me in months," responses that restate the thought in different words might be as follows: "Your son hasn't been around much lately," or "You miss your son's visits." **Restating is used to encourage the patient to continue with information on a topic.**

Reflection is another way to restate the message. The same words the patient has said are reflected back. A patient says, "I'm worried about cancer," and the nurse replies, "You are worried about cancer." The idea is simply reflected back to the speaker in a statement to encourage continued dialogue on the topic.

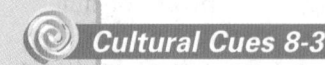

Using Touch to Communicate

Some cultures are more accepting of touch within the health care setting. For example, a Portuguese patient may interpret touch as reassuring. For the patient from Mexico, it may be advisable to touch while you are giving a compliment; touch functions to neutralize the power of the "evil eye." Koreans raised in traditional homes may hug and touch family members or close friends, but touching from strangers is considered disrespectful unless for physical examination purposes. Touching during communication is also not common in the Japanese culture.

Restating and reflection should be used sparingly and skillfully. If overused, the patient will quickly recognize that you are repeatedly saying her words back to her; you do not want to sound like a parrot or an automaton. Patients tend to find that annoying.

CLARIFYING

Clarifying helps verify that the message heard is what the patient intended. It is particularly useful when the dialogue has rambled. If a patient says that family members visited and that they all sat around and drank coffee, and then says that sleeping was difficult last night, the nurse might say, "Are you saying that the coffee kept you awake?" This asks for confirmation that it was the caffeine in the coffee that prevented sleep, and not a problem brought in by the family that might have caused the sleeplessness.

TOUCH

Gentle touch that indicates caring is therapeutic (effective or curative). It may be used to signify support for the person or when appropriate words are hard to find. Touch must be used judiciously, taking into consideration the patient's cultural and personal feelings about being touched by a stranger. You should have verbal or implied permission from the patient for touch to occur. Messages accompanied by touch can add a feeling of caring and comfort. Touching the patient warmly on the shoulder and saying, "I'm glad the medicine has relieved your pain" indicates that you really care. Touch needs to be beneficial for the patient; it should not be done to meet a need of the nurse. The nurse must consider how the patient will perceive and interpret touching before caring is expressed in this manner. Cultural Cues 8-3 presents additionally information about how to use touch with patients from different cultures.

GENERAL LEADS

General leads or broad openings are used to get the interaction under way. If a patient says, "I feel so guilty for breaking my leg," a general lead would be "Tell me more about that." A general lead that is useful first thing in the morning is "Tell me how your night was." General leads are statements or questions that cannot be answered with a "yes" or "no" and require more than a few words in response. "Perhaps you'd like to talk about your chemotherapy," "I noticed the doctor came after I left yesterday; perhaps you'd like to talk about what he said," and "I hear you are being discharged today; what do you think about that?" are other examples.

OFFERING OF SELF

Being available to the patient is one way of offering yourself. Answering call lights quickly or checking on something right away states that you are available to the patient, but this is not always possible. Letting the patient know when you will return or when you will be able to get the desired information conveys availability. Fulfilling such promises to obtain information or return at a particular time helps establish trust. Another form of offering yourself is to tell the patient, "I'll just sit here with you for a while," and then remain with the patient.

ENCOURAGING ELABORATION

Statements such as "You said you have had a difficult time with pain these last few months" or "Tell me more about that" encourage the patient to share feelings about what has been happening. "I'm not certain that I follow what you mean" is another way to encourage the patient to continue. **Encouraging elaboration is used to elicit further information about a topic.** This technique might be used rather than restatement or reflection.

GIVING INFORMATION

Nurses must give patients information about medications, procedures, diagnostic tests, and self-care. Giving information concisely and allowing time for questions is therapeutic for the patient. Pay attention to nonverbal signals and ask for feedback to verify that the patient has understood the information given.

LOOKING AT ALTERNATIVES

Nurses help patients solve problems. To accomplish this, they are sometimes directive in assisting the patient to look at alternative solutions to a problem. Some helpful leads for this purpose are "You might think about...," "Have you thought of your options?" or "What do you think are possible solutions?" The focus is on assisting patients to look at things from their point of view while you refrain from giving advice.

SUMMARIZING

Summarizing what has occurred during the interaction is helpful. A summary of alternative solutions to a problem, decisions made, plans for action, or feelings that have been expressed provides closure to the interaction. "You've indicated that you have a choice between undergoing surgery and trying medication for your problem. We've discussed the potential side effects and benefits of both treatments, and now you want some time to think about it" would be a summarizing statement.

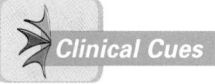
Clinical Cues

To improve your therapeutic communication skills, you will have to practice. Your instructor may ask you to do a process recording. Practice your skills with a real patient, then analyze and think about the patient's behavior and your response. *(See the **Companion CD-ROM** for an example of a process recording.)*

BLOCKS TO EFFECTIVE COMMUNICATION

Just as there are phrases and cues that encourage effective communication, there are phrases that tend to block or terminate interaction. Table 8-2 summarizes blocks to effective communication.

CHANGING THE SUBJECT

When a patient is speaking and you change the subject, it indicates that there is discomfort, disinterest, or anxiety on your part. There is avoidance of listening to a patient's pain, distress, fear, or perception of problems. If you change the subject in an effort to keep the patient's thoughts off unpleasant things, you deny the patient's desire to express feelings. Sometimes the patient will talk about an experience that is similar to something that happened to you. It is tempting to relate your experience, directing the conversation away from the patient. Students often make this mistake. Over time, you'll learn to consider whether the information is of real value to the patient before sharing your personal experiences.

OFFERING FALSE REASSURANCE

Giving reassurance not based on fact is damaging because it discounts the patient's concerns and destroys trust. Saying "Don't worry; everything is going to be fine" when a patient has valid concerns indicates a lack of understanding. The nurse who tells a woman who has just had breast surgery that she should not think that her husband will find her scar distasteful because she is "still a beautiful woman" is offering inappropriate reassurance about someone else's feelings. This type of comment conveys the message that you do not care about the patient's fears and feelings about her new body image and jeopardizes the professional relationship. Reassurance should be based on fact. Informing a patient that there will be some discomfort after a diagnostic procedure but that analgesic medication will be available to relieve that discomfort is much better than saying that it is a simple procedure and not to worry. A realistic approach helps maintain trust.

Table 8-2 **Blocks to Effective Communication**

TECHNIQUE	EXAMPLE	RATIONALE
Changing the subject	Patient says, "I'm so worried about my husband." Nurse says, "It is time for your bath now."	Deprives the patient of the chance to verbalize concerns.
Giving false reassurance	"I'm sure it will turn out fine." "You don't need to worry."	Negates the patient's feelings and may give false hope, which, when things turn out differently, can destroy trust in the nurse.
Judgmental response	"I don't think that was a good thing for you to do considering you have diabetes."	Nurse is judging the patient's action. Implies that the patient must take on the nurse's values and is demeaning to the patient.
Defensive response	Patient says, "My doctor never seems to know what is going on." Nurse says, "Dr. Smith is a very good doctor; he's here every day."	Nurse responds by defending the doctor. Prevents patients from feeling that they are free to express their feelings.
Asking probing questions	"Why were you there at that hour?" "What did you intend to prove?"	Pries into the patient's motives and therefore invades privacy.
Using clichés	"Cheer up, you'll be home soon." "This won't hurt for long." "You have a long life ahead of you."	Negates the patient's individual situation; stereotypes the patient. This type of response sounds flippant and prevents the building of trust between patient and nurse.
Giving advice	"If I were you, I would... ." "I think you should... ." "Why don't you... ."	Tends to be controlling and diminishes patients' responsibility for taking charge of their own health.
Inattentive listening	Turning your back when the patient is sharing feelings or pertinent information; showing impatience with body language (i.e., tapping your foot or having your hand on the door to go out).	Indicates that the patient is not important, that the nurse is bored, or that what is being said does not matter.

GIVING ADVICE

Giving advice is another area that prevents many novice nurses from being more therapeutic. **Giving advice places the focus on the nurse rather than the patient.** Also, many patients often think that they must do what you say because you are the authority figure. Your role is to guide patients to alternative choices for solving their own problems.

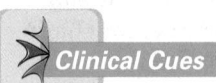 Clinical Cues

You should **not** use phrases such as "Why don't you...," "When that happened to me, I did..," or "I think you should... ." Rephrase to help the patient explore various alternatives. For example, "Have you thought of your options?," or "You might want to think about...," or "Have you considered...?"

DEFENSIVE COMMENTS

Becoming defensive when a patient has a complaint interferes with effective communication. If a patient complains that the call light is not promptly answered in the evenings and you state, "You should realize how short-staffed we are in the evenings," the patient is denied the right to a valid view and complaint. By taking a position opposite to the patient's point of view, you take on the role of adversary rather than helper. Acknowledge the patient's feelings by saying something like, "It's upsetting when no one can get here promptly."

PRYING OR PROBING QUESTIONS

Probing questions may place the patient on the defensive. This occurs when you ask questions about the patient's private business, and these questions have no relation to the treatment or clinical condition. Questioning why the patient did or did not do a particular thing makes the patient defensive about the action and may cause feelings of discomfort. If you ask a patient who has been injured in an automobile accident, "Why were you driving so fast in the rain?," you are inappropriately probing.

USING CLICHÉS

A cliché is an overused expression that may have no real relation to the current situation. Comments such as "You'll be fine," "Don't worry, it will turn out OK," or "There will be a light at the end of the tunnel" are clichés. They show a lack of respect for the patient as an individual. These comments discount what the particular patient might feel. If you use clichés, patients will feel that their individual situations are not being addressed. It is better to express that you are available to listen to the patient's concerns and feelings and to be supportive as needed.

INATTENTIVE LISTENING

Failing to really listen to what the patient has to say is a block to communication. If you continue to straighten the room and turn away while the patient is trying to express feelings or something of importance, your actions express to the patient that you are not interested. **Interrupting or jumping in before the patient has finished speaking also indicates inattentive listening.** Frequently changing the subject or focusing the conversation away from the patient's concerns expresses that you are not interested in listening.

? *Think Critically About* . . . Observe nurses in the hospital as they are communicating with patients. What types of blocks to communication do you see occurring? Speculate as to why these nurses are blocking communication with their patients.

INTERVIEWING SKILLS

An interview is more directed than a therapeutic communication interaction. It is planned and has a definite purpose. It is important to establish rapport (a relationship of mutual trust or affinity) with the patient before beginning an interview (Communication Cues 8-1). Introduce yourself and ask how the patient wishes to be addressed. Include the family in your greeting. Explain the purpose of the interview and provide privacy. Ask patients if they wish their family or friends to remain during the interview by saying, "Would it be better if we are alone for this interview?" Eliminate excess noise by turning off the television or radio. Be certain that the patient is comfortable, draw up a chair to within 3 to 4 feet, and sit down facing the patient (Figure 8-3). Chapter 5 contains more information about the interview.

For an admission interview in which a health history is to be obtained, take control of the interaction and initially ask closed questions that call for specific data. This type of direct interview does not allow the patient to ask questions or discuss concerns until all the necessary information has been collected. Examples of questions might include the following:

- What medications did you take today?
- Do you have pain?
- Do you have any allergies?
- If you have been hospitalized before, what year was it?

After taking the history, use open-ended questions to find out how the patient feels about the hospitalization. Examples of useful open-ended questions include "What brought you to the hospital?" "What are your concerns about this hospitalization?" and "Do you have any questions?" This last question indicates that the interview is coming to an end. A brief summary statement, ending with "I think I have the information I need," closes the interview. Thank the patient for supplying the information collected before leaving the room. An example of the nursing admission history form is found in Chapter 5.

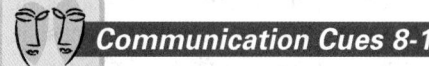
Communication Cues 8-1

Establishing Rapport

To establish rapport with a patient so that you can proceed with the interview or therapeutic interaction, you might use a few of these phrases:

- "Hello, Mr. Sanchez, I'm John; I'd like to know more about you. Can you tell me a little about what you do for a living (or did before you retired)?"
- "Mrs. Jackson, I see that you live alone. Can you tell me a little about your friends and activities?"
- "Ms. Lee, you've had a lot happen to you over the last few weeks; it must be hard to have your life interrupted this way."
- "Mr. Roth, you've been here several days and I don't know what you like to do in your spare time. Do you have any hobbies?"
- "Janice, your mom says you play basketball. It must be hard not being able to play during this part of the season."
- "Joey, it's OK to be angry and cry when you've been hurt. Can you tell me how your leg feels now?"

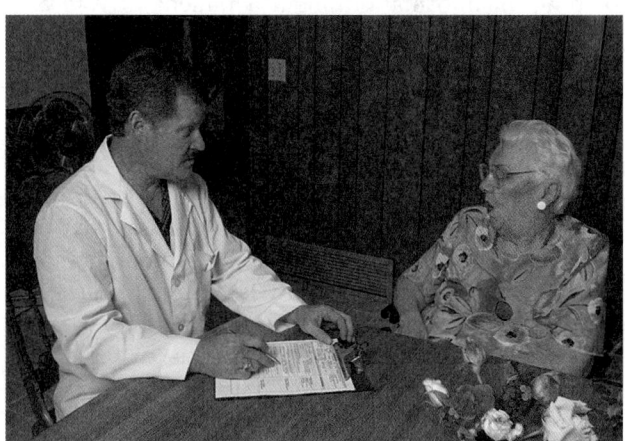

FIGURE **8-3** Interviewing the patient.

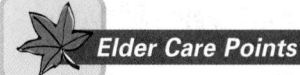
Elder Care Points

When taking a lengthy history from an elderly patient, it may be necessary to redirect the interaction frequently if the patient focuses too long on one illness or hospitalization.

THE NURSE-PATIENT RELATIONSHIP

The nurse-patient relationship focuses on the patient, has goals, and is defined by specific boundaries. The relationship takes place in the health care setting, and boundaries are defined by the patient's problems, the help needed, and the nurse's professional role. When the patient is discharged, the relationship ends.

Good communication skills establish a therapeutic relationship between you and the patient that assists in the patient's healing process. **In this relationship, you are in a helper role rather than a social role.** Interaction between you and the patient should build trust. Without trust, the patient will discount much of what you say.

A social relationship differs from a therapeutic one in that the focus is on both participants and the usual goal is to meet one's own needs. The social relationship is established for mutual enjoyment, and there is considerable sharing of experiences, life events, and thoughts. Social relationships are terminated when one or the other person does not feel that the relationship meets perceived needs any longer.

Characteristics in the nurse that facilitate a therapeutic nurse-patient relationship include effective communication skills, the quality of empathy (ability to understand by seeing the situation from another's perspective), a desire to help, honesty, a nonjudgmental attitude, genuineness, acceptance, and respect for the individual. **Confidentiality on your part must be maintained for trust to endure.** Confidentiality means keeping all information about a patient private and not discussing any patient information with those who are not involved in the patient's care.

EMPATHY

Empathy is the ability to place oneself in another's position. It involves being able to see situations through another person's eyes and perceive them as that person does. If empathy is present, the other person's feeling is understood. Empathy is different from sympathy. With sympathy, concern and perhaps sorrow are felt, indicating that the person is experiencing something difficult. Warmth, a nonjudgmental attitude, and a focus on the patient's feelings are present when empathy is expressed. Be careful about saying "I know how you feel" or "I understand what you are going through" because no one can really know or feel what someone else is experiencing. State an interpretation of the patient's feeling and then seek validation that the interpretation is accurate.

? *Think Critically About* . . . Why is empathy important in the nurse-patient relationship? Discuss incidents where you (or someone you observed) had trouble feeling empathy for a patient. What were the outcomes? What could have been done to alter the situation?

BECOMING NONJUDGMENTAL

Becoming nonjudgmental takes considerable practice and discipline and is directly related to the degree of empathy a person is capable of generating. It is far easier to accept people as they are if things can be truly

seen through their eyes. Patients come from all kinds of backgrounds and have many different sets of values. To be nonjudgmental, you must look at the patient in reference to her values rather than your own.

Be genuine in what is said and done with patients because this helps establish trust. Try to keep promises. A statement such as "I'll be back in 30 minutes" requires that you return to the room at the appointed time. Write down notes on information to be obtained for patients so that the task is not forgotten, and keep interactions focused on the patient. Personal revelations and anecdotes are out of place unless they directly apply to the patient's problems and can be helpful.

MAINTAINING HOPE

Maintaining hope is an important part of the nurse-patient relationship. There is always hope, even if the direction of hope changes. The dying patient can hope for less pain, peace, a pleasant moment, and a good laugh. A patient with cancer can hope for a positive prognosis, a healing outcome from surgery or therapy, or emotional growth from the illness experience. The patient should be helped to establish realistic hopes, but even unrealistic hopes should not be totally dismissed. **Hope is what helps a patient cope in a difficult situation.**

Application of the Nursing Process

Assess the language ability of the patient during the first encounter. Consider the following questions when gathering data about the communication needs of the patient:

- Is English spoken and understood?
- Is the vocabulary level equivalent to that of the average person of this age, or will it be necessary to simplify language to achieve comprehension of communication?
- Does the patient have a neurologic impairment that causes problems with the comprehension of oral or written communication or with the ability to hear or speak?
- What cultural factors affect the way in which this patient is accustomed to interacting verbally?
- How much personal space does the person need in order not to feel threatened or intimidated?
- If the person is unable to speak but can communicate in writing, what provisions need to be made to accommodate this?

Patients who have problems with communication are given the nursing diagnosis of Impaired verbal communication. If the problem is related to difficulty with hearing, the nursing diagnosis of Disturbed sensory perception is used.

Besides writing individual expected outcomes, you must plan appropriate amounts of time with the patient for a communication interaction. An assessment interview should not take more than one-half hour. If the

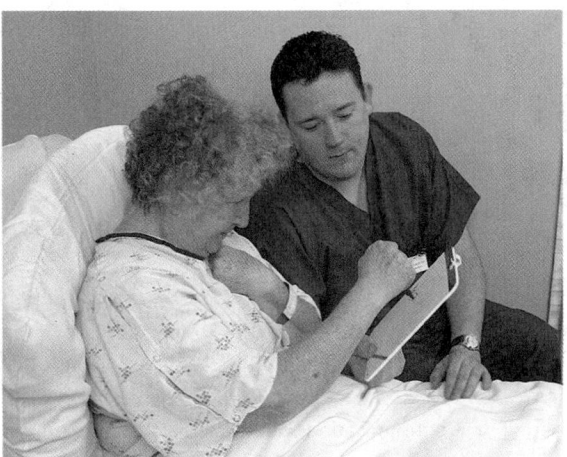

FIGURE **8-4** Communicating with an aphasic patient.

Box 8-1 | *Communicating with the Aphasic Person*

- Make the environment as relaxed and quiet as possible.
- Assume the patient can understand what is heard even though speech is jargon or the patient is mute unless deafness has been diagnosed.
- Speak to the patient on an adult level; do not act as if the patient is mentally incompetent.
- Talk to the patient; do not talk to someone else in the room about the patient.
- Face the patient, establish eye contact, and speak slowly and distinctly without dropping the voice level at the end of sentences; do not shout.
- Give directions with short phrases and simple terms; use pantomime to enhance the words.
- Phrase questions so that they can be answered with a "yes" or "no," and look for nonverbal behavior that agrees with the patient's answer.
- Give the person time to respond to questions; processing may be slower than usual.
- Ask only one question at a time; be patient and wait for an answer.
- If there is a need to repeat something, use the same words the second time. If there is still difficulty, phrase what was said differently.
- Use body language to enhance the message.
- Allow one person to speak at a time.
- Be patient.

---

patient has communication impairment, varying amounts of time will be needed for each interaction. When a patient does not speak English, plan ahead and try to locate an interpreter before beginning an interaction with the patient. If the patient has aphasia (difficulty expressing or understanding language), obtain the assistance of a speech therapist to determine methods that facilitate communication. A white erasable board is handy for those who can write (Figure 8-4).

There are some techniques that can be helpful when communicating with a patient who has aphasia as a result of neurologic damage from a stroke or head injury. The use of appropriate nonverbal gestures some-

times helps. Guidelines presented in Box 8-1 can assist you in communicating more effectively with the aphasic patient. (*See Nursing Care Plan 8-1 on the* **Companion CD-ROM** *for care of the patient with impaired communication.*)

NURSE-PATIENT COMMUNICATION

COMMUNICATING WITH THE HEARING-IMPAIRED PATIENT

When a patient is identified as being hearing impaired, determine how to interact with the patient to promote the best level of communication. If the patient has hearing aids, see that they are used, that the batteries are functioning, and that the device is turned on before trying to communicate. A hearing aid does not guarantee that the individual will hear really well. The following techniques promote comprehension for a hearing-impaired person:

- Speak very distinctly. Do not shout because this can distort speech and does not make the message any clearer.
- Speak slowly and keep the voice pitch at midrange, neither low nor high.
- Get the person's attention, making sure the person is aware that verbalization is going to take place.
- The best distance for speaking to a hearing-impaired person is 2½ to 4 feet. Face the person at eye level. If the person is seated, sit down or bend down. Never speak directly into the person's ear. This can distort the message and hide all visual cues.
- Be aware of nonverbal communication. Facial expressions, gestures, and lip and body movements all give cues to the meaning of the message.
- Use short, simple sentences. If the patient does not appear to understand or responds inappropriately, rephrase the statement. Try to limit each sentence to one subject and one verb. Give the person time to respond to questions.
- Ask for rephrasing to make sure the patient has understood important information.

COMMUNICATING WITH THE ELDERLY

The elderly vary greatly in their communication abilities, interests, and capabilities. Healthy older adults sometimes require more time to think and formulate a response. Other older adults may have hearing, sensory, or motor impairments that interfere with communication. It is best to be certain you have the person's attention before beginning a purposeful interaction. Eliminate outside distractions. Try to introduce one idea at a time. Do not rush the person because this may cause confusion.

It is especially important to obtain feedback from an older adult that the message has been clearly under-

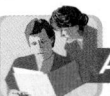

Sharing Communication Tips

Nursing assistants often provide much of the basic activities of daily living (ADLs) care for elderly persons. Share your knowledge about how to communicate with elderly patients and ask the assistants for their input. Also ask them to share their communication success stories.

stood. If people have difficulty comprehending, they may just nod their head, pretending to understand, for fear of appearing dense or forgetful. Many are embarrassed about their hearing deficiency.

Wait for an answer to one question before asking another. Try not to introduce more than one subject at a time in the conversation, and give only one instruction in any one sentence. It is also important for all members of the health care team to communicate in a consistent manner with elderly patients (Assignment Considerations 8-1).

COMMUNICATING WITH CHILDREN

The influence of development on language and thought processes must be taken into account to communicate effectively with children. Young children are very responsive to nonverbal messages. A young child may become frightened by sudden movements or gestures. Approach the child at eye level and use a calm, quiet, friendly voice when communicating.

When interacting with an infant, try to keep the mother within the baby's view. With a toddler or a preschooler, focus on the child's needs and concerns. Use simple, short sentences, and concrete explanations with familiar words.

For the school-age child, give simple explanations and demonstrate how equipment works. Allow the child to handle the equipment if possible. Listen carefully to the child's fears or concerns.

An adolescent needs time to talk. Use active listening, avoid interrupting, and show acceptance. Try not to give advice, and avoid embarrassing questions if at all possible.

Above all, with any child, be honest and tell the child what to expect.

COMMUNICATING WITH PEOPLE FROM OTHER CULTURES

Determine if the person speaks and understands English. If not, obtain an interpreter if possible. Be accepting; do not show impatience with lack of ability to speak English. Most health care agencies have a list of interpreters that can be called for assistance with translation (Figure 8-5).

Follow the patient's lead about the use of eye contact. If the patient is not comfortable making eye con-

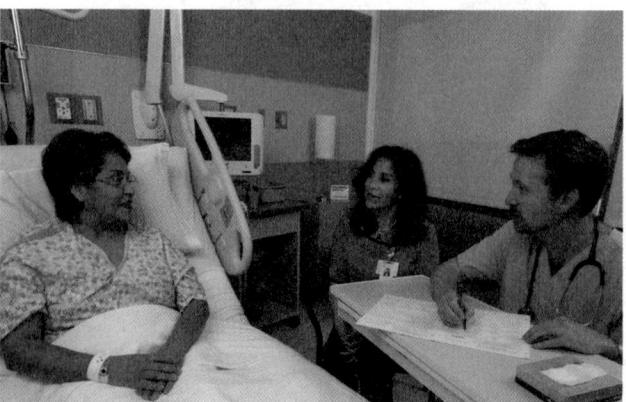

FIGURE **8-5** Communicating with the assistance of a translator.

Cultural Cues 8-4

Assisting Elders from Other Cultures

Remember that in some cultures, it is not usual for an older adult to take instruction from a young person. It may be necessary to enlist the aid of an adult family member who will learn the essentials of self-care for the patient, and then have that person perform the patient teaching. Give the person printed materials and be available to demonstrate or answer questions.

tact, respect this cultural difference. The same is true for the use of distance between you and the patient when speaking. Watch how much distance is maintained between the patient and other people when they interact. Cultural Cues 8-4 presents strategies to use when teaching older adults from other cultures.

For the nurse who is from another culture and whose primary language is not English, it is very important to work on English language skills and correct pronunciation. Your patients are dependent on good communication with you. If you cannot communicate well in English, you may miss catching important signs and symptoms of a change in a patient's condition. Inability to communicate well with the nurse adds further stress to the patient's situation and leads to dissatisfaction with care. Most communities have classes for students who wish to improve their English.

COMMUNICATION WITHIN THE HEALTH CARE TEAM

Communication within the health care team occurs through writing and reading nurses' notes, physicians' orders, the dietitian's notes, and notes and orders of the respiratory, physical, speech, and occupational therapists, as well as listening to and giving a shift report (a verbal communication on the details of a patient's condition and treatment). Filling out a wide variety of forms for the laboratory, radiology, and

Box 8-2 *Information Included in End-of-Shift Report*

- Room number, bed designation; patient name, age, and sex; date of admission; medical diagnoses; and name of primary physician. (If a computer census sheet is used that contains some of this information, then only the room number and name and any missing data are given.)
- Tests and treatments or therapies performed in the past 24 hours with patient response (e.g., computed tomography [CT] scans, surgery, arteriogram); intake and output for past shift.
- Significant changes in patient condition.
- Scheduled tests; consults or surgery; current intravenous solution, flow rate, and amount remaining; next solution to be hung; oxygen flow rate; equipment in use and current settings (e.g., gastric suction on low).
- Current problems (e.g., dehydration, severe pain, anxiety, depression, insufficient rest, or abnormal laboratory values or test results); amount of assistance with activities of daily living (ADLs) needed.
- Scheduled treatments, PRN (as needed) medications given, times given, patient response.
- Concerns, need for order changes, teaching, pertinent family dynamics, and emotional status.

other departments is another method of communication. Entering information on the computer is an essential tool for communication among hospital departments. Clear communication is necessary when consulting with the physician about orders and when delegating tasks to ancillary workers.

END-OF-SHIFT REPORT

Many different formats are used to give a report. Sometimes the report is given as the nurses from the off-going and on-coming shifts walk around from room to room together. This method is termed *walking rounds.* If the report is recorded on an audiotape or if computerized sheets are used, there must be an opportunity to ask and respond to questions. Whatever format is used, the same essential information is necessary for each patient. Get in the habit of organizing the report in the same way each day. A full report on each patient should take about 1 to 3 minutes. Give only essential information. It takes practice to give a logical, organized, concise report on a group of patients. Practicing at home with a tape recorder can help you gain confidence and present information more concisely. Box 8-2 presents the information usually given in an end-of-shift report. One style that can be used for reporting is the SBAR (situation, background, assessment, and recommendation) format (Safety Alert 8-1). If the initial information is handed out on a computer printout, it need not be repeated. The room number and name of the patient are sufficient as a starting point.

Computer-printed Kardex-type information sheets are available at the beginning of the shift for the on-

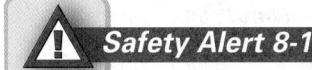

Safety Alert 8-1

SBAR

In accordance with the 2008 National Patient Safety Goals, an end-of-shift report should be conducted in a standardized manner in which caregivers have the opportunity to ask and respond to questions concerning patient care. The **SBAR** format is borrowed from military communication models and has been successfully used in some health care settings. SBAR stands for situation, background, assessment, and recommendation.

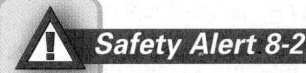

Safety Alert 8-2

Taking Telephone Orders

In accordance with the 2008 National Patient Safety Goals, when taking a telephone order from a physician, you should listen, write down the order, and then read it back to the doctor.

coming nurse in most hospitals. This sheet can be taken and used as a work organization sheet. If notes are added to the sheet during the shift, all the information needed for the report at the end of the shift should be readily at hand.

TELEPHONING PHYSICIANS

Physicians must be telephoned from time to time. Orders may be unclear, the patient's condition may change, the patient may have a particular request, or further information about the patient may be needed from the physician.

If a physician is called regarding a change in a patient's condition or in any situation in which new orders are anticipated, certain steps should be followed. Have current data on the patient at hand, including data from the last vital signs assessment, pertinent laboratory data, information on urinary output, and medications received. Keep the chart handy, have a pencil and paper ready, and anticipate the information that the physician might need to make a decision. Know what allergies the patient has. Perform a quick assessment before calling, and prepare a concise statement of the problem or concern. Document the call, and note the health care provider's statement that the order is correct as read (Safety Alert 8-2).

In addition to its use for the end-of-shift report, SBAR can also be used when communicating with or telephoning physicians (Box 8-3).

The student nurse should have an instructor or another registered nurse standing by to take the new orders from the physician because **students cannot legally take telephone orders.**

| Box 8-3 | *Example of SBAR Communication*

S: Dr. Savoy, this is Nurse Lopez at ABC Extended Care Facility. Mr. Tanglewood is an 85-year-old man with Alzheimer's disease. He tripped in the bathroom and bumped his head on the toilet about 30 minutes ago. One of the nursing assistants saw him trip and there was no loss of consciousness at any time.

B: He is normally alert and oriented to person, and he routinely ambulates independently.

A: His blood pressure is currently 140/83, pulse 75, respirations 16/min. He has a 3-cm laceration and hematoma just superior to his left eyebrow. The bleeding was readily controlled with direct pressure. We have applied an ice pack and pressure bandage over the wound. He is alert and his speech is clear and appropriate to his baseline. He denies any pain, and he does not seem to have tenderness or bruising except on his forehead, but he did extend his right hand to break his fall.

R: Could I get an order to have him transported to the emergency room for additional evaluation and treatment? And do you have any additional orders for Mr. Tanglewood?

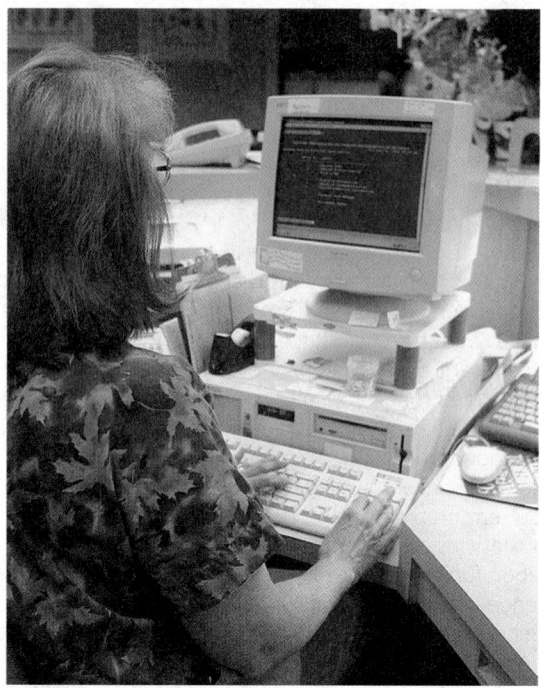

FIGURE **8-6** Communicating by computer.

ASSIGNMENT CONSIDERATIONS AND DELEGATING

You must communicate well in order to assign tasks and delegate (authorize another person to do something) to others effectively. Give clear, concise messages and listen carefully to feedback. Include the desired results and the time constraints for completion of the task. It is better to say "Let me know if Mrs. Hope's noon temperature is above 101.2° F" than to say "Let me know if Mrs. Hope's temperature is high." Ask the person to whom you are assigning a task if there are any questions about what is to be done, and ask for a summary of what is understood about the task to be done.

COMPUTER COMMUNICATION

The computer is used to transmit requests for laboratory, dietary, radiology, physical therapy, respiratory therapy, and other services. Medication orders from the physician are entered into the computer in the pharmacy, and the orders are communicated to the nurse on a patient medication administration record. Supplies for patient care are ordered on the computer, and patient care plans are updated using the keyboard or a touch screen (Figure 8-6). Legal & Ethical Considerations 8-1 includes additional tips regarding computer usage in health care settings.

Many hospitals and home care agencies are converting to a computerized form of charting. In some agencies a hand-held computer is used to note medications given, input (put in information) vital signs, chart assessment data, and record the nurse's observations. The ability to use a computer for communication is essential for today's nurse.

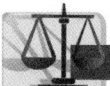 **Legal & Ethical Considerations 8-1**

Computer Usage and Safeguarding Patient Information

Computerized patient information requires extra vigilance to safeguard confidentiality. When you use the computer at the health care facility, remember not to leave a computer screen open when you are finished. Always log out so that someone else cannot access information using your password, and of course do not share your password with others. If your facility uses e-mail to communicate about patient care, it is likely that you will receive training to prevent HIPAA violations. (See Chapter 3 for additional information about HIPAA.)

COMMUNICATION IN THE HOME AND COMMUNITY

Nurses who work in home care often have both a professional role and a social role with their patients and families. Often, the nurse is the only person whom the patient sees on the day of a visit. Because of the social aspects of the visit, it is essential to state when instructions are about to be given so that active listening can occur. Home Care Considerations 8-1 gives additional tips to help you maximize your interview time. Leave written step-by-step instructions with the patient whenever possible. This can prevent many problems. The primary nurse will often call between visits to see how treatment is progressing and to assess for any problems. Safety Alert 8-3 gives additional information that applies to home care phone communication.

Office and clinic nurses often assess patients who call in to see if they have an urgent need for medical

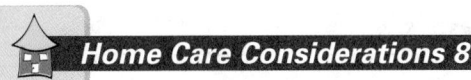

Tips for Efficient Interviewing

Before the initial home visit, ask the home care patient or family to make a list of all medications the patient is taking, including over-the-counter medicines and herbal preparations, and to have the vials and bottles all in one place. Ask that a list of the patient's physicians with phone numbers be ready for you, plus the dates of any recent hospitalization or surgery. This will save you time when doing the interview, and you can take the lists with you for the later completion of your paperwork.

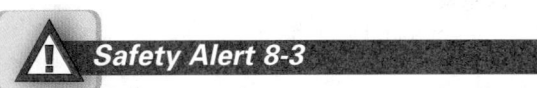

Phone Communication in Home Care Settings

In accordance with the 2008 National Patient Safety Goals, it would be inappropriate for a physician to leave orders for a home care patient on a voice mail message or to ask the family to convey the orders to the nurse. Likewise, a nurse should not leave instructions for a nursing assistant on a voice mail. Exchange of phone information between members of the health care team should follow the format: listen, write, read back, and allow time for questions.

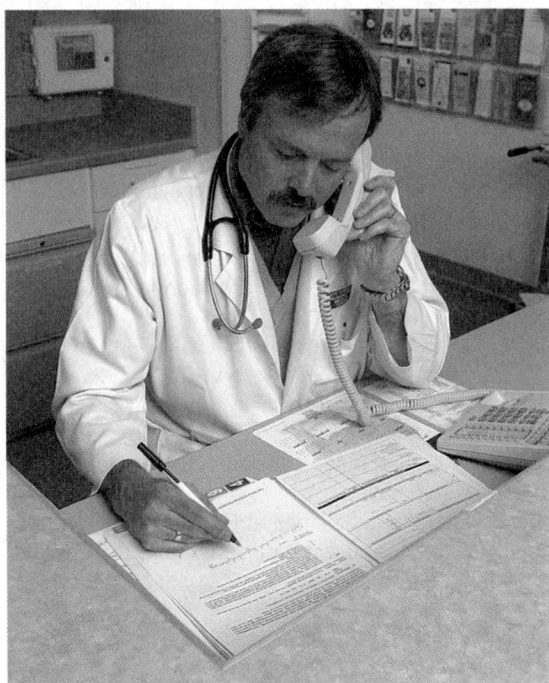

FIGURE **8-7** The nurse instructs a clinic patient over the telephone.

attention. Such assessment requires good communication to obtain the data needed to make such a decision (Figure 8-7). The office nurse gives telephone instructions to patients on how to treat minor illnesses or injuries. It is important in these situations to obtain

feedback so that there is no doubt that the patient understands the instructions.

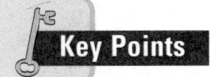

- Communication is a continuous, circular process and occurs in two ways: verbal and nonverbal.
- Culture, past experience, emotions, attitude, mood, and self-concept all contribute to the way people communicate.
- Interpretation of messages is influenced by cultural values, level of education, familiarity with the topic, occupation, and type of previous life experiences.
- An active listener maintains eye contact without staring, gives the patient full attention, and makes a conscious effort to block out other sounds and distractions.
- A period of silence gives the patient time to think and respond.
- Open-ended questions, restating, clarifying, using general leads, offering of self, encouraging elaboration, giving information, looking at alternatives, and summarizing are all therapeutic communication techniques.
- Gentle touch that indicates caring is therapeutic.
- Changing the subject, offering false reassurance, giving advice, making defensive comments, asking probing questions, using clichés, and inattentive listening are blocks to good communication.
- A therapeutic relationship focuses on the patient; helping the patient to maintain hope is important.
- Empathy, a desire to help, honesty, a nonjudgmental attitude, genuineness, acceptance, and respect for the individual also facilitate a therapeutic nurse-patient relationship.
- Special communication techniques are needed for the patient experiencing aphasia (see Box 8-1).
- For patients with a hearing impairment, speak slowly and clearly and face the person.
- The child should be approached at eye level with a calm, quiet, friendly voice when communicating.
- Be accepting and do not show impatience if a patient does not speak English; look for cultural cues regarding eye contact and distance between speaker and listener.
- An end-of-shift report should include patient's name, age, and changes in condition; current concerns; treatments; and response to therapies.
- When taking telephone orders: listen, write, and read back what you have written.
- Protect passwords and log off when using the computer.

 Go to your **Companion CD-ROM** for an Audio Glossary, animations, video clips, and more.

evolve Be sure to visit the companion Evolve site at http://evolve.elsevier.com/deWit/fundamental/ for additional online resources.

NCLEX-PN® EXAMINATION-STYLE REVIEW QUESTIONS

*Choose the **best** answer(s) for each question.*

1. The nurse is using therapeutic communication to establish rapport. The nurse says, "How are you feeling this morning?" Which nonverbal behavior is congruent with the nurse's verbal question?

   1. Looks at patient; stands with a relaxed body position
   2. Nods head up and down; arms folded across chest
   3. Smiles at patient and makes the bed while patient answers
   4. Adjusts IV and evaluates equipment and environment

2. A patient expresses serious concerns about the outcomes of a scheduled surgical procedure. Which of following indicates that the nurse is using active listening while the patient is speaking?

   1. Nurse tells the patient not to worry about the surgery.
   2. Nurse asks the patient to take her medication before continuing.
   3. Nurse asks the patient why she is afraid of the surgery.
   4. Nurse nods his head.

3. The patient says, "I don't know whether chemotherapy or radiation would be best to treat this cancer." Correct restatement would be:

   1. "You think radiation would be best."
   2. "You'd prefer to have the chemotherapy."
   3. "You wondering if chemotherapy or radiation brings the best survival results."
   4. "Tell me what you think about each one of those treatments."

4. A patient says, "I don't know what to do about the problem." The most therapeutic response would be:

   1. "You should define the problem and make a plan."
   2. "What options are you considering?"
   3. "That's not a big problem, you can handle that."
   4. "Have you considered your options?"

5. The patient is aphasic. Which of the following communication strategies would be appropriate in working with this patient? (*Select all that apply.*)

   1. Lean forward and say "Go on... ."
   2. Face the patient, establish eye contact, and speak slowly.
   3. Use pantomime to enhance the words.
   4. Give the person time to respond to questions.
   5. Explain procedures to the family member instead of the patient.
   6. Give directions with short phrases and simple terms.

6. The patient is about to undergo surgery. Which of the following is an example of false reassurance?

   1. "Your surgery will take about 5½ hours."
   2. "You'll come through this procedure just fine."
   3. "Your family will be allowed to see you as soon as you are awake."
   4. "This surgeon has done many of these operations."

7. Which of the following elements characterizes a therapeutic relationship?

   1. Focus is on the patient's needs and there are specific goals.
   2. The patient and the nurse get satisfaction from the relationship.
   3. The patient and the nurse equally exchange information.
   4. The relationship is terminated if needs are not being satisfied.

8. When you are conducting a home care admission interview, time will be saved by:

   1. informing the patient of the purpose of the interview.
   2. calling the patient and asking her to make a list of her medications.
   3. asking open-ended questions to obtain essential data.
   4. including relatives and friends in the interaction.

9. A way to promote trust with a patient is to:

   1. allow family members to visit whenever they want.
   2. assure the patient that her doctor is excellent.
   3. follow through when you say you will do something.
   4. talk with her at length, about her life, likes, and dislikes.

10. A nurse is assigning a task to the nursing assistant. Which of the following is the best example of how to communicate the task to the assistant?

   1. "Please do all the vital signs for my patients, and pay special attention to Mrs. Hondo and Mr. Takedo."
   2. "Please report any abnormal vital signs throughout the day, and keep an eye on Mrs. Hondo and Mr. Takedo."
   3. "Please check Mrs. Hondo's and Mr. Takedo's blood pressure and pulse as ordered by the physician. Call me if you have problems."
   4. "Please do vitals signs at 8 A.M. on Mrs. Hondo and Mr. Takedo, and if the pulse is more than 85 per minute, let me know."

CRITICAL THINKING ACTIVITIES *Read each clinical scenario and discuss the questions with your classmates.*

Scenario A

You are working with a patient who is very quiet and withdrawn. When you walk into her room, she appears tearful and upset, but she tells you that there is nothing wrong. How would deal with this situation?

Scenario B

Consider your own communication style. What three factors do you think have had the greatest influence on the way you communicate?

Scenario C

Develop your own checklist for giving an end-of-shift report. Why is it important for the oncoming nurse to have an opportunity to ask questions?

Patient Teaching for Health Promotion

evolve http://evolve.elsevier.com/deWit/fundamental/

Objectives

Upon completing this chapter, you should be able to:

Theory

1. Discuss the purposes of patient teaching.
2. Describe three ways in which people learn and correlate the importance of these types of learning to teaching.
3. List and differentiate between conditions and factors that can affect learning.
4. Identify adjustments to the teaching plan needed for teaching the very young patient or the elderly patient.
5. Discuss types of resources available to assist in patient teaching.
6. Name three things that must be included in the documentation of patient teaching.
7. Use patient teaching to promote the national goals of health promotion and disease prevention as listed in *Healthy People 2010* and the Canada Health Act.
8. Describe ways in which teaching can be continued following hospital discharge.

Clinical Practice

1. Assess an assigned patient's learning needs.
2. Develop a teaching plan based on the patient's learning needs.
3. Implement the teaching plan at a prearranged time.
4. Evaluate the effectiveness of the teaching and the plan.

Key Terms

Be sure to check out the bonus material on the Companion CD-ROM, including selected audio pronunciations.

affective domain (p. 120)
auditory learning (ăw-dĭ-TŌR-ē, p. 120)
behavioral objectives (bē-HĀV-yŏr-ăl, p. 121)
cognitive domain (KŎG-nĭ-tĭv, p. 120)
feedback (p. 124)
kinesthetic learning (kĭn-ĕs-THĚT-ĭc, p. 120)
psychomotor domain (sī-kō-MŌ-tŏr dōw-MĀN, p. 120)
return demonstration (p. 124)
visual learning (p. 120)

PURPOSES OF PATIENT TEACHING

The ultimate goal of patient teaching is the prevention of illness and the promotion of wellness. **Nurses teach patients about their disease or disorder, including diet, medications, treatment, and self-care.** Preoperative teaching covers the various phases of the surgery, what will be experienced, what can be expected, and the exercises to be done afterward. With hospital stays being so short, patient education has become an even higher priority. **Prior to discharge, the patient must be taught how to care for himself at home.** Because of this, there must be collaboration on the teaching plan among the various health professionals involved in the care, as well as communication with the family and home care nurse, if any.

Patient teaching aids in achieving the goals of *Healthy People 2010*, a program of the U.S. Department of Health and Human Services, and the *Canada Health Act*. The goals of *Healthy People 2010* are to increase the life span and quality of life and eliminate health disparities among different populations. Enabling goals include promoting healthy behaviors, protecting health, ensuring access to quality health care, and strengthening community health prevention programs. Canadian principles include universality, comprehensiveness, accessibility, portability, and public administration.

Discharge planning requires looking ahead in order to meet the patient's ongoing needs at home. **It is a process that begins at the time of admission.** This includes assessing for special needs, learning to identify appropriate teaching moments, and providing learning opportunities that are brief and focused on preparing the patient for self-care. A *teaching moment* occurs when the patient is at an optimal level of readiness to learn and apply a particular piece of information. Take cues from the patient's questions or try to stimulate interest in what he needs to know. Saying, "You'll want to know things you can do to lower your risk of another heart attack" tends to stimulate interest in the recovering myocardial infarction patient.

? *Think Critically About* . . . Can you list three general teaching topics that might be appropriate for most patients under your care?

MODES OF LEARNING

Research has shown that people learn in three ways: (1) visually, through what they see (visual learning); (2) aurally, through what they hear (auditory learning); and (3) kinesthetically, by actually performing a task or handling items (kinesthetic learning). Although most people can learn by any of these routes, one route is usually dominant. For example, if a person is primarily a visual learner, *telling* him everything and not using any written materials or visual examples will make learning much more difficult. Many people do not know how they learn best. It is important to use a variety of teaching techniques so that the patient both sees and hears the information, and performs the action being taught.

? *Think Critically About* . . . Which of the three routes of learning usually works best for you? How have you seen a child learn? An older adult?

During the teaching sessions, listen to how the patient makes responses because the language used may give clues to the person's best learning mode.

Learning can also be categorized by domains. In the cognitive domain, the learner takes in and processes information by listening to or reading the material. In the affective domain, the material is presented in a way that appeals to the learner's beliefs, feelings, and values. For example, people must value cleanliness before you can teach them to wash their hands frequently. In the psychomotor domain, the learner processes the information by performing an action or carrying out a task. All three domains are important to the patient's translation of the learning to desired behaviors.

ASSESSMENT OF LEARNING NEEDS

In order to prepare a teaching plan, you must first know what the patient needs to learn. What does the person need to know about the disease or condition, diet, activity, medications, wound care, treatments, or self-care at home? This information establishes the learning needs.

Patients may require far more complex teaching than can be accomplished in the short time before discharge. In this instance, the basic survival skills are taught first, and after discharge the advanced skills are taught in group or private sessions. Often, a home health nurse will continue with the teaching plan. Make a list of the learning needs and then prioritize them so that you can concentrate first on teaching the essential knowledge needed for safe care at home. Place the identified learning needs on the patient's plan of care.

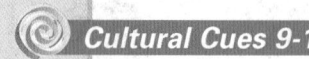 **Cultural Cues 9-1**

Acceptance of Teaching

While planning teaching for male patients of other cultures, find out if the male will be receptive to your teaching. Traditional older Japanese men may not heed what a younger female is trying to teach. This may apply in other cultures as well. Interaction with the family or with the patient himself can provide the needed information.

? *Think Critically About* . . . How would you assess the patient's current understanding to determine where he has knowledge deficits related to his health or self-care?

FACTORS AFFECTING LEARNING

Before beginning to teach, you must assess for factors that might interfere with the patient's ability to learn. Conditions that can affect the learning process include poor vision or hearing, impaired motor function, illiteracy, and impaired cognition. Age may interfere with the strength or dexterity for performing certain tasks. Physical, occupational, or speech therapists can be helpful in assisting the individual to overcome these types of problems so teaching can begin.

Situational factors that interfere with learning include pain, nausea, fatigue, a sense of being overwhelmed by all that is happening, and multiple interruptions.

Cultural Values and Expectations

The patient's cultural values and personal expectations regarding treatment and recovery may differ from those of the nurse and other health care providers. This can interfere with the patient's ability to cooperate and learn needed skills for self-care (Cultural Cues 9-1). **It is necessary to work within the patient's values and cultural system.** The patient may wish to use herb poultices on a wound rather than the medication the physician prescribes. Often a compromise can be worked out, such as alternating the poultice with the medication prescribed (as long as the poultice is not harmful). Patients may practice religious rituals as an aid to healing with which the nurse may not be familiar. In hospitals on American Indian reservations, it is common to see a physician and a tribal shaman working side by side, honoring the strong belief that physical healing must be accompanied by spiritual healing. Such practices rarely conflict with medical treatment and may greatly benefit the patient.

? *Think Critically About* . . . Can you think of a situation in which a patient's culture or value system might prevent his cooperation with learning self-care aspects of his treatment plan?

Confidence and Abilities

Often patients express a lack of self-confidence, saying, "I'll never be able to do that." In such instances you must explore these feelings, being careful to enhance rather than harm the patient's self-esteem. Praise and encouragement go much further than admonishment in promoting needed learning. Teaching may need to be broken down into very small steps (Communication Cues 9-1 on p. 122).

Play techniques can be very successful when teaching younger children. The use of dolls and play equipment is appropriate and helpful. Teaching must be done in short segments to allow for the child's limited attention span. Language must be tailored to the child's level of understanding. Children interpret language literally, so avoid idioms because they can be easily misunderstood.

When teaching the elderly, the pace is slowed to allow more time for processing the information. Patient Teaching 9-1 presents other points to consider.

Never assume that patients are literate. Many adults have gotten through school without learning to read adequately, and they may have spent a lifetime hiding this fact from friends, employers, spouses, and children. A teaching plan using visuals and kinesthetic learning will often be the most effective for these individuals.

Some patients who speak English as a second language may not be able to read English, even if they are fully literate in their original language. When working with a patient for whom another language is primary, offer printed, audiovisual materials in their native language, if available.

When printed materials are used, go over them with the patient and ask questions to determine whether the information has been understood. You should be aware of the patient's educational level so that you can appropriately tailor your vocabulary and teaching materials, but avoid talking down to people. **Assess what patients already know about the skills they need to learn so that you can build upon their current knowledge base.** Do they have a basic knowledge of anatomy and how the body works? What do they already know about their medications? If they are going to give their own injections, have they ever handled a needle and syringe before? Teaching is most effective when you can relate the material to a subject that patients already understand. It can also be very helpful to determine if they have a relative or close friend who is knowledgeable about their health issues and willing to help them after discharge.

Readiness to Learn

You must assess the patient's readiness to learn. Motivation plays a large role in effective learning. The desire to return to independence or to return to the comfort of home is often the motivating factor. **Work with patients to show them the advantages of learning what they need to know.** Teaching sessions will be more successful if the patient is comfortable and rested and there are a minimum of interruptions.

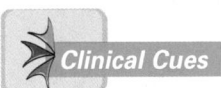
Clinical Cues

If the patient is in a double room and the other patient has several visitors and the noise level is raised, take the patient to the conference room or other location for the teaching session to promote better communication and reduce distractions.

Begin by establishing rapport and developing trust, and maintain a warm, sincere attitude.

Although there are several nursing diagnoses that can be utilized for learning needs, the most commonly used one is Deficient knowledge, with the specific need finishing the statement. Deficient knowledge related to wound care is one example.

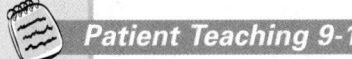
Patient Teaching 9-1

Special Considerations When Teaching the Elderly

When preparing to teach an elderly patient, consider the following:

- Provide good lighting; a light source coming over the shoulder of the patient is excellent.
- Printed materials should be in large type and are visualized best when they are in black type on white nonglare paper.
- Be certain the patient is wearing glasses, if needed, and that the lenses are clean.
- If the patient wears a hearing aid, be certain it is turned on and adjusted.
- Use short sentences and speak slowly; pause frequently to allow time for mental processing.
- Keep medical terms to a minimum and explain those you do use.
- Ask questions at frequent intervals to check for comprehension.

THE TEACHING PLAN

Preparing a teaching plan involves analyzing the assessment data, establishing behavioral objectives or goals, and creating a plan for assisting the patient to achieve these goals in the most timely and effective manner. Behavioral objectives represent the desired changes or additions to current behaviors and attitudes. They state what you are trying to teach the patient to do. "Patient will change the wound dressing using aseptic technique" is a behavioral objective. Behavioral objectives should be stated in terms that make achievement of the objective easy to evaluate. Evalua-

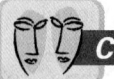 **Communication Cues 9-1**

Teaching the Patient Who Lacks Self-Confidence

Mrs. Dunn, age 72, is to be discharged tomorrow. She has a wound on her left thigh that needs to be cleaned and dressed daily after discharge.

NURSE: "Mrs. Dunn, I've brought the supplies we need to do your dressing change."

MRS. DUNN: "Oh, I don't think I can do it myself; it seems so complicated."

NURSE: "We'll work on it a step at a time. By the time you go home tomorrow, you will feel much better about it."

MRS. DUNN: "Well, I'm willing to try. I do want to go home."

NURSE: "The first step is easy, we just wash our hands."

MRS. DUNN: "Oh, good, I already know how to do that!"

NURSE: "Now, I use gloves here in the hospital, but you won't need to do that."

MRS. DUNN: "I'm glad. Gloves make me so clumsy."

NURSE: "Are you right-handed? OK, remove the old dressing by gently holding the skin smooth with your left hand while pulling the tape up with your right hand."

MRS. DUNN: "That was easy."

NURSE: "Good. Watch me open this package of gauze squares. Open the top and peel back the sides. Stop when you get to the bottom seam. Can you open that one for me?"

The patient picks up the package. She fumbles at first, then manages to grasp the edges and pull them apart as instructed. The nurse does not rush her.

NURSE: "Perfect. Now place it on the table with the paper side down, like this."

The patient places her pack as the nurse has shown her.

NURSE: "Now open the bottle of sterile water like this."

The nurse opens a bottle and sets the cap down on the table upside down.

NURSE: "By laying the cap down this way, the open side stays clean and will not contaminate the bottle when I put it back on. Now, you do it."

The patient picks up the bottle and twists it open, laying the cap on the table like the nurse did.

NURSE: "You're a fast learner, Mrs. Dunn. Now, pour a little on the gauze squares like this."

The patient watches, then pours some water in the middle of her gauze squares.

NURSE: "Now pick up one of the gauze squares and clean the wound just like the nurses have been doing it."

MRS. DUNN: "I'll try, but this is the part that always hurts."

NURSE: "I know, but it usually hurts less when you do it yourself. And if it isn't cleaned out well, it won't heal. You can take some acetaminophen about an hour before you change the dressing. That will help. I'll do the first square, then you do the second, OK?"

The nurse swabs out the wound gently.

NURSE: "Now you try it."

The patient picks up the gauze, squeezes out the excess water, and dabs a couple of times at the wound.

MRS. DUNN: "Like that?"

NURSE: "Yes, that's the idea. See if you can go over the wound a little more slowly from top to bottom with a new gauze square. It's important to use a clean one each time you go back over the area."

MRS. DUNN: "OK. Is this better?"

Mrs. Dunn cleans the area a little more thoroughly.

NURSE: "Yes. I'll give you some acetaminophen before we meet this afternoon and see if that makes it easier for you."

The nurse finishes cleaning the wound.

NURSE: "Now Mrs. Dunn, squeeze a bit of this antiseptic ointment into the wound."

MRS. DUNN: "How much do I use?"

NURSE: "Just a line down the center. It will spread out when the dressing is applied."

The patient squeezes the ointment into the wound.

NURSE: "That's right. Now, for the dressing you want to use a nonadhering pad as the first layer. Cut the one marked 'Telfa' in half. You can cut right through the closed package, and the second half will be in a wrapper waiting for next time."

MRS. DUNN: "Oh, good. I hate to waste things."

Mrs. Dunn cuts the Telfa pad in half.

NURSE: "Now, let's get the tape ready before you take the wrapper off the Telfa. We will be putting gauze over the Telfa and you will need to tape all the way around the edges. If you tear the four pieces of tape and gently stick one end to the table edge, they will be easy to get when you're ready for them."

MRS. DUNN: "OK. This is what I do when I'm wrapping packages."

NURSE: "Then you are a tape pro, Mrs. Dunn. Now, lay the Telfa dressing on the wound and gently press it down. That spreads the ointment and the pad will stick and stay in place while you finish the dressing."

She watches while the patient places the Telfa.

NURSE: "Great. Now open another pack of gauze squares like I showed you. Put those on top of the Telfa and tape everything down."

MRS. DUNN: "It's really important to get the tape ready first. Otherwise, you'd run out of hands!"

NURSE: "Exactly. Now, after each dressing change, you wash your hands again, and then you are done. See how well you did? Do you feel better about doing this now?"

MRS. DUNN: "Quite a bit. I still feel all thumbs, though, and I worry about getting the sore clean enough by myself."

NURSE: "I think having some pain medicine will help. I'll bring your acetaminophen around 1 o'clock, and we'll do the dressing again about 2."

MRS. DUNN: "OK, and thank you. My husband will be here then. Is it okay if he watches?"

NURSE: "Absolutely. He can help you when you get home."

tion of the above objective would be achieved by watching the patient change the wound dressing and determining if correct aseptic technique was used. The teaching plan is part of the care plan. Some agencies use a separate form for the teaching plan so that there is plenty of room to note the specifics (Figure 9-1). In specialty areas there may be a standardized teaching plan. An example would be postpartum teaching plans for self-care after delivery or for basic infant care.

It is essential that the teaching plan be developed collaboratively, with input from all of the disciplines involved in the patient's care. The specifics of the plan should be discussed and agreed upon. Each knowledge deficit is listed as it is identified, and the date is included. The person responsible for providing teaching in each area is also noted. The teacher may be the nurse, physical or occupational therapist, dietitian, speech therapist, or respiratory therapist. The nurse is responsible for overseeing the plan specifics. Even when another person is doing the teaching, the nurse reinforces it. Consistency in teaching is important if the patient is to master and retain the new information.

RESOURCES FOR TEACHING

Many books and articles are available that provide suggested methods and teaching aids for particular topics. Audiovisual materials, pamphlets, and hands-on equipment are also good resources. Become famil-iar with what is available in your facility. Community agencies may also provide these educational tools. Local government agencies often provide printed and online listings of community public service programs. Nursing specialists may be available to assist with information and teaching plans or to do the actual teaching. Hospital social workers and patient representatives are also good sources of information about what is available.

Some of the instructional materials are designed to assist the medical professional and others are directed to the patient. The Internet has a wide variety of resources available for patient teaching. An Internet search by topic will provide links to myriad resources. Leading medical centers and universities across the United States and Canada, as well as governmental agencies such as the National Institutes for Health (NIH), the Centers for Disease Control and Prevention (CDC), and the National Institute of Mental Health (NIMH), provide websites with excellent teaching resources.

IMPLEMENTING THE PLAN

Begin by establishing a time with the patient to begin the teaching. Teaching should be done at a time when visitors, physician rounds, and treatments will not cause interruptions. Teaching can be done one-on-one or in a group setting. Be certain that the room tem-

PATIENT CARE PLAN				Joan Doe - T444333	
Nursing Diagnosis	Dept. or Person Responsible	Nursing Responsibilities/ Plan of Care	Date	Evaluation	Date
1) Deficient Knowledge related to a. Insulin self-administration	Nursing	Teach: Action of regular and NPH insulin	1/4/09 BW	Verbalizes the action of regular and NPH insulin	1/5/09 BW
		How to draw up insulin -2 syringes	1/4/09 BW	Drew up correct dose using 1 syringe for each type of insulin then mixed into one syringe	1/5/09 BW
		-mixed in 1 syringe	1/4/09 BW	Drew up correct amount into one syringe with correct technique	1/6/09 BW
		Self-administer insulin injections	1/4/09 BW	Verbalized location of various injection sites. Practiced injection technique with an orange and normal saline.	1/6/09 BW
				Gave own injection	1/7/09 BW

FIGURE **9-1** Teaching portion of the nursing care plan.

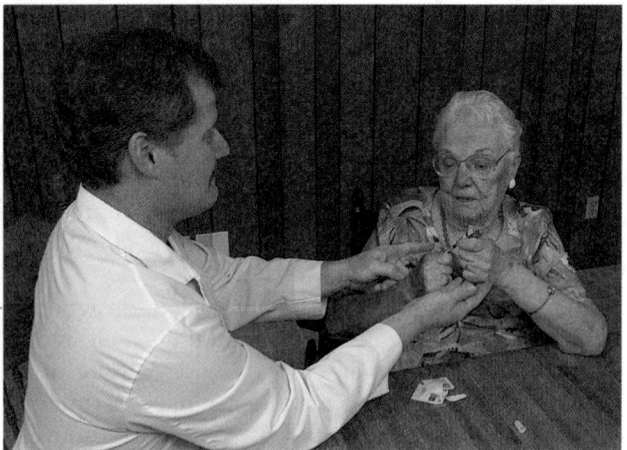

FIGURE **9-2** Nurse teaching patient how to draw up insulin.

perature is acceptable and the patient is comfortable. Medicate the patient prior to the teaching session if pain control is needed. Provide good lighting. Be certain he can hear you and can see adequately.

Keep the teaching session short. Involve the patient in the process; call him by name, and ask for feedback as you progress. If teaching a group, establish eye contact frequently with each person in the group. Pause at intervals and ask if there are questions. When teaching a procedure, talk about the steps of the procedure, demonstrate the procedure, and then talk patients through each step while they perform it (Figure 9-2). Have them write down the steps, or provide them with a written guide they can follow.

At times, you may need to incorporate teaching into daily care. Teaching patients to perform range-of-motion exercises on their weak extremities can be done while bathing. Teaching about wound care can accompany the process of changing the dressing. Reinforcing information about a medication can be done when administering the medication.

The patient needs to receive written or printed information about what has been taught to take home—for instance, a pamphlet or clearly written list of steps to accomplish a procedure, such as performing a blood glucose determination. When possible, this should be in the patient's primary language (Legal & Ethical Considerations 9-1).

Each teaching session should begin with a review of what was previously learned. If the patient was taught a specific skill, such as drawing up insulin, have the patient demonstrate that skill. This is called a return demonstration.

EVALUATION

Evaluating the effectiveness of teaching is critical to the success of the process. It involves obtaining feedback (return of information about the process) from the patient regarding what was taught, then using this feedback to determine whether effective learning has in fact taken place. A return demonstration of a skill is

Legal & Ethical Considerations 9-1

Use of an Interpreter

It is necessary that health care facilities use an interpreter or a telephone interpretation service when obtaining a history or providing necessary patient instruction to someone who does not have a language in common with the health care staff.

one way of evaluating the learning that has occurred. When the learning is not of a skill nature, but is on an information level, asking questions will obtain feedback about retention and comprehension of the material taught. Allow the patient time to think through the answers. Let the patient use any printed materials handed out. This lets you see that the patient can appropriately use the resources you provided.

Allow patients to perform at their own speed. The first step is learning to do the skill correctly. Performance will become more rapid with practice. Learning is a process of many steps, and rushing these steps can cause confusion, frustration, and a sense of failure for both the patient and the nurse.

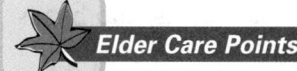

Elder Care Points

Writing down the steps of a procedure helps all learners focus. It is particularly helpful for assisting the elderly person to increase focus and integrate the information. It also aids recall of the information and assists in diminishing any sensory distraction such as background noise.

If the return demonstration or the review questions indicate that the patient has not mastered the skill or material taught, you will need to repeat the instruction and reevaluate performance before going on to a new area of learning. It may also be necessary to alter the method of teaching to more effectively use the patient's strongest learning strategies. The teaching plan should be adjusted and updated according to the evaluation data obtained. New learning needs may also be identified during the teaching and evaluation sessions. These also need to be included in the teaching plan.

DOCUMENTATION

Teaching often occurs informally while performing a nursing task such as administering medications. This makes it a challenge to consistently document patient education. Every staff nurse is legally responsible for providing patient education, and documentation is essential. If the facility does not use a patient education flow sheet, the following information should be entered into the nurse's notes: specific content taught, the method of teaching that was used, and evidence of evaluation with specific results of the teaching. This allows nurses providing continuing care for the patient to follow up and reinforce the teaching.

COORDINATION WITH DISCHARGE PLANNING

Patients may be discharged home before necessary learning is complete. It is important that information regarding the patient's education needs be communicated to the primary physician's office. If the patient is being referred for home health services, it is necessary to also communicate the information to the home care nurse. In addition, the family or significant others who will be caring for the patient may need to be included in some of the teaching sessions Specific learning needs that remain should be discussed with all involved parties, including the patient, and the plan for teaching shared. It is necessary that a printed plan be sent home with the patient. A telephone call to the home health agency or to the physician's office helps provide continuity of teaching.

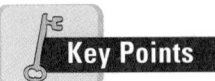
Key Points

- Nurses continually teach patients about aspects of their disease or disorder, diet, medications, treatment, and self-care.
- Patient teaching is a major part of patient care.
- There are three methods of learning: visual, auditory, and kinesthetic.
- The first step in teaching is to assess what the patient needs to know (learning needs, knowledge deficits).
- Many factors can affect learning: physical limitations, situational factors (including pain), readiness to learn, personal values and expectations, age, attitude, and ability to comprehend.
- Environmental factors such as room temperature, noise level, lighting, and interruptions by others can affect learning.
- Establishing rapport and mutual trust are essential to effective teaching.
- A teaching plan is devised and documented based on the patient's learning needs.
- Learning needs must be prioritized to ensure that patients learn those things most important to safe self-care prior to discharge.
- Books, articles, pamphlets, audiovisual materials, and demonstration equipment are good resources for teaching. Nursing specialists are another resource.
- Including the patient in the development of the plan will help keep the patient involved in the education process.
- Teaching may occur one-on-one or in a group setting.
- Evaluating the effectiveness of teaching is critical to the success of the process.
- To evaluate, obtain feedback from the patient either by question and answer or a return demonstration.
- Documentation of patient teaching and the learning achieved is a legal responsibility and should be done consistently.
- Collaboration with other health care professionals involved in the patient's care is essential to the uniformity and the continuity of teaching.

 Go to your **Companion CD-ROM** for an Audio Glossary, animations, video clips, and more.

evolve Be sure to visit the companion Evolve site at http://evolve.elsevier.com/deWit/fundamental/ for additional online resources.

NCLEX-PN® EXAMINATION-STYLE REVIEW QUESTIONS

*Choose the **best** answer for each question.*

1. The primary purpose of patient teaching is to ensure that patients:
   1. can share with others what they have learned.
   2. can reduce the time they are hospitalized.
   3. will follow the treatment plan prescribed.
   4. can provide correct and safe self-care after discharge.

2. There are three types of learning: auditory, visual, and kinesthetic. Learning to apply an ostomy appliance by doing it step by step is an example of _____ learning.
   (Fill in the blank.)

3. A patient newly diagnosed with diabetes has stated that he doesn't understand why he needs insulin. His statement indicates a learning need regarding:
   1. the disease process of diabetes.
   2. the types of insulin available.
   3. the diet a diabetic needs to follow.
   4. the role weight management plays in treatment.

4. When starting the second teaching session for a patient, you should first:
   1. present the new material to be covered in this session.
   2. question the patient about learning from the first session.
   3. review what was taught in the first session.
   4. review the entire teaching plan.

5. When teaching a young child, it is appropriate to:
   1. teach in a group setting.
   2. use play equipment in the teaching process.
   3. do all teaching at one time.
   4. set firm limits on behavior while teaching.

6. When teaching the elderly about a needed diet change, it is best to:
   1. write down the diet instructions.
   2. speak loudly.
   3. show pictures of various foods.
   4. play old tunes in the background.

7. An appropriate patient teaching plan:
   1. is prepared by the nurse based on the patient's diagnosis.
   2. designates 15-minute segments of teaching time.
   3. includes input from all disciplines involved in the care as well as input from the patient.
   4. must be approved by the patient's family members.

CRITICAL THINKING ACTIVITIES *Read each clinical scenario and discuss the questions with your classmates.*

Scenario A
Identify factors that you think might interfere with learning for a patient.

Scenario B
Discuss cultural or religious beliefs that you feel might have a direct impact on the patient's teaching plan.

Scenario C
Assess the learning needs of three patients and then share commonalities of those needs with your clinical group.

10 Delegation, Leadership, and Management

evolve http://evolve.elsevier.com/deWit/fundamental/

Objectives

Upon completing this chapter, you should be able to:

Theory

1. Differentiate among the three different leadership styles discussed in the chapter.
2. Describe four characteristics of an effective leader.
3. Identify management functions of the LPN/LVN working in a long-term care facility, home care, or an outpatient clinic.
4. Compare and contrast examples of effective and ineffective communication.
5. Outline considerations for appropriate delegation of tasks to unlicensed assistive personnel (UAPs).
6. Distinguish the skills and functions of the team leader with those of the charge nurse.
7. Discuss techniques of effective time management.
8. Explain the importance of the "read back" for verbal or telephone orders.

Clinical Practice

1. Determine the leadership style of the charge nurse on the unit to which you are assigned.
2. Appropriately delegate three tasks to a nurse's aide or unlicensed assistive personnel.
3. Create a time-efficient work organization plan for a shift.
4. Demonstrate proficient use of the hospital computer.
5. Accurately and carefully transcribe orders per facility policy.
6. Document accurately for reimbursement.
7. Become aware of the facility's policies and procedures and uphold the standards of nursing practice.

Key Terms

Be sure to check out the bonus material on the Companion CD-ROM, including selected audio pronunciations.

autocratic (aw-tō-KRĂ-tĭk, p. 128)
collaboration (p. 128)
conflict resolution (p. 129)
constructive criticism (p. 131)
delegate (p. 128)
democratic (p. 128)
laissez-faire (LES-a-FAYR, p. 127)
mediate (MĒ-dē-āt, p. 129)
risk management (p. 135)
stat order (p. 133)
unlicensed assistive personnel (un-LI-sĕnst ă -SĬS-tĭv pĕr-sŏ-NĔL, p. 128)

In the current health care delivery system, the LPN and LVN are taking on more and more leadership functions, particularly in the skilled nursing facility. Leadership is a comprehensive process that includes the guidance of staff and effective utilization of resources for the purpose of meeting patient needs. Leadership requires a good grasp of basic management techniques. This chapter discusses the management skills and leadership qualities that the LPN/LVN needs to be effective in those positions that are appropriate for the new nurse during the first year after graduation. More extensive leadership/management positions require considerable experience and advanced management training and skills.

THE CHAIN OF COMMAND

Once you are hired, it is important that you become familiar with the organizational structure of the health facility for which you work. This information is generally provided during your formal orientation to the facility. Be certain you know the chain of command for the area in which you are employed. Who is your immediate supervisor? From whom do you take orders? To whom does your supervisor report? To whom should you report changes in patient condition, signs of complications, and so forth? To whom do you go with concerns or complaints? Who is in charge of scheduling your hours? What is the procedure for calling if you are ill and cannot make it to work?

LEADERSHIP STYLES

Most leaders employ a blend of leadership styles. A permissive or laissez-faire leader does not attempt to control the team and offers little if any direction. This leader assumes that the members of the team are competent and self-directed and will do what needs to be done correctly and efficiently. This leader often has a need to be liked by everyone and therefore avoids any blame for things that go wrong by allowing members to function completely independently. Although this leadership style usually is not effective in the day-to-day management of patient care operations, it can be effective in certain situations involving a highly moti-

Box 10-1 *Attributes that Make a Good Leader*

- Ability to teach
- Active listener
- Articulate
- Assertive
- Calm
- Considerate
- Consistent
- Decisive
- Excellent clinical skills
- Excellent problem solver
- Fair
- Flexible
- Good role model
- Good sense of humor
- Objective
- Open-minded
- Organized
- Responsible
- Sensitive
- Strong character
- Tactful

vated, highly creative group who work well with minimal guidance—for example, a committee.

The authoritarian or autocratic leader tightly controls team members. Staff are rarely consulted when decisions are to be made. Rules are set without input from the staff and directives and orders are given out constantly. This type of leadership style has been described as "my way or the highway." **The leader closely supervises the work of each staff member.** When mistakes are made, they are quickly pointed out. The goal of this leader is accomplishment of tasks without regard to the effect on the people.

The democratic leader frequently consults with staff members and seeks staff participation in decision making. The skills and knowledge of the team members are readily used to ensure that the team functions efficiently. Team members are respected as individuals, and there is an open and trusting attitude overall. The democratic leader is part of the team, not sitting above it, and accepts responsibility for the actions of the team.

There is no one set of qualities that make a good leader. Box 10-1 lists responses that nurses have given when asked what they think makes a good leader. Such a leader instills confidence, trust, and spirit into the team. Appropriate leadership fosters growth among the team members.

Think Critically About . . . With what type of leader do you prefer to work? Why? Is there a situation in which an autocratic leader is needed? Can you explain why?

Safety Alert 10-1

National Patient Safety Goal 2

The Joint Commission has set the following goal for health care facilities: *"improve the effectiveness of communication among caregivers."*

Components of this goal include:

- The requirement of "read back" for verbal orders, telephone orders, or telephone reporting of critical test results.
- Standardization of "Do Not Use" abbreviations, acronyms, symbols, and dose designations by the organization.
- Improvement of timeliness of reporting critical laboratory results and values.
- Implementation of a standard approach to "handoff" communication.

Source: The Joint Commission website: www.jointcommission.org/ PatientSafety/NationalPatientSafetyGoals/08_hap_npsgs.htm.

KEYS TO EFFECTIVE LEADERSHIP

As an LPN/LVN, you will be expected to work with other members of the health care team. Collaboration **(working together) is essential for cost-effective patient care.** Part of your collaborative practice will be learning to work effectively with unlicensed assistive personnel (UAPs). UAPs include unit secretaries, nursing assistants, homemaking aides, housekeeping personnel, and various types of technicians. To be effective in this role, you must learn to delegate (to entrust to another) tasks appropriately and effectively.

EFFECTIVE COMMUNICATION

Leaders use good communication skills. **Communicating in direct, concise terms in a tactful, friendly, non-threatening way is essential to the creation of a supportive work environment.** Obtaining feedback about directions given and listening actively to reports, suggestions, and complaints establishes a pattern for two-way communication. This helps the leader stay in tune with the atmosphere, attitudes, and problems of others on the health care team. The Joint Commission emphasizes the importance of communication by health care providers; it has tailored one of its National Patient Safety Goals specifically toward improving communication (Safety Alert 10-1). SBAR communication (see discussion in Chapter 8) is a streamlined communication tool that many institutions are adopting to improve communication among staff.

Communicating effectively includes taking the time to attend to the person by stopping what you are doing, establishing eye contact with the other person, remembering to be polite by saying "please" and "thank you," and using a warm tone of voice (Figure 10-1). A smile adds warmth to the interaction. Saying,

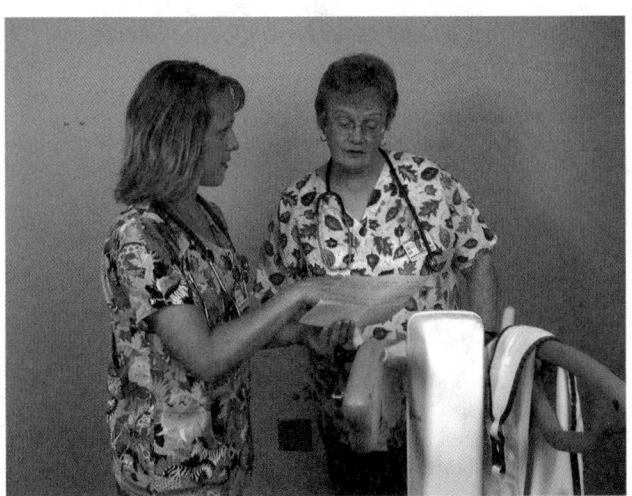

FIGURE **10-1** Charge nurse delegating a task to a staff nurse.

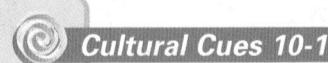

Consider Eye Contact

Remember, of course, that personnel we work with might be from a different cultural background from our own and might be comfortable with more or less eye contact than we are, and more or less personal space than we are. Be careful that your direct eye contact does not turn into a "stare down" of trying to get the other individual to reciprocate. Differences in the gender, age, and culture of the sender and the receiver of instructions can make both parties feel awkward. Your body language and tone of voice go a long way in conveying respect to your team members.

"I would like you to take vital signs on the right side of the hall, please," rather than "Go and take vital signs on that side of the hall," usually enlists better cooperation and a more pleasant attitude toward the task. It is also important to consider the culture of another and how it may affect verbal and nonverbal communication (Cultural Cues 10-1). **Treat others in the manner you prefer to be treated.**

When assigning tasks, be certain to be very specific about what is to be done, how it is to be done, and when the task is to be completed. Inquire if there are questions before ending the interaction. Many a conflict can be avoided by being thorough when giving directions, making a request, or assigning a task. If a conflict does arise, try to remain calm and open and actively listen to the problem. Accept responsibility for any part you played in the development of the conflict. Focus on the issue rather than on the feelings of those involved. Mediate (settle differences) by communicating openly. Sort out the issues involved by identifying key themes in the discussion. Consider the options and weigh the consequences of each option. Choose the option for conflict resolution (resolving a conflict) that offers the best outcome.

CLINICAL COMPETENCE AND CONFIDENCE

As a nurse leader, you must demonstrate competence in the skills of the profession. Confidence in the ability to perform those skills well is essential if you are to have the respect of the other members of the team. Along with this competence and confidence should be sufficient self-esteem to readily admit when a mistake has been made or when you don't know something. Announcing "I don't know, but I will find out" is the best way to handle such a situation. Others will respect you more if you openly admit that you don't know everything. The ability to readily admit such a thing shows that you are human and provides an atmosphere in which others can admit what they don't know and can ask for help.

ORGANIZATION

Being a leader requires good organization. Organizing the work of a unit requires strong time management skills. You should plan each day carefully, and the plan should have some built-in flexibility for unforeseen events and needs. Knowing the strengths of each member of the health care team helps you more effectively divide the workload. Decision-making ability is needed to quickly divide up patients and assign tasks to various personnel.

Problem-solving skills provide the means by which difficult decisions can be made. The problem-solving process is much like the nursing process. The good problem solver first defines the problem (assessment), then looks at the alternatives. The outcomes of using each of the alternatives are estimated (planning), and then one of the alternatives is chosen to be tried as the solution to the problem (implementation). If the alternative chosen does not work to solve the problem, then the whole process is repeated (evaluation). Please see the section Critical Thinking in Chapter 4.

DELEGATION

In beginning the discussion of delegation, it is helpful to first contrast it with the term *assignment*. Assignment of tasks is a method of distributing the workload of the unit, usually by the charge nurse. In assignment, the nurse directs the UAPs to complete tasks within their job description—tasks they are hired and paid to perform. This always occurs at the start of the shift, but may also occur at any time during the shift. In contrast, delegation occurs when a licensed nurse transfers the *authority* to perform a selected nursing duty in a selected patient situation. In delegating a task to a UAP, you are, in essence, "sharing" power with your UAPs. **Many states do not allow licensed practical/vocational nurses to delegate,** and even in a state where it is allowed, you must also be certain that delegation is allowed in your facility of practice before performing it. Furthermore, delegation is done with careful thought—for example, it is not appropriate to simply delegate a nursing duty that you have a dislike of performing. In addition, you must be certain that the individual to whom you are about to delegate is competent to perform such a duty (written evidence of competence is best, to be described shortly), that the patient situation is stable, and that the task to be delegated has a predictable outcome.

You are accountable for the tasks you delegate, if in fact you are permitted by law to delegate. Legally, as a licensed nurse, you are responsible and accountable for the outcome of any task you delegate to another. Delegating appropriately means that you must (1) know the capabilities and competencies of the person to whom you are delegating a specific task; (2) know whether or not the task falls within the domain of tasks that can legally be delegated by you; (3) communicate effectively with the person to whom you are delegating; and (4) understand the patient's needs.

Before any tasks are delegated to a nursing assistant or other UAP, that person should be thoroughly oriented to the facility and the unit on which he is employed. **Competencies of unlicensed personnel must be documented before tasks are delegated to them.** This requires evidence of a training program and *written evidence by a qualified nurse or instructor that the person has demonstrated competence in the task or skill.* If you do not have access to such written documentation, it is best to observe the UAP perform the task or skill the first time you delegate it to verify that a level of competence has been reached. If the task has not been a part of a formal training program for the UAP, then you should demonstrate how the task should be done and ask for a return demonstration.

?
Think Critically About . . . How would you tactfully tell a UAP that you would like to see a particular task performed by him before assigning him to do it on his own?

Be familiar with your state's nurse practice act so that you know what tasks and skills fall within your legal domain. This tells you what you must *not* delegate. In addition, some professional nursing organization websites, such as that of the American Association of Critical Care Nurses (www.aacn.org), have documents that outline examples of tasks that might be appropriate for delegation; however, you must ensure that this matches what is allowed in your state. Your agency should have a job description that spells out what the UAPs can and cannot do. Be certain that you are familiar with the UAP job descriptions before you delegate a task. **It is up to you to know what the UAP cannot do.** The policies and procedures of the agency and the standards of practice for your area of nursing help to define what the UAP is allowed to do (Box 10-2). **Assessment or aspects of the analysis, planning, or evaluation phases of the nursing process must be per-**

Box 10-2 *Delegatable Tasks for Unlicensed Assistive Personnel (UAPs)**

- Applying a condom catheter
- Applying a hearing aid
- Applying cold packs
- Applying elastic stockings
- Applying warm compresses
- Assisting to deep breathe and cough
- Assisting with ambulation
- Giving a bath
- Bed making
- Blood glucose monitoring
- Collecting specimens
- Emptying drainage containers
- Feeding patients
- Filling water pitchers
- Giving a sitz bath
- Giving an enema
- Giving a vaginal douche
- Hair care
- Measuring weight and height
- Oral hygiene
- Performing range-of-motion exercises
- Providing skin care
- Recording intake and output
- Removing a Foley catheter
- Repositioning patients
- Stocking supplies
- Taking specimens to the laboratory
- Toileting patients
- Transferring patient to a chair or bed
- Turning patients
- Vital signs

*May vary from state to state and facility to facility.

---

formed by the registered nurse. These functions cannot be delegated to unlicensed personnel. The majority of tasks that are to be delegated to UAPs are technical, repetitive skills that have a predictable patient outcome. **Interventions that require professional judgment should not be delegated.**

Within the area of general competencies, the UAP should be assessed for competence in patient safety issues such as infection control and moving and positioning patients.

In order to have effective communication with the UAP, you must send clear, concise messages and listen carefully to feedback. It is better to say, "Please take Mrs. Jones' temperature at 2 P.M. and let me know right away what it is so that I can let her physician know," than "Mrs. Jones' temperature needs to be taken at 2 P.M." Likewise, it is better to say, "Tell me immediately if Mr. Hernandez's temperature is above 101.2° F," than "Let me know if Mr. Hernandez's temperature is high." **To delegate effectively you must include the result desired and the time line for completion.** Ask the UAP if there are any questions about what is to be done, and ask for a summary of what he understands is to be done. Asking the person to share with you what you have just said, or asking about his understanding of what you have requested, will verify that your request has been received as intended. Tell the UAP where you will be if a problem or question arises during performance of the task. Be certain that delegation of the task has been accepted by the delegatee, and then give up responsibility for that task to that person. **Remember that when you delegate, you do not give up your responsibility for overall patient care.** You must follow through by verifying that the task has been completed in a timely manner.

Effective delegation includes giving feedback on how the task was performed. Give praise where it is due; share favorable comments from patients about the UAP's work and interactions. If the delegated task did not go as expected, communicate exactly what went wrong in a supportive manner. **Be certain that privacy is provided before giving criticism.** Be tactful. You might share that the patient was upset that it took three tries for the UAP to obtain an accurate blood pressure. Asking "Do you think you need some more supervised practice and suggestions on how to take blood pressures smoothly? Would you like me to demonstrate it again?" allows the UAP a face-saving way to admit that more instruction is needed. Ask what might help the UAP perform better the next time.

When giving constructive criticism, begin by tactfully acknowledging feelings or expressing empathy. Statements such as "I understand that we are one aide short today," begin the interaction on a less threatening note. Next describe the behavior. An example would be "I've noticed that it has been 9:30 three mornings this week before vital signs you took were posted." Then state the expectation for future compliance, such as "It is necessary for the vital signs to be posted no later than 8:30 A.M. from now on." Finally, state the consequences if the expected action does not occur. This can be done by stating something like "The physicians and medication nurses have to track you down when the vital signs are not posted on time. If posting is late again, I will have to document your inability to complete the task on time."

When delegating a variety of tasks, you will probably need to help the UAP prioritize the order in which they should be done. It takes many months for most UAPs to be able to discern which tasks take priority over others.

When performance by a UAP has been poor, documentation of the specific facts (not your opinions) must occur. The unit manager should also be made aware of the performance problem.

The patient must be told when an unlicensed person will be performing some tasks that were formerly only performed by nurses. This is within the domain of a patient's rights. Simply tell the patient that you, the nurse, have primary responsibility for the care given, but that the UAP is your assistant and will be doing certain tasks.

LEADERSHIP ROLES

BEGINNING LEADERSHIP ROLES

Initially, the new LPN/LVN will be performing leadership functions in working with UAPs. This requires appropriate delegation of tasks and supervision of the UAPs' work. Later on, when the new graduate is thoroughly oriented to the facility and its policies, and is functioning competently, team leading may be required. A team leader coordinates and makes assignments for other personnel, assists with patient care, helps resolve conflicts, assists with the writing of policies and procedures, contributes information for evaluation of UAPs, and collaborates with physicians and other health team members.

When working in a medical clinic, the LPN/LVN team leader is often responsible for overseeing the scheduling of patients, performing quality assurance audits, training other staff, evaluating other staff, coordinating the members of the team to accomplish the daily work, assisting with the writing of policies and procedures, attending staff meetings, and resolving staff conflicts (Figure 10-2).

? *Think Critically About . . .* What leadership functions do LPN/LVNs perform in the facility in which you are assigned for clinical experience?

ADVANCED LEADERSHIP ROLES

Eventually the LPN/LVN may become a charge nurse or a supervisor of UAPs in settings such as home care or outpatient clinics. **A charge nurse must have some training and experience in nursing administration and supervision and additional preparation in a specialized area in many states.** A minimum of 1 year of staff nurse experience is often required before taking on

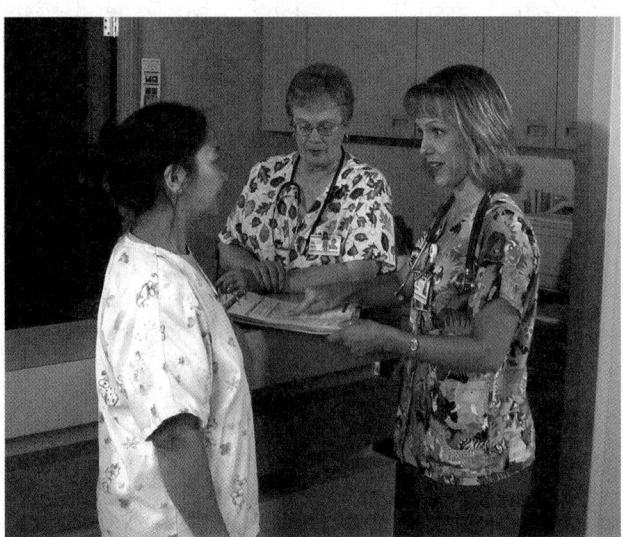

FIGURE **10-2** Charge nurse discussing a new procedure with staff.

charge nurse duties. Sometimes life experience in other roles can expedite assumption of the leadership role.

The ability to recognize significant changes in patient condition and to take necessary action is a primary quality in a charge nurse. The charge nurse is the manager's designee and has all of the manager's authority for the shift; he is **responsible for the total nursing care of the patients on the unit during the shift.**

In a long-term care facility, the charge nurse receives the report from the previous shift, makes patient assignments, makes rounds and assesses all patients, directs the administration of medications and treatments, confers with team members throughout the shift, and reports to the oncoming shift on patient status. Charge nurses also may be responsible for overseeing training of UAPs and for the evaluation of members of the unit's health care team.

MANAGEMENT SKILLS FOR THE LPN/LVN

All nurses are expected to be able to manage time, use a computer, order supplies, transcribe physicians' orders, place phone calls to physicians and families, process verbal orders, and document care appropriately, including for reimbursement of patient costs.

An LPN/LVN working in a home care agency may be asked to assign and supervise nursing assistants and home health aides, in which case he will make patient care assignments, assist with orientation and evaluation, verify that paperwork ensuring reimbursement is correctly completed, and give and receive reports on assigned patients.

TIME MANAGEMENT

Leaders need to use time efficiently. There are techniques that can be learned to assist with time management. Each workday should begin by making a "to-do" list before the shift starts. This just provides a loose structure for the day. One or two general goals for the day should be formulated.

The goal for the home care nurse might be "to complete four visits by lunchtime." Work organization for this nurse involves determining the most efficient order for the visits scheduled for the day, gathering all needed supplies, notifying each patient of the approximate time of the visit, organizing the paperwork to be completed, and making certain the car has gas.

Organizing for the workday in a medical clinic varies depending on the type of clinic and the assigned duties of the nurse. The goals for a clinic nurse might be "to ensure rooms are stocked and set up for treatments, and patients are roomed in an efficient manner." Charts will need to be pulled for patients scheduled to be seen, supplies in examining rooms will need to be replenished, and so forth.

For the staff nurse in the hospital, the shift's goal might be "to ensure that all assigned patients are kept comfortable and safe and that all scheduled treatments and medications are given." After receiving the shift report and obtaining the patient assignments, priorities should be set. To do this, the nurse will identify the patients with the most significant or life-threatening problems. Which patients are physically unstable and need to be checked frequently? Which patients have frequently scheduled assessments or treatments? Which patients are most at risk for complications? Which patients are at risk for injury because they are confused? Priorities are set according to patient need. Unstable patients take precedence over stable patients. Scheduled medications and treatments must be done before tasks that are ordered "three times per day."

The goal for the long-term care nurse might be "to delegate and coordinate care of assigned patients in order to finish all scheduled tasks on time and keep the patients safe and comfortable."

Take a few minutes before making rounds to devise a time schedule for the work of the shift (Figure 10-3). Use a grid that shows each hour of the shift and each patient and room number. Note times you will delegate tasks, assess patients, check intravenous (IV) lines, give treatments, turn patients, document care, perform teaching, prepare for the end-of-shift report, and so on. **Documentation is a critical task in all settings and must be considered a priority to be done as soon as possible when organizing to accomplish the daily workload.**

SAMPLE OF TIME MANAGEMENT TOOL

Initials:
Report notes:
Room #:
Allergies:
Notify MD for:

TIME	ASSESSMENTS	MEDICATIONS	VITAL SIGNS	TREATMENTS/ PROCEDURES
0700				
0800				
0900				
1000				
1100				
1200				
1300				
1400				
1500				

OXYGEN	DIET	IV FLUIDS	ACTIVITY	DRESSINGS	I&O	LABS

FIGURE 10-3 Sample time management tool. Use one page per patient or create your own tool and put several patients on one page.

Use a separate grid to note when medications are due for each patient. Use this sheet to note when you give PRN (as needed) medications. That way you have a quick refresher for charting the PRN medications in the progress notes. As you work throughout the day, you can make small notes on your work organization sheet that will provide data and a guide for charting.

Next consider what has to be done sometime during the shift. Checking the "crash" cart would be such a task. Note on your work schedule when you feel you will have time to do that. Finally, consider things that you would like to do if time permits, such as spending time talking with a lonely patient, giving a back rub, or making a phone call to a patient's family. Note these at the bottom of the work sheet.

Once the work is organized, begin your patient assessment/data collection rounds. This should be done early in the shift. Patient status can sometimes change dramatically during the change-of-shift and report time. Quickly gather data regarding each patient's area of greatest problem (usually the one for which they were admitted). Check all tubes and equipment attached to the patient. You will be able to do more in-depth observations later in the shift. Right now you just need to determine if there are any emergencies, get a feel for the patient's status and needs, and determine what equipment and supplies you will need for each patient during the shift. Inquire about the need for pain medication or other PRN medication while initially in the room. These then can be brought back during early morning medication rounds unless the medication is a badly needed analgesic; this should be administered immediately.

At the end of the workday, you should evaluate the effectiveness of your time management. Did your schedule help? Did it work as well as you had it planned? What took more time to complete than you thought it would take? What would you like to have done differently if you could have a "do over"? This analysis helps you to create a more workable plan the next time. Keep in mind that work plans must be flexible. Even the best plans can be destroyed if one patient's status deteriorates markedly. This happens to all nurses from time to time.

?
Think Critically About . . . Can you design a shift time management sheet for yourself that suits your work style and needs?

USING THE COMPUTER

Computers are used in all health care facilities. The nurse must become proficient in their use in order to perform everyday functions for patient care and unit administration. The computer is used to place orders to the various departments for supplies, medications, diets, laboratory and diagnostic tests, and engineering and housekeeping needs. Surgery and procedures are scheduled by computer. Staffing patterns may be scheduled by computer. Nursing care plans are constructed on the computer and are updated and revised as needed every 24 hours by the nurse. Acuity levels for patients are tracked. The agency census is compiled on the computer. Laboratory results are often sent to the unit via computer. Many hospitals are adopting totally computerized patient records, including medical orders, nursing documentation (nurse's notes, flow sheets), and incident reports.

In order to be a team leader or charge nurse, you must be adept at using the agency's computers in order to efficiently perform all necessary tasks for the job. The computer is used for most communication and coordination within the agency. Also, the HIPAA privacy rule (see Chapter 3 for full discussion) mandates that we take special precautions and safeguard all electronic patient data, just the same as we do with written patient documentation.

TRANSCRIBING WRITTEN ORDERS

When handling newly written orders, first read all of the orders. Then transcribe the "stat" (do immediately) orders first, and verbally communicate them to the nurse responsible for carrying them out. Transfer the orders to the Kardex, computer "care plan," medication and treatment cards (if used), and medication administration record (MAR). Each medication order must include the patient's name and room number, the name of the medication (preferably both generic and trade name), ordered dosage, route of administration, the times the doses are to be given, the date the order was written, and the date it is to be discontinued and/or renewed. **Check off each order as it is transcribed.** Narcotics, anticoagulants, hypnotics, and antibiotics must be renewed every 48 to 72 hours depending on agency policy and state laws. Sign off the order with a red line across the page under the physician's signature and your first initial, last name, and official designation, or according to agency policy. Include the date and the time. Notify the person who will be giving the medication per the new order. The order is transmitted to the pharmacy by phone, fax, or computer and a copy of it is sent to the pharmacy. In some facilities, you may then write "faxed to pharmacy 2PM," with your initials, before returning the original form to the chart.

Dietary orders are transmitted to the dietary department and entered on the Kardex or computer care plan along with notations for any fluid restrictions or requirements for intake and output recording. If intake and output records are required, a recording sheet is placed in the patient's room.

Unclear orders should be clarified directly with the physician who wrote them. When medications arrive on the unit from the pharmacy, they should be checked with the physician's orders before placing them in the patient's drawer or bin. This may be completed by a pharmacy technician. Due to frequent changes in orders, all medication orders on the MAR or Kardex should be verified with the chart orders once every 24 hours.

Positioning, intake and output, treatment requirements, and use of special equipment are noted on the Kardex or on the computer care plan for each patient. **Allergies are noted on the MAR sheet and on the front of the chart to alert all personnel.**

When a medication is discontinued, cross out the item on the MAR/Kardex by using a highlighter over it and write "DC" with the date and time. Some agencies do not use these forms or methods for discontinuation of medications. Check agency policy. Notify the nurse giving the medications for the shift. Alert the pharmacy to the discontinuation order and return leftover doses of the medication to the pharmacy for proper crediting to the patient's account. Sign off the discontinue order on the physician's order sheet.

Orders for laboratory and diagnostic tests require that the order be transmitted to the appropriate department by phone or computer and the correct requisition slip be filled out. The forms and labels for specimen containers are stamped with the patient's addressograph plate. If blood samples are to be drawn when the patient is in a "fasting" state, then an NPO (no food or fluid by mouth) status must be transmitted to the dietary department, to the nurses, and to the patient. An "NPO" sign is posted on the door to the patient's room. The test must be ordered to be drawn before the breakfast hour. A barium enema (BE) and upper gastrointestinal (GI) series are scheduled with the BE before the upper GI series to prevent swallowed barium from interfering with the BE. Laboratory and diagnostic test orders are recorded on the Kardex or computer care plan along with dietary restrictions and pretest medications.

Preoperative orders should include diet/NPO status desired, necessary preoperative treatments, a notation regarding the operative consent and the exact procedure to be performed, laboratory and diagnostic tests to be completed, patient teaching required, and orders for sedatives or preoperative medications. There may also be orders for the type of surgical preparation to be performed and when, insertion of an IV cannula and what solution is to be started, insertion of a Foley catheter, or application of elastic hose. **All orders written preoperatively are considered canceled at the time the patient enters surgery.** Brand new orders must be written in their entirety for the postsurgical patient. "Resume previous orders" is not acceptable by most institutional policies.

Postoperative orders should include a schedule for vital sign measurement; directions for care of tubes, suction, and dressings; IV solutions to be infused; medications to be administered; diet permitted; measurement of intake and output; directions for position-

National Patient Safety Goal 2A ("Read Back")

The Joint Commission International Center for Patient Safety has developed guidelines for accepting and transcribing verbal or telephone orders (National Patient Safety Goal 2A). The Joint Commission requires institutions to verify verbal or telephone orders by having the person receiving the order "read back" the order to the person initiating the order, usually the physician. This "read back" requires that the person accepting the order actually write the order down in the chart in order to be reading it back.

Source: The Joint Commission website: www.jointcommission.org/PatientSafety/NationalPatientSafetyGoals/08_cah_npsgs.htm.

ing, activity, turning, coughing and deep breathing; and time to catheterize if the patient is unable to void and does not have an indwelling catheter. Additional orders may request circulation checks or monitoring of neurologic status.

TAKING VERBAL ORDERS

The practice of taking verbal and telephone orders can be unsafe unless carefully performed. The individual giving the order can misspeak, and the individual receiving the order can mishear, misunderstand, or misinterpret the order due to numerous factors such as distraction/background noise, different pronunciations or accents, cell phone noise, and many others. The Joint Commission discourages the use of verbal and telephone orders unless absolutely necessary because they can be unsafe unless specific guidelines are followed (Safety Alert 10-2). If a physician is present on the unit, he should write orders rather than giving verbal orders. In cases in which implementation of an order is time critical, and the physician is not available in person, a telephone order may be the most appropriate and efficient way to provide expedient care to the patient. At the times when these orders are given, the expectation is that the nurse will write the orders in the chart for the physician to sign later.

The legal ability of the LPN/LVN to take verbal orders from a physician depends on the laws of the state and the written policies of the employing agency. **Verbal orders can only be taken by licensed nurses, and in some states can only be taken by an RN.** Some institutions require that verbal orders may not be taken except in cases of emergency.

If your state and agency allow you to take a verbal or telephone order, follow the guidelines in Box 10-3. The nurse enters it on the physician's order sheet and marks it "V.O." (verbal order) or "T.O." (telephone order) with the date, time, first initial, last name, and professional designation (LVN or LPN). **The physician must sign the written form of the verbal order as soon as possible.**

Box 10-3 | *Guidelines for Taking Telephone Orders*

- Have the patient's medical record open to the appropriate page to accept a new physician order. Have a pen ready.
- Write the order verbatim (word for word) as it is given to you.
- Read it back to the physician as written; verify spelling of medications or diagnostic tests. Do this every time with every physician. Ask for confirmation that the order is correct.
- Document the date and time, and indicate "T.O." for telephone order with your first initial, last name, and LVN or LPN.
- See that the physician signs off on the order when making rounds; this must be done within 48 hours in most agencies.
- If a telephone order is requested during the hours from midnight to 6 A.M., have another person, preferably a nurse, on an extension to verify the order. Physicians awakened from a sound sleep sometimes do not recall the exact order. Have the other nurse initial the order, or have the other person document the order as he heard it given and sign it.
- Make an entry in the nurse's notes describing the circumstances that prompted a telephone order. Include the statement that the orders were read back to the physician and that they were confirmed to be accurate by the physician when read back.

DOCUMENTATION FOR REIMBURSEMENT

All nurses must document care delivered and equipment used for a patient. Reimbursement rates are dependent on the documentation. A charge nurse or supervisor makes certain that all staff are documenting correctly. Each type of agency has guidelines as to the details of care that must be documented and how often each must be noted.

In the long-term care facility, the Minimum Data Set (MDS) must be filled in as accurately as possible in order for the facility to receive the maximum Medicare or Medicaid payment for services rendered. Many facilities use a special MDS coordinator to ensure that these multiple-page forms are filled in correctly. Poor documentation may lead to fines imposed by the Department of Health and Human Services as well as decreased reimbursement.

RISK MANAGEMENT

The increasing occurrence of lawsuits against health facilities, doctors, and nurses has focused attention on risk management (management of areas to decrease risk of harm to patients, occurrence of lawsuits, or excessive damages awards by juries). Risk management practices attempt to prevent adverse events or to mitigate the amount of liability the agency might incur. A key risk management tool is practicing nursing by the accepted standards of the profession and the policies and procedures of the agency. The unit leader must insist that all workers adhere to the facility's written policies and procedures. Nurses must uphold the accepted standards of practice for the area in which they work. Attending to patient complaints and showing concern when patients are upset can help decrease the risk of a disgruntled patient who may sue if something goes wrong. Advising your supervisor when a significant problem has occurred on the unit, along with writing an incident report, is prudent when there has been cause for a patient or the patient's family to be upset with care (see Chapter 3 for a discussion on incident reports). Mediating patient and family complaints is part of the leadership role.

Leadership and management skills develop with practice and continued learning. Professional growth is an important aspect of an evolving career in nursing. Each nurse should seek his own direction and pursue growth opportunities. After a year of experience in direct patient care, enough confidence may have been gained to take on greater responsibility and a leadership role.

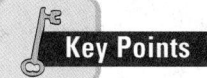

Key Points

- Leadership requires a good grasp of management techniques, effective communication skills, clinical competence, and knowledge of the organizational structure of the agency.
- A laissez-faire leader offers little, if any, direction; autocratic leaders tightly control team members; and democratic leaders frequently consult other staff members and seek participation in decision making.
- Organization of work tasks for the unit is essential; delegation is necessary to accomplish the workload.
- In order to safely and effectively delegate, you must know the capabilities and competencies of the person to whom you are delegating, understand which tasks you can legally delegate, avoid delegating interventions that require professional judgment, and provide feedback.
- Delegation and team leading are beginning leadership functions.
- The charge nurse is responsible for the total nursing care of the patients on the unit during the shift. This position requires training and experience in administration and supervision.
- Computer expertise is necessary for work efficiency; computers are becoming more essential to patient care.
- Risk management techniques include following policies and procedures and showing caring and concern for patients.

 Go to your **Companion CD-ROM** for an Audio Glossary, animations, video clips, and more.

evolve Be sure to visit the companion Evolve site at http://evolve.elsevier.com/deWit/fundamental/ for additional online resources.

NCLEX-PN® EXAMINATION-STYLE REVIEW QUESTIONS

*Choose the **best** answer(s) for each question.*

1. A charge nurse who hands the nurses on one hall the list of patients and tells them to divide the workload evenly among themselves and that hall's nursing assistants according to each person's capabilities is displaying a _____ type of leadership. *(Fill in the blank.)*

2. The ideal type of leadership to be demonstrated by the nurse managing a patient experiencing a cardiac arrest is the _____ type of leadership. *(Fill in the blank.)*

3. A good way to handle conflict is to: *(Select that apply.)*
   1. speak sternly to those involved.
   2. tell those involved to solve the problem.
   3. quickly impose a resolution to the problem.
   4. remain calm and open and listen to all sides.
   5. focus on the issues, not the personalities involved.

4. Delegation of a specific task to a UAP requires: *(Select all that apply.)*
   1. knowledge of the UAP's competencies.
   2. understanding of the nurse practice act.
   3. direct supervision of the performance of the task.
   4. documentation that the task was delegated.
   5. follow-through by verifying the task has been completed.

5. Giving constructive criticism should begin with:
   1. providing feedback on past performance.
   2. stating consequences for the poor performance.
   3. acknowledging feelings or expressing empathy.
   4. asking how you can help improve performance.

6. A first step in time management is:
   1. setting priorities.
   2. seeking assistance.
   3. making patient rounds.
   4. making a time schedule.

7. Verbal orders entered in the medical record should be signed by the physician within:
   1. 8 hours.
   2. 3 days.
   3. 24 hours.
   4. 48 hours.

8. According to The Joint Commission, verbal orders: *(Select all that apply.)*
   1. are potentially dangerous.
   2. are a nice way for the nurse to save the doctor time.
   3. should be avoided unless absolutely necessary.
   4. can be misheard or misunderstood due to different pronunciations or accents.

9. If a patient has a heating pad ordered, but its use is not documented, the insurance company:
   1. will pay because the physician ordered it.
   2. may deny payment because there is no evidence of use.
   3. may request further information.
   4. will request verification from the nurse that the pad was in use.

10. The goal of risk management is to:
    1. minimize agency liability.
    2. minimize the number of risks present in the hospital.
    3. minimize the amount of risk the nursing staff is allowed to take.
    4. increase nursing competence, thereby decreasing risk of patient injury.

11. One risk management technique that is known to often be effective is to:
    1. call family members by their given names.
    2. assign the same nurse to care for the patient all week.
    3. listen empathetically to complaints or concerns.
    4. tell the patient the physician knows best.

CRITICAL THINKING ACTIVITIES *Read each clinical scenario and discuss the questions with your classmates.*

Scenario A
You are assigned eight medical-surgical patients on the day shift. You have one nursing assistant who can help you but who also is assigned to help another nurse. What tasks should you consider delegating to this UAP? How would you verify that the tasks you have delegated have been done and done correctly? Would this method help build team spirit?

Scenario B
You are team leader on one hall. Two of your staff begin to bicker about who should be answering the call light that keeps coming on. How would you handle the situation?

Scenario C
A patient needs to have her blood sugar checked before breakfast. You want the nursing assistant to perform this task and she has been trained to do it. The nursing assistant approaches the patient to perform the procedure, and the patient refuses. How would you handle this refusal?

11 Growth and Development: Infancy through Adolescence

evolve http://evolve.elsevier.com/deWit/fundamental/

Objectives

Upon completing this chapter, you should be able to:

Theory

1. Describe prenatal development.
2. Compare the development of the male and the female.
3. Discuss Freud's theory of personality and the mind.
4. Explain the stages of Erikson's theory of psychosocial development.
5. Explain the stages of Piaget's theory of cognitive development.
6. Discuss moral development according to Kohlberg.
7. Identify the principles of growth and development.
8. Describe the physical development of children.
9. Identify two pros and two cons of early childhood education.
10. Discuss age-appropriate discipline measures for children.
11. Explain the male and female physical changes of puberty.
12. Identify developmental tasks of adolescence.
13. Discuss at least three concerns related to adolescence.

Clinical Practice

1. Explain the importance of regular prenatal health care.
2. Discuss recommended feeding patterns for newborns and older infants.
3. Explain the importance of screening young children for physical development.
4. Provide health promotion teaching to parents and school-age children.
5. Explain how parents and other caregivers can encourage age-appropriate cognitive and psychosocial development.

Key Terms

Be sure to check out the bonus material on the Companion CD-ROM, including selected audio pronunciations.

abortion (p. 142)
autonomy (ăw-TĂ-nō-mē, p. 146)
bonding (p. 145)
cephalocaudal (cĕ-făl-ō-KĂW-dal, p. 144)
cognitive (p. 137)
conception (p. 139)
ego (p. 139)
egocentric (ē-gō-SĔN-trĭk, p. 146)

embryonic (ĕm-brĭ-Ō-nĭk, p. 142)
fetal (p. 142)
gender (p. 141)
gender roles (p. 147)
genes (JĒNS, p. 142)
germinal (JĔR-mĭ-nŭl, p. 142)
id (p. 139)
ideology (ī-dē-Ō-lō-jē, p. 153)
initiative (ĭ-NĬ-shă-tĭv, p. 146)
intelligence (p. 149)
morals (p. 147)
Moro reflex (p. 143)
neonate (NĒ-ō-nāt, p. 143)
peers (p. 147)
prepuberty (prē-PĔW-bĕr-tē, p. 148)
psychosocial (sī-kō-SŌ-shŭl, p. 137)
puberty (p. 151)
reflexes (RĔ-flĕx-ĕz, p. 143)
self-concept (p. 149)
sensorimotor (sĕn-sŏr-ē-MŌ-tŏr, p. 144)
sexual orientation (p. 153)
siblings (p. 141)
social competence (KŎM-pĕ-tĕns, p. 149)
superego (p. 139)
theory (p. 139)
time-out (p. 147)
trimesters (TRĬ-mĕs-tĕrz, p. 142)
vernix caseosa (VĔR-nĭx kă-sē-Ō-sa, p. 143)
viable (VĬ-ă-bŭl, p. 142)
zygote (ZĬ-gōt, p. 142)

The study of human development is fascinating. It is the study of how people change, and stay the same, over time. Each of us is a unique person who continues to develop throughout life. The more you learn about human development, the more you will appreciate the complexity of life. Studying human development may help you better understand yourself and others.

In some ways, people show consistency from one stage of life to another. Some personality traits, for example, appear early in childhood and persist through life. In other ways, such as physical development, people change as they get older. The chapters in this unit focus on three aspects of human development: physical, cognitive (knowledge and thinking processes), and psychosocial (personality, getting along in society). The physical aspect is easy to understand; we can see children

OVERVIEW OF STRUCTURE AND FUNCTION

Prenatal development

What happens in the germinal stage of prenatal development?

- Rapid cell division begins within 36 hours of fertilization. The growing *zygote* travels through the fallopian tube to the uterus. It is now called a *blastocyst*. During the second week, it attaches itself to the uterine wall.

- Supportive tissues essential to the pregnancy are also developing. The *placenta* develops to attach the blastocyst to the uterine wall. The *umbilical cord* carries the fetus' blood to and from the placenta. Nutrients and oxygen pass from the mother's bloodstream through the placenta to the bloodstream of the fetus The blastocyst is surrounded by amniotic fluid and contained in a strong, double-walled membrane called the *amniotic sac*.

- This stage lasts for 2 weeks after fertilization.

What happens in the embryonic stage of prenatal development?

- For the next 6 weeks, the embryo continues to grow rapidly.

- The beginnings of all systems and organs are formed. The nervous system develops most rapidly. The heart begins beating about 3½ weeks after conception.

- Arm and leg buds appear in the fifth week. Eyes and ears begin to take shape.

- Fingers and toes begin developing in the sixth week. The spinal cord is visible on ultrasound at 7 weeks.

- About 95% of body parts are formed by the eighth week.

What happens in the fetal stage of prenatal development?

- Organs and systems become refined and begin functioning. Rapid growth continues. This stage lasts until birth.

- External genitalia appear in the third month. Long bones are visible on radiograph in the fourth month. By the fifth month, the fetus is 11 to 12 inches long and may weigh 1 pound.

- The remaining months are the maturation time for all systems.

What causes multiple births?

- Most multiple births occur when more than one ovum is fertilized; these babies are called *fraternal siblings*. They are like other siblings, who share only some genetic similarities.

- *Identical siblings* occur when a single zygote separates in the early stage of cell division into two or more individual blastocysts. Identical twins account for one fourth to one third of all twin births.

- The use of fertility medications to increase the number of ova released often results in the birth of multiple fraternal siblings.

Adolescent development

How does a girl mature into a woman?

- Girls may begin puberty as early as age 9 or as late as age 17; the average age is around 12. These changes may occur over several years.

- The pituitary hormone *follicle-stimulating hormone* (FSH) stimulates the ovaries to begin producing estrogen hormones.

- Estradiol, from the ovary, is responsible for the appearance of secondary sex characteristics. These include breast development, widening of the hips, the appearance of axillary and pubic hair, and growth of the reproductive organs.

- FSH also stimulates the development of ova, and menstruation begins.

How does a boy mature into a man?

- Boys usually begin puberty a little later than girls; the average age for boys is 14.

- The pituitary hormone *interstitial cell–stimulating hormone* (ICSH) activates the testes to produce testosterone. FSH, also from the pituitary, stimulates the testes to begin producing sperm.

- Testosterone is responsible for the development of male secondary sex characteristics. These include enlargement of the reproductive organs; lowering of the voice; growth of facial, pubic, and axillary hair; thickened bones; and increased size of skeletal muscles.

- Nocturnal emissions occur. For the first year, the concentration of sperm in semen is quite low.

grow. Physical development begins at conception (union of ovum and sperm), continues into young adulthood, and includes the normal changes of later adulthood. Cognitive and psychosocial development also begin early in life and continue throughout the life span.

These three facets of human development, physical, cognitive, and psychosocial, are not separated. Each interacts with the others. Every person is a combination of all three. They are discussed separately for the purposes of study and observation.

People do change over time. **We influence our own development through choices that we make.** Only humans can do that! We are resilient and flexible; we can bounce back, adapt, and get stronger.

AGE-GROUPS

The growth and development of children and adolescents can be divided into these common age groupings:

- Prenatal = conception to birth
- Infancy = birth to 18 months
- Early childhood = 18 months to 6 years
- Middle and late childhood = 7 to 11 years
- Adolescence = 12 to 18 years

These divisions are only for the purpose of study. Each individual's development is unique. You cannot judge someone's development without considering physical, cognitive and psychosocial aspects. Family and cultural factors must also be included when trying to make an assessment. Boundaries of each group should be considered flexible when assessing an individual.

THEORIES OF DEVELOPMENT

A theory (an idea formed by reasoning from facts), especially about human development and behavior, is based primarily on observations. Theories are attempts to explain something; they are always being adapted to new information. More information about the following theorists can be found in psychology references.

Sigmund Freud (1856–1939) made contributions to the understanding of personality development. His psychoanalytic theory has three parts that include levels of awareness, components of the personality or mind, and psychosexual stages of development. The levels of awareness consist of the conscious, subconscious, and unconscious mind. The conscious mind is based in reality and what is sensed, perceived, and thought. The subconscious stores thoughts, feelings, and memories. These are easily brought into the conscious mind. The unconscious level is the part of the mind that is not accessible to one's awareness. The unconscious mind stores memories that are usually painful and are stored here to prevent anxiety and stress. Freud stated that there are three functional components

of the mind. The first is the id (body's basic primitive urges). The id is concerned with satisfaction and pleasure. The pleasure principle, or **libido**, is the main force driving human behavior. At birth we are all id. The ego is considered the "executive of the mind." It emerges in the fourth or fifth month of life. It is the problem solver and reality tester and develops with the person's interaction with the environment and the demands of the id. In this way, the child learns to delay immediate satisfaction of needs. The superego is a further development of the ego and represents the moral component. This is the portion of the mind that judges, controls, and punishes. It dictates what is right and what is wrong and acts much as a conscience. These three components of the mind are constantly in conflict with each other according to Freud. Unrestrained id dominance can lead to a personality breakdown in which the person demonstrates childlike behavior persisting throughout adult life. A harsh superego can cause blocking of reasonable needs and drives and prevent full development of the personality in a healthy way. Table 11-1 shows Freud's stages of psychosexual development.

Erik Erikson (1902–1994) was a psychologist interested in the psychosocial aspect of development. He defined eight psychosocial stages. Each is identified by a psychosocial task that must be successfully mastered before the person can progress to the next stage. This growth aids development of a healthy ego. Erikson also believed that cultural, social, biologic, and environmental factors contribute to development. Table 11-2 summarizes this theory for children, adolescents, and adults. In the names of the stages, the first term listed is the desired psychosocial task to be mastered. The second term listed is the opposite, which Erikson considered a negative result.

Jean Piaget (1896–1980) was a psychologist who developed a theory about how children learn. He said that all people are born with a need to adapt to the environment, and that the ability to use knowledge increases as a child grows. Piaget stressed two principles that allow this to happen: (1) organization—we try to make sense of our world; and (2) adaptation—we discover new information and adjust our thinking patterns. The four stages of Piaget's theory are given in Table 11-3 on p. 141. As children develop, each stage helps them understand the world more thoroughly.

Lawrence Kohlberg (1927–1987) developed a theory of moral development. He defined three levels of moral development occurring along with cognitive growth:

- **Preconventional reasoning.** Young children obey rules to avoid punishment. Moral values are not internalized. Most children are in this stage until about age 9.
- **Conventional reasoning.** At this level, children and adults conform to social standards to avoid disapproval or to avoid guilt. Decisions are based on understanding the social order, laws, justice, and duty. Children begin using conventional rea-

Table 11-1 | *Freud's Psychosexual Stages of Development*

STAGE AND AGE	MAJOR DEVELOPMENTAL TASKS	DESIRED OUTCOMES
Oral (0–1 yr)	Beginning of ego development. Relief from anxiety through oral gratification of needs	Realization that needs can be met and development of trust in the environment
Anal (1–3 yr)	Learning independence and control; focus on the excretory functions Ability to delay immediate gratification	Control over impulses
Phallic (oedipal) (3–6 yr)	Development of sexual identity Beginning of superego development Focus on genital organs	Identification with parent of same sex
Latency (6–12 yr)	Focus on relationships with same-sex peers Growth of ego functions (social, intellectual, mechanical) and the ability to care about and relate to others outside the home	The development of skills needed to cope with the environment and others
Genital (12 yr and beyond)	Emancipation from parents Planning of life goals Development of personal identity Focus on relationships with members of the opposite sex	The ability to find pleasure in love and work and to be creative

Adapted from Varcarolis, E.M., Carson, V.B., and Shoemaker, N.C. (2006). *Foundations of Psychiatric Mental Health Nursing: A Clinical Approach* (5th ed.). Philadelphia: Elsevier Saunders; and Polan, E., & Taylor D. (2007). *Journey Across the Life Span* (3rd ed.). Philadelphia: F.A. Davis.

Table 11-2 | *Psychosocial Development According to Erikson*

STAGE	CHARACTERISTICS	OUTCOMES
Trust vs. mistrust (Birth–1 year)	Caregiver responds in warm, caring manner to child's needs to create trusting environment. If care is inconsistent and unreliable, mistrust develops.	*Positive:* hope, tolerates frustration, can delay gratification, sense of trust *Negative:* suspicion, withdrawal, focus on negative aspect of people's behavior
Autonomy vs. shame and doubt (1–3 years)	Child practices and attains new physical skills, developing autonomy. If not allowed to do things he or she can do, or pushed into doing something when not ready, child may develop sense of shame or doubt.	*Positive:* will, self-control, positive self-esteem, self-confidence *Negative:* compulsion, impulsivity
Initiative vs. guilt (3–6 years)	Initiative is demonstrated when the child is able to formulate a plan of action and carry it out. Believes that desires and actions are basically sound. If the child is punished for expressing his or her desires, then child will develop a sense of guilt.	*Positive:* purpose, enjoys accomplishments, self-starter *Negative:* inhibition, afraid to accept new challenges, guilt over one's actions
Industry vs. inferiority (6–12 years)	Child acquires skills such as reading, writing, and mathematics and social skills. Through acquisition of these skills he or she develops a sense of industry. If always compared to others, or made to believe he or she is inadequate, child will develop sense of inferiority.	*Positive:* competence, enjoys learning about new things, perseverance, takes criticism well *Negative:* inadequacy, inferiority, gives up easily
Identity vs. role confusion (12–19 years)	The adolescent investigates and identifies alternatives regarding his or her vocational and personal future. Premature choices, or the inability to make these choices, will lead to role confusion.	*Positive:* fidelity, confidence in self-identity, optimism, control of one's destiny *Negative:* diffidence, defiance, socially unacceptable identity, sense of purposelessness
Intimacy vs. isolation (19–25 years)	Love relationships are developed. Fear of intimate relationships will lead to a sense of isolation.	*Positive:* love, development of deep interpersonal relationships *Negative:* exclusivity, avoidance of commitment, avoidance of relationships
Generativity vs. stagnation (25–50 years)	Parenting, nurturing others, and fulfilling civic responsibilities are the tasks. The adult finds ways to be productive and of help to others in order to grow personally.	*Positive:* care, concern for future generations of the society, desire to help others *Negative:* stagnated, rejection of others, self-indulgence, self-absorbed, highly critical of others
Ego integrity vs. despair (50 and older)	Reflection on one's life and one's achievements. A sense of pride or despair is developed regarding the accomplishments in life that have been made or were lost.	*Positive:* wisdom, self-satisfaction *Negative:* disdain, disgust, bitterness concerning lost opportunities

From Bowden, V.R., Dickey, S.B., and Greenberg, C.S. (1998). *Children and Their Families: The Continuum of Care* (pp. 207-208). Philadelphia: Saunders.

Table 11-3 *Cognitive Development According to Piaget*

STAGE	AGE RANGE	CHARACTERISTICS
Sensorimotor stage	Birth–2 years	Experiences world through the senses
	1–4 months	Tries to reproduce behavior that was first performed by chance
	4–8 months	Achievement of hand-eye coordination
		Begins to recognize cause and effect—certain actions have certain results
	8–12 months	Demonstrates anticipatory behavior
		Object permanence is developing
		Can solve simple problems
	12–18 months	Beginning of reasoning
		Begins trial-and-error activities
		Understands object permanence
	18–24 months	Views self as separate from others
		Can use symbols mentally
		Understands basics of cause and effect
Preoperational stage	2–7 years	
	2–4 years	Displays egocentrism
		Can form symbolic thought
		Takes instructions literally
		Can imitate others later
	4–7 years	Begins pre-logical reasoning
		Uses language to express thoughts
		Likes socialized play
		Demonstrates illogical reasoning
		Concentrates on one aspect of an object at a time
		Judges by appearance and results
Concrete operations	7–11 years	Begins to logically manipulate symbols
		Demonstrates concrete thinking
		Can reverse thinking
		Demonstrates conservation skills
		Likes to collect and classify objects
		Enjoys a joke
		Can shift attention from one attribute of an object or experience to another
Formal operations	11 years–death	Can logically manipulate abstract and unobservable concepts
		Can use scientific approach to solve problems
		Able to solve complex verbal problems
		Thinks of distant future concretely and sets realistic long-term goals

From Bowden, V.R., Dickey, S.G., and Greenberg, C.S. (1998). *Children and Their Families: The Continuum of Care* (pp. 207-208). Philadelphia: Saunders.

soning at around 11 and may remain in this stage throughout life.

- **Postconventional reasoning.** People at this level have internalized moral principles. They are law abiding and follow their conscience. Kohlberg believes that only a minority of adults operate at this level.

PRINCIPLES OF GROWTH AND DEVELOPMENT

Many factors influence growth and development. Heredity is a major factor, as is the environment. Some developmental psychologists have tried to determine which is more important. So far, there is not much agreement.

Family structure is also important. Are there two parents in the home? What parenting style is seen? What is the family's socioeconomic situation? Some people think that ordinal position (birth order) also plays a part. Even gender (male or female) can influence how a child is raised.

Even with all the variables that can affect growth and development, some basic principles exist:

- Growth occurs in orderly and predictable ways. Patterns and stages can be anticipated.
- The rate of growth and development is individual. Even siblings (brothers and sisters) develop at different rates.
- Development is lifelong. People continue to change throughout life. Physical growth is seen in childhood, but normal changes continue.
- Development is multidimensional. It involves many processes, including physical, cognitive, and psychosocial aspects.
- Development is continual, but may occur at different rates. There may be times when development seems static.

PRENATAL DEVELOPMENT

Prenatal development begins at the time of conception, when the mother's ovum is fertilized by the father's sperm and a new and unique cell is formed. This cell, the zygote (fertilized egg), will, under healthy circumstances, become a baby.

Among the many influences on prenatal development is genetics. Genes (segments of DNA that carry the blueprints of development) pass from parents to child through the sperm and the ovum. The nucleus of the individual cells contains 23 unpaired chromosomes. The chromosomes are filled with tightly coiled strands of DNA. The zygote contains 23 chromosomes from the father and 23 chromosomes from the mother, thus once joined the human cells contain 46 chromosomes. These 46 chromosomes become a unique combination that will almost certainly never occur again. That is why each of us is different from everyone else.

EVENTS IN PRENATAL DEVELOPMENT

There are three stages of prenatal development: germinal (initial), embryonic (early formation), and fetal (late). An overview of prenatal development is provided here.

Pregnancy is divided into three trimesters (periods of 3 months). A full-term pregnancy lasts 40 weeks. Birth within 2 weeks on either side of the estimated date is considered normal. If the baby is delivered earlier than 38 weeks' gestation, it is called *premature*. Premature babies can survive if their systems are mature enough to support life and if the delivery occurs in a safe place. When a pregnancy ends before the fetus is viable (able to survive outside of the womb), it is called an abortion. A naturally occurring abortion is often called a *miscarriage*.

MATERNAL INFLUENCES

The single most important factor in maintaining a healthy pregnancy is early and regular prenatal health care. Visits with health professionals help expectant mothers understand what is happening and how they can contribute to healthy fetal growth. This care also allows the health professional to detect signs of potential problems and intervene before the problems become serious. A healthy outcome for both mother and child is always the goal. Lack of prenatal care is a serious problem for some women. This can occur because of economics, fear, ignorance, lack of access, or other reasons. *Healthy People 2010*'s objective of "increase the proportion of persons appropriately counseled about health behaviors," and the goal of increasing access to health care for all people in the United States, make it imperative to refer pregnant women to an agency that can provide prenatal care regardless of their economic position (Health Promotion Points 11-1).

A second influence in prenatal development is the mother's health. Women with a chronic illness who are pregnant are usually considered high risk. This especially includes women with diabetes or rheumatic heart disease. Contracting a communicable disease

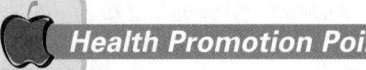

Health Promotion Points 11-1

Prenatal Care

- A female should seek prenatal care as soon as she suspects she is pregnant.
- If planning to become pregnant, she should be certain her intake of folic acid is at least 400 mcg/day, be certain immunizations are up to date for those diseases that could harm the fetus (rubella in particular), and seek control of any chronic disease.

during pregnancy also presents a risk to fetal health. German measles (rubella) is one communicable disease known to cause harm to a fetus.

Another influence can be the mother's age. Pregnancy before the mother reaches her adult growth, at about age 16, can be a high-risk situation. At the other extreme, a woman experiencing her first pregnancy after age 35 is considered high risk. Any pregnancy when the mother is over 40 is also high risk.

A fourth influence is the mother's nutritional state. **Women need to be well nourished before pregnancy begins as well as throughout the pregnancy.** The mother's nutrition is vital for healthy fetal development. A woman who begins a pregnancy at a healthy weight should gain approximately 30 pounds; less than that endangers fetal growth. Excessive weight gain can complicate the delivery and can also make it hard for her to lose weight later. A *Healthy People 2010* objective is to "increase the proportion of mothers who achieve a recommended weight gain during their pregnancies."

Emotional stresses may also influence the pregnancy. Women who experience severe emotional stresses may put the fetus at risk. This is because stress affects the physiology of blood flow and may restrict blood to the placenta. Prolonged stress interferes with adequate nutrition and oxygen to the fetus.

The sixth influence is the use of chemicals. Chemicals known to interfere in some way with fetal development include alcohol, nicotine, caffeine, some medications, and street drugs. As scientists study babies with problems, it is becoming apparent that even casual use of any of these chemicals may be risky. Another *Healthy People 2010* objective is to "increase abstinence from alcohol, cigarettes, and illicit drugs among pregnant women." This will help in the achievement of another goal, to "reduce the occurrence of fetal alcohol syndrome (FAS)."

Think Critically About . . . You have a friend who suspects she is pregnant for the first time, but is postponing seeing a doctor. What will you say to her?

INFANTS

For the first month of life, the baby is a neonate (newborn). This month is a period of adjustment for the infant and the new parents. Infancy extends through the first 18 months (Health Promotion Points 11-2).

APPEARANCE AND CAPABILITIES OF NEWBORNS

At birth, the skin and scalp are often covered with vernix caseosa (a cheesy, waxy substance that protects the skin in fetal life). This wears off in a day or two. Babies' heads appear large in comparison to their bodies, and may be temporarily misshapen. They move their arms and legs aimlessly; the hands and feet may appear slightly cyanotic for a while. Newborns should cry spontaneously after birth. They will usually be quiet when wrapped tightly in a blanket and held as this provides a feeling of security.

A newborn may appear helpless but really has many capabilities. Reflexes (instinctive protective actions) present at birth include blinking, yawning, grasping, stepping, hiccoughing, sucking, and swallowing. The Moro reflex (startle response) can be elicited by making a loud noise near the baby, who will react by arching his or her back and assuming a typical posture with flexion and adduction of the extremities and fingers fanned initially.

Newborns can also express themselves by crying; it usually does not take long for new parents to know the meaning of the different cries they make. Newborns also watch everything and everyone. Their response to people and surroundings is the way they communicate.

A typical newborn sleeps from 16 to 20 hours per day. This time is important for growth and development. Eating and being loved and cared for usually fill the waking hours. Wakefulness increases as they get older. By 1 year of age, most infants need only a morning and afternoon nap.

NUTRITION

Healthy newborns can manage without calories for the first 12 to 24 hours, but usually are breast or bottle fed sooner. After that, they need to have caloric intake to survive. Most pediatricians recommend breast-feeding; breast milk is perfectly designed for the newborn's digestive system. It also provides the newborn with protective antibodies for the first few months. There is a *Healthy People 2010* objective directed at increasing the number of women who breast-feed their infants.

Women who choose to use infant formula, either initially or later, should know that it closely resembles human milk. The physician will recommend the type of formula. Cow's milk is not advised for babies until 11 to 12 months of age because of possible allergic reactions.

The stomach of newborns holds only an ounce or two at first; that is why they need to eat often. Babies grow rapidly; by 1 month they are eating larger amounts. Feeding time should provide emotional closeness. Infants should be held and talked to while being fed.

For the first 6 months, babies need only breast milk or infant formula. The first solids are usually baby cereals, strained vegetables, and strained fruits. It is best to add new foods slowly in order to see how well the baby tolerates them. Older infants enjoy finger foods. Most babies can eat table food by 1 year of age. They should not be given pieces of sausage, peanuts, or hard candies that could be aspirated.

PHYSICAL DEVELOPMENT

The average white newborn weighs 7 to 7½ pounds and is 20 to 21 inches long. Dark-skinned babies may be a little smaller at birth. Newborns between 5½ and 11 pounds are considered equally healthy. There are two categories of low-birth-weight babies. The first is *preterm babies who* are born before 37 weeks of gestation and weigh less than 5 pounds. The second category is *small-for-dates babies.* These infants are born at term but weigh less than 90% of what they should weigh.

All babies should double their birth weight at 5 to 6 months, and triple it by 1 year. They should also grow 11 to 12 inches in the first year (Health Promotion Points 11-3).

The newborn's eyes are dark blue or gray. The permanent eye color will develop by 9 to 11 months. Newborns can see light and darkness, and seem to prefer bright colors. Their vision is focused best at 8 to 15 inches from their eyes. Visual acuity increases in harmony with their growing awareness of their surroundings.

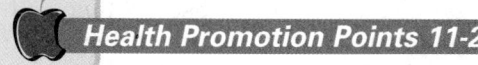

Health Promotion Points 11-2

Infant Health Care

- Regular checkups with the infant's health care provider should occur at 2 months, 4 months, 6 months, 9 months, and 1 year.
- Immunizations for hepatitis B, diphtheria, tetanus, pertussis, *Haemophilus influenzae*, rubella, measles, mumps, polio, pneumococcus, varicella, influenza, and hepatitis A are recommended at birth, 2 months, 4 months, 6 months, and between 12 and 18 months for the infant.

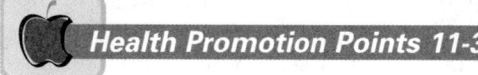

Health Promotion Points 11-3

Indications for Pediatric Evaluation

If a baby is not gaining weight or growing within normal percentiles on the growth chart, or is showing definite developmental delays, further evaluation should be done by a pediatrician.

| Box 11-1 | *Milestones* in Infant Motor Development* |

- **4 to 6 weeks:** Stops crying when held
- **2 months:** Lifts and turns head
- **3 months:** Reaches for and tries to grasp objects
- **4 months:** Sits with support, coos
- **5 months:** Recognizes people, holds own bottle, splashes in water
- **6 months:** Rolls over, sits alone, plays peek-a-boo
- **9 months:** Crawls, knows own name, understands "no"
- **10 months:** Some walk with help
- **12 months:** Most walk alone

*Each infant will develop at his or her own rate. Times given are norms.

Newborns can hear well and are afraid of loud noises. Infants prefer their mother's voice to that of other women, and they often recognize voices of other family members.

The sense of touch is not well differentiated at birth, but babies need to be touched and held. They can feel pain, although it is more generalized than specific for the first few months.

The baby's first teeth, the bottom incisors, usually appear at 5 to 11 months. By 12 months, many babies have six to eight temporary teeth.

The brain grows rapidly in infancy and early childhood. Neurons present at birth are not fully developed. As the baby grows, the neurons continue to extend, grow, and make connections. A newborn's brain weighs 25% of an adult's brain; this increases to 66% in the first year alone. By age 2, the brain weighs 80% of an adult's brain. Infants and young children need a healthy diet, including fats, for brain growth to occur. They also need stimulation for neuron connections to form.

MOTOR DEVELOPMENT

Motor development occurs in a typical pattern. **The pattern is consistent, though the rate may vary from one child to another.**

Cephalocaudal (proceeding from head to tail) development means that babies can lift their head before they can lift their chest. They can sit before they can stand. Development also proceeds from the center of the body toward the outside. They control their shoulders before they control their arms and fingers. Large muscles develop coordination before smaller ones. For example, they can walk before they can draw.

Milestones in motor development are shown in Box 11-1. Parents may need reassurance if one child develops more slowly than another. Children perform motor skills only when they are developmentally ready.

Several environmental factors influence a child's motor development. Children need good nutrition, health care, emotional support, and the opportunity to practice motor skills. Deprivation of any of these factors may cause developmental delay. Safety for the helpless infant is a primary concern (Safety Alert 11-1).

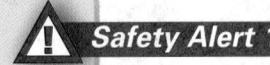 **Safety Alert 11-1**

Infant Safety Factors

- An infant should not be left alone on a surface that does not offer protection against falls.
- The infant should be restrained in a car seat in the back seat of the automobile whenever the vehicle is in motion.
- Bathwater should be tested to see that it is not too hot before an infant is put into the water.
- Small objects should be kept out of reach to prevent entry into the mouth and choking.
- The infant should be placed on its back for sleep, with propping slightly on one side or the other for variation. No infant should be placed on the stomach to sleep.
- An infant should never be left alone in a house or car.

COGNITIVE DEVELOPMENT

According to Piaget's theory of cognitive development, babies actively construct their own cognitive world. They organize experiences and observations and then make adaptations in thinking when new situations occur. Newborns display this process by eagerly sucking on everything that comes near their mouth. Later, they learn that some things, such as a nipple or thumb, are suitable for sucking. These items provide satisfaction, either nutritionally or emotionally. Sucking on a blanket or a toy does not provide the same satisfaction.

The first cognitive stage is sensorimotor. This begins with babies experiencing things about themselves—becoming aware of the sensations of their body, discovering their toes, etc. Then babies move on to learn about other people and objects in their world.

By the time babies are about 8 months old, they realize that an object still exists even when they cannot see it. This is called *object permanence*. It is demonstrated when an infant is shown an object that is then hidden, and the baby looks for it.

Authorities debate whether an infant's intelligence can be accurately measured. One measure that is sometimes used is language development. Most infants begin babbling at 3 to 6 months, the cooing, gurgling stage. Babies learn language by listening to people around them and imitating the sounds they hear. Parents who talk to their babies and spend time with them stimulate language development. Babies often say their first word at 11 to 13 months and begin using two-word sentences at 18 to 24 months. The same sequence exists all over the world.

An infant's efforts at discovery are dependent on the assistance and guidance of the adults in his or her life. **Caregivers can stimulate cognitive development by spending time with the baby, talking, singing, playing, and loving.** Many kinds of experiences should be provided. Babies thrive on receiving lots of attention and being part of family activities (Figure 11-1).

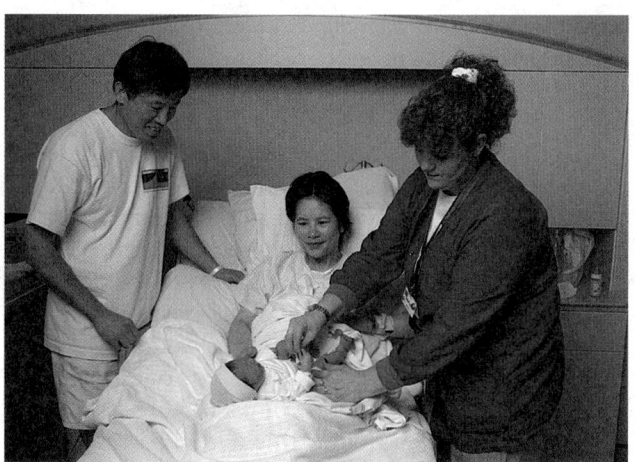

FIGURE **11-1** Every newborn arrives with lots of potential.

PSYCHOSOCIAL DEVELOPMENT

Infants learn to interact with other people by experience with their caregivers. Bonding (sense of attachment between two people) occurs with one or two primary caregivers first, usually the mother and/or father. The infant's need for stimulation and love grows during the first 3 months. Physical contact, caring, and familiarity are important aspects in bonding. By 5 or 6 months, the baby is ready to include other people in relationships.

Bonding gives babies the security they need to develop the sense of trust. Erikson believed that infants learn to trust others when they receive warm, consistent care. To develop trust, infants need to feel comfortable and secure and believe that the caregiver will always meet their needs. Infants who have a sense of trust will have confidence to explore new situations and can usually handle short separations from parents. This will help them develop relationships with other people throughout their lives.

A healthy baby recognizes family members and shows insecurity with strangers by 6 to 7 months of age. Studies show that infants with a secure attachment to another human are happier and less frustrated at 2 years of age than infants with a less secure attachment.

? *Think Critically About . . .* Can a baby develop trust in a foster-care situation?

YOUNG CHILDREN

Young children are defined as those between 18 months and 6 years of age. This group is sometimes divided into toddlers (1 to 3 years) and preschoolers (4 to 5 years). Many developmental milestones occur in these years.

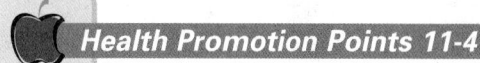

Health Promotion Points 11-4

Health Care for Young Children

- Regular checkups are recommended at least every 2 years to assess growth and development.
- Immunization boosters are recommended between 4 and 6 years of age, and again at 11 or 12 years.
- A test for iron deficiency may be appropriate in the child who is not eating well.
- When a child enters preschool, a physical examination is often required that will include a urinalysis and vision test. The examination may reveal health problems that are not obvious so that early intervention can occur.

PHYSICAL DEVELOPMENT

The rate of growth in early childhood is slower than in infancy. Young children lose their baby fat and appear slimmer as their trunk lengthens. Most young children grow 2 to 3 inches in height and gain 4 to 6 pounds each year. Boys are slightly larger than girls during this period. The size of muscles and bones increases, which can lead to greater strength. Heart and lungs become more efficient, and the child's immunity improves.

Heredity and the environment have been shown to influence this physical development. The primary environmental influence is nutrition. Young children need 1400 to 1800 calories per day. Sometimes when the child doesn't eat much, it concerns parents; at this age some children are fussy about what they will eat. Children over 2 years of age need less fat and sugar in their diets than they are usually fed.

Vision improves during the early childhood years. By 2 years, visiual acuity is usually 20/40. Vision may be checked during a preschool physical exam in the physician's office, but this is usually done during the kindergarten physical examination or at the beginning of the first grade (Health Promotion Points 11-4). Visual screening is often a function of the school nurse.

During early childhood new teeth continue to erupt. A full set of deciduous teeth numbers 24 and should be present by age 3. Supervised toothbrushing and flossing should begin as soon as a child has teeth. The first dental visit may be made when a child is 2 to 3 years old.

A growth chart can monitor the child's physical growth. Height and weight are plotted on the graph and compared with those of the average child. Most children will fall within the guidelines of the curve. A child who falls below the 5th percentile or above the 95th percentile may need further evaluation as something physical may be wrong. **It is important to monitor the child's growth so that any problems can be treated before they become serious.** Growth progress should be steady.

MOTOR DEVELOPMENT

Motor development proceeds as growth occurs. Neuromuscular maturation is needed for motor skills to develop. A milestone of this age-group is toilet training, the age for which varies from culture to culture. Most children are physiologically ready to be bowel trained between 1½ and 2 years, but successful toilet training also depends on psychological readiness. Daytime bladder control usually occurs later than bowel control; nighttime bladder control occurs later than that.

Young children also learn to feed themselves, dress themselves, and become independent in many activities. Improving neuromuscular skills leads to better coordination. For example, at age 2, children usually hold someone's hand to go up a stairway and take only one step at a time. At 3, they can climb stairs using alternate steps, though they may still need to hold on. By age 4, they can climb a stairway alone. At 5, they will run upstairs without even thinking about it.

A commonly used assessment tool is the *Denver Developmental Screening Test,* also known as the Denver II. It is a simple and rapid way to assess developmental maturity of young children before they start school. The test giver spends time with the child to observe gross and fine motor skills, language, and social ability. Some gross motor skills measured include walking, jumping, using a tricycle, throwing and catching a ball, hopping on one foot, and balancing on one foot. Fine motor skills include stacking a pile of blocks, drawing people, and drawing houses.

COGNITIVE DEVELOPMENT

Expanding neuron connections result in increasing learning and thinking skills. Piaget called the ages of 2 to 7 years the stage of *preoperational thought,* defined as learning how to organize thoughts. This stage is subdivided into symbolic function and intuitive thought.

In the *symbolic function substage,* children can think about objects, people, and events in their absence by using mental symbols of them. Watch a child draw a picture or play a game of pretend. The child can think about objects even though they are not currently present.

There are some interesting normal occurrences during these years. Children have vivid imaginations, and many cannot easily distinguish between reality and fantasy. Cartoon characters are real to the young child, and stuffed toys are alive. Young children engage in magical thinking. Because they do not understand cause and effect, they may think that events occur magically.

Another phenomenon is the child's egocentric (I am the center of the world) belief. Young children believe that they are the most important person in the world. They think that their desires should be fulfilled on demand. They also believe that their thoughts influence events, and they cannot grasp another person's viewpoint.

In the *intuitive thought substage,* thinking abilities expand, thoughts are better organized, and early problem solving occurs. Abstractions such as time and numbers often remain hazy.

One highlight in young children's cognitive development is their curiosity. This often surpasses their caution, making safety a concern. The home and play environment should be free of lead contamination to protect against lead poisoning. Children lack the experience and knowledge to understand possible dangers. Childproofing a home (keeping cleaning supplies, medicines, and other potential hazards out of reach) is essential. Health Promotion Points 11-5 presents safety considerations. Children at this age need instruction about dangers: cars, crossing streets, strangers, acceptable ways to touch and be touched. **Parents and other caregivers are primary safety teachers by example and concern.**

Attention spans begin to lengthen during these years. A 5-year-old can sit still much longer for a story than can his or her 2-year-old sister. This makes conversations interesting. A child's memory also improves.

Language develops rapidly during childhood. Most 6-year-olds know 8000 to 14,000 words. Sentence length usually increases proportionately to age. The speed with which a child learns to talk is not necessarily indicative of intelligence. Girls often begin to talk sooner than boys, and firstborn children may talk at a younger age than their siblings.

Young children have lively imaginations. Some develop an imaginary friend who accompanies them everywhere. This friend can conveniently be blamed for minor problems, too. The playmate usually disappears when the child is 5 or 6. Pretend play is also imaginative. Pretending is important between 3 and 8 years, as the child experiments with various roles.

PSYCHOSOCIAL DEVELOPMENT

Erikson's second stage of development occurs from 18 months to 3 years. Autonomy (being independent) develops as children learn to feed themselves and to do other things without help. Children are also more verbal, and can say "no," often with great conviction.

Caregivers who are impatient and do everything for the child may cause feelings of shame and doubt to develop. If parents are overprotective and critical, for example, children may be ashamed of themselves and doubt their ability to accomplish things.

Erikson's stage for ages 3 to 6 is called initiative (willingness to try). Young children are energetic, eager, and curious. They know no fear and want to explore the world. They are also beginning to develop a conscience and to learn what is right and wrong. Will the child be successful in this stage of initiative, or will he or she be plagued by guilt, by not doing the right thing? Parents can aid children through this stage by

Health Promotion Points 11-5

Safety Guidelines for Children

INFANTS AND YOUNG CHILDREN

- Use crib with correct spacing between spindles or slats.
- Never leave the infant alone on an elevated surface, in a high chair, stroller, walker, or other such equipment.
- Secure stairways with safety barrier and keep exit doors closed and/or locked.
- Check toys for loose buttons, long strings, small parts, and rough edges.
- Do not use plastic bags within infant's reach.
- Remove toxic plants from the home; supply chewable objects such as teething rings.
- Do not leave an infant alone in the bathtub at any time.
- Safety-lock doors to appliances, cupboards, and drawers where items are kept that are dangerous, caustic, or toxic.
- Prevent child from chewing on old windowsills or furniture that might have been painted with lead paint.
- Keep the number of the poison control center close to the telephone.
- Avoid using tablecloths that hang over the table within an infant's reach.
- Cover electrical outlets and keep wires and cords out of reach of child.
- Keep household cleaners and medications in childproof containers out of reach of child.
- Avoid giving child hard candies, nuts, popcorn, or small pieces of food that could be easily aspirated.
- Do not drink hot drinks while holding an infant.
- Keep child away from hot surfaces.
- Dress child in flame-retardant sleepwear.

- Use plastic rather than glass or ceramic eating and drinking utensils.
- Supervise play if animals are around.
- Correctly use approved safety seats and restraints for infants and children.
- Supervise play and teach about street dangers.
- Instruct children never to talk to or go anywhere with strangers.
- Keep knives out of reach of children and power tools and guns locked up.
- Keep matches out of reach of children.
- Turn pot handles toward back of stove.
- Fence pool with a locked gate.
- Use garage door with automatic opener adjusted to rise if door strikes an object.
- Keep clothesline above adult head level.
- Mark glass doors with decals.

ADOLESCENTS

- Encourage use of appropriate safety equipment for sports.
- Teach proper warm-up and stretching maneuvers to use before playing sports.
- Educate regarding safe driving.
- Provide education about the dangers of drug use.
- Provide education about safe sex practices, emphasizing abstinence, but including prevention of sexually transmitted diseases and pregnancy.
- Teach water safety and remind not to dive into shallow water or water of unknown depth.

---

giving them freedom to explore within safe limits, by encouraging their questions and ideas, by supporting successes, and by helping the preschooler develop self-esteem.

Young children do need to learn discipline. Many parents find that enforcing **time-out** (quiet time alone without toys) is often effective. It is recommended that 1 minute be used for each year of age. This must occur immediately after the offense or the child will not relate the behavior to the punishment.

Children learn **gender roles** (behaviors and attitudes a culture expects and approves for males or females) during this stage. They observe the behaviors expected of boys and girls and how they differ. By 3, children know their own gender, and by 6 they can usually identify another person's gender by watching appearance and behavior. Some psychologists believe that sex hormones, even in young children, strongly influence a child's behavior. Others believe that the gender roles children adopt are more influenced by their environment. Parents and other adults provide strong influences in the child's gender role adaptation. This occurs through their examples, the toys they provide, and the way they treat children.

Think Critically About . . . Are there gender stereotypes? What examples support your answer? Should gender roles be encouraged? Why is this a concern to some?

A new sibling often arrives in a family during an older child's early years. There is a natural rivalry when children think they must compete for their parents' attention. Parents should make every effort to give adequate attention to each child and to treat each as an individual. A young child can be somewhat prepared for the arrival of a new baby through talking with the parents, reading story books about babies, and participating in special sibling classes. Older children will continue to need much reassurance that they are still loved.

Morals (values of right and wrong) are developed during young childhood. Young children are developing a conscience. They start to understand other people's feelings, which is the beginning of empathy.

The importance of **peers** (others of similar age and background) increases as children get older. The young child is first influenced in the home by parents and

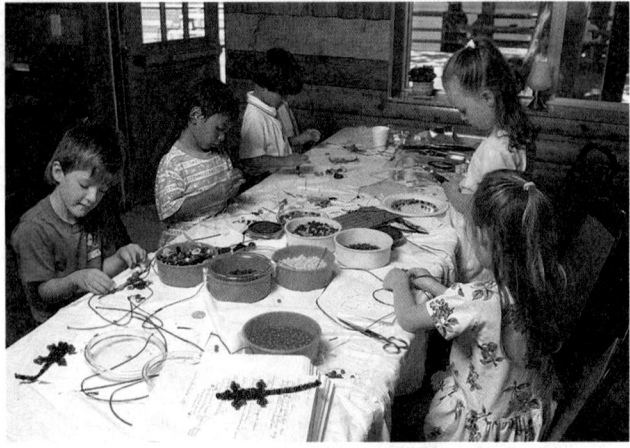

FIGURE **11-2** Preschool children enjoy group activities.

Box 11-2 *Types of Play*

- **Onlooker play:** A child watches others playing, but does not interact. (Ages 1–2)
- **Solitary play:** Playing alone. (Age 1 on)
- **Parallel play:** Children play next to each other but there is little interaction. (18 months–3 years)
- **Associative play:** Children play together, sharing toys and activities and communicating. (Age 2 on)
- **Cooperative play:** Children play together. Games have rules and goals. Groups may have a leader. (Ages 5 on)

---

other family members. By age 3, the child needs exposure to other children. It is important for parents to realize that children naturally begin to seek friendships and experiences outside the home by the time they are 6.

Play contributes to cognitive and psychosocial development. Children's play helps them learn and understand the world around them. Several types of play are shown in Box 11-2. Play should be spontaneous and voluntary. Most preschoolers prefer playing with same-gender children. Children also enjoy playing with adults.

DAY CARE AND EARLY EDUCATION

Many young children in the United States are cared for by adults other than their parents some of the time. According to the U.S. Bureau of the Census (2007), over 10 million American mothers with young children are employed outside of their homes. Child care may be provided in a home setting or in a group setting. Topics considered when choosing appropriate care are the approach to discipline, general child-rearing practices and beliefs, provision of appropriate activities for the child, attention to safety and health, and a nurturing atmosphere. Parents should carefully check a day care situation before entrusting their child to it.

Group settings provide stimulation for the child in areas that may not be available in the home setting. The day care center or preschool also provides an opportunity for the child to adjust to leaving home for a period of time before the beginning of regular school years (Figure 11-2). The child also learns socialization skills. The government provides funds for Head Start, a preschool program for children in lower income families. The child's behavior should be monitored for signs of stress when in a child care setting because some children are maturationally too young to adapt.

? *Think Critically About . . .* How would you counsel parents regarding proper assessment of a day care situation?

MIDDLE AND OLDER CHILDREN

Middle and older children are those from age 7 to 11. Children move through elementary school, join in group activities, and become more grown up. They are filled with energy and enthusiasm. They begin to express their own ideas with confidence and are interesting people.

PHYSICAL DEVELOPMENT

Growth continues to be slow and steady. Children grow an average of 2 to 3 inches in height, and gain 3 to 5 pounds in weight each year. There may be periods of several months without apparent growth, followed by periods of rapid growth. Change is most noticeable in leg length, while the body trunk becomes slimmer. By age 11, some children begin to show signs of prepuberty (beginning sexual development).

Children can run, hit a baseball, swim, and perform many other physical activities. This demonstrates increasing coordination skills.

One health concern for this age-group includes regular dental care, because this is the time when permanent teeth are erupting. Children in this age range often need orthodontic treatment. Immunization boosters are given when the child begins school (Figure 11-3). Vision screening exams are often done for the first time when a child begins formal schooling. Getting adequate sleep is another concern; a child at this age is often energetic and busy. Parents should monitor schedules so that children do not become overly busy. Education about healthy nutrition is also important because habits formed now will influence future diet and health. There has been a large increase in obesity among children related to fast food, calorie-laden juices and sodas, and large servings. **Young people who are properly nourished throughout their childhood tend to be healthier as adults.** There are *Healthy People 2010* objectives directed at increasing the consumption of fruits and vegetables, maintaining weight within recommended limits, increasing calcium consumption to promote healthy

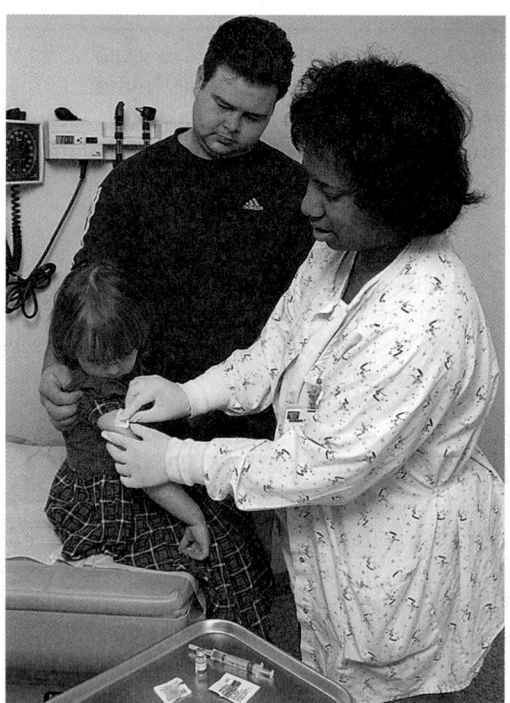

FIGURE 11-3 Prekindergarten immunizations help ensure a healthy start to school.

bones, and diminishing the amount of unhealthy snacks eaten by children.

COGNITIVE DEVELOPMENT

Piaget called this stage of cognitive development *concrete operational thought*. Mental operations are mental activities that can be reversed. Children think in concrete ways about real things, and they draw conclusions based on what they see and know. Ideas are organized and fixed. This demonstrates early problem-solving skills. Children think in black and white; they may have trouble accepting "maybe" situations. They are able to classify things and identify relationships. Children often enjoy collecting things and can spend hours organizing their stamps, rocks, or baseball cards.

Cognition is also apparent in intelligence (a combination of verbal ability, reasoning, memory, imagination, and judgment). No one knows whether heredity or environment is the greater influence on intelligence; certainly both are important. Most children are given some type of intelligence test during their elementary school experience. Scores are given as an *intelligence quotient* (IQ). IQ tests often emphasize language and mathematical skills. The average person has an IQ of 110, with ranges of 80 to 120 considered normal. **Children and their parents need to understand that IQ measurements are only estimates of academic abilities and are not measures of a person's worth or potential for academic success.**

Other tests may be used to measure aspects of intelligence. Most people probably possess many kinds of

---

| Box 11-3 | *Components of Emotional Intelligence* |

- Knowing one's own feelings and using them to make good decisions.
- Managing feelings to keep distress from interfering with the ability to think.
- Motivating oneself despite persistent setbacks.
- Staying hopeful.
- Delaying gratification.
- Empathizing with others.
- Being able to develop rapport with others.

---

intelligence and should be encouraged to discover and nurture their individual strengths and talents. Kinds of intelligence and talent include linguistic, mathematic, spatial, musical, bodily kinesthetic, interpersonal, and intrapersonal.

It is often during the early school years that children with learning problems are identified. Special programs can be helpful for children whose mental development is delayed. Children with an IQ below 70 and who have problems adapting to everyday life are often considered to have special learning needs. This may be an inherited, organic problem, or it may be a result of illness, malnutrition, or lack of mental stimulation.

Numerous types of learning disabilities can be identified through testing and screening procedures. Many children can be aided to develop study habits and alternative learning methods in order to reach their full potential in the education experience.

The other extreme in the range of intelligence is the gifted child, who has an IQ well above the average (140+) and/or possesses a superior talent. Gifted children also need individualized programs. Traditional educational systems may not provide adequate challenge.

Studies of successful adults have led to the concept of emotional intelligence. This consists of six components (Box 11-3). Parents need to model healthy emotional skills. Adults should help children learn to talk about feelings. This requires taking children's feelings seriously and helping them find healthy ways to cope with their feelings.

PSYCHOSOCIAL DEVELOPMENT

Children in the middle years are continuing to develop their self-concept (the way one views oneself). Children need to feel that they are valuable and important. **A comfortable relationship with parents and other adults is vital for development of a healthy self-concept.**

They also begin developing social competence (being comfortable in public, able to get along). They learn to cope with minor stressors. They can see that their behavior may influence others, and they become aware of how they appear to other people.

Erikson called the middle to late childhood psychosocial development stage *industry vs. inferiority*. Children are energetic and capable; they want to accomplish things. They are interested in how things are made and work. Parents and teachers can aid the child through this stage by encouraging ideas, complimenting accomplishments, and helping a little at times. Every child can be complimented on some accomplishment; positive reinforcement helps them thrive. Children need support in facing their problems; they learn that problems can be managed.

The importance of peers increases as children grow. Middle and older children often organize clubs or teams. Belonging to a group builds self-esteem. Group activities are usually with same-gender children. Friendships are vital. Most children have one best friend with whom they share secrets and special times (Box 11-4).

PARENTING

Parents of middle and older children must adjust their expectations and degree of control. It is natural for children to begin spending more time with friends and less with family. Yet parents should remain interested in and involved with their children.

Children at this age can be given more responsibility, including household chores. They need to have opportunities to make decisions. Parents may need guidance in gradually decreasing the amount of supervision.

Some children must spend time alone before and/ or after school because of their parents' schedules. The decision of when this can be permitted will depend on the length of time involved, the child's age and degree of responsibility, and the living situation. Most children under 11 should not be left alone for more than an hour. Each family makes this decision, when necessary, on its own.

Box 11-4 | *Functions of Children's Friendships*

- **Affection:** An emotional relationship outside of the family
- **Companionship:** Playmates who share activities
- **Ego support:** They supply emotional support and encouragement
- **Physical support:** They spend time together
- **Social comparison:** They practice social behaviors
- **Stimulation:** They think of new ideas

? *Think Critically About* . . . How old were you when you were left alone at home? Do you remember how you felt about it? Does your community/state/province have regulations or laws about this?

Middle and older children can no longer be disciplined by a time-out. Denial of privileges is often a better tool. Because of the importance of friends and social events, restricting those activities is often effective.

Three parenting styles have been identified by psychologists: permissive, authoritarian, and authoritative (Table 11-4). The authoritative parent is often considered the ideal.

The reality is that most parents do not use only one style. Two parents in the family may use different styles. Styles may also change with additional children in the family and as the parents mature.

? *Think Critically About* . . . What parenting style do you think your parent(s) used? Was it the same for your siblings? Will you use the same style in raising children? How do people learn to be parents?

CHILD ABUSE

Abuse of children by parents or others can occur at any age. There are many types of abuse: physical, sexual, emotional, neglect, and verbal. Each is damaging to the child's development.

Psychologists have determined that many abusers were themselves victims of abuse and have poor self-concepts. They may not know how to maintain a healthy relationship. This does not excuse their behavior but serves as a warning that the cycle may continue unless someone intervenes. **Health care workers are required, in many states, to report signs of abuse to social agencies or law enforcement authorities** (see Chapter 3).

ADOLESCENTS

The adolescent years begin at age 12 and continue through the teens, to age 18. The actual years are less significant than the experiences and development that

---

Table 11-4 | *Parenting Styles and Outcomes*

STYLE	PARENT BEHAVIORS	CHILD MAY BECOME
Authoritative	Firm, in control, have rules; warm, loving, encouraging	Self-reliant, responsible, socially competent
Authoritarian	Firm, in control, have rules; emotionally distant	Socially anxious
Permissive	Rules, if present, are flexible; may be emotionally warm or not	Impulsive, aggressive, lacking self-control

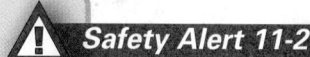

Safety Alert 11-2

Adolescent Safety Factors

- Adolescents should learn safety techniques for the various sports in which they participate. Adequate warm-up and stretching are needed to prevent injury. Bones are growing more rapidly than muscles and tendons at this stage, and injury from sports activities is frequent.
- Safety helmets must be worn when riding a bicycle. Elbow and knee pads, as well as a helmet, should be worn when skateboarding. Scooter riders should wear a helmet also.
- All aspects of water safety should be taught, particularly that one should not swim alone or dive into shallow water or water of unknown depth.
- Once the adolescent is ready to drive, automobile safety must be taught along with the dangers of driving under the influence of alcohol or another drug.

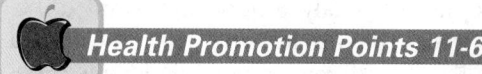

Health Promotion Points 11-6

Sexual Counseling for Adolescents

- If an adolescent is or intends to become sexually active, responsible sexual behavior and birth control need to be addressed.
- Information on contraception options and the nature of sexually transmitted diseases (STDs) and ways to prevent their transmission must be made available.
- Although acquired immunodeficiency syndrome (AIDS) is transmitted in other ways, transmission through sexual intercourse is a real danger, and its incidence by this mode is rising. Although deaths from AIDS are declining, quality of life is greatly affected by it, and deaths do occur.
- Nurses in the school, the clinic, and the physician's office have many opportunities to provide appropriate teaching and counseling regarding sexual behavior.

occur. Because development is different for each individual, some 12-year-olds appear more physically mature than their peers. Another person may be 18 or even a few years older, yet still behave in adolescent ways at times.

Young children often talk about growing up, and older children may express eagerness to become teenagers. Many changes occur and this can be a very confusing time in the young person's life.

PHYSICAL DEVELOPMENT

Adolescents experience major physical changes with the onset of puberty (sexual maturation) which occurs gradually over several years. The normal development of the reproductive system depends on the health of the entire body, especially the endocrine system. **Genetics and nutrition are the primary influences on the age at which puberty occurs.** (See "Overview of Structure and Function" on p. 138 for the physical changes in puberty.)

Puberty also stimulates a growth spurt in adolescents and growth periods may lead to fatigue. Both boys and girls usually continue to gain weight while they are growing in height. Girls usually reach their adult stature by the time they are 18; boys may continue to grow taller well into their 20s.

The difference in the rate of physical development is often a concern to adolescents. Two friends may be the same age, but one may be more developed than the other. Because girls mature at a younger age, they are often taller than boys their age. Adolescents seldom think they compare favorably to their peers. They are preoccupied with their bodies and pay a lot of attention to their appearance. Safety is a concern as adolescents expand their social networks and activities (Safety Alert 11-2).

SEXUALITY

Because the sex hormones also influence thoughts and desires, it is natural that adolescents may seek sexual activity. The media and entertainment industries also encourage sexual thoughts. In 2002, the National Center for Health Statistics reported that 47% of girls and 46% of boys had experienced intercourse by age 18. Reports indicate sexual activity is occurring at younger ages. Although the body is capable of intercourse in adolescence, many young people are not prepared for the emotional aspects of sexual activity (Health Promotion Points 11-6).

Studies show that adolescents actually know much less about sexuality than they pretend or think they know. More sex education is direly needed to prevent early pregnancy and sexually transmitted infection. Parents remain the best teachers, but often they do not take on that role. Schools are often expected to teach about sex. Adolescents need factual information about physical changes and sexual development. Even when adolescents have been taught the basic facts about sexual behavior, they often do not think that such facts will apply to their own circumstances. The United States has a high rate of adolescent pregnancy. Parents, churches, and other organizations can help adolescents develop strategies for saying "no" to sexual activity.

COGNITIVE DEVELOPMENT

Adolescents are learning to think in creative, abstract, logical, and idealistic ways. They begin to examine their own thoughts and try to analyze the thoughts of others. Piaget labeled this stage *formal operations*. Beginning between ages 11 and 14, thought becomes more abstract; the adolescent can think about ideas. Some enjoy becoming quite philosophical.

Young people may analyze how they want to be, how their parents should be, and how the world should be in the future. Sometimes this idealism becomes frustrating for them as they encounter reality. This growth in brainpower is seen in increasing communication skills as they organize their thoughts in logical ways.

Adolescents also become more aware of other people and of what others think about them. They want to fit into society. They also become egocentric again. Young people think that others are as interested in them as they are. They may indulge in attention-seeking behavior.

Another part of egocentrism is believing that their own experiences are unique. They may not realize that other people have faced disappointments and problems, too. Adolescents may also believe that they are immortal. They cannot imagine that anything bad would happen to them, so they may avoid using contraception and lack concern about drinking and driving.

The role of schools in the cognitive development of adolescents remains significant. **Schools that address the individual learning needs of students can aid young people in their search for meaning and identity.** Teachers who understand adolescents can help them figure out the world, as well as stimulate their intellectual growth. School is also important for the social activity it provides.

PSYCHOSOCIAL DEVELOPMENT

The psychosocial development of adolescents can be turbulent. Emotions may be erratic when hormones are newly released. The young person has to learn how to handle those emotions and how to get along with other people.

Change continues to occur in the relationships between adolescents and their families. Teens seek to be autonomous and to be free of parental control. Yet many adolescents also yearn to have rules and to know that parents care about and for them. Parents should gradually allow young people to make more of their own decisions; both parents and teens also have to learn to live with the consequences.

Time spent as a family unit often lessens when the child becomes an adolescent. It is natural for the teen to want to spend more time with peers. Parents should allow more freedom for peer interaction, but should monitor the teen's activities and friends. Parents who try to hold the teen too closely may discover they cause estrangement from their teen. Many people admit only later in their lives that family relationships are important during adolescence.

Serious conflict between parents and teens is most common, when it occurs, during early adolescence. This corresponds to the time of major hormonal shifts and helps explain why the junior high or middle school years may be difficult. When conflict has existed, it usually becomes less acute as the adolescent

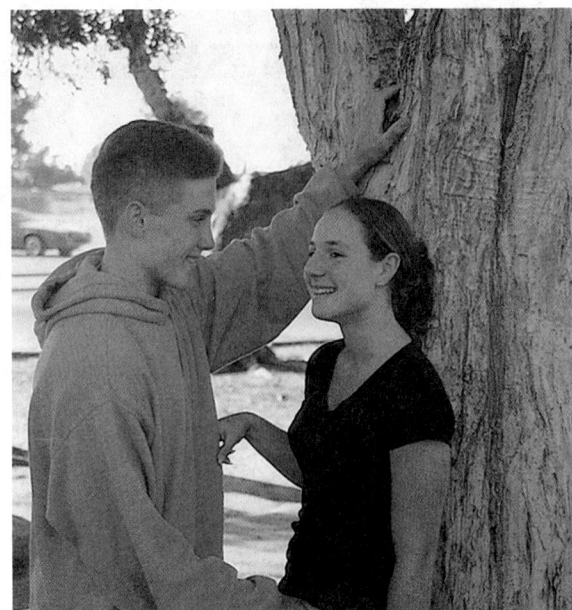

FIGURE **11-4** Dating provides opportunities to help establish values.

matures. By age 17 or 18, relationships with parents often become smoother. The daily negotiations and minor conflicts that occur are natural results of development and help adolescents find their own identity.

Adolescents continue to learn about the world and other people during time spent with their peers. In early adolescence, there is a strong need for young people to conform to a peer group. Young people often want to dress alike, behave alike, and do the same things that their group does.

Dating is an important adolescent experience that also helps young people discover their individual identity. Dating serves many other purposes such as recreation, status, and achievement. Most adolescents become interested in the opposite sex early in puberty (Figure 11-4). The interest grows as they mature. Young people's groups include both boys and girls, gradually evolving into group-dating events.

Erikson's stage for adolescence is *identity vs. role confusion*. The adolescent struggles with questions: Who am I? What am I about? What will I do with my life? The teen who is successful in coping with these questions develops an acceptable sense of self. The teen who is not successful may remain confused, withdraw from society, or passively follow the crowd. Some teens conquer this challenge during adolescence, whereas others struggle longer. A healthy identity is open to change as time goes on.

Some adolescents experiment with a variety of roles in society. This may cause conflicts with parents, as teens explore alternative lifestyles and/or value systems. The types of jobs that adolescents may try can also aid them in discovering who they are. Contemporary theorists agree that the resolution of this identity search may extend into adulthood. This is especially true with young people who continue their education after high school.

Parents of adolescents can aid them in successful psychosocial development by supporting their decisions, acknowledging the struggles that occur, and respecting them as they mature. Parents and teens who have had open communication and mutual respect during their earlier years should navigate this challenging time with less trouble than those whose prior relationship was shaky.

TASKS OF ADOLESCENCE

Discovering their identity is a primary psychosocial task for adolescents. They also begin making decisions that will affect the rest of their lives. One of these is choosing a vocation. Although teens are seldom expected to decide on a lifetime vocation, they should have some ideas about the kind of work they would enjoy.

Ideology (a belief or value system) should be fairly well established by the end of adolescence. A moral code begins to be incorporated. One's sexual orientation (sexual preference) should also be set. Approximately 8% of adolescents have had a sexual encounter with a person of the same sex, but that does not mean they are homosexual. Studies report that about 5% of the population is homosexual (Behrman et al., 2004). All need to accept and understand their own preference.

Some theorists claim that mate selection is also part of adolescent development. In the United States, many young people prefer to postpone marriage until later in their lives.

CONCERNS IN ADOLESCENT DEVELOPMENT

Pregnancy

When an adolescent becomes pregnant, she needs assistance in discussing options. It is difficult to decide whether to place the child up for adoption, to keep the child and remain single, to keep the child and marry, or to abort the pregnancy. Often the father contributes little to the financial and emotional support of the infant of an adolescent mother. Sometimes, adolescents who are unmarried keep the baby, and the grandparents end up with the responsibility of raising the child. This is becoming a significant burden for the older generation. Often the adolescent mother does not continue her education and then has trouble becoming a self-sufficient adult.

The U.S. Bureau of the Census (2007) reported that, in the year 2004, 41,100 girls between ages 15 and 19 delivered babies. This was a 1% decrease from the previous year. It is predicted that 18% of 15-year-olds will have a baby before age 20, and 80% of teens who have a baby will live at the poverty level for 10 years or more (National Coalition for the Protection of Children & Families). Adolescent pregnancy is a high-risk pregnancy, because the young expectant mother is still physically growing. Younger mothers more often have premature babies with low birth weight. Pregnant adolescents must be guided toward early prenatal care, parenting classes, and psychosocial counseling. The social problems generated by adolescent pregnancy are significant as many become single mothers and end up needing welfare for themselves and their child.

Employment

Many adolescents seek part-time work. Most authorities agree that there are positive and negative aspects of adolescent employment. First jobs can be valuable in teaching work ethics and money management. Some adolescents need to work to help supplement the family income. Others want to pay for special clothes or a car. Depending on the number of hours worked, school grades may suffer. Sleep may suffer as well, just when the body needs more sleep for growing, and family interactions also may be affected.

Chemical Abuse

Alcohol is the most common drug used, followed by marijuana and amphetamines. Young people do not achieve positive development in cognitive and psychosocial aspects when they abuse chemicals. Alcohol use contributes to risky sexual behavior and is often a factor in teen pregnancy. Depression may become a problem as the teen isolates from usual activities and school as a result of the chemical abuse.

Eating Disorders

Adolescents who are obsessed with body image (particularly females) may develop severe eating disorders. *Anorexia nervosa* is a disorder in which food intake is severely limited, large amounts of water are consumed, and strenuous exercise may be used to control body weight. The body becomes emaciated and sexual development is delayed. Anorexia nervosa may result in death if left untreated. *Bulimia* is characterized by binge eating followed by inducing vomiting or using laxatives to eliminate the foods from the body. Bulimia may accompany anorexia nervosa or may be a disorder by itself. Bulimic individuals tend to maintain a more normal weight. Both disorders are psychological illnesses that present as physical symptoms, and both can have long-term negative physical effects. Growing up in a dysfunctional family may contribute to the development of eating disorders.

Depression

Mental health disorders are sometimes undiagnosed in adolescence. Untreated depression may be the cause of attempted or successful suicide. At other times, depression seems to be a sudden reaction to a change in one's life (Safety Alert 11-3).

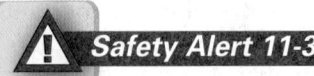

Safety Alert 11-3

Depression in Adolescents

- Any adolescent who exhibits signs of depression should be evaluated by a mental health professional who is used to working with young people.
- Suicide is a far too frequent occurrence among depressed teens.
- Signs of adolescent depression include declining school grades, chronic melancholy, alcohol or other drug use, and expressions of feeling down or blue.

Early Deaths

Causes of death among adolescents in the United States, in order of frequency, are accidents, homicide, suicide, and AIDS.

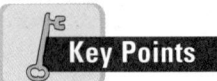

Key Points

- Growth and development begin at conception and continue throughout life. Development includes physical, cognitive, and psychosocial aspects.
- Development of children is commonly divided into five stages: prenatal, infancy, early childhood, middle and late childhood, and adolescence.
- Freud's theory has three parts that include levels of awareness, components of the personality or mind (the id, ego, and superego), and psychosexual stages of development (see Table 11-1).
- Erikson's theory of psychosocial development identifies certain tasks that should be accomplished at each stage (see Table 11-2).
- Piaget's theory of cognitive development identifies ways that children learn to think and to understand the world (see Table 11-3).
- Kohlberg's theory of moral development identifies stages in the development of moral behavior.
- Early and regular prenatal health care is essential for optimal development of the fetus.
- Newborns have many capabilities at birth, but are dependent on caregivers to meet their needs.
- An infant's cognitive development is enhanced by adults who provide a variety of appropriate stimulation.
- Bonding is important in the psychosocial development of babies.
- Growth should be monitored by health care providers in order to detect any concerns as early as possible.

- Young children are naturally curious but are not aware of possible dangers in their world.
- Health promotion and safety are important throughout childhood and adolescence.
- Parents who use day care providers should be selective about the caregivers chosen. Preschool education can help prepare a child for school and teach important socialization skills.
- Good nutritional habits learned in childhood will contribute to health throughout life.
- There are many different kinds of intelligence.
- Children in the middle years are industrious and need to be successful in some activities to increase their self-worth.
- Childhood friendships provide important stimulation and help children learn to get along with other people.
- Three different parenting styles have been identified: permissive, authoritarian, and authoritative. Children will develop differently with different parenting styles (see Table 11-4).
- Discipline measures change as a child grows. Young children are often given time-outs. Older children may need to be denied an activity.
- The physical and emotional changes of puberty can be upsetting for the adolescent.
- Sexual thoughts and desires increase during adolescence.
- Adolescents' cognitive development becomes abstract, idealistic, and more adult-like.
- Adolescents are concerned about discovering their own identity and finding their place in the world.
- Conflicts between adolescents and their parents are not unusual as teens experiment with adult roles and behaviors.
- Dating is an adolescent ritual important in psychosocial development.
- Adolescents should determine their ideology and sexual orientation, and they should have some ideas about vocational direction, by the end of this stage.
- Concerns of adolescence include pregnancy, employment, chemical abuse, eating disorders, depression, and early death.

 Go to your **Companion CD-ROM** for an Audio Glossary, animations, video clips, and more.

evolve Be sure to visit the companion Evolve site at http://evolve.elsevier.com/deWit/fundamental/ for additional online resources.

NCLEX-PN® EXAMINATION-STYLE REVIEW QUESTIONS

*Choose the **best** answer(s) for each question.*

1. According to Freud's theory, the part of the mind that acts as one's conscience is the _____ _____. *(Fill in the blank.)*

2. Milestones in infant development indicate that infants begin using two-word sentences at:
   1. 10 to 13 months.
   2. 12 to 16 months.
   3. 18 to 24 months.
   4. 24 to 36 months.

3. When considering the principles of growth and development, remember that:
   1. although development occurs in an orderly sequence, the rate may vary between individuals.
   2. development occurs evenly, with periods of no growth occurring every third year.
   3. all children should grow at the same rate; all 4-year-olds should weigh within 11 pounds of each other.
   4. most children can run before they can walk.

4. The purpose of play during infancy is to:
   1. aid exploration of the environment.
   2. promote toilet training.
   3. generate self-discipline.
   4. promote brain development.

5. According to Erikson, a sense of initiative is best explained as:
   1. establishing trust.
   2. the ability to express one's needs.
   3. trying new roles without feelings of guilt.
   4. finishing tasks started.

6. In Piaget's theory, using language to express thoughts occurs at age _____. *(Fill in the blank.)*

7. Bonding is necessary for the child to develop:
   1. appropriate personal boundaries.
   2. a sense of security.
   3. eventual independence.
   4. a sense of trust.

8. Parents of children ages 3 to 6 may need guidance in:
   1. making the child feel secure when a newborn arrives.
   2. helping the child cope with peers.
   3. methods of toilet training that are effective.
   4. allowing the child to make more of his own decisions.

9. A parent who insists that the child stay in his room for the full 11-minute time-out and then smiles and hugs the child when the time is up is showing a parenting style that is:
   1. authoritative.
   2. passive.
   3. authoritarian.
   4. punitive.

10. Growth and development should be monitored regularly for every child in order to:
    1. provide statistics needed for proper research.
    2. detect abnormal growth patterns so that early care and treatment of problems can begin.
    3. provide data to establish norms for growth and development at various ages.
    4. reassure to parents that their children are healthy.

11. An effective discipline measure for adolescents is:
    1. restricting social activities for a limited time.
    2. grounding them to the house for several weeks.
    3. assigning extra chores that must be done.
    4. fining them a portion of their allowance.

12. Egocentrism as a characteristic of adolescence is displayed by the teen feeling that:
    1. parents only have to be obeyed when it is convenient.
    2. a big disappointment like what just happened has never happened to anyone else in this way.
    3. his peers are much smarter than his parents.
    4. he can visualize a world in the future that will be far better than the world now.

13. The adolescent who is thinking in logical and abstract ways as he completes a term paper shows:
    1. aspects of industry.
    2. identity confusion.
    3. appropriate cognitive development.
    4. appropriate psychosocial development.

CRITICAL THINKING ACTIVITIES *Read each clinical scenario and discuss the questions with your classmates.*

Scenario A
A single mother whose 7-year-old daughter has a bad cold brings the child to the clinic where you are working. The child is smaller than average. As you interview them you learn that because of the mother's work schedule, the girl is home alone every school morning for 2 hours and does not always eat breakfast. What concerns about this situation might you have?

Scenario B
The math teacher at the high school told the parents of 17-year-old John that he is surly in class, falls asleep often, is not consistently handing in homework, and made a "D" on the last test. John's mother has asked you what to do. When she tried to talk with John, he became sarcastic and walked out. John has a part-time job at the local fast-food restaurant.

Objectives

Upon completing this chapter, you should be able to:

Theory

1. List three stages of adulthood.
2. Explain Schaie's theory of cognitive development in young and middle adults.
3. Discuss Erikson's stages of psychosocial development in young and middle adults.
4. Describe the physical and psychosocial development and changes of young and middle adults.
5. List at least three functions of families.
6. Describe the effects of divorce on involved persons.

Clinical Practice

1. Identify at least three health concerns of young adults.
2. Identify at least four health concerns of middle adults.
3. Design an educational program to help adults maintain a healthy lifestyle.
4. Explain how caring people can nourish the cognitive and psychosocial development of adults.

Key Terms

 Be sure to check out the bonus material on the Companion CD-ROM, including selected audio pronunciations.

achievement stage (p. 156)
baby boomers (p. 162)
boomerang children (BOO-mĕr-ăng, p. 160)
career (p. 157)
empty nest syndrome (SĬN-drōm, p. 164)
executive substage (ĕx-Ĕ-kĕw-tĭv, p. 157)
generativity (jĕn-ĕr-ă-TĬ-vĭ-tē, p. 157)
intimacy (ĬN-tĭ-mă-sē, p. 157)
libido (lĭ-BĒ-dō, p. 163)
maturity (mă-TŬR-ĭ-tē, p. 158)
menopause (MĒ-nō-păwz, p. 163)
mentors (p. 165)
presbycusis (prĕs-bē-KŪ-sĭs, p. 162)
presbyopia (prĕs-bē-Ō-pē-ă, p. 162)
responsibility stage (rĕ-spŏn-sĭ-BĬ-lĭ-tē, p. 157)
sandwich generation (p. 165)
stagnation (stăg-NĀ-shŭn, p. 157)
vocational (p. 160)

THEORIES OF DEVELOPMENT

Do you remember wanting to be a "grown-up" so that you would have all the answers to life's questions? Young children, especially, pretend to be grown-ups as they play; older children become a little more skeptical, and adolescents often think adults are not very bright. It can be a surprise to realize one day that you *are* an adult and you *still* don't know the answers!

Chapter 11 discussed growth and development from conception through adolescence. This chapter continues the story of our maturation as young and then as middle adults. Chapter 13 tells about development of older adults. It will help you appreciate your patients' attitudes and behaviors when you can identify their stage of life and the kinds of challenges they may be facing.

ADULTHOOD AS CONTINUING CHANGE

Adulthood usually begins around the age of 19, although people may continue some adolescent behaviors into their 20s. Adults continue to grow and develop throughout the life span. As their bodies change, they become more susceptible to health disorders and must work harder to maintain health. Thinking patterns and life goals also change as time goes on.

For the purposes of study, adulthood will be divided into three segments. The first is young adulthood, which is ages 19 to 45. Second is middle adulthood, ages 46 to 64 years of age. Older adulthood is the third stage, 65 to 75 years of age. Advanced age is 76 to death (see Chapter 13). As with younger people, the boundaries should be considered flexible when considering an individual.

SCHAIE'S THEORY OF COGNITIVE DEVELOPMENT

Piaget thought that adolescents and adults think in the same ways (see Chapter 11). Contemporary theorists believe that formal operational thinking becomes more refined in adulthood. Several stages of cognitive development in adults were identified by K. Warner Schaie, who expanded on Piaget's ideas.

Schaie called the young adult stage of cognitive development the achievement stage (needing to learn and successfully use your abilities). He felt that young adults are optimistic and strive to improve themselves. They want to use what they have learned, continue learning, prove their competence, and increase their choices of career (work that requires specific training).

The responsibility stage (concerned with real-life problems, in charge of self and others) occurs in middle adulthood. He stated that these adults are responsible for themselves, a job, often a family, and perhaps some aspect of the community. This includes attention to the needs of a spouse, children, co-workers, and others.

For some middle adults, Schaie identified the executive substage (responsible for major corporations, the country). He states that many middle adults with multiple responsibilities learn to function as executives in their lives. They delegate appropriately, juggle roles, and manage complex situations.

ERIKSON'S STAGES OF ADULT PSYCHOSOCIAL DEVELOPMENT

Erikson called the young adult stage intimacy (close, meaningful relationships) versus isolation (see Table 11-2). Intimacy means more than only sexual relationships. Young adults want to give of themselves and to be committed to others. They establish close, intense relationships with other people. Close family ties is another positive example.

Generativity (guiding the lives of younger people) versus stagnation (inactivity, self-absorption) is the psychosocial stage of development seen in middle adults. Many are willing and eager to help young people, their own children and grandchildren, and others in their community. Middle adults are productive people who accept the interdependence necessary for satisfactory living. People who are stagnant may have trouble keeping a job, are not interested in volunteering, and are self-involved.

FAMILIES

Because people are social beings, one cannot study an individual's development without knowing about the family environment that influences it. "Family" is defined as a group of individuals who care about and for each other (Figure 12-1).

Families are important because in families children learn basic values and how to relate to other people. Functions of families are listed in Box 12-1. A family's cultural and ethnic background also influences children. **The support of family remains important throughout the life span.**

TYPES OF FAMILIES

There have always been different kinds of families, but there is more awareness of differences as we move into the 21st century. Some types of families are given in Box 12-2.

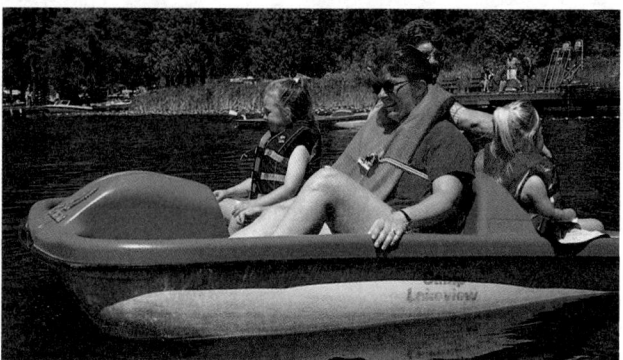

FIGURE **12-1** Exercising together helps keep everyone healthy.

Box 12-1 *Functions of the Family*

- **Physical maintenance:** Providing essentials for life
- **Protection:** Creating an atmosphere for health and safety
- **Nurturance:** Providing loving care and guidance
- **Socialization:** Interacting appropriately with others
- **Education:** Teaching about values and the world
- **Reproduction:** Continuing the species
- **Recreation:** Having fun together

Box 12-2 *Types of Families*

- **Nuclear:** One or two parents and children.
- **Extended:** Parents, children, grandparents, and other relatives.
- **Step:** One parent and child(ren) and a new parent.
- **Blended:** Mom and her children, dad and his children.
- **Single Parent:** Woman or man in separate household with child(ren) as a result of divorce, death, desertion, or individual preference.
- **Partner:** Parents are the same gender. Children are from previous relationships, artificial insemination, or adopted.
- **Cohabitation:** Couples who live together with their children but remain unmarried.

Think Critically About . . . What kind of family did you have as a child? Did you ever wish it were different? What kind of family do you have now?

HISTORICAL CHANGES IN FAMILIES

Sociologists have identified many changes in American family life in the past 50 years. Varieties of families are one example. Others include

- **Urbanization:** Rural families of the past were more self-sufficient than today's city dwellers. Only a small percentage of the population now lives on farms.
- **Mobility:** Many families do not stay in one community, usually because of a changing job mar-

ket. Some children attend four or five schools before they finish high school. This also affects relationships among the extended family.

- **Size:** The average size of families is decreasing. As living expenses increase, people realize they can't afford as many children as their parents or grandparents raised. The use of contraception helps people plan family size.
- **Use of paid caregivers:** Nearly 70% of two-parent families have two wage earners. Most single parents are employed. Children are cared for by others for part of every workday.
- **Fathers' roles:** Since the 1980s, men are taking a greater role in their children's lives. Whether married or single, many men enjoy participating in child care. It is also more common for single fathers to be custodial parents than it was in earlier decades.
- **Increased longevity:** Health care advances contribute to longer life spans. Some families have four or five living generations.

DIVORCE AND FAMILIES

Divorce ends nearly 36% of marriages, according to 2006 U.S. Bureau of the Census figures. People expect a great deal from marriage; partners expect each other to be best friends, confidantes, and perfect lovers. Some factors that increase the risk of divorce are listed in Box 12-3. It is easy to see that some factors may coexist.

Divorce early in a marriage, especially before there are children, may seem the least harmful. However, the people involved may be deeply affected. There may have been abuse or infidelity. Often, counseling is necessary for a person ending a difficult relationship.

Studies have shown that divorce is usually harder on children than it is on their parents. Young children may feel that they are to blame for the family breakup; they often harbor guilt feelings. They may fantasize about reuniting the family.

Older children and adolescents can sometimes understand that their parents' problems are not the fault of the young person, but they are still affected by the divorce. It may influence the way they relate to other people, especially as they begin dating, and may affect their ability to trust others.

Some couples discover that they have little in common after their children are grown. Approximately 25% of divorces occur among couples over 40 years of age. Their adult children often have trouble understanding why this happens.

Divorce also affects the parents and other relatives of the divorcing couple. Sometimes grandparents lose opportunities to be with their grandchildren. The increasing incidence of divorce in the latter half of the 20th century is viewed as a major cause of poverty because so many divorced women have low incomes. **Divorce occurs between two people, but the effects ripple into their extended families and their community.**

YOUNG ADULTS

The 2 to 8 years after high school are a time of transition for young people. Most are completing adolescent developmental processes and moving into the roles and responsibilities of young adults. Several major events usually occur during this time. Decisions young adults make during these years will influence the rest of their lives.

In our culture, there are two significant milestones signaling that a person is a young adult. The first is *economic independence,* which usually happens when a person is employed full time. Many young people in college or technical education programs cannot reach this milestone until later. The second is *independent decision making.*

Some theorists say that maturity (being fully developed) is a significant marker of reaching adulthood. It is probably more accurate to say that we are all growing toward maturity. **Mature people have established a philosophy of life based on their own belief system and personal ethics.** Other characteristics of mature behaviors are listed in Box 12-4.

Box 12-3 | *Risk Factors for Divorce*

- Bride and groom younger than 20
- Low economic circumstances
- Cohabitation before marriage
- Premarital pregnancy
- Having children from a previous marriage
- Either partner has been previously divorced
- Knowing each other for only a short time before marriage
- One or both did not finish high school
- No religious affiliation or practicing different faiths
- One or both have divorced parents

Box 12-4 | *Behaviors Indicating Maturity*

The ability to:
- acknowledge and express feelings with restraint
- laugh at yourself
- accept responsibility for your own actions
- tolerate frustration
- accept diversity and individuality in others
- trust others
- display self-confidence
- cope with stress
- discipline yourself
- handle problems without losing sight of goals

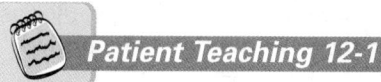

Patient Teaching 12-1

Health Habits for Young Adults

Young adults should be provided health teaching regarding the following topics:

- Muscle development and fat accumulation contribute to changes in body shape.
- **The dietary and exercise habits a person develops during this stage will influence weight management for many years.**
- Regular exercise is also important to increase endurance, strength, flexibility, and muscle tone.
- The young adult should be encouraged to maintain weight within normal limits, reduce fat to less than 30% of caloric intake, and establish and maintain a regular exercise program.

PHYSICAL DEVELOPMENT

Most young adults are physically at their peak. Their strength, endurance, and energy are at high levels. Most report their general health as good; very few have chronic health concerns. Young adults usually have fewer colds and minor illnesses than when they were children. Good physical health at age 30 is considered an indicator of good physical health in later years as well (Patient Teaching 12-1).

Skeletal development is completed when young adults reach their full stature. For women this often occurs by age 18 or 19; men continue to grow until their later 20s. The physical differences between men and women are significant. Generally men are taller, heavier, and stronger than women. They have broader shoulders, narrower hips, and larger hands and feet.

Dental maturity is achieved with the eruption of wisdom teeth. Regular dental care is important to maintain healthy teeth and gums.

Physical growth of the brain continues into the mid-20s, peaking during these years, and memory is acute. Learning seems easier for young adults because they often can learn quickly. Growth of neural connections continues into later years. Middle and older adults continue to learn but often at a slower pace.

The early young adulthood years, ages 19 to 26, are physically the best years for reproduction. Many young adults choose to delay childbearing until they are economically and emotionally prepared for parenting.

The validity of studies about sexual behavior is often questioned because the results are based on self-reporting. During young adulthood, sexual preferences are identified and there may be numerous partners. Promiscuity increases the risk of sexually transmitted diseases, especially human immunodeficiency virus (HIV).

HEALTH CONCERNS OF YOUNG ADULTS
Risky Behavior

Because young adults are generally healthy and feel well, they may feel invincible and engage in risky behaviors. Examples of such behaviors include chemical abuse, overeating, inadequate sleep, an inactive lifestyle, and sexual promiscuity. The abuse of chemicals often contributes to other risky behavior.

Young adults die primarily because of accidents, suicide or homicide, and acquired immunodeficiency syndrome (AIDS). Motor vehicle accidents are the primary cause of death for white males; homicide is the leading cause of death for African American males.

Stress-Related Illness

Some stress-related illnesses are headaches, gastric ulcers, and hypertension. The incidence of these conditions increases as people get older. **Young adults over 30 begin to be affected by these illnesses.** Sometimes people use alcohol and/or other drugs in unhealthy attempts to relieve stress.

Early Disease

The third health concern for young adults is development of diseases, especially cancer. Young women should learn to examine their breasts and perform monthly breast self-examinations. They should see a physician if they find any changes. Mammograms every 2 years are recommended for all women beginning at age 40; women with breast cancer in their family should have annual mammograms beginning at age 35. Women should also have annual pelvic examinations, including a periodic Papanicolaou (Pap) test to screen for cervical cancer.

Men should learn and perform regular self-examination of the testicles. They should see a physician if they detect any growths or changes.

Both men and women should have annual physical examinations to screen for hypertension and assess weight management (Figure 12-2). Periodic Mantoux tests are advised to screen for tuberculosis. Immunizations should be kept current.

COGNITIVE DEVELOPMENT

In the achievement stage of Schaie's theory, young adults apply their intelligence to higher education and to early career development. Young adults are no longer egocentric. They are more able to reason, solve problems, and set reasonable goals (Patient Teaching 12-2).

Cognitive development of young adults is aided by the support of others. Young adults may need guidance to identify their goals clearly and continue striving toward them. Helping them understand their stage of development may provide encouragement.

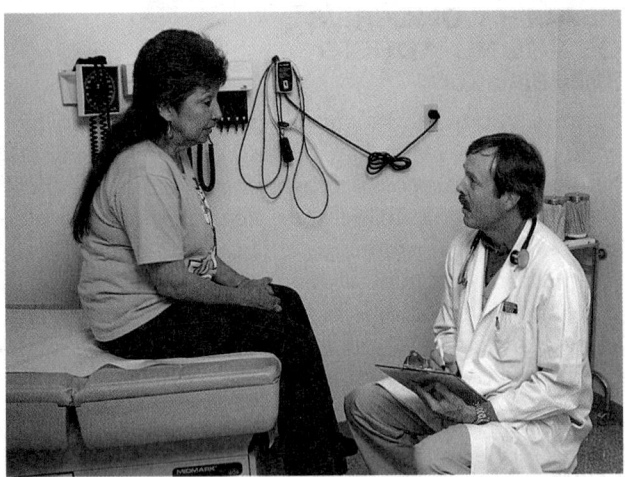

FIGURE **12-2** Regular physical checkups monitor health status.

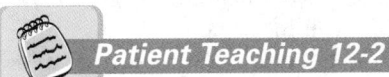

Teaching Young Adults

The following points should be kept in mind when teaching young adults:
- It is best to build on previous knowledge and skills.
- The goals of teaching should be made clear.
- Indicate how the new knowledge can be applied and how it is of personal benefit.
- Use interactive, problem-oriented methods that relate to daily tasks at home, work, or school.

Continuing Education

Many young adults continue their education after high school. Higher education can help people understand their world, learn to manage their time, and prepare for a career.

It is generally believed that 1 or 2 years of higher education, even if career goals are unclear, can help young adults learn more about themselves and the world. Not everyone wants to continue school once high school is finished, however. Many kinds of careers are best learned on the job or in vocational/technical schools and do not require college degrees.

Careers and Work

The ability to earn a living is an important accomplishment of young adulthood. Working provides the means of personal, social, and financial survival. It can also give a person a sense of identity and increase self-worth and respect. Some view their work as a service to others.

Exploration of vocational (trade, profession, or occupation) choices is expected in late adolescence and early adulthood. Some counselors encourage young adults to try several kinds of jobs to better select one that will provide satisfaction. It is common for individuals to have up to seven different jobs throughout their work life. Disillusionment about the ideal job is frequent as realities of the work world are identified.

> **?** *Think Critically About . . .* How many kinds of jobs have you had? Why have you left jobs in the past? What are you looking for in a career? Is a career different from a job?

What do young adults want from their work? Of course adequate money must be considered, but it is not always most important. A main priority is that they want the work to be interesting. They also want the opportunity to use their skills and abilities. The fourth concern is the chance for advancement.

Unemployment can be the result of many factors, but is often viewed as personal failure. Prolonged and unwanted unemployment can cause financial crisis, loss of self-esteem, and depression.

The roles of employed women in the United States continue to stimulate discussion. *Gender equality* is the movement for equal opportunity and equal pay for women and men. Young women often have a dilemma when choosing a type of work. Some may prefer to be full-time homemakers and mothers. That option may be impossible because of the economic pressures facing young families.

Concerns about career versus family may cause personal or family conflict. Family-friendly employment policies are becoming more common and benefit both women and men. The kinds of work available to women remain restricted in some fields. The U.S. Bureau of the Census stated that the earning power of women overall in 2007 continues to be about 75.7% of what men earn in similar work (McCombs School of Business, 2007).

PSYCHOSOCIAL DEVELOPMENT

Independence from the parental family is a primary achievement during young adulthood. This is interpreted as living on your own and making your own decisions. The trend toward young adults being boomerang children (children who return to the parental home for a period of time) has grown considerably as children find it difficult to make sufficient money to establish a successful home of their own. Sometimes returning young adults bring their children along. This is commonly due to economic hardship.

Erikson called the young adult stage of psychosocial development *intimacy vs. isolation.* It is important that people continue the development of meaningful relationships with others. If this task of developing intimacy is not accomplished, the young adult might not trust others and may be hesitant to share himself or herself. This could lead to withdrawal and depression.

According to Erikson, adolescents should find identity, which helps them become more independent. Independence precedes the need for developing intimacy and sometimes may conflict with it. A secure and independent person is ready to be intimate with another and can allow the other person to be independent.

Personality development continues throughout the life span. Most theorists agree that your early life is significant in forming your basic personality. Major personality changes in adulthood are not likely to occur. The person who is usually happy will remain so; the opposite is also true. **Changes that a person wants to make require self-analysis and a lot of work.**

DEVELOPMENTAL TASKS
Marriage

Deciding whether to marry is a major concern in young adulthood. Ninety-five percent of Americans do eventually try marriage. The average age at first marriage is 25.1 for women and 26.7 for men (U.S. Bureau of the Census, 2006). These ages are increasing as more people choose to delay marriage. Selection of a marriage partner is a critical decision; there are no foolproof rules for mate selection. **Although opposites may attract, successful marriages often involve partners who share basic values and philosophies about life.** Young love is romantic and intense. Marriage requires mutual respect, sharing, and commitment. The fear of making a poor choice is one reason people decide to cohabit before or instead of marrying. Married people are generally healthier and happier throughout their lives.

Single adults include those who have never been married and those who are widowed, separated, or divorced. In the United States, approximately 26% of adults of all ages live alone, according to government figures. The role of single adults in society is another aspect of adult development.

Many singles live full, happy lives. There are positive and negative aspects to living alone. Single people can be independent with their time and money; they don't have to be concerned about a partner's ideas or desires. However, they have no one to depend on when trouble occurs. They have to be responsible for their own decisions. Many single adults report that they are often lonely.

Think Critically About . . . What are some of the challenges facing a young adult who is also a single parent? What kinds of guidance might be needed from a health care provider?

Parenting

Becoming a parent occurs for many people during young adulthood. Some couples carefully discuss and plan decisions about having children. Others choose not to use birth control measures. U.S. Bureau of the Census 2003 data demonstrate that the average age of first-time mothers is about 25.1 years, although many women have a child when they are younger.

Some women delay having children in favor of career development. There might then be concerns about their "biologic clock" running out, meaning they may have trouble conceiving after age 30 as fertility lessens. The option of in vitro fertilization is available then, but is very expensive. By age 40, a woman is statistically at high risk during a pregnancy. Technological developments have made it possible for some women to become pregnant in their mid-40s and 50s.

Childbearing is only the beginning of parenting. The issues of day care, discipline, and other child-rearing aspects continue for years. Many young parents discover they imitate their own parents in dealing with their children. Most people learn about parenting from the examples seen in childhood.

Think Critically About . . . If you have a child, are you aware of how you are parenting? Is it similar to or different from the way your parents raised you? If you do not have a child, what kind of parent do you think you would be? Would you want to use the model of your parents?

In the past, young families were often geographically near older relatives and had the emotional support of extended family. Many young families today don't live near other family members and may struggle with child-rearing issues. Some areas have developed Early Childhood and Family Education (ECFE) programs through schools or community organizations where young adults can share concerns and learn about successful parenting.

Home Management

The tasks involved in making life run smoothly need regular attention. Having groceries on hand, keeping things in order, and remembering to have the oil changed in the car are examples of home management. Money management, laundry, and cleaning the refrigerator are tasks.

Developing a Social Group

Having friends who share values is vital for socialization. Friendships beyond the extended family are valuable. For young adults, this can be a challenge when they go away to school or take a job in a new locale. They may have always lived in one area until this stage, and now have to make new friends in a new part of the world. Young adults who are confident, outgoing, and willing to be active in their community have a good chance of being successful.

Community Responsibility

Beginning involvement in community affairs is another mark of young adulthood, as people begin to think about the world beyond their family. Examples of this include joining a service organization, being involved in a religious community, or becoming active in local government. Young adults with healthy psychosocial development begin to reach beyond their own needs to be concerned with others. Sharing your expertise in a voluntary way is good for society as a whole.

MIDDLE ADULTHOOD

People ages 46 to 64 are categorized as middle adults. Images of middle age are varied. Middle adults are viewed as in the best years of their life; they are the wise, powerful leaders. Negative generalizations are also made about middle age. Stereotypes about people growing older begin to appear. Life is portrayed as all downhill and unhappy. Some people are reluctant to admit they are middle aged because of such negative views. These can be challenging years, too, as people expand their personal and social involvement.

The oldest baby boomers (people born between 1946 and 1964) reached middle age in the 1990s. This large group of people (76 million) has had a major impact on U.S. society at every stage of their development. They have challenged traditional beliefs and forged new ways of thinking about and living every stage. Their viewpoints about middle and older adulthood may become quite different.

PHYSICAL DEVELOPMENT

Physical changes that may be considered declines begin to appear during the middle years of life. **The rate of change, even changes of aging, varies among individuals.** Not every middle adult will experience all of these changes; most normal changes occur so slowly that they may be unnoticed for years. Middle adults often seek ways to slow the aging process. Individuals who exercise regularly, eat sensibly, and take care of their bodies can often delay some of these changes (Complementary & Alternative Therapies 12-1).

During the middle adult years there is a natural redistribution of body weight, which changes the contours of the body, even if weight remains fairly constant. Men commonly add inches around the waist as body fat increases by about 30%. Women's body fat increases by nearly 40% and is often added to hips and thighs. It becomes more difficult to lose weight. Some middle adults may try to look and act younger to deny their aging.

One common occurrence is presbyopia (decreased flexibility of the eye lens). This makes near vision more difficult, and leads to the need for reading glasses. By age 60, some people may have retinal damage as a result of lessened blood flow, which leads to visual problems. Cataracts may develop during the middle years. Regular eye examinations and the use of corrective lenses can help maintain vision.

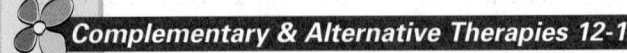

Complementary & Alternative Therapies 12-1

Herbs and Supplements to Help Slow Various Problems of Aging

- Black cohosh (*Cimicifuga racemosa*), used to lessen signs and symptoms of menopause
- Garlic (*Allium sativum*), recommended to reduce blood pressure and cholesterol and to prevent blood clots
- Vitamin E, to possibly prevent or slow dementia; may help prevent heart attacks
- Glucosamine and chondroitin sulfate, used to help maintain cartilage and decrease arthritis
- Evening primrose (*Oenothera biennis*), recommended to treat signs and symptoms of dry skin and menopause
- Ginkgo (*Ginkgo biloba*), used to improve blood flow to the brain and decrease forgetfulness

These remedies have been historically used for the various problems, but are not FDA approved. They may work in some patients, but not others.

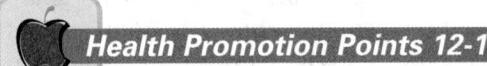

Health Promotion Points 12-1

Hearing Loss in Middle Adults

- The person who thinks hearing acuity is decreasing should have the hearing tested.
- It is much easier to adapt to a hearing aid when hearing loss is in the early stages than when it has progressed for several years.

Presbycusis (loss of hearing) begins in early adulthood, but rarely becomes apparent until later (Health Promotion Points 12-1). The ability to hear higher-pitched sounds is lost earlier than the ability to hear lower sounds. Men seem to lose this sense at younger ages than women. **Noisy work settings and loud music can contribute to eventual hearing loss by causing damage to auditory nerve endings.**

Gradual compression of the spinal column occurs as intervertebral disks shrink; this can cause the loss of up to 1 inch of height by age 60. It may surprise middle-aged people to realize that they have suddenly become shorter (Health Promotion Points 12-2).

Muscles throughout the body lose tone and elasticity during these middle years. Fatigue arrives earlier with physical labor. Reaction time may also slow. Muscle changes also affect internal muscles; heart and lungs become less efficient. Blood pressure increases when arteries become less elastic. The skin becomes less resilient and wrinkles appear. Changes in the muscles of the digestive system may cause disturbances and food intolerances.

Many people in middle age begin to have graying hair. Thinning of scalp hair can occur in both genders. Increased hair growth in men is seen in bushier eye-

Health Promotion Points 12-2

Bone Health in Middle Adults

- Women with a family history of osteoporosis should begin regular bone density screening at age 45.
- Anyone who has experienced a loss of height of 2 inches since age 20 should be screened for osteoporosis.
- Calcium intake should be 1200 mg/day prior to menopause and should be increased to 1500 mg/day after menopause.
- Obtaining sufficient vitamin D from sunlight or supplementation is also important.

Box 12-5 | *Signs and Symptoms Occurring with Menopause*

- Decreased vaginal lubrication
- Emotional lability
- Fatigue
- Flushing and hot flashes with heavy sweating
- Headache
- Heart palpitations
- Insomnia

brows and hair occasionally in noses and ears. These events may be related to heredity.

Both males and females produce sex hormones. Women produce greater amounts of estrogens, and men produce greater amounts of testosterone. As middle age proceeds, this balance shifts slightly as hormone production slows. This is most obvious in women; the decrease in estrogen production causes menstrual changes and eventually menopause (cessation of menstruation).

The average age of menopause is 51. This ends the reproductive years and may be accompanied by minor physical and/or psychological signs and symptoms (Box 12-5). Some women see menopause as a natural event and the beginning of new freedoms and choices; other women have a negative view. Women can learn about their bodies and the natural changes from a variety of sources. They can discuss their feelings with others in order to better understand and cope. Many women seek new ways to contribute to their profession and/or their community.

The shift in hormone balance also occurs in men, although there is not as obvious a physical change. Sexual ability does not decline in either sex. Some people report a lessening of libido (the sex drive). People who are concerned about this should discuss it with a physician.

HEALTH CONCERNS

Health status becomes a greater concern in middle adulthood. Lifestyle, heredity, and use of the health care system are major influences on the state of health. People who make efforts to take care of them-

Health Promotion Points 12-3

Blood Pressure Control in Middle Adults

- Adults should keep their blood pressure within the normal range of 110/70 to 120/80 mm Hg and ideally keep it to no higher than 110/70.
- Decreasing sodium intake can help lower the blood pressure.
- Drinking minimal alcohol helps control blood pressure.

Health Promotion Points 12-4

Cognitive Stimulation in Middle Adults

Working crossword or Sudoku puzzles, playing bridge, playing board games that require strategy, studying some new subject, using computer programs such as "Brain Age," and other activities that stimulate the mind all help maintain mental crispness.

selves are generally healthier than those who do not. This includes controlling one's diet and remaining physically active. Health screening for diabetes, risk factors for heart disease, hypertension, colon cancer should occur at regular intervals (Health Promotion Points 12-3).

Leading causes of death in the 50s and 60s are heart disease, cancer, vascular disease, and accidents. The major health problems of middle adults include accidents, alcohol abuse, obesity, diabetes, heart disease, hypertension, and mental illness. Healthy stress management at all ages contributes to improved general health.

COGNITIVE DEVELOPMENT

Schaie's stage of responsibility is seen as middle adults manage the complexities of their lives. Studies show that intellect remains stable in middle adulthood. Early signs of illnesses may cause the impression of slight mental declines. People who are active and use their intellect remain bright and interested in life.

Creativity is believed to peak during middle adulthood. However, there are many examples of people who are creative and productive in their older years as well. Creative people are often creative throughout their lives. Men and women are equally creative and intelligent.

One aspect of cognition that may change in midlife is memory. Middle adults often need to work harder at remembering things, and many find lists and notes helpful. It is easier to remember important information than incidental information (Health Promotion Points 12-4). Older persons should not be overly concerned about forgetfulness; it is more likely related to a busy life than to cognitive problems.

Work Life

Satisfaction with work is a part of cognitive development. It appears to increase throughout life for both men and women. Many people spend more of their time in work-related activities when they reach the middle years. Increased income and responsibilities accompanying career growth explain increased satisfaction. Most career advancement occurs during the 50s.

Middle adults may make a conscious decision to make a midlife career change. Some begin evaluating their desires and accomplishments. If a dream is unfulfilled, perhaps a change will help it come true. Middle adults begin to realize that their own life spans are limited, and they want to try new areas of interest while they have time. Some adults are willing to change their lives entirely by starting a new career. The changes occurring in midlife are handled best when the person has a good support system.

Some middle adults change careers because of labor market demands. Job loss resulting from downsizing, and the need for retraining, are serious concerns. Changes in technology may create new work opportunities. Middle adults forced to make changes may have a difficult time adjusting.

> **?** *Think Critically About* . . . Do you know anyone who has made a midlife career change? Was it by choice? Was the result satisfactory?

Past studies report differences between men and women regarding career paths and responsibilities. Many of those studies have focused on white men. As more women and minorities move into leadership positions, previous differences should become less significant. Women, and more recently men, who choose to place family concerns ahead of career goals may find their career advancement is slowed since they are not totally focused on the job.

Many baby boomers are finding that as retirement age approaches, they have not saved the financial reserves necessary to support them and they must continue working. Some do retire and then run short of money and have to try to reenter the job market.

The use of leisure time is also important. Middle adults should develop interests outside their work. Leisure activities can be healthy ways to reduce stress. Hobbies can also help people prepare for retirement by providing fulfillment

Lifelong Learning

Many adults discover that returning to college is rewarding and challenging. They may enroll in one or two classes, or may undertake an entire program of study. There can be many reasons for this. It may fulfill a lifelong goal, it may be to keep a job, or it may be to prepare for a career change.

Women who chose to raise a family prior to developing a career are especially likely to prepare for new jobs and new lives in midlife. Rather than think of this stage as downhill, they think of it as an opportunity to try another path.

> **?** *Think Critically About* . . . Do you know anyone who returned to or began college after the age of 40? How did they feel about it? What kind of support did they need?

PSYCHOSOCIAL DEVELOPMENT

Relationships with other people remain the focus of psychosocial development in middle adults. People in these years also begin to think more globally about life and their roles.

Marriage

The marital relationship often grows from romance and passion into the affectionate love of middle adults. The steady companionship of a partner is important for social and psychological support. Some marriages improve as children leave home and child-rearing responsibilities lessen. Couples may find more time for each other. It is vital that they have and develop mutual interests and activities.

A couple who has been unhappy for years may decide to divorce when the children are gone. A woman who had been at home when children were younger may discover a new world if she begins a job or returns to school. Changing roles and responsibilities can create or intensify marital problems.

The empty nest syndrome (children have left home, causing a sense of loss and sadness) affects some middle adults who have centered their lives on their children. They may need guidance in finding additional interests. Conversely, many adults look forward to more freedom when children are no longer dependent on them.

Friendships

Whether single or married, middle adults need to have close friends. Friendships that have endured for years continue to be vital. Many middle adults find new importance in relationships with siblings. Friends and siblings find more time for each other once the time-consuming work of parenting is past.

Parenting

Most studies of middle adults involve those whose children are leaving or have left the parental home. Couples who had children later in life will enter midlife with children who are younger. Therefore, parenting concerns will vary.

Those with adult children can find this stage rewarding. Parents gain satisfaction in realizing that

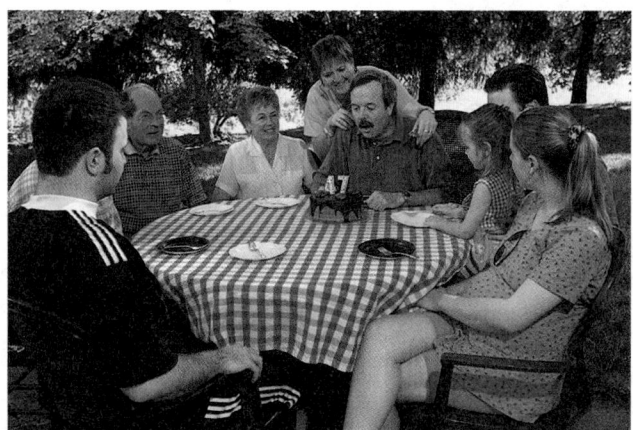

FIGURE **12-3** Family gatherings contribute to our sense of belonging.

their child is a responsible young adult. If grandchildren arrive in the family, another dimension is added. Grandparents usually enjoy baby-sitting at times and inclusion in the younger family's life (Figure 12-3).

Caring for Parents

The relationship with aging parents is another concern in midlife. If the relationship has been mutually supportive, these can be satisfying years. As adults mature, they may become more appreciative of the struggles their own parents experienced. Family ties will sometimes improve as children realize the sacrifices and guidance their parents provided.

Some middle adults find themselves in the sandwich generation (dependent children at home, dependent elders needing caregiving). As longevity increases, more older adults will need assistance and support, usually from their own children. Daughters and daughters-in-law often become primary caregivers for elderly parents.

Caring for aging parents can be stressful when combined with personal careers and family responsibiltiies. Families must make important decisions. Open communication within the family can ease the necessary adjustments. Community resources are available to assist families who need support and help with caregiving.

Generativity

Erikson's middle adult psychosocial stage of *generativity vs. stagnation* is most easily seen in parents whose children have become young adults. However, people who are not parents, or those whose children live far away, often get involved in the nurturing of younger people. Most middle adults are self-confident regarding the knowledge they have accumulated. They are concerned for others and want to contribute to the community. They may do this through social activities, leadership roles in community or religious organizations, and career involvement. Middle adults are often mentors (teachers or coaches) to younger adults in these settings.

? *Think Critically About . . .* Do you have a mentor? Are you a mentor? How did that relationship develop?

Some adults are said to experience a midlife crisis. Most psychologists say that is not true. There are many changes in midlife, and some of them may create a crisis situation for some people, but there is no single event that causes a crisis for all middle adults.

Middle adults realize that they are no longer young. They begin to evaluate their self-concept and their role in the world. There may be times of pain or stress due to physical decline or financial problems. They must explore many questions in order to continue healthy development. **Middle adults accept that life is not simple and that instances occur over which they have little control.**

In every stage of life, the sincere listening and caring of other people can help individuals develop to their full potential. Education about the changes people experience as life evolves helps everyone understand and aids in coping with challenges. There are support groups for people in all kinds of crises, such as chemical abuse, divorce, and parenting issues. Learn about such groups in your locality and make necessary referrals when needed.

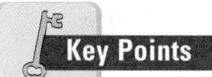

Key Points

- Adulthood is a time of continuing change and growth. Young adulthood is considered ages 19 to 45, whereas middle adulthood is considered ages 46 to 64. Ages 65 to 75 is later adulthood, and after age 76 is advanced age.
- Schaie's theory of cognitive development calls the young adult stage that of achievement; middle adults are in the stage of responsibility.
- Erikson's theory calls the young adult stage that of intimacy versus isolation. Middle adults are in the stage of generativity versus stagnation.
- Families are groups of interacting individuals who care about and for each other. It is in families that children learn basic values.
- Approximately 50% of marriages end in divorce. Divorce affects many people besides the couple involved.
- Maturity is a goal. Mature people demonstrate responsibility, confidence, trust, and self-discipline, as well as other characteristics.
- Young adults are generally healthy and in the best years for reproduction.
- Health promotion practices help adults achieve and maintain health.
- Career exploration is common during early young adulthood. Work provides many benefits economically, socially, and developmentally.

- Personality does not change significantly during the life span. People who want to change must work hard at it.
- Marrying and establishing a family are typical goals of young adults, although they may be postponed until a career is established.
- Married people are generally happier throughout their lives.
- Young adults expand their concern for other people and for the community.
- Gradual physical changes related to aging begin in the 30s and continue during middle adulthood.
- Menopause means the end of the reproductive years for women. Some women find it a time of new freedom and challenges.
- A person's lifestyle, especially diet and exercise habits, is a major influence on her health. Heredity also contributes, as does use of the health care system. Stress management at all ages contributes to improved health.
- Leading causes of death in the 50s and 60s are heart disease, cancer, vascular disease, and accidents.

- Work satisfaction seems to increase through life for most people. Middle adults often have greater responsibilities and may earn more money. Many become mentors.
- Many adults find returning to school challenging and rewarding. Learning should be a lifelong activity.
- Relationships with others remain the focus of psychosocial development. Marriage, extended family, and friendships are valued.
- Some middle adults become involved in caring for their elderly parents. This can be stressful for families; open communication and community support can help.

 Go to your **Companion CD-ROM** for an Audio Glossary, animations, video clips, and more.

evolve Be sure to visit the companion Evolve site at http://evolve.elsevier.com/deWit/fundamental/ for additional online resources.

NCLEX-PN® EXAMINATION-STYLE REVIEW QUESTIONS

*Choose the **best** answer(s) for each question.*

1. Types of families include nuclear, extended, step, blended, and partner. Because of the high incidence of divorce and remarriage, many more _____ families have emerged. *(Fill in the blank.)*

2. Young adults are likely to spend leisure time in activities that are:
   1. calm and quiet, alone or with only one or two others.
   2. inclusive of their parents and grandparents.
   3. physically and mentally demanding and competitive.
   4. ways to earn extra money.

3. The psychosocial task for the young adult is to seek:
   1. identity.
   2. intimacy.
   3. industry.
   4. generativity.

4. Failure to develop through Erikson's stage of young adulthood will cause the person to be:
   1. unable to form meaningful relationships.
   2. unsuccessful in further education.
   3. unable to keep a job.
   4. unsure of how to raise children.

5. The "sandwich generation" refers to:
   1. couples who care for both children and grandchildren.
   2. elderly who prefer sandwiches over a hot meal.
   3. people who do not have time to cook.
   4. people caring for both elderly parents and their own children.

6. People who eat nutritiously, rest adequately, and exercise regularly can:
   1. live to be more than 100 years old.
   2. continue to bear children until they are 60 or 70.
   3. postpone many of the effects of gradual aging.
   4. maintain their youthful vigor for their entire life.

7. When working with depressed middle-aged adults, and following Erikson's theory, you encourage them to find meaning in life by:
   1. developing intimate relationships with spouses.
   2. caring for their elderly parents.
   3. contributing to the development of younger people.
   4. volunteering as a hospital aide.

8. A 58-year-old man complains that he has difficulty remembering everything he wanted to buy when he gets to the store. Your best response would be:
   1. "Forgetting some things is a common occurrence with aging."
   2. "Do your siblings have similar problems?"
   3. "You should always take a list with you to the store."
   4. "Life is so busy that everyone forgets things now and then."

9. The psychosocial task of generativity refers to:
   1. the task of procreation.
   2. achieving one's career goals and ambitions.
   3. how one achieves economic stability.
   4. assisting and guiding the next generation.

10. Successful coping with midlife changes are likely when the individual:
    1. has children still at home.
    2. has a good support system.
    3. is married.
    4. is established in a career.

CRITICAL THINKING ACTIVITIES *Read each clinical scenario and discuss the questions with your classmates.*

Scenario A

As a clinic nurse, you are interviewing a new patient, a 34-year-old high school French teacher who complains of irregular menstrual periods. She has been married for 2 years and has no children.

1. What are some of the health concerns this patient might have? How can you help her understand the workings of her reproductive system?
2. What kinds of questions can you ask to help determine whether this patient is within the parameters of expected cognitive and psychosocial development?

Scenario B

Another clinic patient is a 52-year-old man who has recently been diagnosed with type 2 diabetes mellitus. He is 5'11" tall and weighs 245 pounds. His BP is 160/100 at this time. He works as a computer consultant and travels about 3 days each week.

1. How will you begin exploring any health concerns he may have? What will you say to determine how much of his diagnosis he understands? How can you encourage him to follow the prescribed regimen for maintaining or improving his physical health?
2. What is his expected stage of cognitive development? Where would you expect him to be in the occupational cycle? What are some questions you might ask?
3. You learn that he is divorced and shares custody of three adolescent children. How can you tactfully determine whether he is at the appropriate stage of psychosocial development?

Promoting Healthy Adaptation to Aging

evolve http://evolve.elsevier.com/deWit/fundamental/

Objectives

Upon completing this chapter, you should be able to:

Theory

1. Compare the biologic theories of aging.
2. State how a person might behave in response to the psychosocial theories of aging.
3. Identify four factors that contribute to longevity.
4. Discuss physical changes that occur as adults get older.
5. Explain Schaie's theory of cognitive development in the older adult.
6. Explain Erikson's stage of psychosocial development in the older adult.

Clinical Practice

1. Identify at least six signs and symptoms of normal aging.
2. Design an educational program to help older adults maintain physical health.
3. State three ways the nurse could help older adults maintain cognitive health.
4. Identify nursing problems related to changes in psychosocial health.
5. Guide the older adult's family members regarding signs that the older person needs assistance.

Key Terms

Be sure to check out the bonus material on the Companion CD-ROM, including selected audio pronunciations.

ageism (Ā-jĭsm, p. 173)
aging (p. 168)
benign senescence (bē-NĪGN sĕ-NĔ-sĕns, p. 170)
biologic theories (p. 171)
centenarians (sĕn-tĕn-ĀR-ē-ănz, p. 170)
dementia (dē-MĔN-shē-ă, p. 171)
demographic (dē-mō-GRĂ-fĭk, p. 170)
ego integrity (p. 174)
elder abuse (p. 174)
gerontologists (jĕr-ŏn-TŌ-lŏ-jĭsts, p. 168)
life span (p. 169)
longevity (lŏng-JĔ-vĭ-tē, p. 169)
psychosocial theories (SĪ-kō-SŌ-shăl, p. 169)
reminiscence (rĕ-mĭ-NĬ-sĕns, p. 174)
wisdom (p. 172)

OVERVIEW OF AGING

Aging (a continual process of biologic, cognitive, and psychosocial change) begins at conception. Although there is no way to escape it, we can learn to live with it. As a nurse, you will care for people of all ages. In most health care settings, many of your patients will be older adults. You are also aging, as are family members and friends. Knowing about normal development in the later years of life will help you in many ways.

Older adults are not all alike. Some are active, busy, and healthy; others are inactive because of illness and may be dependent on others. Being an older adult means different things to different people; **it is your perception of aging that influences your definition of being old.**

Because Americans are living longer than they did a few generations ago, scientists are interested in learning how a healthy body can be achieved into advanced years. Research about healthy aging is ongoing, and results are changing our ideas. Many older adults have the ability and potential for years of interesting and productive living. For them, the later years of life are exciting and rewarding. Most people do not mind growing older, especially if they are relatively healthy. Some, however, fear that the later years of life will be painful, boring, and filled with illness and despondency. Box 13-1 contains the *Healthy People 2010* major goals and objectives for older adults. Overcoming the myths about aging (Box 13-2) can be a challenge for nurses when working with middle and older adults.

? *Think Critically About . . .* When are people considered old? What does it mean to be old? How do older adults view life? What are the concerns of older people?

THEORIES OF AGING

There are numerous theories about aging. Some gerontologists (specialists in the study of aging people) claim that aging is primarily determined by genetics, whereas others are just as certain that environment and lifestyle play important roles. It is obvious that

Box 13-1 **Healthy People 2010** *Goals and Objectives for Older Adults*

- Increase the life span and the quality of life by focusing on wellness, prevention of illness, and treatment of disease.
- Increase to at least 80% the receipt of home food services by people ages 65 and older who have difficulty in preparing their own meals or are otherwise in need of home-delivered meals.

Box 13-2 *Myths about Old People*

- Old people are sick.
- Old people cannot learn new things.
- It is too late for lifestyle changes to improve health.
- Genetics are the main factor in longevity.
- Old people are not sexual.
- Old people are a drain on society.
- Old people are senile.
- Most old people are isolated from their families.
- Most old people live in nursing homes.
- Old people are poor.
- Old people are unhappy.

those factors interact, along with other things, to determine how long a person lives.

Biologic theories (theories based on cellular function and body physiology, or *apoptosis*) provide ways to look at the physical aging process. The *biologic clock* is one of these theories; this states that body cells are programmed to function for a specific length of time, after which they break down and die. When too many cells quit functioning, the person eventually dies.

Advocates of the *free-radical theory* believe that cells are damaged by toxins, ions break off from ion pairs, and the resulting free radicals are unstable. This occurs in the environment, in waste products of metabolism, and from disease. These toxins are causes of free radicals, or oxidizing substances in the body; the use of antioxidant vitamins and lotions is supposed to counteract the harmful chemicals. The *wear-and-tear theory* states that body cells and organs eventually wear out, like machinery.

In the *immune system failure theory*, the system loses its ability to protect the body from disease. Older persons become more susceptible to diseases such as influenza, which may kill them. The *autoimmune theory* is similar; here the body no longer recognizes itself, and begins to attack itself and break down, as occurs in some types of arthritis.

Think Critically About . . . Can you think of other health problems that could be examples of the biologic theories of aging?

There are also psychosocial theories (theories related to socialization and life satisfaction). The *disengagement theory,* since rejected, suggests that it is normal for older people and society to withdraw from each other. Most gerontologists no longer give credence to this concept.

The *activity theory* states that people who remain interested and active will continue to enjoy life and to live longer. Conversely, people who make no effort to contribute become less and less involved and shorten their life as a result.

In the *continuity theory,* each individual continues to live and develop as the unique person he or she is. Individuals' basic personalities do not change, and they will cope with aging in ways similar to the ways in which they coped with other stages of life.

LONGEVITY

The life span (the maximum years a species is capable of living) for human beings is 115 to 130 years. Longevity (length of life) has been increasing. In 1900, the average length of life in the United States was 47 years. In 2004, the U.S. Bureau of the Census projected the average life span to be 77.9 years. What caused this increase?

A major contributor to longer life is that people are healthier throughout their lives now than they were 100 years ago. Principles of hygiene have helped eliminate many illnesses. Health care has improved, anti-infective drugs are in common use, and technology allows surgeons to perform intricate procedures and replace more body parts. Improved nutrition is also another factor in longer life.

Education also contributes to longevity. People who are better educated seem to be more aware of how their bodies work and make more efforts at staying healthy. These people practice preventive health care and may seek treatment earlier in the course of an illness.

Lifestyle makes a significant difference in longevity. A healthy diet and regular exercise are crucial. Nonsmokers usually live longer than smokers; people who abuse chemicals risk shortening their lives. People who are married tend to live longer. Stress management is part of a healthy lifestyle, too.

A person's personality seems to affect the length of life as well as its quality. **The optimistic, happy person generally lives longer.** This is true even when a chronic illness is present.

Gender has been a contributing factor to longevity in the past; women in the 20th century lived 6 to 7 years longer than men. Currently, if a man reaches age 75, he dies only 2 years sooner than the average woman. The final factor in longevity is genetics. Gerontologists had claimed that heredity determined 50% of longevity, but recent research lowers that to about 30%.

? *Think Critically About . . .* How long did your ancestors live? Has the longevity of your family been increasing? How long do you think you will live?

DEMOGRAPHICS

Demographic (statistics about populations) studies show that there are more older people in the United States every year. In 2000, there were nearly 35 million people over 65, only 12.4% of the total population. U.S. Bureau of the Census experts predict that by 2030, nearly 66 million people, or 25.6% of the population, will be over 65.

For purposes of study, the older adult or elderly population is often divided into three distinct groups: the "young old" are 65 to 74 years of age, the "middle old" are 75 to 84, and the "very old" are 85 and beyond. Sixty-five years is used because the federal Social Security system uses the 65th year as a marker for retirement. As people live longer, the government may change that marker to 67 or even 70.

The young old are those who remain fairly healthy and active. You may not even recognize them as old when you see them in the shopping mall, restaurant, or theater. Many continue to contribute to their community and may remain employed, at least part time. They are not much different from middle adults.

The middle old are in a transition time. As people approach 80, they often become more frail and are thus less able to be as active. The very old are the most rapidly growing group, and this group will continue to increase in the future. These are also the most dependent older adults.

Centenarians (people 100 years old or older) are becoming more common. About 72,000 people were 100 years old in 2000. It is projected that there will be 129,000 centenarians by 2010, and the U.S. Bureau of the Census projects that by 2050, that figure will rise to 834,000 (U.S. Bureau of the Census, 2004).

Living a long and better life is everyone's goal. The ancient Greeks are credited with being the first to say they wanted to "die young, as late in life as possible." Most people who have become centenarians have been in good health at least into their 90s. To live to be very old, you have to be healthy for most of your life. **People are becoming healthier, better educated, and actively involved in their own health care, and are therefore living longer.**

? *Think Critically About . . .* Do you know any centenarians? What are they like? What does this mean for nursing and other health care providers?

Physical declines happen to everyone. Benign senescence (normal physical changes of aging) begins occurring early in adulthood, but often goes unnoticed until a problem develops. Changes mentioned in Chapter 12 continue. Table 13-1 summarizes the physiologic changes that occur with aging. Heart and lungs gradually become less efficient. Bones become more fragile and posture becomes bent.

Table 13-1 | *Physiologic Changes of Aging*

BODY SYSTEM	SOME TYPICAL CHANGES
Cardiovascular	Increased heart size
	Decreased cardiac output, causing less blood flow to all organs
	Thickened heart valves and blood vessels
	Less elasticity of blood vessels
	Slower blood cell production
	Slower immune response
Respiratory	Thickened alveolar walls, causing less elasticity
	Weakened respiratory muscles
	Decreased vital capacity and tidal volume
	Decreased number of cilia
Musculoskeletal	Thinned intervertebral disks
	Decreased bone calcium
	Smaller muscle mass
	Less elasticity of ligaments and tendons
	Degeneration of cartilage
Integumentary	Thinner, drier skin
	Loss of subcutaneous fat
	Slowed rate of hair and nail growth
Urologic	Decreased bladder capacity and tone
	Loss of nephrons, slowed function of remaining nephrons
	Decreased sphincter control
Neurologic	*Vision:* presbyopia, slowed accommodation, cataract development, decreased peripheral vision and depth perception
	Hearing: presbycusis, thicker eardrum, increased wax production, decreased hair cells in inner ear
	Taste, smell, touch: decreased number of receptors
	Balance: may be affected by decreased circulation
	Reflexes: slowed reaction time
	Slowed autonomic system responses
Endocrine	Slowed production of all hormones
	Decreased metabolic rate
	Delayed insulin response
Gastrointestinal	Decreased secretion of saliva and other digestive enzymes
	Slowed peristalsis
	Slowed liver and pancreatic functions
	Reduced absorption of nutrients
Reproductive	Decreased hormone production
	Atrophy of ovaries, uterus, vagina
	Benign prostatic hypertrophy
	Slowed sexual responses

The skin is thinner and more fragile; a reduced amount of subcutaneous tissue causes older adults to complain of feeling cold. Older people often have smaller appetites. Vision continues to deteriorate; night driving becomes difficult.

Hearing deficits may become more pronounced. Nearly 75% of the population over age 75 has some hearing loss. Various types of hearing aids can be very helpful. The earlier a person with hearing difficulty obtains a hearing aid, the better the brain can adjust to it and provide a good quality of hearing.

Changes in the brain also occur with normal aging. There may be less blood flow. Chemicals vital for nerve functions may be imbalanced. Because brain cells do not easily regenerate, losses caused by injury or illness will affect the body's functions. The brain can adapt by growing more dendrites up to age 90 if the person is reasonably healthy. Brain changes are also important in trying to understand cognitive changes in older adults, such as sensory and memory losses.

Think Critically About . . . What kinds of health problems can you relate to the typical changes identified in Table 13-1? What nursing responses could be helpful?

HEALTH CONCERNS

Most people over 75 have at least one chronic health problem. Hypertension is the most common; 51% of older adults have hypertension. Arthritis is second, with 48% of older adults have some joint stiffness. Heart disease is third, with 31% of older adults having some cardiac problem. Obesity contributes to joint problems by causing increased stress on joints; it also contributes to hypertension. For many older adults, these conditions do not seem to prevent living active and full lives.

Other common concerns include anemia, diabetes, influenza, cancer, malnutrition, cirrhosis, and mental illness. The leading causes of death are heart disease, cancer, stroke, lung disease, accidents, diabetes, and Alzheimer's disease (National Center for Health Statistics, 2004).

Older people are often concerned about falling, especially about breaking a hip, and about being dependent on others (Health Promotion Points 13-1). Accidents may happen because of changes in depth perception, changes in gait, and slower reaction times. It is important to teach older people safety measures to prevent falls (see Chapter 40).

Mental health in the older adult may be difficult to evaluate. Many physical conditions, such as malnutrition, dehydration, infection, and misuse of medications, can lead to impaired cognition. A thorough examination should be done to make an accurate diagnosis. About 6% of older adults are clinically de-

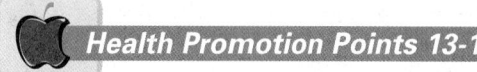
Health Promotion Points 13-1

Fitness for the Older Adult

- A fitness program to promote strength and balance is an excellent way to decrease the risk of a fall and to promote the ability to stay independent.
- Many communities have special fitness programs for the older adult.

pressed, whereas 37% have depressive symptoms (National Institute of Mental Health, 2007). Depression can often be treated successfully with medications and counseling.

Dementia (degeneration of brain tissue) occurs in a small percentage of older adults. The incidence rises as aging progresses. Confusion, memory loss, and disordered thinking are early signs. There are numerous causes of this problem, from malnutrition to ministrokes to Alzheimer's disease. (Alzheimer's disease is covered in Chapter 41.) Table 13-2 compares the memory decline that is age-related with depression-related and dementia-related memory problems. Between 6% and 10% of older adults have dementia; two thirds of that number have Alzheimer's disease.

HEALTH PROMOTION BEHAVIORS

One behavior that helps delay physical aging is eating a healthy diet. Older adults should be encouraged to learn about nutrition and meal planning. Additional seasonings can counter the loss of taste buds. Some physicians encourage a daily multivitamin. Eating is a social experience for many, so they should find opportunities to share meals with others. Many communities offer communal dining; prepared meals can also be delivered to a home.

Physical activity also postpones many effects of aging. Many older adults participate in regular exercise groups. Daily activity, whether walking, biking, or swimming, keeps the body functioning. Older adults also benefit from weight training. The *Exercise Guide for Older People,* in English or Spanish, is available free from the National Institute on Aging. It describes appropriate exercises to keep fit and promote good balance.

Another positive behavior is having regular physical examinations to monitor chronic conditions and to screen for new problems. Older adults may need encouragement to participate in their own health care management. The cost of health care is a concern to some, but there are programs designed for older adults that will help provide regular care.

Older adults who smoke should be encouraged to quit. They may have been smoking for years, but the health benefits of quitting are significant, even in advanced years. The use of nicotine patches and a support group may be helpful. Alcohol use should also be

Table 13-2 *Memory Decline as the Result of Normal Aging, Depression, or Dementia*

NORMAL AGE-RELATED MEMORY DECLINE	DEPRESSION-RELATED MEMORY PROBLEMS	DEMENTIA-RELATED MEMORY PROBLEMS
Onset age specifically identifiable	Onset with depression	Hard to establish onset
Slow progression of symptoms	Rapid or sudden progression of symptoms	Slow or stepwise progression
History of depression less common	History of depression more common	History of depression less common
Complains about memory loss	Complains about memory loss	Usually unaware of memory loss
May emphasize disability	May emphasize disability	Conceals disability
May decrease or increase efforts to perform	Decreases efforts to perform	Struggles to perform
Uses notes and other memory aids	May not try to keep up	Needs instruction to use memory aids
No lasting mood change associated	Consistent depressive mood	Emotional lability and shallowness
Behavior may or may not change	Behavior change is greater than impairment	Behavior change may be appropriate
Nocturnal drop in performance unusual	Nocturnal drop in performance unusual	Nocturnal drop in performance common
"Don't know" answers common	"Don't know" answers common	Guesses or "near miss" answers common
Recent and remote memory losses are equal	Recent and remote memory losses are equal	Recent memory impaired, remote is intact
	Memory gaps for specific events common	Memory gaps for specific events unusual

From Leifer-Hartson, G., & Hartson, H. (2004). *Growth and Development Across the Lifespan: A Health Promotion Focus,* Philadelphia: Saunders.

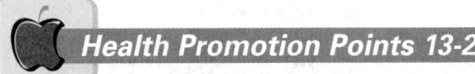

Health Promotion Points 13-2

Medication Regimen Aids for Older Adults

- Using a pill-minder box with a compartment for each day of the week, or for different times of each day for a week, is very useful for helping the older adult to remember to take required medications on time and regularly.
- The box is refilled once a week, and a list can be made for the person to follow when filling the box.

limited as its effects may be greater in the elderly and it may interfere with prescribed medications. Some adults may need guidance in taking prescribed medications correctly (Health Promotion Points 13-2).

COGNITIVE ASPECTS OF AGING

Schaie's stage of cognitive development for older adults is called the *reintegrative stage.* This states that older adults are more selective about how they will spend their time. They will take time for interesting things, but not for things that seem irrelevant. A woman who regularly hosts family meals on special occasions may try new recipes and enjoy a cooking class. However, someone who lives alone and rarely entertains may not be interested in such activities.

Discovering the interests of older persons can provide clues to ways to stimulate and maintain their cognitive abilities. One person may enjoy crossword puzzles and another may enjoy reading mysteries.

Healthy adults can maintain intelligence into advanced years. The speed of thinking may slow, but thinking processes remain intact. Many older adults who are ill or who have vision or hearing deficits do not suffer cognitive dysfunction. They should be certain that glasses and/or hearing aids are in place before interacting with other persons.

WISDOM AND LEARNING

Wisdom (having good judgment based on accumulated knowledge) is often credited to older adults because of their wealth of life experiences. Younger people can benefit by listening to the advice of older people.

Because older adults sometimes think more slowly, some people assume they can no longer learn. This is not true. Subjects of interest can fascinate the older learner (Patient Teaching 13-1). They have more patience for learning. Many have learned to operate computers and enjoy using that technology. Elder hostel programs, often operated by colleges, provide stimulating opportunities to learn and sometimes travel with other older adults.

MEMORY ISSUES

Some older adults have problems remembering recent events; this is short-term memory loss. They may not recall much of yesterday. However, long-term memory remains intact. They can remember many details of their younger life. Memory aids such as making lists or notes on a calendar can help keep life orderly (Health Promotion Points 13-3).

The more severe memory losses and dementias of aging are often the result of circulatory changes. Per-

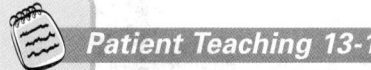

Patient Teaching 13-1

Teaching the Older Adult

Keep the following points in mind when attempting to teach the older adult:

- Provide motivation for the content to be learned.
- Keep the topic relevant to the learner.
- Assess readiness to learn and take advantage of "teaching moments" (when the learner is most receptive).
- Use visual aids in large print and bright colors.
- Good lighting in the room and on the materials is essential.
- Be certain the individual has needed reading glasses and that the hearing aid is turned on if one is worn.
- Speak clearly, distinctly, and slowly in a normal tone.
- Obtain feedback at intervals about what has been taught.
- Relate learning to better autonomy, health, and activity.

Health Promotion Points 13-3

Cognitive Stimulation in Older Adults

Regular exercise of at least 30 minutes five times a week is thought to decrease mental decline by 35%. Encourage elderly patients to engage in some sort of exercise program even if it is just walking in the neighborhood. Exercise classes at the senior center or Parks and Recreation Department are available in many communities. Dancing is excellent exercise. If ballroom dancing is not appealing, contra dancing or any country dancing is very good exercise and can be done as a "single."

sons experiencing memory changes and their family members should not assume that such changes are inevitable. The older adult should be evaluated for nutritional status, hypertension, arterial health, an endocrine disorder, and specific neurologic problems. Sometimes underlying conditions can be treated and the memory problems will also be resolved.

EMPLOYMENT AND RETIREMENT

The ability and desire to keep a job is an individual decision, depending partially on the cognitive ability of the older adult. Some types of work maintain a mandatory retirement age, particularly if the work involves public safety. In other situations, retirement is a matter of preference.

Think Critically About . . . What are some suggestions you could give to assist an older adult to remain active after retirement?

Some people are eager to leave a regular job and may retire in their 50s or early 60s. Some continue to work because they need the income. Retiring early requires planning for finances and other concerns. Other

people enjoy working and want to continue beyond a traditional retirement age. According to the U.S. Bureau of Census statistics, about 10% of older adults have incomes that place them in the poor or near-poor category (*Senior Journal*, 2005). About 5 million older adults are employed at least part time.

Workers who lose their jobs a few years before retirement may find it hard to obtain other employment at similar wages. Ageism (discrimination because of age) is illegal in the United States. A worker who has lost a job in favor of a younger person has recourse through the government and the courts.

Think Critically About . . . Do you know anyone who lost a job in their 50s or early 60s? Were they able to find other employment at a comparable income? How did they feel about that experience?

Retirement brings with it major changes in many aspects of lifestyle: no alarm clock, no set schedule, no coffee break with co-workers, no need to dress neatly, no paycheck. People who have adequate finances may feel comfortable about retiring. Some will travel extensively if health and finances permit.

Many early retirees discover they have time on their hands and begin a second career. Older adults may continue to work in family businesses. Others volunteer to keep themselves busy and involved. The contributions of older adults should not be underestimated. About 7% of grandparents are providing extensive care for grandchildren; 1 out of 15 of those are putting in enough hours for it to qualify as a full-time job (*Senior Journal* Editors, 2007). Again, attitude is important. People whose lives revolved around their work may have difficulty adjusting to retirement. Sometimes people without other interests become disillusioned with retirement and find another job. Other people become depressed, withdraw, feel useless, and die. Recent retirees should be encouraged to set small daily or weekly goals until the adjustment has been made.

HEALTH PROMOTION BEHAVIORS

Behaviors that help with successful cognitive aging are the same behaviors that are encouraged throughout life. Having a positive attitude remains important. Some people are unhappy with their lives and unwilling to try to change; it is not easy for health care workers to accept that. Encouragement is always appropriate. For example, you can remind them of their past accomplishments, of their success in raising children, or even the accomplishment of living a long life.

Active involvement in a job and community during earlier adulthood often carries into continuing involvement in hobbies, religious and service groups, and volunteerism in older adulthood. Older adults can be reminded of how much they have to offer their community because of their broad experience.

Using the brain by reading, doing puzzles, using a computer, and writing keeps the neural connections active and healthy. A computer game called "Brain Age" has been shown to improve cognition in the elderly. The brain is like a muscle in one way: it should be exercised regularly. Even the older adult who is physically limited can maintain mental stimulation with a little effort.

PSYCHOSOCIAL ASPECTS OF AGING

Erikson's stage of development for older adults is called ego integrity (state of being complete) versus despair (see Table 11-2). Older persons naturally spend time thinking about their lives. If they find their lives have been good, then they are satisfied and have ego integrity. However, if they are unhappy about the way life has evolved, they will despair. Resolution to ego integrity may occur if you can help the person find enough areas of satisfaction to outnumber the areas of regret.

LIFE REVIEW

This is the time for reminiscence (reviewing one's life). If individuals accept that they have had good lives, and that they have contributed to others, then they are satisfied. People who were not successful at working through a developmental stage when younger may find unhappiness with the way their lives progressed. Sometimes it is enough to realize that one did the best one could under the circumstances.

Many psychologists consider this stage of life review important as a person faces mortality. **Being content with past accomplishments is important for self-worth at any stage of life.** The older adult simply has more years about which to reflect.

FAMILY RELATIONSHIPS

Families continue to be important in older adulthood. Married people seem to live longer than those who are alone (Figure 13-1). Widows usually adjust better than do widowers. According to the U.S. Bureau of the Census (2002), 43% of all women over 65 are widows; 14% of men are widowers (Administration on Aging, 2005). Many widowed, divorced, or single older adults may continue to date, and some will remarry.

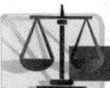 *Think Critically About . . .* Widowers frequently die within 1 year of their wife's death. Why do you think that is true?

The majority of older adults who have children live within 40 miles of one child. Contact with that child usually occurs at least weekly. One reason this is im-

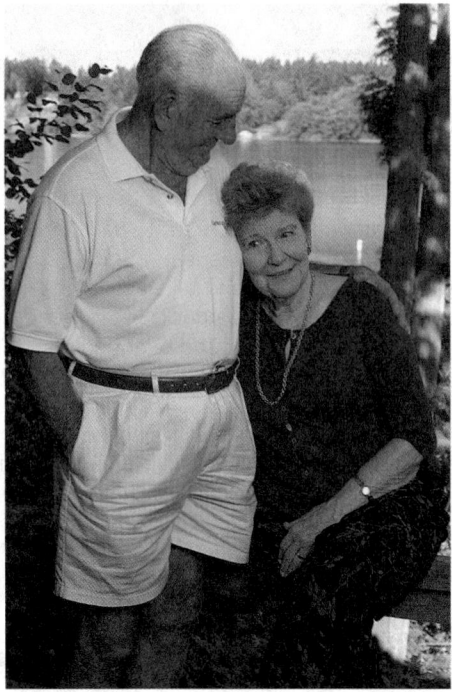

FIGURE **13-1** Romance can exist in later life.

Legal & Ethical Considerations 13-1

Reporting Elder Abuse

All licensed professionals are required to report any signs of or suspected abuse to a law enforcement agency. Social services personnel or law enforcement officials will conduct an investigation.

portant is that the older parent may need assistance with one or more aspects of daily life.

The active older adult may contribute to extended family life by helping with child care of grandchildren or great-grandchildren. Sometimes retired adults end up raising grandchildren. Adult children may have died or may be imprisoned, hospitalized, or otherwise unable to care for the children. This arrangement can bring both benefits and problems for the children and for the older adults.

Nearly 2.1 million older adults are affected by elder abuse (any type of abuse of the elderly). Those over age 80 have the greatest incidence, with the primary type being neglect. This is a 15.6% increase since 2004 (National Center on Elder Abuse, 2006). When it occurs in a family, it is for many of the same reasons abuse happens to children or spouses. Elder abuse may occur in a long-term care setting (Legal & Ethical Considerations 13-1).

SOCIAL ACTIVITY

Community involvement was discussed earlier relative to cognitive development; it is also important for psychosocial health. **Older adults need to feel needed; this contributes to their self-concept and emotional**

health. Some volunteers and part-time workers choose those activities primarily for the social activity.

Older adults experience a gradual loss of their peer group as friends and siblings die. These can be difficult times for the survivors; they continue to need support from their family and community. Those who have cultivated friendships with younger people fare best.

LIVING ARRANGEMENTS

Many older adults prefer to live in their own homes as long as they are physically able. Others choose to rent an apartment when they cannot maintain a house and yard. About half of older adults (54.7%) lived with a spouse in 2004 (Administration on Aging, 2005). About 30.8% live alone; many of these need some assistance at times. About 671,000 grandparents age 65 or over maintained households in which grandchildren were present in 2004. That number continues to grow.

According to the U.S. Bureau of the Census, only 4.5% of all people over age 65 lived in long-term care settings and 5% lived in senior housing in 2000 (U.S. Bureau of the Census, 2000). This percentage increases with age, with nearly 18.2% of people over age 85 residing in long-term care settings.

As more people live to be older adults, it is important for them to remain healthier longer. This is beginning to happen. People over 85 remain the most frail and will probably continue to need help with daily activities. As that group grows, more nurses and other health care workers will be needed to give care.

HEALTH PROMOTION BEHAVIORS

Older adults have several psychosocial challenges to face. They need to accept and adjust to a changing body. Family roles change, especially if one spouse becomes ill or dependent on the other, or dies. There are changes in the use of time as a result of retirement. Finally, older adults have to face their own mortality.

The helpful behaviors for these adjustments continue to revolve around maintaining an optimistic outlook, staying as physically fit as possible, and remaining involved with others. **Those who face the future with a hopeful, positive attitude will cope better with aging.**

Older adults should be encouraged to make a living will and to designate someone to make health care decisions for them in case they cannot. Completing a durable power of attorney for financial arrangements is recommended. Each state has guidelines and forms that can be obtained from lawyers or health clinics. The office of the patient's physician should be given a copy of the documents.

Older adults with children should involve them in planning. If there are no children, another relative, a younger friend, or a trusted lawyer can be named as their trustee.

WHEN A PARENT NEEDS HELP

It is not easy for adult children to admit that a parent needs their assistance. Sometimes the nurse can help stimulate a conversation about the future and offer resources for the family.

Some older adults recognize that they will need help and will initiate discussion with their children or others (Figure 13-2). They may decide when to move to a smaller apartment or into an assisted living arrangement. Others will deny their aging and resist making any changes until a crisis arises. This denial is an understandable way of maintaining their dignity and self-esteem.

PLANNING AHEAD

Experts suggest that adult children keep communication lines open with their parents. The parent may need encouragement to discuss alternative living arrangements or other changes that may be needed. Adult children should try to do the following:
- **Plan ahead:** Discuss possibilities and make plans with the parent before a crisis occurs. This way decisions will be mutually agreeable and less traumatic.
- **Include everyone:** Siblings should share in planning and decisions. No one adult child should be made to feel wholly responsible.
- **Find important information:** This includes knowing about the parent's financial situation, the medical care presently received, medications used, and alternative housing possibilities. If parents are reluctant to discuss changes, it sometimes helps to allow more time for them to think about it. Consider the choices and seek resources.

OBSERVING CHANGES

Safety is a basic need. Adult children will have to make decisions for parents who are no longer able to safely care for themselves. If older adults show signs

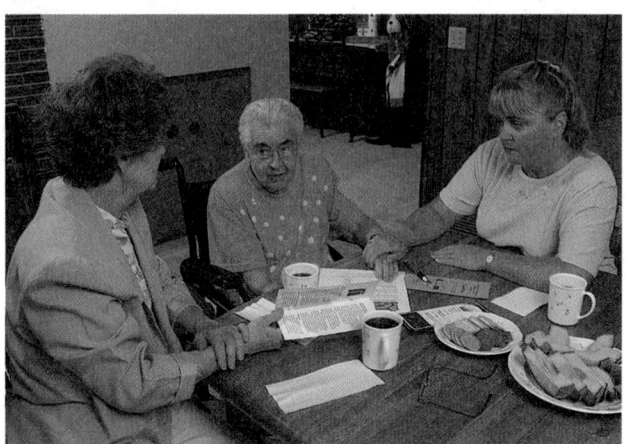

FIGURE **13-2** A family gathers to consider options for the older adult.

Box 13-3 *Signs that an Older Person Needs Help*

- Neglected personal hygiene, irregular dressing, and soiled clothing
- Changed eating habits in last year resulting in weight loss; having no appetite, or missed meals
- Home neglect and less than desirable sanitary conditions
- Inappropriate behavior, such as being unusually loud or quiet, paranoid, or agitated, or making phone calls at all hours
- Frequent falls, burns, injury marks
- Social isolation and cessation of previous activities that were important
- Altered relationship patterns such that friends and neighbors express concern
- Inability to find the right words
- Forgetfulness resulting in unpaid bills, unopened mail, missed appointments, or hoarding money
- Confusion about medications
- Making unusual purchases, such as more than one subscription to the same magazine, increased buying from television advertisements

---

of deteriorating behavior, it is time for adult children to make some of those decisions for them (Box 13-3).

RESOURCES FOR FAMILIES

Many communities provide services for older adults, including adult day services, chore services, transportation, counseling, companionship programs, exercise and rehabilitation programs, and telephone reassurance services. To learn what is available in your community, begin with the yellow pages in the phone book. Your state agency on aging coordinates information. The federal Administration on Aging and the Internet can also provide information. AARP (the American Association of Retired Persons) can provide information about services for older adults.

Some websites for information are www.aoa.gov, www.aarp.org, www.cdc.gov/aging, and www.caregiver911.com.

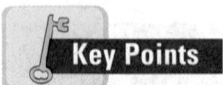

Key Points

- Most older Americans are in reasonably good health and living independently. Americans are living longer.
- There are biologic theories of aging and psychosocial theories of aging.

- Many factors contribute to longevity. Genetics, maintaining a healthy lifestyle, appropriate use of the health care system, and education are some factors.
- Young old adults are ages 65 to 74; middle old adults are ages 75 to 84; very old adults are 85 and beyond. Centenarians are people 100 and older.
- Leading causes of death in older adults are heart disease, cancer, strokes, lung disease, diabetes, and cirrhosis.
- Exercise for increasing strength and balance helps prevent falls and promotes longer independence.
- Older adults can benefit by improving their diets and increasing their physical activity. A positive attitude helps all aspects of development.
- Schaie's stage for older adults is the reintegrative stage; older adults are careful about how they spend their time and only take time for things that are of interest to them.
- Short-term memory may weaken with age, but memory aids can help. Although mental processing slows, given time, the older adult can do as well as a younger adult.
- The age of retirement varies widely. About 5 million older adults are employed at least part time, whereas others volunteer.
- Erikson's stage for older adults is ego integrity versus despair. Older adults reminisce, and if life has been satisfactory, they have ego integrity.
- Family relationships remain important. Role changes occur when a spouse becomes ill or dependent, or dies.
- Many older adults prefer living in their own home as long as possible.
- Adult children of older adults should remain aware of their parents' status and be prepared to help if the parents are no longer able to safely care for themselves.

 Go to your **Companion CD-ROM** for an Audio Glossary, animations, video clips, and more.

evolve Be sure to visit the companion Evolve site at http://evolve.elsevier.com/deWit/fundamental/ for additional online resources.

NCLEX-PN® EXAMINATION-STYLE REVIEW QUESTIONS

*Choose the **best** answer(s) for each question.*

1. Demographers in the United States predict that there will continue to be more older people because: *(Select all that apply.)*
   1. the baby boomers are healthier as they get older than were previous generations.
   2. medical technology is extending life for many, especially those with heart disease.
   3. most people today are much happier than were those of previous generations.
   4. there are more wealthy people who can afford good health care.
   5. more vitamins and supplements are available to delay aging.

2. The biologic clock theory of aging states that:
   1. body systems eventually wear out.
   2. body cells are destined to live a specific period of time.
   3. no one can live more than 110 years.
   4. there is little one can do to change one's life span.

3. The majority of older Americans live in:
   1. long-term care facilities.
   2. special senior housing.
   3. the home of relatives.
   4. their own homes.

4. To fulfill Erikson's psychosocial stage, older adults can be encouraged to:
   1. play with their grandchildren.
   2. continue with hobbies and light exercise.
   3. remain employed as long as is possible.
   4. review their lives, recalling accomplishments.

5. The important behaviors that can help an older adult to age successfully include:
   1. moving closer to a child.
   2. remaining physically and mentally active.
   3. limiting exercise to conserve strength.
   4. eating at least 2000 calories daily.

6. In order to help parents plan for possible future changes, adult children should:
   1. investigate alternative housing arrangements.
   2. keep communication lines open within the family.
   3. choose a nursing home for the parent.
   4. consult with the parent's physician.

7. The U.S. government defines old age as the time when full Social Security benefits become available, which is after age
   1. 55.
   2. 65.
   3. 75.
   4. 85.

8. Signs of elder abuse include: *(Select all that apply.)*
   1. fear of caregivers.
   2. bruises and cuts in various stages of healing.
   3. timid and withdrawn behavior.
   4. forgetfulness.
   5. disheveled appearance.

9. When trying to teach an older adult, a very important aspect is to:
   1. provide good illumination in the room.
   2. present only one point per teaching session.
   3. speak loudly and point as you talk.
   4. use very simple language.

CRITICAL THINKING ACTIVITIES *Read each clinical scenario and discuss the questions with your classmates.*

Scenario A
One of your home care patients is an 82-year-old woman with arthritis and adult-onset diabetes. She had a hip replacement 3 months ago after a fall and has recently returned to her apartment after rehabilitation in a long-term care setting. You are to assist her with her hygiene needs and monitor her medications.

1. What are some observations you could make to assess her cognitive abilities and stage of development?
2. How might you assess her psychosocial development?
3. What could you do to assist her in adjusting to this stage of her life?

CHAPTER 14

Cultural and Spiritual Aspects of Patient Care

Objectives

Upon completing this chapter, you should be able to:

Theory

1. Describe how culture influences health and health care choices.
2. Identify three beliefs or values affecting health care that might be found among patients from the following cultural groups: Hispanic American, Asian American, American Indian, African American, and European American.
3. Plan ways to support the spiritual needs of patients of various religions.
4. Compare ethnic differences of Hispanic Americans and Middle Eastern Muslims.
5. Discuss the ways in which poverty often impedes adequate health care within our country.
6. Describe how religious beliefs and practices may affect health and health care choices.
7. Incorporate major differences in dietary and nutritional choices among cultural and religious groups into patients' plans of care.

Clinical Practice

1. Demonstrate cultural competence when caring for a culturally different patient.
2. Plan nursing interventions for a patient whose culture is different from your own.
3. Discuss ways to protect patients' rights when their culture does not permit the use of a medical intervention.
4. Identify signs of spiritual distress in a patient and plan three interventions to relieve it.
5. Discuss boundaries of professional care for a patient whose religious beliefs are different from yours.

Key Terms

Be sure to check out the bonus material on the Companion CD-ROM, including selected audio pronunciations.

agnostic (ăg-NŎS-tĭk, p. 179)
atheist (Ā-thē-ĭst, p. 179)
baptized (p. 180)
beliefs (p. 179)
bias (BĪ-ăs, p. 184)
chi'i (CHĒ, p. 186)
circumcision (sŭr-kŭm-SĬ-shŭn, p. 182)
communion (p. 180)
cultural awareness (KŬL-chŭr-ăl a-WĀR-nĕs, p. 184)

cultural competence (KŎM-pĕ-tĕns, p. 184)
cultural sensitivity (sĕn-sĭ-TĬ-vĭ-tē, p. 184)
culture (p. 178)
curandero (kŭr-ăn-DĒ-rō, p. 186)
dialects (DĪ-ă-lĕkts, p. 184)
egalitarian (ē-găl-ĭ-TĂR-ĭ-ăn, p. 185)
ethnic (p. 183)
ethnocentrism (ĕth-nō-SĔN-trĭsm, p. 184)
faith (p. 179)
generalization (jĕn-ĕr-ăl-ĭ-ZĀ-shŭn, p. 184)
holistic (p. 186)
kosher (KŌ-shŭr, p. 182)
matriarchal (MĀ-trē-ăr-kăl, p. 185)
patriarchal (PĀ-trē-ăr-kăl, p. 185)
personal space (p. 184)
prejudice (PRĔ-jŭ-dĭs, p. 184)
race (p. 183)
religion (p. 179)
rituals (p. 179)
shaman (SHĀ-măn, p. 187)
spiritual distress (SPĬR-ĭ-tū-ăl, p. 189)
spirituality (p. 179)
stereotype (STĔR-ē-ō-tĭp, p. 184)
subcultures (p. 183)
transcultural nursing (p. 183)
values (p. 179)
worldview (p. 178)
yang (p. 186)
yin (p. 186)

CULTURE, RELIGION, AND SPRITUALITY

Culture and religion have a strong impact on health care because they influence the ways in which people think and behave. Lifestyle choices related to nutrition, exercise, stress management, smoking, and alcohol or drug use are all influenced by culture. Religion or spiritual practice has a definite role in recovery of health for many people.

Culture consists of the values, beliefs, and practices shared by the majority within a group of people. Culture includes the attitudes, roles, behaviors, and religious or spiritual practices accepted and expected by the cultural group. Cultural traditions are carried out and passed on from generation to generation. A group's worldview is the way in which the group's people explain life events and view life's mysteries. This view

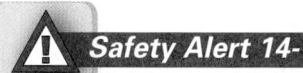

Safety Alert 14-1

Cultural Diversity and Medication Safety

- Asian and Hispanic patients may stop taking medications due to side effects without telling their health care provider. This can be accounted for by their deference to doctors and a natural reluctance to share very personal information.
- African Americans and Native Americans may doubt the need for medications when symptoms ease, and may discontinue drugs such as antibiotics or antidepressants before the prescription is finished or when it is supposed to be ongoing.
- Vietnamese patients may take only half of the prescribed dose of a medication, believing it is too strong.
- Asians and Eskimos need lower doses of anxiolytics than whites. Asians, Indians, and Pakistanis should be prescribed lower doses of antipsychotic drugs and lithium. Hispanics may do better with lower doses of antidepressants (*Nurse Advise-ERR* Editors, 2005).

directs the formulation of values, which are those ideas and perceptions seen as good and useful.

Immigration has brought increasing cultural diversity within the United States and Canada, as is seen in the different languages, physical characteristics, skin tones, and attire of people, and the ethnic restaurants and foodstuffs encountered in most cities. Patients from many different cultures are encountered in all types of health care settings (Safety Alert 14-1).

Although the terms *religion* and *spirituality* are often used interchangeably, there is a difference. Both have to do with attempting to understand one's place in the world and life's meaning or purpose. Spirituality concerns the spirit, or soul, and is an element of religion. It is intangible and may include a belief in a higher power, creative force, or divine being, or a belief in spirits of departed people and the supernatural. Religion is a formalized system of belief and worship. Rituals (ceremonial acts) or practices related to health, illness, birth, and death, and prescribed behavior are part of organized religion and sometimes spirituality. Beliefs are convictions or opinions that one considers to be true. Faith is a belief that cannot be proven, or for which no material evidence exists. A person who does not believe in the existence of God is an atheist. An agnostic is a person who doubts the existence of God, because it cannot be proved or disproved.

Spiritual and religious beliefs (or nonbelief) are learned in the family or culture of a child. Over time, faith matures into a way of thinking that influences lifestyle, behavior, attitudes, and beliefs about life, health, illness, and death. Religious and spiritual beliefs change over time and may be especially affected by changes in health. **During illness, and especially in the face of death, religious and spiritual beliefs may be strengthened, questioned, or rejected.** Health care decisions may be influenced by beliefs regarding health as a gift, or illness or disease as a punishment. There also may be religious prohibitions or requirements for treatment. Some people with spiritual beliefs may see illness or disease as displeasure of the spirits that requires special rituals and ceremonies to remove the displeasure. Prayer and meditation often are used along with a scientific medical regimen by spiritual and religious people.

MAJOR RELIGIONS IN THE UNITED STATES AND CANADA

Many different religions flourish in the United States and Canada. People who identify themselves as Christians are the majority. Until recently, people of the Jewish faith were the second largest group, but rapid increases in the numbers of people who are Muslims now make that religion second largest. All three religions have a faith in one God who created the world and has revealed himself at some point in history. Smaller numbers of people in the United States and Canada, particularly among the Southeast Asian, Chinese, Korean, Indian, and Japanese populations, may believe in the religions of Buddhism, Hinduism, Confucianism, or Taoism (Daoism). Religious beliefs and rituals are interwoven into a group's culture. However, not all members of a particular cultural group are of the same religion. **It is important to inquire about the spiritual life of each individual patient.**

CHRISTIANITY

The largest religion in the world is Christianity, with its three main divisions: Roman Catholic, Eastern Orthodox, and the Protestant faiths. Christians believe in eternal life, as promised in the New Testament of the Bible in the message of Jesus. Death is viewed as a transition to a life with God. The administration of the sacraments, particularly the sacraments of baptism and Holy Communion, is very important to most Roman Catholics. A priest or a religious leader should be called if the patient desires a sacrament. Catholic and Eastern Orthodox beliefs related to health care are presented in Box 14-1.

Protestant denominations began when a rift developed between King Henry VIII of England and the Roman Catholic Church and when religious leaders such as Martin Luther objected to some practices of the Roman Catholic Church. The Anglican and Lutheran churches and other Protestant denominations were founded. There are a great many Protestant denominations. The Protestant religious leader is usually called a minister or pastor. Some denominations with considerably different beliefs and practices are Christian Science, Jehovah's Witnesses, The Church of Jesus Christ

---

Box 14-1 *Roman Catholic and Eastern Orthodox Beliefs and Health Care*

ROMAN CATHOLIC

Birth: Infants must be baptized soon after birth because of the belief that babies not baptized will not go to Heaven. Even aborted fetuses must be baptized. If a priest is not immediately available, the nurse may baptize by pouring holy water on the head and saying "I baptize you in the name of the Father, of the Son, and of the Holy Spirit." Chart the information in the nurse's notes, and inform the priest and the family.

Holy Communion: Patients receiving communion must not have anything to eat or alcohol to drink 1 hour before receiving the Host, if at all possible. Medicine and fluids may be taken any time.

Sacrament of the sick: When the patient is ill, the priest is called to give this sacrament. He applies holy oil to the patient's forehead and hands. This sacrament may also be done after death. The nurse records this in the nurse's notes.

Diet: When hospitalized, the Catholic patient is excused from dietary rules.

Death: Catholics must receive the sacrament of the sick and make a confession. All body parts must be buried or cremated.

Birth control: Natural family planning is the only acceptable birth control. Nurses may teach family planning.

Sterilization is forbidden unless needed for medical reasons.

Organ donation: Donation and transplants are acceptable.

Religious articles: Rosary beads are used to pray. Medals and other objects are important to the patient and should be kept visible and secure.

EASTERN ORTHODOX

Birth: The baby must be baptized by 40 days after birth. A priest or deacon must baptize the child with holy water or by moving the baby in the air in the sign of the cross.

Holy Communion: Call the priest if the patient wants to receive communion.

Sacrament of the sick: The priest will do this at the bedside.

Diet: Hospitalized patients are excused from fasting from meat and dairy products on holy days.

Holidays: Christmas is celebrated January 7, and New Year's Day on January 14.

Death: The priest must be called by the nurse while the patient is conscious for the patient to receive the last rites (anointing of the sick). The Orthodox Church discourages assisted deaths, autopsy, cremation, and organ donation.

Adapted from Carson, V. (1989). *Spiritual Dimensions of Nursing Practice.* Philadelphia: Saunders.

---

of Latter-day Saints (Mormon), Unitarian Universalist Association, and the Unification Church. The Bible provides guidance and solace for Christians.

Most Protestant patients seek and accept health care. However, because of the diversity of denominations and their beliefs, it is essential to perform a spiritual assessment to ascertain what needs and concerns the patient might have. Prayer, reading of scripture and devotionals, and attendance at church services are the main religious activities of Protestant patients.

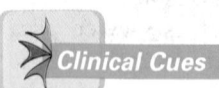
Clinical Cues

Quiet time for reading of the scriptures or devotionals should be offered. Do not interrupt the patient for procedures during these quiet times.

Many Protestant patients may wish to have Holy Communion while hospitalized. Some denominations believe in the anointing of the sick. The pastor or minister should be contacted for the patient desiring these sacraments. Abortion is generally opposed by most Protestant denominations except if the mother's life is in danger. Birth control decisions are generally left up to the individual family. The religious groups whose beliefs differ from some of the main beliefs described and in specific areas relevant to health care are presented in Table 14-1. Some protestant denominations forbid the use of alcohol, tobacco, tea, coffee, and caffeine substances because they are considered drugs.

Beliefs of individuals within each denomination vary, and specific spiritual assessment regarding the various issues relevant to health care is essential.

Think Critically About . . . From the information in Table 14-1, you know that Jehovah's Witnesses will not accept a blood transfusion. How would you react if a 24-year-old female accident victim who is a Jehovah's Witness says that she will refuse to accept a blood transfusion, even though she knows she is likely to die without it? How would you handle this situation?

ISLAM

Islam is one of the fastest growing religions in the world. It is most prevalent in the Middle East, Africa, South Asia, and parts of Eastern Europe. It emphasizes equality of the races and social classes and attempts to promote brotherhood for all. The prophet Muhammad, who made Mecca the focal point of this religion, is believed to have received revelations from God through the angel Gabriel during meditation in the seventh century. Muhammad began preaching that there is only one God, Allah. Visions experienced by Muhammad during his life were written in the Koran and include instructions and guidance about how to live a good life and thereby achieve salvation. An *imam* is a Muslim religious prayer leader, and the main place of worship is the mosque (Figure 14-1).

Table 14-1 *Protestant Beliefs Affecting Health Care*

DENOMINATION	BELIEFS
Christian Science	• Do not normally seek traditional health care; have own midwives and nurses. • Believe that sickness, evil, and sin are not of God but of the mind. Illness and sin can be changed by altering thoughts rather than by medical intervention. • Illness and sin are overcome through prayer, which alters thoughts. • When ill, a practitioner may be called to minister to the sick person to provide spiritual healing. May seek the services of an orthopedic surgeon to set a fracture. • Do not take medications.
Jehovah's Witness	• Abortion is forbidden. • Taking blood into the body is prohibited, and transfusion of blood or blood products is not permitted. Transfusion with dextran or blood expanders is permitted. • An organ transplant may be accepted, but the organ must be cleansed with a non-blood solution before transplantation. • Only meat that has been drained of blood may be eaten. • The body must be buried with all its parts, which prevents donation of tissues.
Church of Jesus Christ of Latter-day Saints	• A church elder should be notified in the event of death. • Natural means of birth control are recommended. • Cleanliness is of vital importance. A sacred undergarment may be worn that should only be removed in an emergency. If removed, the garment should be put back on as soon as possible.
Seventh-Day Adventist	• The Sabbath is observed on Saturday. • Many are vegetarians, and most avoid eating pork.
Unitarian Universalist Association	• Strong belief in woman's right of choice regarding abortion. • Advocate donation of organs and body parts for transplant and research.
Mennonite	• Women may wish to wear head covering while hospitalized.

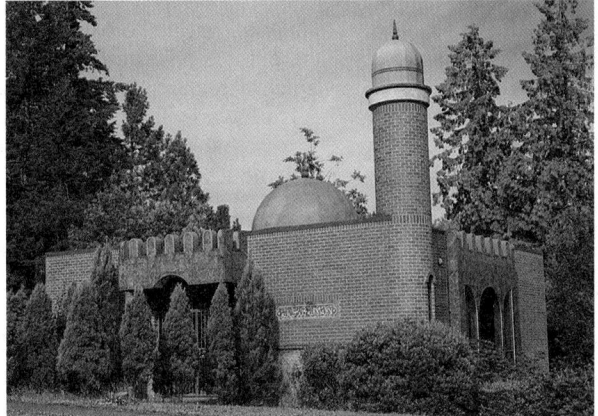

FIGURE **14-1** The main place of worship for Muslims, the mosque.

Women may not have the independence in a traditional Islamic family that the American assumes as a norm, and some women may not be allowed to make decisions about their health care. Sometimes the woman's husband or father must be present to give consent for treatment. Beliefs and practices related to health care are listed in Box 14-2.

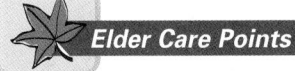

Elder Care Points

The elderly Muslim patient may insist on a same-sex caregiver because of the strong taboo regarding touching nonfamily members of the opposite sex.

Box 14-2 *Muslim Beliefs and Health Care*

Birth: After birth, the baby is bathed immediately and then given to the mother. Circumcision is performed within the first 7 days of life or at least before puberty. A baby born prematurely but at least of 130 days' gestation is treated the same as a full-term infant.

Diet: No pork or alcoholic beverage is allowed. All meat animals must be killed and blessed in a special way. Many may not eat traditional African American foods such as cornbread or collard greens.

Death: Patients must face Mecca and confess sins and beg forgiveness in the presence of the family. If family is unavailable, any practicing Muslim can provide this support. After death, the body should not be touched until the family has washed and prepared it and positioned it facing Mecca. Burial is performed as soon as possible. Cremation is forbidden. Autopsy is prohibited except for legal reasons. Body parts may not be removed or donated for transplantation unless a donor card is signed or organs are willed.

Birth Control: Many feel that artificial birth control interferes with God's will; others feel that women should only have as many children as the husband can afford, and contraception is permitted.

Abortion: Abortion is generally prohibited, but may be permitted in special cases.

Other Practices: Washing is required at prayer time. Privacy must be provided for prayer. The Koran should not be touched by anyone ritually unclean, and nothing is to be placed on top of it. Muslim women are very modest and usually wear clothing that covers all of the body.

Box 14-3 *Jewish Beliefs and Health Care*

ORTHODOX JUDAISM

Birth: Babies are named by the father. Male children are named 8 days after being born, when circumcision is done. Female babies are usually named while the Torah is read. Nurses need to be sensitive to the needs of those parents of an ill infant who has not been named.

Care of women: The woman is thought to be unclean during her menses or after the birth of a child until she has bathed in a pool called a mikvah. Nurses need to be sensitive to the needs of the woman. The Orthodox Jewish man cannot help the woman with her care; the nurse will need to help with her care.

Dietary: Kosher rules include no mixing of milk and meat, using separate utensils for milk and meat, not eating any animal not slaughtered according to Jewish law, fasting during the Yom Kippur holiday, not eating raised breads during Passover, and saying thanksgiving before and after meals. Nurses will help by giving the patient time and quiet for this practice.

Sabbath: From sunset Friday to sunset Saturday, the laws say not to ride in a car; smoke; or use lights, money, or television. Even surgery or other medical treatments or care is avoided until a later time if possible.

Death: Death happens when there are no respirations and circulation, and this cannot be corrected. Orthodox Jews forbid assisted deaths. It is the duty of the family and friends to visit, and someone needs to be with the patient when he or she dies, and when the soul leaves the body. Nurses need to allow for the family to be with the dying and the dead patient until burial. The dead are buried within 24 hours. The body may not be touched for 8 to 30 minutes and then only by an Ortho-dox person. On the Sabbath, a body must not be handled. The nurse may do basic care while wearing gloves. All body parts removed during autopsy must be buried with the body because it is believed that the entire body must be returned to the earth.

Birth control/abortion: Birth control is discouraged, and vasectomies are forbidden. Abortion is allowed only to save the mother's life.

Organ transplantation: This may be allowed with the rabbi's approval.

Shaving: The beard is a sign of holiness, and no blade must touch the skin. Scissors or an electric razor may be used.

Hats: Orthodox men wear skull caps (yarmulkes) all the time, and women cover their hair after marriage.

Prayer: Prayer to God is required. Nurses need to allow a quiet environment for prayer.

REFORM JUDAISM

Birth: Orthodox practice may or may not be observed, but circumcision may be practiced.

Care of women: The beliefs do not follow the rules about not touching women.

Dietary: Kosher diets are usually not observed.

Sabbath: There is worship on Fridays in temples but no other rules.

Death: The beliefs allow life support but no heroic measures. Cremation is allowed, but it is preferred that the ashes be buried in a Jewish cemetery.

Organ transplantation: This is allowed with the rabbi's approval.

Hats: Praying is usually done without yarmulkes.

From Carson, V. (1989). *Spiritual Dimensions of Nursing Practice.* Philadelphia: Saunders.

JUDAISM

Judaism has several branches: Orthodox, Conservative, Reform, and Reconstructionist. The religious leader in Judaism is called a *rabbi,* and the main place of worship is the synagogue (temple). Judaism began when the one God revealed himself to the nomadic tribes of the Middle East (in the region that is now Israel) thousands of years before the birth of Christ. Strict rules regarding hygiene, diet, sexual mores, and religious ceremony were passed down orally and later written down in the Torah, which is the basis for the Christian Old Testament. Orthodox Jews follow the most strict interpretation of Jewish law. Food is prepared according to Jewish dietary laws during slaughter, processing, and packaging and is then labeled kosher. Jewish religious laws may be relaxed during illness, but it is still very important to consult with the patient to be sure that nursing care does not cause spiritual distress. There are rituals regarding care of a dead body and burial, and the rabbi should be consulted.

Circumcision is a Jewish religious ritual performed by a man called a *mohel* on the eighth day of a boy's life. It involves the ceremonial removal of the penile foreskin. Box 14-3 presents the major Jewish beliefs to be considered when planning health care.

HINDUISM, BUDDHISM, AND TAOISM

Many Hindus are vegetarians because most believe that eating meat involves harming a living creature, which is contrary to their beliefs. Illness or disease is seen as the result of the misuse of the body or a consequence of sin committed in a previous life. There is a strong belief that life is controlled by God and that the individual has little control over what happens. Within the family, the eldest woman is considered the authority on health and healing matters. She should be consulted and included in any patient teaching. *Ayurvedic* medicine, founded in India, follows principles of "hot" and "cold" to balance the diet as needed for the season and the disease state.

Buddhists do not believe in healing through faith, but believe spiritual peace and liberation from anxiety through following Buddha's teachings are important in promoting health and recovery. Taoists believe that illness or disease is due to an imbalance in yin and yang.

Table 14-2 | *Religious Dietary Practices*

RELIGION	DIETARY PRACTICES
Hinduism	Some sects are vegetarians.
Buddhism	Consumption of beef is prohibited. Some are vegetarians, and many will not use alcohol or tobacco and may hesitate to use drugs. Many will fast on Holy Days.
Islam	Prohibits consumption of pork and alcohol. Fasting is done during the month of Ramadan.
Judaism	Some observe the kosher dietary restrictions of avoiding pork and shellfish and not preparing and eating milk and meat at the same time.
Christianity	Some Baptists, Evangelicals, and Pentacostals discourage the use of alcohol, caffeine, and tobacco. Some Roman Catholics may fast during Lent, Ash Wednesday, Good Friday, and 1 hour before receiving Communion.
Jehovah's Witnesses	Members may avoid food prepared with or containing blood.
Mormonism	Members abstain from alcohol, caffeine, and tobacco.
Russian Orthodox	Followers must observe fast days as well as a "no meat" rule on Wednesdays and Fridays. During Lent, all animal products, including dairy products and butter, are forbidden.
Native American	Food practices are influenced by individual tribal beliefs.

From Potter, P.A., & Perry, A.G. (2005). *Fundamentals of Nursing* (6th ed., p. 561). St. Louis: Elsevier Mosby.

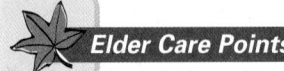

Elder Care Points

- Elderly patients may be particularly upset with interruptions in their religious practice caused by illness or hospitalization.
- Providing time for prayer, reading scripture to them, or contacting their religious leader may assist in decreasing spiritual distress.

The Asian diet consists of less meat and more vegetables than that of other Americans. Meats are sliced, diced, or shredded and added in small quantities to vegetables. A variety of sauces and spices are used in cooking. "Hot" or "cold" foods are consumed during illness or disease to regain balance within the body (see Nutrition, p. 185). Many religions have dietary rules (Table 14-2).

CULTURAL GROUP CHARACTERISTICS

The main characteristics that differentiate cultural groups from one another are nationality, race, color, gender, age, and religious affiliation (Purnell and Paulanka, 2003). Race is a biologic way of categorizing people. Race is based on physical characteristics such as skin color and texture, facial characteristics, and body proportions. Although there has been considerable blending of race in various parts of the world, there are three basic races: white (people from Europe, western Russia, North Africa, the Middle East, and southwest Asia), Negro (most Africans), and Mongoloid (northern and eastern Asians, Pacific Islanders, and some American Indians). Various ethnic groups are found within a race; these groups are usually differentiated by geographic, religious, social, or language differences (Purnell and Paulanka, 2003).

Major cultural groups within the United States and Canada are European Americans, American Indians, African Americans, Hispanic Americans, Asian/Pacific Islander Americans, and Arab Americans. Subcultures are smaller groups within the culture whose members have similar views and goals in addition to or in place of those of the main culture. A subculture may be based on a variety of characteristics such as socioeconomic status, education, occupation, political beliefs, sexual orientation, or residence in a rural versus urban area. Those living in poverty, a socioeconomic state, become a subculture because of the shared beliefs and practices of the poor. Their orientation is day-to-day survival with little hope for the future. There may be unstable family relationships, alcohol and drug abuse, and often elderly grandparents caring for young children. Emotional and physical disorders may prevent some within this group from meeting their basic needs for shelter, food, and clothing and they become homeless.

The poor and the homeless are more likely to suffer from illnesses and diseases such as malnutrition and tuberculosis, and chronic disorders may become worse because they go untreated. Because of lack of funds, lack of transportation, and/or lack of access to health care, the poor do not attend to preventive health practices and may not receive care for acute illnesses.

TRANSCULTURAL NURSING

Transcultural nursing is a term used by Dr. Madeline Leininger to describe care that recognizes cultural diversity and is sensitive to the cultural needs of the patient and family. It is based on the fact that although there is diversity or differences among cultures, there are also universal patterns of behavior. **Dr. Leininger described human caring as what all people need most to grow, remain well, avoid illness, and survive or face death** (Leininger, 1991). Thus human caring is part of every culture, but it may be expressed in different ways.

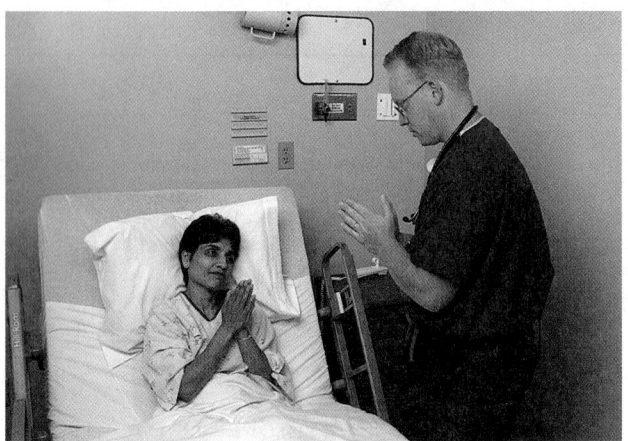

FIGURE **14-2** Nurse giving traditional greeting to a Hindu patient. This method of greeting honors the spirit within each of us.

DEVELOPING CULTURAL COMPETENCE

Nurses must develop cultural awareness and cultural sensitivity in order to deliver culturally competent care. Cultural awareness involves knowledge of a people's history and ancestry and an appreciation for their artistic expressions, foods, and celebrations. Cultural sensitivity is refraining from using offensive language, respecting accepted patterns of communication, and refraining from speaking in ways that are disrespectful of a person's cultural beliefs (Figure 14-2). Cultural competence involves knowing yourself, examining your own values, attitudes, beliefs, and prejudices. Keeping an open mind and trying to look at the world through the perspectives of culturally diverse peoples is another aspect of cultural competence. Learn all you can about other cultures. Literature written by authors from other cultures can provide a wealth of information and insight into others' views of the world. Respect differences among people, recognizing that every group has its strengths and weaknesses. Be willing and open to learning by getting to know people. Learn to communicate effectively, being sensitive to the affect, body movements, use of personal space, and gestures of others (Narayan, 2003). Don't make judgments about cultural behaviors and practices that are different from yours. Be resourceful and creative in fitting nursing interventions into the belief system of the patient. Consider your nursing actions carefully when interacting with a patient from another culture (Cultural Cues 14-1).

Care must be taken not to let ethnocentrism affect one's attitude toward a patient. Ethnocentrism is the tendency of human beings to think that their ways of thinking, believing, and doing things are the only way or the only right way. Beliefs that greatly differ from one's own are seen as strange and are therefore considered wrong.

A generalization identifies common trends, patterns, and beliefs of a group. Generalizations may be true for the group, but not necessarily for a particular

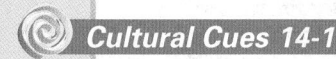

Cultural Cues 14-1

Cultural Aspects to Consider

The following should be considered when caring for a patient from a different culture:
- Form of address considered appropriate within the culture
- Whether an interpreter is needed
- Whether eye contact is considered polite or rude
- Amount of space between speakers considered appropriate when conversing
- The meaning of nonverbal gestures such as head nodding, smiling, and hand gestures; unacceptable gestures
- When, where, and by whom touch is acceptable
- Who the traditional decision makers are within the culture and family
- Manner and attire of a person considered a "professional," one whose instructions are valued

individual in the group. Additional information must be sought from the individual patient to determine whether the generalization is true. It is also essential not to stereotype a patient. A stereotype is a set opinion or belief about the group that is applied to an individual. "Hispanics like hot peppers" is a stereotype. Although many Hispanics may like hot peppers, this is not true of all Hispanic people. **Stereotypes can be negative or positive, but they all ignore the uniqueness of the patient.**

Bias or prejudice (positive or negative attitude or opinion that is unsupported by evidence) should not affect the quality of care a patient receives. **All patients should be given the same level of care regardless of race, socioeconomic status, gender, age, spiritual/religious orientation, or personal habits.**

CULTURAL AND ETHNIC DIFFERENCES

Particular areas in which cultural difference is evident are communication, view of time, organization of the family, nutrition, issues related to death and dying, and health care beliefs (Purnell and Paulanka, 2003).

COMMUNICATION

An obvious cultural difference among people is language. In a large city, there may be many different languages spoken by various groups as well as differing dialects (regional variations of the language with different pronunciation, grammar, or word meanings). Nonverbal communication patterns differ among cultural groups—for example, degree of eye contact that is acceptable, amount of personal space (space acceptable between two people when conversing) that is appropriate, acceptable touching, and meaning of gestures such as head nodding. The Vietnamese avoid eye contact when talking with someone they consider an authority figure or who is older (Lindsay, Narayan, and Rea, 1998). The American Indian may find sustained direct eye contact rude or disrespectful. In European American culture, 18 inches is the usual space between people that is comfortable when they are talking together. Asians, people from the Middle East, and Hispanics tend to stand closer together when they converse. In some cultures, it is not acceptable to disagree with a superior, which may result in an outward appearance of agreement by people even though they do not agree with what is being said.

Learning key phrases in other languages frequently encountered, or using translation lists of common questions or symptoms, is helpful. A skilled interpreter is needed, however, to obtain assessment data and convey instructions. Most health agencies have people available to interpret when needed. **A good interpreter knows the language and the customs of the patient and is knowledgeable about the health care system.** One should avoid the use of family members as interpreters whenever possible because the patient may be reluctant to talk through a family member because of modesty or because of privacy concerns. AT&T has a language line service for over-the-phone interpretation of more than 140 languages. It is available 24 hours a day, 7 days a week at 1-800-752-6096. This is not as good a solution as an interpreter who is present, but it helps until one can be found.

VIEW OF TIME

Orientation to time varies from one culture to another, and attitudes about time can cause misunderstanding. An orientation toward the future is a European American dominant cultural value in the United States. There is a sense of time urgency (not enough time), and importance is placed on punctuality and schedules. Other cultures, notably the Hispanic American and the African American, do not have this same view of time. The focus in these cultures is on the here and now, and there is not a feeling of urgency to be someplace right on time. Generally, this applies to social occasions rather than business or medical appointments.

A second consideration of time is whether the culture is mostly concerned with the past, present, or future. Past-oriented cultures attach considerable importance to traditions. Ancestor worship may occur. Some people believe the past is unimportant and the future unpredictable; they live in the present. Future-oriented cultures place a high value on change where their circumstances will be improved. A balance of all three views is prevalent for many individuals. **It is important to know the patient's view of time.**

ORGANIZATION OF THE FAMILY

Family households may be male dominated (patriarchal), may be female dominated (matriarchal), or may share equality between men and woman (egalitarian).

Knowing the family dominance pattern is important because the head of the household usually plays a role in the health care decisions for the patient. There are very specific roles within some cultures for men and women. Men may be expected to provide for the family and protect its members, manage the finances, and deal with issues in the outside world. The expected female role may be to take care of the children, maintain the home environment, and perform all household tasks. These cultural differences must be respected without trying to impose an egalitarian viewpoint, which is prevalent in the United States.

The position of the elderly varies considerably from one culture to another. In some cultures, the elderly are considered wise and are revered. They are provided for by their children when they are no longer able to care for themselves. In other cultures, although the elderly are loved, when self-care becomes a problem, they may be cared for outside the home.

Extended family members may all live together in some cultures, and there may be several generations under the same roof. In other cultures each couple, with or without children, has its own living space apart from the extended family members.

NUTRITION

What people eat or avoid is influenced by culture. Food has much symbolic and social meaning. People learn from their family culture what foods are "good for you" or should be avoided or used for specific illnesses or diseases. Certain foods are associated with celebrations, and others with comfort and nurture. When a patient is in a health care facility, food choices may be very limited, and changes from the usual time and rituals of eating may occur. Foods are categorized in some cultures (Asian, Hispanic, Middle Eastern) as "hot," "cold," or "cool," based not on their temperature, but on their effect in the body. Each culture has its own set of foods that are viewed as "hot" or "cold." That effect is used to counteract illness or disease—cold foods are used to treat "hot" illnesses or diseases, and hot foods are used to treat "cold" illnesses or diseases. Because of these beliefs, many patients would not think of drinking ice water when ill.

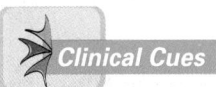
Clinical Cues

It is culturally sensitive to check with the patient before leaving a pitcher of ice water at the bedside.

Family members can often provide food for the patient that fits within the medical orders. Such additions to the health care facility diet not only meet nutritional needs but also provide security and belonging for a patient who may feel frightened and ill at ease in the health care facility setting.

? *Think Critically About . . .* What food and drink do you seek or avoid when you have the following illnesses: nausea or vomiting, a severe cough and stuffy nose, diarrhea? What are the foods that calm you when you are stressed or upset?

DEATH AND DYING

It is important to become knowledgeable about rituals concerning death and bereavement so that cultural taboos can be avoided. In some cultures, the body must be buried whole; for others, cremation is preferred. Pacific Islanders leave a window open when someone dies, so that the soul can leave (Lester, 1998). Learn cultural views about autopsy before approaching a family on this issue. There may be cultural rituals for preparing the body for burial. Expressions of grief are also culturally based. In some cultural and ethnic groups it

is appropriate to display emotions, and in others one is expected to bear the grief of the loss in silence.

HEALTH CARE BELIEFS

Beliefs about health, disease, illness, and treatment are culturally based. In cultural groups who believe the world is dominated by supernatural forces, people feel that one's fate depends on the action of a god or gods. They are at the mercy of the spiritual force. Religion is an integral part of culture and often plays a very important part in the treatment of the patient.

All cultures have an element of folk or home remedy medicine that is handed down through families for treatment of common illnesses. Folk medicine relies on home remedies and self-care practices. Folk medicine is often used first before consulting a health care professional, or it may be used along with seeking professional assistance for an illness. Treating a cough with a particular type of tea with honey and lemon is an example of a folk medicine remedy. The

---

Table 14-3 | *Common Cultural Values, Practices, and Beliefs*

Asian/Pacific Islander Americans	• Value self-control, age, authority, and harmony (avoidance of conflict). • Maintain a **holistic** (attention to mental, social, spiritual, and physical aspects) view of health and illness in which nature is a dominant force. Health is dependent on the flow of **chi'i** (universal life force or energy). If chi'i is out of balance or in disharmony, illness may result. • **Yin** (negative, dark, cold, feminine) and **yang** (positive, light, warm, masculine) are the names given other balancing forces affecting health; when they are out of balance with each other, illness may occur. • *Acumassage* (manipulating the energy flow), *acupressure* (compressing the flow), and *acupuncture* (inserting needles to interrupt the energy flow) are treatments used to restore balance between yin and yang. • May believe that a misdeed leads to illness or that disease or accident is due to misdeeds in a previous life. • Often are reluctant to express emotion to others. Tend to be stoic about pain. • Consider it disrespectful to disagree with those in authority. May be overly agreeable in attempt to maintain harmony. • Buddhism, Taoism, Hinduism, and Christianity are prominent faiths.
Hispanic Americans	• Value the family over the individual; family system is patriarchal (head of family is father). • Individuals must actively develop their potential through strength of will and volition. • Health is seen as a gift from God; maintain health by achieving equilibrium. • Equilibrium is achieved through prayer, religious objects, rituals, and use of herbs and spices, and by treating others fairly and with respect. • Often seek help within the family first when ill. Some may seek the services of a **curandero** (folk healer). • May believe in use of "hot" and "cold" foods to restore equilibrium (certain foods have hot or cold properties unrelated to temperature of food). • May be superstitious; some believe that staring at an infant or commenting on its beauty brings *mal de ojo* (the evil eye). May wear an amulet to ward off *mal de ojo*. • Wearing of religious objects and their placement in the home is common. • Expect a thorough examination when visiting a health professional. Often expect a prescription for treatment. • Consider it acceptable to be vocal about illness or pain. • Touch on the arm, shoulder, or back is comforting and helps promote rapport. • Expect health care personnel to dress professionally, listen attentively, and answer questions patiently. • Spiritual dimension of life is very important. • Health requires being in harmony with the supernatural forces and the Creator.
African Americans	• Among new immigrants or among lower socioeconomic families, health and illness may be intertwined with religion and with good and bad forces. • Families are often multigenerational, close, and supportive. Members of the church may also be considered "family." • Family structure is often matriarchal (mother is head of family). • May believe that all illness is preventable if they are attentive to their relationship with God, nature, and other persons. • Folk or home remedies and faith healers may be used as well as professional health care. • Christianity and Islam are prominent faiths.

Table 14-3 | *Common Cultural Values, Practices, and Beliefs—cont'd*

American Indians	• Majority of tribes share a present orientation, a respect for the aged, and an inclination to work cooperatively with avoidance of individual gain. • Believe in keeping a natural harmony between humans and the universe. The universe is made up of the individual, the family, the community, the tribe, the environment, and the spirit world. • Each individual has a physical and a spiritual dimension, each of which is governed by different laws. Living by both sets of laws results in a balanced, healthy, and happy life. • Believe illness occurs when there is disharmony in some aspect of the individual, the environment, or the spirit world. • Believe in the cyclic nature of birth, life, and death. • Periods of silence and avoidance of eye contact show respect. • Health care practices are linked to spirituality and living in harmony with the universe. • Harmony is achieved by respecting the earth and all living things, honoring the spirits, and appeasing them when they are angry. • Treatment of illness includes herbal medicines, rituals, fasting, massage, and consultation with the shaman (medicine man). • The family and community provide strength and spiritual support in times of illness.
European Americans	• Value youth, attractiveness, cleanliness, order, punctuality, individualism, education, and hard work. Future oriented. • Value self-care and self-improvement and use preventive health practices. • Maintain scientific view of health and illness in which life is controlled by physical and biochemical processes that can be altered by human intervention. • Often use home remedies before seeking professional health care. • Use medical technology and health care professionals to diagnose and treat illness. • Extended family support often disrupted by geographic distance. • Elderly may need care outside the family because of lack of family proximity or the demands of family's employment. • Christianity and Judaism are prominent religious faiths.
Arab Americans	• Value family and affiliation with others; may have daily gatherings of extended family. • Food plays a central role in life. Caring is shown by offering food. Muslims do not eat pork or drink alcohol. • Common bonds of group are the Arabic language and the Islamic religion, although many Arab Americans are Christian. • Touch is generally only acceptable between members of the same sex except within the family. • Considered rude to pass things with the left hand as it is considered "unclean." • Considered rude to sit with the sole of the shoe within view of someone. • Professional occupations are favored, and most are well educated. • Expect an effective cure from health care rather than personal care. • May be reluctant to disclose detailed information about themselves to strangers.

use of the tea may be continued even after going to the clinic and receiving a prescription for antibiotics for a lung infection. Knowing how a patient's family usually treats the type of illness the patient has is important in understanding any reluctance the patient has in following the professionally prescribed regimen for the illness. Although the scientific view of health care is the majority view in the United States, it may not be the belief of a person raised in another culture. Table 14-3 presents values, practices, and beliefs of various cultures.

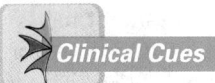 *Clinical Cues*

Not all people of a particular culture have these values, beliefs, or practices. Because there are so many variables in what people believe about health and illness, it is essential to assess what each patient believes about the cause of the present illness or disease and the way to health.

Methods of treatment of illness or disease from cultures that believe in holistic health care are slowly becoming integrated into the Western science-based practice of medicine. Alternative therapies such as massage, acupuncture, and chiropractic adjustment are being recommended along with the use of prescription medications and other standard medical treatments. More and more evidence is pointing to a connection between mind and body that influences health, and more emphasis on the use of prayer and meditation is beginning to occur (Patient Teaching 14-1).

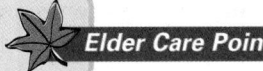 *Elder Care Points*

• The older patient is more likely to value long-held cultural patterns.
• Conflicts may arise among the generations when the children have adopted the modern cultural view and seek to impose it on their elderly parents.

Patient Teaching 14-1

Meditation

Meditation can be used as part of spiritual practice for clearing the mind and focusing, or simply as stress relief. There are various types of meditation. Here is a basic meditation technique that can be taught to patients. Meditation creates a relaxation response and can reduce daily stress.

- Choose a quiet place in which to meditate.
- Plan a session of 20 minutes while learning; time can be extended to an hour later if desired.
- Choose the floor, a portion of the bed, or a chair in which to sit while meditating.
- Assume a comfortable position with legs either crossed in front or flat on the floor. Try to keep your back straight. Position your hands so that the right index fingertip touches the tip of the left thumb. (This is so that, if you start to fall asleep, the pressure on the thumb will awaken you.)
- Close your eyes, but remain awake and relaxed.
- Begin slow, deep, abdominal breathing. Think of breathing in light and joy and breathing out troubles and stress.
- Focus on a low humming sound, a single thought of a bright light, or an image of a bright red-orange ball.
- Do not fight thoughts creeping into your mind, but dismiss them and return to your focus.
- You may have a clock close by and can slowly open your eyes to see the time toward the end of the meditation period.
- When the time is up, open your eyes and stay in position for a few minutes to adjust to the outer world again.
- Get up slowly and evaluate the positives of the experience.

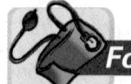

Focused Assessment 14-1

Cultural and Spiritual Assessment

To assess cultural aspects that may affect health care, ask the following questions:
- What do you think has caused this illness?
- What problems has the illness created for you?
- What has been done to treat the illness so far?
- What do you fear about this illness or its treatment?
- What type of treatment do you think is appropriate?
- What benefits do you expect from treatment?
- What traditional remedies or rituals might be used in your culture to treat this illness?

Some simple questions can identify spiritual aspects that need further exploration or referral to a spiritual or religious counselor:
- Are you a member of a religious or spiritual group?
- Is there anything we (the nursing staff) should know about your religious practices or your spiritual needs?
- Are there any foods that your religion forbids?
- What do you do to nurture your spirituality?
- Does prayer help in your life? Do you meditate?
- Is there a spiritual or religious leader (priest, rabbi, pastor, imam) with whom you would like to meet? Would you like to talk with the chaplain?
- Tell me about the beliefs in your faith that are important to you: What helps you cope with this illness? What worries you, or frightens you?

learn about various disorders that are predominant in a particular group.

APPLICATION of the NURSING PROCESS
Assessment (Data Collection)

Consider the general aspects of the patient's culture and spiritual orientation before beginning the assessment. What are the social customs of this culture? What are the nonverbal communication patterns? Is eye contact considered polite or rude? Is touch acceptable? What taboos are there regarding touch? What is the appropriate personal space between people when talking in this culture? Begin the introduction in English unless you speak the patient's language. Obtain an interpreter if one is needed, and then begin the general assessment (Focused Assessment 14-1).

A frequently overlooked area of assessment has to do with spiritual/religious assessment. Observe for the presence of religious or spiritual objects such as a cross, Star of David, Bible, rosary beads, prayer shawl or cap, feathers or amulets, crystals, or books on spirituality. Listen for references to church, temple, or mosque; religious or spiritual activities; or God. See Focused Assessment 14-1 for an assessment of the spiritual dimension of the patient.

SUSCEPTIBILITY TO DISEASE

Certain diseases are passed from parent to child through the genes that determine a person's characteristics. Nurses should be alert for signs of disorders that are common to a particular culture or race. People of African or Mediterranean background are predisposed to sickle cell trait or sickle cell anemia, a blood disorder that is passed from parents to child. Keloid formation (abnormal scar tissue formation) and sarcoidosis (fibrous nodules that can interfere with function) are also more common in African Americans. People of Eastern European Jewish ancestry may carry the trait for a fatal neurologic disorder of infancy called Tay-Sachs disease. Lactase deficiency—the absence of an enzyme needed to digest lactose, a sugar found in milk and milk products—is common in people of Hispanic, African, Chinese, Thai, and American Indian origin.

Diabetes is more common among the Hispanic and American Indian populations because of a genetic susceptibility. Hypertension is prevalent among the African American group and some Pacific Islanders. A part of obtaining knowledge for cultural competence is to

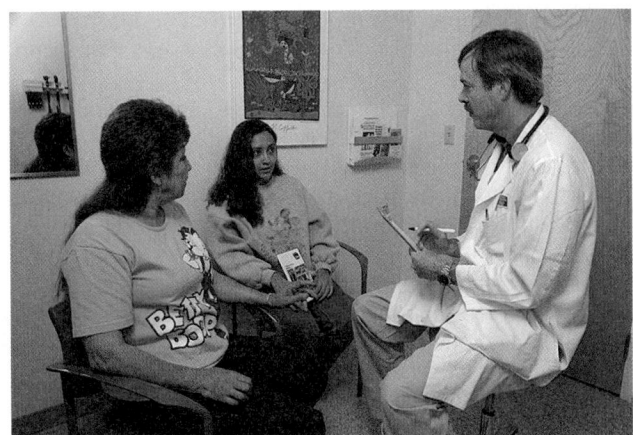

FIGURE **14-3** Observe and respect the way in which extended family members view being involved in the health care decision making.

Nursing Diagnosis

Some nursing diagnoses specifically related to cultural and spiritual problems or differences might be as follows:

- Impaired verbal communication
- Decisional conflict
- Spiritual distress

Spiritual distress may be related to feelings of guilt and unworthiness if the patient views illness as punishment for wrongdoing or sin. Other aspects of spiritual distress are feelings of abandonment, anger, despair, or hopelessness as the patient questions the presence of God. Fear of death also causes spiritual distress. The need to seek forgiveness, either from significant people in the patient's life or from God, is often expressed. Spiritual distress may also be related to a conflict between one's religious or spiritual beliefs and medical treatment or the inability to attend or actively participate in religious services or spiritual rituals.

Planning

While planning, consider the patient's family and social support system as well as the belief in culturally traditional health care practices. Write individual expected outcomes for the selected nursing diagnoses. Integrate the patient's cultural practices related to the illness and treatment into the planned interventions as much as possible. Expected outcomes related to the above nursing diagnoses might be that the patient will:

- Express comfort with the designed plan of care.
- Express needs and opinions through an interpreter.
- Cope with cultural differences of agency routines.
- Develop, reestablish, or continue the spiritual practices that nurture a relationship with God or a higher power.
- Express comfort with her relationship to God and significant others.
- State that she feels at peace.

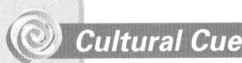

Culturally Sensitive Nursing Interventions

- Secure a skilled interpreter for history taking or important teaching.
- If needed, use "flash cards" with common phrases or questions in the patient's language or a phrase book.
- Assist the patient and the family in designing a therapeutic diet with culturally indicated or preferred foods.
- Involve the extended family in formulating the treatment plan for the patient.
- Advocate for the right of the patient to choose treatment, or refuse treatment.
- Provide quiet, private time for prayer or meditation.
- Contact religious or spiritual leader for the patient.
- Incorporate religious or spiritual ceremonies that are significant to the patient into the plan of care.

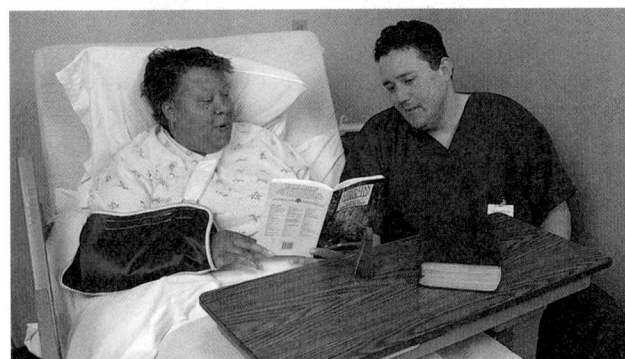

FIGURE **14-4** Attending to the patient's spiritual needs.

- Identify and employ spiritual supports: prayer, reading, visits from religious/spiritual representative, engagement in religious/spiritual rituals.

Implementation

Implement care with consideration of the patient's usual cultural and spiritual practices. Enlist various family members to assist with the patient's care if that is desirable within the culture (Figure 14-3). Show courtesy and respect for the patient as an individual (Cultural Cues 14-2).

Developing a therapeutic caring relationship permits patients to express their fears, concerns, and distress and allows the nurse to identify spiritual interventions. **One's own spiritual or religious beliefs must be set aside when they differ from those of the patient.** One helpful intervention is to assist the patient to use prayer and meditation to reduce spiritual distress. At the patient's request, praying with or for the patient can be very comforting. Reading scripture is also calming for many. The Psalms are particularly supportive and are part of the Christian, Jewish, and Islamic traditions.

Religious objects may be very important to the patient. Be sure that items such as a medal or crucifix, rosary beads, Bible, Koran, prayer shawl and cap, or prayer rug are respected and within reach (Figure 14-4). If these must be removed during surgical procedures, assure the patient that they will be restored as soon as possible after the surgery. In some hospitals, special arrangements can be made to keep the item with the patient throughout the surgery or procedure.

Think Critically About . . . How do you feel about reading scripture or praying aloud with a patient? How would you respond to a patient if you were asked to do these things and are not comfortable doing either of them? How can you still meet the patient's spiritual needs if you are not able to read from scripture or pray with the patient?

Evaluation

Evaluation is based on achievement of the expected outcomes and should not be based on whether treatment is successful from the standpoint of the nurse's cultural orientation. Transcultural nursing is successful when a mutual understanding and trust develop between the patient and the nurse. Nurses must be sensitive to the cultural and spiritual aspects of their patients in order to give holistic care. Nurses can contribute to a positive health care experience for all people when they seek to learn about the patient as a unique individual and advocate for the rights of patients to choose health care practices that fit with their cultural or spiritual background.

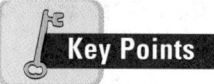 **Key Points**

- Culture includes the values, beliefs, behaviors, and religious or spiritual practices of the majority within a group of people.
- Patients from many different cultures are encountered in all types of health care settings.
- Lifestyle choices related to nutrition, exercise, stress management, smoking, and alcohol or drug use are all influenced by culture.
- Religion or spiritual practice has a definite role in recovery of health for many people.

- Cultural competence requires learning about the various religions of the world and their beliefs related to health care.
- Nationality, race, color, gender, age, and religious affiliation are the main characteristics that differentiate cultures one from another.
- People within the subculture of poverty may have a difficult time meeting their health care needs.
- Transcultural nursing is nursing care that recognizes cultural diversity and is sensitive to the cultural needs of the patient and family.
- Cultural awareness and cultural sensitivity are necessary for delivery of culturally competent nursing care.
- Areas in which cultural difference is evident are communication, view of time, organization of the family, nutrition, issues related to death and dying, and health care beliefs (see Table 14-3).
- Certain cultural groups of people are more susceptible to particular diseases and disorders than other cultural groups. Nurses should be familiar with the major potential health problems of each cultural group in order to assess for signs of those diseases and disorders.
- Cultural sensitivity is essential during the assessment process.
- Spiritual/religious assessment should be included.
- Nursing diagnoses are chosen based on the assessment data.
- Specific expected outcomes are written for each nursing diagnosis.
- Interventions that demonstrate cultural sensitivity can be included in the nursing care plan.
- Nurses must be sensitive to the cultural and spiritual aspects of their patients in order to give holistic care.
- Evaluation is based on achievement of the expected outcomes.

 Go to your **Companion CD-ROM** for an Audio Glossary, animations, video clips, and more.

evolve Be sure to visit the companion Evolve site at http://evolve.elsevier.com/deWit/fundamental/ for additional online resources.

NCLEX-PN® EXAMINATION-STYLE REVIEW QUESTIONS

*Choose the **best** answer(s) for each question.*

1. Culturally competent care is best defined as:
   1. generalized care that will not offend any particular cultural group.
   2. care delivered by nurses who have a thorough understanding of their own cultural heritage.
   3. care adapted to the patient's cultural beliefs and values.
   4. care that only imposes the nurse's own cultural norms when they will not interfere with the patient's.

2. Which of the following cultural groups is likely to believe in treating "hot" illnesses with "cold" foods and vice versa?
   1. Native Americans
   2. Hispanics
   3. African Americans
   4. Eastern Europeans

3. Of the following cultural groups, which is likely to use the services of *curanderos?*

   1. African Americans
   2. Arab Americans
   3. Asian Americans
   4. Hispanic Americans

4. A patient who is Islamic says she cannot sign the surgical consent form without her husband's consent. You would respond:

   1. "Only you, the patient, can sign the surgical consent."
   2. "But, you said he agreed that you should have the surgery."
   3. "I have to ask you to sign this consent form now."
   4. "Call me when your husband gets here and you have talked with him."

5. An elderly Japanese patient who does not speak English is admitted to the surgical unit after major abdominal surgery, with no family member present. The nurse cannot speak the patient's language. To assess for pain, the nurse should:

   1. look for nonverbal indicators of pain: grimacing, moaning, or restlessness.
   2. obtain the services of a translator to devise question-and-answer cards regarding pain.
   3. wait for the family to come to ask the patient about pain.
   4. use pantomime and gestures to get the patient to indicate his pain level.

6. A person who is an Orthodox Jew may be hesitant to eat hospital food because:

   1. hospital food tastes terrible.
   2. kosher-prepared foods are served in this hospital.
   3. special foods are used to treat specific diseases.
   4. separate dishes and utensils are used for meat and milk foods, and there is concern that the hospital may not keep separate sets of dishes and utensils for this purpose.

7. A patient who is Roman Catholic asks to have the priest come to hear her confession and administer communion before she goes to surgery. The priest arrives the evening before the patient is scheduled for the operating room but after normal visiting hours. The nurse should:

   1. suggest that the priest return after surgery because the patient has been medicated and is drowsy.
   2. provide privacy for the priest to hear confession and administer communion.
   3. inform the priest that the patient has not attended confession for a long time.
   4. offer to stay with the patient and the priest during the visit to assist the priest.

8. Hindus believe that illness or disease is caused by: *(Select all that apply.)*

   1. a lack of piety and attention to the rituals of Hinduism.
   2. misusing the body in some way.
   3. sin committed in a former life.
   4. eating the wrong foods.
   5. misusing natural resources.

9. A patient says to the nurse, "Is God punishing me with all this pain?" To continue with a spiritual assessment, the nurse could best respond:

   1. "God often punishes people for sins. What sins have you committed?"
   2. "God doesn't punish people with pain—you have cancer of the bone that is causing your pain."
   3. "I'll see if the doctor will order more pain medication. You don't need to suffer with this pain."
   4. "Tell me what you believe about God."

10. When an Islamic Arab American dies in the hospital, you know: *(Select all that apply.)*

    1. to thoroughly wash the body before wrapping it.
    2. not to touch the body before the family bathes it.
    3. to position the body facing north.
    4. turn the bed so that the body faces Mecca.

CRITICAL THINKING ACTIVITIES *Read each clinical scenario and discuss the questions with your classmates.*

Scenario A
Rosa Souza is a 76-year-old patient of Mexican origin preparing for surgery of an abdominal tumor for which she had previously been treated by a *curandero.* She is Roman Catholic, wears religious medals, and reads from her Spanish Bible. Her family (husband, two daughters, one son, and several grandchildren) is often present, surrounding the bedside. She will be having surgery in several days.

1. What assessments are important for Mrs. Souza from a cultural or spiritual viewpoint? What questions would you ask?
2. What religious activities might be important for Mrs. Souza.? How can you determine these?
3. Discuss the significance of limiting visitors to allow Mrs. Souza to rest versus accommodating large numbers of family at the bedside.

Scenario B
Esther Sommes is a 33-year-old patient being treated for end-stage kidney failure and diabetes. She is aware that her disease is terminal. On her admission record she indicated "none" for religion.

1. What is the difference between religion and the spiritual dimension of a person?
2. What assessment of Ms. Sommes' spirituality is indicated?

Scenario C
You are assigned an Arab American male as a patient.

1. In what ways could you demonstrate culturally sensitive care for this Arab American patient?
2. How could you accommodate the family's need to visit in groups and to supply him with special food?

Objectives

Upon completing this chapter, you should be able to:

Theory

1. Describe the stages of grief and of dying, with their associated behaviors and feelings.
2. Discuss the concept of hospice care.
3. Identify four expected symptoms related to metabolic changes at end-of-life stages.
4. Identify three common fears a patient is likely to experience when dying.
5. List the common signs of impending death.
6. Explain the difference between the patient's right to refuse treatment and assisted suicide.
7. Explain how the *Code for Nurses* provides guidelines for the nurse's behavior regarding the patient's right to refuse treatment, euthanasia, and assisted suicide.

Clinical Practice

1. Identify ways in which you can support or instill hope in the terminally ill patient and his family.
2. Demonstrate compassionate therapeutic communication techniques with a terminally ill patient and/or his family.
3. Describe one nursing intervention for comfort care that can be implemented in a hospital or a nursing home for a dying patient for each of the following problems: pain, nausea, dyspnea, anxiety, constipation, incontinence, thirst, and anorexia.
4. Explain the reason for completing an advance directive to a terminally ill patient, and what "health care proxy" and "DNR" mean in lay language.
5. Prepare to provide information regarding organ or tissue donation in response to family questions.
6. Prepare to perform postmortem care for a deceased patient.

Skills and Steps

Skills
Skill 15-1   Postmortem Care

Key Terms

Be sure to check out the bonus material on the Companion CD-ROM, including selected audio pronunciations.

acceptance (p. 196)
advance directive (p. 202)
anticipatory grieving (ăn-TĬ-sĭ-pă-tō-rē, p. 193)

assisted suicide (SŪ-ĭ-sīd, p. 203)
autopsy (p. 204)
bargaining (p. 196)
bereavement (bĕ-RĒV-mĭnt, p. 193)
brain death (p. 194)
Cheyne-Stokes respirations (SHĀN-stōks rĕs-pĭ-RĀ-shŭns, p. 202)
closure (KLŌ-shŭr, p. 202)
comfort care (p. 197)
coroner (KŎR-ō-nĕr, p. 204)
death (p. 194)
denial (p. 196)
durable power of attorney for health care (DŪ-ră-bŭl, p. 202)
dysfunctional (dĭs-FŬNK-shŭn-ăl, p. 193)
euthanasia (active, passive) (ū-thă-NĀ-zhē-ă, ĂK-tĭv, PĂ-sĭv, p. 203)
grief, grieving process (p. 193)
health care proxy (PRŎX-ē, p. 202)
hope (p. 197)
hospice (HŎS-pĭs, p. 195)
loss (p. 193)
obituary (ō-BĬ-chū-ĕr-ē, p. 202)
palliation (păl-ē-Ā-shŭn, p. 197)
postmortem (pōst MŎR-tĕm, p. 204)
rigor mortis (RĬ-gŏr MŎR-tĭs, p. 205)
shroud (SHRŎWD, p. 205)
thanatology (thăn-ă-TŌL-ō-jē, p. 196)

Loss, grief, and death are well-known and universal parts of life. Loss involves change, and some loss is necessary for normal growth and development; for example, a child loses baby teeth to make way for permanent teeth. Other losses do not seem to have positive outcomes, such as loss of health, loss of a significant other, or loss of life. People adjust to loss through the grieving process, and coping with loss is learned from childhood on. **A person's reaction to loss is influenced by the importance of what was lost and the culture in which the person is raised.**

According to the National Center for Health Statistics (2007), life expectancy recently increased to 77.9 years, mainly because of advances in treatment of heart disease, cancer, AIDS, and stroke. Heart disease and cancer are responsible for 50% of all deaths. HIV/

AIDS is no longer one of the 15 leading causes of death. Alzheimer's disease has moved from 11th to 7th place. Accidents rank number 5 and diabetes number 6. Life expectancy for white females is highest (80 years), followed by African American females (76.5 years), white males (75.7 years), and African American males (69.8 years). The most recent death statistics indicate approximately 2,448,017 deaths in the United States annually (National Vital Statistics Report, 2008).

Death is a universally shared event. In all cultures and religions, there are beliefs and rituals to explain and cope with death, loss, and grief. It is common in American society to avoid talking about death, and to be unable to imagine our own death. Expressions such as "passed away," or "went to his reward" are used instead of "died." Children are often kept away from funerals, and most people have little contact with the dying. Many adults can state they have never seen a dead body, and more can say they have not been present during a death. Only in recent years has there been a move away from silence and denial toward a willingness to examine a universal life event: death.

Nurses and other health care professionals may have similar fears and anxieties about the end of life. Because so many deaths occur in hospitals and nursing homes, health care workers see more of death and dying than other people do. They are responsible for providing the best care possible to their dying patients. However, to meet the emotional and physical needs of patients and their significant others, nurses must first take the time to look at their own views of death and come to terms with its reality.

?
Think Critically About . . . What are your earliest memories of death—a pet, a relative, a friend? How was the death explained to you? Was it frightening, confusing, reassuring?

LOSS AND GRIEF

LOSS

Loss is to no longer possess or have an object, person, or situation. It is a familiar occurrence in everyday life, for example, losing money, a job, one's health, or life. One's own death is often described as the most difficult loss for a person to accept. A loss can be physical, such as the amputation of a leg, or inability to speak or walk after a stroke. A loss can also be psychosocial. Disfiguring surgery or scarring from burns may result in an altered self-image and emotional problems. A person may lose the ability to carry out the role of homemaker or wage earner as a result of illness. A familiar environment and independence may be lost with a move to a nursing home. Very often loss con-

sists of both physical and psychosocial aspects. Loss can be viewed as ranging from minor to catastrophic. A person's reaction to loss depends not so much on the size of the loss but on the person's value of what has been lost plus the influence of previous experiences and the ability to cope. **Only the person experiencing the loss can define the value of the loss**—you must put aside your own values regarding loss and accept the patient's meaning of loss.

GRIEF

Grief is the total emotional feeling of pain and distress that a person experiences as a reaction to loss. The grieving process occurs over a period of time. A person adapts to the feelings and moves through the pain and associated symptoms toward recovery or acceptance. People who are dying as well as their loved ones experience loss and grief when faced with a terminal diagnosis. Bereavement is the state of having suffered a loss by death. A person who is grieving may experience physical and emotional symptoms, such as crying, fatigue, changes in appetite, sleep disturbances, loneliness, and sadness (Box 15-1). When a person thinks or knows that a loss is going to occur in the future, anticipatory grieving may occur before the loss actually happens. This happens when patients and their families face a serious or life-threatening illness, and it is believed to improve coping with the loss when it occurs.

Grieving may also be dysfunctional when it falls outside normal responses. In prolonged grieving, the person seems trapped in a stage and unable to prog-

---

Box 15-1 *Symptoms of Grief*

- Depression, sadness, crying, mood swings
- Fatigue, apathy, lack of interest and motivation, inability to concentrate, inability to complete tasks
- Loneliness, isolation
- Sleep alterations: sleep more, insomnia (unable to sleep)
- Loss of appetite, weight loss or weight gain, nausea
- Change in sexual interest
- Anxiety, shortness of breath, chest pains, rapid heartbeat, sighing, heaviness in chest
- Feelings of helplessness, restlessness, anger, guilt, irritability
- Forgetfulness, tendency to make mistakes, accident prone
- Confusion, disorientation (especially in the elderly), indecisiveness
- Symptoms of the same illness that the deceased suffered
- Sensing the loved one's presence, hearing the voice, seeing the face, expecting the person to walk in the door
- A need to tell and retell and remember things about the loved one, and the death experience

ress. However, there is no actual time frame for completion of grieving, and a major loss may result in grieving for 1 to 2 years. Visible absence of grieving may be viewed by others as a good adjustment, but it often results in later psychosomatic illness.

STAGES OF GRIEF

It has long been thought that the grieving person goes through stages: denial, anger, bargaining, depression and acceptance. Each stage has identifying behaviors and feelings, and each person moves through the stages at his own pace, and may skip or return to an earlier stage. Nurses have always been taught to recognize the great individuality of the grieving person and offer supportive care for the symptoms or behavior the person demonstrates, rather than anticipating what grieving response is the right one.

Until recently, the hypothesis of these stages had not been investigated empirically. However, the stages of grief theory was put to the test by Maciejewski and others (2007). Examination of the stage theory of grief has revealed that denial is not the first grief indicator. Instead, the loss is readily accepted, and yearning is the dominant grief indicator. This is followed by anger and depression. The five grief indicators—denial, yearning, anger, depression, and acceptance—peak within 6 months after the loss. The nurse should reevaluate and create additional nursing plans for patients who continue to score high in these areas after 6 months.

You can assist persons who are grieving by accepting their feelings and behaviors and validating their loss. To *validate* the loss is to reassure the grieving person that the loss was important and understood. Quiet presence, a warm caring concern for the person's wellbeing, and the ability to listen to the person speak about the pain and loss are supportive (Figure 15-1). Encourage grieving individuals to tell you what the person (or lost object) was like, and what the loss means to them. Avoid the use of clichés like "You'll forget all about this after awhile," and do not minimize the loss. Observe the nonverbal communication of the patient, and be aware of and use appropriate nonverbal language such as a smile or a gentle touch. Crying may be embarrassing for the patient, and a simple act of handing a tissue acknowledges the acceptability of weeping. You should never tell a patient "Don't cry." You may be uncomfortable in a situation in which you feel like crying along with the patient. The patient will not be offended by your crying, and may draw support from a shared experience. You can acknowledge feelings of sadness and loss, but should avoid saying "I know just how you feel," because this minimizes the patient's feelings.

As a person moves through the stages of the grieving process, there is a continuing decline in function as the person attempts to adjust to the loss. With the stage of acceptance, there is gradual improvement in the

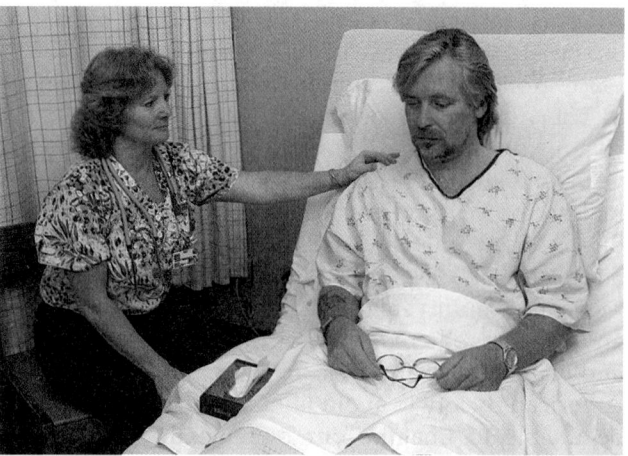

FIGURE **15-1** The nurse provides caring and comfort to the patient who experiences grief.

level of daily function. Successful movement through the grieving stages allows the person to emerge with realistic memories of the event and the deceased, find renewed energy, a sense that life has meaning, and an ability to again experience pleasure, social relationships, and activities. The time it takes to move through the stages will depend on the loss and its meaning to the person.

DEATH AND DYING

THE NATURE OF DEATH

Death is an event marked in different ways. The absence of a heartbeat and breathing was and is a historic and widely accepted definition of death. In today's high-tech hospital environment, a ventilator can support the patient's breathing and thereby provide oxygen to the heart when it would not continue unassisted. So, a definition of death that has been used since the 1970s is brain death (the permanent stopping of integrated functioning of the person as a whole as evidenced by the absence of EEG waves).

Except for suicide, a person has no control over when or how death occurs. Death may be sudden, unexpected, and instant, as when a person is killed in an accident or dies of a massive heart attack or stroke. Death may also be the end of a long battle against a chronic disease such as cancer or heart disease, or simply the diminished function of multiple systems in old age. Death is also encountered in situations in which the outcome could be either death or survival, as in an acute severe infection or trauma. Nurses who work in an emergency room, intensive care unit, medical-surgical unit, nursing home, or hospice will each have different experiences of patients' death and dying (Cultural Cues 15-1). In these different cases and situations, the individuals who die and those who care about them will experience different emotions and physical reactions.

Cultural Cues 15-1

Cultural Views About Disclosure

Many people feel they have the right to know if they are dying, and nurses often do not like it if that fact is being hidden from a patient. However, cultural factors need to be considered. For example, Mexican Americans and Korean Americans are less likely to want to be told if they have a terminal illness. They also feel that the family, not the patient, should make decisions about life-sustaining treatments. These beliefs need to be considered before speaking to a patient about a terminal prognosis.

Box 15-2   Standards of Care for the Terminally Ill

1. You must consider the terminally ill patient's preferences, personality, and lifestyle when planning care. Rigid rules, routines, and agency regulations should not be automatically applied.
2. Every effort is made to maintain functional capacity and to relieve discomfort through the control of symptoms, regardless of the expected length of time until death.
3. Pain control is a major goal of treatment.
4. The patient's preferences and intentions regarding health care as set out in an advance directive, or by durable power of attorney for health care, will take precedence as far as the law will allow.
5. The patient should feel safe and secure with the care that is provided and with the level of communication regarding this care.
6. The patient will have ample opportunities to finish business with loved ones and to say goodbyes.
7. Opportunities will be provided for the dying patient to spend final moments in a personally meaningful way with people who are important to the patient.
8. Family members and significant others will have opportunities to discuss the patient's imminent death and their emotional needs with the staff.
9. Family members and significant others will be provided with private time with the patient before and after death as desired.
10. Family members will be allowed to perform rituals and carry out cultural customs regarding the body after death.

Each death and dying experience is unique, although there are commonalities that can help you to provide truly satisfying care to the patient and the family (Box 15-2).

END-OF-LIFE CARE WITHIN THE HEALTH CARE SYSTEM

The focus in our health care system has been one of cure and the development of diagnostic, technical, and chemical interventions to treat disease and injury that often have been fatal in the past. As a result, patients may be viewed as failures of the system if they die in spite of the

Box 15-3   Rights of the Dying Patient

The person who is dying has the right to:
- be treated as a person until death.
- caring human contact.
- have pain controlled.
- cleanliness and comfort.
- maintain a sense of hope, whatever its focus.
- participate in his care or the planning of it.
- respectful, caring medical and nursing attention.
- continuity of care and caregivers.
- information about his condition and impending death.
- honest answers to questions.
- explore and change religious beliefs.
- maintain individuality and express emotions freely without being judged.
- make amends with others and settle personal business.
- say goodbye to family members and significant others in private or with the assistance of the nurse.
- assistance for significant others with the grief process.
- withdraw from social contact if desired.
- die at home in familiar surroundings.
- die with dignity.
- respectful treatment of the body after death.

best efforts of the health care team. Those with terminal illness who refuse life-prolonging (or death-delaying) treatment may feel as though their needs will not be met in the acute care environment (Box 15-3).

HOSPICE AND PALLIATIVE CARE

Hospice is a philosophy of care for the dying and their families. It developed in England in the early 1960s as a reaction to the needs of dying people for care and comfort. After World War II, hospitals rather than the home had become the place where people died. Nurses provided around-the-clock care, and families were relieved of that burden. However, many of the needs of the dying were not being met in the hospital setting. A *hospice* originally was a medieval guest house or stopping place for travelers. Now the name "hospice" is also used to describe the specialized care provided to the dying in small clinics, houses, or the patient's (or patient's family's) own home. Currently, a hospice is not necessarily a special facility but rather a program of care to meet the needs of the terminally ill and their families in their home or a health care facility.

The hospice philosophy is based on the acceptance of death as a natural part of life and emphasizes the quality of remaining life. The medical, nursing, social, psychological, and spiritual needs of the patients and their significant others are met through a team approach. The team provides *palliative care*. Palliative care is concerned with treating symptoms, providing comfort measures, and promoting the best quality of life possible day by remaining day (see Nursing Care Plan 15-1). Nurses who care for the dying patient have a unique opportunity to become an intimate part of the patients' lives. Nurses can support the dying patient physically and emotionally while maintaining a professional role.

Whether assisting the patient in the hospital or at home, certain comfort measures are required. Palliative care requires a specialized body of knowledge and skills that can be difficult to learn since it isn't focused on "cure." Family members are involved in this planning, and necessary support is provided to meet the needs of all those affected by the impending death (Figure 15-2). RNs and LPNs or home health aides provide nursing and personal care; trained volunteers are used to provide a variety of respite (relief) or socialization services. Hospice care may be provided in the patient's home, nursing home, hospital, or hospice unit. Follow-up of the family during the year following the death provides assistance with the grieving process.

Palliative care is a fairly new field, and many nurses have chosen to undertake this specialty. The palliative care nurse is an important element for the patient's and family's comfort during this transition. In September 2004, a certification examination for LPNs and LVNs was launched by the National Board for Certification of Hospice and Palliative Nurses (NBCHPN).

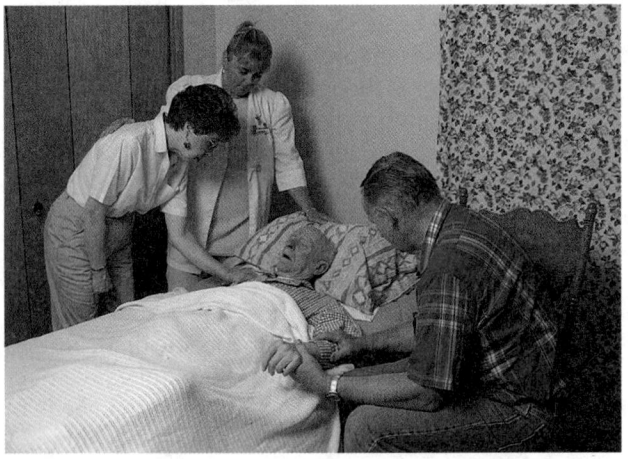

FIGURE **15-2** The hospice nurse assists the family in saying goodbye to the dying patient.

Detailed information is available by calling (888) 519-9901 or visiting www.nbchpn.org.

THE DYING PROCESS
Kübler-Ross and the Five Stages of Coping with Impending Death

In the late 1960s, Dr. Elisabeth Kübler-Ross, a psychiatrist, began talking with terminally ill patients and identifying their needs. She also began educating medical students, nurses, and doctors about death and the stages through which she saw terminally ill patients progress. She transformed the way the health care community and much of the public view death, and she promoted much additional research into the areas of loss and death. As a result of her pioneering work, nurses and doctors are much more sensitive to the needs of the dying patient and family. Other researchers have added to her work, and the field of **thanatology** (the study of death) continues to grow.

Dr. Kübler-Ross' identification of the stages a dying person moves through has been the foundation for understanding the dying process. Five stages, similar to those of the grief process, are described as being characteristic of dying: denial, anger, bargaining, depression, and acceptance (Table 15-1). The stages overlap, and as with the grieving process, the patient may move back and forth or even skip stages. In some cases, the patient may "get stuck" in one stage and not move through to acceptance. Family members are often at different stages from the patient and each other. Nurses, too, will move through the stages when they care for patients who are dying.

Other Theories of the Dying Process

Theories of the dying process have identified other emotions that are commonly seen during the dying process: fear of dying, yearning, guilt, hope, despair, and even humor. Some professionals point out that an individual's reaction to the threat of death is consistent with the way the person has coped with difficulties in the past, and that rather than experiencing stages, a person reacts with denial, anger, bargaining, hope, de-

Table 15-1 *Kübler-Ross's Stages of Coping with Death*

STAGE	DESCRIPTION
Denial	"No, not me." The person cannot believe the diagnosis or prognosis. It serves as a buffer to protect the patient from an uncomfortable and painful situation. A patient may seek other opinions or believe there has been an error.
Anger	"Why me?" The person looks for a cause or fixes blame. Doctors and nurses are often the target of displaced anger, as well as family and even God. Powerlessness to control the disease and events is an underlying issue.
Bargaining	"If I'm good, then I get a reward." The wish is for extension of life, or later for relief from pain, and the person knows from past experience that "good behavior" is often rewarded.
Depression	"It's hopeless." There is a sense of great loss, of the impending loss of being. People mourn losing family, possessions, responsibilities, all they value.
Acceptance	"I'm ready." The pain is gone, the struggle is over, the patient has found peace. There is withdrawal from the engagement of everyday activities and interests. Verbal communication is less important, and touch and presence are most important.

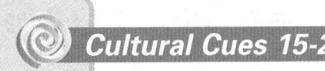

Cultural Cues 15-2

Cultural Views About Death

Certain cultures believe that talking about death can bring it on. This belief is found in some people from Greece, China, Italy, Korea, Mexico, and the southern African nations. American Indian culture includes a fear of death, and it is thought that truth-telling about a terminal prognosis violates traditions and taboos, and can lead to harmful outcomes (Mitty, 2001). The nurse needs to consider the cultural orientation of the patient before broaching the subject of death or terminal illness.

spair, and so forth in a fluctuating pattern. Coping with death takes many forms and is not limited to the dying person. It involves all who are connected with the dying person's experience: family, friends, and caregivers. Coping with death may also involve tasks or actions that the dying person must work on in the areas of physical, social, psychological, and spiritual being (Cultural Cues 15-2). An example of a physical task would be to minimize physical distress such as pain. A social task might be to enhance or restore a relationship that is important to the dying person. Another example would be updating a will, making amends, and saying good-bye to friends and loved ones.

Hope and the Dying Process

Hope is an inner positive life force, a feeling that what is desired is possible. It takes many forms and changes as the patient declines. At first there is hope for cure, then a hope that treatment will be possible, next a hope for the prolonging of life, and finally hope for a peaceful death. Open-ended questions such as "What are you hoping for from this admission?" or "What are you hoping for today?" can allow patients to talk about their needs. You can always be supportive of hope by recognizing and affirming the wish the patient is expressing.

NURSING AND THE DYING PROCESS

Patients express many fears when they know they are dying: fear of pain, loneliness, abandonment, the unknown, loss of dignity, and loss of control. There may also be unfinished business that occupies the patient's thoughts. The concept of comfort care is focused on identifying symptoms that cause the patient distress and adequately treating those symptoms. Palliation is the relief of symptoms when cure is no longer possible, and treatment is provided solely for comfort. **This concept can be applied in any health care setting.** Prevention of many symptoms is possible by anticipating their likelihood. The application of the nursing process to care of the dying patient uses skills and knowledge from physical, emotional, social, and spiritual contexts.

Throughout the nursing process, therapeutic communication is an important skill the nurse uses to promote communication. Beginning students and new graduates are often fearful of not knowing what to say or of saying the wrong thing. The first step in addressing these fears is for you to become comfortable with your own beliefs, values, and attitudes about death and dying. Second, read and learn about the actual dying process and observe experienced nurses talking with dying patients and grieving relatives. Third, be open to the difficult questions of life and death that permit patients to discuss their feelings and needs. Patients are usually very sensitive as to how caregivers (and family members) react to uncomfortable subjects. Often, a patient will not bring up a subject with family members or staff who avoid conversations that are painful or anxiety provoking. Time and experience are the best teachers. Chapter 8 discusses specific therapeutic communication skills in greater detail.

A trusting relationship with the patient occurs as you are able to meet the identified needs. Listening skills, observation, and use of nonverbal communication, touch, and presence all contribute to the patient's sense of acceptance. Fears of isolation or loneliness decrease with nursing care that seeks to treat the patient with compassion and individuality. The family's anxiety decreases as they see the patient responding to the care and attention of the team.

Think Critically About . . . What questions that a dying person might ask would be most difficult for you to respond to? Think about what you might say in response to such questions.

APPLICATION of the NURSING PROCESS

Assessment (Data Collection)

A baseline assessment and continuing data collection are essential to identify the problems and needs of the patient and his family. An admission history should determine what they have been told by the physician regarding the illness and its expected course. Asking "What has your doctor told you about your condition?" may lead to identifying knowledge the patient needs in order to make informed decisions. Questions about advance directives regarding treatment options, resuscitation, advanced life support, and organ donation can provide information about the patient's attitude toward death and the stage of his grief or dying reaction (denial, anger, etc.). Asking questions about religious beliefs and practices, as well as asking directly "What do you hope for during this admission?" and "What are your concerns?" provides data for the provision of comprehensive comfort care. **At no time should the patient be pushed to discuss something he is obviously avoiding.** A question such as "Is there

Safety Alert 15-1

Use Analgesia Cautiously

Does your patient have renal or hepatic dysfunction? Administration of opioid pain medication may need to be altered to avoid respiratory depression, hypotension, or central nervous system (CNS) toxicity. Consider the recommendations given in Table 15-2 when a patient with renal dysfunction is prescribed an opiate.

anything else you'd like to talk about?" opens the door to issues the patient may wish to discuss.

An assessment of the patient's *physical* condition would include such measures as weight (with attention to usual weight), mobility and the ability to perform activities of daily living, weakness or energy level, appetite (nausea, indigestion, gas), bowel and bladder function, and respiratory function (Safety Alert 15-1). Special attention should be paid to assessing pain: location, nature, and what relieves it or makes it worse. Pain should then be assessed using a 0-to-10 scale or similar method of measuring the patient's report of pain. The frequency of pain assessment will depend on many factors, such as the severity of pain and whether pain is increasing or well controlled on the current treatment regimen (see Chapter 31).

The patient's *emotional* condition can often be observed during the interaction, and symptoms such as anxiety, agitation, confusion, or depression may be obvious. Validating your observation with the patient allows him to speak about his feelings. Stating "Tell me how you are coping with all this" begins to identify strengths and needs. *Spiritual* assessment can begin with questions about the patient's religious affiliation, and whether he would like to meet with a spiritual advisor (chaplain, rabbi, religious leader). Even when a patient indicates "none" for religious affiliation, spiritual needs may be present. Clues regarding spiritual distress may be found in questions such as "Why is God punishing me?" or what the meaning in his life has been.

Nursing Diagnosis

Nursing diagnoses for the dying patient will be varied, depending on the disease process. For example, a patient dying of end-stage renal disease will have problems with fluid excess, whereas a patient dying of chronic obstructive lung disease (COPD) will have problems with ineffective airway clearance. Certain nursing diagnoses are common at some point to most dying patients (Box 15-4).

Planning

It is very important to include the patient and his family in the planning of care, and in establishing the goals or outcomes. Planning should be a team effort, with all members of the team aware of the patient's

---

| Box 15-4 | *Nursing Diagnoses for the Patient Who Is Dying* |

- Activity intolerance
- Death anxiety
- Deficient knowledge
- Fatigue
- Fear
- Grieving
- Imbalanced nutrition: less than body requirements
- Impaired physical mobility
- Impaired skin integrity
- Pain
- Risk for loneliness
- Self-care deficit

---

goals and needs. **Giving the patient control is a first priority at a time when it seems that he has no control.** As far as possible, agency rules and routines that are geared toward cure should be relaxed to recognize that the goal is comfort. These would include relaxing restrictive visiting hours, eliminating routine vital signs and lab work, and avoiding rigid schedules for getting up, bathing, or sleeping.

Implementation

The nurse promotes self-care as long as the patient is able. Family members can derive much satisfaction in learning to provide physical care when the patient is no longer able to be independent. Be sensitive to patient or family member reluctance to provide (or receive) what is uncomfortable for either one, such as performing perineal care for a parent.

Common Problems of the Dying Patient and Nursing Management

Anticipatory Guidance. Anticipating the death assists in preparing the family and patient by giving them guidance about physical changes, symptoms, and complications that may arise. This may also aid the patient and family in deciding about possible hospice care.

End-Stage Symptom Management. There are many expected symptoms, such as pain, gastrointestinal distress, dyspnea, fatigue, cough, death rattle, and delirium, that are related to metabolic changes at the end of life. The last few days of patient life have been studied extensively. The nurse must recognize these symptoms and be able to either alleviate them or help explain them to the patient and family.

Pain Control. Although nursing research has demonstrated safe and effective principles of pain control, many terminally ill patients unnecessarily die with uncontrolled pain. It is perhaps the first fear patients have regarding dying. Several myths still contribute to inadequate pain relief. The patient may fear becoming an addict, or that the medication will not work when he needs it if he takes it for minimal pain. Another fear that nurses have is that the pain medicine will result in hastening the patient's death by depressing respirations. Still a third is the reliance on PRN (as-needed) medication for end-of-life pain rather than around-the-clock dosing. **A truly compassionate nurse studies and learns about pain management and applies those principles in daily practice.**

Pain can be controlled (eliminated) in almost all cases when the medical and nursing team work together (Nursing Care Plan 15-1). **Regularly scheduled pain medication with PRN backup for breakthrough pain is one of the most effective methods of control-**

NURSING CARE PLAN 15-1

Care of the Dying Patient

SCENARIO Mrs. Rodney is in the palliative care unit, actively dying from breast cancer with metastases. She is receiving pain medication, complains of thirst, and is expressing considerable pain.

PROBLEM/NURSING DIAGNOSIS *Pain is not adequately controlled/*Pain related to breast cancer process and metastases.
Supporting Assessment Data: *Subjective:* Pain at a level of 8/10. *Objective:* Grimacing with movement, holding body rigid; advanced breast cancer with metastases.

Goals/Expected Outcomes	Nursing Interventions	Selected Rationales	Evaluation
Patient and family will verify patient has adequate pain control. Patient will verbalize relief/control of pain.	Assess characteristics of pain: location, severity on a scale of 1-10, frequency, precipitating factors, and factors that relieve the pain.	Pain management is most successful when the underlying cause of pain is identified and treated.	*Is pain controlled adequately?* Patient reports adequate control of pain and does not have increased BP, P, or R; no diaphoresis, dilated pupils, guarding, facial mask of pain, crying/moaning, abdominal heaviness, or cutaneous irritation.
	Eliminate factors that precipitate pain (e.g., excessive noise, wrinkled bed sheets, joint discomfort from positioning, thirst, wet bed, gown, cluttered environment, interrupted rest).	Pain may be aggravated by many factors.	
	Offer analgesics on a set round-the-clock schedule per physician orders. Teach patient to request more analgesia before breakthrough pain becomes severe.	Scheduled dosing controls pain better than PRN dosing. It is easier to prevent severe pain than to curtail it once the cycle begins.	Gave additional analgesia at 3:30 P.M. for escalating pain.
	Explore nonpharmacologic methods for reducing pain and promoting comfort: • back rubs • foot rubs • slow, rhythmic deep breathing • imagery exercises • relaxation exercises • repositioning • diversional activities such as music, TV, games • restful intervals between care or treatments	Combination of analgesia and nonpharmacologic measures yields the best pain control.	Using imagery and breathing techniques. Refused back rub. Repositioned every hour. Watching TV. Body posture more relaxed. Continue plan.

? CRITICAL THINKING QUESTIONS

1. What are some ways to help Mrs. Rodney with her pain? Should she be given additional pain medication (opioids)?

2. Some of the family members are afraid that additional opioids will hasten Mrs. Rodney's death. What can you say to the family members?

Key: *BP,* Blood pressure; *P,* pulse; *PRN,* as needed; *R,* respirations.

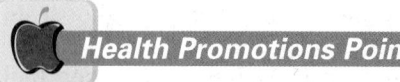

Health Promotions Points 15-1

WHO's Three-Step Ladder for Pain Relief

The World Health Organization (WHO) has developed a three-step ladder to follow for adequate pain relief. According to this ladder:

1. Start with nonopioid drugs +1 adjuvant therapy.
2. If pain persists or increases, add an opioid designated for mild to moderate pain.
3. If pain persists or increases, change to an opioid designated for moderate to severe pain.

The pain ladder is additive to the first step. In other words, when changing from one step to the next, always continue the previous step(s) as well.

Table 15-2 *Opioid Use in Patients with Renal Impairment*

DRUG	RECOMMENDATION
Morphine	Use cautiously with dose adjustment and careful monitoring
Hydrocodone	Use cautiously with dose adjustment and careful monitoring
Oxycodone	Use cautiously with dose adjustment and careful monitoring
Codeine	DO NOT USE
Methadone	Safe
Fentanyl	Appears safe, reduce dose
Meperidine	DO NOT USE
Propoxyphene	DO NOT USE

ling pain. Carefully assess pain location, intensity, and response to medication every 2 to 4 hours, or more often if needed, to determine the necessity for increases in dosage (Health Promotion Points 15-1). **There is no concern for addiction or of reaching a safety or effectiveness limit when narcotics are increased in response to pain for the dying patient.** Patients with severe pain can receive huge doses of narcotics without respiratory depression or tolerance when the dose has been increased in response to increasing pain. Since comfort is the goal of palliative care, administering only oral medications, when feasible, is the preferred choice. However, this may not be possible as death draws near, and it is also the goal to allow a pain-free death. In some cases it may be possible to administer transdermal and/or rectal pain medications. The oral route and long-acting transdermal patches can also avoid the necessity of injections. Even when the patient is no longer taking fluids by mouth, small amounts of concentrated pain medication can be inserted in the buccal cavity (cheek) (Table 15-2). Transdermal fentanyl has helped eliminate the burden of pain at the end of life. Sometimes this regimen is supplemented with rescue doses of morphine if pain isn't controlled. Whatever the regimen for pain control, studies have shown that pain relief, either total or at least to a level that is tolerable, is possible 75% to 97% of the time.

Nonchemical approaches to pain relief may include visualization and guided imagery, relaxation and breathing exercises, massage, music therapy, meditation, religious healing, biofeedback, hypnosis or self-hypnosis, the use of transcutaneous electrical nerve stimulation (TENS), and hydrotherapy (e.g., whirlpool). Teach the patient these simple techniques as an adjunct to drug therapy. Provide a quiet environment and assist the patient as necessary (see Chapter 31).

Constipation, Diarrhea. Constipation is predictable for a patient receiving opiates, experiencing decreased fluid intake and mobility, and having certain abdominal diseases. In addition to classic nursing measures for preventing constipation (increasing fiber, fluids, and exercise; see Chapter 30), consult with the physician for orders for stool softeners and a standing laxative order. Suppositories and enemas, or manual disimpaction, can be avoided in most cases with careful monitoring and adherence to a laxative schedule.

Anorexia, Nausea, Vomiting. *Anorexia*, or loss of appetite, may be due to nausea, drug side effects (especially a sore mouth), the disease process, or the slowdown that occurs naturally in the dying process. Antiemetics are the first choice to eliminate nausea and vomiting. Small servings, home-prepared food favorites, and attention to eliminating unpleasant sights and odors at mealtime may stimulate a poor appetite. A bad taste can be improved by frequent oral care, mouthwashes, or hard candies (sour balls). A nutritionist may be very helpful in suggesting food choices that are appealing as well as easily digested. You can do a great deal to support the patient and the family with an explanation of the dying process: that decreased intake is more comfortable for the patient than having food to digest and move through a system that is slowing down. There is also some evidence to suggest that starvation decreases the patient's awareness of pain by producing chemicals that act as pain relievers. Weight loss is commonly seen in dying patients, but few patients complain of feeling hungry. *Dysphagia* (difficulty swallowing) may also be a problem. Moistening the mouth with fluids or artificial saliva may be helpful. Additional care of the dysphagic patient is presented in Chapter 27.

Dehydration. As death nears, patients spend more time sleeping or in a semiresponsive state. They take in fewer and fewer fluids until the question arises about providing intravenous (IV) fluids or tube feedings out of concern for dehydration. Research has shown that dehydration results in less distress and pain and that hydration does not improve comfort. Dry mouth and thirst are the most common complaints, which may be induced by the drugs being administered, and these can be alleviated by small sips of fluids, ice chips, and lip lubrication. Resulting decreased urine output means less effort to use a commode or less incontinence. This is an issue that is best discussed before it arises, at the time advance directives are being established. It is an emotional issue, and families often have a difficult time accepting that withholding fluids is more comforting than administering them. Families can be comforted with an explanation of how the dying person is indeed made more comfortable by withholding fluids. The nurse must help educate the patient and family as to both the benefits and burdens of hydration. Many times the course is for patients to choose what to take and be allowed to refuse further nourishment. This is referred to as "patient-endorsed intake."

Dyspnea. Difficult breathing may be seen early in the dying process in certain lung or heart disorders. It is also seen shortly before death, when respirations may become noisy, irregular, or labored. Secretions in the lungs accumulate and block the airways to contribute to noisy or rattling respirations. The patient is usually not responsive, or not aware of the dyspnea, but it is very upsetting to family members. Suctioning is not effective in clearing the secretions, but medications such as a scopolamine patch or morphine can decrease secretions and ease breathing. Administering oxygen by nasal prongs may provide comfort.

Death Rattle. Noisy respirations are heard when patients can no longer clear their throats of normal secretions. Family members are often alarmed and are afraid the patient will choke to death. In these cases, scopolamine or atropine, drugs that are known to reduce secretions, may be used to quiet the patient and bring breathing back to normal.

Delirium. Dying patients may experience hallucinations and/or altered mental status. Nurses must first search for causes such as pain, positional discomfort, or bladder distention and address those physical problems. Next, the nurse should discuss the delirium with the patient's family and encourage the family to talk to the patient in quiet tones while remaining calm.

Impaired Skin Integrity. Weight loss, decreased nutrition, incontinence, and inactivity all contribute to the risk of skin breakdown. Turn and position the patient, use protective measures such as an air pressure mattress, heel or elbow protectors, and sheepskin or foam pads, and keep the skin clean and dry. An indwelling or condom catheter may be indicated to conserve the patient's dwindling energy as well as to prevent skin breakdown.

Weakness, Fatigue, Decreased Ability to Perform Activities of Daily Living. Increasing weakness eventually results in the patient's becoming bed-bound. Accept the patient's wishes regarding walking, sitting up in a chair, or remaining in bed. **The dying patient is not going to get stronger or better; he gets weaker and weaker, not because he is lying in bed, but because he is dying.** Allow the patient to do as much as possible for himself, and provide physical care when he is no longer able.

Anxiety, Depression, Agitation. Emotional or psychological symptoms may be treated with appropriate drugs with good effect. Listen and use good therapeutic communication skills to allow the patient to express his fears, feelings, and needs, and to convey nonjudgmental acceptance (see Chapter 8). Skillful assessment of these symptoms may identify physical pain or spiritual distress that can be treated.

Spiritual Distress, Fear of Meaninglessness. Each person needs to believe that his life has had meaning, and this is the essence of the spiritual nature of the dying process. A life review allows the patient to put his life in perspective. Reminiscing is one way of starting a life review. Encourage the patient to tell about family photographs or albums. Ask "What was it like when you were a child (or worked on the farm, lived in the city, met your wife)?" **It is more important to listen than to talk.**

Evaluation

Evaluation is based on the specific expected outcomes written for the patient. These will depend on which nursing diagnoses are pertinent to the patient's situation. In most cases, the degree of comfort obtained for the patient by the nursing interventions will need to be evaluated. Was pain adequately controlled? Was tissue integrity protected? Were actions to facilitate the patient's and family's grieving process effective? Was the patient's fear alleviated? Did interventions for a self-care deficit make the patient more comfortable? Answers to these questions will help determine whether expected outcomes have been met. If the plan of care is not effective, the plan must be revised.

SIGNS OF IMPENDING DEATH

PHYSICAL SIGNS

As death approaches, the patient grows physically weaker and begins to spend more time sleeping. Body functions slow, appetite decreases, and the patient may refuse even favorite foods and later fluids as well. Explain to the patient and the family what to expect. Moistening the patient's lips and mouth, and providing oral hygiene, will be more comforting than "pushing" food or fluids.

Urine output decreases and urine becomes more concentrated. There may be edema of the extremities or over the sacrum. Incontinence may occur as patients become less aware of their surroundings. However, be alert to the possibility of urinary retention and the need for catheterization.

Vital signs change as death approaches. The pulse increases and becomes weaker or thready. Blood pressure declines, and the skin of the extremities becomes mottled, cool, and dusky. Respirations become shallow and irregular. There may be pooling of secretions in the lungs that causes respirations to sound moist. Often at the time of death, a "death rattle" of those secretions occurs. Cheyne-Stokes respirations may be noted: respirations that gradually become shallower and are followed by periods of *apnea* (no breathing). Body temperature may rise, and the patient (if responsive) may complain of feeling hot or cold, although the extremities will be cool to the touch as circulation slows. Blankets should be used as the patient desires.

PSYCHOSOCIAL AND SPIRITUAL ASPECTS OF DYING

As outlined in Kübler-Ross' stages of coping with dying, it is hoped that the patient will have reached the stage of acceptance as death draws closer. It is during this time that the patient will talk about making funeral arrangements and "putting my affairs in order." To die with closure is to say goodbye to those people and things that are important. It may also involve saying "I'm sorry, forgive me," "I forgive you," and "I love you." It is a time when the patient may give to family and friends special memories or possessions. A life review can assist patients to tell their story and put their life in perspective. Assisting the patient to write or share his life story with significant others allows them to keep special memories of their loved one.

As individuals approach death, their spiritual needs take on greater importance. As patients ponder the meaning of their life, their beliefs about what happens to them in death take on new meaning. Religious practices and rituals have great significance for some patients. It is important for you to be familiar with those beliefs (see Chapter 14). **Rather than impose your own religious beliefs on dying patients and family, you should assist patients to find comfort and support in their own belief systems.** An assessment of the spiritual needs of the patient is outlined in Chapter 14, and when indicated, you may collaborate with the patient's religious representative or hospital chaplain to provide spiritual care.

As life ebbs, the patient becomes less verbal and more withdrawn. Everyday activities and news are not of interest, and nonverbal communication becomes most important. Sitting with patients and using touch, such as holding their hand or stroking their hair, will be most meaningful. Even when patients appear to be sleeping or nonresponsive, physical touch and presence are comforting. **Always be aware of remarks you make in the presence of an unresponsive patient because they DO hear. Hearing is believed to be one of the last senses to be lost before death, and "dying" patients have awakened to report conversations by family and health care workers that they were not meant to overhear.**

Dying patients may exhibit confusion and disorientation. They may report dreams or visions of deceased relatives, and they usually are not frightened by these experiences. Often this is comforting, and they may speak of preparing for a journey to join loved ones. At times patients may become restless and agitated. Adequate pain and anxiety medication can ease the distress of these symptoms. Keep soft lights on in the room. Assurance that it is "okay to go" and that family members will take care of each other may ease dying individuals' anxiety about leaving their responsibilities.

? *Think Critically About . . .* What would you wish to include in your obituary (a notice of the death published in newspapers)? Write your own obituary, imagining at what age you would die, and what will have happened in your life (education, jobs, family) between now and the time of your death. What funeral arrangements will you make?

LEGAL AND ETHICAL ASPECTS OF LIFE AND DEATH ISSUES

The health care system is still grappling with care of the dying. Recognizing the patient's right to make decisions about end-of-life situations, advance directives, and the designation of a health care proxy have gained legal and public acceptance.

ADVANCE DIRECTIVES

An advance directive spells out patients' wishes for health care at that time when they may be unable to indicate their choice. A durable power of attorney for health care is a legal document that appoints a person (health care proxy) chosen by the patient to carry out his wishes as expressed in an advance directive. Discussing advance directives with patients opens the communication path to establish what is important to them, and what they view as promoting life versus prolonging dying. Patients determine under which situations they would agree to *do-not-resuscitate* (DNR) orders. Their choices regarding artificial feeding and fluids, ventilators, and administration of antibiotics are documented.

Elder Care Points

- When competent elderly individuals have not completed an advance directive before admission, even though it may be very difficult to communicate with them, they should be included in discussions and decisions about end-of-life care.
- Confusion about time or place does not automatically make patients incapable of expressing their wishes and preferences.

Much of the debate in health care today deals with end-of-life decisions such as euthanasia, assisted suicide, adequate pain control, and death with dignity. Nurses must be active in keeping up to date on legal decisions regarding these issues, and continue to learn

Table 15-3 **Legal and Ethical Considerations for Euthanasia**

VOLUNTARY EUTHANASIA	INVOLUNTARY EUTHANASIA
ARGUMENTS FOR	
Respects individual liberty and rights	Reduces depletion of financial resources
Provides more dignified death	Allows the patient dignity
Reduces suffering	Reduces suffering
Demonstrates mercy	Demonstrates mercy
Supports constitutional right to privacy	Supports right to die
Demonstrates right of self-determination	
Upholds right to autonomy	
ARGUMENTS AGAINST	
Exploits the terminally ill	Ignores informed consent
Breaks the Hippocratic oath	Violates right to life
Unnecessary—nature will take its course	Unnecessary
Morally wrong	Morally wrong

LEGAL CONSIDERATIONS

The courts have approved the withholding of treatment in both voluntary and involuntary euthanasia cases if the parties can demonstrate that it is in the best interest of the patient and the family requests it. However, be aware that "assisted suicide" is illegal in most states and legal consequences may follow. In addition, active euthanasia is never legal or permissible.

and apply new nursing theory and procedures regarding end-of-life care. They must also deal with their own feelings and values regarding patient choices to seek life-prolonging or death-seeking treatment.

EUTHANASIA

Euthanasia is the act of ending another person's life to end suffering, with (voluntary) or without (involuntary) his consent. It may be called "mercy killing." Some distinction is also made between active and passive euthanasia. Passive euthanasia occurs when a patient chooses to die by refusing treatment that might prolong life. An example would be withholding artificial feeding or parenteral (IV) fluids when the patient is unable to take them orally. It would also include not treating pneumonia with antibiotics. **Honoring the refusal of life-prolonging treatment of a patient with a terminal illness is legally and ethically permissible.** Active euthanasia is generally defined as administering a drug or treatment to end the patient's life. **Active euthanasia is not legal or permissible in the United States**. The arguments for legal and ethical considerations regarding euthanasia are presented in Table 15-3.

Assisted suicide is distinguished from active euthanasia. It is making available to patients the means to end their life (such as a weapon or drug) with knowledge that suicide is their intent. **Both active euthanasia and assisted suicide are considered to be a violation of the American Nurses Association's** *Code for Nurses.* Their position statements regarding active euthanasia state that "the nurse does not act deliberately to terminate the life of any person" (American Nurses Association, 1994, p. 2) and that "nurses must . . . not participate in assisted suicide" (American Nurses Association, 1995, p. 6).

Assisted suicide has generated a great deal of debate and dialogue in health care as nurses witness firsthand the despair, pain, and debilitation of their patients. As-

sisting the patient's death may be seen as a compassionate and humane response. Although an individual case may be compelling, there is a larger potential for abuse of this solution for difficult care problems, especially for the elderly, the disabled, and the poor. Oregon passed a law legalizing assisted suicide in 1998. However, the courts in other states continue to decide cases involving assisted suicide and active euthanasia that may change the legal status of such acts.

ADEQUATE PAIN CONTROL

Adequate pain control is another issue that affects the comfort of the dying and has to do with the reluctance of physicians to prescribe large enough doses of pain medication for fear of legal action under the Controlled Substances Act. There is also concern that they may be viewed as prescribing lethal doses in an assisted suicide effort. National legislation (the Lethal Drug Abuse Prevention Act of 1998) had been proposed to prevent physicians from prescribing controlled substances for the purpose of assisting suicide. The bill failed. If passed into law, it could have had a negative effect on the physician's willingness to prescribe adequate pain medication.

Nurses must be advocates for compassionate end-of-life care. Knowledgeable and skillful symptom management, the relief of suffering, and the promise of presence, of not abandoning the patient, become the cornerstones of end-of-life care that can eliminate the need for a person to choose euthanasia or suicide.

ORGAN AND TISSUE DONATION

Kidneys, livers, hearts, and lungs are organs that can be transplanted from one person to another. Other tissues such as corneas, bone, and skin can also be transplanted. The need for organs and tissues exceeds the supply. Every day people die waiting for a transplant. People can indicate their wish to be donors on their driver's license or in advance directives, but permission to remove the organs or tissues of a dead person must be given by the next of kin. Organs such as hearts, lungs, and livers can only be obtained from a person who is on mechanical ventilation and has suffered brain death but still has perfusion to the organs. Other tissues can be removed for several hours after death, such as after a massive heart attack or stroke. The donor must be free of infectious disease and cancer. The criteria are set by the United Network for Organ Sharing (UNOS). Physicians are usually the people to request organ donation from family members, but you may be in a position to answer questions the family raises about organ donation. You should know that donation of organs does not delay funeral arrangements, that there is no obvious evidence that the organs were removed when the body is dressed, and there is no cost to the family for the removal of organs donated.

POSTMORTEM (AFTER DEATH) CARE

When the patient stops breathing, the heart may continue to beat for several minutes. (It is when the heart stops that death is said to have occurred, unless the person is on a ventilator.) When a patient is being mechanically ventilated, brain death must be established to determine death. In a hospital or nursing home, a physician is usually designated as the person responsible for pronouncing the death. However, in some institutions midlevel providers, such as physician assistants and nurse practitioners, may perform this function. When a patient dies at home, the pronouncement of death may be delegated to an undertaker, registered nurse, or coroner. A coroner is a person with legal authority to determine cause of death. Any deaths that occur under suspicious circumstances are investigated by a coroner. These would include deaths that result from injury, accident, murder, or suicide. Any death within 24 hours after admission to the hospital, during surgery, or death of a person who has not been under a physician's care, is reported to the coroner. In the health care setting, if a death is a coroner's case, no tube or line is removed from the body to prevent removal of evidence of wrongdoing. IV lines and associated tubing are simply cut, tied off, and the catheters left in place.

A death certificate is completed by the physician, the undertaker, and a pathologist if an autopsy is done. An autopsy is an examination of the body, organs, and tissues to determine the cause of death. Consent for autopsy must be obtained from the next of kin, except in a coroner's case, when no permission is needed.

As the nurse, you are responsible for postmortem (after death) care of the body. Family members may wish to assist with or perform the preparation of the body as their last service to the patient, especially if they have been present throughout the dying process.

If family members were not present when the patient died, the body may be prepared for the family to come to say goodbye and for removal to the morgue or undertaker (Skill 15-1). It is comforting for the family to have you indicate such things as "he died very peacefully," and to explain the final care the patient received. Ask if the family wishes to be left alone with the body for their final goodbyes. You should return any personal belongings of the patient to the family, especially jewelry or valuables. The family members' reactions become your focus, and a private quiet place should be provided for them to begin the grieving process until they are able to leave. Unused drugs are returned to the pharmacy according to agency policy. Unused drugs are never given to the family. It is not recommended to flush the drugs down the toilet.

Nurses can gain a great deal of satisfaction in caring for the dying patient and his family. Helping patients to attain their goal of dying with dignity, without pain, and with a sense of closure is a tremendous challenge, but one that is rewarding. You should realize that you will also grieve for the dying patient. Many hospitals and health care agencies provide for support sessions after a particularly difficult death or when a unit has a succession of unexpected or challenging losses. You will need to take care of yourself in order to continue taking care of your patients, and this includes recognizing the normal feelings that occur with loss, and allowing yourself to move through the grief rather than trying to avoid it. Talking with the chaplain, coworkers, and other experienced nurses can support and heal the grief. Seeking professional assistance may be indicated if grieving becomes dysfunctional.

Key Points

- Loss is to no longer possess or have a person, object, or situation. Grief is a normal reaction to loss. Death is the most difficult loss human beings experience.
- The grieving process consists of feelings and acts that move to eventual recovery. The symptoms of the grieving process include crying, depression, loss of appetite, changes in sleep, loneliness, and sadness. The grieving person may be the patient, loved one, or caregiver.
- Each person who grieves does so in a unique way that depends on the value of the loss to them, their previous experiences with loss, and their learned coping skills.
- Nurses assist the grieving person through validation of the loss, teaching of adaptive coping skills, and caring support.
- Therapeutic communication techniques—active listening, avoiding clichés, and attention to nonverbal communication—are invaluable in dealing with the person who is experiencing loss.
- Death may occur in different ways, and each person's reaction to death will also be different.

Skill 15-1 | Postmortem Care

After death, you will prepare the body for transport to the morgue or to the funeral home. Always check records to see if the patient is a designated organ donor. If so, initiate the organ donation process according to agency policy.

■ Supplies

- ✓ Shroud (sheet used to wrap body after death) pack
- ✓ Death care kit (shroud, gauze 4 × 4 dressings, and protective pads if not in shroud pack)
- ✓ Gloves
- ✓ Bag for belongings
- ✓ Valuables list
- ✓ Bathing supplies
- ✓ Comb and brush
- ✓ Tape and large safety pins
- ✓ Body tags or labels
- ✓ Gurney or morgue cart

Review and carry out the Standard Steps in Appendix 3.

■ Assessment

1. **ACTION** Verify the patient's identification.

   RATIONALE Ensures that the patient is properly identified.

2. **ACTION** Determine whether an autopsy will be done; check for signed autopsy consent.

   RATIONALE Drainage or other tubes are not removed if an autopsy is planned.

3. **ACTION** Determine if the family wishes to assist with bathing or caring for the body, or if they wish to view the deceased after the nurse prepares the body.

   RATIONALE Family may gain closure from this last act of care for their loved one.

■ Planning

4. **ACTION** Gather equipment, and prepare the working space by raising the bed to proper height and positioning the over-the-bed table for use.

   RATIONALE Promotes work efficiency and prevents back strain.

5. **ACTION** Close the door and/or privacy curtains.

   RATIONALE Protects privacy and dignity.

■ Implementation

6. **ACTION** Perform hand hygiene and don gloves.

   RATIONALE Protects you from contact with body fluids.

7. **ACTION** Position the patient in supine position with a pillow under the head and the head of the bed elevated 15 to 20 degrees. Close the eyelids if necessary.

   RATIONALE Raising the head prevents pooling of blood, which might discolor the face. Closing the eyelids protects the eyeballs.

8. **ACTION** Replace the dentures if they are out of the mouth if hospital policy requires it. Close the eyelids and mouth. A small rolled towel may be placed under the chin if needed to keep the mouth closed. Depending on agency policy, dentures may be placed in a labeled denture cup without water and sent with the body so that the mortician does not have to remove the dentures again to embalm the body.

   RATIONALE Closing the eyelids and mouth protects the eyes and keeps the face in the most natural position during rigor mortis (rigidity of muscles that occurs after death).

9. **ACTION** Remove any jewelry and clothing. List all personal articles on the valuables list. Place in bag to be returned to the family and handle according to agency policy.

   RATIONALE This provides for return of personal property to the family.

10. **ACTION** Wash all areas of the body soiled with blood, feces, urine, or drainage. Place protective pads under rectum and between the legs to protect from drainage from rectum, vagina, or urethra.

    RATIONALE After death, sphincter muscles relax, allowing leakage of stool, urine, or body fluids.

11. **ACTION** Comb the hair and arrange neatly.

    RATIONALE Combing the hair improves the appearance of the body, and prevents matting or tangling.

12. **ACTION** Deflate any balloons and remove all tubes (IVs, catheters, nasogastric) unless an autopsy is planned, if this is agency policy. Otherwise, convert IV catheters to intermittent locks. To secure tubes left in place, remove the drainage bag or IV fluid container, cut the tubing, and fold over twice. Secure with a rubber band.

    RATIONALE Properly deflating balloons before tube removal prevents tissue damage. Leaving the IV catheter in place prevents leaking during embalming. Prepares body for coroner/undertaker.

Continued

Skill 15-1 | **Postmortem Care**—cont'd

13. **ACTION** Change any soiled dressings and remove adhesive marks with appropriate solvent.

 RATIONALE Improves appearance of the body.

14. **ACTION** Dress the body in a clean gown if family will be viewing the body, and remain with them unless they wish to be alone. The gown may be removed before wrapping the body.

 RATIONALE Dressing the body preserves dignity, and remaining with the family provides emotional support.

15. **ACTION** After the family leaves, attach identifying tags, usually on the big toe or ankle and the wrist.

 RATIONALE Proper identification ensures that the body will be transported to the correct mortuary.

16. **ACTION** Place padded ties around the ankles; crisscross the wrists over the abdomen and secure; and place a gauze tie or chin strap under the jaw to keep the mouth closed. Some mortuaries prefer that the limbs not be tied together. In this case, position the arms in a natural position at the sides of the body and keep the legs straight and together.

 RATIONALE Ankles and wrists are sometimes secured to prevent the arms and legs from being damaged during transport. However, the ties can damage the skin and make embalming more difficult.

17. **ACTION** Place the body on the shroud or in the morgue bag and check for placement of drainage pads. Fold the shroud according to agency procedure using the numerical order indicated. Secure the shroud at the chest, waist, and knees, and place an identification (ID) tag on the outside.

 RATIONALE The shroud covers the body and prevents unnecessary exposure. The ID tag ensures correct disposal of the body. Some mortuaries prefer the body not be shrouded.

18. **ACTION** Transfer the body to the stretcher or morgue cart. Secure the body with straps that are secure but not so tight as to cause bruising. Remove gloves and perform hand hygiene. Transport the body to the morgue in the service elevator unless the mortuary will come to the room to transport it.

 RATIONALE Transport to the morgue is done quickly and with as little notice as possible, as it may be upsetting to other patients or visitors to see the body. Doors to patient rooms may be closed, and the elevator held ready for transport. In some agencies, the face may be left uncovered so pas-

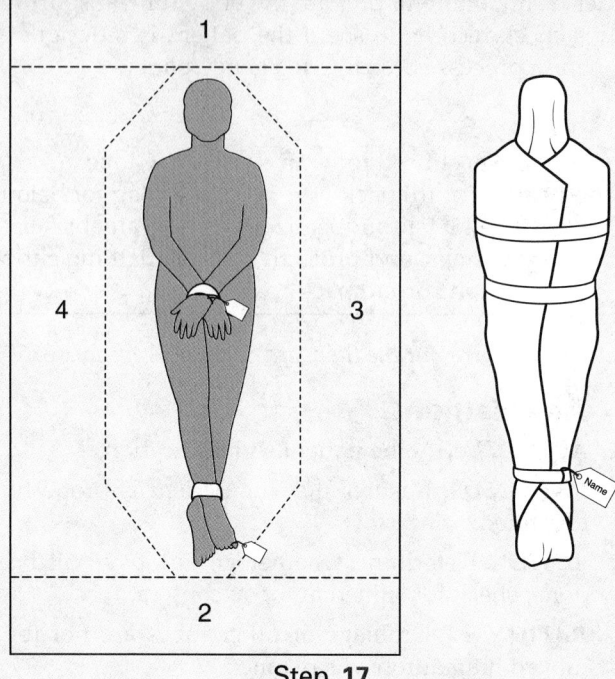

Step 17

sersby think the person is just unconscious. Some mortuaries come directly to the room to transport the body.

■ **Evaluation**

19. **ACTION** Ask yourself: Was the procedure carried out in a quiet, respectful way? Was the family supported and helped to say goodbye? Did the deceased appear clean, peaceful, and well cared for?

 RATIONALE Determines if expected outcomes have been met. Indicates whether the way in which the procedure has been carried out needs to be changed.

■ **Documentation**

20. **ACTION** Note the care provided in the chart.

 RATIONALE Documentation is legal proof of the nursing care provided.

Documentation Example

2/17 1030 Pt stopped breathing. 1033 No apical pulse detected. Dr. Grover notified. 1040 Pronounced dead by Dr. Grover. Family present and assisted in washing and preparing the body for transport to morgue. Foley catheter removed. ID tags attached to right toe, right ankle, and outside of shroud. Transported to morgue at 1120.

_____

(Nurse's signature)

❓CRITICAL THINKING QUESTIONS

1. Catherine Baumgartner has just died from complications as a result of extensive drug-resistant tuberculosis. The patient has been in isolation with minimal visitor contact, and the family has had to follow isolation precautions in order to visit the patient.

   a. Would you perform postmortem care differently than you would for a patient who died from cancer? If so, what would you do differently?
   b. The family wants to spend time alone with the patient, bathing and preparing the body for burial. What would you tell the family? How would you proceed with family activities?

- Hospice is a concept of care for the dying and their families that focuses on symptom control, comfort measures rather than cure, and a team approach to meeting the expressed needs of the patient and the family.
- Kübler-Ross's theory of the stages of dying includes denial, bargaining, anger, depression, and acceptance.
- The dying person may experience fear of pain, of the unknown, and of loss of control as well as guilt, hope, and despair.
- Hope is a positive life force that can be nurtured in different ways for the dying.
- Palliative care is a concept of providing care that relieves symptoms when cure is no longer possible. This concept can be applied in any setting.
- The nursing process identifies the physical, emotional, social, and spiritual aspects of the dying patient's care and provides a comprehensive team approach.
- Patients may have tasks to complete before death, such as saying goodbye, making amends, reconciling with family or friends, and doing a life review.
- Research and practice provide effective ways of controlling pain and managing symptoms of nausea, constipation, anorexia, dyspnea, anxiety, or spiritual distress.
- Terminal dehydration has been shown to be palliative in reducing pain. Intravenous hydration is not indicated unless it is a patient's choice.
- Signs of impending death include decreasing level of consciousness, decreasing urine output, mottling of skin, cool extremities, Cheyne-Stokes respirations, death rattle, and incontinence. Hearing and touch are among the last senses to be lost before death.
- Nurses must be aware of patients' religious beliefs and assist them in the practice of those religious rituals that are important to them.
- Advance directives indicate a patient's choices about end-of-life decisions such as DNR orders and artificial hydration or tube feedings.
- Euthanasia and assisted suicide are legal and ethical issues for health care professionals.
- Assisted suicide is ethically not acceptable for health care professionals. Legally it is being tested in the courts, and new laws are constantly being proposed.
- Donation of organs from a dying person is possible if relatives give permission. Nurses have an important role in explaining the aspects of organ donation.
- Nurses are responsible for care of the body after death (except in some religions).
- Caring for patients in the final stage of life can be rewarding and satisfying. Nurses will recognize signs of grieving in themselves after the death of a patient.

 Go to your **Companion CD-ROM** for an Audio Glossary, animations, video clips, and more.

evolve   Be sure to visit the companion Evolve site at http://evolve.elsevier.com/deWit/fundamental/ for additional online resources.

NCLEX-PN® EXAMINATION-STYLE REVIEW QUESTIONS

*Choose the **best** answer(s) for each question.*

1. A patient who has been recently diagnosed with cancer says to the nurse, "If I can just live until my son graduates from college, I'll donate 10% of my estate to the church." The patient is in a stage described by Dr. Kübler-Ross as:
   1. acceptance.
   2. denial.
   3. bargaining.
   4. anger.

2. A therapeutic response the nurse could make when a patient says, "I don't want to die" is:
   1. "I'm sure you don't want to die."
   2. "You have an excellent physician, maybe you won't die."
   3. "None of us wants to die."
   4. "I'm sorry you are going through this; would you like to talk about it?"

3. A clinical sign that a patient is close to death would be:
   1. nausea that occurs after meals.
   2. pain that is well controlled with small doses of morphine.
   3. increasing blood pressure, pulse, and respirations.
   4. periods of apnea and irregular respirations.

4. Comfort care for a terminally ill patient would include:
   1. a magnetic resonance image (MRI) to determine if metastases were causing bone pain.
   2. use of medication to relieve nausea.
   3. insertion of an intravenous line to provide fluids.
   4. a gastrostomy tube to provide nutrition when the patient is unable to eat normally.

5. The priority of palliative care is to:

   1. control symptoms and promote comfort without the hope of cure.
   2. prevent the recurrence of cancer when it is first diagnosed.
   3. control costs of terminal illness by avoiding expensive treatments or drugs.
   4. keep the patient at home rather than in a hospital or nursing home.

6. Validation of loss can be of great comfort to a grieving individual. A patient states, "I am so depressed! I didn't know it would be so difficult to cope after losing my mother." To validate the loss, you respond:

   1. "Yes, but time is a great healer and you will eventually adjust."
   2. "I am sorry you are having such a hard time. Tell me a little about your mother and what she meant to you."
   3. "Would it help to see a grief counselor?"
   4. "Have you ever lost a loved one before?"

7. Certain cultures believe that talking about bad things like "death" can bring it on. Your patient is an American Indian with advanced breast cancer whose family is at her bedside. The family has asked that you only discuss plans for a cure, and not discuss palliative measures. How do you plan for the patient's care during the final stages of her illness?

   1. You ignore end-of-life issues and continue to treat the patient for a cure, even though the treatment is painful.
   2. You discuss palliative measures with the family, being careful to discuss "comfort" and not "death."
   3. Tell the family that their family member cannot receive hospice care if she does not know about her impending death.
   4. If the family asks you questions, refer them to the physician.

8. An assigned patient has prostate cancer and is declining rapidly. He is frightened by the progression and asks you if there is any hope. What is your response?

   1. "Your prostate cancer is incurable. We have exhausted our treatment measures, but I can discuss comfort measures with you."
   2. Would you like me to call a chaplain for you? Maybe it's time to put your trust in a higher power."
   3. "There is always hope. Let's look at how we can address your issues together. What is it that you are hoping for at this point?"
   4. "You cannot give up! A positive attitude helps effect a cure."

9. A patient with terminal cancer has accepted his impending death and so has his family. They have asked for palliative care. You know that this involves:

   1. moving the patient to a hospice because that is the only place palliative care is appropriate.
   2. keeping the patient in the hospital, which is the only place he can receive pain medicine in large doses.
   3. moving the patient home, where he can be in familiar surroundings, even though his access to medicines and nursing care will be limited.
   4. helping the patient and his family arrange for a setting that is comfortable to them.

10. After receiving palliative care for several months, your patient has died. The family is feeling deep grief. You feel saddened also, and you know that:

    1. crying is inappropriate because you are not even a family member or a close friend.
    2. it is appropriate for you to shed some tears also, allowing yourself to move through the grief rather than trying to avoid it. You may also need to seek professional assistance.
    3. you need to ignore your feelings and stay strong for the family so you can provide better nursing care.
    4. you should avoid the family and allow them to grieve in private. You are no longer needed, and your presence just reminds them of their loss.

CRITICAL THINKING ACTIVITIES *Read each clinical scenario and discuss the questions with your classmates.*

Scenario

Lynn Nuñez, a 45-year-old woman with advanced breast cancer that has spread to her lungs and bones, is admitted to your unit for terminal care and palliation. She has draining sores on her left breast. She is experiencing a great deal of pain when she moves, but she does not want to be "sedated." Her wish is to spend her last days with her family, which includes her husband, mother and father, and two teenage daughters. The family is close and supportive, but is having a very hard time seeing Lynn suffer. She is Roman Catholic, and the parish priest has visited daily. She has indicated she does not wish to have extraordinary measures, including feeding tubes, IVs, or antibiotics. She is DNR.

1. What would you think are Lynn's prioritized needs for care?
2. If she were assigned to you for care, what do you think you might suggest for
   - Frequency of vital signs measurement
   - Personal care: bathing, mouth care, skin care
   - Feeding: what, when, how much
   - Activity level
3. What might your response be if Lynn were to ask you, "Why do I have to suffer like this?"

16 Infection Prevention and Control: Protective Mechanisms and Asepsis

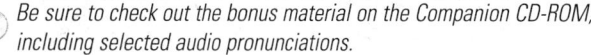
http://evolve.elsevier.com/deWit/fundamental/

Objectives

Upon completing this chapter, you should be able to:

Theory

1. List the types of microorganisms that can cause infection in humans.
2. Discuss the links in the infection process and give an example of each.
3. Discuss factors that make the elderly more susceptible to infection.
4. Explain how the body's protective mechanisms work to prevent infection.
5. Explain how the inflammatory and immune responses protect the body.
6. Identify means for removal or destruction of microorganisms on animate and inanimate objects.
7. Compare and contrast medical asepsis and surgical asepsis.
8. Describe accepted methods of disinfection and sterilization.

Clinical Practice

1. Discuss the surveillance, prevention, and control of infections in hospitalized patients.
2. Demonstrate proper hand hygiene technique.
3. Consistently demonstrate application of Standard and Transmission-Based Precautions while caring for patients.
4. Prepare to teach a home care patient with a wound infection how to prevent the spread of infection to family members.

Skills and Steps

Skills
Skill 16-1   Hand Hygiene
Skill 16-2   Using Personal Protective Equipment (PPE): Gown and Mask

Steps
Steps 16-1   Removing Gloves

Key Terms

Be sure to check out the bonus material on the Companion CD-ROM, including selected audio pronunciations.

antibiotic (p. 211)
antimicrobial (ăn-tĭ-mĭ-KRŌ-bē-ăl, p. 211)
antiseptic (ăn-tĭ-SĔP-tĭk, p. 230)
asepsis (ā-SĔP-sĭs, p. 219)
aseptic (ā-SĔP-tĭk, p. 214)
bacteria (băk-TĒ-rē-ă, p. 211)
contaminated (p. 213)
debris (dĕ-BRĒ, p. 215)
disinfectants (dĭs-ĭn-FĔK-tănts, p. 230)
fungi (FŬN-jī, p. 212)
helminths (HĔL-mĭnths, p. 212)
immune response (ĭ-MŪN rē-SPŎNS, p. 218)
interferon (ĭn-tĕr-FĒR-ŏn, p. 216)
medical asepsis (p. 219)
microorganism (mī-krō-ŌR-găn-ĭz-ĕm, p. 209)
pathogens (PĂTH-ō-jĕnz, p. 209)
personal protective equipment (PPE) (p. 220)
prions (p. 211)
protozoa (prō-tō-ZŌ-ă, p. 212)
rickettsia (rĭ-KĔT-sē-ă, p. 212)
Standard Precautions (p. 220)
sterile (p. 213)
sterilization (stĕr-ĭ-lĭ-ZĀ-shŭn, p. 213)
surgical asepsis (p. 219)
viruses (p. 211)

An **infection** is the entry into the body of an infectious agent, a microorganism (organism only visible with a microscope) that then multiplies and causes tissue damage, and may result in illness and disease. Health care professionals work to eliminate infection from the body and to prevent its spread to others. Careful hand hygiene is essential to prevent **cross-contamination.** Box 16-1 presents vocabulary related to infection. Microorganisms that are capable of causing disease are called pathogens (Figure 16-1). Nonpathogenic organisms that are prevalent on and in the body are called *normal flora* (Table 16-1). These normal flora prevent more harmful microorganisms from colonizing and multiplying within the body. They do this by occupying receptor sites on cells, monopolizing the nutrients, and secreting substances that are toxic to other

Box 16-1 | Vocabulary Related to Infection

Aerobic: Needing oxygen to live and grow

Anaerobic: Able to live and grow only when oxygen is absent

Colonization: Microorganisms take up residence and grow

Cross-contamination: Transmission of infectious microorganisms from one person or object to another

Culture: Propagation of living organisms or tissue in special media conducive to their growth

Endotoxin: A heat-stable toxin associated with the outer membranes of certain gram-negative bacteria that is released when the cells are disrupted

Exudate: Fluid in or on tissue surfaces that has escaped from blood vessels in response to inflammation that contains protein and cellular debris

Gram-negative: Bacteria that lose the stain in Gram's method of staining

Gram-positive: Bacteria that retain the stain in Gram's method of staining

Hospital-associated infection: Infection acquired during hospitalization

Host: An animal or plant that harbors and provides sustenance for another organism (a parasite)

Infection: Invasion and multiplication in body tissues of microorganisms that cause cellular injury

Inflammation: Localized response caused by injury or destruction of tissues that serves to contain the injurious agent and injured tissue

Leukocytosis: Increase in the number of leukocytes in the blood, resulting from infection or other causes

Phagocytes: Cells capable of ingesting particulate matter (e.g., macrophages)

Phagocytosis: The engulfing of microorganisms and foreign particles by phagocytes

Spores: Oval bodies formed within bacteria as a resting stage during the life cycle of the cell; characterized by resistance to environmental changes (heat, humidity, or cold)

Toxin: A poison; a poisonous protein produced by certain bacteria

Vector: Carrier that transports an infective agent from one host to another, such as animals, insects, and rodents

Virulence: Degree to which a microorganism can cause infection in the host or invade the host

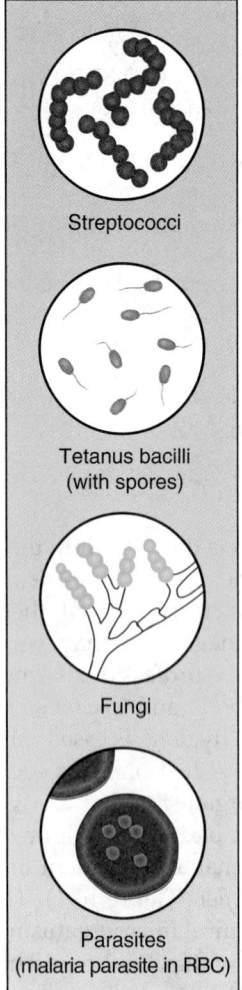

FIGURE **16-1** Pathogenic microorganisms. (Key: *RBC,* Red blood cell.)

Streptococci

Tetanus bacilli (with spores)

Fungi

Parasites (malaria parasite in RBC)

Table 16-1 | Normal Flora of the Body*

SITE	NORMAL FLORA
Upper respiratory tract (nose, mouth, throat)	Staphylococci
	Corynebacteria
	Streptococcus pyogenes (group A)
	Neisseria sp.
	Streptococci (*viridans* group)
	Enterobacter sp.
	Haemophilus
	Klebsiella sp.
	Lactobacilli
	Various types of anaerobes
Skin	*Staphylococcus aureus*
	Staphylococcus epidermidis
	Corynebacteria
	Yeasts
Small bowel and colon	*Enterobacter* species (coliforms)
	Bacteroides species
	Streptococcus faecalis (enterococci or group D)
	Clostridium perfringens
	Anaerobes
Vagina	*Lactobacillus* sp.
	Staphylococcus epidermidis
	Alpha-hemolytic streptococci
	Enterococci
	Enterobacteriaceae
	Many types of anaerobes

*The lower respiratory tract, central nervous system, bladder, and upper urinary tract are normally sterile (no microorganisms present).

microorganisms. Some pathogenic microorganisms produce harmful **toxins** and others release **endotoxins.** Endotoxins are responsible for the symptoms seen in botulism, tetanus, diphtheria, and *Escherichia coli* infection.

INFECTIOUS AGENTS

Bacteria

Bacteria are single-cell microorganisms lacking a nucleus that reproduce anywhere from every few minutes up to several weeks. Bacteria are classified according to their need for oxygen, their shape, and their Gram-staining properties. **Aerobic bacteria need oxygen to grow and thrive. Anaerobic bacteria can grow only when oxygen is not present.** The Gram stain technique helps classify bacteria. For a Gram stain, bacteria placed on a slide are stained and then treated with a contrasting dye; those retaining the stain are **gram positive** and those losing the stain and taking up the counterstain are **gram negative.** Many gram-negative bacteria are more dangerous than gram-positive bacteria because they may produce an endotoxin that can cause hemorrhagic shock and severe diarrhea and can alter resistance to other bacterial infection. Classification of bacteria according to their shape, or *morphology,* is based on whether they belong to one of three main groups. *Cocci* are round, *bacilli* are rod-shaped, and *spirochetes* are spiral or corkscrew-shaped. Some grow in chains (streptococci), some in pairs (diplococci), and some in clusters (staphylococci).

Final identification is by chemical testing of the bacteria grown by **culture.** To culture the bacteria, the infected body secretion is transferred to a medium in which it can grow. Sensitivity tests are then performed to determine which antibiotic (chemical substance that can kill or alter the growth of microorganisms) is most effective against the bacteria.

When culture results show that a drug-resistant organism is responsible for an infection, extreme care must be taken to prevent the spread of the organism. The four most common multidrug-resistant organisms are (1) methicillin-resistant *Staphylococcus aureus* (MRSA); (2) vancomycin-resistant *Enterococcus* (VRE); (3) extended-spectrum beta-lactamase–producing (ESBL) gonorrhea (*Neisseria gonorrhoeae*); and (4) *Clostridium difficile* (C. diff). There is a new quick test, the BD GeneOhm StaphSR Assay, that identifies MRSA bacterium in 2 hours. It is performed on a blood sample. Penicillin-resistant *Streptococcus pneumoniae* causes pneumonia. These organisms, and especially MRSA, are being contracted outside the hospitals now and are an increasing problem (Health Promotion Points 16-1). Patients must be educated about the correct use and possible misuse of antimicrobial (killing or suppressing growth of microorganisms) agents. Encourage each patient to take the entire antibiotic prescription as ordered by the heath care provider

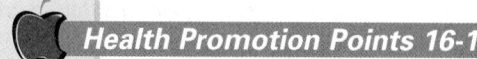
Health Promotion Points 16-1

Preventing Spread of MRSA

To prevent the spread of methicillin-resistant Staphylococcus aureus *(MRSA) in your community:*
- Wash hands frequently; use an alcohol-based rub when not close to running water.
- Keep cuts and abrasions clean and covered with a bandage until healed.
- Avoid sharing personal items such as razors, towels, make-up, etc.
- Avoid contact with other people's bandages or wounds.

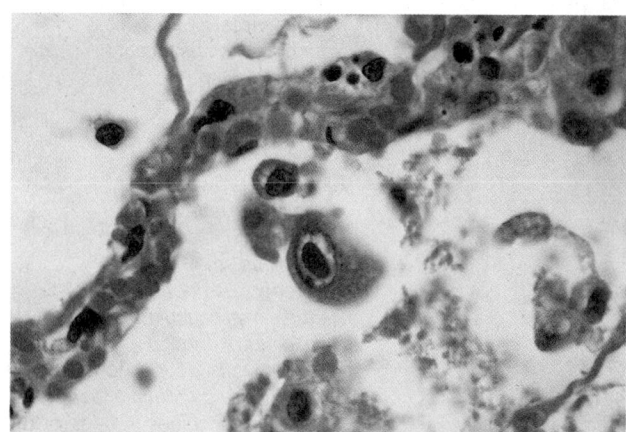

FIGURE **16-2** Electron microscope view of viruses.

for an infection. Taking only part of the prescription prevents the killing of all of the microorganisms responsible for the infection. This gives them a chance to mutate and develop drug resistance. Consistent use of Standard Precautions plus any Transmission-Based Precautions (e.g., Contact or Droplet Precautions) is essential, especially when a drug-resistant organism is present.

Prions

Prions are protein particles that lack nucleic acids and are not inactivated by usual methods for destroying viruses. They do not trigger an immune response, but cause degenerative neurologic disease such as variant Creutzfeldt-Jakob disease (mad cow disease).

Viruses

Viruses are extremely small and can be seen only with an electron microscope (Figure 16-2). They are composed of particles of nucleic acids, either DNA or RNA, with a coat of protein, and in some cases a membranous envelope. **Viruses can grow and replicate only within a living cell.** Once inside cells, viruses can trigger an immune reaction or damage cells in other ways. Their survival and multiplication are dependent upon host tissue. Viruses are identified in the laboratory by fluorescent techniques, electron microscopy, and tissue culture.

Table 16-2 *Disease-Producing Organisms (presented in order of increasing complexity)*

ORGANISM CLASS	COMMON EXAMPLES	COMMON DISEASE MANIFESTATIONS
Bacteria	*Staphylococcus* sp.	Superficial skin infections, osteomyelitis, pneumonia, bacteremia
	Streptococcus sp.	Pharyngitis, skin infections, pneumonia
	Neisseria meningitidis	Meningitis
	Escherichia coli	Urinary tract infection
	Pseudomonas aeruginosa	Skin infection, otitis, urinary tract infection
Prions		Bovine spongiform encephalitis (BSE)/Creutzfeldt-Jakob disease, Kuru*
		Possible role in Alzheimer's disease, Parkinson's disease, and amyotrophic lateral sclerosis (ALS)†
Viruses	Poliovirus	Poliomyelitis
	Hepatitis A virus	Hepatitis
	Rhinovirus	Common cold
	Influenza A virus	Influenza
	Mumps virus	Mumps
Protozoa	*Entamoeba histolytica*	Diarrhea, colitis
	Plasmodium sp.	Malaria
	Leishmania sp.	Fever, weight loss, cutaneous lesions
	Toxoplasma gondii	Chorioretinitis, encephalitis
Rickettsiae	*Rickettsia rickettsii*	Rocky Mountain spotted fever
	Rickettsia prowazekii	Typhus
	Coxiella burnetii	Q fever
Fungi	*Candida albicans*	Thrush, vaginitis
	Aspergillus sp.	Sinusitis, brain abscess
	Cryptococcus neoformans	Meningitis, pneumonia
	Histoplasma capsulatum	Pneumonia
	Coccidioides immitis	Pneumonia
	Pneumocystis jiroveci (formerly *carinii*)	Pneumonia
Helminths	*Ancylostoma duodenale* (hookworm)	Anemia
	Ascaris lumbricoides (roundworm)	Intestinal obstruction
	Enterobius vermicularis (pinworm)	Anal pruritus
	Schistosoma sp. (blood flukes)	Hydronephrosis
	Taenia solium (pork tapeworm)	Epilepsy from cysticercosis
Chlamydiae	*Chlamydia trachomatis*	Trachoma, lymphogranuloma venereum, conjunctivitis
	Chlamydia psittaci	Psittacosis (parrot fever)
Mycoplasmas	*Mycoplasma pneumoniae*	Pneumonia
	Ureaplasma urealyticum	Urethritis
	Mycoplasma hominis	Pyelonephritis, pelvic inflammatory disease

From Ignatavicius, D.D., & Workman, M.L. (2006). *Medical-Surgical Nursing: Critical Thinking for Collaborative Care* (5th ed., p. 508). Philadelphia: Elsevier Saunders.
*Mastrianni, J.A., & Roos, R.P. (2000). The prion diseases. *Seminars in Neurology, 20,* 337-352.
†Prusiner, S. (1999). Nobelist believes prions may be at root of Alzheimer's, Parkinson's, ALS. *Reuter's Health,* October 20. Available at www.reutershealth.com. (Dr. Stanley Prusiner is a 1997 Nobel Prize winner for the discovery of prions.)

Protozoa

Protozoa are one-celled microscopic organisms belonging to the animal kingdom. Protozoa that are pathogenic to humans include the *Plasmodium* species that causes malaria; *Entamoeba histolytica,* which causes amebic dysentery; and other strains capable of causing diarrhea.

Rickettsia

Rickettsia are small round or rod-shaped microorganisms that are transmitted by the bites of lice, ticks, fleas, and mites that act as **vectors.** They multiply only in host cells. Rocky Mountain spotted fever and typhus are caused by rickettsias.

Fungi

Fungi are tiny, primitive organisms of the plant kingdom that contain no chlorophyll. Yeasts and molds are members of this group. Fungi feed on living plants and animals and decaying organic material and thrive in warm, moist environments. Fungi reproduce by means of **spores.** In humans, fungal infections are called *mycoses.* When the balance of normal flora is altered by antibiotic therapy, fungal infection may occur. Common fungal infections are vaginal candidiasis and athlete's foot (*tinea pedis*).

Helminths

Helminths are parasitic worms or flukes and belong to the animal kingdom. Pinworms, which mostly affect children, are the most common helminths worldwide. Roundworms and tapeworms are other helminths.

Other Infectious Agents

Several types of organisms differ enough in structure to fall outside the above classifications. Mycoplasmas are very small organisms without a cell wall. They cause infections of the respiratory tract or the genital tract. *Mycoplasma pneumoniae* is an example. *Chlamydia*, another type of organism, affects the genitourinary and reproductive tract and has become increasingly more common in the last 20 years. In countries where hygiene is poor, *Chlamydia trachomatis* is responsible for trachoma, an eye disease that can cause blindness. In this country, the same organism causes a significant amount of sexually transmitted infection (Table 16-2).

PROCESS OF INFECTION

The process by which an infectious disease is spread from one person to another can be thought of as a continuous chain. Each link must be present in its proper order for the chain to remain intact and for the infection to be passed on to someone else. Figure 16-3 shows how the links of the chain connect and infection occurs.

CAUSATIVE AGENT (LINK ONE)

A causative agent is any microorganism or biologic agent capable of causing disease. These agents include bacteria, viruses, protozoa, rickettsia, fungi, and helminths.

Some microorganisms are more virulent than others. Characteristics that affect **virulence** are ability to (1) adhere to mucosal surfaces or skin, (2) penetrate mucous membranes, (3) multiply once in the body, (4) secrete harmful enzymes or toxins, and (5) resist **phagocytosis** (destruction by white blood cells). Microorganisms differ in structure and characteristics (see Figure 16-1).

Pathogenic microorganisms must be destroyed or rendered harmless in order to remove this link from the chain. Disinfection and sterilization (process of destroying all microorganisms and pathogenic products) are methods used to destroy pathogens. Procedures for disinfection should be utilized in all areas in which patients are receiving treatment.

The most effective means for destroying viruses and all other kinds of microorganisms is to expose them to moist heat at a high temperature for 16 to 20 minutes. This is accomplished by using a special machine called an autoclave.

The Centers for Disease Control and Prevention (CDC), a government agency (www.cdc.gov), provides a wealth of information on all aspects of infectious diseases and their prevention and control.

RESERVOIR (LINK TWO)

Reservoirs are places in which microorganisms are found. Reservoirs can be infected wounds, human or animal waste, animals and insects, contaminated (made unclean) food and water, and the person with an infection. Assorted precautions are used to prevent the spread of infection from the reservoir. Good hand hygiene is one of the most effective ways to prevent

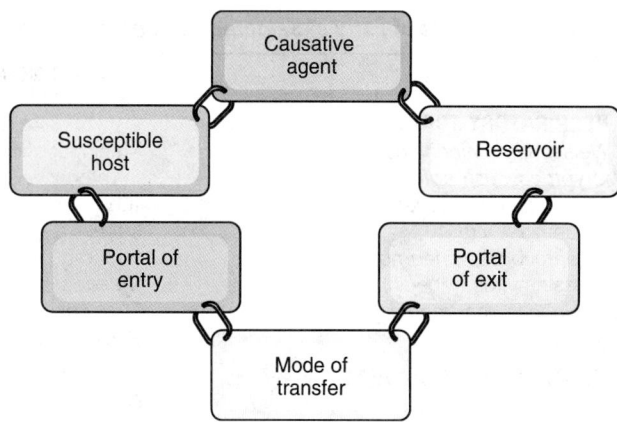

FIGURE **16-3** The infection chain.

the spread of microorganisms. Using sterile (without pathologic organisms) technique to insert an indwelling urinary catheter helps prevent the transfer of normal flora from the skin and mucous membranes into the sterile bladder, where it could cause an infection.

PORTAL OF EXIT (LINK THREE)

The portal of exit is the route by which a pathogen leaves the body of its host. An example of a portal of exit is the gastrointestinal tract, through which the feces may transport the typhoid bacillus from an infected person. The respiratory tract can be a portal of exit when microorganisms are released with coughing or sneezing. Measles, mumps, pulmonary tuberculosis, and influenza can be transmitted by exit from the respiratory tract. The skin and mucous membranes can also serve as a portal of exit when an open wound exists.

Portal-of-exit transmission can be interrupted by identifying and treating patients who are infected with pathogens. Isolation techniques and barrier precautions that include the proper handling and disposal of secretions, urine and feces, and **exudate** can prevent transfer of pathogens. CDC recommendations for Transmission-Based Precautions and isolation techniques are based on scientific evidence that has proven how various pathogens are transmitted. Chapter 17 contains the specific recommendations.

MODE OF TRANSFER (LINK FOUR)

Modes of transfer of pathogens include (1) direct personal contact with body excreta or drainage from an ulcer, infected wound, boil, or chancre; (2) indirect contact with contaminated inanimate objects (called *fomites*), such as needles, drinking and eating utensils, dressings, and hospital equipment; (3) vectors such as fleas, ticks, mosquitoes, and other insects that harbor infectious agents and transmit infection to humans through bites and stings; (4) droplet infection, or contamination by the aerosol route through sneezing and coughing; and (5) spread of infection from one part of the body to another.

Table 16-3 | *Portals of Entry of Selected Pathogenic Organisms*

INFECTING ORGANISMS	RESULTANT DISEASES
RESPIRATORY TRACT	
Neisseria meningitides	Meningococcal pneumonia, meningococcal meningitis, meningococcemia
Cryptococcus neoformans	Cryptococcal meningitis, cryptococcal pneumonia
Mycobacterium tuberculosis	Tuberculosis
Influenza A virus	Influenza
Streptococcus pneumoniae	Pneumococcal pneumonia
Measles virus (rubeola)	Measles
Legionella pneumophila	Legionnaires' disease
Varicella-zoster virus	Chickenpox
GASTROINTESTINAL TRACT	
Salmonella enteritidis	Gastroenteritis
Salmonella typhi	Typhoid fever
Clostridium botulinum	Botulism
Poliovirus	Poliomyelitis
Hepatitis A virus	Hepatitis A
Escherichia coli O157:H7	Possibly, hemolytic uremic syndrome
GENITOURINARY TRACT	
Neisseria gonorrhoeae	Gonorrhea
Chlamydia trachomatis	Lymphogranuloma venereum, cervicitis, urethritis, endometritis
Enterobacteriaceae (*E. coli, Klebsiella* sp., *Serratia* sp., *Proteus* sp.)	Urinary tract infections
INTACT SKIN OR MUCOUS MEMBRANES	
Rhinovirus	Common cold
Respiratory syncytial virus	Pneumonia, bronchiolitis, tracheobronchitis
Schistosoma sp.	Schistosome dermatitis (swimmer's disease)
Herpes simplex virus	Oral or genital herpes
BLOODSTREAM	
Hepatitis B or C viruses	Hepatitis B or C
Plasmodium sp.	Malaria
Clostridium tetani	Tetanus
Human immunodeficiency virus	Acquired immunodeficiency syndrome

From Ignatavicius, D.D., & Workman, M.L. (2006). *Medical-Surgical Nursing: Critical Thinking for Collaborative Care* (5th ed., p. 509). Philadelphia: Elsevier Saunders.

The mode of transmission can be interrupted by effective hand hygiene, proper disinfection and sterilization of medical equipment, use of aseptic (free of microorganisms) technique in performing procedures and diagnostic tests, and use of Standard Precautions to prevent contamination. Teaching patients to cover the mouth when sneezing or coughing, to dispose of soiled tissues correctly, to wash the hands after contact with potentially contaminated items, and to avoid people who have an infection can reduce transmission of pathogens.

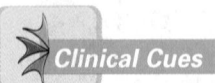
Clinical Cues

Current CDC recommendations are to sneeze or cough into the bended elbow rather than covering the mouth with the hands. This way spread of the respiratory droplets is prevented and the hands that will be touching things are not contaminated.

Controlling insects with abatement programs, such as for mosquito control, and air filtration in health care facilities are other methods of reducing transmission of pathogens.

? *Think Critically About . . .* Hepatitis A is spread through the oral-fecal route. In what ways could hepatitis A virus be spread in a restaurant if one of the employees is the reservoir?

PORTAL OF ENTRY (LINK FIVE)

Pathogens can enter the body through the eyes, mouth, nose, trachea, skin, and mucous membranes. Consuming food or water that is contaminated with disease-causing microorganisms is an example of how entrance can occur. Breathing in droplets containing pathogens and contracting a virus through broken skin or abraded mucous membrane are examples for portals of entry. Table 16-3 shows some of the pathogenic organisms that enter through the various body portals.

Using only sterile and clean items when caring for patients reduces the entry of pathogens. Barrier precautions (gloves, masks, condoms), safe handling of food and water, good personal hygiene, avoidance of high-risk behaviors, and protection from insect bites and stings can prevent entry of microorganisms.

Table 16-4 *Factors that Increase Susceptibility to Infection*

FACTOR	CONSEQUENCE
Age	The elderly and the very young are more susceptible to infection, probably because of declining or immature immune function, respectively.
Malnutrition	Poor nutrition interferes with cell growth and replacement, which contributes to decreased immune function.
Excessive stress or fatigue	These states seem to interfere with the body's normal defense mechanisms.
Low leukocyte (WBC) count	Fewer white blood cells (WBCs) are available to fight infection.
Altered defense mechanisms	Body damage from trauma disrupts the natural defense mechanism of the skin and mucous membranes, allowing entry to microorganisms.
Alcoholism	Has an inhibiting effect on the immune system.
Chronic illness	Upsets the normal homeostatic balance within the body, impairing the normal defense mechanisms. Serious illness taxes the immune system, causing greater susceptibility to other pathogens.
Indwelling tubes or equipment	Fracture pins, catheters, intravenous (IV) cannulas, feeding tubes, heart valves, and hip prostheses all provide either a portal of entry for microorganisms or a place for colonization of microorganisms.
Immunosuppressive treatment, chemotherapy, or corticosteroid treatment	Immunosuppressive treatment or chemotherapy depresses the immune system or harms the bone marrow, decreasing the number of leukocytes and macrophages. Corticosteroids depress the inflammatory response, inhibiting one of the body's defense mechanisms.

SUSCEPTIBLE HOST (LINK SIX)

A human **host** may be susceptible by virtue of age, state of health, or broken skin. Measures are used to prevent exposure to infectious agents and to improve a person's state of health by teaching good health and hygiene habits. Immunization to help protect against influenza or pneumococcal pneumonia is another means of decreasing susceptibility.

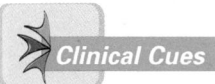

Clinical Cues

Influenza immunization is recommended yearly for all health care workers, the elderly, the very young, and those who have chronic illnesses.

Susceptible hosts can be protected by using aseptic techniques, barrier precautions, and protective isolation (see Chapter 17). Proper nutrition and a healthy lifestyle also increase resistance to infection. Table 16-4 lists factors that increase susceptibility to infectious agents. Table 16-5 shows ways in which the chain of infection can be broken at each link.

Susceptibility of the Elderly

Many factors can place the elderly person at higher risk of infection. Poor nutrition, poor mobility, poor hygiene, chronic illness, and physiologic changes all contribute to this risk. Table 16-6 presents the physiologic factors involved. Elderly persons are hospitalized more frequently for problems due to a chronic illness or for treatment after a fall than younger people. This places them at higher risk for a health care–associated infection. **Health care–associated infections** are acquired by patients in health care facilities when microorganisms are transferred to the patient by contaminated objects or infected people.

? Think Critically About . . . Which organisms are you most frequently exposed to that could cause disease? How can you protect yourself against disease-causing organisms?

BODY DEFENSES AGAINST INFECTION

The body has many natural defenses against invasion of pathogens. Intact skin serves as a *first line of defense* against harmful agents in the environment. It functions as a protective barrier for the underlying tissues. Through excretion of sweat as well as lactic and fatty acids from the sebaceous glands, growth of bacteria is inhibited.

Secretions from the mucous membranes lining the respiratory, gastrointestinal, and reproductive tracts contain an abundance of the enzyme *lysozyme*, which is bactericidal. This enzyme is also found in tears and saliva. Cilia, which line the respiratory tract, trap microorganisms and debris (dead tissue or foreign matter) and propel them up and out of the body with a wavelike action. The bones protect the more delicate and vital organs from outside trama. The bone marrow produces defensive blood cells.

The Kupffer cells in the liver destroy bacteria that have found their way into the portal liver circulation. Only about 1% of bacteria that enter the portal circulation from the intestines pass through the liver into the general circulation. The intestinal system is a major por-

Table 16-5 | *Breaking the Chain of Infection*

LINK	WAYS TO BREAK THE CHAIN	INTERVENTIONS
RESERVOIR		
Infected patient	Prevent transfer of microorganisms	Proper hand hygiene
		Use of gloves
		Use of Standard Precautions
		Isolation techniques
PORTAL OF EXIT		
Secretions	Prevent contamination	Thorough hand hygiene
Feces		Use of Standard Precautions
Blood		Not recapping needles
Urine		Handling sharps correctly
Sputum		Containing contaminated materials
		Disinfection
		Following medical aseptic practices
MODE OF TRANSFER		
Hands	Prevent contamination	Use of Standard Precautions
Contaminated food	Eliminate vectors	Proper hand hygiene
Contaminated supplies and		Sterilization, proper cleaning, and refrigeration of foods
other objects		Disinfection
		Proper disposal
		Surgical asepsis
		Isolation techniques
		Pest control
ENTRANCE		
Mouth	Put only clean things in mouth	Keeping objects out of mouth
Break in skin	Protect skin	Good hygiene practices
Mucous membranes	Protect mucous membranes	Good skin care
		Thorough cleansing of skin before an invasive procedure
		Covering skin breaks
		Use of Standard Precautions: goggles, face shield, or mask; gloves; gown
HOST		
Susceptible person	Protect natural body defenses by	Assessing for degree of risk of infection
	• Good nutrition	Promoting natural body defenses
	• Good hygiene	Protective isolation
	• Adequate sleep	Use of Standard Precautions
	• Decreased stress	Proper hand hygiene

tal of entry for pathogens, and the liver is an essential part of the body's defense system. The liver also detoxifies harmful chemicals by isolating various substances and facilitating their breakdown and excretion from the body.

Gastric secretions such as hydrochloric acid easily destroy ingested pathogens. Evacuation of feces flushes bacteria from the intestine, and the formation and elimination of urine flushes the urinary system.

The body's *second line of defense* helps destroy pathogens that escape the first line of defense. This includes the mechanisms of fever, leukocytosis, phagocytosis, inflammation, and the action of interferon (biologic response modifier that affects cellular growth).

The body automatically raises its temperature in response to infection. Fever, because of the effect of heat, slows the growth of many pathogens until other body defenses can be mobilized.

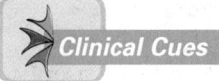 **Clinical Cues**

A fever should not be treated right away unless it is dangerously high. In many instances, it is not desirable to lower the body temperature to normal. Rest and increased fluids are the correct treatment for the first few days. Fever is a natural defense mechanism.

Leukocytes, which are white blood cells (WBCs), are released in response to microorganisms, particularly bacteria, entering the body. This increased production or release of leukocytes is termed **leukocytosis.** They travel through the capillary walls out into the tissues to engulf the invader. The **phagocytes,** located in the lymphatic tissue, the alveoli of the lungs, the gastrointestinal system, the spleen, and the liver, work to destroy or inactivate them. The macrophages assist in this process by removing cellular debris, engulfing

Table 16-6 | *Increased Susceptibility of the Elderly to Infection*

The elderly are at higher risk of infection than the younger adult. Any elderly person with a chronic illness is experiencing increased stress on the body and a strain on the body's defense mechanisms from that disease; this makes the person more susceptible to other infections. The following factors also increase the risk of infection. You can institute certain interventions to try to decrease that risk.

AREA	FACTOR	NURSING INTERVENTION
Homeostasis	Lose homeostatic state more easily than younger adult as a result of loss of functioning cells in all body organs with aging.	Protect from exposure to pathogens. Promote good nutrition, exercise, and adequate rest to boost resistance to disease.
Immune function	Both immediate and delayed immune response are decreased or altered.	Protect from exposure to pathogens. Immunize against influenza and pneumonia. Promote good nutrition to boost immune system.
Respiratory function	Impaired cough mechanism and impaired function of cilia decrease ability to expel foreign substances and mucus from the lungs, predisposing the person to respiratory infection.	Discourage smoking. Encourage deep breathing and intake of fluid to keep lung secretions thinned.
	Decreased macrophage activity in the lungs.	Encourage good oral hygiene to decrease potential for colonization of trachea and lungs with microorganisms.
	Less ability to expand the thorax predisposes to atelectasis after surgery.	Assist postoperative patients to maintain a semiupright position (semi-Fowler's) to aid lung expansion. Encourage use of incentive spirometer, deep breathing, and coughing. Ambulate as soon as possible.
Skin	Decreased elasticity, increased dryness, and decreased vascular supply make the skin susceptible to injury or breakdown and slower to repair. Breaks allow entry of microorganisms.	Instruct in appropriate skin care. Keep skin well lubricated. Prevent abrasions by using a lift sheet or a trapeze bar for positioning. Inspect skin each shift for pressure areas.
Gastrointestinal system	Decreased secretion of stomach acid and therefore decreased destruction in the stomach of microorganisms ingested in food and drink.	Promote good oral hygiene to prevent swallowing pathogenic microorganisms.
	Pancreatic enzyme secretion is decreased, causing less destruction of microorganisms in the gastrointestinal (GI) tract.	Instruct in proper preparation and storage of food to prevent GI infection.
Urinary tract	Prostatic hypertrophy, cystocele, rectocele, and degeneration of nerves to bladder cause urine stasis in bladder as a result of incomplete emptying. Stasis predisposes to urinary tract infection.	Encourage intake of sufficient fluid to keep urine dilute. Encourage intake of cranberry juice and other foods that keep urine acidic, which will discourage the growth of microorganisms.

and destroying bacteria and viruses, and removing metabolic waste products. Some phagocytes are called *tissue macrophages;* others, which are concerned with immunity, are the *lymphocytic cells.* Phagocytosis is part of the inflammatory response, another defense mechanism of the body. When infection and resultant leukocytosis occur, the WBC count is elevated. If the neutrophil count is decreased on the differential WBC count, while the monocyte count and lymphocyte counts are elevated, the cause of infection is probably viral. Increase in the percentage of basophils may indicate parasitic infection. A large increase in the percentage of monocytes often indicates a bacterial infection.

Interferons are produced in response to viral invasion of the cell. They stimulate antiviral proteins that prevent replication of viruses. Interferons can attack a wide variety of viruses, inhibiting or destroying them. The interferons stimulate the immune system, increase resistance to viral invasion, and interfere with viral replication.

INFLAMMATORY RESPONSE

Inflammation is an immediate response of the body to any kind of injury to its cells and tissues. The inflammatory response can be induced by any mechanical, chemical, or infectious disease–producing factor that injures cells of the body. **Inflammation is a localized protective response brought on by injury or destruction of tissues.** The blood vessels dilate, bringing more blood to the damaged area, causing redness, warmth, and edema. The basic purposes of the inflammatory response are to (1) neutralize and destroy harmful agents, (2) limit their spread to other tissues in the body, and (3) prepare the damaged tissues for repair. The chemicals *histamine* and *serotonin* are released. These chemicals act on the walls of the capillaries, making them more permeable so that

Local inflammation

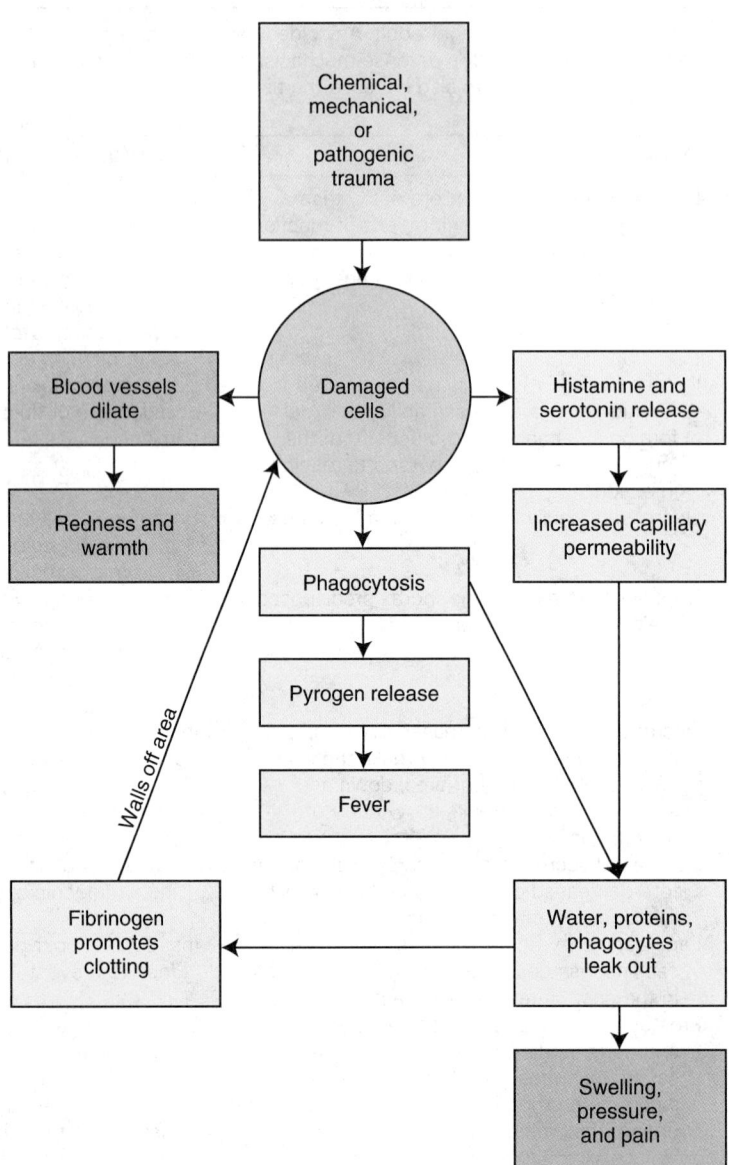

CONCEPT MAP **16-1** The inflammatory response.

water, proteins, and defensive cells can pass out of the blood and into the fluid surrounding the damaged cells. This leakage of fluid is responsible for localized swelling, which in turn causes increased pressure and pain. Fibrinogen promotes clotting, blocking the lymphatic vessels. This results in a walling off of the area that delays spread of bacteria, toxins, and other harmful agents to other parts of the body (Concept Map 16-1). *Pus,* the debris that sometimes results from the inflammatory process, may accumulate at the site. Phagocytes attracted to the damaged tissue begin their work.

IMMUNE RESPONSE

The immune response is the *third line of defense* against pathogenic organisms. Microorganisms and other substances that do not belong in the body, such as pollen, are recognized as foreign invaders and trigger an immune response (reaction of the body to substances

interpreted as nonself). For example, macrophages in the lungs engulf bacteria, dust particles, and any other foreign material that might threaten to damage the lung tissues. If the foreign particles are not digestible, the leukocytes and later macrophages in the alveoli help wall them off, thereby preventing their spread to other tissues. An example of this process is the localizing of tubercle bacilli that have not been destroyed by the body's other defenses. Pulmonary tuberculosis bacilli are walled off, preventing their dissemination.

The immune system response is specific to the type of invader. There are unique antigens on the surface of an individual's cells that aid the immune system in distinguishing *self* from *nonself* (invaders) so it can destroy foreign material *(antigens).* Once exposed to a microorganism, the body will produce *antibodies* against that invader. In this way, *naturally acquired immunity* occurs. Every antigen stimulates formation of a specific type of

Table 16-7 | *Comparison of Medical Asepsis and Surgical Asepsis*

FACTOR	MEDICAL ASEPSIS	SURGICAL ASEPSIS
Patient	Has infection, lowered resistance to other infections	Potential host; lowered resistance makes more susceptible
Reservoir of infection	The patient	Other people and the environment
Objective of barriers	Confine organisms to the room, unit, or locale	Prevent organism from reaching patient or area
Equipment and supplies	Disinfect, sterilize, or dispose of after contact with patient; use clean materials	Disinfect or sterilize before contact with patient; use sterile materials
Nurse's protective attire: gown, mask, gloves	Use clean attire to protect worker from organisms; discard after contact with patient	Sterile attire to protect patient; remedy if contaminated
Goal of nursing action	Confine organisms and prevent spread of infection to others	Reduce number of organisms and prevent spread of infection to patient
	(Medical asepsis reduces the number of microorganisms or contains them to reduce risk of transmission.)	(Surgical asepsis keeps an area or objects free of all microorganisms for a period of time.)

antibody. The next time that same microorganism invades the body, the antibodies respond and attempt to destroy it. Some types of naturally acquired immunity last a lifetime, but others last only a short time.

Passive acquired immunity occurs when a person is given an antitoxin or antiserum that contains antibodies or antitoxins that have been developed in another person. Tetanus antitoxin is an example of a substance that provides passive immunity. It protects a person from the current invasion of microorganisms but does not provide lasting immunity.

Naturally acquired passive immunity occurs when the fetus receives antibodies from the mother through placental blood before birth. This type of immunity is also acquired by the breast-feeding infant. The immunity is temporary and lasts only until the infant's own immune system matures enough to function properly.

Artificially acquired immunity is achieved through injection of vaccines or immunizing substances that contain dead or inactive microorganisms or their toxins. The vaccine prompts the body to produce antibodies. Vaccinations against polio, measles, hepatitis B, influenza, tetanus, and diphtheria provide this type of immunity.

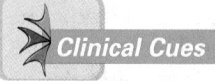
Clinical Cues

All patients should be asked during a health assessment whether they have had a tetanus immunization within the past 10 years. If they have not, seek an order for the immunization as long as the patient is healthy enough to receive it. Tetanus can be deadly.

Artificially acquired passive immunity is provided by injection with antibodies derived from the infected blood of people or animals. Serum immune globulin is often used for this purpose and is given to people who have been exposed to hepatitis A virus or mumps and have not been previously immunized. The injection provides antibodies that will protect the person for a short period of time.

? *Think Critically About . . .* What alterations could you make in your lifestyle to make yourself less susceptible to infection?

ASEPSIS AND CONTROL OF MICROORGANISMS

MEDICAL ASEPSIS AND SURGICAL ASEPSIS

Asepsis is the practice of making the environment and objects free of microorganisms. Two types of asepsis are practiced within health care agencies. The first, medical asepsis, is the practice of reducing the number of organisms present or reducing the risk for transmission of organisms. It prevents reinfection of the patient and the spread of infection from person to person. It involves cleanliness and is accomplished by protecting items in the environment from contamination and by disinfecting items that have been contaminated. Medical asepsis is referred to as *clean technique* because most, but not all, microorganisms are destroyed.

Surgical asepsis is the practice of preparing and handling materials in a way that prevents the patient's exposure to living microorganisms. Surgical asepsis is referred to as *sterile technique*. It involves sterilization of all instruments and inanimate equipment, as well as use of sterile supplies and sterile technique for procedures that invade the body and for wound care. Most microorganisms are destroyed. Timed hand scrubs may be used by the personnel working in the operating room to reduce the number of microorganisms on the skin, or a hand rub with an alcohol-based product may be used instead. Barrier garments are used to prevent spread of microorganisms between the health care personnel and the patient. The air in the operating room is filtered and exchanged at least 15 times an hour. The operating room must be thoroughly disinfected after each use. Table 16-7 compares medical and surgical asepsis. Techniques for surgical asepsis are covered in Chapter 37.

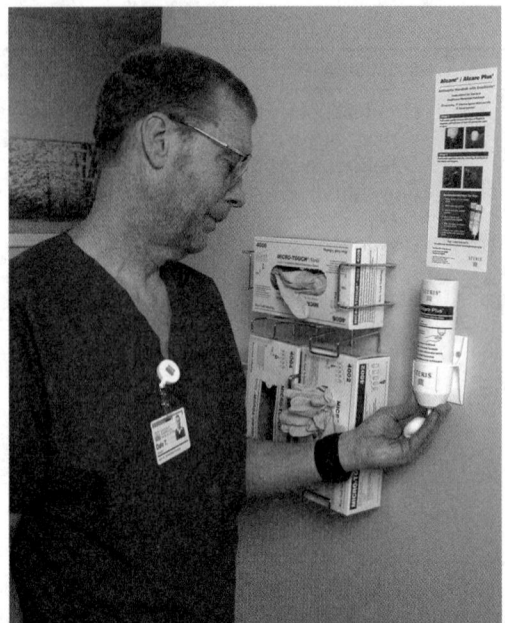

FIGURE **16-4** Nurse using an alcohol hand rub to cleanse the hands of microorganisms.

HAND HYGIENE

Hand hygiene is one of the most effective ways to reduce the number of microorganisms on the hands, thereby preventing the transfer of microorganisms from one object to another or from person to person by the nurse. Any person may harbor microorganisms that are harmless to that person but may be potentially harmful to another person if they gain a portal of entry.

Gloves should be used to prevent contact with any body fluids. **Health care workers must perform hand hygiene before and after giving care to a patient.** In 2005, the CDC concluded from research that alcohol hand rubs can be more effective than handwashing in ridding the hands of microorganisms (Centers for Disease Control, 2005). Many hospitals and health care agencies are providing alcohol hand rubs for personnel to use when hands **are not visibly contaminated** (Figure 16-4). Box 16-2 provides the overview of the new CDC Hand Hygiene Guidelines.

When hands are visibly soiled, the CDC recommends at least a 15-second vigorous washing using soap and friction under running water. The hands should be wet before adding the soap. Drying the hands thoroughly is very important. Skill 16-1 provides the steps for correct hand hygiene. For a surgical scrub, the hands are washed with soap and water first and then scrubbed with an FDA-compliant antimicrobial scrub agent or an FDA-compliant alcohol-based antiseptic hand rub agent. The procedure for surgical hand antisepsis is presented in Chapter 17 (Health Promotion Points 16-2).

You should not wear jewelry when you are providing patient care because microorganisms become lodged in the settings of stones, in the grooves of rings,

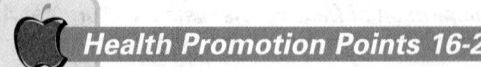

Basics of Hand Hygiene

Everyone should perform hand hygiene before eating and after using the bathroom, bedpan, or commode. Hands should be washed thoroughly after handling raw meat. Most supermarkets are providing sanitizing wipes to clean the grocery cart handle before using it. It is wise to perform hand hygiene after handling money.

and on the skin beneath the jewelry. The only exceptions are a plain wedding band and a watch with an expandable band that allows it to be pushed up above the wrist area for hand hygiene. Fingernails should be kept clean and short, both for patient safety and because it is easier to clean fully beneath a short nail. Polish, if used, should not be chipped because it could then harbor bacteria. No artificial nails, nail wraps, or nail jewelry should be worn. Proper hand care includes prevention of hangnails and skin abrasions, which provide a point of entry for bacteria into the body.

STANDARD PRECAUTIONS

Infectious disease can be controlled by interrupting the chain of infection at any link. This breaks the transmission cycle. Standard Precautions have been developed by the CDC to facilitate breaking the chain of infection. **These precautions protect both the nurse and the patient and are to be used for every patient contact;** they are listed in Box 16-3 on p. 225 and include the use of hand hygiene and personal protective equipment (PPE). PPE includes gloves, gowns, masks, protective eyewear, shoe covering, and hair covering.

Gown

A clean barrier gown that is impermeable to fluid is worn when there is a chance of being splashed with blood, body fluid, or other potentially infectious materials, or when these fluids may be aerosolized. The gown must be impermeable to water. The gown is removed after use, being careful not to contaminate the skin or clothing. Skill 16-2 on p. 226 explains how to put on and take off a barrier gown.

Mask

A mask is applied before entering the room if there is a chance that the nurse will be in contact with an airborne pathogen or splashed body fluids, such as when a patient is coughing or the nurse is performing endotracheal suctioning. The mask is placed over the nose and mouth and is secured in place by an elastic band or ties (Figure 16-5, p. 228). An N95 respirator mask is worn when entering an area where pulmonary tuberculosis or other dangerous airborne microorganisms are known to be present. N95 respirator masks must

Box 16-2 *Overview of CDC Hand Hygiene Guidelines*

The Centers for Disease Control and Prevention (CDC) recently released new recommendations for hand hygiene in health care settings. *Hand hygiene* is a term that applies to either handwashing with soap and water, use of an antiseptic alcohol-based hand rub, or surgical hand antisepsis (water and antiseptic agent). Evidence suggests that hand antisepsis—the cleansing of hands with an antiseptic hand rub—is more effective in reducing health care–associated infections than washing the hands with soap and water.

FOLLOW THESE GUIDELINES IN THE CARE OF *ALL* PATIENTS:
- Continue to wash hands with either a non-antimicrobial soap and water or an antimicrobial soap and water (see Skill 16-1, p. 222) whenever the hands are visibly soiled.
- Use an alcohol-based hand rub to routinely decontaminate the hands in the following clinical situations: (Note: if alcohol-based hand rubs are not available, the alternative is hand hygiene with soap and water.)
  - Before and after direct patient contact
  - After contact with a patient's intact skin (e.g., when taking a pulse or blood pressure or lifting and moving a patient)
  - Before donning sterile gloves when inserting central intravascular catheters
  - Before performing invasive procedures (e.g., urinary catheter insertion, nasotracheal suctioning) that do not require surgical asepsis
  - After contact with blood, body fluids, excretions or other potentially infectious materials, mucous membranes, nonintact skin, and wound dressings
  - If hands will be moving from a contaminated body site to a clean body site during patient care
  - After contact with inanimate objects (including medical equipment) in the immediate vicinity of the patient
  - After removing gloves
- Before and after eating and after using a restroom, wash hands with a health care facility–approved alcohol-based hand rub or soap and water.
- Antimicrobial-impregnated wipes (i.e., towelettes) are not a substitute for using an alcohol-based hand rub or antimicrobial soap.
- If contact with spores (e.g., *Clostridium difficile* or to *Bacillus anthracis*) is likely to have occurred, hands must be washed with soap and water. The physical action of washing and rinsing hands is recommended because alcohols, chlorhexidine products, iodophors, and other antiseptic agents have poor activity against spores.

- Do not wear artificial fingenails or extensions if duties include direct contact with patients at high risk for infection and associated adverse outcomes (e.g., those in ICUs or operating rooms)

METHOD FOR DECONTAMINATING HANDS:
When using an alcohol-based hand rub, apply product to palm of one hand and rub hands together, covering all surfaces of hands and fingers, until hands are dry. Follow the manufacturer's recommendations regarding the volume of product to use. Note how many applications of the product are permitted before handwashing with soap and water must be performed. Most products state no more than 5 applications before washing the hands with soap and water.

FOLLOW THESE GUIDELINES FOR SURGICAL HAND ANTISEPSIS:
- Surgical hand antisepsis reduces the resident microbial count on the hands to a minimum. See Skill 17-1, p. 244, for the surgical hand scrub procedure.
- The CDC recommends using an antimicrobial soap, and to scrub hands and forearms up to the elbows for the length of time recommended by the manufacturer, usually 2 to 5 minutes. Refer to agency policy for time required.
- When using an alcohol-based surgical hand scrub product with persistent antimicrobial activity, follow the manufacturer's instructions. Before applying the alcohol solution, prewash hands and forearms with a non-antimicrobial soap, clean under the nails, and rinse and dry hands and forearms completely. After application of the alcohol-based product as recommended, allow hands and forearms to dry thoroughly before donning sterile gloves.

GENERAL RECOMMENDATIONS FOR HAND HYGIENE
- Use hand lotions or creams to minimize the occurrence of irritant contact dermatitis associated with hand antisepsis or hand hygiene.
- Do not wear artificial fingernails or extenders when having direct contact with patients at high risk (e.g., those in intensive care units or operating rooms).
- Keep natural nails tips less than ¼-inch long.
- Wear gloves when contact with blood, body fluids, or other potentially infectious materials, mucous membranes, and nonintact skin could occur.
- Remove gloves after caring for a patient (see Steps 16-1, p. 229). Do not wear the same pair of gloves for the care of more than one patient, and do not wash gloves between uses with different patients.

Modified from Centers for Disease Control and Prevention. (2008). *Standard Precautions*. Retrieved from www.cdc.gov/ncidod/dhqp/gl_isolation_standard.html.

be approved by the Occupational Safety and Health Administration (OSHA). They prevent passage of 95% of particulate matter. There are several styles of both types of masks. Masks should be removed, handling only the elastic band or ties, and discarded when not in use; they should not be left hanging around the neck. **The mask should be changed any time it becomes moist.**

Protective Eyewear

Protective eyewear is worn to prevent fluid from entering the eye area and coming in contact with the mucosa or surface of the eye through splattering or aerosolization. Eyewear may be in the form of goggles, a face shield, or glasses with side and top pieces. Protective eyewear may be disposable or durable. If of the durable variety, the eyewear should be disinfected after each

Text continued on p. 228

Skill 16-1 | Hand Hygiene

Hand hygiene is performed at the beginning of the shift, before and after caring for each patient, before performing procedures, after toileting, before and after eating, before entering special care areas, and whenever the hands have become visibly soiled. Before beginning the shift, the hands should be washed vigorously for at least 15 seconds (30 seconds if in specialty care areas), or according to agency policy. Thereafter, hand hygiene either by washing with soap and water or by use of an approved alcohol-based rub product may be utilized. The CDC recommends that no artificial nails, nail wraps, tips, or nail jewelry should be worn and that natural nails should be kept no longer than ¼ inch past the fingertips.

■ Supplies

✓ Sink with warm running water
✓ Facility-approved liquid soap
✓ Disposable paper towels
✓ Trash can
✓ Facility-approved hand lotion
✓ Approved alcohol-based hand rub product
✓ Handwashing

Review and carry out the Standard Steps in Appendix 3.

■ Assessment (Data Collection)

1. **ACTION** Determine correct agent to be used and length of time needed for handwashing according to task at hand or degree of soiling.

   RATIONALE The longer the washing with the approved agent, the more microorganisms are removed.

■ Planning

2. **ACTION** Check that soap and towels are at hand before beginning.

   RATIONALE Saves time.

3. **ACTION** Activate the towel dispenser so that towels are ready to tear off when needed before beginning, or set roll on end so towels can be torn off without contaminating the hands. Push wristwatch up the arm.

   RATIONALE Activating the towel dispenser prevents contamination of clean, wet hands by the dispenser after washing. Two to four towels are necessary. Pushing the wristwatch up the arm protects the watch.

■ Implementation

4. **ACTION** Turn on water and adjust to a comfortable temperature with medium water force. Keep body away from sink.

   RATIONALE Warm, continuously running water aids in the removal of organisms. Medium water force should be used because splashing can cause contamination. Leaning against the sink may contaminate your clothes.

5. **ACTION** Wet your hands with water, pointing your fingers toward the bottom of the sink.

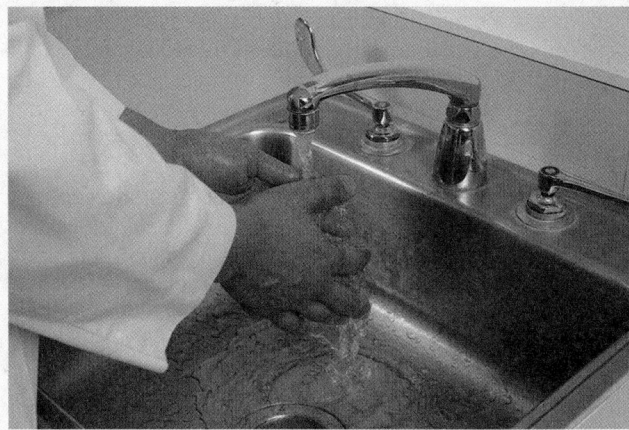

Step 5 Wetting the hands.

RATIONALE Water will drain from the wrists to the fingertips, carrying organisms away.

6. **ACTION** Apply a small amount of liquid soap (2 to 4 mL).

   RATIONALE Using liquid soap rather than a soap bar helps prevent transfer of microorganisms.

7. **ACTION** Wash your hands:

   a. **ACTION** Use 10 circular strokes for the palms while applying friction.

   RATIONALE Friction helps work up a lather and removes organisms.

   b. **ACTION** Wash the back of each hand with 10 circular motions.

   RATIONALE Vigorous rubbing removes organisms. Ten strokes should dislodge the organisms.

   c. **ACTION** Wash the fingers with 10 circular motions; rub the palms together, slide the back of one hand up the palm of the other while encircling the fingers with the opposite hand, and circle the thumb of opposite hand; run the hand over the back of other hand and around the wrist, alternating hands; and interlace the fingers of one hand with those of the other and with friction rub back and forth 10 times to clean the spaces between the fingers. Repeat as needed for the full length of the scrub.

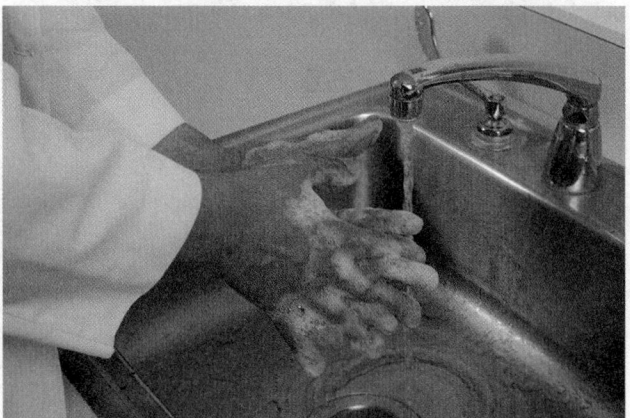

Step 7 Scrubbing the hands.

RATIONALE All surfaces of the hands and wrists are washed.

8. *ACTION* Rinse the wrists, hands, and fingertips, keeping the fingers pointed downward. Avoid touching any part of the sink or faucet.

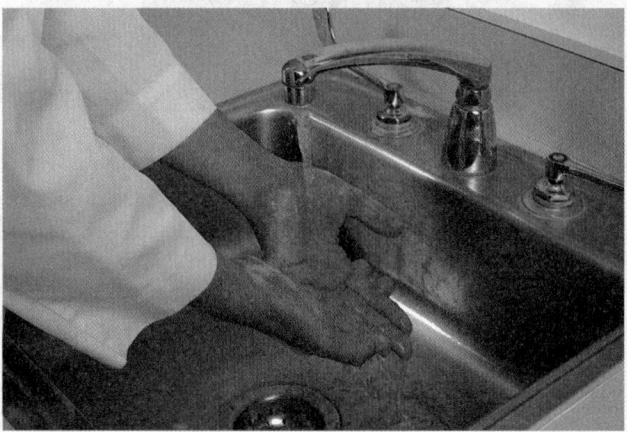

Step 8 Rinsing the hands.

RATIONALE Pointing hands and fingers downward moves debris downward rather upward onto cleaner areas. Touching the sink would contaminate the newly washed area of the hand or fingers.

9. *ACTION* Remove towels from the dispenser, and dry the hands and wrists thoroughly, beginning at the fingertips and working up the hand. Pat rather than rub.

RATIONALE Dry gently but thoroughly to prevent chapping of the skin. Use a clean towel for each combined wrist and hand.

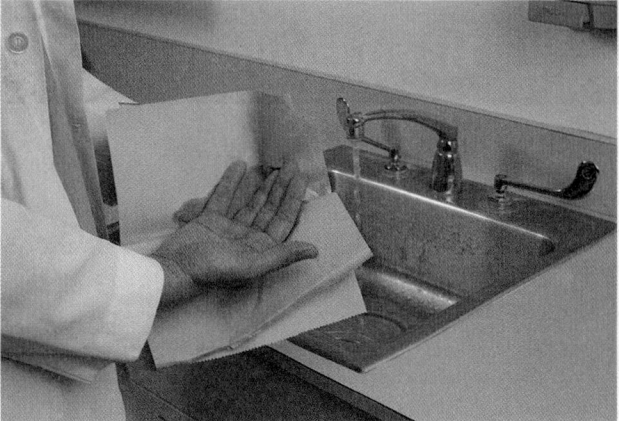

Step 9 Drying the hands.

10. *ACTION* With a dry paper towel, being careful not to touch the handles with the bare hand, turn off the water if hand controls are present. Discard towel in trash receptacle.

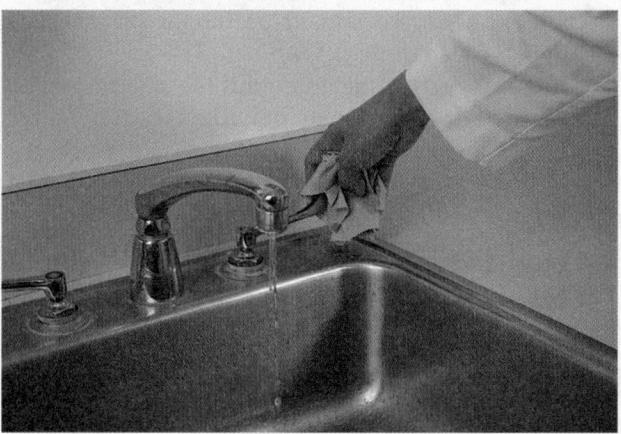

Step 10 Turning off the water.

RATIONALE Using a clean towel prevents recontamination of freshly washed hands.

11. *ACTION* Apply hand lotion if subject to chapping.

RATIONALE Lubricates skin and keeps it soft; prevents cracking of the skin.

■ **Evaluation**

12. *ACTION* Check to see that hands are clean and dry and have been washed the proper length of time. Assess for breaks in the skin.

RATIONALE Ensures that hands are clean. Breaks in the skin provide a point of entry for microorganisms.

■ **Documentation**

Hand hygiene does not ordinarily need to be documented.

Continued

Skill 16-1 | Hand Hygiene—cont'd

■ Special Considerations

✓ Visibly soiled hands must be washed with soap and water.

✓ Wait until lotion has been absorbed before donning latex gloves because not waiting could increase the risk of developing latex allergy.

✓ For surgical asepsis scrubs, hands are held upward throughout the scrub and the rinse. Sinks are used that accommodate this position. When possible, rinse hands with fingertips higher than the wrist.

✓ When working in a patient's home, a clean hand towel may be used in place of paper towels if no paper towels are available.

✓ Home care nurses should carry a container of liquid soap, and alcohol-based hand rub, in their bag.

✓ Caregivers and family members who have contact with the patient should be taught proper hand hygiene technique.

✓ If the rim or perimeter around the sink is wet, use a folded dry towel to dry it without contaminating your hands.

✓ If fingernails are dirty, clean with nail of other hand or with an orange stick.

■ Hand Hygiene with Alcohol-Based Hand Rub–Approved Product

13. *ACTION* Dispense the required amount of hand rub into the palm of one hand. Using both hands, disperse the product over the entire surface of the hands and fingers to the wrists.

    RATIONALE Follow the manufacturer's written instructions regarding amount of hand rub to use and the number of times it may be used before handwashing with soap and water is required. Different products require different amounts to be used for hand hygiene. Often after 4 or more uses of the hand rub, hands should be washed with soap and water. Product must make contact with all parts of the skin to eliminate microorganisms.

14. *ACTION* Continue to rub hands together over all surfaces until the hands are dry.

    RATIONALE Contact with the skin until dry assists with elimination of microorganisms.

■ Special Considerations

✓ When working with a patient who has active pulmonary tuberculosis, hands must be washed with soap and water rather than using a hand rub product. Hand rub products do not kill tuberculosis spores.

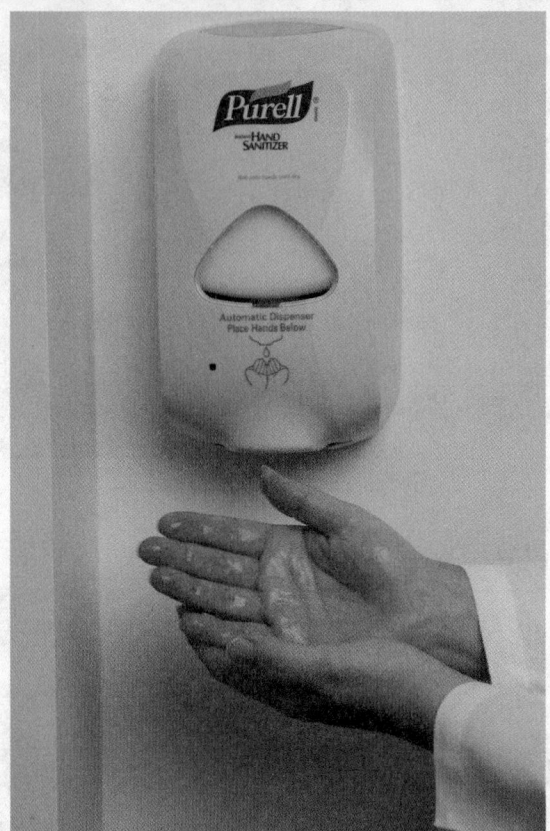

Step 14 Using hand rub for hand hygiene.

✓ When working with a patient who has diarrhea, wash hands with soap and water because the diarrhea may be caused by *Clostridium difficile*, which is not eliminated by alcohol-based hand rub products.

❓CRITICAL THINKING QUESTIONS

1. When assigned to care for two patients, one of whom has diarrhea and the other of whom is undergoing chemotherapy for metastatic cancer, how long would you wash your hands when you have left the room of the patient with diarrhea before entering the room of the chemotherapy patient?

2. If you just used an alcohol-based hand cleanser and you enter the room of a patient to perform a physical assessment and the patient states, "I didn't see you wash your hands," what would you do?

Box 16-3 | *CDC Standard Precaution Guidelines*

Use Standard Precautions, or the equivalent, for the care of all patients. *Category IB*

A. Hand hygiene

(1) Wash hands after touching blood, body fluids, secretions, excretions, and contaminated items, whether or not gloves are worn. Perform hand hygiene immediately after gloves are removed, between patient contacts, and when otherwise indicated to avoid transfer of microorganisms to other patients or the surrounding environment. It may be necessary to wash hands between tasks and procedures on the same patient to prevent cross-contamination of different body sites. *Category IB*

(2) Use a plain (nonantimicrobial) soap for routine hand hygiene. *Category IB*

(3) Use an antimicrobial agent or a waterless antiseptic agent for specific circumstances (e.g., control of outbreaks or hyperendemic infections), as defined by the infection prevention and control program. *Category IB*

B. Gloves

Wear gloves (clean, nonsterile gloves are adequate) when touching blood, body fluids, secretions, excretions, and contaminated items. Put on clean gloves just before touching mucous membranes and nonintact skin. Change gloves between tasks and procedures on the same patient after contact with material that may contain a high concentration of microorganisms. Remove gloves promptly after use, before touching noncontaminated items and environmental surfaces, and before going to another patient, and wash hands immediately to avoid transfer [of] microorganisms to other patients or environments. *Category IB*

C. Mask, Eye Protection, Face Shield

Wear a mask and eye protection or a face shield to protect mucous membranes of the eyes, nose, and mouth during procedures and patient-care activities that are likely to generate splashes or sprays of blood, body fluids, secretions, and excretions. *Category IB*

D. Gown

Wear a gown (a clean, nonsterile gown is adequate) to protect skin and to prevent soiling of clothing during procedures and patient-care activities that are likely to generate splashes or sprays of blood, body fluids, secretions, or excretions. Select a gown that is appropriate for the activity and amount of fluid likely to be encountered. Remove a soiled gown as promptly as possible, and wash hands to avoid transfer of microorganisms to other patients or environments. *Category IB*

E. Patient-Care Equipment

Handle used patient-care equipment soiled with blood, body fluids, secretions, and excretions in a manner that prevents skin and mucous membrane exposures, contamination of clothing, and transfer of microorganisms to other patients and environments. Ensure that reusable equipment is not used for the care of another patient until it has been cleaned and reprocessed appropriately. Ensure that single-use items are discarded properly. *Category IB*

F. Environmental Control

Ensure that the hospital has adequate procedures for the routine care, cleaning, and disinfection of environmental surfaces, beds, bedrails, bedside equipment, and other frequently touched surfaces, and ensure that these procedures are being followed. *Category IB*

G. Linen

Handle, transport, and process used linen soiled with blood, body fluids, secretions, and excretions in a manner that prevents skin and mucous membrane exposures and contamination of clothing, and that avoids transfer of microorganisms to other patients and environments. *Category IB*

H. Occupational Health and Bloodborne Pathogens

(1) Take care to prevent injuries when using needles, scalpels, and other sharp instruments or devices, when handling sharp instruments after procedures; when cleaning used instruments; and when disposing of used needles. Never recap used needles, or otherwise manipulate them using both hands, or use any other technique that involves directing the point of a needle toward any part of the body; rather, use either a one-handed "scoop" technique or a mechanical device designed for holding the needle sheath. Do not remove used needles from disposable syringes by hand, and do not bend, break, or otherwise manipulate used needles by hand. Place used disposable syringes and needles, scalpel blades, and other sharp items in appropriate puncture-resistant containers, which are located as close as practical to the area in which the items were used, and place reusable syringes and needles in a puncture-resistant container for transport to the reprocessing area. *Category IB*

(2) Use mouthpieces, resuscitation bags, or other ventilation devices as an alternative to mouth-to-mouth resuscitation methods in areas where the need for resuscitation is predictable. *Category IB*

I. Patient Placement

Place a patient who contaminates the environment or who does not (or cannot be expected to) assist in maintaining appropriate hygiene or environmental control in a private room. If a private room is not available, consult with infection control professionals regarding patient placement or other alternatives. *Category IB*

From Garner, J.S. (1996). *Guideline for Isolation Precautions in Hospitals.* Hospital Infection Control Practices Advisory Committee. Atlanta: Centers for Disease Control and Prevention. (Last modified April 1, 2005.)

Skill 16-2 | Using Personal Protective Equipment (PPE): Gown and Mask

An isolation/barrier gown is most often an impermeable paper gown with cuffs, although a treated fabric gown may be provided. A gown is used whenever the nurse's clothing might be contaminated with body substances or airborne microorganisms from a patient who is undergoing isolation precautions. A mask is required when a patient is infected with an organism that can be transmitted by airborne particles. A mask is also necessary when entering a protective isolation unit to act as a barrier between the nurse and the patient. It is helpful if nurses speak to patients from the doorway and let the patients see their faces before donning the masks. Remember that protective eyewear is to be used anytime there is a possibility of being splashed by body fluids. All PPE items must be carefully removed after use to prevent transfer of microorganisms.

■ Supplies

✓ Head cover   ✓ Eyewear   ✓ Shoe covers
✓ Mask   ✓ Isolation gown   ✓ Gloves

Review and carry out the Standard Steps in Appendix 3.

■ Assessment (Data Collection)

1. **ACTION** Determine PPE equipment necessary and assess cart for available supplies.

   RATIONALE Ensures that items needed are present. (Assume that a gown, mask, gloves, and eyewear are needed.)

■ Planning

2. **ACTION** Check supplies to see that sufficient numbers of each item are on the cart or in the anteroom for the entire shift.

RATIONALE Prevents you from having to run to the supply room for an item when you are trying to deliver care.

■ Implementation

3. **ACTION** Remove a gown from the supply on the cart or in the anteroom of the isolation unit. Hold it by the neck area and allow it to unfold with the opening in the back toward you.

   RATIONALE Allows entry into the gown. A clean gown is used every time the patient's room is entered.

4. **ACTION** Slip arms into the sleeves and tie the ties at the back of the neck and the waist.

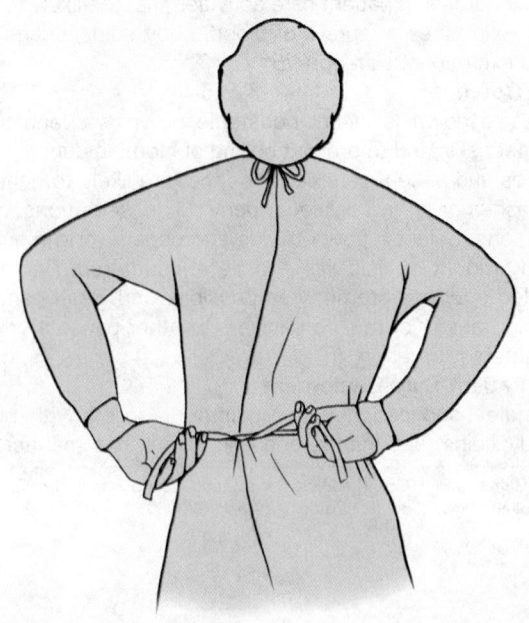

Step 3 Donning a non-sterile gown.

Step 4 Tying the gown.

RATIONALE The tied gown will prevent contaminants from coming in contact with your clothing.

5. *ACTION* Remove a mask from the cart or ante-room and place the mask with the metal band on the outside at the nose. Cover both the mouth and the nose. Secure the mask to the head with the elastic band or tie the ties above the ears and around the neck.

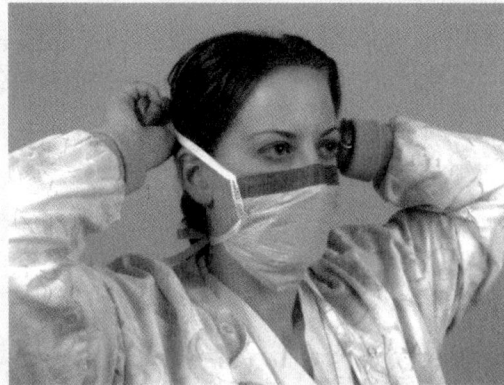

Step 5 Putting on a mask.

RATIONALE A mask protects against airborne infection. Accordion-type masks should cover the nose, mouth, and chin. Pinching the metal band so the mask conforms to the shape of your nose helps keep it from slipping. The mask should fit close to the face without gaps. When a special respirator mask is needed, use only an N95 respirator variety. A mask must be replaced if it becomes moist.

6. *ACTION* Put on protective eyewear if such is not attached to the mask.

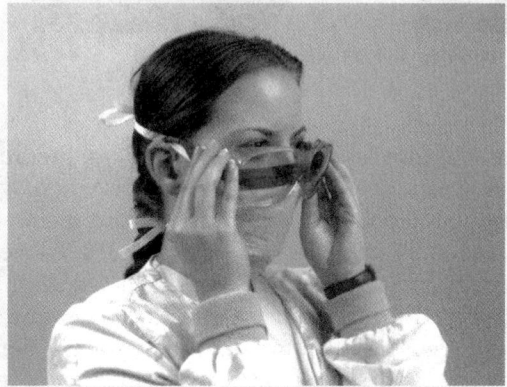

Step 6 Putting on eyewear.

RATIONALE Eyewear that has a full face shield that curves around the face, or top and side pieces to protect the eye area, keeps droplets and splashes from entering the mucosa of the eye.

7. *ACTION* Shoe covers and head cover are worn if there is danger of contamination of the shoes and/or hair or for protective isolation.

RATIONALE Disposable shoe covers and head cover protect the shoes and hair from contamina-

tion and from carrying microorganisms out of the isolation room.

8. *ACTION* Gloves are donned last.

RATIONALE Glove cuffs are pulled up over the gown cuffs. This prevents any gap of unprotected skin at the wrists.

Removing PPE

9. *ACTION* Remove the gloves without contaminating your hands (see Figure 16-6 and Steps 16-1).

RATIONALE If the skin of the hand touches the contaminated surface of the glove, microorganisms can be transferred.

10. *ACTION* Remove the protective eyewear without touching your face and place disposable face covering in the trash. Place reusable eyewear in an impervious container so it can be disinfected.

RATIONALE Careful handling of the contaminated eyewear prevents transfer of microorganisms.

11. *ACTION* Remove the face mask by untying the lower strings first, then the upper ones; or remove it by the elastic band. Discard the used mask in the proper receptacle.

RATIONALE Reduces transfer of microorganisms. A used face mask should never be allowed to dangle around the neck when not in use.

12. *ACTION* Unfasten the waist tie on the gown, then the neck ties. Place your hands inside the neckline, and pull the gown down off the shoulders and over your upper arms. Slip your hands up inside each sleeve. Pull out your arms and hands and place the gown's outside surfaces together so it is turned inside out. Handle only the inside of the gown. Discard it in the proper receptacle.

RATIONALE Prevents further contamination of the hands. Reduces transfer of microorganisms.

13. *ACTION* Perform hand hygiene.

RATIONALE Removes microorganisms.

■ Evaluation

14. *ACTION* Ask yourself if the PPE was effective. Would you do anything differently the next time?

RATIONALE Evaluates technique of garbing in PPE.

■ Documentation

15. *ACTION* Document use of PPE for patients in isolation.

RATIONALE Verifies that correct protective procedure was used.

Continued

Skill 16-2 | Using Personal Protective Equipment (PPE): Gown and Mask—cont'd

Documentation Example

10/12 1020 Wound irrigated with 10 mL NS; gown, mask, goggles, and gloves worn.

_____
(Nurse's signature)

?CRITICAL THINKING QUESTIONS

1. What articles of personal protective equipment should you wear if you enter the room of a patient who has undergone a bone marrow transplantation after full-body irradiation that severely depletes immune function?

2. What items of personal protective equipment do you need to put on when you are going to irrigate an infected wound?

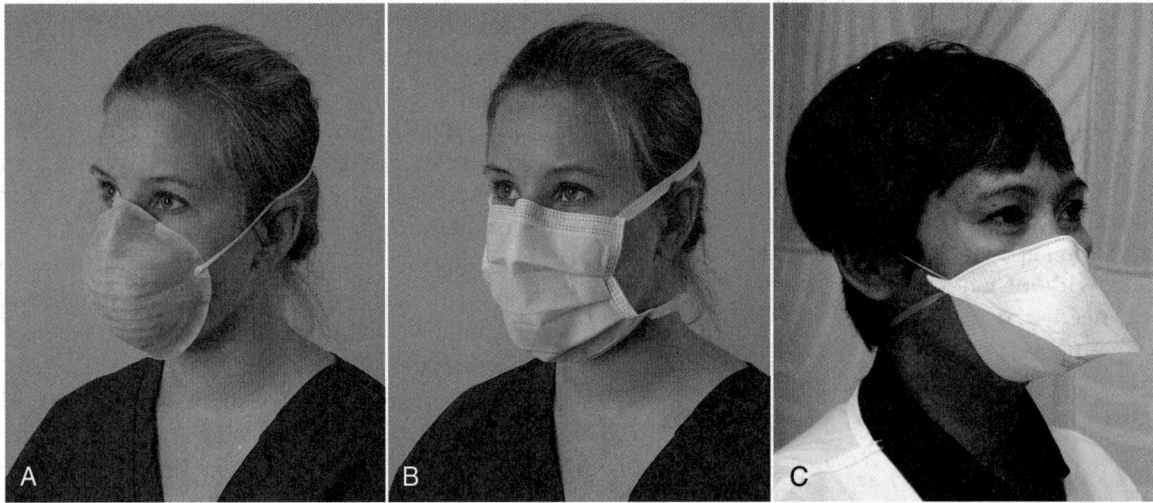

FIGURE **16-5 A,** Preformed mask. **B,** Accordion mask with ties. **C,** N95 respirator mask.

use. Eyewear is worn when performing oral, nasotracheal, or endotracheal suctioning (unless a closed system is used); for performing wound irrigations; and whenever performing or assisting with procedures in which blood might splatter. An example of such a procedure is the insertion of a central venous line.

Head Cover

A cap or head cover is placed on the head if there is danger of contamination of the hair or if microorganisms resident in the hair might endanger the patient. The cap is removed by slipping the fingers beneath the elastic and handling only the inner surface of the contaminated head cover to prevent hand contamination.

Shoe Covers

Skin around the ankles should be covered by appropriate protective covers whenever there is a chance of splashing body fluids during a procedure. **Shoes are covered so that pathogens are not carried out of the room; the covers are removed when exiting the room in the same manner as the head cover.**

Gloves

Disposable gloves are used for Standard Precautions and are worn when there is a chance that there will be contact with blood or body fluids, mucous membranes, nonintact skin, or secretions or excretions. Gloves are also used for handling items contaminated with these substances. They are put on after the other pieces of personal protective equipment have been donned. Gloves reduce the possibility of transmission of microorganisms between the nurse and the patient. **Hand hygiene is performed before gloving and immediately after removing the gloves because no glove is 100% protective.** Gloves are contaminated once they are used and must be discarded before doing the next task or caring for the next patient. Steps 16-1 show how to properly remove contaminated gloves (Figure 16-6). The gloves are immediately placed in a trash receptacle, and hand hygiene is performed. **Gloves are never reused or washed.** When a gown is worn, gloves are pulled up over the cuffs of the gown.

Latex Allergy. Since the adoption of Standard Precautions, the use of latex has dramatically increased in

Steps 16-1 Removing Gloves

Nonsterile gloves are used for Standard Precautions and most isolation procedures. After use, the contaminated gloves are removed in a manner that prevents the spread of microorganisms.

1. *ACTION* Grasp the cuff of the glove of one hand and slide the glove off the hand, folding the outside of the contaminated glove to the inside.

   RATIONALE Care must be taken not to touch the skin of the wrist or hand with the contaminated gloved hand or microorganisms may be transferred.

2. *ACTION* Hold the glove removed in the palm of the other gloved hand, and slip the ungloved hand under the band of the second glove. Roll the glove off, turning it inside out over the first glove.

   RATIONALE Being careful not to touch the contaminated glove with the bare hand reduces transfer of microorganisms.

3. *ACTION* Touching only the inside surface of the rolled-up gloves, drop them in the trash.

   RATIONALE Rolling the contaminated gloves together with only the uncontaminated inner surface exposed helps prevent the transfer of microorganisms. Disposing of gloves properly helps reduce the spread of infection.

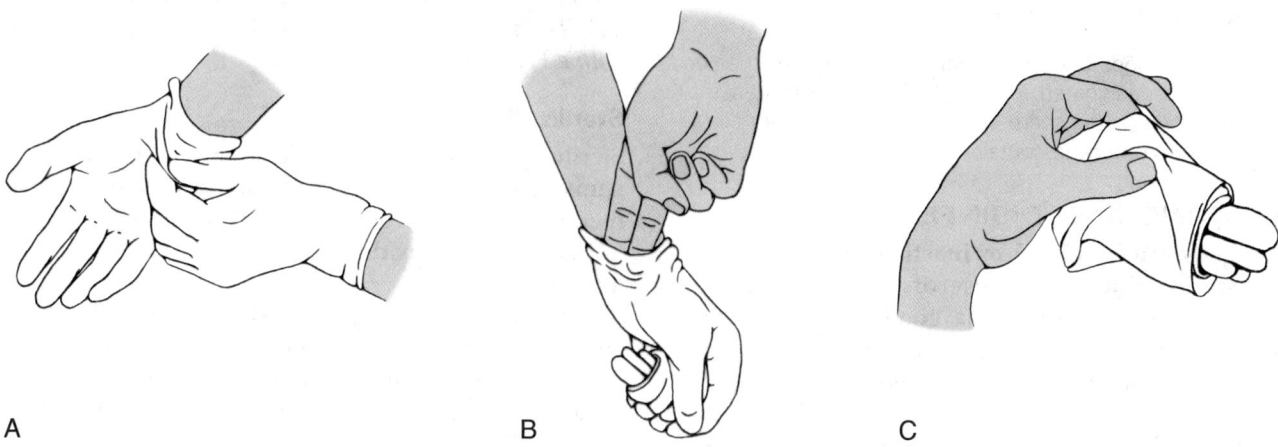

A   B   C

FIGURE **16-6** **A,** Removal of the right glove. **B,** Removal of the left glove. **C,** Method of holding the removed gloves.

health care. Because of the greater exposure through glove use, more people have developed sensitivity or allergy to latex. Exposure may cause redness, local inflammation and pruritus of the hands, and anaphylaxis. People who have had multiple surgical procedures; who have food allergies to bananas, kiwis, or avocados; or who have had histories of reactions to other latex-containing products are at risk for the development of this allergy. If a health care worker has a latex allergy, by law the employer must supply an alternative type of glove. Measures to help prevent latex sensitivity include using gloves in appropriate situations and not for routine tasks in which a blood, body fluid, or microorganism contact exposure is unlikely. Gloves are removed directly over a trash receptacle without "snapping" them off. Do not use petroleum-based lotions under latex gloves because they attract latex proteins from the gloves, which can increase the risk of developing the allergy.

Disposal of Sharps

Disposable sharp instruments, referred to as "sharps," are placed directly into a special red, puncture-resistant sharps biohazard container immediately after use (Figure 16-7). All needles, intravenous (IV) cannulas, and items that are sharp or might cause a skin break are placed in the sharps container (Safety Alert 16-1). Sharps containers should be replaced when they are three-quarters full.

Contaminated Waste

Items contaminated with infectious material must be disposed of in sealed, impermeable, plastic bags marked "Hazardous Waste" or "Biohazard." This includes soiled dressings, used sanitary pads, suction drainage containers, and any other item that has been in contact with body fluids. Contaminated linens are handled in a like manner unless all linen in the facility is treated as a contaminated biohazard. Soiled linens should be gathered carefully and bagged at the site of use.

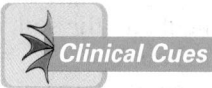
Clinical Cues

Keep used linens away from your uniform. Do not put them on the floor or chair because microorganisms from the patient can be spread this way. Place them directly into the linen hamper.

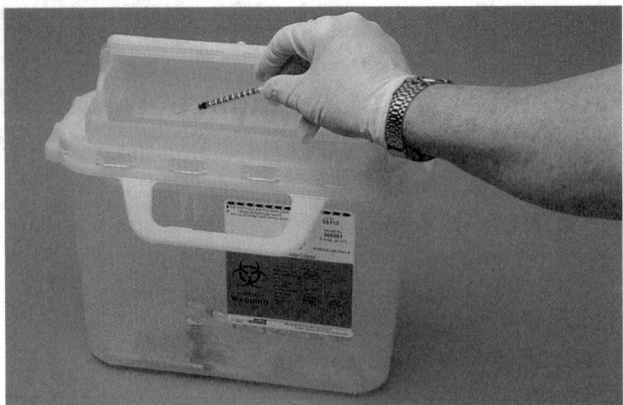

FIGURE **16-7** Deposit a used syringe and needle in a sharps container.

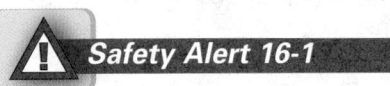

Disposing of Sharps

Drop used syringes and other sharps into the container or onto the area designated for sharps disposal and then trip the lever, dropping the sharp into the container. Never allow your fingers to enter the container.

CLEANING AND DISINFECTION

Pathogens can be killed or inactivated by disinfection, sterilization, or the use of sanitizing agents. Eliminating the reservoir is a good way to prevent transmission. Water, sewage treatment, and rodent control eliminate reservoirs for pathogens.

Appropriate cleaning removes and inhibits the growth of microorganisms. Always wear gloves when cleaning visibly soiled objects or whenever performing wound care. Whether in the hospital, a long-term care facility, or a home setting, certain steps should be followed for cleaning objects:

1. Rinse the object with cold water to remove organic material. Hot water coagulates protein contained in organic material, making it adhere to the item.
2. Once all visible organic material has been removed, wash the object in hot, soapy water. Soap's emulsifying action reduces surface tension and helps remove soil. (How the object is washed and the agent used depends on the object and the manufacturer's recommendation for cleansing and sanitizing.)
3. Use a stiff-bristled brush or abrasive to clean equipment with grooves and narrow spaces. Friction helps dislodge soil.
4. Rinse the object well with moderately hot water.
5. Dry the object; it is now considered clean, but not sterile.

Always disinfect the cleaning equipment and the sink when you have finished cleaning soiled objects.

Disinfectant agents can be used to eliminate some types of organisms that are left after cleansing. Disinfectants are solutions containing chemical compounds such as phenol, alcohol, or chlorine that kill or inactivate

nearly all microorganisms. These chemicals can be caustic to the skin and are used only on inanimate objects. A recommended disinfectant is chlorine bleach and water at a ratio of 1:10. Before disinfection, items must be thoroughly rinsed after cleaning because soap may react with the disinfectant, preventing its killing properties from working. An antiseptic is a chemical compound that is used on skin or tissue to inhibit the growth of or to eliminate microorganisms. Disinfectants and antiseptics have bactericidal or bacteriostatic properties. A *bactericidal* solution destroys bacteria; a *bacteriostatic* solution prevents the growth and reproduction of some bacteria. Povidone-iodine is an example of an antiseptic. Items that cannot be sterilized, such as skin, can be disinfected with antiseptic agents.

Wounds are cleansed using sterile normal saline or an antiseptic solution. Often a bacteriostatic cream or ointment is applied before the wound is dressed (Nursing Care Plan 16-1). (*Also refer to the **Companion CD-ROM** for Nursing Care Plan 16-2: Care of the Patient with a Foot Wound.*)

Sterilization

Sterilization is the best method of eliminating microorganisms from equipment and supplies. There are five methods of sterilization: steam/moist heat, dry heat/hot air, ethylene oxide, low-temperature gas plasma, and radiation.

Moist heat is most often used as steam under pressure in a device called an *autoclave*. Steam under pressure attains temperatures higher than the boiling point. Under pressure, steam reaches temperatures of 250° to 275° F (121° to 135° C).

Ethylene oxide gas is effective against microorganisms and spores. It is used for heat-sensitive items and where good penetration is essential.

For cleansing items in the home, boiling in water is the easiest method. Items should be boiled for a minimum of 16 minutes. Items that cannot be boiled or disinfected by running them through the dishwasher's "sanitize" cycle can be exposed to direct sunlight for several hours. The heat and ultraviolet rays will kill exposed microorganisms.

Radiation. Ultraviolet light can be used for disinfection. Ionizing radiation is used to sterilize drugs, foods, and other items that would be damaged by heat. Radiation is being considered as a way to ensure a safer food supply in the United States.

ASEPSIS IN THE HOME ENVIRONMENT

Precautions are not as stringent in the home as in the hospital because the ordinary home does not contain the many pathogens found in a hospital environment. The number and degree of home precautions are based on whether there is an infected person in residence and what microorganism is involved. Contaminated dress-

NURSING CARE PLAN 16-1

Care of the Patient with Abrasions and Splenectomy

SCENARIO Terry Jackson, age 32, was admitted to the emergency room after a motorcycle accident in which he skidded and was thrown into a telephone pole. He has many abrasions on his legs and forehead and underwent a splenectomy for a ruptured spleen.

PROBLEM/NURSING DIAGNOSIS Incision/Impaired skin integrity related to surgical incision and multiple abrasions. *Supporting Assessment Data: Subjective:* "These scrapes sting." *Objective:* Abdominal surgical incision covered with a dressing; abrasions on both legs and on forehead.

Goals/Expected Outcomes	Nursing Interventions	Selected Rationale	Evaluation
Surgical incision will heal within 2 wk without signs of infection. Abrasions will heal within 2 wk without signs of infection.	Change dressing as ordered using sterile technique.	Sterile technique will decrease likelihood of microorganisms entering the wound.	*Are incision and abrasions healing without signs of infection?* Yes, although the forehead abrasion is draining serous fluid.
	Inspect for signs of infection every shift.	Monitoring temperature, pulse, and WBCs and inspecting wounds for redness, drainage, warmth, and pain helps detect infection.	Temperature 99.0° F (37.2° C), pulse 78, WBCs 10,090. Incision clean and dry; abrasions beginning to scab. *Wound care performed?*
	Apply antiseptic ointment to abrasions and dress q day.	Antiseptic ointment will decrease microorganisms at wound site. Dressing will prevent further microorganisms from entering the wound.	Yes, ointment and fresh dressing applied daily.

PROBLEM/NURSING DIAGNOSIS Surgical incisions/Risk for infection related to abdominal surgery, splenectomy, and abrasions. *Supporting Assessment Data:* **Objective**: Spleen was removed after it was lacerated in motorcycle accident. Several abrasions sustained in accident.

Goals/Expected Outcomes	Nursing Interventions	Selected Rationale	Evaluation
Patient will not contract tetanus from introduction of microorganisms from road surface.	Administer 0.5 mL tetanus toxoid IM. Monitor for malaise or fever.	Tetanus toxoid vaccine provides antibodies to tetanus bacillus.	*Tetanus toxoid given?* Yes.
Patient will not contract hospital-related infection before discharge.	Discourage visitors who have an active infection.	Patients without a spleen are more susceptible to infection.	*Any signs of infection?* No.
	Maintain strict aseptic technique when handling IV lines and catheter, and performing wound care.	Aseptic technique reduces the introduction of microorganisms to the patient.	*Aseptic technique maintained?* Yes. IV site clean, dry, and without redness. Catheter draining clear urine without foul odor.
	Perform appropriate hand hygiene before touching patient, tubes, or dressings.		Hand hygiene performed rigorously.
	Assess for signs of surgical wound infection: chills, redness, swelling, increased pain in area, foul odor from wound, elevated WBC count, purulent drainage.	Serious infection may be averted if early signs of infection are noted.	*Any sign of surgical wound infection?* No; incision clean and dry without redness, swelling, or increased pain. WBC count 10,090. Continue plan.

? CRITICAL THINKING QUESTIONS

1. What causes tetanus? Why is it a particular concern for Terry with this injury?

2. What other complications could occur if the surgical wound becomes infected?

3. Why are people who have lost their spleen more susceptible to infection?

Key: *IM,* Intramuscular; *IV,* intravenous; *WBC,* white blood cell.

ings and other disposable supplies are secured in plastic zip-closure bags before disposal. Linens contaminated with blood or body secretions should be placed in a sealed plastic bag until laundered. They should be rinsed in cold water as soon as possible and then washed in hot, soapy water. Hot water causes protein to coagulate, making cleaning more difficult.

A 1:10 solution of chlorine bleach and water can be used to disinfect counters and bathrooms if they become soiled with body secretions. Running the dishwasher on the "sanitize" cycle or scalding eating utensils with boiling water will reduce microorganisms.

Frequent "damp" dusting and vacuuming decreases the number of microorganisms in the environment. Exposing bedding and other items the patient uses that cannot be disinfected to 6 to 8 hours of sunshine may reduce the number of microorganisms on them. Tissues containing expectorated sputum or nasal secretions of an infected patient should be disposed of in a sealable plastic bag.

Forceps, scissors, and other small implements used for dressing changes can be washed with hot water and detergent, and then soaked in a bleach solution. They should be rinsed, drained, allowed to air dry, and then stored in a covered container. Drainage bags can be cleansed, disinfected, dried, and reused.

INFECTION CONTROL SURVEILLANCE

Within each health care agency, there is an infection control practitioner who is responsible for ensuring infection prevention and control measures are followed. When a patient is known to have an infection, the information is typically reported to the infection control professional. This person works with the health care staff to ensure they understand which patient care and environmental cleaning measures are to be used. This professional also assesses for spread of infection. All hospital patients are at risk for health care–associated infection, and each nurse must be vigilant in watching for signs of infection in each patient under his care. Patients at high risk for infection are those who (1) are weakened by injury or severe illness; (2) have another chronic illness; (3) have a central venous catheter, IV cannula, or indwelling drainage tube; (4) are very young or very old; (5) have an open wound; (6) have a surgical incision; or (7) have a compromised immune system from chemotherapy or immunosuppression. Whenever an infection is suspected, additional precautions are taken to prevent the possible spread of microorganisms.

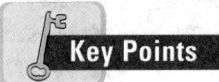

Key Points

- Microorganisms are abundant in our environment, and many can cause infection if not controlled.
- Pathogens include bacteria, viruses, protozoa, rickettsia, fungi, and helminths.
- There are more than 30,000 strains of viruses. They are very small, and some are difficult to control or kill.
- The most effective way to destroy many kinds of microorganisms is to expose them to moist heat at a high temperature for 16 to 20 minutes.
- Standard Precautions are to be used for all patients to prevent the spread of microorganisms.
- The spread of infection is prevented by breaking one of the six links of the infection chain (see Figure 16-3).
- The elderly are typically more susceptible to infection due to the effects of natural aging on the body (see Table 16-6).
- Body defenses against infection are intact skin, the inflammatory process, and the immune response.
- The purposes of the inflammatory response are to neutralize and destroy harmful agents, limit their spread, and prepare damaged tissue for repair.
- There are five types of immunity: naturally acquired, passive acquired, naturally acquired passive, artificially acquired, and artificially acquired passive.
- Medical asepsis, or *clean technique*, reduces the number of microorganisms present and decreases the risk of transmission of microorganisms from one person to another.
- Surgical asepsis, or *sterile technique*, is a method of preparing materials in such a way that microorganisms cannot be transferred from them to a person.
- Hand hygiene is the most effective way to prevent the transfer of microorganisms.
- Hand hygiene is performed before and after caring for each patient.
- Personal protective equipment is used to carry out Standard Precautions and includes items such as gloves, masks, gowns, protective eyewear, head cover, and shoe covers.
- Infection prevention and control is the responsibility of all health care workers.
- Pathogens can be killed or inactivated by disinfection, by sterilization, or by the use of antimicrobial agents.
- There are five methods of sterilization: steam/moist heat, dry heat/hot air, ethylene oxide, low-temperature gas plasma, and radiation.
- Asepsis is not as stringent in the home environment as found in a health care agency, but patients and families must be taught infection prevention and control techniques.

 Go to your **Companion CD-ROM** for an Audio Glossary, animations, video clips, and more.

evolve Be sure to visit the companion Evolve site at http://evolve.elsevier.com/deWit/fundamental/ for additional online resources.

NCLEX-PN® EXAMINATION-STYLE REVIEW QUESTIONS

*Choose the **best** answer(s) for each question.*

1. The most common method of microorganism transfer from one person to another in the hospital setting is prevented by:
   1. disinfecting instruments in special solutions.
   2. filtering the air in the hospital.
   3. changing bed linens daily.
   4. performing hand hygiene thoroughly and frequently.

2. The skin is the first line of defense and protects the body by: *(Select all that apply.)*
   1. repelling microorganisms.
   2. providing an intact physical barrier.
   3. secreting bactericidal substances.
   4. releasing macrophages.
   5. shedding dead cells.

3. The reason for lengthening hand hygiene time when hands are contaminated is to:
   1. render the skin totally free of microorganisms.
   2. mechanically remove as many microorganisms as possible.
   3. increase the circulation in the hands.
   4. provide a thicker layer of soap foam.

4. Means to decrease *susceptibility* of individuals to infection include: *(Select all that apply.)*
   1. discouraging visitors who have an infectious illness.
   2. using gloves and hand hygiene techniques properly.
   3. giving antibiotics prophylactically at the time of surgery.
   4. providing immunization as available.
   5. promoting good nutrition and adequate rest.

5. Drug-resistant organisms are a problem within the community as well as within the hospital. Reasons for this include: *(Select all that apply.)*
   1. overprescription of antibiotics by health care providers.
   2. lack of proper sanitation within communities.
   3. discharging patients with infected wounds before treatment is complete.
   4. patients stopping taking antibiotics before all of the prescription is gone.
   5. mutation of microorganisms in response to commonly used antibiotics.

6. When applying PPEs before entering a patient's room, if a gown, gloves, mask, and eyewear are required, indicate the proper sequence for putting them on: _____, _____, _____, and _____ .
   1. gown
   2. gloves
   3. mask
   4. eyewear

7. Malnutrition contributes to the susceptibility to infection because:
   1. there is little energy for healing.
   2. it decreases immune function.
   3. it prevents sufficient exercise.
   4. it upsets homeostatic balance in the body.

8. Passive acquired immunity is obtained by:
   1. exposure to a disease.
   2. immunization with antibody response.
   3. recovering from a disease.
   4. giving an antitoxin or antiserum.

9. Medical asepsis differs from surgical asepsis in that medical asepsis is aimed at:
   1. sterilizing all equipment.
   2. killing all microorganisms.
   3. preventing transmission of microorganisms.
   4. preventing entry of microorganisms into the body.

10. Considering the chain of infection, a vector might be:
    1. an uninfected patient.
    2. *Staphylococcus* bacteria.
    3. a tick carrying Lyme disease.
    4. a contaminated water supply.

CRITICAL THINKING ACTIVITIES   *Read each clinical scenario and discuss the questions with your classmates.*

Scenario A
Discuss specific ways in which a person with a cold who goes to the movies can transmit the virus to others.

Scenario B
You are assigned to care for a patient who has viral pneumonia, a disease of the respiratory tract. What precautions would be necessary?

Scenario C
A parent asks you why her child should be immunized against tetanus when she is still a baby. How would you respond?

Scenario D
An elderly neighbor keeps complaining about getting respiratory infections and small infected wounds. He asks you what he could do to prevent this. What would you tell him?

Infection Prevention and Control in the Hospital and Home

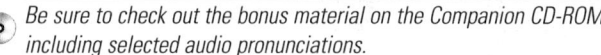

Objectives

Upon completing this chapter, you should be able to:

Theory

1. List the stages of an infectious process.
2. Identify five ways to decrease the occurrence of health care–associated infections (HAIs).
3. Explain how Transmission-Based Precautions are used with Standard Precautions.
4. Describe how procedures for Airborne Precautions differ from those for Droplet Precautions.
5. Discuss the special requirements for Airborne Precautions when the patient has pulmonary tuberculosis.
6. List techniques for handling of specimens; disposal of dirty linen, trash, and sharps; and the cleaning of equipment in the isolation setting.
7. Compare infection prevention and control procedures appropriate for the hospital with those used in the home.
8. Give three examples of nursing measures used to provide for the psychosocial care of a patient in isolation.
9. State the four rules of surgical asepsis.

Clinical Practice

1. Use Standard Precautions when caring for patients.
2. Utilize Transmission-Based Precautions when caring for patients.
3. Properly bag and remove soiled linens and trash from an isolation room.
4. Demonstrate performance of a surgical scrub.
5. Teach a patient or family member how to properly dispose of soiled items at home.

Skills and Steps

Skills

Skill 17-1 Performing Surgical Hand Antisepsis: The Surgical Scrub

Skill 17-2 Performing Surgical Hand Antisepsis: The Surgical Hand Rub

Skill 17-3 Opening Sterile Packs and Preparing a Sterile Field

Skill 17-4 Sterile Gloving and Ungloving

Steps

Steps 17-1 Pouring Sterile Liquids

Key Terms

Be sure to check out the bonus material on the Companion CD-ROM, including selected audio pronunciations.

Airborne Precautions (p. 237)
Contact Precautions (p. 237)
convalescent (p. 235)
Droplet Precautions (p. 237)
health care–associated infections (HAIs) (p. 235)
human immunodeficiency virus (HIV) (ī-mū-nō-dĕ-FĬ-shŭn-sē, p. 236)
impervious (p. 236)
incubation period (ĭn-kū-BĀ-shŭn, p. 234)
infection prevention and control (p. 235)
isolation (ī-sō-LĀ-shŭn, p. 235)
leukocytosis (lēw-kō-sī-TŌ-sĭs, p. 235)
malaise (mă-LĀZ, p. 235)
prodromal period (prō-DRŌ-măl PĚR-ē-ŏd, p. 235)
Standard Precautions (p. 236)
Transmission-Based Precautions (p. 236)

T his chapter will build on concepts learned in Chapter 16, including how microorganisms are spread, the body's defense mechanisms against infection, and the use of Standard Precautions, including hand hygiene and personal protective equipment (PPE), to protect both patients and health care workers from disease-causing organisms.

INFECTION

STAGES OF INFECTION

Infection occurs when pathogenic microorganisms invade the body and multiply. There are four stages in the infectious process: the incubation period, prodromal period, illness period, and convalescent period. The length of each is influenced by many factors, including the organism itself, the overall health of the host, and the environment in which infection has occurred.

The incubation period begins when the organism firsts enters the body and lasts until the onset of symptoms. During this period the organism multiplies, and the duration of the period varies depending on the type of microorganism. In many viral diseases, the infection can be transmitted during the incubation period.

The prodromal period is the short time from the onset of vague, nonspecific symptoms to the beginning of specific symptoms of infection. The patient may be irritable and experience fatigue, malaise (not feeling "right"), and elevated temperature. This period lasts a few hours to a few days. **Microorganisms are most likely to be spread during this highly infectious stage.** Typically, precautions against spreading the infection are not taken because people do not realize that they are ill until the more specific symptoms of infection appear.

During the **illness period,** localized and systemic signs and symptoms appear. The individual may have fever, headache, and malaise. Other specific signs of infection may be detected, such as rash, swollen lymph nodes, leukocytosis (increased white blood cells), purulent wound exudate, diarrhea, and vomiting. **The severity of the symptoms and the duration of the illness depend on the virulence of the pathogen and the person's susceptibility to the causative microorganism.** It is in this phase that people perceive they are ill and may seek professional care.

The convalescent (recovery) period begins when the symptoms begin to subside and extends until the patient has returned to a normal state of health. This can take days to weeks, depending on the microorganism and the overall state of health of the affected individual.

HEALTH CARE–ASSOCIATED INFECTIONS (HAIs)

Infections that are transmitted to a person while receiving health care services are called health care–associated infections (HAIs). A health care worker can also contract an HAI (e.g., head cold, flu, staphylococcal skin infection). The Centers for Disease Control and Prevention (CDC) estimate that HAIs just in hospitals cause at least 2 million infections, 90,000 deaths, and $4.5 billion in excess health care costs annually.

Many invasive procedures predispose patients to infection either because the integrity of the skin or mucous membrane is altered, or because an illness reduces the body's ability to defend itself against invading microorganisms. Patients at greatest risk for HIAs include those with

- Surgical incisions with or without drains
- Artificial airways, including endotracheal tube or tracheostomy
- Urinary catheters
- Intravenous (IV) lines, particularly central venous or arterial lines
- Implanted prosthetic devices (such as heart valves, vascular grafts, or orthopedic joints, rods, and screws)

- Repeated injections or venipunctures for lab specimens
- Immune compromise from such things as chemotherapy, HIV, or long-term steroid use

---

INFECTION PREVENTION AND CONTROL

Infection prevention and control uses medical and surgical asepsis, Standard Precautions, and Transmission-Based Precautions to prevent or control the spread of microorganisms. The strict use of aseptic technique for all diagnostic and therapeutic procedures involving the use of catheters, IV therapy, endotracheal and tracheostomy tubes, drainage tubes, and wound care reduces the incidence of HAIs. Health Promotion Points 17-1 presents some specific ways to help avoid HAIs in your patients. The current guidelines for infection precautions are delineated in Box 17-1 on p. 237. Isolation is a means of preventing contact between a patient and others to prevent the spread of infection. **Emphasis is placed on containing microorganisms and preventing their spread.**

 Health Promotion Points 17-1

Specific Ways to Prevent Health Care–Associated Infections (HAIs)

- Perform proper hand hygiene before and after caring for the patient, before donning gloves, and after their removal.
- Cleanse hands and change gloves between procedures that involve contact with mucous membranes, the perineal or perianal area, feces, wound drainage, or other contaminated matter.
- Keep urinary catheter drainage bags below the level of the bladder at ALL times (even when transferring a patient). Not all drainage bags have a fail-proof one-way valve.
- Clean residual urine off the catheter bag drainage tube after emptying the bag; do not let the tube touch the collection container.
- Assist all patients on bed rest to turn, deep breathe, and cough effectively every 2 hours.
- Assess intravenous line sites for signs of infection whenever you enter the patient's room.
- Use correct aseptic technique for cleansing the skin before performing an invasive procedure.
- Cleanse from the urinary meatus toward the rectum. Never cleanse from the rectal area to the urinary meatus.
- Clean incontinent patients promptly. Carefully cleanse feces from surface of indwelling catheters as well as the skin and mucous membranes.
- Always use aseptic technique when suctioning the airway.

? *Think Critically About . . .* What do you think might be the most common types of health care–associated infections? Why do you think this?

Infection prevention and control involves the following:

- Monitoring diagnostic reports related to infection
- Observing patients for signs of infection
- Implementing procedures to contain microorganisms when infection is suspected
- Properly handling, sterilizing, or disposing of contaminated items and equipment
- Utilizing approved sanitation methods
- Recognizing individuals at high risk for infection and implementing appropriate protection

The infection prevention and control practitioner receives a report from the laboratory every time a culture is performed for an infectious organism. A report is also sent from the nursing unit whenever a patient is identified as having an infectious disease or local infection. Appropriate precautions are then initiated for the type of organism present. The practitioner also investigates all HAIs, looking at possible causes, including breaks in the use of approved precautions; and provides ongoing education regarding infection prevention and control for the health care staff.

Infection prevention and control techniques have undergone many changes over the past three decades. In the United States, current precautions are based on guidelines and regulations developed by the CDC and the Occupational Safety and Health Administration (OSHA). Initially, isolation techniques focused on hospitalized patients, but the evolution of human immunodeficiency virus (HIV), hepatitis strains, and a variety of drug-resistant bacteria have caused a broadened focus. Infection prevention and control practices are now focused on protecting patients, health care workers, family members, and social contacts in all settings.

There are two premises underlying the current system of isolation. One is that **infection may be present before the diagnosis is made.** The second is that the **greatest risk of transmitting infection from most organisms comes from direct contact with the organism by the caregiver's hands or equipment and supplies that have been soiled by blood, body fluids, and other potentially infectious materials.** It is known that all body substances may harbor microorganisms and be infectious, and contact with body substances must therefore be avoided.

Current standards consist of two tiers developed by the Hospital Infection Control Practices Advisory Committee (HICPAC) of the CDC. Tier 1 is Standard Precautions, and Tier 2 is Transmission-Based Precautions. Standard Precautions delineate methods for avoiding direct contact with all body secretions except sweat, whether or not visible blood is present. This includes the mucous membranes and all nonintact skin. Standard Precautions were presented in Box 16-3. Transmission-Based Precautions are based on interrupting the mode of transmission by identifying the specific secretions, body fluids, tissues, or excretions that might be infective. **Transmission-Based Precautions are used alone or in combination but are always used in addition to Standard Precautions.** Box 17-1 lists Transmission-Based Precautions requirements.

? *Think Critically About . . .* Standard Precautions are to be used when there is possible or expected exposure to which body fluids?

CDC and OSHA guidelines have also brought about the development of needleless IV connection systems, and syringes with readily activated protective shields to cover needles immediately following use. These systems decrease opportunities for needle-stick injuries, one of the major factors in health care worker exposure to pathogenic organisms. Use of these devices has significantly reduced the number of needle-stick injuries.

Although Standard Precautions and Transmission-Based Precautions can seem overwhelming at first, the concepts are actually relatively simple. For example, never touch with bare hands anything that contains fluids from a body surface or cavity. Gloves are worn for all contact with body fluids of any sort, including blood, saliva, urine, and feces. The only time gloves are not worn is for contact with intact skin or unsoiled articles. Hand hygiene is performed well and often, paying close attention to areas around and under the fingernails and between the fingers.

Another precaution is the wearing of impermeable gowns when clothing may become soiled with body substances while providing patient care. Masks are worn when contact with respiratory droplet secretions is anticipated, and during suctioning. Protective eyewear is added when there is the possibility of splashing body fluids. All sharps are to be disposed of in puncture-resistant containers located in the patient's room, with the protective shield activated before disposal. Trash and used linens are placed in impervious, or moisture and particle-proof, plastic bags (Figure 17-1).

Elder Care Points

- The elderly are at greater risk for infection because their immune system is not as active as that of a younger person.
- An elderly person hospitalized for one infection has an increased risk of developing a second, health care–associated infection because the body's available defenses are already working to fight the first infection.

Box 17-1 | *Transmission-Based Precautions Requirements*

STANDARD PRECAUTIONS
Use for the care of all patients

AIRBORNE PRECAUTIONS
Use in addition to Standard Precautions for patients with known or suspected serious illnesses transmitted by airborne droplet nuclei. Examples of such diseases are:
- Measles
- Varicella (including disseminated zoster)
- Pulmonary tuberculosis

DROPLET PRECAUTIONS
Use in addition to Standard Precautions for patients with known or suspected serious illnesses transmitted by large-particle droplets. Examples of such illnesses are
- Invasive *Haemophilus influenzae* type b disease, including meningitis, pneumonia, and epiglottitis
- Invasive *Neisseria meningitidis* disease, including meningitis, pneumonia, and sepsis
- Other serious bacterial respiratory infections spread by droplet transmission, including diphtheria (pharyngeal), *Mycoplasma* pneumonia, pertussis, and pneumonic plague
- Streptococcal (group A) pharyngitis, pneumonia, or scarlet fever in infants and young children
- Serious viral infections spread by droplet transmission, including adenovirus, influenza, mumps, parvovirus B19, and rubella

CONTACT PRECAUTIONS
Use in addition to Standard Precautions for patients with known or suspected serious illnesses easily transmitted by direct patient contact or by contact with items in the patient's environment. Examples of such illnesses include
- Gastrointestinal, respiratory, skin, or wound infections or colonization with multidrug-resistant organisms
- Enteric infections with a low infectious dose or prolonged environmental survival, including *Clostridium difficile*
- For diapered or incontinent patients: enterohemorrhagic *Escherichia coli* O157:H7, *Shigella,* hepatitis A, or rotavirus
- Respiratory syncytial virus (RSV), parainfluenza virus, or enteroviral infections in infants and young children
- Skin infections that are highly contagious or that may occur on dry skin, including diphtheria (cutaneous), herpes simplex virus (neonatal or mucocutaneous), impetigo, major (noncontained) abscesses, cellulitis, decubitus ulcers, pediculosis, scabies, staphylococcal furunculosis in infants and young children, and zoster (disseminated or in the immunocompromised host)
- Viral/hemorrhagic conjunctivitis
- Viral/hemorrhagic infections (Ebola, Lassa, or Marburg virus)

Adapted from Centers for Disease Control and Prevention. (2007). Guideline for Isolation Precautions: Preventing Transmission of Infectious Agents in Healthcare Settings. Available at: www.cdc.gov/ncidod/dhqp/gl_isolation.html.

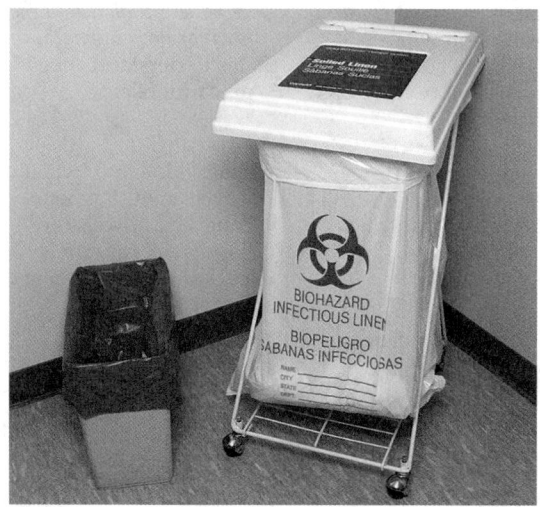

FIGURE **17-1** Biohazard trash and linen containers.

APPLICATION of the NURSING PROCESS

Assessment (Data Collection)
At the first encounter with the patient, assess for signs of infection that may require Transmission-Based Precautions. Wounds should be assessed each shift for signs of infection. Monitor the patient's temperature.

Admission lab studies may also give indications of possible infection, such as an increased white blood cell count or a urinalysis that is positive for bacteria. If cultures are ordered, check the reports to see if any microorganism has been identified. Frequent voiding of small amounts, pain on urination, or a decrease in overall output may also indicate infection.

Nursing Diagnosis
The nursing diagnosis would be Infection, risk for, related to surgical wound, open wound, or weakened condition.

Planning
Expected outcomes would include "No health care–associated infection is evident." When using Transmission-Based Precautions that require putting on personal protective equipment, you must prepare before each entry into the patient's room. For example, will you need more linen? Are all the dressing supplies in the room? Does the patient need pain medication? Are there routine medications due at this time? Is there ice and drinking water in the room? Speaking to the patient in advance via the intercom can help ensure you will have everything necessary when you don your protective clothing and enter the room.

Implementation

A patient with an infection will need teaching about the disease process, modes of transmission, and precautions necessary to prevent spread of the infection (Nursing Care Plan 17-1). Standard and Transmission-Based Precautions will need to be explained.

Standard Precautions are to be used for each contact with every patient, regardless of whether or not infection is known to be present. **Transmission-Based Precautions are implemented based on the individual patient's infection status.**

Hand Hygiene

Hand hygiene is the most important action in preventing the transmission of infection. Guidelines for cleaning one's hands were presented in Chapter 16. Hand hygiene is required before and after contact with a patient, wound care, or any invasive procedure.

Frequent hand hygiene is performed when caring for patients susceptible to infection. Patients with decreased immune status are often placed in protective isolation to reduce exposure to infectious organisms. People providing care for these individuals must wear gowns, gloves, and masks, and the patient needs to be in a private room. Specific guidelines vary with the facility and the degree of immune deficiency. Know and follow your agency's policies and procedures.

Hand hygiene is to be performed before donning gloves and after removing them. Although tasks such as interviewing the patient do not require hand hygiene, if a patient is coughing or sneezing during the interview, hand hygiene should be performed before leaving the room (Safety Alert 17-1).

NURSING CARE PLAN 17-1

Care of the Patient Under Airborne Precautions

SCENARIO Doug Gamble, age 18, has pulmonary tuberculosis. He is in a private isolation room. It is his second day of hospitalization. He has just told the nurse he is feeling rejected because everybody wears a mask when they come in to see him.

PROBLEM/NURSING DIAGNOSIS *Does not understand infection precautions*/Knowledge, deficient related to infection and mode of transmission.

Supporting Assessment Data **Subjective:** States he can't understand why he has to stay in his room and why people have to wear masks to visit. **Objective:** PPD skin test positive. Sputum culture positive for acid-fast bacilli. Radiologic studies: cavitations in apex of right lung. Medical diagnosis: Active pulmonary tuberculosis.

Goals/Expected Outcomes	Nursing Interventions	Selected Rationales	Evaluation
Patient will voice understanding of the pathogen and need for Transmission-Based Precautions.	Teach regarding pathogen that causes pulmonary TB, transmission of the organism, and need for masks and staying in room.	Understanding of disease transmission will help patient adhere to transmission precautions.	*Does patient understand the need for precautions?* States understands need for precautions.
	Teach specifics of good hand hygiene and respiratory etiquette, including covering mouth when coughing and containment of used tissues and sputum.	Hand hygiene and proper respiratory etiquette will help prevent transmission of pathogen.	Attentive to hand hygiene. Covers mouth when coughing, disposes of tissues appropriately. Expected outcome being met.

PROBLEM/NURSING DIAGNOSIS *Under visitor precautions*/Social interaction, impaired related to transmission precautions.

Supporting Assessment Data **Objective:** In private isolation room for Airborne Precautions. Visitors must wear a mask when in the room. No visitors except parents since admission.

Goals/Expected Outcomes	Nursing Interventions	Selected Rationales	Evaluation
Patient will have visits of family or friends at least twice a day.	Speak with parents about the need for social interaction. Remind that people may visit if they wear a mask in the room.	Understanding may promote cooperation and obtain visitors for patient.	*Are visitors coming?* Parents state they understand.
	Ask parents to call patient's friends and ask them to visit and arrange a visiting schedule.	A schedule for visiting will promote properly spaced visits that may increase social interaction without tiring the patient.	Mother is working on a visitor schedule. Continue plan.

NURSING CARE PLAN 17-1

Care of the Patient Under Airborne Precautions—cont'd

PROBLEM/NURSING DIAGNOSIS *Feels rejected*/Situational low self-esteem.
Supporting Assessment Data Subjective: States he feels rejected and dirty because people have to wear a mask when close to him. *Objective:* Standard Precautions call for a mask whenever in the room.

Goals/Expected Outcomes	Nursing Interventions	Selected Rationales	Evaluation
Patient will adjust to Transmission-Based Precautions requirements by showing less anxious behavior when someone with a mask enters the room.	Remind him of the route of transmission of the organism. Assure that the wearing of masks simply protects the visitors and caregivers.	Understanding the virulence of the organism and that it is transmitted by airborne droplets will help him understand the need for masks to prevent transmission to others.	*Is patient less anxious?* States understands the danger of the organism and how it is transmitted.
	Ask that each health care person entering the room show her face at the door before donning a mask.	Showing the patient the face behind the mask makes the interaction more personal and friendly.	Each caregiver is showing face and introducing self at the door.
	Show warm interest in the patient as a person. Include ordinary conversation during interactions so he knows he is seen as a person, not a disease.	Interest in the patient bolsters feelings of self-esteem.	Talking with patient about his interests appears to decrease feelings of isolation and help him cope. Progressing toward expected outcome.

? CRITICAL THINKING QUESTIONS

1. How would you assess Doug's understanding of his illness?
2. Why is it important to schedule rest between activities for Doug?

3. Why is it important to keep Doug well nourished and hydrated?

Key: *PPD*, Purified protein derivative; *TB*, tuberculosis.

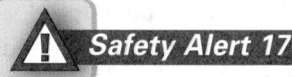

Safety Alert 17-1

Hand Hygiene

Hand hygiene must always be performed after the nurse touches the patient or anything in the patient's room. Methicillin-resistant *Staphylococcus aureus* (MRSA) and other pathologic organisms can survive for varying periods of time on almost any surface.

Personal Protective Equipment

Standard Precautions guidelines state when personal protective equipment (PPE) is to be worn (see Chapter 16). Clean disposable gloves are used for most general care, such as bathing, perineal care, IV site care, and most dressing changes. Masks are worn when working within 3 feet of a patient under Droplet Precautions. (*Refer to the companion CD-ROM for Nursing Care Plan 17-2: Care of the Patient Under Droplet Precautions.*) The nurse who is coughing should wear a mask when in contact with patients. CDC guidelines state that if full PPE is required, it is donned in the following order: gown, followed by the mask or respirator, then goggles or face shield, and finally gloves. The sequence for removing PPE is gloves, followed by face shield or goggles, then the gown, and finally the mask or respirator.

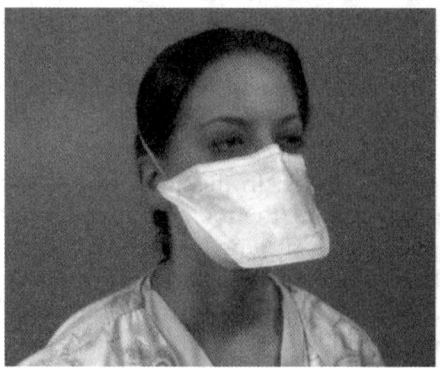

FIGURE **17-2** The particulate filter mask.

Skill 16-2 shows the correct procedure for putting on a gown and mask. Skill 17-4 on pp. 253-255 shows the correct procedure for putting on and removing sterile gloves. Hand hygiene is always performed after removing gloves or any combination of PPE.

When the patient has known or suspected pulmonary tuberculosis, a special particulate filter mask called an N95 mask must be worn (see Figure 16-5, C). The same type of mask is used when caring for patients with known or suspected rubeola or varicella unless the nurse is immune to these diseases (Figure 17-2).

? *Think Critically About* . . . What personal protective equipment would you don to take the vital signs of someone under Airborne Precautions?

General Guidelines for Isolation Precautions

Specimen Preparation and Transportation. Label the specimen container with the patient's name and medical record number plus the type of specimen before entering the patient's room. Place the label on the container itself, not the lid, because once the lid is removed in the lab, the specimen is unlabeled. Collect the specimen and carefully place it in the leak-proof container without contaminating the outside of the container. Be sure the lid is fully tightened. Clean or disinfect containers that are visibly contaminated before sending them to the laboratory. Both OSHA and the Clinical Laboratory Improvement Act (CLIA) require that specimens be transported to the laboratory in a plastic bag marked "Biohazard."

Linens. Soiled linen is handled as little as possible. Roll it up and place it inside the patient's linen hamper in the room. When the bag is two-thirds full, tie it closed and send it to the laundry according to agency policy. Double bagging is not necessary.

Trash. Disposable soiled equipment and supplies are placed inside the plastic bag lining the waste receptacle in the patient's room. Red bags marked with a biohazard symbol are for biohazardous waste only. Ordinary trash is to be placed in standard trash bags and disposed of in the routine manner. Biohazardous waste requires special disposition that is very costly, and non-biohazardous trash should never be mixed in with it. The bag is sealed when it is two-thirds full, removed, and sent to waste collection. The only time double bagging is necessary is if the plastic bag is soiled on the outside. In this instance, another nurse standing just outside the room doorway holds open a second plastic bag, placing her hands under the edge of the bag, which is folded outward to cover the nurse's gloved hands. This further protects her hands from soiling. The nurse in the patient's room then places the first bag carefully inside the second one. The nurse outside the room ties the bag closed, being careful not to touch the inner first bag.

Sharps. Needles are not to be recapped before disposal. All used needles, scalpel blades, IV cannulas, suture needles, and other sharp items are dropped into a puncture-resistant sharps biohazard container. *Never put your fingers inside the opening of the sharps container.* Shake the container gently to settle the contents and make more room if necessary. Sharps containers should be replaced when they are two-thirds full. The full sharps container is sealed and sent to the biohazard waste storage area for later removal.

Federal policy and The Environment of Care guidelines of the Joint Commission require that sharps con-

tainers be secured in patient care areas, and that holding areas for biohazards must be accessible by staff only.

Other Equipment. Reusable equipment is cleaned if it is visibly soiled and then sent to central supply to be disinfected. A stethoscope and blood pressure cuff are issued to the isolation patient, and only these are used within the isolation room. When the patient is discharged, these items are returned to central supply for disinfection as needed. No special treatment is necessary for dishes. Some agencies use paper dishes and trays for patients under Transmission-Based Precautions but this is not a CDC requirement. Box 17-2 presents other general principles.

? *Think Critically About* . . . What types of trash would you place in a red biohazard bag?

Natural Defenses. You should institute measures to protect and enhance the natural body defenses of the patient. These defenses were discussed in Chapter 16. In particular, you should protect intact skin and mucous membranes, promote a balanced diet and sufficient fluids, provide opportunity for adequate sleep and rest, and decrease stress as much as possible.

Patient Placement. A patient in need of Transmission-Based Precautions is usually placed in a private room. An exception can be made if another patient has the same type of infection. Then they can be cohorted in the same room. If the patient is under Airborne Precautions, a private room with negative air flow or a portable HEPA (high-efficiency particulate matter) filter machine is essential. The door to the room must remain closed except when someone is entering or leaving. This helps ensure the organism remains contained and does not enter the rest of the unit. Box 17-3 presents recommended isolation precautions for hospitals.

Transporting the Patient. Transporting the isolation patient is avoided unless absolutely necessary. If transporting is unavoidable, the patient is given a standard mask to wear while out of the room. For a patient under Droplet Precautions, measures are taken to prevent soiling of the environment. The unit or department receiving the patient must be notified ahead of time that a patient under this particular type of Transmission-Based Precautions is coming to the area. Information about any additional precautions required must be shared with those receiving the patient.

Infection Prevention and Control in the Home

The patient at home has less exposure to HAIs, but can still be at risk. The emphasis in the home environment is on containing pathogens and preventing transmission to health care personnel, caregivers, and others in the household. The home health nurse must teach patients and families to dispose of dirty supplies in a safe manner.

Box 17-2 | *General Principles Regarding Isolation*

- Floors are contaminated. Anything dropped on the floor is contaminated and must be discarded or cleaned carefully before reuse.
- Patients with communicable diseases should be grouped according to the epidemiology of transmission:
  - Contact through respiratory spread
  - Transmission by the gastrointestinal tract
  - Direct contact with wound or skin infection
- Keep the dust down. Sweeping compounds or wet mops with disinfectants and damp dusting must be used for this purpose.
- Protect the patient from drafts.
- Establish contaminated and clean zones. The clean areas should include those used by the health care worker. Items such as telephones outside the unit should not be used by the patient. There should be a clean area in the isolation unit where no contaminated articles are permitted. Items not in the clean area are considered contaminated.
- Anything that is brought into the isolation area must not be removed except in proper containers, which are then placed in an outside container labeled "Hazardous Materials—Biohazard."
- Never rub your eyes or nose or put your hands near your mouth when taking care of a patient in an isolation unit.
- Never shake linen when removing it or placing it on the bed.
- Change gloves and perform hand hygiene after handling contaminated items.
- Provide a clean area for placement of supplies by putting a paper towel or square of paper on a dry surface.
- Keep a water pitcher and glass in the room. Ice and fresh water are brought to the door and transferred.
- Faucets should be turned on and off using a paper towel to protect the hands.
- The same nursing procedures are carried out for these patients as for any patient, but you must use the appropriate barrier precautions.
- Use the room clock for taking the patient's pulse and respirations. If the room does not have a clock, your watch can be taken in by putting it in a clear plastic bag. When leaving the room, it can be emptied onto a clean paper towel.
- You should monitor your own level of resistance to infection and report to the unit director or charge nurse any skin lesion, sore throat, or other evidence of infection you may have. (You may be reassigned to protect yourself and the patient.)

Box 17-3 | *Recommended Isolation Precautions in Hospitals: Transmission-Based Precautions (Tier 2)*

AIRBORNE PRECAUTIONS
Use the Tier 1 precautions (Standard Precautions) as well as the following:
1. Place the patient in a private room that has negative air pressure: 6 to 12 air exchanges per hour and discharge of air to the outside or a filtration system for the room air.
2. If a private room is not available, place the patient with another patient who is infected with the same microorganism.
3. Wear a respiratory device (N95 respirator) when entering the room of a patient who is known to have or suspected of having primary tuberculosis.
4. Susceptible people should not enter the room of a patient who has rubella (measles) or varicella (chickenpox). If they must enter, they should wear a respirator.
5. Limit movement of the patient outside the room to essential purposes. Place a surgical mask on the patient if possible.

DROPLET PRECAUTIONS
Use the Tier 1 precautions (Standard Precautions) as well as the following:
1. Place the patient in a private room.
2. If a private room is not available, place the patient with another patient who is infected with the same microorganism.
3. Wear a mask if working within 3 feet of the patient.
4. Transport the patient outside of the room only when necessary, and place a surgical mask on the patient if possible.

CONTACT PRECAUTIONS
Use the Tier 1 precautions (Standard Precautions) as well as the following:
1. Place the patient in a private room.
2. If a private room is not available, place the patient with another patient who is infected with the same microorganism.
3. Wear gloves as described in Standard Precautions.
   a. Change gloves after contact with infectious material.
   b. Remove gloves before leaving the patient's room.
   c. Cleanse hands immediately after removing gloves. Use an antimicrobial agent.
   d. After hand hygiene, do not touch possibly contaminated surfaces or items in the room.
4. Wear a gown when entering a room if there is a possibility of contact with infected surfaces or items, or if the patient is incontinent or has diarrhea, a colostomy, or wound drainage not contained by a dressing.
   a. Remove gown in the patient's room.
   b. Make sure clothing does not contact possible contaminated surfaces.
5. Limit movement of the patient outside the room.
6. Dedicate the use of noncritical patient care equipment to a single patient or to patients with the same infecting microorganisms.

From Hospital Infection Control Practices Advisory Committee (HICPAC). (2007). Guidelines for Isolation Precautions in Hospitals. Available at: www.cdc.gov/ncidod/dhqp/gl_isolation.html.

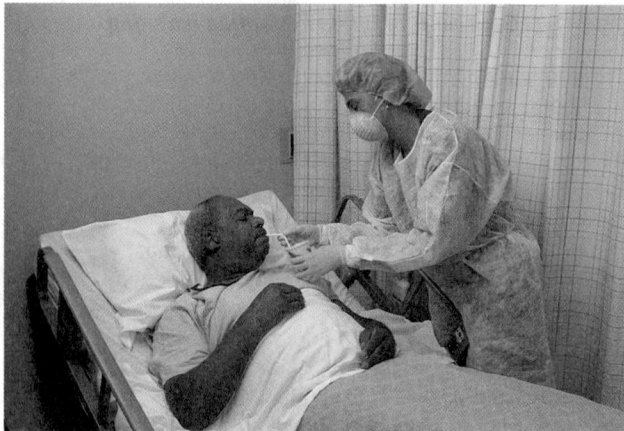

FIGURE **17-3** Nurse in personal protective equipment caring for patient in protective isolation room.

Home Care Considerations 17-1

Infection Prevention and Control Precautions for Patients in the Home Setting

- Patients and families must be taught the importance of hand hygiene. Stress that hands must be cleansed before caring for the patient and after care is finished. Gloves are needed in addition to hand hygiene for tasks such as tracheal suctioning and tracheostomy care; dressing changes and wound or drain care; tube feedings; and cleansing of personal areas of the body.
- Used dressings, tissues, wound-cleaning supplies, and any other item contaminated with body fluids should be discarded into a plastic bag and sealed before being placed in the household trash for pickup.

When the patient has an infection, care should be taken that his towels, sheets, and clothes are kept away from contact by others until they can be washed. The patient's clothing and linens can in most cases be laundered with the rest of the household wash. Washing in warm water with standard laundry detergent is usually sufficient. Items should be thoroughly dried prior to use, either in a dryer or outside in the sun.

The patient is taught to perform correct hand hygiene and to dispose of any paper towels or facial tissues in an appropriate container. Other family members must be instructed to perform hand hygiene frequently as well. The bathroom should be cleaned daily with standard household chemicals or a 1:10 solution of chlorine bleach and water. Dishes should be washed on the hot cycle of the dishwasher or soaked in scalding water after washing and allowed to air dry. The patient's laundry should be washed separately, using hot water and bleach if possible.

Soiled dressings and wound care supplies should be disposed of in plain, unlabeled plastic bags that are tied up securely and stored in an appropriate trash receptacle for pickup with the rest of the household trash. Trash marked with the biohazard symbol cannot be placed in the household trash pickup. Handling or transporting biohazard trash requires special permits.

A heavy plastic jug with a secure top can be used to contain needles and syringes and other sharp objects used in the patient's care. Placing a 1:10 solution of chlorine bleach and water in the container helps kill microorganisms. Disposal of the jug is subject to local regulations in the city, county, or province where the patient lives.

Clean gloves are used for wound care unless there is an order for sterile dressing changes. Patients and family members should be taught to properly remove and dispose of contaminated gloves. It should be stressed that hands are to be cleansed before putting on gloves, and again after the gloves are discarded. Reinforce that gloves should not be reused.

The patient's room should be cleaned frequently, with dust kept to a minimum. Fresh air should be allowed to circulate in the room. Sunshine through the windows can elevate the patient's mood and decrease the presence of some microorganisms. Trash, newspapers, and clutter should be kept to a minimum to discourage transfer of microorganisms. Clean supplies should be kept in one area, well away from any contaminated items or trash (Home Care Considerations 17-1).

Protective Isolation

When a patient is immunocompromised, it is very important to protect him from exposure to potential pathogens. The patient is placed in a special isolation room with its own ventilation system. No one with an active infection is allowed in the patient's room. Until recently, the degree of isolation was as absolute as possible, extending even to sterile dishes and having anyone who entered wear full protective equipment. Recent studies in major medical centers throughout the world are indicating that environments can be less stringent without increasing the rates of HAIs, and that PPE is not required for routine entry into the room. It is important, therefore, to remain aware of your facility's policies and procedures regarding protective isolation and to follow them at all times (Figure 17-3).

Psychological Aspects of Isolation

The patient in Transmission-Based Isolation precautions is at risk for both decreased self-esteem and sensory deprivation. This is particularly true for young children, who under normal circumstances are rarely alone, and are often used to highly stimulating and entertaining environments. The elderly, too, can find isolation particularly trying, and it may lead to confusion secondary to the lack of normal stimulation and interaction. Assessment for sensory deprivation needs to be ongoing. The signs can include boredom, slowness of thought, disorganized thoughts, excessive sleeping during the day, anxiety, hallucinations, or panic attacks.

Having visitors at intervals can be very helpful in preventing sensory deprivation. They can talk with the patient about interests they share, and a visitor at mealtime often encourages improved nutritional intake by making mealtime more enjoyable. The nurse should learn about the patient's interests and provide appropriate activities. These can include games, books, puzzles, phone calls, radio or TV, a video, or a craft project. However, avoid overtiring the patient by also allowing periods of rest between activities.

Sensory deprivation may occur if visitors are intimidated by the isolation precautions. There may be decreased interaction with the health care team because of the need to put on personal protective equipment to enter the room. All of this can lead to a loss of self-esteem because the patient begins to feel that he is somehow unclean or unworthy of attention.

Listen to the patient's feelings. Make positive comments on efforts at grooming or self-amusement (Cultural Cues 17-1). Try to engage the patient in conversation that is meaningful by asking about particular interests or hobbies. Assisting visitors to feel welcome and to understand that the patient benefits greatly from their presence can also help. Addressing self-esteem needs is very important for complete recovery.

?
• *Think Critically About . . .* How might you reassure a patient with pulmonary tuberculosis under Airborne Precautions who states that he feels everyone is avoiding him because he is "dirty"?

Infection Prevention and Control for the Nurse

OSHA regulations protect health care workers from occupational exposure to blood-borne pathogens in the workplace. In Canada, the Occupational Health and Safety Act addresses worker safety. The three main modes of occupational exposure to blood-borne pathogens are as follows:

- Puncture wounds from contaminated needles or other sharps
- Skin contact, allowing blood, body fluids, and other potentially infectious materials to enter through damaged or broken skin
- Mucous membrane contact, allowing infectious materials to enter through the mucous membranes of the eyes, mouth, and nose

Actions that decrease the nurse's risk for infection include good hand hygiene and other general medical asepsis techniques, the wearing of personal protective equipment, using needleless IV equipment and needles with guards, and avoiding carelessness in the clinical area.

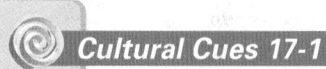
Cultural Cues 17-1

Cleanliness

People in the United States and Canada generally place a high value on cleanliness. The idea of being "contaminated," "soiled," or "dirty" can make the patient feel at fault or inferior. The patient may place blame on himself. The nurse can help overcome this with a warm, caring, and accepting attitude, and by avoiding displaying any irritation about the precautions or any evidence of distaste in dealing with the infection.

It is also recommended that health care workers be immunized if they are not shown to have an active immune status to certain diseases. These include hepatitis B, influenza, mumps, measles, rubella, varicella (chickenpox), tetanus, diphtheria, pertussis, and meningococcal disease.

Surgical Asepsis

Surgical asepsis is another method used to prevent infection. Surgical asepsis is practiced in the operating room, obstetric areas, special diagnostic areas, and for procedures such as administering injections, changing wound dressings, performing urinary catheterization, and administering intravenous therapy. In the operating room, strict surgical asepsis is practiced, and head coverings, sterile gowns, masks, and gloves are worn. To perform a sterile dressing change outside the operating room, sterile gloves, a mask, and a sterile field are used. Talking during the dressing change is discouraged.

The four rules of surgical asepsis are as follows:
1. Know what is sterile.
2. Know what is not sterile.
3. Separate sterile from unsterile.
4. Remedy contamination immediately.

The goal in surgical asepsis is to keep an area free of microorganisms. You must constantly be aware of which items and areas are sterile, clean, or contaminated to maintain surgical asepsis. The importance of maintaining sterility must become ingrained, and you must consistently maintain principles of surgical asepsis to protect the safety of patients (Box 17-4). By being constantly sensitive as to what is sterile, what is clean, and what becomes contaminated, breaks in sterile technique are caught and rectified before microorganisms are transferred to the patient.

Surgical Scrub. The surgical scrub is more lengthy and vigorous than normal handwashing. Its purpose is to remove as many microorganisms as possible without damaging the skin of the hands. Skill 17-1 presents the steps for the traditional surgical scrub. Water, a nail stick, an antiseptic agent, a scrub brush or sponge pad, and friction are used to mechanically cleanse the hands and forearms. The scrub begins at the hands and ends 2 inches above the elbows. All rinsing is done under

Box 17-4 *Principles of Aseptic Technique*

These principles form the basis of surgical asepsis:

1. A sterile surface touching a sterile surface remains sterile.
2. A sterile surface touching an unsterile surface becomes contaminated.
3. Sterile materials must be kept dry; moisture transmits microorganisms and contaminates.
4. Only sterile items are used within the sterile field.
5. A sterile barrier must be considered contaminated after it has been penetrated.
6. The edges of a sterile package or container are considered contaminated after it is opened.
7. When there is a doubt about the sterility of any item, it must be considered not sterile.
8. Reaching across or above a sterile field with bare hands or arms or with other nonsterile items must be avoided.
9. Coughing, sneezing, or unnecessary talking near or over a sterile field must be avoided.
10. When wearing sterile gloves, hands must be kept in sight, away from all unsterile objects, and above waist level.
11. Gowns are considered sterile only in front from shoulder level to table level and the sleeves to 2 inches above the elbow.
12. The wrapper of a sterile pack must be opened away from the body, the distal flap first, the lateral flaps next, and the proximal flap toward the body last, thus making it unnecessary to reach over the sterile field.
13. Only the horizontal surface of a table is considered sterile.
14. An area of 1 inch surrounding the outer edge of the sterile field must be considered unsterile.
15. The sterile field must be kept in sight at all times. Do not turn away from it or leave it. If this happens, you cannot be sure that it is still sterile.
16. The floor must be recognized as the most grossly contaminated area. Clean or sterile items that fall on to the floor should be discarded or decontaminated.

Skill 17-1 Performing Surgical Hand Antisepsis: The Surgical Scrub

The purpose of the surgical hand scrub is to remove dirt, skin oil, and microorganisms from the hands and lower arms and to reduce the microorganism count to as near zero as possible. The antiseptic residue remains on the skin to prevent the growth of microorganisms for several hours. A timed scrub is performed for the interval recommended by the manufacturer of the antiseptic agent used. Some agencies may allow a counted-stroke scrub.

A surgical scrub is performed before entering the operating room, the labor and delivery area, the newborn nursery, or the neonatal intensive care unit (NICU). The scrub is repeated prior to the next surgical procedure or delivery, or any time that the hands become contaminated. A 5-minute scrub is presented here.

A brushless surgical scrub using an antimicrobial agent that is at least 60% alcohol may be substituted in some hospitals for the traditional surgical hand scrub (see Skill 17-2).

■ Supplies

✓ Sterile towels
✓ Foot faucet control
✓ Running water
✓ Antiseptic soap in dispenser with foot control
✓ Scrub brush or sponge pad
✓ Nail stick

Review and carry out the Standard Steps in Appendix 3.

■ Assessment (Data Collection)

1. *ACTION* Determine whether all supplies needed are available before beginning.

   RATIONALE Missing supplies can mean interrupting the scrub to collect them, and then having to start the scrub over.

■ Planning

2. *ACTION* Remove rings and watch.

   RATIONALE These items are unsterile and cannot be worn during a sterile procedure. Fasten them with a large safety pin inside a pocket of your scrub clothes on the front of the scrub shirt or gown. Jewelry harbors microorganisms. No objects may be touched after beginning the surgical scrub.

■ Implementation

3. *ACTION* Adjust the water to a comfortable temperature using the foot control.

   RATIONALE The water remains running during the scrub and should be comfortably warm.

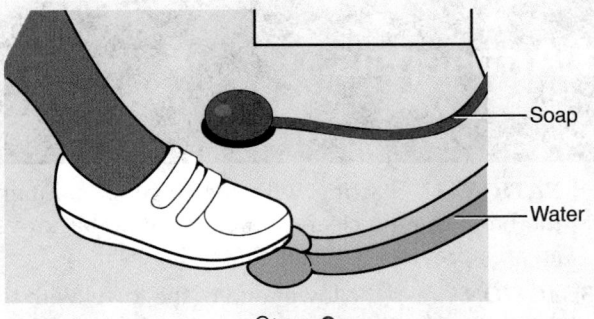

Step **3**

4. **ACTION** Wet your hands and arms from above the elbows to the fingertips, with the hands kept higher than the elbows throughout the scrub.

   RATIONALE Moisture will aid the formation of the cleansing lather. Keeping the hands higher than the elbows prevents microorganisms from draining over the cleansed hands.

5. **ACTION** Dispense the soaping agent onto the palms using the dispenser foot control and rub hands together to work up a lather. Clean the fingernails with a nail stick. Wash the hands and forearms to a point at least 2 inches above the elbow.

   RATIONALE The soaping agent assists in cleaning dirt from under the nails.

6. **ACTION** When using a prepackaged scrub brush or sponge pad, open the package, remove the nail cleaner, and clean the nails. The nail stick is held until the nails have all been cleaned, and then it is discarded. Remove the brush or pad from the package and discard the package. Do not set down the brush or pad once the scrub is begun. If the brush or sponge pad is not impregnated with the cleansing agent, moisten the brush or pad and dispense the antiseptic agent onto it.

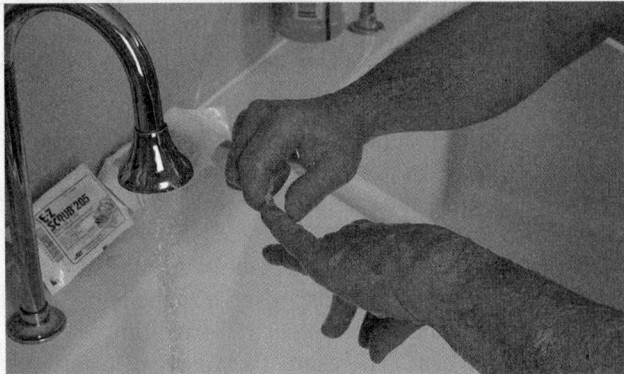

Step **6**

   RATIONALE Putting the brush or pad down during the scrub contaminates it. It must remain in the hands until the scrub is complete, then discarded.

7. **ACTION** Start at the fingertips and, with a circular motion, work around each finger and between each finger, holding the scrub brush or sponge pad perpendicular to the fingers and nails. Use light to

moderate friction. Scrub the back of the hand, the palm, and then the wrist with circular strokes. Scrub each hand and arm for 2½ minutes. Care should be taken to not abrade the skin.

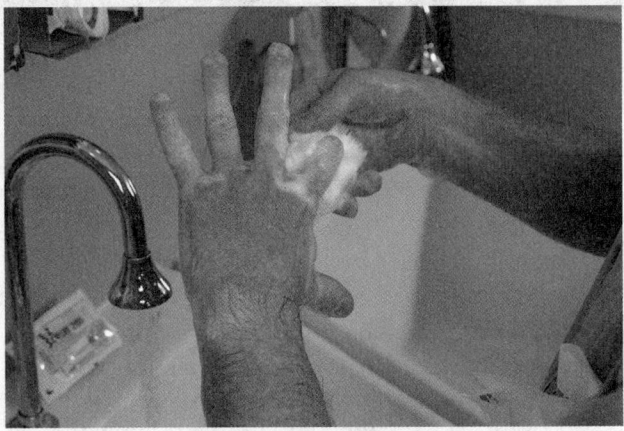

Step **7**

RATIONALE Achieving the desired degree of skin asepsis requires an extended cleansing time. Excessive pressure can injure the skin and should be avoided.

8. **ACTION** Continue up the arm to the elbow using circular scrub strokes on all surfaces, holding the brush or sponge pad parallel to the arm.

   RATIONALE Dirt and microorganisms need to be removed from portions of the arm that will be working in the surgical field even though these skin areas will be covered by a sterile gown and sterile gloves.

9. **ACTION** Rinse each hand and arm thoroughly, holding the hand above the level of the elbow and allowing the water to run from the fingertips down

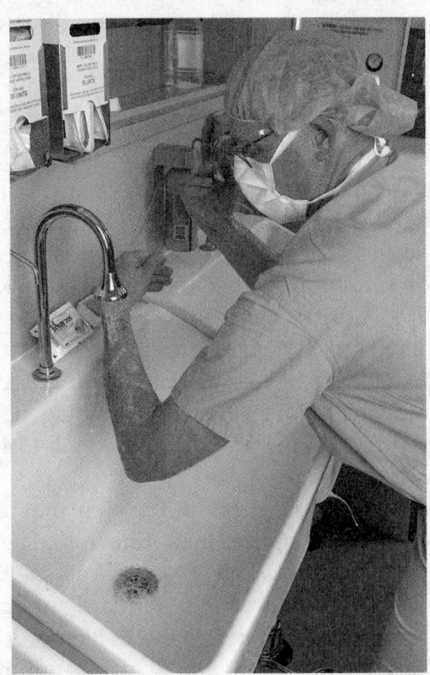

Step **9**

Continued

Skill 17-1 | Performing Surgical Hand Antisepsis: The Surgical Scrub—cont'd

the hand to the wrist, then the forearm, and off the elbow area.

RATIONALE Maintains the hands as the cleanest area by not rinsing dirt from above over them.

10. *ACTION* Turn off the faucet using the foot control.

RATIONALE Prevents contamination of the hands from the faucet handle. Maintains the sterility of the scrub.

11. *ACTION* Dry the hands with a sterile towel. Step away from the sterile field, lean slightly forward from the waist and unfold the towel, holding it by a corner and allowing it to unfold downward. Do not let the towel reach below waist level, or to come in contact with the body or any object in the room.

RATIONALE When the towel is taken from a sterile field, it is lifted straight up and away from the sterile field, which keeps water from dripping on the sterile field. Maintaining the arms and hands above waist level and the hands above the elbows protects the scrubbed area. The hands are dried away from the sterile field. When working in the operating room or delivery room, the hands are dried upon entering that room.

12. *ACTION* Keep the arms and hands above waist level and away from the body with the hands and fingers pointed up. Use the top half of the towel to blot the opposite fingers and hand dry, and move to the forearm. Use a rotary motion to move the towel from the forearm to the elbow. Do not go back over an area already dried.

RATIONALE Starting with the fingers, maintains the hands as the cleanest area. Moving back over an area previously dried contaminates it.

13. *ACTION* Grasp the lower end of the towel with the dried hand, and use the same procedure to dry the other hand and forearm. Discard the towel by dropping it into the proper receptacle when finished. Keep your hands and arms above waist level.

RATIONALE Touching a damp part of the towel with the dried hand will contaminate that hand. Gowning and gloving are done next.

■ Evaluation

14. *ACTION* Ask yourself the following questions: Did the hands refrain from touching any part of the sink during the scrub? Were the hands higher than the elbows throughout the scrub? Was each hand and arm scrubbed for a full 2½ minutes? Were the hands dried without breaking technique?

RATIONALE If the answer is yes to all of the questions, the scrub is complete. If contamination occurred, the scrub is done over from the beginning.

Documentation

No documentation is required for this procedure.

?CRITICAL THINKING QUESTIONS

1. Why should you avoid excessive pressure on the skin during the scrub?

2. If you are finished with the surgical scrub and are rinsing your hands and arms and accidentally touch the faucet spout, what would you do?

flowing water, not in a container of water (Figure 17-4). The timing for the scrub does not include the rinsing time. Some agencies allow the use of the counted-stroke method of scrubbing rather than by-the-clock timing (Figure 17-5). Current standards regarding the time for the traditional scrub are based on the recommendations of the antiseptic agent manufacturer, and consequently the recommended time varies from one agency to another, depending on the product in use. A 2- to 4-minute scrub is average.

A newer brushless technique, which may be done with or without water, uses an antimicrobial agent that is at least 60% alcohol. This method was shown to be equally effective compared to a standard surgical scrub in a research study (Gruendemann & Bjerke, 2001). For the brushless scrub technique, 2 mL of antimicrobial agent are dispensed into the palm of one hand. With the fingertips of the opposite hand, some of the alcohol-based agent is worked under the nails. The remaining portion of the agent is spread over all surfaces of the hand and arm to just above the elbow. Another 2 mL of the antimicrobial agent is dispensed into the palm of the other hand and the procedure is repeated on the opposite hand and arm. There are variations in technique depending on the product used. *Check the manufacturer's directions for the correct technique.* The hands and arms must be allowed to dry before gloving (Skill 17-2).

Opening Sterile Packs and Packages and Setting Up a Sterile Field. Many sterile supplies are prepared commercially and are disposable or one-time use items. The package, set, or kit provides all the items commonly required in a variety of nursing procedures, such as catheterization, suture removal, dressing change, and irrigation. Individually wrapped items can be obtained to supplement the packs as needed.

Packs and kits are opened by removing the outer plastic or paper covering, taking out the inner package, and aseptically unfolding the wrapper to form a sterile field (Figure 17-6). The principles of asepsis apply regardless of whether the package is disposable or a wrapped tray is prepared by the central supply department of the hospital. Skill 17-3 shows the steps for opening sterile packs and preparing a sterile field.

The principles to observe when opening sterile packages are as follows:
- Perform hand hygiene.
- Open the sterile package away from the body.
- Touch only the outside of the wrapper.
- Do not reach across a sterile field; go around the sterile field if necessary to reach the other side.
- Always face the sterile field, even when moving to the other side.
- Allow sufficient space (at least 6 inches) between the body and the sterile field.

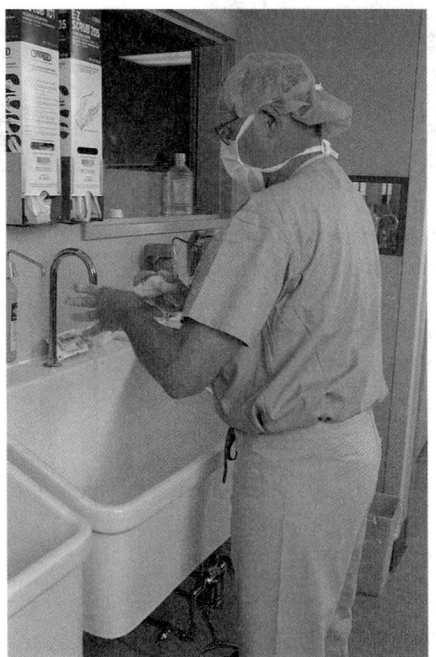

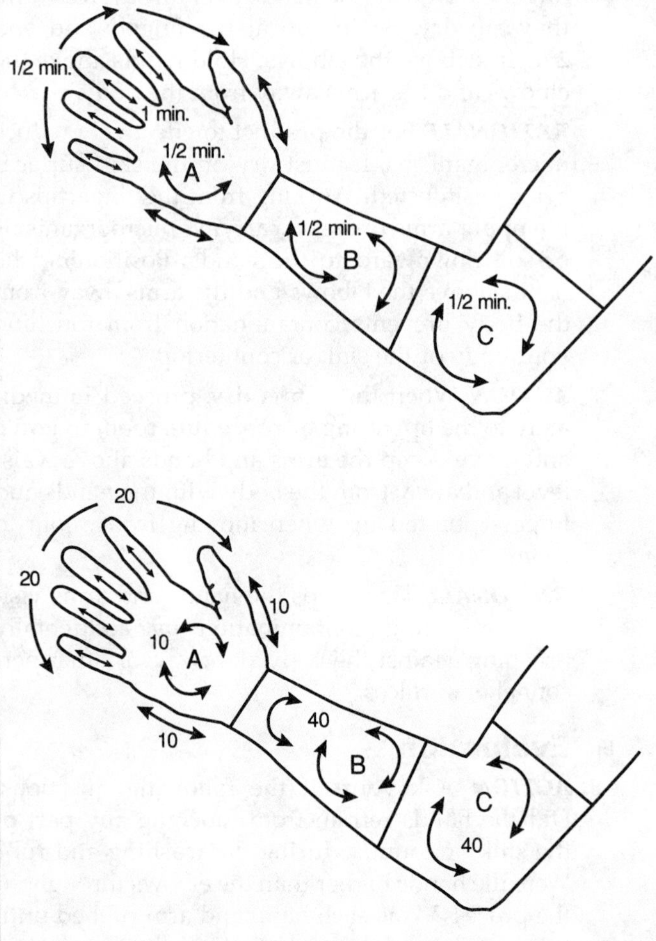

FIGURE **17-4** Nurse performing surgical scrub.

ANATOMIC TIMED SCRUB METHOD

AREA	TIME
1. Nails (A)	30 seconds w/brush
2. Fingers, each side and web space (A)	1 minute w/sponge
3. Palmar surface (A)	15 seconds w/brush
4. Dorsal surface (A)	15 seconds w/sponge
5. Forearm, divided in half to 2" above elbow (B and C)	1 minute w/sponge (30 seconds each half)
6. Repeat process for other hand	

COUNTED BRUSH STROKE METHOD

AREA	TIME
1. Nails (A)	20 strokes w/brush
2. Fingers, each side and web space (A)	10 strokes w/brush
3. Palmar surface (A)	10 strokes w/brush
4. Dorsal surface (A)	10 strokes w/sponge
5. Forearm, divided in half to 2" above elbow (B and C)	40 strokes each half (10 strokes each side w/sponge)
6. Repeat process for other hand	

FIGURE **17-5** Surgical scrub techniques.

Skill 17-2 | Performing Surgical Hand Antisepsis: The Surgical Hand Rub

The surgical hand rub is an approved alternate method for removing dirt, skin oil, and microorganisms from the hands and lower arms, and to reduce the microorganism count to as near zero as possible. Antiseptic residue remains on the skin to prevent the growth of microorganisms for several hours.

A surgical hand rub is performed before entering the operating room, the labor and delivery area, the newborn nursery, or the NICU. The rub is repeated prior to the next surgical procedure or delivery, or any time that the hands become contaminated. It uses an antimicrobial agent that is at least 60% alcohol.

■ Supplies

- ✓ Sterile towels
- ✓ Foot faucet control
- ✓ Antiseptic soap
- ✓ Running water
- ✓ Antiseptic rub in dispenser with foot control
- ✓ Scrub brush or sponge pad
- ✓ Nail stick

Review and carry out the Standard Steps in Appendix 3.

■ Assessment (Data Collection)

1. *ACTION* Determine whether all supplies needed are available before beginning.

   RATIONALE Missing supplies can mean interrupting the scrub to collect them, and then having to start the scrub over.

■ Planning

2. *ACTION* Remove rings and watch.

   RATIONALE These items are unsterile and cannot be worn during a sterile procedure. Fasten them with a large safety pin inside a pocket of your scrub clothes on the front of the scrub shirt or gown. Jewelry harbors microorganisms. No objects may be touched after beginning the surgical scrub.

■ Implementation

3. *ACTION* Adjust the water to a comfortable temperature using the foot control.

   RATIONALE The water remains running during the prewash and should be comfortably warm.

4. *ACTION* Wash hands and forearms arms thoroughly with antimicrobial soap and running water; cleanse under nails with nail stick.

   RATIONALE Removes surface soiling and dirt that might provide a barrier for microorganisms.

5. *ACTION* Rinse hands and arms under running water with hands held above the elbows. Dry thoroughly with paper towels.

   RATIONALE Removes soil loosened in the washing process without washing the soap down over the hands and possibly carrying microorganisms from the upper arms to the hands. Excess water on the skin may interfere with the action of the rub solution.

6. *ACTION* Dispense the antiseptic rub onto the palms using the dispenser foot control and spread over hands and arms per manufacturer's instructions, which may vary depending upon the product. Make sure that all surfaces are fully covered, paying particular attention to the thumbs and fingers. Rub with the hands over all surfaces until they are dry. Begin rub at the fingers and end 2 inches above the elbows. Hold hands above the elbows and the arms away from the body.

   RATIONALE For the product to effectively reduce microorganisms, it must dry on the skin surfaces being disinfected. Working from the fingertips to the upper arms prevents carrying microorganisms or soil downward to the hands. Positioning the hands above the elbows and the arms away from the body prevents contamination from touching your body or the sink or countertop.

7. *ACTION* When the rub is dry, proceed immediately to the operating or procedure room to gown and glove. Keep the arms and hands above waist level and away from the body with the hands and fingers pointed up when moving from room to room.

   RATIONALE This keeps the hands and arms visible, preventing contamination by accidentally brushing against the body, doorway, or other personnel or surfaces.

■ Evaluation

8. *ACTION* Ask yourself the following questions: Did the hands refrain from touching any part of the sink or counter during the washing and rub? Were the hands higher than the elbows throughout the process? Was each hand and arm rubbed until the surface was fully dry? Were the hands and arms in full view and kept away from contact dur-

ing the movement from the scrub area to the procedure/operating room?

RATIONALE If the answer is yes to all of the questions, the rub is complete. If contamination occurred, the rub is done over from the beginning.

Documentation

No documentation is required for this procedure.

?CRITICAL THINKING QUESTIONS

1. Why should you pay particular attention to the fingers and thumbs during the procedure?
2. If you are finished with the surgical hand rub and accidentally brush your elbow against the door frame when moving into the procedure/operating room, what would you do?

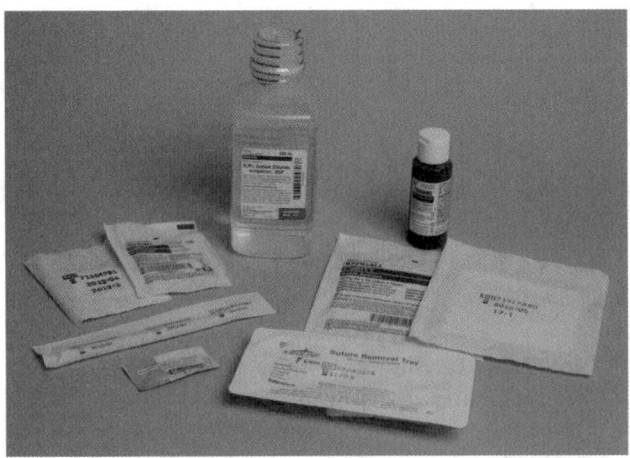

FIGURE **17-6** Types of expiration dates on sterile supplies.

Most sterile items are available as individually wrapped or separate items, such as sterile packages of cotton-tipped applicators, tongue blades, 4 × 4 gauze dressings, ABD (abdominal) dressings, alcohol swabs, syringes, needles, Foley catheters, sterile gloves, and intravenous catheters. Instructions often appear on the outside of the package directing you where to open it, indicating the direction in which to tear, or showing where to peel at a certain point. Follow these instructions to avoid contaminating the contents.

When sterile supplies have been brought to the patient's bedside, they should never be returned to the unit stock shelves. The outsides of these items are contaminated, and returning such supplies carries organisms from the patient's room back to the store of sup-

Skill 17-3 | Opening Sterile Packs and Preparing a Sterile Field

When sterile procedures are to be performed, sterile equipment and supplies are set up on a sterile field. Commercial disposable sterile sets of equipment and supplies are available for most standard procedures. Hospitals also wrap reusable equipment and cloth towels in packs that are sterilized prior to use. Hospital-prepared sterile packs are dated and are returned for re-sterilization if not used by the expiration date. Check the date before using a hospital-prepared prepared sterile pack. Commercially prepared packs may also have expiration dates that need to be checked prior to use.

A sterile field is set up by using the inside of the wrapper on the sterile pack or by opening and draping a tabletop or instrument tray with sterile drapes and then placing the sterile items to be used on the field. The field is considered sterile to within 1 inch of its horizontal, or flat, border. The portion of the sterile drape that falls over the table or tray edge is always considered unsterile.

■ Supplies

✓ Sterile disposable equipment and supply tray

or

✓ Hospital-prepared sterile pack and sterile drapes

Review and carry out the Standard Steps in Appendix 3.

■ Assessment (Data Collection)

1. **ACTION** Select a dry tabletop or instrument tray that is above waist level.

   RATIONALE Moisture can travel upward from the surface and contaminate the sterile field and supplies. Anything below waist level is considered contaminated according to principles of surgical asepsis.

■ Planning

2. **ACTION** Obtain the equipment tray and supplies to be used for the procedure and explain the procedure to the patient if appropriate.

   RATIONALE Ensures that all needed equipment is on hand before scrubbing and gloving. Ensures patient is prepared for the procedure.

Continued

■ Implementation

3. **ACTION** Perform hand hygiene.

   RATIONALE Removes microorganisms.

4. **ACTION** Remove the plastic outer wrap, leaving the inner wrap in place. If a hospital-prepared pack does not have a plastic wrap, remove the tape holding it closed. When setting up a field at the bedside, the plastic wrapper can be used for discards. Place the pack so that the flap that opens to the back of the table is on top.

   RATIONALE The outside of the sterile pack is not considered sterile and can be touched. The first flap is to be opened away from the nurse's working area.

5. **ACTION** Facing the table, move to the far side and open the initial flap by lifting it upward away from the pack, then outward and down over the edge of the table. If the pack is small enough, this can be done by reaching around the pack and opening the distal flap rather than moving to the other side of the field.

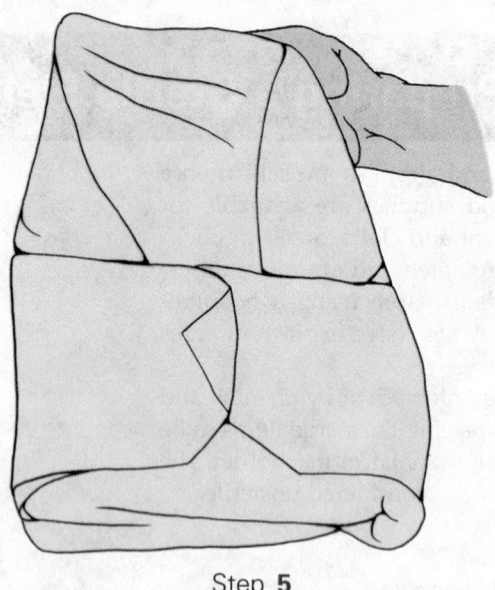

Step **5**

   RATIONALE Opening the distal flap first prevents contaminating the pack by reaching over the exposed sterile contents after the other flaps are opened.

6. **ACTION** With the left hand, move the flap on the left up and laterally away from the package. Pull edge down over the edge of the table. Then open the right flap with the right hand in the same manner. Be careful to touch only the outside of the wrapper and not to reach across any area of exposed sterile supplies.

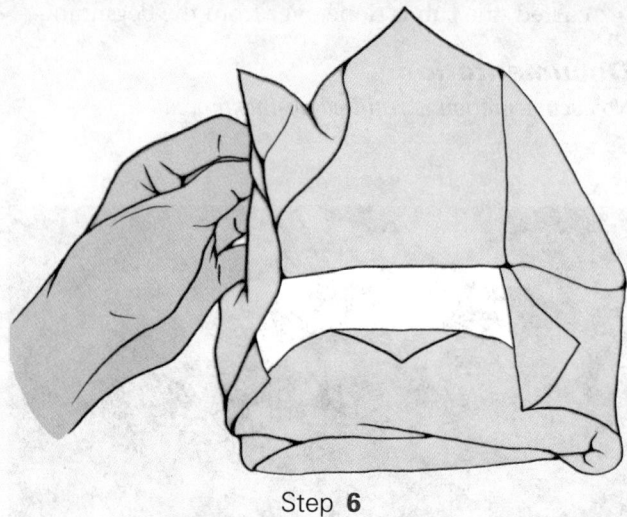

Step **6**

   RATIONALE Maintains the sterility of the inside of the pack and its equipment and supplies. Pulling the drape edges downward over table edges ensures that the wrap does not fall back over the field and contaminate it.

7. **ACTION** Lift the front (proximal) flap up and toward you, handling only the outside of the wrapper or pull-tabs. If the entire pack is to be handed off to someone in sterile gown and gloves, grasp the contents firmly in one hand from the underside and pull each flap down over the hand that is grasping the contents of the package. Secure the flaps with your other hand when offering the pack contents to the sterile person who needs them. If the pack has an inner wrap, this is sterile and need not be opened before handing off the tray.

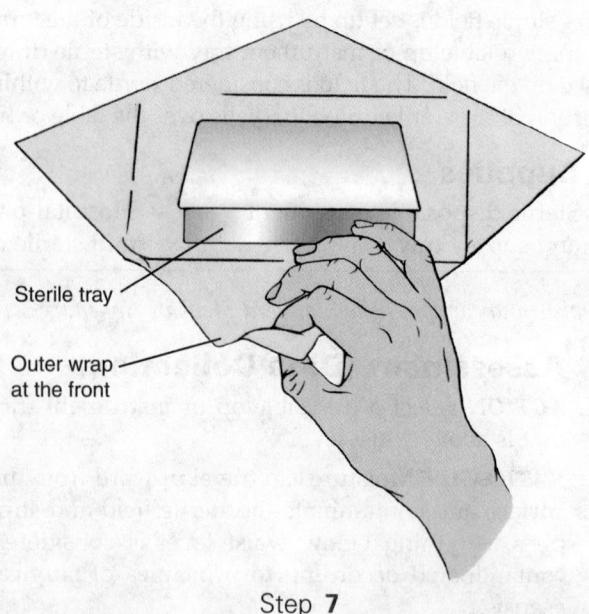

Sterile tray

Outer wrap at the front

Step **7**

RATIONALE Maintains the sterility of the pack contents. Holding back the flaps prevents them from falling forward and touching the gloved hands of the sterile person, or the hands of the nonsterile person from touching the sterile gloves.

8. *ACTION* The inside of the outer wrap is used as the sterile field. Using gloves and/or sterile forceps, arrange the equipment and supplies on the sterile field in the order in which they will be used. Keep all items at least 1 inch from the edge boundary.

   RATIONALE The inside of the wrapper that has not been touched is still sterile. Only sterile items may touch or move over the sterile field, or it will be contaminated. The outside 1-inch edge of the horizontal surface of the wrapper or field is considered contaminated because the edge is in contact with an unsterile surface or is hanging below waist level and subject to contact contamination. The entire field must remain dry to maintain sterility. You must continue to face the field. If your back is turned to the field or it is outside your line of vision, it is considered contaminated because it was not within your visual limits and something nonsterile could have fallen on it or touched it.

Adding Supplies or Equipment to the Sterile Field

9. *ACTION* Inspect the disposable package to see which edge is to be opened. Bring both hands together, and grasp the small flaps at the edge to be opened.

   RATIONALE Establishes the grip to open the package at the intended point.

10. *ACTION* Peel the two parts of the package apart by turning the hands outward to separate the sealed edges.

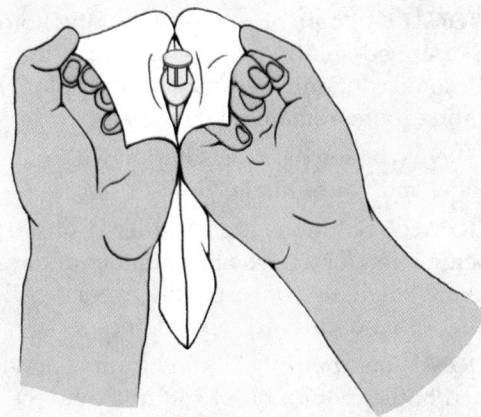

Step **10**

RATIONALE Opens the package, exposing the sterile contents. Allows the sterile person to extract the sterile contents of the package without being contaminated, or allows you to gently toss the sup-

ply item or piece of equipment onto your sterile field without contaminating it.

11. *ACTION* Alternately, for supplies you will use yourself, after starting the peeling process, lay one side of the package flat on a clean, dry surface and peel the top part of the package all the way back.

   RATIONALE The bottom inside of the package serves as a sterile field until the item is used.

12. *ACTION* Perform the sterile procedure, maintaining the principles of surgical asepsis (see Box 17-4).

   RATIONALE Any break in sterile technique contaminates the field, supplies, and equipment.

■ Evaluation

13. *ACTION* Ask yourself: Was the pack opened while maintaining sterile technique? Has the sterile field been within my line of vision during the whole procedure? Have I added supplies to the field in an aseptic manner?

   RATIONALE Answers will determine if the field has been kept sterile.

■ Documentation
Example

9/17 1435   Straight catheterization performed using sterile technique with 14-Fr catheter. No problems encountered; 190 mL clear, yellow urine drained; sterile specimen obtained.

_____
(Nurse's signature)

■ Special Considerations

✓ In the operating room, supplies are added to the field by being opened by the nonsterile (circulating) nurse and handed off to the sterile (scrub) nurse as described in point 10 above.

✓ In the patient's room, after the kit for a procedure is opened, extra supplies can be opened and positioned around the outside of the sterile field on their own wrappers, where they will be within reach.

✓ When offering a peeled package of supplies, keep the opened flaps over your hands so that the sterile person will not touch your nonsterile skin or the nonsterile flaps

?CRITICAL THINKING QUESTIONS

1. You have opened a sterile Foley catheter kit and are gloved. While cleansing the meatus (the hand touching the patient is now nonsterile, the hand with the swab is sterile), you accidentally contaminate the glove on your sterile hand. What do you do if you are there alone? What do you do if you have someone assisting you?

2. What do you do if a package of 4 × 4s you have opened and dropped into the field lands right at the edge of the field?

plies for the unit. Do not stockpile supplies in the patient room to avoid costly waste.

The procedure for pouring sterile liquids is listed in Steps 17-1.

Sterile Gloving. Sterile gloves must be used for sterile procedures. These gloves are made of various substances, including latex and nitrile, and are less permeable than the disposable plastic gloves. The method of donning and removing sterile gloves is presented in Skill 17-4.

Correcting Breaks in Asepsis. Whenever it becomes apparent that a break in surgical asepsis has occurred, you must rectify the error. A scrub is begun again if the hands touch the sink, which is always considered contaminated; sterile gloves are discarded and new gloves donned when any part of a glove touches a nonsterile area or item. Sterile supplies are discarded or put aside for re-sterilization if they become contaminated, and new packs or packages are opened aseptically to replace them.

It is up to every nurse to point out breaks in sterile technique that occur when others seem un-aware that they have contaminated themselves or the sterile field. Surgical asepsis is used in every aspect of nursing.

Evaluation

If the patient is recovering without additional instances of infection from other organisms, or infection of other body areas with a resident organism, goals are being met. Evaluation also includes assessing whether the patient's infection has been transmitted to any health care worker or any other patient on the unit or in the hospital. The infection prevention and control practitioner monitors for this and, if it occurs, usually works in conjunction with the unit manager to ensure that staff members are correctly implementing infection prevention and control procedures.

Infection prevention and control is the responsibility of each and every nurse. The principles and techniques learned here will protect you and your patients from harmful microorganisms.

Steps 17-1 | Pouring Sterile Liquids

Sterile liquids are used during surgical procedures, for wound irrigations, and for cleansing during sterile procedures.

1. *ACTION* Perform hand hygiene and, using sterile technique, set up the sterile field with a sterile container for the solution. Properly opened, the wrapper from a sterile kit such as an irrigation kit makes an appropriate sterile field at the bedside.

   RATIONALE Prepares an area where the sterile solution can be safely poured.

2. *ACTION* Check the solution label to verify that it is the ordered solution. Check the expiration date.

   RATIONALE Prevents using the wrong solution or an outdated solution. Sterile solutions are not considered sterile if the expiration date has passed.

3. *ACTION* Unscrew and remove the bottle cap without touching the inside of the cap or the opening of the bottle.

   RATIONALE The inner surface of the cap is considered sterile.

4. *ACTION* Place the cap with the inner surface facing up on the table outside the sterile field.

   RATIONALE Prevents contamination of the inside of the cap.

5. *ACTION* With sterile gloved hands or sterile transfer forceps, move the empty sterile container for the solution to 1 inch inside the edge of the sterile field.

   RATIONALE Positioning the container to 1 inch inside the edge of the sterile field allows you to pour the liquid without moving your arm or hand over the sterile field, while keeping the sterile container within the sterile field.

6. *ACTION* Hold the bottle about 6 inches above the empty sterile container and pour liquid into the container in a steady stream, preventing splashing of the liquid onto the sterile field.

   RATIONALE Pouring the liquid from this height and maintaining a steady stream prevents splashing. If splashing occurs, the field is contaminated, and a new sterile field must be prepared.

7. *ACTION* When pouring is completed, pick up the cap by the outside and recap the bottle. Set it down outside the sterile field.

   RATIONALE In patient rooms and in the home setting, recapped solutions may be used if they have not become contaminated during recapping. In the operating room, remaining solution is discarded.

8. *ACTION* Write the date the solution was opened on the label and your initials.

   RATIONALE Solutions are considered unsterile after being open for a particular number of days, and some are single use only. Follow agency policy regarding discard dates for open solutions.

9. *ACTION* When pouring liquids from a previously opened bottle, pour a bit of solution over the lip of the bottle into a discard container, and then pour the solution into the sterile container.

   RATIONALE This washes the edge of the bottle and aids in preventing contamination of the solution.

Skill 17-4 | Sterile Gloving and Ungloving

Sterile gloves are used for performing sterile procedures and handling sterile equipment and supplies. Sterile gloves are to be removed and replaced any time they become contaminated when performing a sterile procedure.

■ Supplies
✓ Package of sterile gloves in correct size

Review and carry out the Standard Steps in Appendix 3.

■ Assessment (Data Collection)
1. **ACTION** Determine what size gloves are needed.

   RATIONALE Gloves should fit snugly, but not be so tight that they are extremely difficult to put on.

■ Planning
2. **ACTION** Select a clean, flat, dry surface above waist level on which to open the glove package.

   RATIONALE Glove package should remain stationary and easily accessible while putting on the gloves to decrease chance of contamination from contact with surface of table. A wet surface will contaminate the gloves.

■ Implementation
Gloving
3. **ACTION** Place the package of correctly sized gloves on the flat surface. Perform hand hygiene.

   RATIONALE Hands must be clean and dry before gloving to reduce the transfer of microorganisms.

4. **ACTION** Peel open the outside wrapper, exposing the sterile glove package.

   RATIONALE The outer package keeps the inner pack sterile until opened.

5. **ACTION** Position the package so that the designation of right ("R") and left ("L") is visible right side up if this is indicated on the package.

   RATIONALE This places the gloves in correct association with the right and left hand, facilitating proper gloving. Some gloves can be used on either hand; those packages will not be marked R and L.

6. **ACTION** Use sterile technique, and open the glove package, handling only the outer wrapper. Handle the wrapper by the underneath part of the folded-back flaps. Pinch the corners of the flaps after pulling them open so that they remain open.

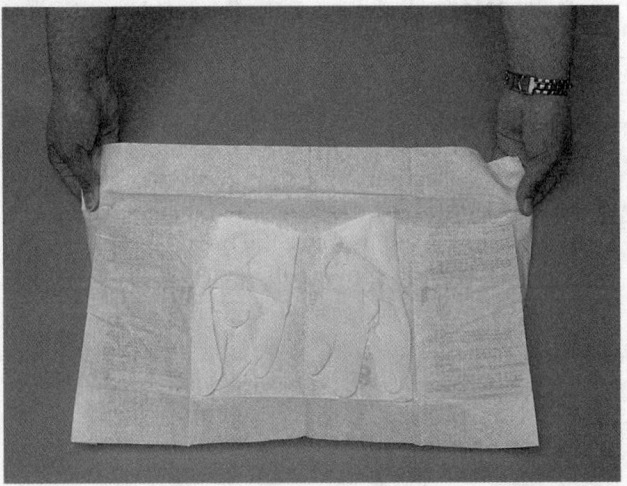

Step **6**

RATIONALE Handling the outside of the wrapper only prevents contamination of the inner surface and the gloves. Allowing the wrapper to fall back on the gloves contaminates them.

7. **ACTION** Pick up one glove by slipping the thumb into the opening and grasping the glove with the thumb and fingertips at the folded-over cuff edge, and lift it up at least 12 inches off the wrapper, being careful not to touch the glove to yourself or any surrounding objects.

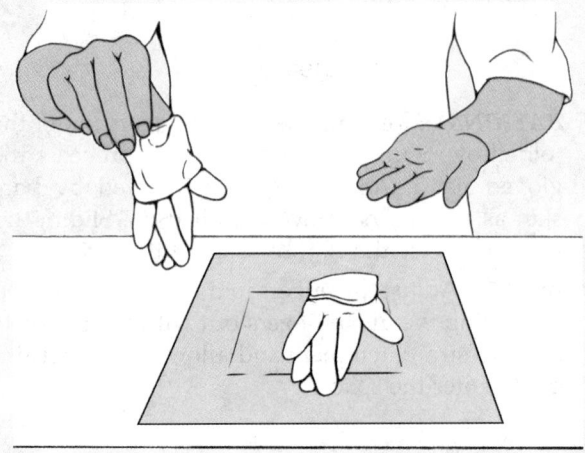

Step **7**

Continued

Skill 17-4 | Sterile Gloving and Ungloving—cont'd

RATIONALE Only the inside of the glove, which will be against the skin, is touched, leaving the outside sterile.

8. *ACTION* Insert the fingers of the other hand into the glove, and extend and hold the fingers slightly apart. Pull the cuff outward as you slip your hand into the glove.

   RATIONALE Touching only the inside surface of the glove prevents contaminating the outside sterile surface.

9. *ACTION* Pick up the second glove by placing the (sterile) gloved fingers under the cuff fold; slip the bare hand into the glove, being careful not to touch the outside of the glove or the other gloved hand with your bare skin. Once the hand is settled in the glove, slide the glove cuff up carefully over the wrist.

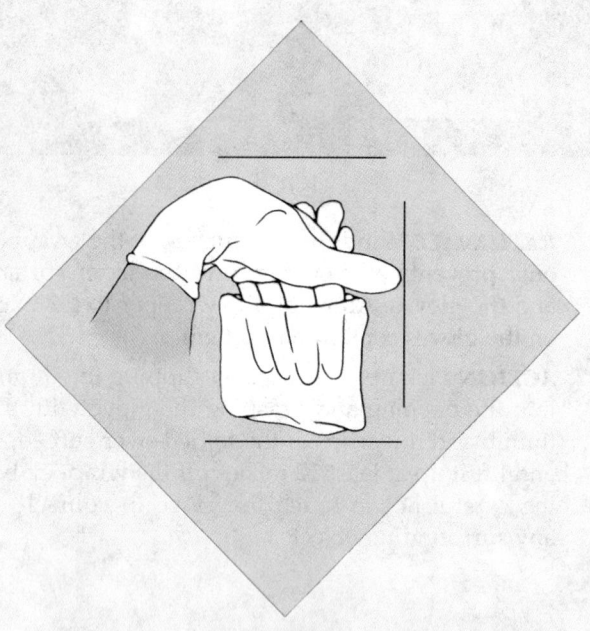

Step **9**

RATIONALE Keeping the gloved fingers under the folded-over cuff of the second glove prevents the gloved hand from being contaminated by bare skin as the second glove is pulled on. Sliding up the cuff covers the exposed skin of the wrist.

10. *ACTION* Adjust the fingers in the gloves as needed by pulling the glove fingers out with the opposite hand to straighten them and allow the proper finger to enter the space.

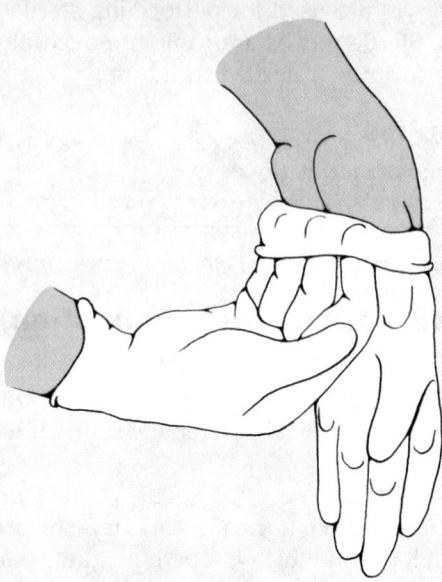

Step **10**

RATIONALE Fingers must be situated correctly to permit hand dexterity while performing the procedure.

Ungloving

11. *ACTION* When finished with the sterile procedure, unglove by grasping the outside surface of one glove about 2 to 3 inches below the cuff edge with the opposite gloved hand.

    RATIONALE Grasping the glove in an area away from exposed skin prevents contaminating the skin with the now contaminated glove.

12. *ACTION* Pull the glove off the hand while turning it inside out, and rolling it into the palm of your other gloved hand.

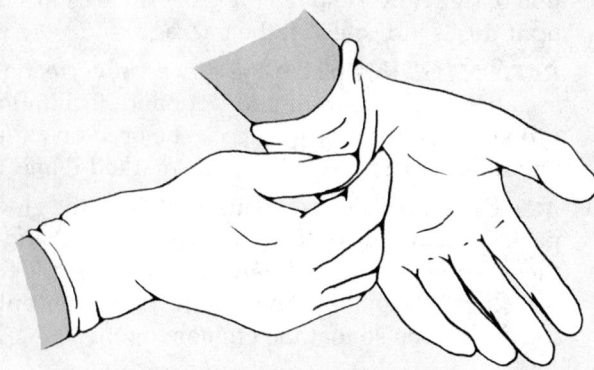

Step **12**

RATIONALE This technique prevents organisms on the contaminated gloves from coming into contact with your skin.

13. **ACTION** Still holding the first glove in the remaining gloved hand, place the fingers of your ungloved hand under the cuff of the remaining glove next to your skin. Slide the glove off, turning it inside out as you remove it.

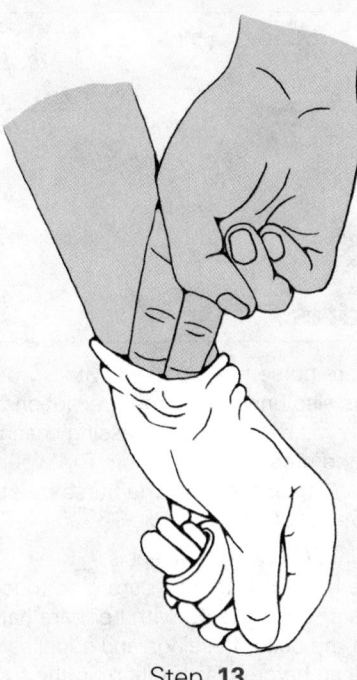

Step **13**

RATIONALE Touching only the skin of the hand with your bare hand prevents contaminating yourself with the outside of the now contaminated glove. The first glove's contaminated surface is now encased in the second.

14. **ACTION** Dispose of the contaminated gloves in the proper receptacle.

RATIONALE Because the contaminated surfaces of the gloves are on the inside of the gloves, they can be discarded in the trash.

15. **ACTION** Perform hand hygiene.

RATIONALE This removes glove powder, if present, and removes any organisms that might have traveled through the gloves. Hand hygiene after removing gloves is required by Standard Precautions.

■ Evaluation

16. **ACTION** At all times during the wearing of sterile gloves, ask yourself: Have I touched a glove surface to an unsterile object? Have my gloved hands dropped below waist level? Do I need to reglove?

RATIONALE If hands drop below waist level, they are considered contaminated because they are generally out of the field of vision.

■ Documentation

No documentation is required for this procedure.

?CRITICAL THINKING QUESTIONS

1. You are preparing to do a dressing change with the patient in bed, and set up the sterile field and supplies on the over-the-bed table. Where would you place the sterile glove pack to don the sterile gloves?

2. When donning sterile gloves, in what ways might the gloves become contaminated?

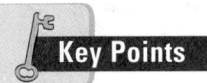 **Key Points**

- Illness progresses through an incubation period, a prodromal period, an illness period, and a convalescent period.
- Infection prevention and control curtails the spread of disease through the use of Standard Precautions, Transmission-Based Precautions, and medical and surgical asepsis.
- Standard Precautions are to be used for all contact involving potential exposure to bodily fluids regardless of the patient's infection status.
- The present system of infection prevention and control consists of two tiers: Standard Precautions, to be used for all patients, and Transmission-Based Precautions, to be used for patients who have an organism that is transmissible.
- Transmission-Based Precautions are always used along with Standard Precautions.
- Personal protective equipment (PPE) is used to protect patients and health care workers. The mode of transmission of a microorganism determines which PPE is necessary.

- Hand hygiene is the best method of preventing health care–associated infection.
- Personal protective equipment includes head covering, protective eyewear, masks, gowns, gloves, and shoe covers.
- A special respirator (N95) mask is necessary to care for a patient under Airborne Precautions who has or may have pulmonary tuberculosis, varicella, rubeola, or severe acute respiratory syndrome (SARS).
- Laboratory specimens are labeled and bagged before removal from an isolation room.
- Linens and trash are deposited in specially marked biohazard bags before removal from an isolation room.
- Sharps are placed in a puncture-resistant sharps container marked "Biohazard." *Fingers are never inserted into the opening of a sharps container.*
- Patients under Transmission-Based Precautions are placed in a private room or with a roommate who is infected with the same organism.
- If an isolation patient must be transported, a mask is worn by the patient under Airborne Precautions.
- Special measures are taken to prevent soiling of the environment for the patient under Droplet Precautions.

- Emphasis in the home environment is on preventing the transmission of microorganisms to others and on containing pathogens.
- Protective isolation is used for severely immunocompromised patients. Full use of PPE is required for all persons entering the patient's room.
- The nurse should oversee appropriate activities and opportunities for contact with friends and family to prevent adverse psychological consequences for the isolation patient.
- Nurses must be knowledgeable about and strictly follow the principles of surgical asepsis and the use of sterile technique.

 Go to your **Companion CD-ROM** for an Audio Glossary, animations, video clips, and more.

evolve Be sure to visit the companion Evolve site at http://evolve.elsevier.com/deWit/fundamental/ for additional online resources.

NCLEX-PN® EXAMINATION-STYLE REVIEW QUESTIONS

*Choose the **best** answer(s) for each question.*

1. The nurse is delivering a meal tray to a patient who is under Droplet Precautions for bacterial pneumonia. Which articles of personal protective equipment (PPE) need to be worn?
   1. Gown, mask, gloves, shoe covers
   2. Special filtration mask and gloves
   3. Only a mask is needed
   4. No PPE required

2. The nurse is preparing to assist a patient with his bath. He has an infected, draining wound. What PPE would be required for these tasks? *(Select all that apply.)*
   1. Gown
   2. Mask
   3. Eyewear
   4. Gloves

3. Which of the following steps are to be taken when preparing a sputum specimen to go to the laboratory? *(Select all that apply.)*
   1. Label the container.
   2. Collect the specimen and secure the lid.
   3. Place the container in a sealed plastic bag marked "Biohazard."
   4. Place the biohazard bag in another plastic bag.
   5. Place the completed lab slip in the pocket on the bag.
   6. Put the container in the rack for the lab courier.

4. A nurse is working in a small hospital with a combined med-surg unit. The only beds available are in two-bed rooms, and each room already has a patient. The recovery room nurse is about to send a 25-year-old female who just had her tonsils removed. Who would be the most appropriate roommate?
   1. A 60-year-old woman newly diagnosed with bacterial pneumonia
   2. A 23-year-old woman with a draining wound
   3. A 15-year-old girl who had oral surgery yesterday
   4. A 50-year-old woman recovering from an alcohol overdose

5. A home care nurse has a patient with a wound infection who is also under Airborne Precautions. The patient's wife will be doing the dressing change on the days that the nurse does not visit. The wound must be cleansed and then dressed. The nurse must teach the wife to: *(Select all that apply.)*
   1. maintain strict surgical asepsis.
   2. cleanse her hands and be careful to touch only the corners of the dressing with her bare hands.
   3. contain the used dressings and supplies in a sealed plastic bag before placing them in the trash.
   4. wear a mask as well as gloves when changing the dressing.

6. A patient under Contact Precautions wants to know if he may have visitors. The nurse tells him that:
   1. visitors may come but they must wear a mask and gown.
   2. there are no special requirements for people visiting a patient under Contact Precautions.
   3. visitors may come but should wear gloves if they touch the patient.
   4. visitors may come but should wash their hands before and after socially touching the patient.

7. When performing a sterile dressing change on a patient, correct technique must be regarded as broken if: *(Select all that apply.)*
   1. supplies are placed touching the edge of the sterile field.
   2. a gloved hand touches the dressing table below tabletop surface.
   3. a sterile glove touches one of the sterile dressings on the field before the procedure is begun.
   4. the nurse reaches over the sterile field when placing a swab used to clean the wound in the discard bag.

8. Standard Precautions are used:
   1. for all patients.
   2. for all patients unless they are under Transmission-Based Precautions.
   3. for all patients except those in protective isolation.
   4. for any patient the nurse believes might be infectious.

9. The correct actions when donning a pair of sterile gloves include: (*Select all that apply.*)

   1. picking up the first glove by placing the fingers of the opposite hand under the cuff.
   2. smoothing the first glove over the hand before putting on the second.
   3. picking up the first glove by grasping it on the fold of the cuff.
   4. holding the glove with its fingers downward.

10. When making up the bed in an isolation room, the nurse: (*Select all that apply.*)

    1. places and unfolds linen carefully.
    2. wears gloves.
    3. checks on items the patient might need before entering the room.
    4. places dirty linens on the floor until finished.

CRITICAL THINKING ACTIVITIES *Read each clinical scenario and discuss the questions with your classmates.*

Scenario A
You are caring for a 43-year-old man who has an infected leg wound following a hiking accident. He is to keep his leg elevated and is under Contact Precautions. He has recently retired from the military and has just moved to the area. He is bored and restless. How would you help meet his psychosocial needs?

Scenario B
What would you do if you observed the physician's glove become contaminated during a sterile procedure and the physician appears unaware that this has occurred? Be specific

Scenario C
Your home care patient is an older man with a large abdominal wound that needs daily dressing changes. He lives with his wife, but she has severe arthritis in her hands and is unable to perform the procedure. You are scheduled for three visits per week. How would you solve the problem of getting his daily dressing change done on the days you are not scheduled to visit?

Objectives

Upon completing this chapter, you should be able to:

Theory

1. Describe the anatomy and function of the musculoskeletal system.
2. Explain the importance of proper body mechanics, alignment, and position change for both patient and nurse.
3. Discuss the principles of body movement and positioning, giving an appropriate example for each principle.
4. Identify ways to maintain correct body alignment of the patient in bed or in a chair.
5. Describe the proper method for transferring a patient between wheelchair and bed.

Clinical Practice

1. Correctly position a patient in the following positions: supine, prone, Fowler's, and Sims'.
2. Assist patients to sit up in bed.
3. Demonstrate complete passive range-of-motion (ROM) exercises for a patient.
4. Correctly transfer a patient from a wheelchair to a bed.
5. Transfer a patient from a bed to a stretcher.
6. Demonstrate the correct techniques for ambulating a patient and for breaking a fall while ambulating.

Skills

Skill 18-1	Positioning the Patient
Skill 18-2	Moving the Patient Up in Bed
Skill 18-3	Passive Range-of-Motion (ROM) Exercises
Skill 18-4	Transferring the Patient to a Wheelchair
Skill 18-5	Transferring the Patient to a Stretcher
Skill 18-6	Ambulating the Patient and Breaking a Fall

Key Terms

 Be sure to check out the bonus material on the Companion CD-ROM, including selected audio pronunciations.

alignment (ă-LĪN-mĭnt, p. 258)
ambulate (ĂM-bŭ-lāt, p. 263)
bone (p. 259)
bursa (BŬR-să, p. 259)
cartilage (CĂR-tĭ-lĭj, p. 259)
contractures (kŏn-TRĂK-chŭrz, p. 262)
dangling (p. 277)
Fowler's position (FŎW-lĕrs, p. 264)
gait (p. 263)

gait belt (p. 282)
joint (p. 259)
kinesiology (kĭ-nē-sĭ-Ŏ-lō-jē, p. 258)
lateral position (p. 264)
ligaments (LĬG-ă-mĕntz, p. 259)
logrolling (LŎG-rō-lĭng, p. 272)
necrosis (nē-KRŌ-sĭs, p. 262)
pivot (PĬV-ŏt, p. 262)
pressure ulcers (PRĔ-shŭr ŬL-sĕrz, p. 262)
prone position (PRŌN, p. 264)
semi-Fowler's position (SĔ-mĭ FŎW-lĕrs, p. 264)
shearing force (SHĒR-ĭng, p. 262)
side-lying (lateral) position (SĪD-ly-ĭng/LĂ-tĕr-ăl, p. 264)
Sims' position (p. 264)
skeletal muscles (p. 259)
supine position (SOO-pĭn, p. 263)
symmetry (SĬM-ĭ-trē, p. 262)
tendons (p. 259)
transfer belt (p. 282)

Lifting, moving, and positioning patients is an integral part of your workday. In order to provide the best patient care and to prevent self-injury, you must know the principles of body mechanics. Coordinated movement involves using the bones, joints, and skeletal muscles properly. Some hospitals and institutions are moving to a policy of "no manual lifting" or to the use of a lift team. The goal of this change is to decrease health care worker back injuries from repetitive lifting. The shift in policy is slowly occurring across the United States. Until equipment or lift teams are in place in all health care institutions, there will be instances when a nurse must lift a patient without assistance or use of a mechanical device. The following principles and practices serve as guides to help prevent injury.

PRINCIPLES OF BODY MOVEMENT FOR NURSES

Kinesiology is the study of the movement of body parts (also called body mechanics). There are two main reasons why the use of good body movement is important for you and your patient. The first reason is that the body functions best when it is in correct anatomic position or alignment (arrangement in a straight line, bringing a line into order). Correct body align-

OVERVIEW OF STRUCTURE AND FUNCTION OF THE MUSCULOSKELETAL SYSTEM

Which structures are involved in positioning and moving patients?

- The musculoskeletal system contains skeletal muscles, ligaments, tendons, bones, joints, and cartilage.

- Bone is a dense and hard type of connective tissue. There are four basic types of bones—short, long, flat, and irregular—and they are made up of compact and spongy bone.

- A joint is the place of union of two or more bones in the body.

- There are freely movable, slightly movable, and immovable joints in the body.

- Bursae are small fluid-filled sacs that provide a cushion at friction points in freely movable joints.

- Skeletal muscles are striated muscles that are made of bundles of muscle fibers surrounded by a connective tissue sheath.

- Tendons are cords of fibrous connective tissue that connect a muscle to a bone to allow for joint movement.

- Ligaments connect bones or cartilage to provide support and strength.

- Cartilage is a fibrous connective tissue that acts as a cushion.

What are the functions of bones for positioning and moving patients?

- Bones provide the scaffolding or framework to the body (Figure 18-1).

Continued

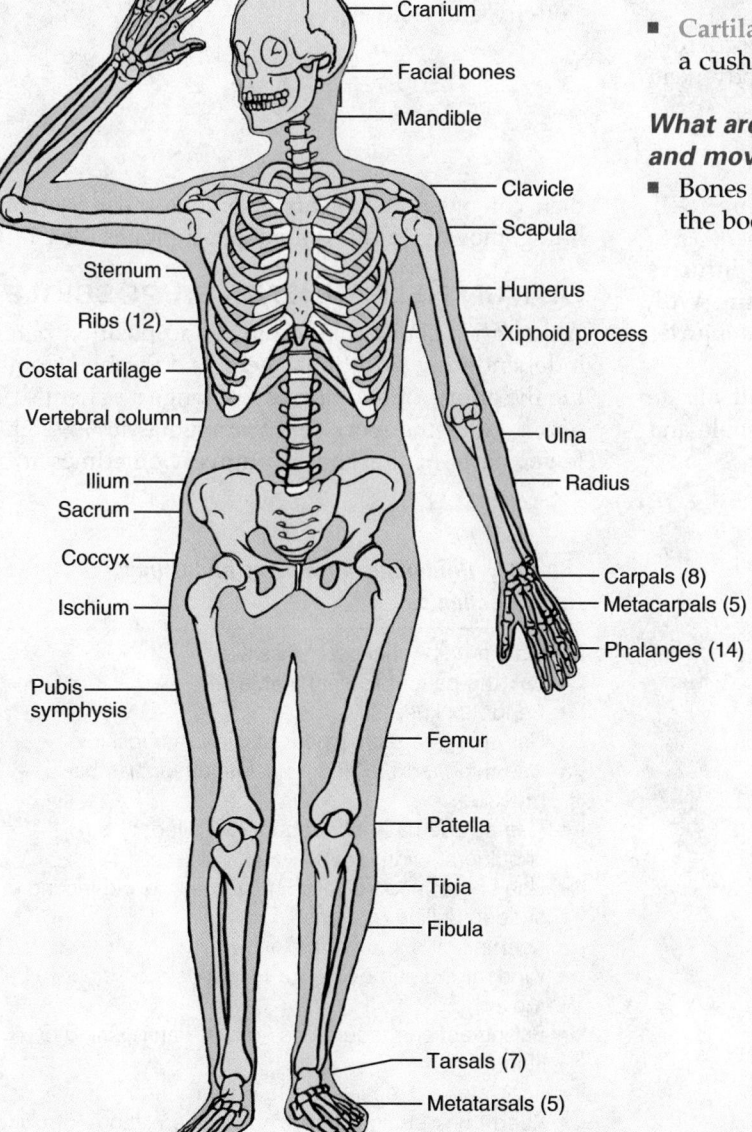

Cranium
Facial bones
Mandible
Clavicle
Scapula
Sternum
Ribs (12)
Costal cartilage
Vertebral column
Humerus
Xiphoid process
Ilium
Sacrum
Coccyx
Ischium
Ulna
Radius
Pubis symphysis
Carpals (8)
Metacarpals (5)
Phalanges (14)
Femur
Patella
Tibia
Fibula
Tarsals (7)
Metatarsals (5)
Phalanges (14)

FIGURE **18-1** Anterior view of a normal skeletal system.

OVERVIEW OF STRUCTURE AND FUNCTION OF THE MUSCULOSKELETAL SYSTEM—cont'd

- The skeleton gives the body shape and supports the internal organs and skin.

- The bones provide places for the ligaments and tendons to attach, thereby allowing movement.

- The primary function of a joint is to provide movement and flexibility to the skeleton.

What are the functions of muscles for positioning and moving patients?

- Muscles can be stimulated electrically, which allows them to contract, stretch, or extend elastically.

- Skeletal muscle contraction is accomplished through the stimulation of its many muscle fibers.

- The contraction of skeletal muscles provides movement, stabilizes joints, produces body heat, and maintains posture.

What changes in the system occur with aging?

- Bone strength and mass are lost because of the resorption of minerals. This may lead to osteoporosis, which is more common in women.

- The loss of bone density predisposes the elderly patient to fractures. The fractures do not heal as quickly because of the decreased uptake of minerals.

- Muscle cells are lost and replaced by fat. This leads to a loss of muscle strength and endurance.

- The elasticity of muscle fibers is decreased or lost, which causes a loss of flexibility.

- Joint motion may decrease, limiting mobility, activity, and exercise.

ment is generally called "good posture" (Figure 18-2). The second reason for proper body movement is to prevent injuries. **One of the most common injuries for health care workers is lower back strain.** With proper use of body mechanics, many of these injuries can be avoided.

In today's health care environment, more patients are being cared for at home. In order for these people and their caregivers to be safe, everyone must use correct lifting, moving, and positioning techniques (Box 18-1).

OBTAIN HELP WHENEVER POSSIBLE

Although it is possible to move and position patients independently, additional help is desirable. Combining the efforts of two nurses to change a patient's position divides the work. Each nurse has less weight or fewer parts of the body to move. Sometimes it may

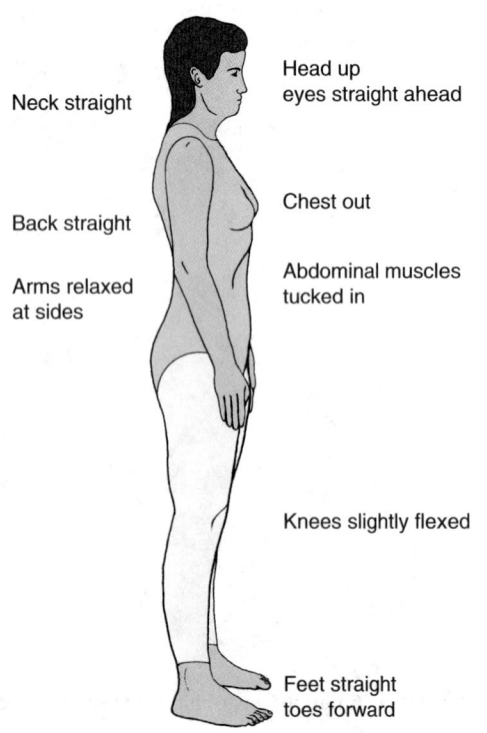

Neck straight

Head up
eyes straight ahead

Chest out

Back straight

Arms relaxed
at sides

Abdominal muscles
tucked in

Knees slightly flexed

Feet straight
toes forward

FIGURE **18-2** Correct standing body alignment.

Box 18-1 *Guidelines for Moving and Lifting: Body Mechanics*

- Obtain help whenever possible.
- Ask the patient to help if able.
- Bend/flex knees.
- Use the greatest number of muscles possible.
- Use thigh, arm, or leg muscles rather than back muscles.
- Use a wide base of support. Keep feet about shoulders' width apart.
- Use smooth coordinated movement; avoid jerking or sudden pulling motions.
- Keep elbows and work close to your body.
- Work at the same level or height as the object to be moved.
- Pulling actions require less effort than pushing or lifting.
- Face in the direction of the movement.
- Keep trunk straight; don't twist when lifting or pulling.
- Use arms as levers when pulling the patient toward you. Lock the elbows and rock back on your heels, using the weight of your body to move the patient.

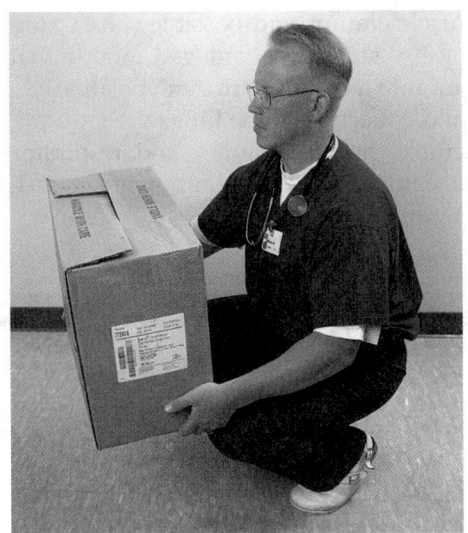

FIGURE **18-3** Using leg muscles to prevent back strain.

seem difficult to find another staff person to assist you. It is always better to wait for help than to risk injury to yourself or the patient. Encourage the patient to assist when transferring and moving if possible. Use devices such as mechanical lifts and transfer or roller boards where available. Properly used, these items decrease the workload and prevent injury.

USE YOUR LEG MUSCLES

In positioning and transferring, use the muscles in your legs as much as possible. Instead of bending over at the waist to pick up something from the floor, bend at the knees and lower yourself until you can pick up the item without straining your back (Figure 18-3). Use the greatest number of muscles possible when lifting or moving an object. For instance, when turning a patient in bed, flex your knees and use the muscles in your legs as well as your arms. Without the power in your legs, there will be more work for the muscles

in your arms. It is far better to use thigh, arm, and leg muscles rather than back muscles.

PROVIDE STABILITY FOR MOVEMENT

Keep your feet about shoulders' width apart. This establishes a wide base of support and provides stability for movement. Think how easy it is to sway if you stand with your feet together and your eyes closed. Yet, if you spread your feet apart and close your eyes, you do not sway.

USE SMOOTH, COORDINATED MOVEMENTS

Use smooth, coordinated movements instead of jerking or sudden pulling motions. To coordinate effort, tell the patient and other staff members to move, lift, or pull "on the count of 3." This will help to ensure that everyone is working at the same time to maximize the effort and decrease the individual load.

KEEP LOADS CLOSE TO THE BODY

Keep your elbows and work close to your body. This keeps the work load close to your waist and center of gravity. Pick up your textbook and hold it close to your body. Although it is a heavy book, it is easily managed close to your center of gravity. Slowly start to extend your elbows forward. This moves the book farther from the center of gravity and it becomes increasingly heavier. Do not fully extend your elbows or you will put stress and strain on your back muscles.

KEEP LOADS NEAR YOUR CENTER OF GRAVITY

Work at the same level or height as the object to be moved (Figure 18-4). This way your work load is near your center of gravity. Changing bed linens is a good example of this principle. In most institutions, the bed's height may be adjusted. When changing linen or

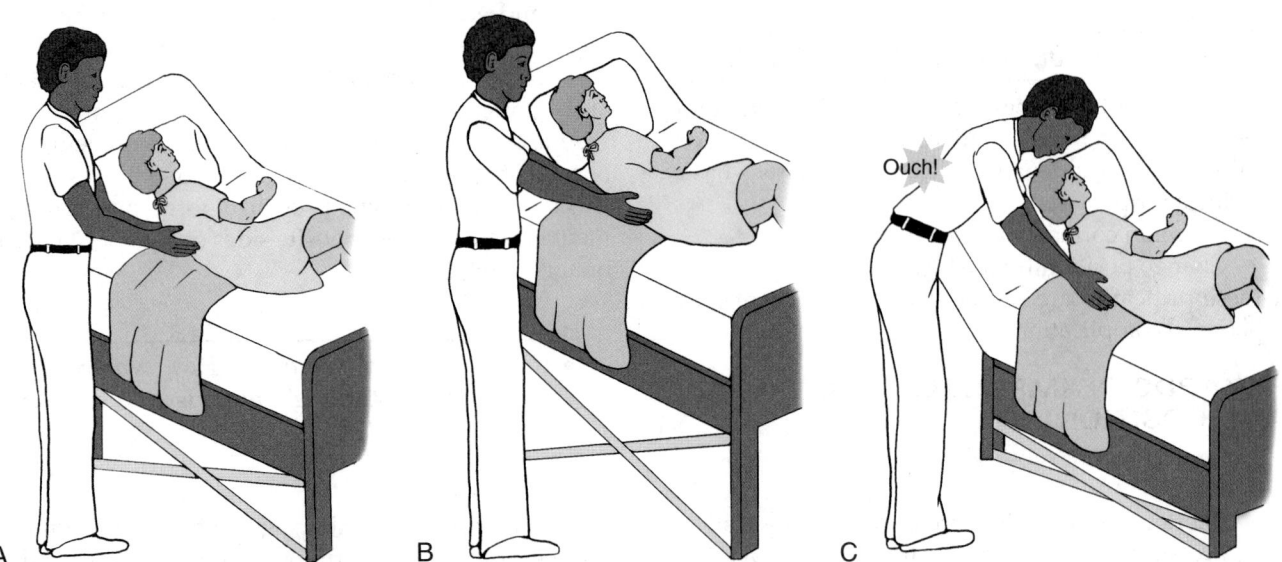

FIGURE **18-4** **A,** Correct working height. **B,** Work is too high. **C,** Work is too low.

moving a patient, raise the bed to about waist level to keep the work near your center of gravity. Injuries are more likely to occur the farther away the work is from the center of gravity.

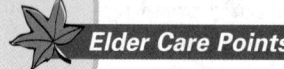

Elder Care Points

The elderly may need to be reeducated on how and what they may safely lift. As the body ages, there is a change in body posture and usually a decrease in muscle mass. Items that could be lifted safely during youth often cannot be lifted safely in the later years. Consideration should be given as to whether the elderly person has a spinal deformity or osteoporosis when considering how much weight is safe to lift.

PULL AND PIVOT

Pulling actions require less effort than pushing or lifting. Whenever possible, use pulling motions. When transferring a patient to a stretcher, two nurses should stand on the far side of the stretcher to pull the patient toward them onto the stretcher. This movement is easier than pushing because it brings the patient closer to each nurse's center of gravity. **Face in the direction of the movement.** It is much easier to move an object if you are facing in that direction. For example, place an object on the floor. Stoop down with the object in front of you and move the object forward. Fairly easy. Now place the same object on the floor, stoop down, only this time with the object to the side. Moving the object forward is not as easy in this instance.

In order to move the object at your side forward, you would need to twist to the side. To maintain proper body mechanics, keep your trunk straight when lifting or pulling. Twisting should be avoided. Instead, if turning is needed, pivot (turn or change direction with your feet while remaining in a fixed place). Pivoting prevents twisting, which can lead to back strain and injury.

PRINCIPLES OF BODY MOVEMENT FOR PATIENTS

Body movement and alignment are also important for patients. Many patients are unable to change position or move in bed independently. There are two basic principles for patients:

- Maintain correct anatomic position.
- Change position frequently.

If these principles are not observed, the patient may experience complications.

HAZARDS OF IMPROPER ALIGNMENT AND POSITIONING

The hazards of improper alignment and positioning include

- Interference with circulation, which may lead to pressure ulcers (ulcers that form from local interference with circulation)

- Muscle cramps and possible contractures (resistance to stretch in damaged muscle that pulls a joint into a fixed or "frozen" position)
- Fluid collection in the lungs

Contractures, muscle cramps, and respiratory problems as complications of immobility are discussed more thoroughly in Chapter 39.

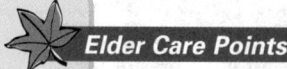

Elder Care Points

The elderly have a greater risk for skin breakdown than younger patients because they have decreased muscle mass and less moisture in their skin, and their capillaries are more fragile. Handle elderly patients very carefully.

Pressure Ulcers

Pressure ulcers, also known as decubitus ulcers or bedsores, occur from pressure on the skin. This pressure causes a local area of tissue necrosis (local death of tissue from disease or injury). Most often the area of pressure occurs between a bony prominence and an external surface. Besides pressure, the other main factor in the development of pressure ulcers is a shearing force. Shearing is an applied force that causes a downward and forward pressure on the tissues beneath the skin. Shearing forces occur when a patient slides down in a chair, if bedclothes are pulled from beneath the patient, or the patient is slid up to the head of the bed without lifting the body. More information on pressure ulcers may be found in Chapter 19.

APPLICATION of the NURSING PROCESS

Assessment (Data Collection)

When assessing the standing patient's body alignment, begin by noting the head position in relation to the rest of the body (see Figure 18-2). Is the head centered and erect? Are the shoulders and hips parallel? Are the knees and ankles slightly flexed and parallel to the hips and shoulders? Do the arms hang comfortably at the patient's side? Are the feet slightly apart to provide a base of support? During the assessment, also observe for any muscle weakness or paralysis, and check symmetry (equality in size, form, and arrangement of parts on the opposite sides of a plane; a mirror image) of extremities.

Think Critically About . . . How would you describe your posture right now? Is your body in correct alignment?

When a patient is sitting, again observe for symmetry (Figure 18-5). Determine if the patient's head is erect and centered over the shoulders. Are the but-

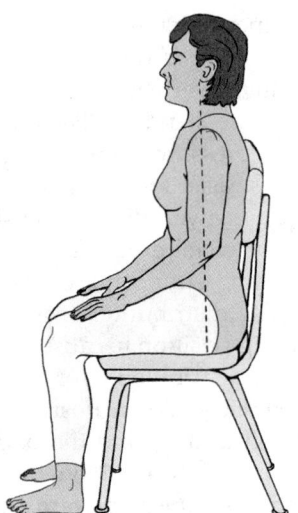

FIGURE **18-5** Correct sitting body alignment.

tocks in the same plane as the shoulders and are the thighs in line with the shoulders? The patient's weight should be distributed evenly over the buttocks and thighs. The knees should be flexed at about 90 degrees with the feet resting comfortably on the floor. Provide a footstool if the feet do not reach the floor. The arms should lie comfortably in the lap or be supported by the chair armrests.

Patients often lie on their back when in bed. It is important that this position be changed frequently to prevent the problems associated with immobility. Support the head with one pillow so the neck is not hyperflexed. The vertebral column should be centered and in alignment and there should not be any observable curves. The mattress should support the body in this position.

Assess the patient's ability to ambulate (walk) and to change position independently. (A physician's order is needed for a patient to be out of bed.) Observe the patient walking. Is the head centered over the vertebral column? Is the gait (style of walking) even and unlabored? Is the patient balanced? Is there any weakness or favoring of one side? This will determine the patient's ability to ambulate independently or determine the type of assistance needed.

Nursing Diagnosis

Nursing diagnoses commonly used for problems with body movement are as follows
- Risk for injury
- Impaired physical mobility
- Risk for impaired skin integrity
- Impaired walking

The defining characteristics for the patient are added to the nursing diagnosis stem to individualize the care plan. Nursing diagnoses for patients with problems of immobility are covered more extensively in Chapter 39.

Planning

The data collected during the assessment phase give information about how to best promote independence or assist the patient. If the patient is not able to move independently, then the patient's position will need to be changed at least every 2 hours to avoid complications. Your assessment will indicate whether you can move the patient independently or you will need assistance. During planning, decide how to change the patient's position and whether you can delegate this task to assistive personnel.

The home setting must also be considered when planning care for the patient. Will the family be able to turn or assist in turning the patient correctly after discharge? Will the patient or family need any assistive devices, and do they know how to use them? Will extra pillows need to be purchased to assist with positioning? Will the patient be able to get around in and out of the home independently? Assessment and planning will answer these questions.

Expected outcomes are written for each nursing diagnosis. Examples related to the above nursing diagnoses might be as follows:
- Patient will experience no musculoskeletal injury.
- Former level of mobility will be reattained within 6 months.
- Skin integrity will remain intact.
- Patient will not experience an injury while ambulating.

Implementation

Positioning

Basically, changing position accomplishes four things: (1) it provides comfort; (2) it relieves pressure on bony prominences and other parts; (3) it helps prevent contractures, deformities, and respiratory problems; and (4) it improves circulation. It is essential to know how to correctly support and position the patient while maintaining good body mechanics.

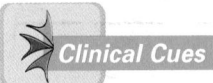

It is essential to maintain the patient's privacy through draping while changing positions. Many positions can leave a patient feeling vulnerable, and draping demonstrates respect for the patient and supports privacy.

Common Positions and Their Variations

While in bed, there are three basic positions for the patient: supine, side-lying, and prone.

The supine position is when patients are resting on their back. It is recommended after spinal surgery and after the administration of some types of spinal anesthetics. The supine position is similar to proper standing alignment except that the body is in the horizontal as opposed to the vertical plane.

Variations of the supine position are Fowler's, semi-Fowler's, and low Fowler's positions. Fowler's position is arranged by elevating the head of the bed 60 to 90 degrees. Semi-Fowler's position is an elevation of 30 to 60 degrees, and low Fowler's is an elevation of 15 to 30 degrees. Unless contraindicated, the knees can be raised 10 to 15 degrees in these positions. Alternatively, a footboard can be placed at the bottom of the bed to brace the patient's feet in correct alignment. Cardiac output and respiration are improved and urinary and bowel elimination are promoted in these positions. Do not place a patient who had abdominal surgery in a Fowler's position unless ordered. Elevation of the knees above 15 degrees is contraindicated in elderly and postoperative patients because it is associated with decreased circulation of the lower extremities; check the orders. Fowler's position may help the patient who has had a stroke and has paresis to swallow food and secretions.

Dorsal recumbent and *dorsal lithotomy positions* are other variations of the supine position. In the dorsal recumbent position, patients are on their back with knees flexed and soles of the feet flat on the bed (Figure 18-6). This is used for a variety of procedures and examinations. The dorsal lithotomy position (Figure 18-7) is used for examining the pelvic organs. It is like the dorsal recumbent position except the feet are usually placed in stirrups and the legs are spread farther apart and abducted. Patients with joint problems or arthritis may have difficulty assuming this position.

The side-lying or lateral position is achieved by having patients rest on their side. It alleviates pressure from bony prominences on the back. The major portion of the patients' weight is on the dependent shoulder and hip. Maintain the vertebral column in proper alignment as if they were standing. The oblique side-lying position removes pressure from the dependent shoulder and hip and is easier for patients to maintain.

Sims' position is a variation of the side-lying position. It is used for rectal examinations, administering enemas, or inserting suppositories, or for an unconscious patient. The distribution of weight is different from the side-lying position because in the Sims' position the weight is distributed over the anterior ilium, humerus, and clavicle. When positioning on the left side, place the left arm behind the patient and draw the right knee and thigh up above the left lower leg. Tilt the chest and abdomen forward so the patient is resting on them as well.

The prone position is when the patient is lying face down. It provides an alternative for patients who are on prolonged bed rest or are immobilized. Spinal cord–injured patients often use this position. The position is generally not well tolerated because it is boring. In the prone position, for patients who have not had a spinal cord injury, turn the head to one side or the other and support with a small pillow. If the head is not turned, or the patient is not on a special bed with a removable piece at the head, the patient would not be able to breathe.

The *knee-chest position* is a variation of the prone position (Figure 18-8). The patient is face down on the bed with the head turned to one side. The chest, elbows, and knees rest on the bed and the thighs are perpendicular to the bed. The lower legs rest flat on the bed. This is used for rectal examinations and as a method to restore the uterus to a normal position. Do not leave the patient alone in the knee-chest position because the patient may become dizzy, faint, or fall. A patient with arthritis or joint abnormalities may not be able to assume this position.

Skill 18-1 describes how to place the patient in many of the above positions.

Positioning Devices Devices used for positioning include pillows, boots or splints, footboards, cushioned boots or high-top sneakers, a trapeze bar (Figure 18-9, *A*, p. 269), sandbags, hand rolls, trochanter

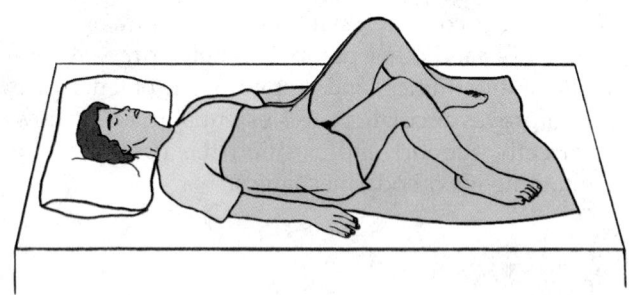

FIGURE **18-6** Dorsal recumbent position.

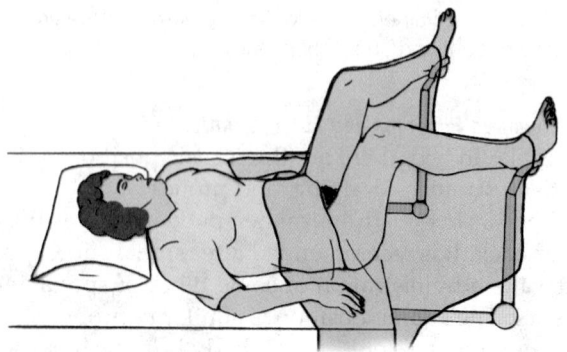

FIGURE **18-7** Lithotomy position.

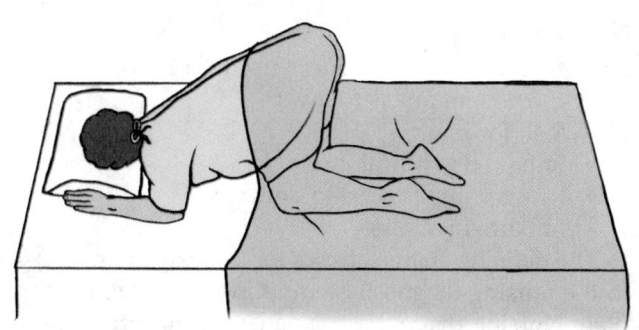

FIGURE **18-8** Knee-chest position.

Skill 18-1 | Positioning the Patient

Correct positioning of patients is essential for maintaining proper alignment. Many patients, because of injury, disease, helplessness, or therapeutic devices, need assistance with repositioning. Change the position of the bed patient at least every 2 hours. Obtain help to prevent injury to yourself and the patient.

■ Supplies

Positioning devices as needed for each position:
✓ Pillows
✓ Boots

✓ Trochanter rolls
✓ Hand rolls
✓ Trapeze bar
✓ Splints
✓ Side rails

✓ Sandbags
✓ Bed board
✓ Footboard or high-top sneakers

Review and carry out the Standard Steps in Appendix 3.

■ Assessment (Data Collection)

1. **ACTION** Assess for any restrictions to placing patient in particular positions.

   RATIONALE Provides baseline data and indicates positions that are contraindicated.

■ Planning

2. **ACTION** Gather positioning supplies.

   RATIONALE Provides easy access to equipment.

3. **ACTION** Explain what the patient is expected to do.

   RATIONALE Decreases fear and prepares patient to assist when possible.

4. **ACTION** Raise level of bed to a comfortable working height and raise far side rail.

   RATIONALE Promotes safety and reduces back strain.

5. **ACTION** Remove positioning devices before beginning.

   RATIONALE Readies patient for move.

6. **ACTION** Get help if necessary.

   RATIONALE Promotes safety.

7. **ACTION** Provide privacy during the position change.

   RATIONALE Demonstrates respect and reduces embarrassment.

■ Implementation

8. **ACTION** Perform hand hygiene.

   RATIONALE Reduces transfer of microorganisms.

9. **ACTION** Move patient to head of bed (see Skill 18-2).

   RATIONALE Prepares patient to be repositioned properly in the bed.

Supine Position

10. **ACTION** Place patient on back with bed in flat position if not contraindicated.

    RATIONALE Promotes working with gravity.

11. **ACTION** Place a pillow under the patient's head, neck, and upper shoulders.

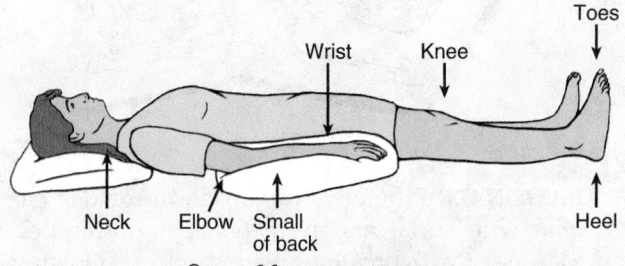

Step **11** Body alignment.

RATIONALE Prevents flexion contractures of neck.

12. **ACTION** If needed, place sandbags or trochanter rolls parallel to the lateral aspect of the thighs.

    RATIONALE Prevents external rotation of the hips.

13. **ACTION** Use heel pads or a small pillow or rolled towel under the ankles to lift the heels off the mattress.

    RATIONALE Decreases chance of pressure ulcer formation.

14. **ACTION** Maintain upper arms parallel with body and place pillows under pronated forearms.

    RATIONALE Prevents extension of elbows and decreases internal shoulder rotation.

15. **ACTION** Place hand rolls or towels in patient's hands if needed to maintain correct slightly flexed position.

    RATIONALE Promotes thumb adduction and finger flexion.

Continued

Skill 18-1   Positioning the Patient—cont'd

Fowler's and Semi-Fowler's Positions

16. **ACTION** For Fowler's, elevate head of bed 60 to 90 degrees. For semi-Fowler's, elevate head of bed 30 to 45 degrees.

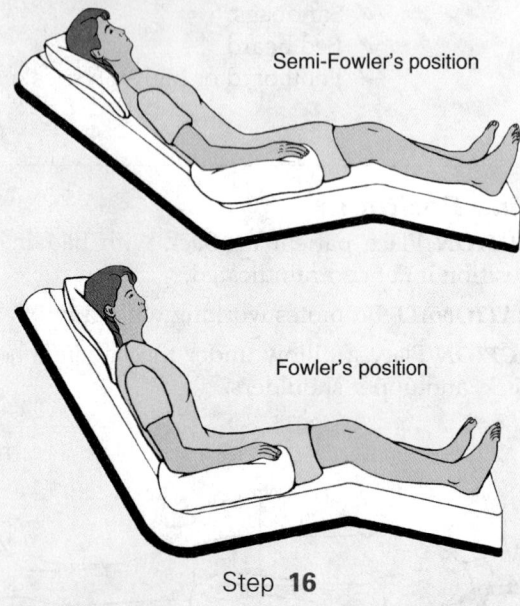

Semi-Fowler's position

Fowler's position

Step **16**

RATIONALE Promotes comfort and provides patient with social and recreational opportunities. May assist with breathing, eating, and swallowing for patient with problems in these areas.

17. **ACTION** Place head and neck against small pillow on bed.

RATIONALE Prevents cervical flexion.

18. **ACTION** Support arms and hands with pillows if needed.

RATIONALE Prevents flexion contracture of hands and wrists and shoulder dislocation from pull of arms and hands.

19. **ACTION** Place small pillow or towel roll under thighs.

RATIONALE Provides comfort without hyperextension of the knees or occlusion of popliteal artery.

20. **ACTION** Protect heels by using a small pillow, rolled towel, foam boots, or heel pads under patient's ankles.

RATIONALE Decreases the chance of pressure ulcer formation.

Side-Lying Position

21. **ACTION** Place patient on back on flat bed, if not contraindicated, or with bed as low as patient can tolerate. Move patient slightly to far side of bed,

starting with the head, torso, and then feet; align the body correctly.

RATIONALE Promotes easy access and working with gravity. Body will be centered in the bed when in new position.

22. **ACTION** Stand on side of bed to which you will turn the patient.

RATIONALE Pulling requires less effort than pushing.

23. **ACTION** Flex the patient's far knee across the near thigh.

RATIONALE Supports and prevents injury to joints.

24. **ACTION** Ask patient to raise the near arm above the head. Place one hand on patient's far shoulder and the other hand on patient's far hip and roll patient toward you with a smooth motion, or use a lift sheet to smoothly turn patient onto her side.

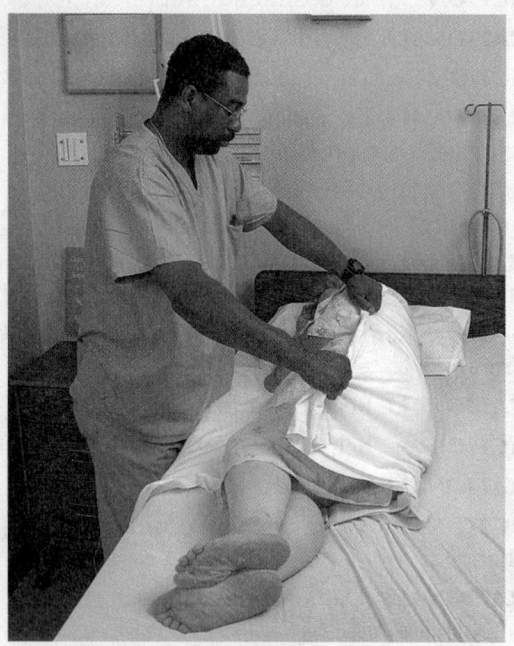

Step **24**

RATIONALE Supports and prevents injury to joints.

25. **ACTION** Fold pillow lengthwise; tuck upper edge under patient; roll the pillow against the patient's back, rolling it toward the mattress. Place a lengthwise pillow between the flexed knees from knee to foot.

RATIONALE Supports and promotes alignment. Prevents pressure ulcer formation. Prevents patient from rolling back to prior position.

For Side-Lying Oblique Position

26. **ACTION** Move shoulder blade against the bed forward toward you.

   RATIONALE Disperses weight so it is not centered on shoulder.

27. **ACTION** Flex the arm next to the mattress; raise hand so that it is even with top of patient's head.

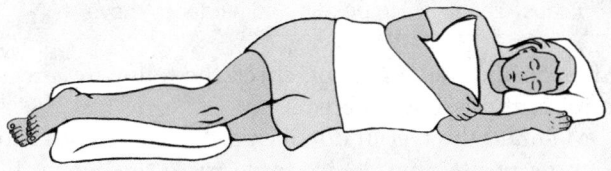

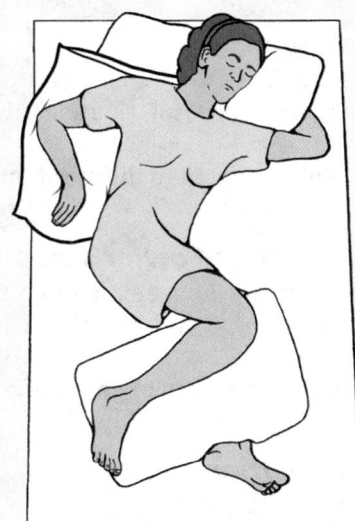

Step **27**

   RATIONALE Places less pressure on the shoulder and promotes comfort and flexibility of the elbow.

28. **ACTION** Support other arm with pillow placed level with the shoulder.

   RATIONALE Promotes chest expansion and decreases adduction and internal rotation of shoulder.

29. **ACTION** Reach under hip area and pull the hip slightly forward.

   RATIONALE Decreases pressure on the hip by placing the body at an oblique angle.

30. **ACTION** Slightly flex knees and support upper leg from thigh to ankle with pillow(s) folded lengthwise.

   RATIONALE Supports the leg joints and decreases adduction and internal rotation of hip and thigh. Decreases pressure on bony prominences.

Sims' Position

31. **ACTION** Position patient in complete side-lying position, but move slightly to the far side of the bed that back is facing. Partially roll patient forward partly on abdomen.

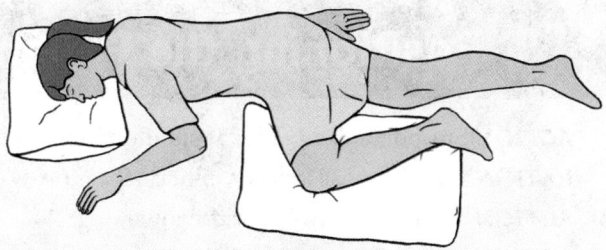

Step **31**

   RATIONALE Patient will be centered in bed when repositioned. Rolling patient partly onto abdomen promotes even weight distribution.

32. **ACTION** Slightly flex arm next to mattress behind patient.

   RATIONALE Prevents extension of elbow. Promotes comfort, and weight is not focused on shoulder joint.

33. **ACTION** Support flexed uppermost arm and leg with pillows so that the hand is level with the shoulder.

   RATIONALE Promotes chest expansion; decreases adduction and internal rotation of shoulder.

Prone Position

34. **ACTION** Lower head of bed to a flat position; place patient in supine position; and move to opposite side of the bed.

   RATIONALE Promotes working with gravity.

35. **ACTION** Put a small pillow on the patient's abdomen, below the diaphragm.

   RATIONALE Positions pillow for support after turn. Aids respirations by decreasing pressure on the diaphragm. Decreases hyperextension of lumbar vertebrae.

36. **ACTION** Place arms close to the body with elbow extended and hand under the hip.

   RATIONALE Maintains alignment for turning.

37. **ACTION** Roll patient toward you and place on abdomen (pillow is between patient's abdomen and the bed). Patient should be centered in bed.

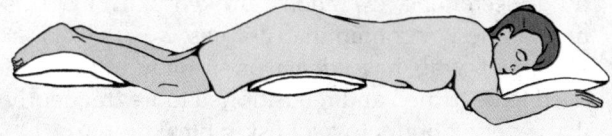

Step **37**

   RATIONALE Maintains alignment.

38. **ACTION** Place a small pillow under patient's head; turn head to one side, and be sure ear is flat against the pillow.

   RATIONALE Decreases flexion of neck.

Continued

Skill 18-1 | Positioning the Patient—cont'd

39. **ACTION** Support flexed arms at shoulder level.

    RATIONALE Decreases risk of joint dislocation.

40. **ACTION** Place a pillow under the lower legs.

    RATIONALE Promotes dorsiflexion of ankles and knee flexion.

Completing Care

41. **ACTION** Lower the bed and restore the unit. Perform hand hygiene.

    RATIONALE Makes patient comfortable and promotes safety. Performing hand hygiene reduces transfer of microorganisms.

■ Evaluation

42. **ACTION** Observe the newly positioned patient. Is the patient in proper alignment? Are positioning devices correctly placed? Is the patient comfortable? Check Special Considerations for common trouble areas with each position.

    RATIONALE Detects if patient is in proper body alignment and position.

■ Documentation

43. **ACTION** Document on the flow sheet or in the nurse's notes, depending on agency policy. Note date, time, position, and positioning devices used.

    RATIONALE Provides for consistency among personnel and validates actions provided.

Documentation Example

3/6 0800 Placed in supine position. Correct alignment maintained with pillows, hand rolls, and foot splints.

_____
(Nurse's signature)

■ Special Considerations

✓ Gloves should be worn when moving or positioning a patient if you will be touching blood, body fluid, secretions, excretions, broken skin, mucous membranes, or contaminated items.

✓ A patient who has edema or is dehydrated will need to be turned and repositioned more frequently than every 2 hours to avoid skin breakdown.

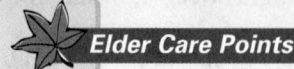

Elder Care Points

When repositioning an elderly person, you must move slowly and carefully to avoid hurting the patient. Arthritis may cause the joints to be stiff and harder to move.

After positioning a patient, check the following areas to prevent possible problems.

✓ Maintain the feet in dorsiflexion; you may need to use a positioning device to decrease the chance of footdrop.

Supine Position

✓ If the patient complains of lower back pain, place a small pillow or rolled towel under the patient's lumbar spine.

✓ Pressure points common to this position are the occiput, lumbar vertebrae, elbows, and heels.

Fowler's and Semi-Fowler's Positions

✓ Check to see that the lower extremities have palpable pulses, verifying that the popliteal artery is not occluded.

✓ Pressure points common to this position are the scapula, sacrum, elbows, and heels.

Side-Lying Position

✓ Avoid lateral flexion of the neck.

✓ Pressure points common to this position are the ankles, knees, trochanter, ilium, and ear.

Sims' Position

✓ Check to see that the hip and shoulder are supported properly to prevent internal rotation and adduction.

✓ Pressure points common to this position are the clavicle, humerus, ilium, knees, and ankles.

Prone Position

✓ Feet must be positioned in dorsiflexion. Sustained extension with plantar flexion is undesirable.

✓ Pressure points common to this position are the ear, chin, hips, and knees.

? CRITICAL THINKING QUESTIONS

1. If you use a pillow, you do not need to check for pressure points in that area. Is the statement true or false? Why?

2. What are some of the advantages of having a trapeze on a bed when the patient has a broken leg?

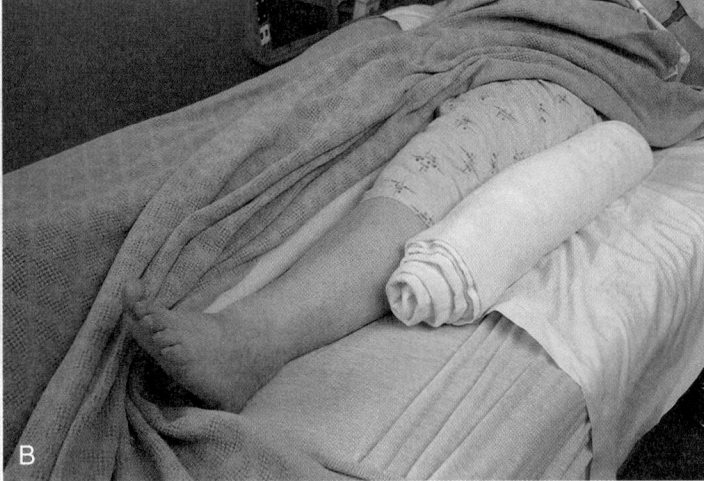

FIGURE **18-9** Positioning devices. **A,** Trapeze bar. **B,** Trochanter roll.

rolls (Figure 18-9, *B*), side rails, and bed boards. Pillows are used to support the body or extremities and elevate body parts. Boots or splints help to maintain dorsiflexion of the feet and may help to prevent heel pressure. Footboards and high-top sneakers are other devices used to maintain foot dorsiflexion. Trochanter rolls prevent external rotation of the hips and legs when a patient is lying in a supine position. Sandbags immobilize an extremity, provide support, and maintain correct body alignment. Hand rolls and splints for the hands and wrists help to prevent contractures of the hands, promote thumb adduction, keep the fingers slightly flexed, and prevent dorsiflexion of the wrist. A trapeze bar allows a patient to adjust position by enabling the trunk and buttocks to be raised off the bed. The patient may use it to help with moving up in bed or transferring from bed to wheelchair and to strengthen upper extremities. Side rails assist the patient to change position and turn in bed. Bed boards are boards that are placed under the home mattress to give more support to the mattress and thereby improve vertebral alignment.

Moving Patients Up in Bed

Patients need different amounts of help moving in bed. After proper instruction, many are able to reposition and move themselves up in bed independently. Other patients are able to provide assistance after they are told what is expected of them. Totally dependent patients rely on the nursing staff for this procedure. Before moving a patient up in bed, one of the most important steps is to determine how much help will be needed. If lift equipment is available, use it. When manually lifting, if there is any doubt about whether a patient is too heavy or immobile to be moved by you, at least one other person's help should be enlisted. Skill 18-2 describes how to move patients up in bed.

Skill 18-2 | Moving the Patient Up in Bed

Many healthy patients can reposition themselves in bed independently after proper instruction. Others, because of injury, disease, helplessness, or therapeutic devices, may be able to help somewhat or will be totally dependent on you. It is always easier for two people to assist any patient to move up in bed. If the patient is large or heavy, use lift equipment or a slide board if available instead of manually lifting. Check the agency policy.

■ Supplies

✓ Lift sheet or slide board for the patient who is dependent or requires assistance

Review and carry out the Standard Steps in Appendix 3.

■ Assessment (Data Collection)

1. *ACTION* Assess alignment, muscle strength, activity tolerance, and mobility.

   RATIONALE Indicates how much patient can assist.

■ Planning

2. *ACTION* Gather positioning supplies and lift sheet if needed.

   RATIONALE Promotes easy access to equipment.

3. *ACTION* Explain what you wish the patient to do.

   RATIONALE Prepares patient and decreases fear.

Continued

Skill 18-2 | Moving the Patient Up in Bed—cont'd

4. **ACTION** Raise level of bed to a comfortable working height.

   RATIONALE Promotes proper body mechanics and reduces back strain.

5. **ACTION** Remove positioning devices for patient's current position.

   RATIONALE Removes obstacles.

6. **ACTION** Get help if possible or needed.

   RATIONALE Provides safety.

7. **ACTION** Provide privacy during the position change.

   RATIONALE Protects the right to privacy and reduces embarrassment.

■ Implementation

8. **ACTION** Perform hand hygiene.

   RATIONALE Reduces transfer of microorganisms.

9. **ACTION** Lock bed wheels and lower rail, if up, on side closest to you.

   RATIONALE Prevents bed from rolling and provides access.

10. **ACTION** Place pillow upright against headboard.

    RATIONALE Prevents the patient from striking head against the headboard.

For the Patient Who Can Assist

11. **ACTION** Place the patient on back. Ask the patient to flex both knees, reach back with one or both arms, and grab the side rails (or hold trapeze bar if present), place chin on chest, then push down on the bed with both feet, lift the buttocks off the bed, and push upward.

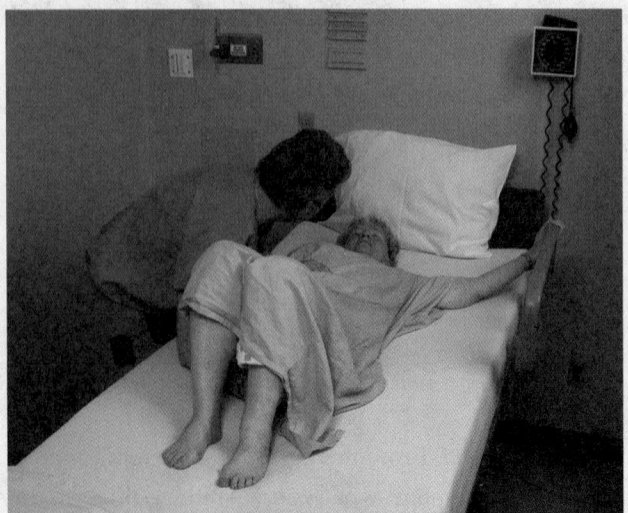

Step **11** Moving patient up in bed.

RATIONALE Allows the patient control while promoting exercise and independence. The chin on the chest prevents neck strain and decreases friction on the back of the head.

For the Patient Who Needs Assistance (1 or 2 Nurses)

12. **a. ACTION** Place the patient on back. Face the head of the bed and, with a broad stance, place one foot in front of the other with the back foot closest to the bed.

    RATIONALE Prevents twisting and strain of back. Provides a good base of support.

    b. ACTION Unless contraindicated, ask the patient to flex both knees, or flex them for the patient.

    RATIONALE Decreases resistance of dragging legs.

    c. ACTION Place the patient's arms across the chest.

    RATIONALE Decreases resistance of dragging arms.

    d. ACTION Place one hand and forearm under the patient's shoulder, support neck, and place the other hand and forearm under the patient's upper thighs. If you have help, each person holds the patient in this way on opposite sides of the bed.

    RATIONALE Supports the patient's heaviest parts. Having two people decreases effort needed.

    e. ACTION With rocking motion of hips and legs, and on the count of 3, shift body weight forward, moving patient toward the head of the bed. Push with the arms as the patient lifts buttocks and pushes with both feet.

    RATIONALE Coordinates movement; helps to overcome forces of inertia.

For the Immobile Patient (1 Nurse)

13. **a. ACTION** Place patient supine.

    RATIONALE Promotes working with gravity.

    b. ACTION Stand diagonally next to the patient's legs in a broad stance with one foot in front of the other and the back foot closest to the bed; slide arms under the legs.

    RATIONALE Prevents strain or twisting of back and provides a good base of support.

    c. ACTION Flex knees and hips so arms are level with patient's legs. Slide patient's legs diagonally toward head of bed.

    RATIONALE Allows a pulling motion and legs are easier to move.

d. ACTION Stand next to patient's hips; place one arm under patient's thighs and the other arm under patient's lower back. Slide the patient's hips diagonally toward head of bed.

RATIONALE Maintains body alignment for you and aligns patient's hips and feet.

e. ACTION Place your arm nearest the head of the bed under patient's neck; support head and patient's other shoulder. Place other arm under patient's chest. Slide trunk, shoulders, neck, and head toward head of bed. Patient is now in alignment on one side of the bed.

RATIONALE Supports the patient's body weight during movement. Patient is aligned on one side of the bed.

f. ACTION Raise side rail. Switch sides of bed and repeat as necessary until patient reaches desired place in bed.

RATIONALE Promotes safety and moves patient while maintaining alignment.

g. ACTION Center patient in bed, moving the body in the three sections.

RATIONALE Maintains alignment.

For the Immobile Patient (2 Nurses with a Lift Sheet)

14. a. ACTION Obtain a lift sheet.

RATIONALE Less effort is needed to move patient on a sheet than to move with hands.

b. ACTION With patient on side, place the lift sheet under patient by rolling up the edge of the sheet close to the patient and placing it firmly against the patient.

RATIONALE Allows sheet to be pulled easily out from under the patient once turned. Supports the heaviest part of the patient.

c. ACTION Roll the patient back to the other side over the lift sheet. Pull sheet through. Place patient on back; with a nurse on each side of the bed, roll or fan-fold the sheet close to each side of the patient.

RATIONALE Decreases risk of injury. If the patient is large, more than two nurses may be needed to safely transfer the patient.

d. ACTION Each nurse places one foot slightly in front of the other, about shoulders' width apart, to form a broad base of support.

RATIONALE Increases balance.

e. ACTION With hips and knees slightly flexed, and back straight, grasp the sides of the rolled or folded sheet as close as possible to patient. On the count of 3, lift patient to the head of the bed.

RATIONALE Enables you to shift body weight in direction of movement, decreasing force needed to lift patient. Maintains proper body movement, decreasing chance of injury.

Completing Care

15. ACTION Smooth out lift sheet under patient. Position patient in desired position, raise side rails, lower bed, and replace call bell.

RATIONALE Maintains alignment and promotes safety.

16. ACTION Restore the unit and perform hand hygiene.

RATIONALE Promotes comfort and safety. Performing hand hygiene reduces transfer of microorganisms.

■ Evaluation

17. ACTION Observe patient's level of comfort, position, body alignment, and potential pressure points.

RATIONALE Maintains support to body and decreases risk of injury.

■ Documentation

18. ACTION Repositioning for comfort and body alignment is charted on the flow sheet or in the nurse's notes according to agency policy. Note date, time, procedure, and position.

RATIONALE Documents position changes and validates they have been done.

Documentation Example

3/6 0900   Feet over end of mattress; moved to head of bed with assistance; repositioned supine for comfort; placed in proper alignment. Bed down, call bell within reach.

_____
(Nurse's signature)

❓CRITICAL THINKING QUESTIONS

1. Explain how positioning yourself correctly when moving a patient up in bed aids the process.
2. Describe complications, other than development of a pressure ulcer, that can occur from improper alignment and positioning.

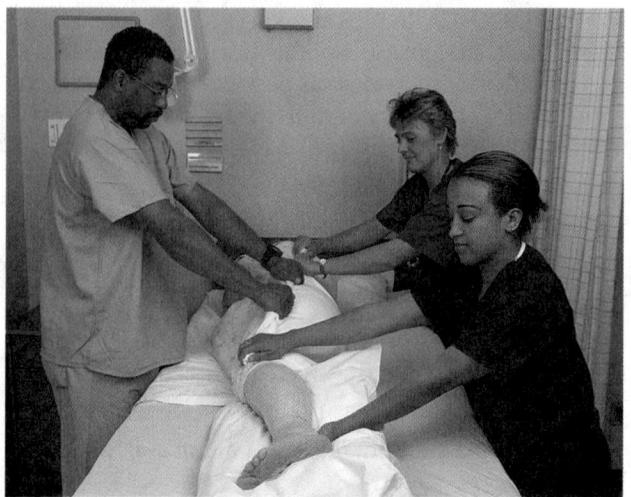

FIGURE **18-10** Logrolling a patient using a lift sheet.

One of the techniques to move patients in bed is called logrolling. Logrolling is turning the patient as a single unit while maintaining straight body alignment at all times. Logrolling is often used for patients with injuries or surgery to the spine and for those who must avoid twisting. The linens for an occupied bed are often changed by using the logrolling turn. Logrolling can be done either with or without a lift sheet. If a lift sheet is used, two or three people are needed to accomplish the move, depending on the size of the patient (Figure 18-10). It takes at least two other people to assist when logrolling a patient without a lift sheet (Figure 18-11).

When using a lift sheet, you and preferably two other assistants stand on opposite sides of a locked, flat bed at waist level. Leave a pillow under the patient's head and lower the side rails. Place a pillow or two, if needed, between the patient's legs. All the nurses face the bed with one foot slightly in front of the other. Roll the lift sheet close to the patient's body and, on the count of 3, lift the patient to one side of the bed, keeping the body in straight alignment. By lifting the patient to one side of the bed first, the patient should be centered in the bed after being logrolled.

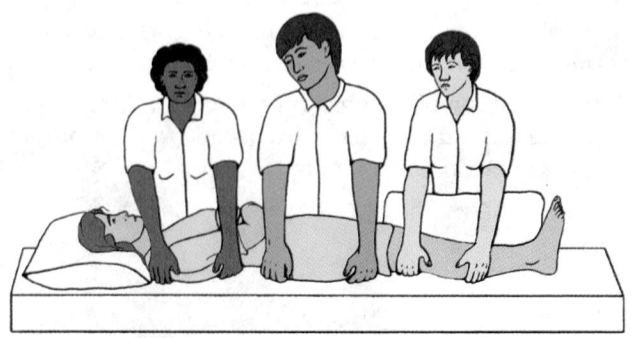

FIGURE **18-11** Logrolling a patient without a lift sheet.

The tallest nurse is positioned on the far side of the bed and should be at the middle portion of the patient. The other two nurses are positioned one at the shoulders and neck and one at the legs and feet of the patient so that they can control movement of these parts. The nurse on the far side of the bed grasps the lift sheet. Again, the sheet is held as close to the patient's body as possible, and on the count of 3 the patient is rolled in one smooth, coordinated, even motion with the body in straight alignment. The pillow is rearranged under the patient's head and any other positioning devices are placed before lowering the bed and putting the call bell within the patient's reach.

Logrolling without a lift sheet is accomplished in a similar manner. Three nurses are evenly spaced along one side of a locked, flat bed at waist level. One nurse supports and rolls the head, neck, and shoulder region; one supports and rolls the waist and hips; and the third supports and rolls the thighs and lower legs.

Therapeutic Exercise

Physical therapy is often ordered for the patient who is immobilized for an extended period of time. The physician indicates the patient's problems, and the therapist performs an evaluation and then designs an exercise program to help the patient and to prevent further musculoskeletal problems from occurring. If a physical therapist is not available, you will need to assist your patient in performing these exercises. The family and/or significant other can also be shown how to assist the patient with exercise.

Full range-of-motion (ROM) exercises should be performed either actively or passively several times a day. Active ROM exercises are used for the patient who independently performs activities of daily living but for some reason is immobilized or limited in activity or is unable to move one extremity due to injury or surgery. Passive ROM exercises are performed on the patient who cannot actively move. This patient

---

Box 18-2 *Principles Guiding Range-of-Motion (ROM) Exercise*

- Move the body part to stretch the muscles and keep the joint flexible, but avoid movement to the point of discomfort.
- ROM exercises of the joints of helpless or immobile patients are performed at least twice a day, or more often if tolerated.
- Support the limb above and below the joint when performing passive exercises of arms and legs.
- Each movement should be performed a minimum of three to five times for each exercise.
- Involve patients in planning their exercise program and encourage active performance of the exercises if allowed and capability returns.

cannot contract muscles, so muscle strengthening cannot be accomplished. All muscles over a joint are maximally stretched to achieve or maintain flexibility of the joint. This is accomplished by moving the muscles to the point of slight resistance but not beyond. To prevent joint injury in performing passive ROM exercises, support the limb to be exercised above and below the joint. Principles related to carrying out ROM exercises for patients are listed in Box 18-2. Skill 18-3 describes how to provide passive ROM exercises.

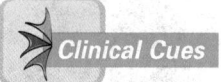
Clinical Cues

Watch the patient's face as you perform passive ROM so that you will know if you are causing pain. If the patient is expressing pain, you are moving the joint too far.

Lifting and Transferring

Lifting and transferring patients also require the use of proper body mechanics and positioning principles. Some patients may be independent or need minimal

---

Skill 18-3 | Passive Range-of-Motion (ROM) Exercises

Many patients are paralyzed or have limited mobility of the extremities. To prevent joints from becoming rigid and immovable and to prevent contractures, it is necessary to provide motion to the joints on a regularly scheduled basis. Each exercise is repeated three to five times per session. Remainder of the patient is kept draped while one extremity is exercised.

■ Supplies

✓ Blanket or top sheet

Review and carry out the Standard Steps in Appendix 3.

■ Assessment (Data Collection)

1. **ACTION** Check the orders for any contraindication to performance of ROM.

   RATIONALE Prevents injuring the patient with ROM exercise.

2. **ACTION** Assess the patient for areas of weakness or paralysis.

   RATIONALE Indicates which joints need passive ROM and which can be actively exercised.

■ Planning

3. **ACTION** Be certain wheels of bed are locked and that the bed is raised to working height.

   RATIONALE Prepares area for the procedure and prevents injury.

■ Implementation

4. **ACTION** Place patient in supine position, remove the pillow, and drape with sheet or blanket.

   RATIONALE Positions patient for the procedure. A drape provides privacy for the patient.

5. **ACTION** Perform passive ROM of the head and neck:

   • Support the head with your hands, and bring the head forward until the chin touches the chest.

   • Extend the neck by elevating the chin and having the patient look upward. Return the head to the neutral position.

• Support the head with your hands, and turn it toward the right shoulder and then toward the left shoulder. Pause in a neutral position.

• Bend the head laterally to the right shoulder and then to the left. Return the pillow under the head.

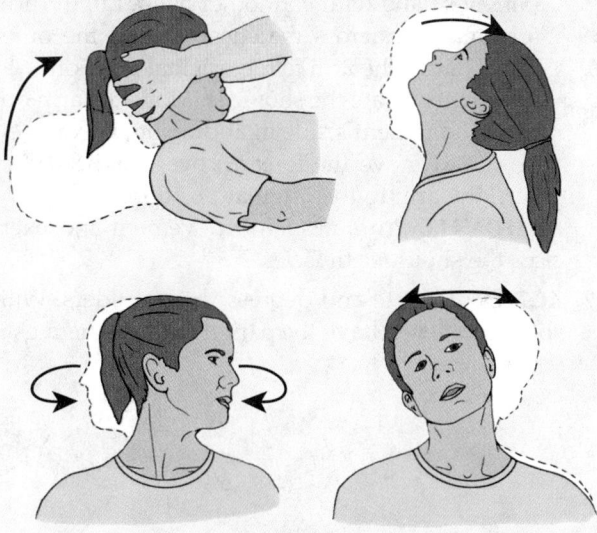

Step **5**

RATIONALE Exercises the neck and trapezius muscles. Promotes cervical spine mobility. Pillow makes patient more comfortable.

6. **ACTION** Flex and extend the shoulder and elbow:

   • Supporting the elbow with one hand, grasp the wrist with your other hand. Bring the arm straight up over the head, then lower it and bend the elbow. Return the arm to the patient's side.

Continued

Skill 18-3 | **Passive Range-of-Motion (ROM) Exercises**—cont'd

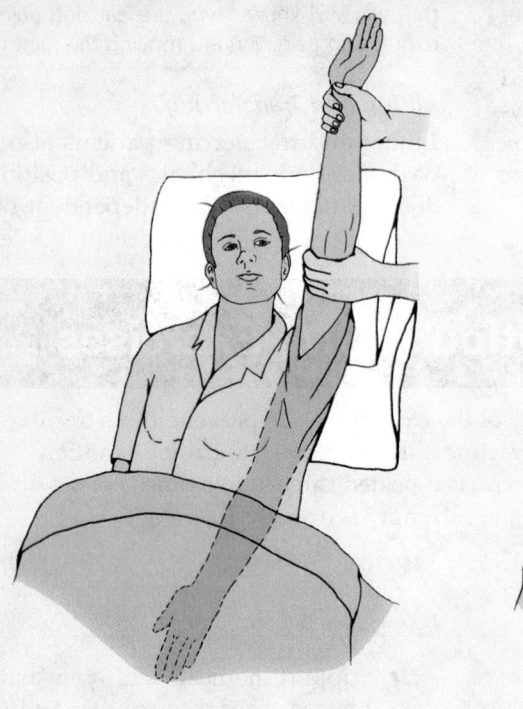

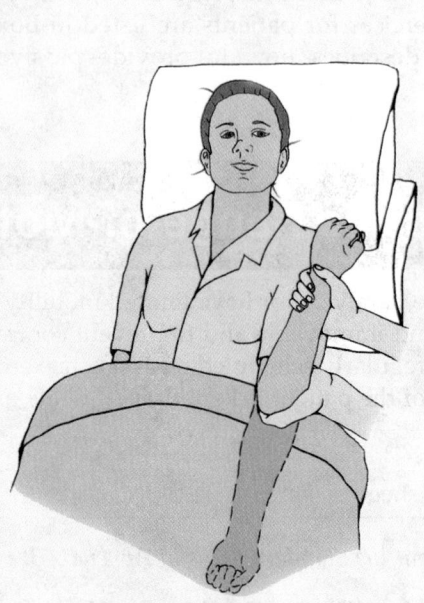

Step **6**

- Internally rotate the shoulder. Place one hand on the patient's arm above the elbow, and grasp the patient's hand with your other hand. Lift the arm and move it across the chest toward the other side. Return the arm to the original position.
- Externally rotate the shoulder. Move the arm out from the patient's side in abduction. Flex the elbow, and move the forearm over the head. Return the arm to the original position.
  RATIONALE Promotes joint movement and exercises the shoulder muscles.

7. **ACTION** Elevate and depress the shoulders. With shoulders level, have the patient elevate them as if shrugging. Have the patient lower the shoulders as far as possible and then return to a level plane.
   RATIONALE Loosens the shoulder joints and promotes relaxation.

8. **ACTION** Flex the wrist:
   - Hold the patient's wrist with one hand and the palm of the hand with your other hand, keeping the patient's fingers straight. Hyperextend the wrist by bending it backward. Extend the wrist by straightening.
   - Flex the wrist by bending the hand forward and closing the fingers to make a fist. Perform circumduction of the hand and wrist. Hold the

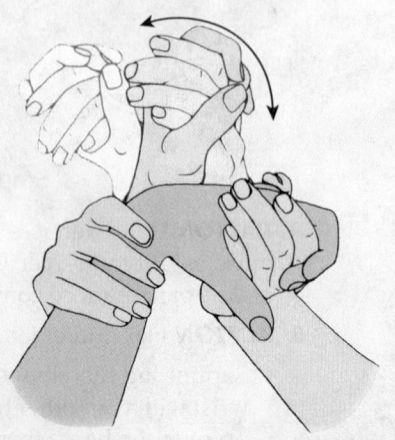

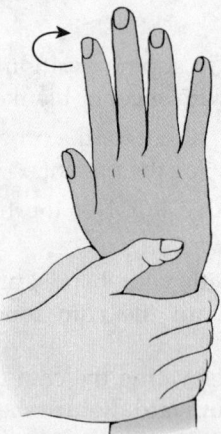

Step **8**

patient's wrist with one hand and the palm of the hand with your other hand, keeping the patient's fingers straight. Bend the wrist forward, and move it in a circular motion.

- Rotate the wrist and hand. Grasp the wrist in both of your hands. Rotate the wrist by turning the palm toward the patient's face for supination and then toward the feet for pronation.

RATIONALE Exercises the wrist. Circumduction promotes joint flexibility and prevents contractures. Rotation promotes joint flexibility and movement.

9. *ACTION* Exercise the thumb and fingers:

- Hold the patient's hand with one hand, and grasp the thumb with your other hand. Avoid pressing on the nail bed. Flex the thumb and then the fingers by bending them onto the palm.
- Extend the fingers by returning them to their original position. Abduct the fingers by spreading them.
- Adduct the fingers by returning them to a closed position. Circumduct the fingers and thumb by moving them in a circular motion.
- Oppose the thumb by touching it to each of the fingers in turn.

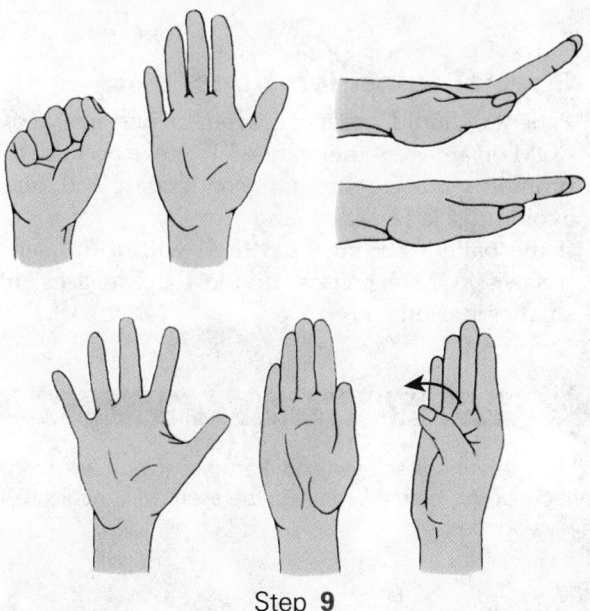

Step **9**

RATIONALE Promotes opposition of thumb and grasp for other fingers needed to perform activities of daily living.

10. *ACTION* Exercise the hip and knee:

- Place one hand under the knee, and cup the heel in your other hand. Flex the leg by bending the knee and moving the leg toward the chest as far as it will go without causing pain. Extend the leg by lifting the foot upward and then lowering the leg to the bed.
- Abduct the hip joint by keeping the leg straight and slowly moving the entire leg toward the

edge of the bed. Adduct the hip joint by moving the leg back to the original position.

- Rotate internally by keeping the leg flat on the bed, and roll the leg inward with toes pointed in toward the opposite foot. Rotate externally by keeping the leg flat on the bed; roll the leg outward with toes pointed away from opposite foot.

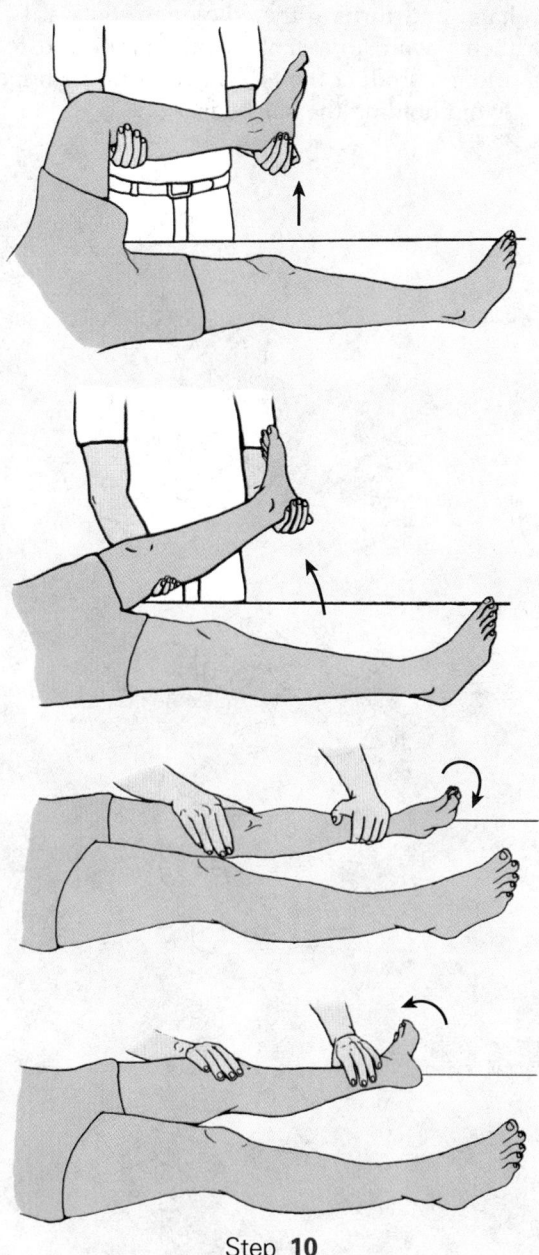

Step **10**

RATIONALE Promotes successful mobility when the patient is able to resume ambulation and prevents hip contracture.

11. *ACTION* Exercise the ankle and foot:

- With the patient's leg on the bed, place one hand on the ball of the foot; then place the other hand just above the ankle.
- Perform dorsiflexion by pushing the foot forward toward the body and pushing down on the heel at the same time.

Continued

Skill 18-3 Passive Range-of-Motion (ROM) Exercises—cont'd

- Perform plantar flexion by pushing the toes away from the body while pushing down on the heel. Circumduct by holding the ankle with one hand and turning the whole foot outward and then inward in a circular motion. Flex, extend, and circumduct the toes as you did the fingers. Avoid holding the nail beds.

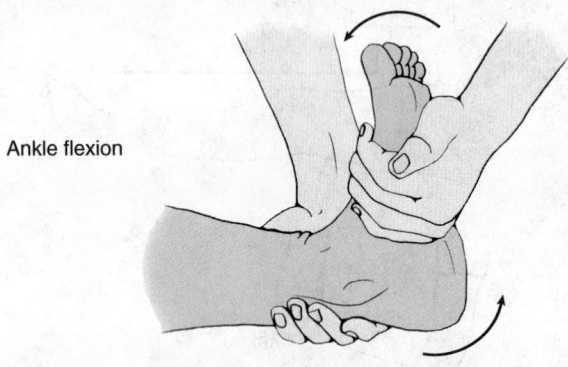

Ankle flexion

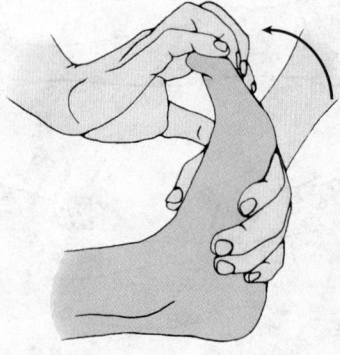

Dorsiflexion

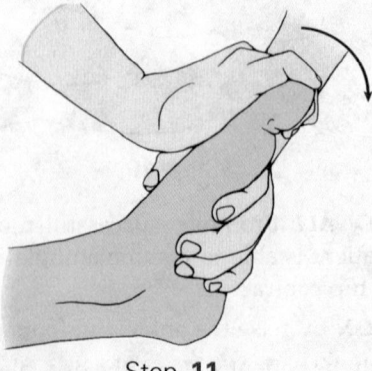

Plantar flexion

Step **11**

RATIONALE Prevents footdrop and promotes mobility when the patient is able to resume ambulation.

■ Evaluation

12. ***ACTION*** Ask the following questions: Was each joint exercised with three to five repetitions? Did the patient experience pain? Does any joint show diminished range of motion?

    RATIONALE Answers to these questions provide data to determine if expected outcomes are being met.

■ Documentation

13. ***ACTION*** Document the performance of ROM and any problems encountered.

    RATIONALE Validates that ROM was performed and any problems encountered.

Documentation Example

3/8 0900   Passive ROM exercises carried out to all extremities, head, and neck. No evidence of contractures. Slight discomfort noted with left ankle flexion. All other motions carried out with ease.

_____
(Nurse's signature)

■ Special Considerations

✓ Patients should be encouraged to perform active ROM on any joint they can safely move because this promotes muscle strength contraction and helps avoid muscle weakness and atrophy.
✓ If the patient becomes too tired with a full set of passive ROM exercises, divide the exercises into smaller sessions.

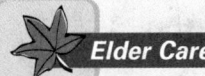 **Elder Care Points**

Elderly patients often have some arthritic joints. Ask the patient about this before beginning the exercises; medicate for pain as needed.

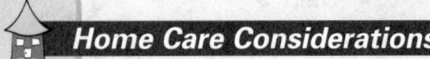 **Home Care Considerations**

Instruct the caregiver with the home patient on how to do the exercises and leave a written schedule form for tracking performance.

❓CRITICAL THINKING QUESTIONS

1. Your patient asks you why she needs to perform active ROM exercises. What would you tell her?
2. What benefits do you think will occur if you involve the patient in her exercise plan?

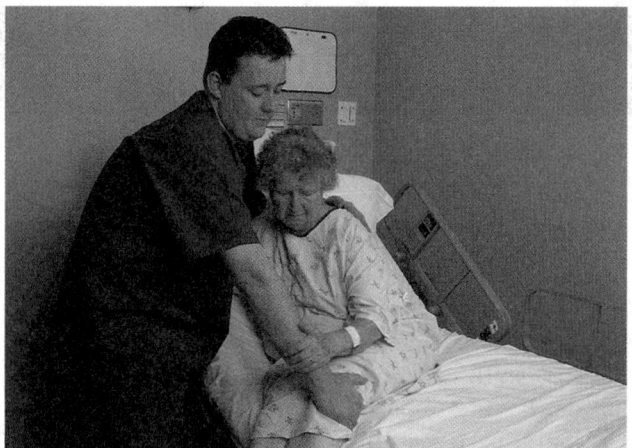

FIGURE **18-12** Assisting the patient to dangle at the side of the bed.

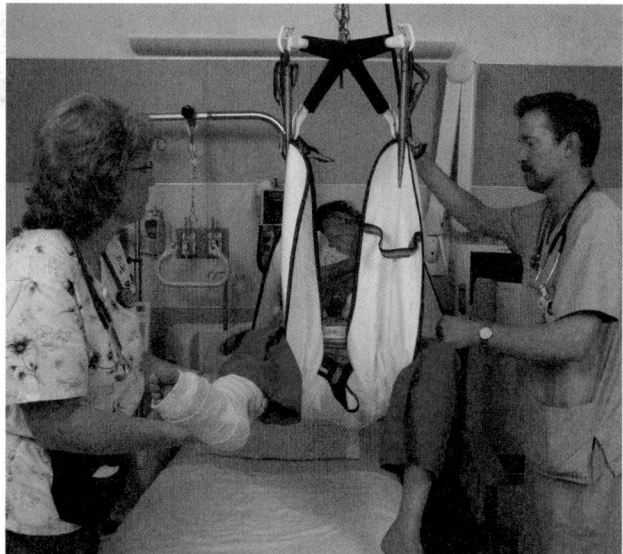

FIGURE **18-13** Nurse using lift equipment to transfer a patient from bed to chair or chair to bed.

assistance to ambulate. Others may need to be transferred to a chair, wheelchair, or stretcher.

Before transferring a patient to a wheelchair, have her dangle her legs over the side of the bed first (Figure 18-12). Dangling is the term used for the patient position of sitting on the side of the bed with the legs and feet over the side. **The feet are either on the floor or supported on a footstool.** Dangling is often the first step before sitting in a chair or ambulating. The purpose is to gradually accustom the body to the position change. While the patient is dangling, assess the patient's balance, and monitor for orthostatic hypotension, dizziness, or nausea before getting the patient out of bed. If a patient has been on prolonged bed rest,

she may only be strong enough to dangle for a few minutes and then will need to lie down again.

Wheelchairs are often used to transport an ambulatory patient to different areas for tests and procedures, or for the patient who is unable to walk or tolerate the fatigue associated with the effort. Either lift equipment or two nurses should transfer a patient to a wheelchair if the patient is unsteady, weak, or heavy (check agency policy) (Figure 18-13). Transferring a patient to a wheelchair is described in Skill 18-4.

Skill 18-4 | Transferring the Patient to a Wheelchair

A patient is often transported to another area of the facility by wheelchair. Patients may be transferred to a wheelchair to provide greater independence. A similar procedure is used to transfer a patient to a chair. If the patient is large or heavy, use lift equipment for the transfer if available. Check agency policy.

■ Supplies
✓ Bed
✓ Wheelchair

✓ Safety jacket if patient is unstable when sitting

✓ Transfer belt if necessary
✓ Slippers/nonskid socks and robe

Review and carry out the Standard Steps in Appendix 3.

■ Assessment (Data Collection)

1. *ACTION* Assess patient's size, ability to assist in move, and ability to follow instructions.

   RATIONALE Provides baseline data; indicates what is needed for a safe transfer.

■ Planning

2. *ACTION* Gather wheelchair and transfer belt if needed.

   RATIONALE Provides easy access to equipment.

3. *ACTION* Maintain privacy by closing door and/or curtain.

   RATIONALE Protects right to privacy and reduces embarrassment.

4. *ACTION* Get help if needed.

   RATIONALE Provides safety for you and patient.

5. *ACTION* Explain the procedure and what the patient is to do.

   RATIONALE Decreases fear of the unknown and prepares patient.

Continued

Skill 18-4 | Transferring the Patient to a Wheelchair—cont'd

■ Implementation

6. *ACTION* Perform hand hygiene.

   RATIONALE Reduces transfer of microorganisms.

7. *ACTION* Place wheelchair parallel to the side of the bed. Lock wheelchair.

   RATIONALE Promotes easy reach and access. Locking wheelchair promotes safety.

8. *ACTION* Place transfer belt on patient if patient is weak or paralyzed on one side.

   RATIONALE Decreases the risk of a fall during transfer and prevents pressure on patient's axillae.

9. *ACTION* Lower bed and side rail if elevated. Elevate the head of the bed to the highest level the patient can tolerate.

   RATIONALE Decreases the work for you and patient and promotes safety.

10. *ACTION* Assist the patient to turn onto side. Support the patient's shoulders with one arm, and with the other arm at the patient's thighs, help the patient sit up and move the legs over the edge of the bed. Help patient move forward on bed until feet rest on the floor and allow the legs to dangle.

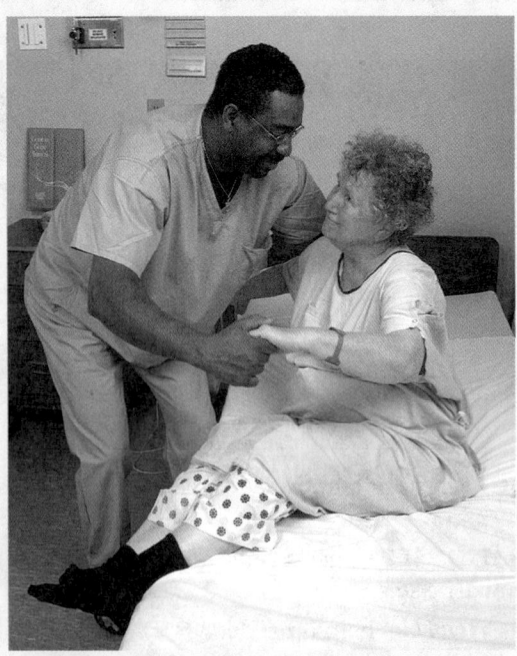

Step **10**

   RATIONALE Maintains alignment and proper body mechanics.

11. *ACTION* Assist patient in donning robe.

   RATIONALE Provides privacy.

12. *ACTION* Place slippers or nonskid socks on patient.

   RATIONALE Prevents patient's feet from slipping during transfer.

13. *ACTION* Reposition wheelchair closer if necessary so the patient can stand, pivot, and sit without having to back up to chair. Place the chair so that it is closest to the patient's strongest side.

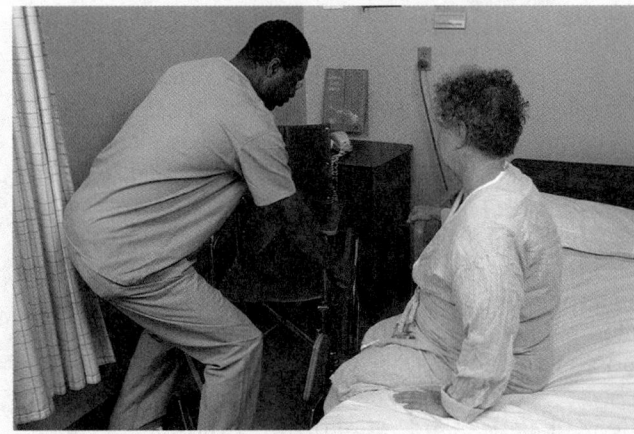

Step **13**

   RATIONALE Reduces distance the patient must travel to sit safely in the chair.

14. *ACTION* Check that both wheels are still locked on wheelchair.

   RATIONALE Maintains safety because unlocked wheels allow chair to back away from patient as she sits. This can lead to patient's falling and possible injury for both parties.

15. *ACTION* Assist the patient to stand by assuming a moderately wide stance in front of the patient; brace the patient's legs with your knees, which are slightly flexed.

   RATIONALE Provides base of support, maintains alignment, and prevents back injury.

16. *ACTION* Place your arms under the patient's axillae and your hands on the patient's scapula. If the patient is not able to push self off of bed, have patient place arms around your shoulders (not your neck). If the patient is able to help push up from the bed, have patient place hands on the bed.

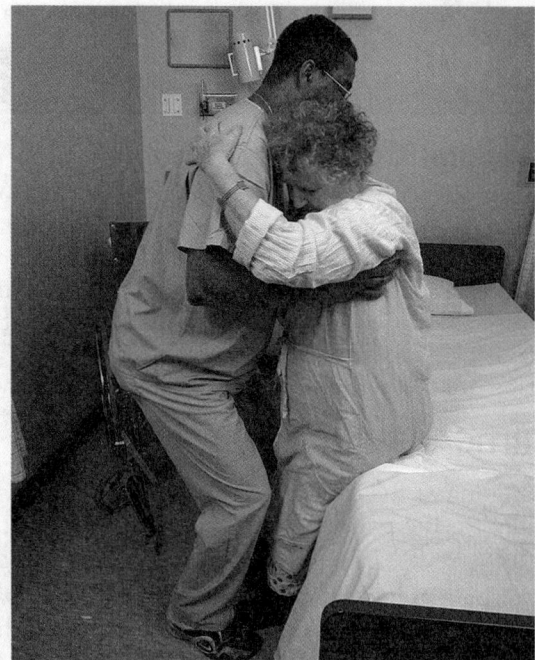

Step **16**

RATIONALE Brings patient close to your center of gravity and provides a point of leverage for lifting.

17. **ACTION** On the count of 3, have the patient push on the bed and lift patient upward while maintaining correct alignment in your back. Depending on your assessment of the patient's ability, a transfer belt or another nurse on the opposite side may be needed.

RATIONALE Uses leverage to raise patient to a standing position. Assistance helps maintain safety.

18. **ACTION** Pivot 90 degrees so the patient's back is toward the seat of the chair. Have the patient reach back and grasp the arms of the chair, if able. Be

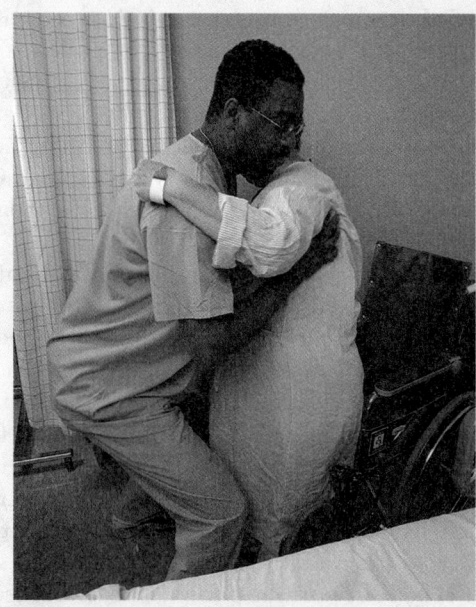

Step **18**

sure patient's legs are against seat of chair and lower the body into the chair. Flex your knees as patient lowers into the chair.

RATIONALE Pivoting allows patient to sit down without twisting. Having legs against seat places the patient's weight directly over the chair, providing safe support during sitting. Flexing your knees prevents self-injury.

19. **ACTION** Assist the patient to place the feet on the footrests. Avoid striking the patient's ankles while fixing the footrest. Apply a protective device if ordered. Position patient in the chair in correct alignment—hips should be back in chair. If needed, assist patient to reposition farther back in chair. Provide support for weak or paralyzed extremities.

RATIONALE Maintains alignment and prevents injury.

Transferring the Patient Back to the Bed (a Reversal of the Procedure)

20. **ACTION** Check to ensure the brakes are locked on the wheelchair. Have patient grasp both arms of the chair and push up and out of the chair to a standing position. Assist patient by placing one arm under the axilla and the other under the elbow.

RATIONALE Maintains safety. Patient assists with lifting. Hands under the axilla and elbow stabilize the patient.

21. **ACTION** Assist the patient to pivot 90 degrees so the back is next to the bed. When able to stand unassisted, remove the robe. Have patient place hands on bed and lower to sit on bed.

RATIONALE Pivoting allows patient to sit without twisting. Having patient stand aids in removal of robe because patient is not sitting on robe.

22. **ACTION** Remove slippers. Have patient lean against the elevated head of the bed, and assist in swinging legs up into bed, maintaining good body mechanics.

RATIONALE Positions patient at head of bed so patient will not need to be moved up in bed.

23. **ACTION** Cover the patient, raise side rail if necessary, and place call bell within reach.

RATIONALE Maintains privacy, and institutes safety measures.

■ Evaluation

24. **ACTION** Assess patient's position, alignment, and comfort level. Modify as necessary.

RATIONALE Maintains support of body and decreases chance of injury resulting from poor positioning or movement.

Continued

Skill 18-4 | Transferring the Patient to a Wheelchair—cont'd

■ Documentation

25. ACTION Document, noting date, time, position, length of time patient was out of bed, and how patient tolerated the procedure. If the patient was transported to another area for a test, include this information. Note number of personnel needed to complete the transfer.

RATIONALE Validates effectiveness of nursing care and activity of patient, and provides data for transferring patient.

Documentation Example

3/8 1000 By one nurse, assisted out of bed to wheelchair by standing and pivoting. No weakness or difficulty noted during transfer. Returned to bed after 30 minutes.

_____
(Nurse's signature)

Stretchers may also be called litters, gurneys, or carts. They are used for transporting a patient who is unable to sit in a wheelchair or is having certain tests or procedures done—for example, surgery. Stretchers have side rails and a safety belt that should be secured before moving the patient (Safety Alert 18-1).

 Think Critically About . . . Your 39-year-old patient has been on bed rest for 1 week. She has not been out of bed yet and needs to go to the x-ray department for a chest x-ray. Do you use a wheelchair or a stretcher to send her? Why?

Moving a wheelchair or a stretcher is an exception to a principle of body mechanics discussed earlier in this chapter. Both devices are pushed rather than pulled. To pull a wheelchair or stretcher would cause back strain and twisting.

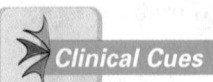 **Clinical Cues**

When transferring a patient into or out of a wheelchair, check feet and arms for positions where they will not hit the parts of the chair or the bed. The footrests should be positioned where they won't interfere with the feet during transfer. Many skin injuries occur when transferring patients into or out of wheelchairs.

Transferring Devices

Devices that may be used in lifting and transferring patients include mechanical lifts, lift or pull sheets, roller boards, slide boards, and transfer or gait belts.

■ Special Considerations

✓ When transferring a patient to a wheelchair, you may need to help the weak patient readjust position in the wheelchair. To do this, stand behind the wheelchair with your knees flexed. Place your arms under the patient's axillae and lift the patient up and back by using your leg muscles. Reposition and place call bell within patient's reach.

? CRITICAL THINKING QUESTIONS

1. Dangling at the side of the bed is important, especially for the patient who has not been out of bed. Why?

2. Your patient had a right stroke with left-sided paresis. In transferring the patient to the wheelchair, which side of the patient should be closest to the chair? Why?

⚠ Safety Alert 18-1

Lock the Wheels

Remember to lock the wheels on the wheelchair and the bed or stretcher before attempting to transfer a patient into a wheelchair or stretcher or onto the bed. Otherwise, the wheelchair or stretcher could roll away from you, and you and the patient could be injured.

Mechanical lifts are discussed in Chapter 39. Lift sheets are often used to move and transfer a patient. Transferring a patient to a stretcher is discussed in Skill 18-5. Lift sheets may be used alone or with the following devices to help maintain the patient's alignment during a transfer.

A _roller board_ consists of several roller bars between fixed end bars. The bars are enclosed in a vinyl covering that allows the bars to turn when something or someone is pulled over top of the roller board. It works similar to a conveyor belt.

To use a roller board to transfer a patient to a stretcher, turn the patient to one side and place the roller board and lift sheet underneath the patient. Return the patient to a supine position and place the stretcher against the bed with the side rail down. Lock the stretcher wheels. One or more nurses are on the far side of the bed and you and another nurse are on the far side of the stretcher. The lift sheet is held as close to the patient as possible. On the count of 3, the patient is pulled across the roller board. The nurse(s) on the far side of the bed support the patient's head and feet and help guide the patient to the stretcher. A _slide board_

Skill 18-5 | Transferring the Patient to a Stretcher

Patients are transferred to a stretcher to be moved from place to place in the hospital for diagnostic tests or surgery. Care must be taken to prevent injury to the patient and yourself during this task. As with any skill, it is important to have the correct number of staff members to transfer the patient safely. Observe proper body movement and alignment to prevent injury. Three staff members or more are needed depending on patient size. Use a roller board or slide device if available.

■ Supplies
✓ Bed
✓ Stretcher
✓ Bath blanket or sheet
✓ Second bath blanket or sheet
✓ Roller board or slide board

Review and carry out the Standard Steps in Appendix 3.

■ Assessment (Data Collection)

1. *ACTION* Assess patient's size and ability to assist in move (e.g., folding arms on chest).

   RATIONALE Provides baseline data and indicates the number of additional staff needed for transfer.

■ Planning

2. *ACTION* Gather stretcher and other supplies needed for the transfer.

   RATIONALE Promotes access to equipment for safe transfer.

3. *ACTION* Maintain patient's privacy by closing door and/or curtain.

   RATIONALE Protects the patient's right to privacy and reduces embarrassment.

4. *ACTION* Get other staff members needed to help with transfer.

   RATIONALE Provides for a safe transfer.

5. *ACTION* Explain the procedure to the patient.

   RATIONALE Decreases fear of the unknown and prepares patient for what will occur.

■ Implementation

6. *ACTION* Perform hand hygiene.

   RATIONALE Reduces transfer of microorganisms.

7. *ACTION* Lock the wheels of the bed and raise it level with the height of the stretcher.

   RATIONALE Prevents the patient from falling between bed and stretcher. Level surfaces allow maintenance of proper body movement and alignment.

8. *ACTION* Fold the top covers to the foot of the bed, making sure feet are uncovered. Remove any positioning devices from bed. Cover patient with bath blanket or sheet.

   RATIONALE Moving covers prevents feet from becoming tangled in bed linen during transfer.

Removing positioning devices prevents obstruction during transfer. Covering the patient provides privacy during transfer.

9. *ACTION* Check for any tubes (e.g., intravenous [IV], nasogastric, urinary catheter, or chest tube), and position them so they will not be pulled out or dislodged during transfer.

   RATIONALE Prevents patient injury and loss of access, as with an IV.

10. *ACTION* Lower the side rail of the bed on the side where the transfer will take place if raised, and have one nurse remain at the bedside to protect the patient from falling.

    RATIONALE Improves access to patient and provides for safety.

11. *ACTION* Place the lift sheet and/or slide device under the patient as described in Skill 18-2. The slide device is placed beneath the lift sheet.

    RATIONALE Lift sheet aids transfer. Slide device makes transfer much easier.

12. *ACTION* Place patient on back; have both nurses grasp the edge of the sheet, and on the count of 3, move patient to the open edge of the bed.

    RATIONALE Decreases the risk of injury by using more people. If the patient is large, more than three nurses may be needed to safely transfer the patient.

13. *ACTION* Place the stretcher firmly against the open side of the bed and lock its wheels.

    RATIONALE Maintains safety and prevents patient from falling.

14. *ACTION* Two nurses stand with a correct stance on the far side of the stretcher. The third nurse stands or kneels on the other side of the bed to assist in guiding the patient from the bed to the stretcher. On the count of 3, the two nurses pull and the third nurse lifts and guides the patient to the stretcher.

Continued

Skill 18-5 | Transferring the Patient to a Stretcher—cont'd

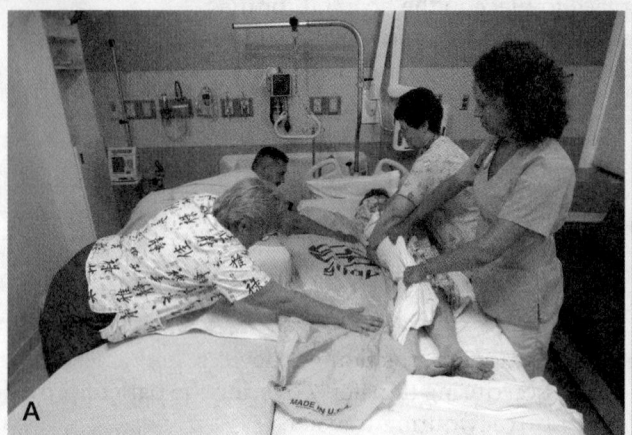 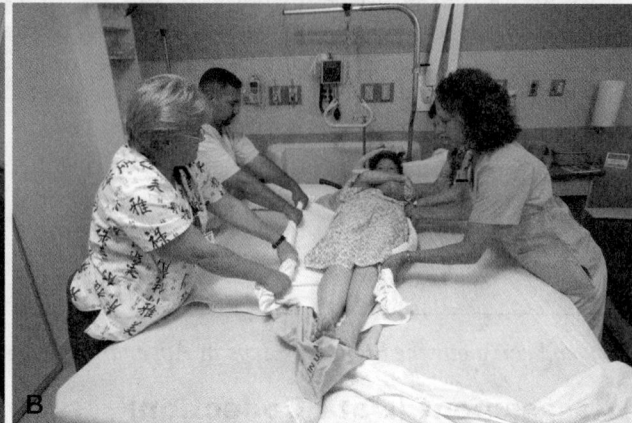

Step **14**

RATIONALE Pulling is easier than pushing, and it promotes a smooth transfer.

15. *ACTION* Smooth out the lift sheet under the patient. Check and straighten the patient's body alignment. Fasten the safety belt securely over the patient and raise the side rail of the stretcher.

RATIONALE Provides safety.

16. *ACTION* Cover the patient for more warmth if needed and put a pillow under the patient's head.

RATIONALE Provides comfort.

17. *ACTION* Unlock the wheels, move the stretcher away from the bed, and raise the opposite stretcher rail.

RATIONALE Allows patient to be moved to site of test or procedure.

18. *ACTION* Remake or straighten the patient's bed in preparation for patient's return.

RATIONALE Conserves time because bed is ready for patient upon return.

■ Evaluation

19. *ACTION* Assess patient's position, alignment, and comfort level. Modify as necessary.

RATIONALE Maintains support of body and decreases chance of injury resulting from poor positioning or mechanics.

■ Documentation

20. *ACTION* Document the transfer: date, time, type of transfer, number of personnel necessary, and how patient tolerated the procedure. If the patient was transported to another area for a test, include this information.

RATIONALE Notes patient transfer off unit.

Documentation Example

3/18 1330   To x-ray. Transferred from bed to stretcher by three staff members using a pull sheet without incident. Safety belt applied.

_____

(Nurse's signature)

? CRITICAL THINKING QUESTIONS

1. Why are two nurses placed on the side to which the patient is being moved onto the stretcher?

2. What purpose does a roller board serve in transferring your patient to the stretcher?

works similarly to a roller board except that it does not roll. It has a slippery surface that allows the patient on a lift sheet to be slid across it to a stretcher or to a wheelchair.

A transfer belt or gait belt may be used to ambulate and/or transfer the weak or unsteady patient. It is made of a tightly webbed canvas material and is very sturdy. Place and buckle the belt around a patient's

waist before having the patient stand. It needs to be tightened just enough to allow space for your hand to grasp it from the rear. **Insert your hand into the belt from the bottom so that, if the patient falls, you will be able to support the weight.** If you hold the belt from the top, it could slip out of your hand from the patient's weight during a fall. Skill 18-6 discusses how to assist a patient to ambulate and how to break a fall.

Skill 18-6 | Ambulating the Patient and Breaking a Fall

A patient may need assistance with ambulation due to being unsteady from illness or trauma, becoming weak from prolonged bed rest, or needing to manage therapeutic equipment such as drains or intravenous lines. Sometimes during ambulation a patient may begin to fall unexpectedly. It is important to know how to properly ambulate the patient and break a patient's fall to prevent injury to both the patient and yourself. The patient must be able to stand unassisted before attempting to ambulate.

■ Supplies
✓ Robe
✓ Socks
✓ Slippers or shoes
✓ Transfer or gait belt (if necessary)

Review and carry out the Standard Steps in Appendix 3.

■ Assessment (Data Collection)

1. *ACTION* Check the patient's written activity order.

   RATIONALE A written order is required to get the patient out of bed.

2. *ACTION* Assess patient's comfort level, coordination, activity tolerance, strength, and balance.

   RATIONALE Provides baseline data and informs you if more than one staff member will be needed.

■ Planning

3. *ACTION* Gather patient items and transfer belt if necessary.

   RATIONALE Provides easy access.

4. *ACTION* Get additional help if necessary.

   RATIONALE Promotes safety.

5. *ACTION* Explain the procedure to the patient.

   RATIONALE Decreases fear of the unknown and prepares patient for what will occur.

■ Implementation
Ambulating the Patient

6. *ACTION* With the patient seated on the side of the bed with robe and socks and slippers on, place patient's feet firmly on the floor. Position yourself in front of the patient with feet apart and outside the patient's feet. Place your arms under the axillae and hands over both scapulae, and assist the patient to a standing position. (Alternative: For the weak patient, use a transfer or gait belt. Hold belt behind the patient with one hand from underneath.) Support the patient's arm/elbow on the side closest to you. Check and secure all tubes.

   RATIONALE Forms a support base for you and the patient and provides leverage for lifting. Maintains patient's center of gravity midline. Transfer or gait belt enables you to support the patient's weight. Tubes must not be pulled on or trip the patient.

7. *ACTION* Move to the patient's side, and provide support as the patient balances before walking. Allow to stand for a couple of minutes. Check patient's posture, and encourage patient to walk with head up and eyes open, looking forward.

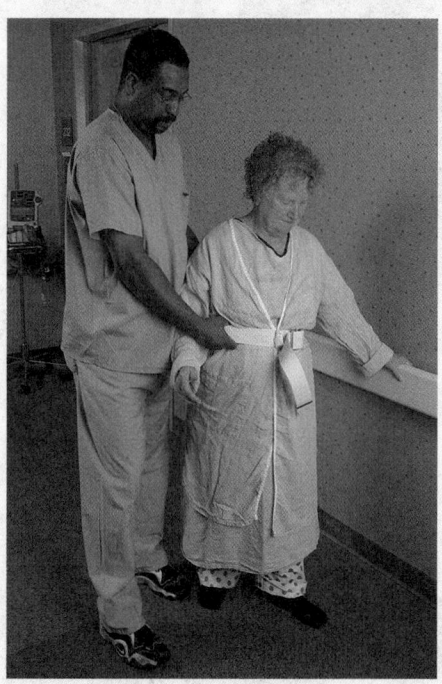

Step 7

   RATIONALE Promotes balance.

8. *ACTION* Walk at the patient's side. Match your gait with the patient's. The patient may hold your elbow or hand for stabilization.

   RATIONALE Conveys caring as well as stability, thus encouraging the patient to achieve greater mobility. Support prevents loss of balance and falling.

Continued

Skill 18-6 | Ambulating the Patient and Breaking a Fall—cont'd

Breaking a Patient's Fall

During ambulation, a patient may unexpectedly stumble or begin to fall.

9. **ACTION** If the patient begins to fall, stand with your feet apart slightly behind the patient, and grasp the patient's body firmly at the waist or under the axilla.

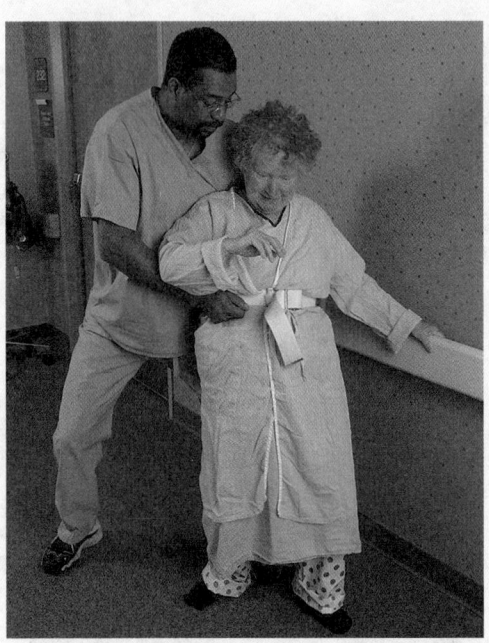

Step **9**

RATIONALE Provides a broad base of support.

10. **ACTION** Extend your near leg against the patient's leg, and slowly slide the patient down your leg to the floor, keeping your body in straight alignment.

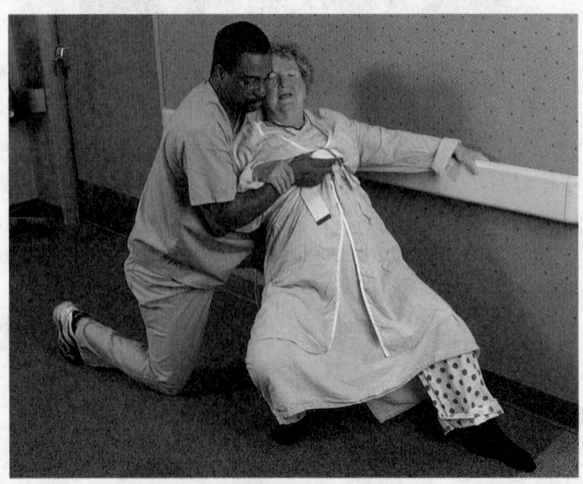

Step **10**

RATIONALE Slows the rate of descent, decreasing the risk of injury. Straight alignment keeps your line of gravity within your base of support.

11. **ACTION** As the patient slides, bend your knees to lower your body while continuing to support the patient.

RATIONALE Maintains weight within your center of gravity.

12. **ACTION** Call for additional help, check the vital signs, and examine the patient for any injuries incurred as a result of the fall before allowing the patient to rise.

RATIONALE Prevents any further injury or discomfort to the patient.

Assisting the Patient Back to Bed After Ambulating

13. **ACTION** Walk to the side of the bed and have patient turn her back to the bed. Patient reaches back for the mattress with both hands for support. Reconnect tubing that was disconnected for ambulation; secure all tubing appropriately. Continue to assist the patient back to bed as described in Skill 18-4.

RATIONALE Mattress provides support and security. Alignment is maintained. Intravenous (IV) tubing, urinary catheter, drainage tubes, and suction must be re-secured and checked for patency.

■ Evaluation

14. **ACTION** For ambulating: Note patient's posture during ambulation, effort, tolerance, comfort level, and the distance ambulated.

RATIONALE Provides data for comparison and modification if necessary.

15. **ACTION** For breaking a fall: Note difficulty encountered and if injury occurred and physician was notified. Did patient stumble or feel dizzy? Was the patient hypotensive?

RATIONALE Provides data for prevention of fall and highlights necessary modifications.

■ Documentation

16. **ACTION** For ambulating: Record distance ambulated, patient's tolerance of procedure, and assistive devices or personnel necessary.

    RATIONALE Records effectiveness of nursing care and provides for consistency of care among personnel.

Documentation Example

3/18/09 1430   Assisted to ambulate the length of the hall. Walked slowly with minimal assistance. No complaint of weakness or dizziness. Back to bed, placed in a semi-Fowler's position for comfort. Bed down, call bell in reach.

_____
(Nurse's signature)

17. **ACTION** For breaking a fall—Document the fall and its consequences per institutional policy. Note any perceived or patient-stated cause of fall, any injury sustained, and measures taken.

    RATIONALE Documents incident, presents assessment findings and care provided.

Documentation Example

3/18 1030 While ambulating in hallway, patient stated became dizzy and began to fall. Fall broken and patient gradually supported in slide to the floor. Checked for injuries. No cuts, bruises, or abrasions noted. B/P, 110/76; pulse, 92; respirations, 24. Complains of no discomfort, only weakness. Assisted to wheelchair and back to bed. Bed down, call bell in reach. Physician and charge nurse notified.

_____
(Nurse's signature)

■ Special Considerations

✓ Assess for signs and symptoms of orthostatic hypotension when the patient is dangling at the side of the bed.

✓ If the patient is weak or partially paralyzed on one side, support the patient on the opposite, unaffected side.

✓ Only suction tubing and oxygen cannula should be disconnected when ambulating the patient out of the room. The IV line needs to be checked for the correct drip rate after the patient is returned to bed. All tubes should be checked for kinks and to determine patency.

✓ Do not overtire the patient when ambulating.

✓ Support the patient's head when breaking a fall.

✓ For minimal support, hold the patient's arm with your hand.

✓ For moderate support, encircle the patient's waist with your near arm and use the other arm to support the patient's near arm and hand.

✓ For maximal support, have another person help you so that support can be provided on each side of the patient.

? CRITICAL THINKING QUESTIONS

1. What steps would you take to avoid having a patient fall during ambulation?

2. On which side do you support a patient who has left-sided weakness? Why?

Evaluation

During evaluation, determine whether the expected outcomes and goals from the planning phase have been met. Evaluate your own use of proper body mechanics. Feedback from the patient and other personnel should be obtained regarding positioning and transfers. Did you position the patient safely and correctly? Was the patient comfortable when you finished, or did you need to readjust the position? Did pressure areas develop on the skin? If the plan needs to be changed, document the changes for other personnel. Record the progress achieved in meeting the goals and outcomes (Nursing Care Plan 18-1).

Practicing the techniques of proper body mechanics and alignment will increase your confidence in being able to safely move and position any patient. Using your muscles and these techniques correctly will help protect your back. Preventing back injuries is a major concern for all health care professionals.

NURSING CARE PLAN 18-1

Care of the Patient at Risk for Injury

SCENARIO Darla Porter, age 74, a patient on your orthopedic unit, sustained a proximal fracture of the right tibia during a motor vehicle accident. Mrs. Porter has a long leg cast and a history of arthritis in her hands. You implement this plan of care.

PROBLEM/NURSING DIAGNOSIS *Leg in cast*/Risk for injury related to inability to change position independently.
Supporting Assessment Data Subjective: States since car accident is unable to move in bed without help.
Objective: Arthritis in her hands makes using a trapeze bar difficult. She is not able to shift her position independently.

Goals/Expected Outcomes	Nursing Interventions	Selected Rationales	Evaluation
Patient will remain free of injury until able to move independently.	Inspect skin for signs and symptoms of impaired integrity q 2 hr.	Patient at risk for development of pressure ulcer because of inability to independently move.	*Has any injury occurred?* No redness, blanching, or pallor noted on skin pressure points.
	Encourage the patient to perform ROM exercises twice a day; assist as necessary.	ROM exercises help to maintain joint mobility.	ROM performed 1 time this shift.
	Inspect the musculoskeletal system for joint contractures every day.	Early detection is key for intervention, thus avoiding contractures.	No contractures noted.
	Reposition patient at least every 2 hours using appropriate devices such as pillows, footboard, etc., to maintain anatomic alignment.	Adjusting position at least every 2 hours helps to prevent skin breakdown. Positioning devices help to maintain anatomic alignment and therefore decrease chance of injury.	Correct anatomic alignment maintained.
	Encourage the patient to cough and deep breathe every hour.	Coughing and deep breathing help to avoid collection of fluid in the lungs.	Expected outcome is being met.
	Teach patient and family correct transfer techniques	Correct transfer techniques protect the patient and the family member from injury.	

? CRITICAL THINKING QUESTIONS

1. What are some other possible nursing diagnoses this patient might have? Construct a care plan for one or two of those diagnoses using some of the above information.

2. Describe the benefits of using positioning devices.

Key: *ROM*, range-of-motion.

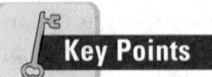

Key Points

- The musculoskeletal system is involved in positioning and moving patients.
- The body functions best when it is in anatomic alignment.
- Observing proper body alignment and mechanics helps prevent injuries. Lower back strain is one of the most common injuries for health care workers.
- Get help whenever necessary before moving or positioning a patient.
- Observing these principles helps to prevent the hazards of improper positioning: pressure ulcers, muscle contractures, and fluid collection in the lungs.

- Pressure and shearing force are the main factors in developing pressure ulcers.
- There are three basic positions: supine, side-lying, and prone. Other positions include Fowler's, semi-Fowler's, low Fowler's, and Sims'.
- Common positioning devices include pillows, boots, splints, high-top sneakers, trochanter rolls, sandbags, trapeze bars, side rails, and bed boards.
- Logrolling is a technique in which the patient is turned as a single unit.
- A lift sheet supports a patient from the shoulders to below the buttocks and facilitates transferring.
- While the patient is dangling, monitor for orthostatic hypotension, dizziness, or nausea before getting the patient out of bed.

- The wheels on stretchers and wheelchairs must be locked before transferring patients; otherwise, injury may result.
- Transferring devices include mechanical lifts, roller boards, slide boards, lift or pull sheets, and transfer or gait belts.
- Pulling motions are better than pushing motions, except that wheelchairs and stretchers are pushed to maintain alignment.

 Go to your **Companion CD-ROM** for an Audio Glossary, animations, video clips, and more.

evolve Be sure to visit the companion Evolve site at http://evolve.elsevier.com/deWit/fundamental/ for additional online resources.

NCLEX-PN® EXAMINATION-STYLE REVIEW QUESTIONS

*Choose the **best** answer(s) for each question.*

1. An elderly person may need to be reeducated on how to lift safely because: (*Select all that apply.*)
   1. muscles and bones lose strength as one ages.
   2. bone density is decreased.
   3. decreased muscle mass and changed posture.
   4. she has forgotten how to lift things.

2. When moving the patient up in bed:
   1. place one foot in front of the other.
   2. use only those muscles absolutely necessary.
   3. pushing is better than pulling as your weight helps.
   4. lock the knees before moving the patient.

3. Forgetting to reposition a patient in a wheelchair for more than 1 hour may lead to:
   1. the beginning of a pressure ulcer.
   2. muscle atrophy.
   3. pooling of lung secretions.
   4. skin abrasions from shearing forces.

4. When preparing to move a patient up in the bed who can assist, you would *first*:
   1. pull the bed covers down to the foot of the bed.
   2. raise the bed to a good working height.
   3. ask the patient to grab the upper guard rails.
   4. ask the patient to bend the knees and plant the feet on the mattress.

5. The oblique side-lying (lateral) position is helpful because:
   1. the patient does not need to be repositioned as often.
   2. it takes pressure off of the trochanter and shoulder.
   3. all areas of the lung will drain secretions to the bronchus.
   4. the shoulder is rolled to a forward position.

6. When placing the elderly patient in Fowler's position, you must:
   1. raise the head of the bed to 45 degrees.
   2. use at least five pillows for positioning.
   3. protect joints by placing a pillow between the legs.
   4. refrain from raising the knees more than 15 degrees.

7. When changing the patient's position:
   1. use only those muscles absolutely necessary.
   2. stand with feet close together for greater strength.
   3. work at the same level or height as the patient.
   4. pushing is better than pulling as your weight helps.

8. A common pressure point for a patient in the supine position is the:
   1. trochanter.
   2. malleolus
   3. humerus.
   4. scapula.

9. When performing passive range-of-motion exercises:
   1. help patients who are independently performing these activities.
   2. avoid moving the joint to the point of discomfort.
   3. perform each exercise at least 15 to 20 times.
   4. support the extremity above the joint to promote movement.

10. When a patient falls, you document in the nurse's notes:
    1. your best guess about what happened.
    2. a statement concerning how you believe the hospital was negligent.
    3. any patient-stated cause of fall.
    4. nothing, as you do not provide any written documentation of the event.

CRITICAL THINKING ACTIVITIES *Read each clinical scenario and discuss the questions with your classmates.*

Scenario A
You are to get a patient who has left-sided paresis out of bed and into a chair for the first time. The patient has been in this country only a short time. How would you go about doing this? Would you need assistance?

Scenario B
You and three other nurses are logrolling a patient. You are 5 feet 6 inches tall and the other nurses are all at least

3 inches taller. How high do you position the bed to logroll the patient?

Scenario C
Your patient became weak while walking and you broke her fall and assisted her to the floor. What would you do next? What procedures would need to be followed?

Assisting with Hygiene, Personal Care, Skin Care, and the Prevention of Pressure Ulcers

evolve http://evolve.elsevier.com/deWit/fundamental/

Objectives

Upon completing this chapter, you should be able to:

Theory

1. Describe the structure and function of the integumentary system.
2. Describe factors that influence personal hygiene practices.
3. Recall skin areas most susceptible to pressure ulcer formation.
4. Discuss risk factors for impaired skin integrity.
5. Discuss the purposes of bathing.
6. Describe how hygienic care differs for the younger and older patient.

Clinical Practice

1. Perform a complete bed bath and back rub.
2. Briefly describe how to prevent and stage a pressure ulcer.
3. Provide oral care for an unconscious patient.
4. Prepare to provide personal care for a patient, including nail care, mouth care, perineal care, and shaving.
5. Assist a patient with the care of contact lenses.
6. Instruct a patient in ways to prevent buildup of cerumen in the ears.

Skills and Steps

Skills

Skill 19-1 Administering a Bed Bath and Perineal Care
Skill 19-2 Administering Oral Care to the Unconscious Patient
Skill 19-3 Denture Care
Skill 19-4 Shampooing Hair

Steps

Steps 19-1 Providing a Tub Bath or Shower
Steps 19-2 Shaving a Male Patient

Key Terms

Be sure to check out the bonus material on the Companion CD-ROM, including selected audio pronunciations.

blanch (p. 290)
caries (KĀ-rēz, p. 304)
cerumen (sĕ-RŪ-mĕn, p. 289)
dermis (DĔR-mĭs, p. 289)
diaphoresis (dī-ă-fō-RĒ-sĭs, p. 290)

epidermis (p. 289)
eschar (ĔS-kăr, p. 292)
exacerbation (ĕg-zăs-ĕr-BĀ-shŭn, p. 302)
halitosis (p. 304)
hygiene (HĪ-jēn, p. 288)
induration (ĭn-dū-RĀ-shŭn, p. 292)
integumentary (ĭn-tĕ-gū-MĔN-tăr-ē, p. 289)
maceration (mă-sĕr-Ā-shŭn, p. 290)
melanin (MĔL-ăw-nĭn, p. 289)
reactive hyperemia (rē-ĀK-tĭv hī-pĕr-Ē-mē-ă, p. 290)
sebaceous (sē-BĀ-shŭs, p. 289)
sebum (SĒ-bŭm, p. 289)
syncope (SĬN-kō-pē, p. 301)

This chapter discusses assisting patients with hygiene and personal care. Hygiene is the practice of cleanliness that is conducive to the preservation of health. Assisting the patient with hygiene and personal care activities is an essential nursing function. The skin is the largest organ of the body and must be kept clean to prevent skin disorders and pressure ulcers. Proper care of the skin, hair, teeth, and nails promotes good health by protecting the body from infection and disease. In turn, this promotes a sense of well-being for your patient. You are responsible for maintaining safety, privacy, and warmth when providing or assisting patients in hygiene practices. You must also encourage patients to function at their highest level of independence.

APPLICATION of the NURSING PROCESS

Assessment (Data Collection)

The bath provides an excellent opportunity for assessment of the patient. Assess the individual factors affecting the patient's hygiene as well as his ability to perform self-care. During a bath, assess the condition of the patient's skin as well as his overall physical appearance, emotional and mental status, and learning needs.

Factors Affecting Hygiene

Hygiene practice is affected by such variables as sociocultural background, economic status, knowledge level, ability to perform self-care, and personal preference.

OVERVIEW OF STRUCTURE AND FUNCTION OF THE INTEGUMENTARY SYSTEM

What is the structure of the skin?

The integumentary system contains the skin, hair, nails, and sweat and sebaceous glands. The skin, the largest organ in the body, has two main layers—the epidermis and the dermis (Figure 19-1).

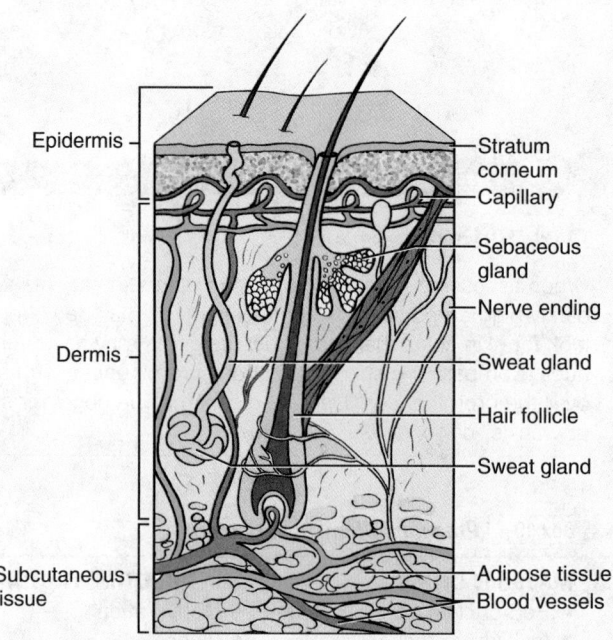

Epidermis — Stratum corneum
— Capillary
— Sebaceous gland
— Nerve ending
Dermis — Sweat gland
— Hair follicle
— Sweat gland
Subcutaneous tissue — Adipose tissue
— Blood vessels

FIGURE **19-1** Cross section of the skin.

- The epidermis (outer, thicker layer) consists of stratified squamous epithelial tissue and does not contain blood vessels. It receives its nutrition by diffusion from vessels in underlying tissues. It is also called the *stratum corneum*.

- The bottom layer of the epidermis contains melanocytes that secrete melanin, the main determinant of skin color.

- The dermis (inner, thinner layer) is made of dense connective tissue that gives the skin strength and elasticity. It is also called the *corium*.

- The dermis contains blood vessels, nerves, fibroblasts, the base of hair follicles, and glands; the nails are derived from the epidermis. Fibroblasts produce new cells to heal skin after injury.

- Hair and nails are made of keratin and have no nerve endings or blood supply.

- Sebaceous glands secrete an oily substance called sebum. Sweat glands secrete sweat, and ceruminous glands (modified sweat glands) secrete a waxy substance called cerumen.

- Mucous membranes, although not strictly part of the integumentary system, line the cavities or passageways of the body that open to the outside, such as the mouth, digestive, respiratory, and genitourinary tracts. Like skin, they are made of a surface layer of epithelial tissue over a deeper layer of connective tissue.

What are the functions of the skin and its structures?

- There are four main functions: protection, sensation, temperature regulation, and excretion and secretion.

- The skin is the first line of defense in protecting the body from bacteria and other invading organisms. It protects tissues from thermal, chemical, and mechanical injury.

- The sebaceous glands produce sebum, which helps make the skin waterproof by preventing water loss from underlying tissues and too much water absorption during bathing and swimming.

- Melanin absorbs light and protects against ultraviolet rays. When exposed to ultraviolet light, the skin makes vitamin D, which is needed for absorbing phosphorus and calcium.

- The skin has sensory organs for touch, pain, heat, cold, and pressure.

- The skin regulates temperature by dilating and constricting blood vessels and activating or inactivating sweat glands.

- Sweat glands assist maintenance of homeostasis of fluid and electrolytes. They serve as excretory organs because sweat contains nitrogenous wastes. As sweat evaporates, it produces a cooling effect. Sweat glands in the axillae and external genitalia also secrete fatty acids and proteins.

- Sebum lubricates the skin and hair, keeping these structures softer and more pliable. It also decreases the amount of heat lost and bacterial growth.

- Mucous membranes protect against bacterial invasion, secrete mucus, and absorb fluid and electrolytes.

What changes in the system occur with aging?

- Skin wrinkles and sags from the loss of elastic fibers and adipose tissue in the dermis and subcutaneous layers. This causes the skin to be thinner and more transparent.

Continued

OVERVIEW OF STRUCTURE AND FUNCTION OF THE INTEGUMENTARY SYSTEM—cont'd

- The loss of collagen fibers in the dermis makes the skin more fragile and slower to heal.

- Dry and itchy skin is caused by the decreased activity of the sebaceous glands.

- Temperature control is altered by the decreased sebaceous gland activity and the loss of density of the skin. This results in intolerance to cold and puts the person at risk for heat exhaustion.

- Hair becomes thin and grows more slowly because the number of hair follicles decreases. Hair loses its color from the loss of melanocytes at the hair follicles.

- Nail growth decreases and the nails thicken.

One of the most basic factors is a patient's sociocultural background. **Different cultures have different views on hygiene practices.** In some cultures, people do not use deodorant products or bathe daily. Other cultures consider the use of deodorant products and a daily bath essential. The economic status of a patient may affect that patient's hygiene because the money for supplies may or may not be available. The patient may have a lack of knowledge of a particular aspect of hygiene. The ability to perform self-care may be affected by the patient's mental or physical condition, which may be temporarily altered because of illness or injury. The last factor affecting hygiene practice is personal preference. One patient may prefer to bathe at night, whereas another may prefer to bathe every 2 days.

> **?**
> • *Think Critically About . . .* Your patient is elderly and complains of being cold. What safety concern would you have with him preparing his own bath water?

Self-Care Abilities

You need to assess your patient's ability to provide self-care by assessing cognitive and physical function. Are there any factors such as poor vision, decreased sense of touch, or limitations in range of motion that interfere with self-care? Are coordination, muscle strength, and balance adequate? A patient with limitations in these areas may need additional, if not total, help with hygiene.

Skin and Pressure Ulcers

Chapter 18 states that a pressure ulcer is an ulcer that forms from a local interference with circulation. The interference with circulation causes the skin to blanch (turn white or, in darker skin, become pale). If the pressure is relieved at this point, the skin will become red or a darker color because of vasodilation (Cultural Cues 19-1). This process in which the blood rushes to a place where there was a decrease in circulation is called reactive hyperemia.

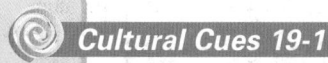
Cultural Cues 19-1

Dark Skin Assessment

When assessing for stage I pressure ulcers in patients with darkly pigmented skin, use natural light or a halogen lamp to look for skin color changes. Pressure areas may have purple hues. Compare the skin around bony prominences with skin over the prominences. Damaged skin may be boggy or stiff, or warmer or cooler (AHRQ, 2007).

Box 19-1 *Pressure Ulcer Risk Factors*

MAJOR FACTORS	CONTRIBUTING FACTORS
• Bed or chair confinement	• Dehydration
• Inability to move	• Obesity
• Loss of bowel or bladder control	• Excessive diaphoresis
• Poor nutrition	• Extreme age causing fragile skin
• Lowered mental awareness	• Edema

Risk Factors for Pressure Ulcers. Chapter 18 also notes that pressure and shearing forces can cause the development of pressure ulcers. The Agency for Healthcare Research and Quality (AHRQ) (formerly known as the Agency for Health Care Policy and Research) lists five risk factors in the development of pressure ulcers (Box 19-1).

The first two risk factors deal with a patient's mobility. If a patient is confined to a bed or chair, the same areas of the body sustain pressure. This also happens if a patient cannot independently change position, such as a patient who is paralyzed, is unconscious, or has recently had a major orthopedic procedure.

Incontinence (loss of bowel and/or bladder control) puts the patient at risk for ulcer development. Skin that is frequently wet leads to maceration (the softening of tissue that increases the chance of trauma or infection). Diaphoresis (perspiration) or not drying a patient properly after a bath also places a patient at risk due to moisture.

A balanced diet is necessary to prevent ulcer development. Without proper nourishment, the body's cells, capillaries, and tissues are easily damaged.

Lowered mental awareness may predispose a patient to pressure ulcers. Patients with impaired cognition may not realize they have been in the same position for a prolonged period because they have lost the concept of time. Lowered mental awareness may be caused by medication, anesthesia, or health problems.

?
Think Critically About . . . Why do you think an obese patient might be more prone to problems of tissue integrity?

Skin Assessment for Pressure Ulcers. Perform a skin assessment for pressure ulcer risk upon admission. A commonly used tool is the Braden Scale for Predicting Pressure Sore Risk (Figure 19-2). After the initial assessment, reassess every 24 hours. This may be done while you are bathing your patient. Pay attention to the skin over bony prominences (Figure 19-3). Check

the areas that had pressure when turning and repositioning your patient.

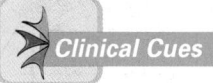
Clinical Cues

As of October 1, 2008, Medicare will not reimburse payment for "reasonably preventable" pressure ulcers. Pressure ulcers present on admission must be thoroughly and accurately documented. Presence of stage III or IV will be reimbursed at a higher rate if documented in the medical record within 2 days of inpatient admission (Stokowski, 2008).

The AHRQ states that redness can normally be expected to be present for one half to three fourths as long as the pressure prevented blood flow. If the redness subsides during this time, or the area blanches from fingertip pressure, then damage to the tissues is not expected. For example, your patient has been in a supine position for an hour and is now turned to a right side-lying position. You notice a 1-inch diameter area of redness on the sacrum. If there has not been damage, then you expect the redness to subside in

---

Braden Scale
FOR PREDICTING PRESSURE SORE RISK

Patient's Name _____   Evaluator's Name _____   Date of Assessment

	1	2	3	4			
SENSORY PERCEPTION ability to respond meaningfully to pressure-related discomfort	**1. Completely Limited:** Unresponsive (does not moan, flinch, or grasp) to painful stimuli, due to diminished level of consciousness or sedation. OR limited ability to feel pain over most of body surface.	**2. Very Limited:** Responds only to painful stimuli. Cannot communicate discomfort except by moaning or restlessness. OR has a sensory impairment which limits the ability to feel pain or discomfort over 1/2 of body.	**3. Slightly Limited:** Responds to verbal commands, but cannot always communicate discomfort or need to be turned. OR has some sensory impairment which limits ability to feel pain or discomfort in 1 or 2 extremities.	**4. No Impairment:** Responds to verbal commands. Has no sensory deficit which would limit ability to feel or voice pain or discomfort.			
MOISTURE degree to which skin is exposed to moisture	**1. Constantly Moist:** Skin is kept moist almost constantly by perspiration, urine, etc. Dampness is detected every time patient is moved or turned.	**2. Very Moist:** Skin is often, but not always moist. Linen must be changed at least once a shift.	**3. Occasionally Moist:** Skin is occasionally moist, requiring an extra linen change approximately once a day.	**4. Rarely Moist:** Skin is usually dry, linen only requires changing at routine intervals.			
ACTIVITY degree of physical activity	**1. Bedfast:** Confined to bed	**2. Chairfast:** Ability to walk severely limited or non-existent. Cannot bear own weight and/or must be assisted into chair or wheelchair.	**3. Walks Occasionally:** Walks occasionally during day, but for very short distances, with or without assistance. Spends majority of each shift in bed or chair.	**4. Walks Frequently:** walks outside the room at least twice a day and inside room at least once every 2 hours during waking hours.			
MOBILITY ability to change and control body position	**1. Completely Immobile:** Does not make even slight changes in body or extremity position without assistance.	**2. Very Limited:** Makes occasional slight changes in body or extremity position but unable to make frequent or significant changes independently.	**3. Slightly Limited:** Makes frequent though slight changes in body or extremity position independently.	**4. No Limitations:** Makes major and frequent changes in position without assistance.			
NUTRITION <u>usual</u> food intake pattern	**1. Very Poor:** Never eats a complete meal. Rarely eats more than 1/3 of any food offered. Eats 2 servings or less of protein (meat or dairy products) per day. Takes fluids poorly. Does not take a liquid dietary supplement. OR is NPO and/or maintained on clear liquids or IV's for more than 5 days.	**2. Probably Inadequate:** Rarely eats a complete meal and generally eats only about 1/2 of any food offered. Protein intake includes only 3 servings of meat or dairy products per day. Occasionally will take a dietary supplement. OR receives less than optimum amount of liquid diet or tube feeding.	**3. Adequate:** Eats over half of most meals. Eats a total of 4 servings of protein (meat, dairy products) each day. Occasionally will refuse a meal, but will usually take a supplement if offered. OR is on a tube feeding or TPN regimen that probably meets most of nutritional needs.	**4. Excellent:** Eats most of every meal. Never refuses a meal. Usually eats a total of 4 or more servings of meat and dairy products. Occasionally eats between meals. Does not require supplementation.			
FRICTION AND SHEAR	**1. Problem:** Requires moderate to maximum assistance in moving. Complete lifting without sliding against sheets is impossible. Frequently slides down in bed or chair, requiring frequent repositioning with maximum assistance. Spasticity, contractures or agitation leads to almost constant friction.	**2. Potential Problem:** Moves feebly or requires minimum assistance. During a move skin probably slides to some extent against sheets, chair, restraints, or other devices. Maintains relatively good position in chair or bed most of the time but occasionally slides down.	**3. No Apparent Problem:** Moves in bed and in chair independently and has sufficient muscle strength to lift up completely during move. Maintains good position in bed or chair at all times.				
Key: at risk, 15-18; Moderate risk, 13-14; High risk, 10-12; Severe risk, 9.				Total Score			

FIGURE **19-2** Braden Scale for Predicting Pressure Sore Risk. (Key: *IV,* Intravenous; *NPO,* nothing by mouth; *TPN,* total parenteral nutrition.)

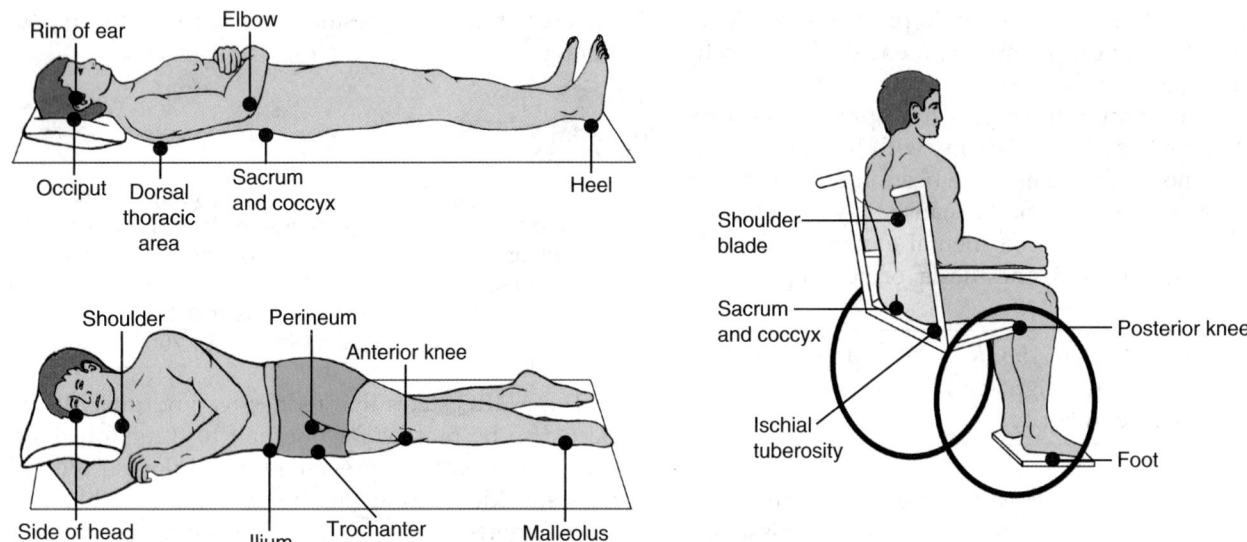

FIGURE **19-3** Pressure points where pressure ulcers often occur.

30 to 45 minutes. If the redness persists after that time, then the pressure has damaged the skin and the underlying tissues because they have not received an adequate supply of blood, oxygen, and nutrients. Unrelieved, the damage eventually will lead to tissue necrosis and a pressure ulcer.

If you note a reddened area when repositioning, reassess later to check to see if reactive hyperemia is present. If the redness remains and the skin does not blanch to fingertip pressure, then the patient has a stage I pressure ulcer.

The National Pressure Ulcer Advisory Panel (2007) has issued an updated staging system for pressure ulcers (Figure 19-4):

Suspected Deep Tissue Injury: Localized discolored intact skin that is maroon or purple or a blood-filled blister resulting from damage to underlying soft tissue from pressure or shear. The area may be painful, firm, mushy, boggy, warmer, or cooler when compared to adjacent tissue.

Stage I: An area of red, deep pink, or mottled skin that does not blanch with fingertip pressure. In people with darker skin, discoloration of the skin, warmth, edema, or induration (area feels hard) may be signs of a stage I pressure ulcer.

Stage II: Partial-thickness skin loss involving epidermis and/or dermis. It may look like an abrasion, blister, or shallow crater. The area surrounding the damaged skin may feel warmer.

Stage III: Full-thickness skin loss that looks like a deep crater and may extend to the fascia. Subcutaneous tissue is damaged or necrotic. Bacterial infection of the ulcer is common and causes drainage from the ulcer. There may be damage to the surrounding tissue.

Stage IV: Full-thickness skin loss with extensive tissue necrosis or damage to muscle, bone, or supporting structures; sinus tracts may be present.

Infection is usually widespread. The ulcer may appear dry and black, with a buildup of tough, necrotic tissue (eschar), or it can appear wet and oozing.

Unstageable: Loss of full thickness of tissue. The base of the ulcer is covered by eschar (tan, brown or black) in the wound bed, or the base of the ulcer contains slough (yellow, tan, gray, green, or brown).

The AHRQ states that during staging, it is important to be aware of the following:

- Stage I ulcers may be just superficial, or may be a sign of deeper tissue damage.
- Stage I pressure ulcers are not always accurately assessed in people with darker skin.
- When eschar is present, the ulcer cannot be staged accurately. **Eschar must be removed to stage the ulcer.**
- It may be difficult to assess pressure ulcers if your patient has a cast or other orthopedic device, or support stockings. Extra care is necessary to assess ulcers in these instances.

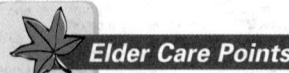

Elder Care Points

- Older adults have an increased risk of developing impaired skin integrity from the changes of normal aging. They have decreased subcutaneous fat, sebaceous gland activity, and elasticity in their skin. This makes them less able to tolerate pressure, shearing, and friction forces.
- Document the location of any abnormality, its color and size, and reaction to the blanch test. Add other descriptive terms as they apply, such as induration, blisters, drainage, odor, or eschar. Some institutions use forms with an outline of a body so you may draw the location of the area(s) involved. A Braden score of 18 or below indicates pressure ulcer risk.

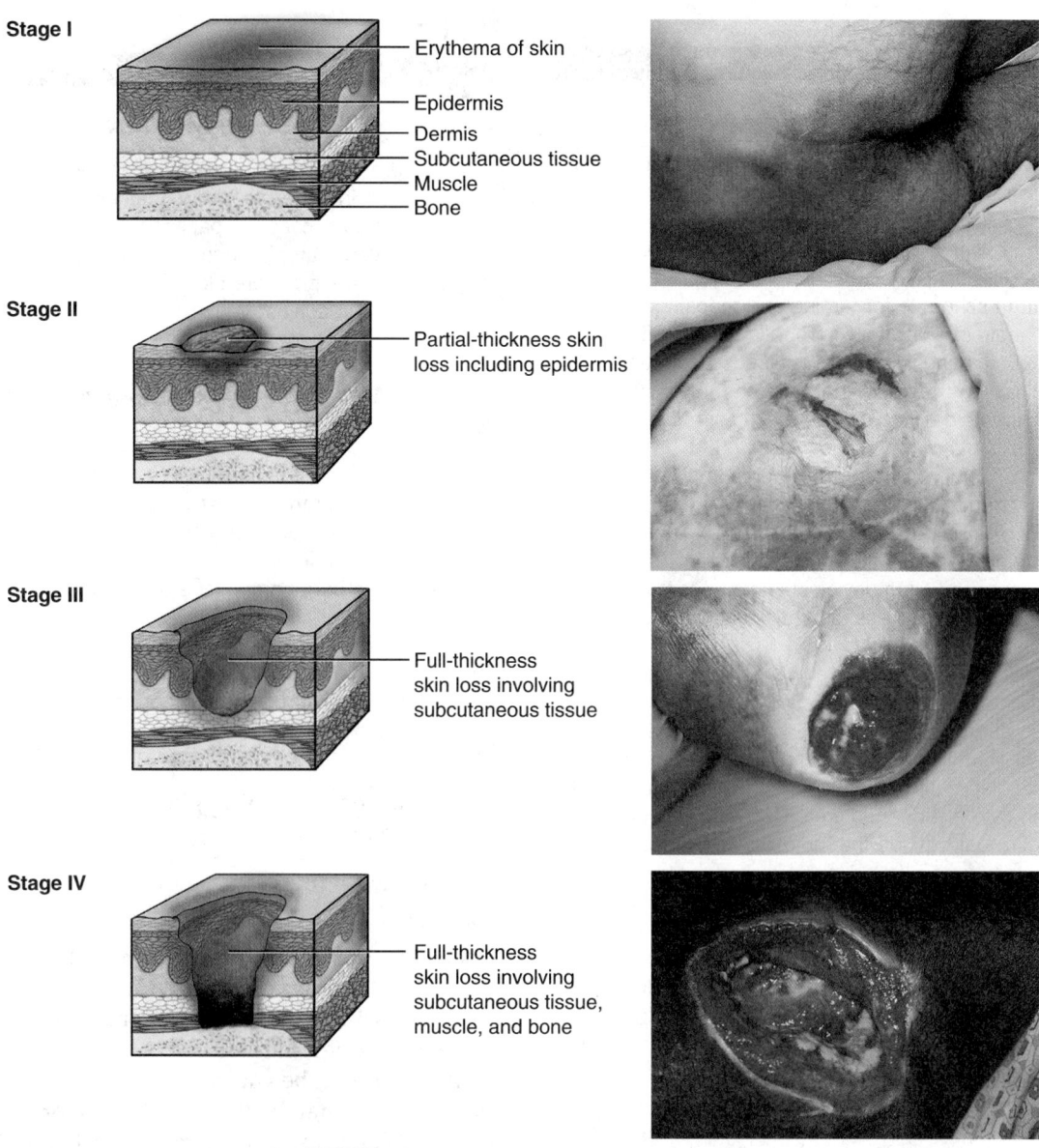

FIGURE **19-4** Four stages of pressure ulcers.

Healing pressure ulcers are not "reverse staged." The ulcer is called a "healing stage—pressure ulcer." Document by objective description and measurement.

Prevention of Pressure Ulcers. **Excellent nursing care is the main factor in the prevention of pressure ulcers.** It is your responsibility to be aware of any risk factors your patient may have and attempt to lessen them. Safety Alert 19-1 describes measures helpful in preventing pressure ulcers. **Prevention is less time-consuming and less costly than pressure ulcer treatment** (Legal & Ethical Considerations 19-1).

Treatment and Care for Pressure Ulcers. The AHRQ states that the most effective method of pressure ulcer treatment is through a team approach. The team should consist of the patient, the family or caregivers, and health care providers. Treatment options should be explained, and the patient should be encouraged to be an active participant. The plan needs to be con-sistent with the individual patient and family prefer-ences, goals, and abilities. Include education on how pressure ulcers develop and how to prevent addi-tional ulcers.

The initial care of a pressure ulcer involves débride-ment, wound cleansing, and the application of dress-ings. In many cases, the ulcer is infected and antibiotic therapy is used. Surgery is needed to repair some pres-sure ulcers. Wound care is discussed in more depth in Chapter 38.

Nursing Diagnosis

Nursing diagnoses for a patient who might have problems with hygiene and/or skin integrity are listed in Box 19-2. To individualize the care plan, add the defining characteristics to the nursing diagnosis stem based on the information you obtained regard-ing your patient.

Safety Alert 19-1

Prevention of Pressure Ulcers

- Observe the color of the skin carefully and frequently. Skin that is red, blue, or mottled indicates impaired circulation.
- Change the patient's position at least every 2 hours when in bed.
- Use a written schedule for turning and repositioning.
- Keep the heels of the totally immobile patient off the bed. Use positioning devices as described in Chapter 18.
- Avoid positioning the patient directly on the trochanter. Use an oblique side-lying position with appropriate wedges to maintain the position.
- Minimize skin injury caused by friction and shear forces by using proper positioning, transferring, and turning techniques. The use of cornstarch, creams, protective films, dressings, and padding reduces friction.
- Use a pressure-reducing device such as a foam pad, pressure-reducing mattress, or alternating-pressure pad when in bed.
- Use a pressure-reducing device in the chair for chair-bound patients. Reposition at least once an hour or return the patient to bed after 1 hour. Encourage self–weight shifting every 15 minutes.
- Restore circulation to a deprived area by rubbing around rather than over a reddened area. Use a circular outward motion, start just outside the red area, and move in an ever-widening circle.
- Do not massage reddened skin as it has already suffered temporary damage. Do not massage directly over bony prominences.
- Wash and dry the incontinent patient promptly and thoroughly because urine and feces are irritating to the skin.
- Avoid mechanical and/or physical injury from improperly fitting splints, braces, casts, and prostheses.
- Avoid burns caused by excessively hot or cold applications such as hot water bottles, ice bags, heating pads, and heat lamps.
- Provide adequate nutrition and fluid intake.

Planning

The data collected during the assessment will give you information you need to plan hygiene care. Include the patient's ability to perform the hygiene tasks and any personal preferences or habits. Efforts should be made to help the patient maintain body image. Educational needs and the home environment must also be considered.

Nursing goals for hygiene might include the following:

- The patient's skin integrity will be maintained.
- The patient's hair is clean and neatly styled each day.
- The patient's mouth is intact and free from odor.

Planning must include the times during the day that care will be needed. Box 19-3 describes common

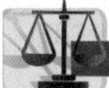

Legal & Ethical Considerations 19-1

Document Preventive Measures

All measures taken to prevent pressure ulcers should be documented in order to show that all possible measures were instituted in case the patient develops a pressure ulcer in spite of your care. This can protect you from charges of negligence if the pressure ulcer doesn't heal and the patient brings a lawsuit against you.

Box 19-2 | Nursing Diagnoses for Hygiene and Skin Integrity Problems

- Chronic low self-esteem
- Imbalanced nutrition: less than body requirements
- Impaired physical mobility
- Impaired skin integrity
- Ineffective peripheral tissue perfusion
- Pain (acute or chronic)
- Risk for impaired skin integrity
- Self-care deficit, bathing/hygiene
- Self-care deficit, dressing/grooming
- Sensory perception, disturbed (visual)

times and the types of hygiene care provided during the course of a day.

Implementation

Bathing

There are four basic purposes for bathing: (1) cleanse the skin, (2) promote comfort, (3) stimulate circulation to all areas of the body, and (4) remove waste products secreted through the skin.

Water should be warm but should not burn the patient (approximately 105° F [40.5° C], or according to policy). When water cools, replace it. Bed rails must be up when away from that side of the bed since the bed is raised to working height. Fully draw curtains around the bed to maintain privacy. There should not be any gaps that may expose the patient to others in the room. Place a sign on the outside of the door to indicate that a bath is in progress. Appropriately drape the patient; only the part of the body being bathed should be exposed at any one time. Draping prevents chills and promotes warmth and comfort. Closing the patient's door and windows provides warmth by decreasing drafts. Encourage the patient to be independent, but offer assistance as needed. Depending on the patient's ability and activity level, you may need to give either a partial or complete bath.

Types of Baths. A bath may be cleansing or therapeutic, and complete or partial. A complete bath is when all areas of the patient's body are washed. The term *partial bath* has two different meanings depending on your institution. In one case it means only certain parts of the body are bathed, such as the face, hands, axillae, back,

Scheduling Hygiene Care

Each patient will have different needs and abilities, but in general care is provided on the following basis. Individual needs are always addressed while encouraging the patient to perform to an optimal level of functioning.

EARLY-MORNING CARE
- Offer bedpan or urinal or provide help to the bathroom or bedside commode.
- Wash hands and face.
- Clean and clear the over-the-bed table.
- Provide oral care.
- Prepare for tests or surgery (e.g., enemas, shaves).

A.M. CARE OR MORNING CARE
Generally occurs after breakfast and is the main hygiene care.
- Offer bedpan or urinal, etc.
- Provide oral care.
- Bathe—complete or partial bed bath, shower, or tub bath.
- Give back rub.
- Shave and provide hair care.
- Care for nails.
- Dress.
- Straighten patient unit.

AFTERNOON CARE
- Provide care after any diagnostic or special test as needed; for example, electroencephalography (EEG) may leave electrode paste in the patient's hair.
- Offer bedpan or urinal, etc.
- Provide oral care.

HOUR-OF-SLEEP (HS) CARE (BEDTIME)
- Offer bedpan or urinal, etc.
- Wash hands and face.
- Provide oral care.
- Change to gown if needed.
- Give back rub.
- Help/adjust patient position in bed.
- Straighten patient unit.

Linens are straightened and/or changed as needed throughout the day.

 **Elder Care Points**

- Because of decreased sweat and sebaceous gland activity, a full bath is not needed every day. Personal preference must be considered.
- Because of thinner skin and decreased subcutaneous fat, chilling is more likely during the bath. Prevent this by pre-warming the bath area and providing adequate draping.
- The elderly have less subcutaneous fat and their skin is more fragile and drier. Use warm (not hot) water and minimal amounts of mild soap, rinse thoroughly, and pat dry well to minimize skin irritation. Bath oils may be used, but special care needs to be taken to prevent slips and falls.
- Moisturize the skin immediately after the bath with a lotion or cream. Apply this while the skin is still damp to trap additional moisture.
- Evaluate the home environment for safety aids such as nonskid tub or shower mats, safety bars, and shower or bench chairs if appropriate.

---

and perineal area. In the other case a partial bath means a complete bath is done—partially by the patient (the areas that can be reached) and partially by you (all other areas) (Assignment Considerations 19-1).

Cleansing Baths. The most common type of bath is a cleansing bath. It is generally provided in either a bed, tub, or shower. Bed baths are given to patients who are unable to use a tub or shower. Skill 19-1 details how to administer a bed bath.

Steps 19-1 on pp. 300-301 explain the procedures for providing a tub bath or shower. Offer the use of the toilet before running the bath water or placing the patient in the tub or shower. A shower chair or bath

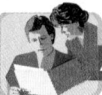 **Assignment Considerations 19-1**

Baths

When assigning baths to the UAP, be explicit in which type of bath or shower the patient is to have. Ask that the skin be inspected and any lesions or problems be reported to you. Remind the UAP to abide by cultural practices of the patient and explain what is needed. Ask that the patient be allowed to perform as much self-care as possible, but to not tire the patient excessively.

---

bench and grab bars are used for the patient who is weak or not ambulatory (Figure 19-5, p. 301). If the patient does not have a problem with balance, assist the patient into a tub that is half filled with warm water. Once the patient is in the tub/shower, add warmer water as desired. A call bell should be within easy reach of the independent patient. Check on this patient every 5 minutes and inform the patient that the bath should not exceed 15 to 20 minutes (Communication Cues 19-1, p. 301).

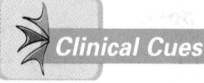 **Clinical Cues**

If the patient is weak, do not leave the bathroom and provide assistance with the bath.

Provide a towel for the patient to drape the genital area while in the tub to decrease embarrassment. Nursing Care Plan 19-1 on p. 302 presents one plan for hygienic care.

Skill 19-1 Administering a Bed Bath and Perineal Care

A complete bed bath is given when the patient is dependent and unable to provide hygiene self-care. Examples of such instances are patients with severe pain, injuries, or diseases that limit movement, or when the physician has ordered that the patient not expend the energy to self-bathe. In some instances, special perineal care is ordered.

■ Supplies

✓ Basin of warm water
✓ Soap
✓ Towels and washcloths
✓ Bath blanket
✓ Clean linen for bed

✓ Clean gown
✓ Body lotion
✓ Toilet articles
✓ Hamper or bag for soiled linen
✓ Bedpan, urinal, toilet paper

For Perineal Care
✓ Underpad
✓ Gauze pads or washcloths
✓ Pitcher and water or ordered solution

Review and carry out the Standard Steps in Appendix 3.

■ Assessment (Data Collection)

1. *ACTION* Assess patient's preferences, including cultural factors.

   RATIONALE Demonstrates respect for patient preference and encourages participation in care.

■ Planning

2. *ACTION* Gather supplies.

   RATIONALE Provides easy access to equipment needed for hygiene and personal care bathing.

3. *ACTION* Explain the procedure to the patient.

   RATIONALE Decreases fear of the unknown and prepares patient.

4. *ACTION* Prepare environment for bathing—close doors and windows, adjust room temperature if necessary, pull curtains around bed, and place a sign ("Bath in progress") on the door.

   RATIONALE Promotes comfort by warming room and decreasing chance of drafts. Placing sign on door provides privacy.

5. *ACTION* Offer bedpan or urinal.

   RATIONALE Provides comfort and decreases chance of interruption during bath.

■ Implementation

6. *ACTION* Perform hand hygiene. Wear gloves if you or patient has any broken skin. Gloves must be worn while cleansing perineal area.

   RATIONALE Reduces transfer of microorganisms.

7. *ACTION* Raise the side rails and raise the level of bed to a comfortable working height. Lower rail on side closest to you and position patient in a comfortable position close to you.

   RATIONALE Promotes proper body alignment because work is at your center of gravity. Provides comfort for patient.

8. *ACTION* If a bath blanket is available, fan-fold the blanket horizontally and place it across patient's chest. Ask the patient to hold the top edge of the bath blanket. Pull the blanket and the covers to the foot of the bed. Remove the top covers out from underneath the bath blanket. Use the top sheet if a bath blanket is not available for a drape.

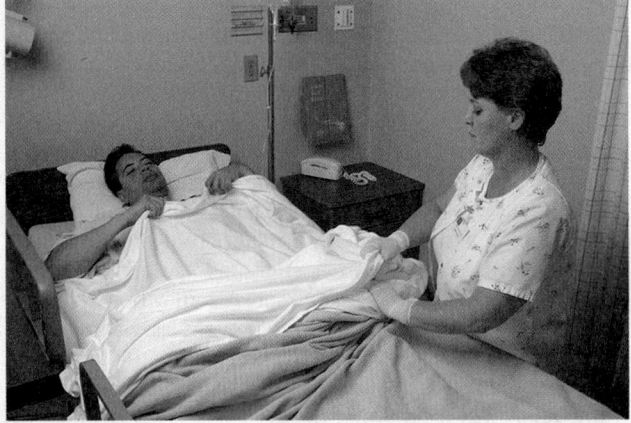

Step **8**

   RATIONALE Drapes patient, protecting privacy.

9. *ACTION* Remove linens as directed in Skill 20-2.

   RATIONALE Prepares linens to be replaced on bed.

10. *ACTION* Remove patient's gown, being careful to keep patient draped. If the patient has an intravenous (IV) line in place, remove the gown by gently pulling the gown off the patient's arm over the IV line without pulling on the line or disturbing the IV cannula. Lift the IV bag and tubing and thread them through the sleeve from the outside toward the inside of the gown to free the gown.

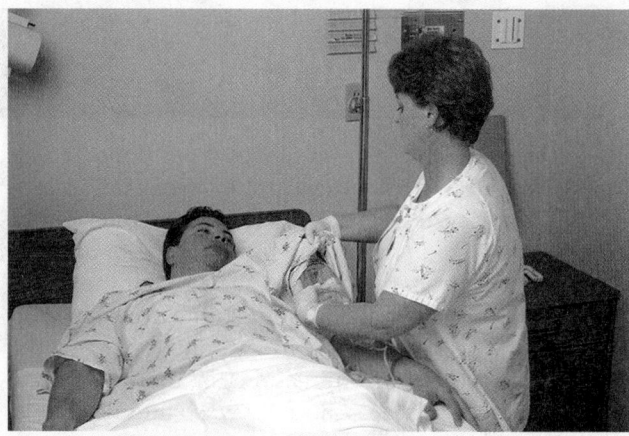

Step **10**

RATIONALE Prepares patient for bathing. Careful removal of gown protects the IV site.

11. *ACTION* Raise the side rail while preparing the bath water. Water should be warm and checked with either a bath thermometer or the inside of your wrist. Do not leave the soap in the water. Change water when it cools or becomes soiled, or a soap film develops.

RATIONALE Provides for safety. Warm water is soothing, and maintaining warm clean water is comforting.

12. *ACTION* Lower rail and remove the pillow under the patient's head or place a towel over the pillow. Make a bath mitt by grasping the washcloth at an edge and folding one third of it over your fingers. Bring the opposite edge across your fingers and hold it with your thumb. Bring the top end of the cloth down to your palm and tuck that end under the lower edge.

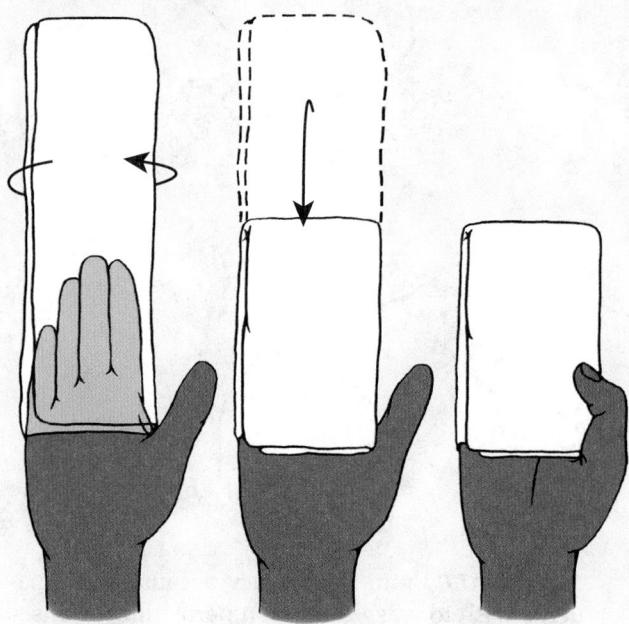

Step **12**

RATIONALE Provides better control of the washcloth; loose ends do not drag across patient. Loose ends cool quickly and chill the patient.

13. *ACTION* Fold drape to expose only the area being cleaned. Spread a towel across the patient's chest.

RATIONALE Protects patient privacy and prevents chills.

14. *ACTION* Ask the patient about preference of using soap on the face. Moisten the bath mitt with water and wash one eye area from the nose to the outer edge near the ear; use a separate part of the mitt to wash the other eye area. Do not use soap near eyes. Wash patient's face and neck. Dry well. Rinse cloth and wash forehead from the center to each side; wash the rest of face, using a circular motion around the mouth. Rinse and dry the face well. Wash, rinse, and dry each ear and the neck. Patient may wash own face if able.

RATIONALE Using different parts of the cloth to wash eye area prevents moving bacteria from one eye to the other. Rinsing well prevents the soap from drying the skin.

15. *ACTION* Place a towel under the far arm, make a bath mitt, use soap, and wash the entire arm with long, sweeping strokes from distal to proximal (toward the axilla). Give special care to the axilla with extra soaping. Rinse and pat dry well. Wash the hands and fingers, rinse, and dry. Move the towel, and wash and dry the near arm and hand in the same manner.

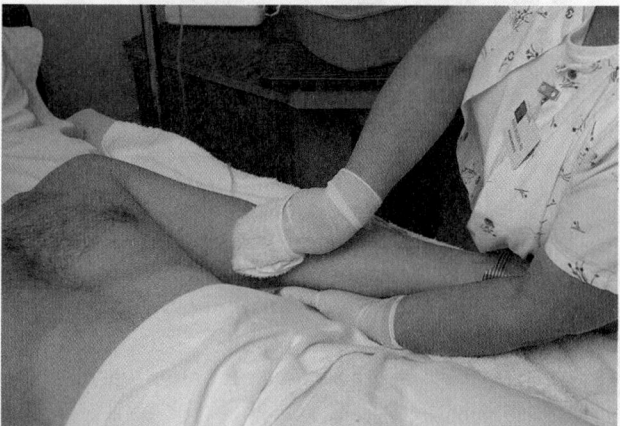

Step **15**

RATIONALE Towel protects the mattress from getting wet and is available for drying. Washing distal to proximal promotes circulation. Bacteria collect in the sweat gland areas, and extra cleansing of axilla is needed to remove secretions and decrease body odor.

16. *ACTION* Keep the towel in place over the patient's chest and pull the drape down to the waistline. Make a bath mitt and wash under the towel over the entire chest; wash breasts with a circular movement. Wash skin folds under the female patient's

Continued

breasts by lifting each breast. Rinse and dry well, paying special attention to skin fold areas. Fold the drape to the top of the pubic bone and wash the lower abdomen; rinse and dry well.

RATIONALE Washing in sections provides privacy and protects the patient from chills.

17. **ACTION** Expose the far leg, and tuck the bath blanket around the patient to prevent chilling. Flex the leg and place a towel lengthwise on the bed. Wash from the foot to the knee with long sweeping strokes and then from the knee to the hip in the same manner. Rinse and dry the leg well. Place the bath basin on the towel and lift the foot, placing your hand under the heel, and place it into the water. Wash the foot and dry it. Dry each toe separately, and place the leg and foot under the drape. Wash the near leg in the same manner.

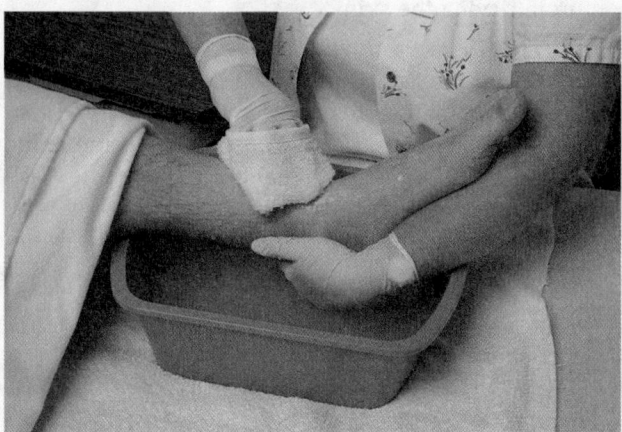

Step **17**

RATIONALE Tucking bath blanket around patient keeps the patient warm. Stroking from distal to proximal encourages venous return. Placing the foot into warm water is soothing and comforting to the patient.

18. **ACTION** Change the bath water after washing the legs and feet.

RATIONALE Prevents using water that has been used on the feet on other parts of the body.

19. **ACTION** Turn the patient to the side, place a towel lengthwise along the back, and wash the back with long, sweeping motions. Rinse and dry well. Then wash the folds of the buttocks and anus well. Wear gloves if patient is incontinent of stool or has diarrhea. Offer a back rub at this time.

RATIONALE Towel protects mattress from moisture.

20. **ACTION** Change water and washcloth. Provide privacy for the patient to wash the genital area. If

patient is unable, put on gloves if not done in Step 6; place an underpad beneath the perineum to protect the mattress and wash the area thoroughly, rinse well, and pat dry carefully. For the female patient, wash from the front to the back. For the uncircumcised male patient, retract the foreskin and clean the head of the penis, rinse, and reposition the foreskin. Lift the scrotum and clean the area well. If a catheter is in place, carefully wash around it with soap and water, and rinse the area. Dry the penis and scrotum. Remove the underpad.

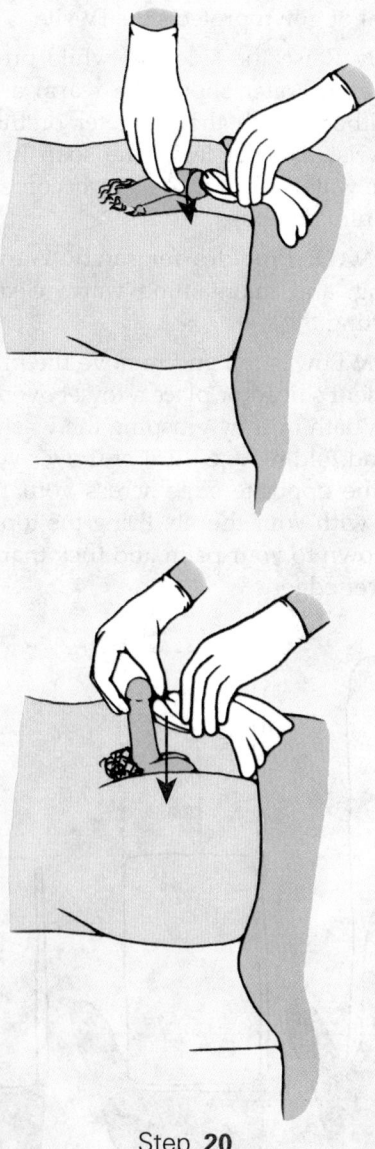

Step **20**

RATIONALE Promotes privacy because many patients wish to wash their own perineum. Cleanses areas patient cannot manage. Washing around a catheter removes body secretions.

For Specially Ordered Female Perineal Care

21. **ACTION** Place the patient in the dorsal recumbent position in bed. Drape with a bath blanket diagonally (it should look like a diamond resting on the patient). Take the point of the bath blanket by the patient's feet and fold it up to the pubic area. Place the outer sides of the bath blanket over the patient's knees and wrap the corners around each foot.

    RATIONALE Provides privacy and prevents chills.

22. **ACTION** With gloves in place, remove any peripad or dressings and observe characteristics of the drainage. Discard soiled items in a sealable plastic bag.

    RATIONALE Standard Precautions must be used when handling items soiled with body substances.

23. **ACTION** Slip underpad under the patient's hips and position patient on the bedpan as described in Chapter 29. Raise the head of the bed slightly or use pillows to support the patient's head.

    RATIONALE Underpad prevents soiling the linens and mattress. Positioning patient prevents back strain by supporting the head and shoulders.

24. **ACTION** Carefully pour warm water or the prescribed solution over the perineal area to rinse off urine, feces, or vaginal drainage.

    RATIONALE Cleanses outer perineum.

25. **ACTION** Use nondominant hand to separate the labia majora, and, with downward strokes from the pubic area to the rectum, cleanse the skin folds with cotton balls, gauze pads, or a washcloth. Use only one downward stroke with each gauze pad, cotton ball, or portion of the washcloth. Rinse and pat area dry with clean towel or fresh gauze pads. Remove the underpad and replace peripad or redress as needed.

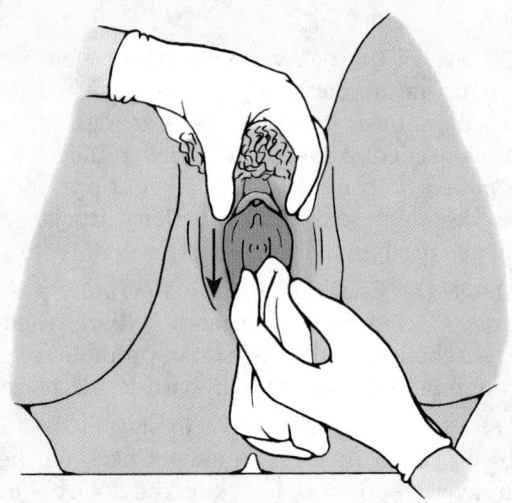

Step **25**

RATIONALE Cleaning with downward strokes prevents carrying bacteria from the dirty rectal area up to the vaginal area and urinary meatus. Peripad or dressing provides for collection of secretions.

Completing Care

26. **ACTION** Put a clean gown on the patient. If the patient has an IV in place, lift the IV bag and line and put it through the sleeve of the gown from the inside of the gown to the outside, *just as the arm will go through the sleeve.* Then, carefully place the patient's arm through the sleeve of the gown. If a patient has a weak or paralyzed side, dress this extremity first.

    RATIONALE Maintains IV site and prevents the IV cannula and tubing from coming apart. Dressing is more comfortable and easier for the patient and you.

27. **ACTION** Complete personal care by combing the patient's hair, caring for fingernails and toenails, and permitting the male patient to either shave himself or be shaved (see Steps 19-2).

    RATIONALE Increases patient's sense of well-being and self-esteem.

28. **ACTION** Lower the bed, lower unneeded side rails, and restore the unit. Empty, rinse, and wipe out the basin before returning to storage.

    RATIONALE Makes patient comfortable and safe. Cleaning basin prepares it for next use; wiping removes soap scum that rinsing alone leaves behind.

29. **ACTION** Make the occupied bed if needed (see Skill 20-2).

    RATIONALE The patient who needs a bed bath may not be able to get out of bed.

■ Evaluation

30. **ACTION** Observe the newly bathed patient. Is the patient comfortable? Did the bath tire the patient? Are there any modifications you would make in providing future hygiene care for this patient?

    RATIONALE Determines if any changes are needed.

■ Documentation

31. **ACTION** Document on the flow sheet or in the nurse's notes depending on agency policy. Note type of bath performed or given, the patient's tolerance of the procedure, any teaching done, and any abnormalities found during the bath.

    RATIONALE Validates effectiveness of nursing care and notes teaching provided.

Documentation Example

6/25/09 0930   Complete bed bath given and back rub performed. Reddened area 2 cm in diameter found on sacrum. Repositioned on right side in correct body

Continued

Skill 19-1 | Administering a Bed Bath and Perineal Care—cont'd

alignment and maintained with pillows. Informed patient of the importance of avoiding pressure on the sacral area. Bed down. Call bell in reach.

_____
(Nurse's signature)

■ Special Considerations

Home Care Considerations

• Close doors and windows to prevent drafts during the bath.
• Ascertain that safety bars and nonskid tub and shower pads are in place in the home bathing area.
• Caution patients to always check the water temperature before entering the bathtub or shower.
• Trim nails after bathing while the nails are soft.
• Check fingernails and toenails once a week to decide if they need to be trimmed.
• Inform patients that many hairdressers will come to the home for those with an extended illness.
• Refer the patient to an appropriate agency if there is a need for bathing assistance at home.
• Instruct the patient and/or the caregiver to assess the perineum for signs or symptoms of infection, such as redness, drainage, odor, burning, or itching. Explain the importance of checking the skin integrity of the perineal area.

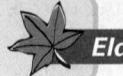
Elder Care Points

• Soap is not generally used on the elderly person's skin every day. On alternate days, use soap only on areas visibly soiled.
• Elderly women who cannot reach and bend easily need to have the nurse perform perineal care. Rather than giving this patient a choice, say, "I'm going to clean the areas that are difficult to reach." If the patient protests, allow her to wash herself.

?CRITICAL THINKING QUESTIONS

1. You are a male nurse and scheduled to care for a mature woman patient from southern Asia (India or Korea). Does your patient's culture have any implications for you? Why or why not?

2. The patient in your assignment is the same age as you but of the opposite sex. You will need to provide special perineal care to this patient. What is the best approach in completing this task?

3. Describe three things you would do to promote the comfort of your patient during a complete bed bath.

Steps 19-1 | Providing a Tub Bath or Shower

When inpatients can safely bathe by themselves, the bathing area is prepared and then patients are readied for the bath or shower. Patients must be checked on frequently while in the tub or shower.

1. **ACTION** Schedule use of tub or shower room. Clean according to institution's policy. Place towel on floor outside of tub/shower and nonskid mat in tub/shower.

   RATIONALE Scheduling ensures area is available when patient is ready. Cleaning prevents spread of microorganisms. Towel provides a dry warm area for the patient to step on and the mat decreases chance of falls.

2. **ACTION** Gather supplies and assist patient to area. Completely drape patient or have in robe and slippers.

   RATIONALE Assisting the patient promotes safety. Draping or robing decreases chance of chills and provides privacy.

3. **ACTION** Place "occupied" sign on door; demonstrate use of call bell system.

   RATIONALE Maintains privacy and promotes safety.

4. **ACTION** Fill tub halfway with warm water; check the temperature per policy and adjust as needed. If using the shower, turn on water and adjust temperature as needed. A hand-held sprayer allows you or the patient to control water flow and prevents you from becoming soaked. Place toiletry articles within patient's reach. Assist patient as needed.

   RATIONALE Checking water temperature prevents burns. Placing toiletry articles within reach decreases chance of falls. Assistance promotes hygiene through helping patient with hard-to-reach areas.

5. **ACTION** Instruct patient not to stay in the tub or shower longer than 20 minutes. Check on the patient every 5 minutes; knock on the door before entering. Remain within calling distance if the patient

has a history of syncope (fainting), light-headedness, or dizziness, or is taking a shower or bath for the first time after surgery or illness.

RATIONALE Time limit decreases chance of light-headedness or dizziness resulting from vasodilation from the warm water. Checking on patient and remaining within calling distance provide privacy and promote safety.

6. *ACTION* Assist patient out of tub/shower. Encourage the use of safety bars during transfer. Assist with drying and dressing. Transport back to room.

RATIONALE Promotes safety. Drying and dressing patient maintain warmth by preventing chills.

7. *ACTION* Clean tub/shower per institution's policy.

RATIONALE Prevents transfer of microorganisms.

8. *ACTION* Document type of bath taken, tolerance of procedure, condition of skin, and amount of assistance needed by patient.

RATIONALE Promotes continuity of care.

FIGURE **19-5** Shower bench and grab bar assist the weak patient.

? *Think Critically About . . .* Your patient does not want a bath now, but your instructor expects the bath to be done by 10 A.M. What do you do?

Therapeutic Baths. Therapeutic means having healing or medicinal qualities. Therapeutic baths are performed to achieve a desired effect and include several types. A whirlpool bath is done in a bathtub or special whirlpool tub that has a device that agitates the water. The heat of the water and agitation gently massage the skin. Whirlpools are used to cleanse, stimulate peripheral circulation, and provide comfort. Starch or oatmeal baths are used for patients with dermatitis. Plain instant oatmeal is added directly to the bath water until the desired consistency is reached. Commercial products are also available and are added according to package directions. The skin is patted dry after the bath so the nerve endings are not stimulated by rubbing.

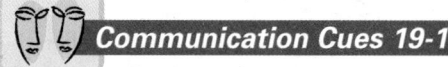

Communication Cues 19-1

Assisting the Weak Patient

Bob Rodriguez is 59 years old and was admitted to the hospital yesterday for a right-sided cerebrovascular accident (CVA). He has some upper extremity weakness on his left side but no other deficits. Mr. Rodriguez has just pushed his tray onto the floor. His nurse, Mary, enters his room after hearing the crash.

NURSE: *"Mr. Rodriguez, I heard your tray fall to the floor. Are you all right?"*

MR. RODRIGUEZ: *"No! I am not sure if I will ever be all right again."*

NURSE: *"You're not sure if you'll be all right . . . what do you mean?"*

MR. RODRIGUEZ: *"I am left-handed and got disgusted trying to feed myself."*

NURSE: *"Using your right hand to feed yourself breakfast was very frustrating for you, wasn't it?"*

MR. RODRIGUEZ: *"Yes! I just don't know how I will ever be able to take care of myself."*

NURSE: *"You're worried and I understand your concern. It is still too early to tell how much weakness will remain on your left side. The therapists from physical and occupational therapy and I will work with you to teach you how to care for yourself while you are here in the hospital."*

MR. RODRIGUEZ: *"Do you really think that I will be able to feed and bathe myself at home?"*

NURSE: *"Yes. There are many techniques and devices available to help people care for themselves independently. Would you like something else to eat? I could call the kitchen for another tray."*

MR. RODRIGUEZ: *"Thank you, Mary, but I don't really want anything right now."*

NURSE: *"Would you like to start your bath? I could begin teaching you some of the techniques now, if you are ready for me to help you with your bath. What do you think?"*

MR. RODRIGUEZ: *"Yes, I would like to learn. Thank you, Mary."*

Sitz baths are used to apply moist heat and clean the perineal or anal area (Figure 19-6). The bath promotes healing and relieves pain and discomfort. It is commonly used after birth and vaginal or rectal surgery. Body soaks are usually indicated to cleanse open

---

NURSING CARE PLAN 19-1

Care of the Patient with a Self-Care Deficit

SCENARIO Herman Gray, age 67, has a diagnosis of exacerbation (an increase in the severity or symptoms of a disease) of chronic obstructive pulmonary disease. Mr. Gray is widowed and lives alone. He was admitted to your unit this morning, and you devised the following plan for hygiene care.

PROBLEM/NURSING DIAGNOSIS *Fatigue*/Self-care deficit in bathing/hygiene related to intolerance to activity. *Supporting Assessment Data* *Subjective:* States "I get too tired standing at the sink to wash myself." *Objective:* Visibly tired with minimal activity. Becomes short of breath with exertion.

Goals/Expected Outcomes	Nursing Interventions	Selected Rationales	Evaluation
Patient will participate in hygiene care each day.	Gather supplies for patient.	Patient participation in self-care will maintain/increase self-esteem.	*Participating in hygiene care?* Washed face and hands. Bathing after A.M. rest period.
	Plan hygiene care when the patient is well rested.	Provides more energy for the patient to actually perform the self-care.	
Patient completes hygiene care without fatigue by discharge.	Provide a chair for the patient to sit by the sink for bathing.	Sitting in a chair takes less energy than standing and will allow patient to complete more of own care.	*Experiencing fatigue with hygiene care?* Some fatigue noted, but less than yesterday.
	Assist with hygiene when patient becomes tired.	Assisting with care helps patient conserve energy for self-care he deems most important.	
	Suggest scheduling hygiene activities throughout the day, to minimize fatigue. If patient has a PRN oxygen order, have patient use oxygen during bath.	Breaking up care preserves patient energy and allows patient to complete more of own care in smaller increments. Enhances self-esteem as able to provide for self.	Patient is able to participate in care when done in increments throughout the day. Outcome met.
	Advise patient of assistive devices available for bathing, such as long-handled sponge and shower chair or bench.	Assistive devices may help conserve energy by making hard-to-reach areas easier to clean and minimizing exertion. Chairs or benches also help preserve patient safety.	
Patient makes decisions about obtaining hygiene care at home before discharge.	Refer to visiting nurses association or home health agency for home care if needed.	Provides care after discharge.	*Have decisions been made?* No referral necessary at this time. Patient has applicable phone numbers and contacts.

? CRITICAL THINKING QUESTIONS

1. When thinking of Mr. Gray caring for himself at home, what other self-care activities might be a problem based on his statement?

2. On discharge, it is noted that Mr. Gray is able to perform his own hygiene activities. What devices do you think he should have at home to perform these tasks?

Key: *PRN*, As needed.

---

wounds or apply medicated solutions to an area. Feet and arms are the parts of the body most often soaked. Cooling sponge baths are also known as tepid sponge baths. An order is usually needed before this type of bath may be used to bring down a fever. A cool sponge bath can be soothing but also may be uncomfortable if the patient's fever is high.

Variations of the Bed Bath. A bag bath is a variation of the bed bath. Instead of using a basin, a self-contained bag with several premoistened disposable cloths is used. The cloths are moistened with a cleansing agent that does not need rinsing. They may be heated or used directly from the bag. The bag contains many cloths, so a different cloth may be

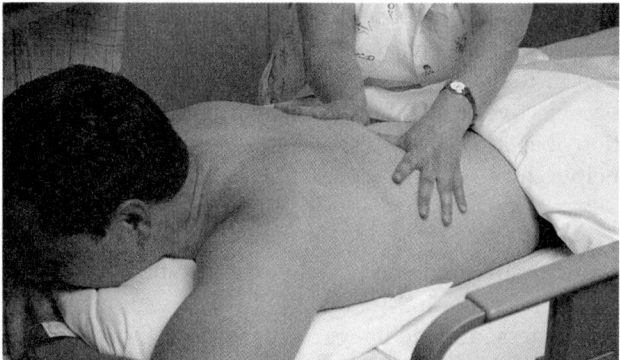

FIGURE **19-7** A back rub is soothing and relaxing.

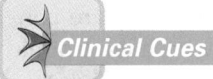

FIGURE **19-6** Sitz bath.

used for different body parts. The major disadvantage to this system is that it is more costly.

Clinical Cues

Keep in mind these key points when bathing a patient:
- Maintain safety.
- Provide privacy.
- Prevent chills.
- Encourage independence.

Back Massage

A back massage is an important part of hygiene care and involves the sense of touch. Benefits of the back rub include the following:
- Communicates caring
- Fosters trust in the nurse-patient relationship
- Provides an opportunity to assess the skin on the back
- Stimulates circulation of blood to the area
- Reduces tension and promotes relaxation

Box 19-3 notes that a back rub should be performed with morning care and at bedtime. It is essential to provide one to patients confined to bed. Oils, lotions, or powder may be used according to patient preference and the skin's condition. Avoid open wounds and areas of pressure injury while performing a back rub.

Use more pressure on the up strokes toward the head and less pressure on downward strokes. The pressure should be firm but should not cause tensing or discomfort for the patient. After a few minutes, rub in any remaining lotion using short circular strokes, paying particular attention to the shoulders and neck. During the back rub, remember the following safety/comfort issues:
- Move the patient close to you to maintain proper body mechanics to prevent self-injury.

- Raise the bed to an appropriate height and lower only the rail on the side where you are standing during the back rub.
- Make sure your hands are warm and relaxed before beginning. If using lotion or oils, warm them in your hands before placing them on the patient. Cool hands and cold lotions cause the patient to tense and pull away.

An effective back rub should last approximately 3 to 5 minutes (Figure 19-7).

Perineal Care

Usually a patient will accept your assistance with perineal care, although a few will try to avoid it because they feel embarrassment. Perineal care may cause embarrassment to you and the patient as a result of your close contact with the genital area. Proper draping helps promote comfort with the procedure (Figure 19-8). You can reduce your feelings of embarrassment if you re-

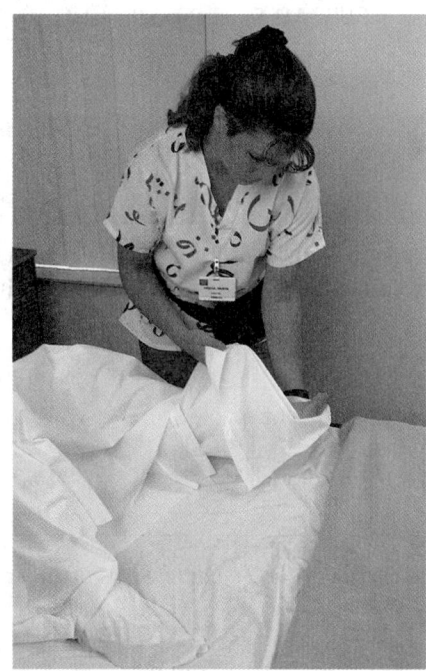

FIGURE **19-8** Draping the female patient in the lithotomy position for perineal care.

member your purpose is to assist the patient. Explain the procedure to reassure the patient and gain cooperation in the task. Maintain a matter-of-fact attitude and be objective; avoid any sexually suggestive conversation or actions. A professional and dignified attitude can help reduce any embarrassment.

Mouth Care

Mouth care removes food particles and secretions, which prevents halitosis (bad breath), feelings of uncleanliness, and dental caries (cavities). Oral hygiene promotes a better appetite and maintains the healthy state of the mouth, gums, teeth, and lips. It must be provided on a regular basis; ideally, offer it four times a day as noted in Box 19-3.

Mouth Care for the Conscious Patient. To assist a patient with mouth care, raise the head of the bed 45 to 90 degrees. Wear gloves when providing or assisting with mouth care. If the patient is unable to sit up, turn the patient to the side facing you. Place a towel under the chin. Moisten the toothbrush with water or mouthwash and spread it with toothpaste or tooth powder. Brush from the gum line to the edge of the teeth. All surfaces of each tooth should be brushed (Figure 19-9). Have the patient rinse the mouth and spit the solution

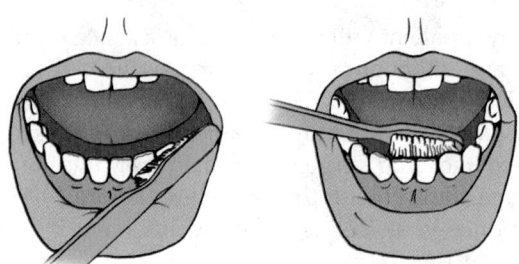

FIGURE **19-9** Brushing the teeth.

into the emesis basin. Repeat as desired or necessary. Provide the patient with a cloth or tissue to wipe the mouth when finished.

To assist the patient to floss the teeth, obtain 12 to 15 inches of floss. Loosely wrap the ends of the floss around the index finger on each hand and work the floss between each tooth. Slide the floss gently down to the gum line, pulling the floss back and forth. If toothpaste is applied before flossing, then the fluoride can come into direct contact with the tooth surfaces to prevent dental caries. Rinse and wipe the mouth again. Report any excessive bleeding of the gums after flossing.

Mouth Care for the Unconscious Patient. **A patient who is unconscious should be provided full mouth care at least once every 8 hours.** If the patient is mouth-breathing, care should be done every 4 hours. Mouth-breathing causes the tongue to dry and become crusty. The dry secretions need to be removed because they cause halitosis and may obstruct airflow. Moist swabbing of the mouth is done every 2 hours or as needed to maintain the integrity of the oral cavity. Mouth care of the unconscious patient is described in Skill 19-2.

Denture Care. Patients with dentures who are confined to bed, comatose, or weak or who have trouble with hand and finger dexterity may need you to assist with or provide care for their dentures. Dentures should be cleaned to prevent irritation to the gums and infection. A patient may use an adhesive for a better fit. Usually, a patient who uses adhesive does not like to remove the dentures during the day. Care should then be provided in the morning and at bedtime. Do not place dentures on a meal tray because they are often lost when the trays are removed. **When not in the mouth, dentures should be kept in a labeled denture container containing water or normal saline.** Skill 19-3 details how to clean dentures.

Skill 19-2 | Administering Oral Care to the Unconscious Patient

Unconscious patients require frequent mouth care. Cleansing is especially important for these patients because they often breathe through their mouths, which leads to dryness and crusting of the area.

■ Supplies

✓ Toothbrush and toothpaste
✓ Mouthwash
✓ Mouth suction device
✓ Gloves

✓ Hydrogen peroxide
✓ Water-soluble lubricant
✓ Water
✓ Paper towels
✓ Tongue blade and gauze 4 × 4s

✓ Towel or toothettes
✓ Emesis basin
✓ Irrigation syringe

Review and carry out the Standard Steps in Appendix 3.

■ Assessment (Data Collection)

1. *ACTION* Assess for gag reflex.

   RATIONALE Identifies risk of aspiration.

■ Planning

2. *ACTION* Gather supplies and place on paper towels on the over-the-bed table.

   RATIONALE Provides easy access to equipment. Paper towels keep table clean.

3. ***ACTION*** Explain the procedure to the patient.

   RATIONALE Provides stimulation as unconscious patients may be able to hear.

4. ***ACTION*** Close door or pull curtain.

   RATIONALE Provides privacy.

■ Implementation

5. ***ACTION*** Raise bed level to comfortable working height. Turn patient laterally on side of bed nearest you. Lower side rail.

   RATIONALE Promotes good body mechanics; work is at your center of gravity.

6. ***ACTION*** Turn on the suction and place the suction device under the corner of the pillow near you. Put a towel under the patient's head and the emesis basin beneath the patient's mouth and chin.

   RATIONALE Readying suction device provides for immediate use of suction in case patient gags. Towel and basin keep gown and linens clean.

7. ***ACTION*** Wear gloves. Use toothettes or toothbrush and toothpaste to cleanse the teeth and mouth. Use hydrogen peroxide (half strength) and mouthwash or water to clean the interior of the cheeks, roof of the mouth, teeth, and tongue. A 4 × 4 gauze pad may be wrapped around an index finger or tongue blade to remove crusts. Repeat as necessary.

   RATIONALE Observes Standard Precautions. Hydrogen peroxide and mouthwash or water are good cleansing agents. Removing crusting and debris maintains a healthy mouth.

8. ***ACTION*** Floss by holding a 12- to 15-inch piece of floss with the ends wrapped around the middle finger of each hand. Using index fingers and thumbs, gently work floss between each tooth, moving down to gum line and back up to tooth edge.

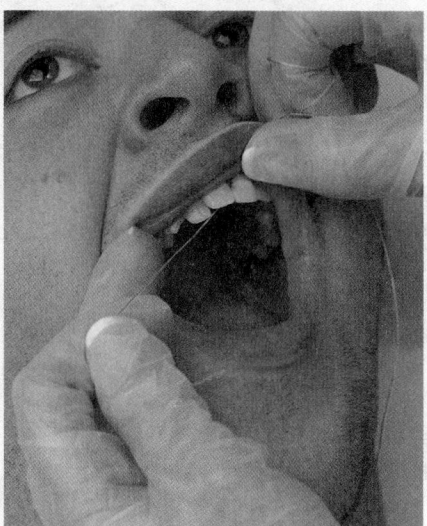

Step **8**

RATIONALE Removes tartar and plaque.

9. ***ACTION*** With the patient's head turned to the side, intermittently rinse the mouth by gently squirting water in with the syringe; use the suction device to remove water and debris.

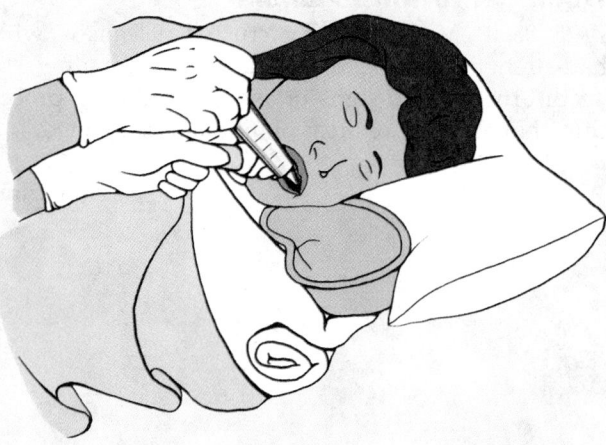

Step **9**

RATIONALE Using small amounts of water and turning the head to the side to promote drainage reduce risk of aspiration.

10. ***ACTION*** Wipe the patient's mouth and lubricate the lips and corners of the mouth with water-soluble lubricant.

    RATIONALE Prevents drying of lips and cracking.

11. ***ACTION*** Explain to the patient that you have finished the procedure.

    RATIONALE Provides stimulation because unconscious patients may be able to hear.

12. ***ACTION*** Remove gloves and dispose of them properly. Reposition patient, raise side rail, and lower bed.

    RATIONALE Proper removal and disposal of gloves prevents spread of microorganisms. Repositioning patient and restoring unit promote safety and comfort.

13. ***ACTION*** Clean supplies and tidy unit.

    RATIONALE Readies equipment for next use and straightens patient's environment.

■ Evaluation

14. ***ACTION*** Put on gloves and inspect mouth to check effectiveness of procedure.

    RATIONALE Determines if other actions are needed.

■ Documentation

15. ***ACTION*** Note procedure done and assessment of mouth before and after care.

    RATIONALE Notes any abnormalities.

Continued

Skill 19-2 | Administering Oral Care to the Unconscious Patient—cont'd

Documentation Example

7/28 0800 Mouth heavily crusted. Cleansed with half-strength hydrogen peroxide and mouthwash. Teeth brushed. No signs of aspiration during procedure. No bleeding or areas of inflammation noted.

_____
(Nurse's signature)

?CRITICAL THINKING QUESTIONS

1. Complete oral care is necessary for the patient who is comatose. What precautions will you take to ensure this patient's safety and your own?

2. Every 8 hours, complete oral care is needed for the comatose unconscious patient. Will you perform any other actions between the full care? If so, what?

3. What purpose does talking to the patient during the procedure serve?

Skill 19-3 | Denture Care

Dentures must be cleaned at least twice a day to maintain oral hygiene and promote oral health. If the patient is unable to perform this task independently, then you must provide assistance or clean the dentures.

■ Supplies

✓ Denture brush or toothbrush
✓ Denture adhesive
✓ Denture cup
✓ Denture powder or paste
✓ Emesis basin
✓ Gloves
✓ Optional: denture soak
✓ Small towel or washcloth

Review and carry out the Standard Steps in Appendix 3.

■ Assessment (Data Collection)

1. **ACTION** Ask the patient how the dentures fit and if they are comfortable.

   RATIONALE Poor fit causes mouth irritation.

2. **ACTION** Explain the procedure.

   RATIONALE Promotes cooperation and understanding, decreases any anxiety over procedure.

■ Planning

3. **ACTION** Arrange supplies on over-the-bed table or near sink.

   RATIONALE Provides access to equipment.

4. **ACTION** Pull curtain and close door.

   RATIONALE Provides privacy. Many patients are reluctant to be seen without their dentures in place.

5. **ACTION** Ask patient to remove dentures. If unable, put on gloves and remove upper denture by grasping the front teeth with the thumb and index finger. Move denture up and down slightly to break the vacuum seal. Turn slightly and slip it out of the mouth. Place in the emesis basin. Grasp the lower denture with thumb and index finger and pick it up; turn slightly and carefully remove it from the mouth without stretching lips. Place in the emesis basin.

   RATIONALE Allows full access to mouth.

6. **ACTION** Assess the mouth and gums.

   RATIONALE Detects any irritation, redness, or swelling.

■ Implementation

7. **ACTION** Take emesis basin to the sink and place a washcloth or small towel in the sink. Fill sink with tepid water to about 1 inch in depth.

   RATIONALE Placing towel in sink decreases chance of breaking if dentures are accidentally dropped. Tepid water prevents the dentures from becoming softened or deformed.

8. **ACTION** Brush all surfaces with brush and paste or powder. Dentures may be soaked first in a commercial cleansing soak.

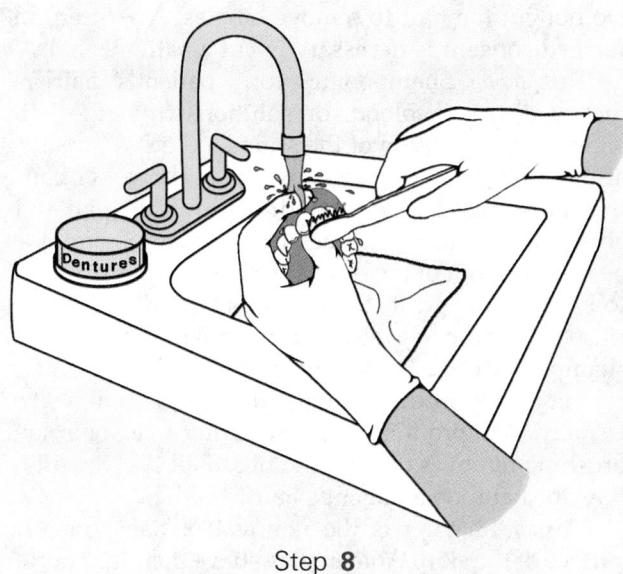

Step **8**

RATIONALE Prevents accumulation of food and bacteria, thereby reducing odor and stains.

9. *ACTION* Rinse well in tepid water and place in denture cup or emesis basin that is half-filled with cool water.

   RATIONALE Rinsing removes toothpaste or powder, bacteria, and food. Placing dentures in cup keeps dentures safe until needed.

10. *ACTION* Clean the patient's mouth (gums, palate, and tongue) with a soft brush and toothpaste.

   RATIONALE Promotes oral hygiene by removing debris and stimulating circulation.

11. *ACTION* Assist the patient to replace moistened dentures or replace them yourself. Use a dental adhesive if requested or needed. Insert the top denture first by reversing removal procedure (tilt slightly and push up onto gum), press into place. Insert lower denture.

   RATIONALE Wetting dentures aids insertion and provides comfort. Adhesive promotes a better seal and provides a feeling of increased comfort because some patients prefer an adhesive. Upper denture is easier to place first because it is larger. Pressing into place creates a seal against the roof of the mouth.

12. *ACTION* Store dentures in a labeled denture cup in cool water if they are not being replaced immediately in the mouth.

   RATIONALE Prevents loss because cup is labeled. Most patients do not sleep with their dentures in place.

13. *ACTION* Clean equipment and tidy unit.

   RATIONALE Readies supplies for next use and straightens patient's environment.

■ Evaluation

14. *ACTION* Ask patient if the dentures are comfortable.

   RATIONALE Determines if the dentures were inserted correctly or if there is any irritation.

■ Documentation

15. *ACTION* Document on flow sheet or nurse's notes per policy. Note any areas of irritation or abnormality and action taken.

   RATIONALE Validates care and promotes continuity. Indicates if there are any problems or abnormalities.

Documentation Example

7/28 2200   Dentures cleaned; c/o small area of irritation on front gum line of lower denture; 1-cm diameter area of redness noted. Mouth swished with half-strength hydrogen peroxide. Dentures left in labeled denture cup on the bedside stand; reassess area in A.M.

_____

(Nurse's signature)

?CRITICAL THINKING QUESTIONS

1. Many people feel self-conscious when they remove their dentures. What can you do to make the patient more comfortable for this task?

2. What is the purpose of placing a washcloth or small towel in the sink before cleaning dentures?

3. After removing your patient's dentures, you note an area of irritation on the right lower gum. What do you do?

Hair Care

Hair care should be given regularly during illness. It consists of brushing and combing, shampooing, shaving, and mustache and beard care. Morale and body image are improved when the patient is comfortable with his appearance. Hair care is usually provided after the morning bath. Brushing and combing the hair stimulates circulation, which helps to promote hair growth, prevent hair loss, distribute oil along hair shafts, and bring nutrients to the roots (Cultural Cues 19-2).

Brushing and Combing. Use a clean brush or comb to brush from the scalp toward the hair ends to decrease pulling. Separate the hair into three sections; then each of those sections may be split into smaller sections. It is easier and more comfortable for the patient to brush or comb small sections of hair at a time. Be sure to be gentle when providing hair care.

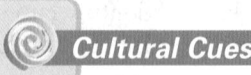
Cultural Cues 19-2

Caring for African American Hair

The hair of African Americans tends to be much drier than the hair of whites. It should only be washed with shampoo every 7 to 10 days. It can be rinsed daily. This type of hair breaks easily, and a wide-toothed "pick" comb should be used to comb out tangles. The hair should be combed while wet. A leave-in type of conditioner may be used daily. Heat should not be used on the hair to dry it. A satin pillowcase or scarf or cap may be desired for sleep to decrease tangling. Alternatively, the hair may be plaited or tied back for sleep. Style is a matter of individual preference.

A patient may have tangled or matted hair. To decrease pain, hold the hair between the scalp and the area you are brushing or combing. Braiding the hair helps to reduce tangles. Ask your patient's permission before braiding. Alcohol, astringents, or water may be used to loosen hair strands that are tangled or matted.

Do not cut the hair to remove tangles. **A written, informed consent is necessary to cut a patient's hair.**

Shampooing. Shampooing your patient's hair removes dirt, soil, blood, or solutions from the hair; stimulates circulation of the scalp; and eases brushing and combing. A patient who is able to shower or bathe may be shampooed without difficulty. If the patient is able to be out of bed in a chair, the shampooing may be done in front of the sink. The shampooing will need to be done in bed if the patient is bedridden. Dry or rinseless shampoo is available for cleaning hair, as is a shampoo cap such as "Ready Bath" shampoo. The benefit of this product is that it does not require water. Usually, the product is sprayed into the hair and brushing removes the dirt and oils. Skill 19-4 describes how to shampoo a patient's hair in bed.

Shaving. Shaving is the removal of hair from the surface of the skin. Women may shave their leg and/or axillary hair, whereas men may shave their facial hair. Some patients may not want to shave or be shaved. Respect the patient's request in this instance.

Skill 19-4 | Shampooing Hair

Assistance is given for shampooing the hair when the patient is unable to perform this procedure and the hair needs to be shampooed.

■ Supplies

✓ Shampoo
✓ Comb and brush
✓ Hair dryer
✓ Pitcher
✓ Waterproof pad
✓ Basin or pail for waste water
✓ Rinse (optional)
✓ Shampoo tray or plastic trough
✓ Washcloth
✓ Bath blanket
✓ Bath towels (2-4)

Review and carry out the Standard Steps in Appendix 3.

■ Assessment (Data Collection)

1. *ACTION* Assess need for shampoo. Assess for contraindications to performing hair wash.

   RATIONALE Prevents injury to patient.

2. *ACTION* Check written order to see if a special shampoo is ordered.

   RATIONALE Medicated shampoos may be ordered in cases of dandruff, head lice, or other abnormalities.

■ Planning

3. *ACTION* Gather supplies.

   RATIONALE Provides easy access to equipment.

4. *ACTION* Explain the procedure to patient.

   RATIONALE Decreases fears and anxiety over procedure.

■ Implementation

5. *ACTION* Wear gloves if patient's scalp has lesions, cuts, or infestation, or there is dried blood in the hair.

   RATIONALE Prevents spread of microorganisms.

6. *ACTION* Raise the bed, lower the near side rail, remove the pillow, and move the patient to the near side of the bed. Place a waterproof pad under the patient's shoulders and head. Drape patient with a bath blanket. Place a towel around patient's shoulders.

   RATIONALE Promotes proper body alignment and mechanics. Waterproof pad keeps linens dry. Drape prevents chills, and towel helps to keep patient dry.

7. *ACTION* Brush or comb patient's hair.

   RATIONALE Removes tangles.

8. *ACTION* Place basin or pail on chair at the head of the bed to collect the waste water. Place the shampoo tray under the patient's head. Lower bed and obtain warm water.

   RATIONALE Shampoo tray keeps runoff water in basin or pail and protects bed from moisture. Using warm water promotes comfort.

9. *ACTION* Raise bed and lower near rail. Offer patient a folded washcloth to cover the eyes. Pour a small amount of water through patient's hair, start-

ing at the front hairline and moving to the back of the head; wet entire hair surface completely. Apply shampoo and lather. Use your fingertips to massage all parts of the scalp. Again, start from the front and work to the back. Lift the head slightly to fully massage and wash the back of the head. Add water as needed to maintain lather.

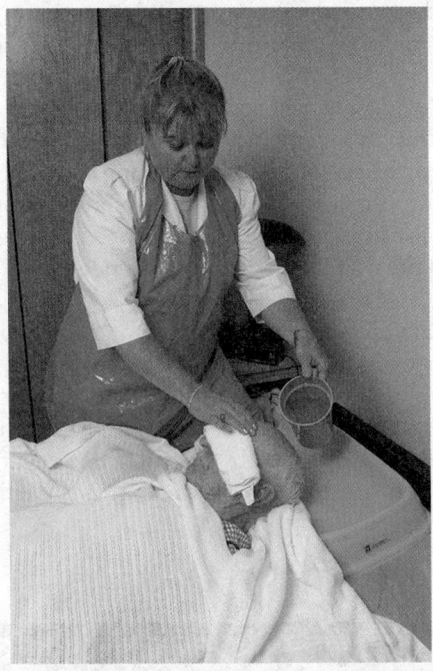

Step **9**

RATIONALE Promotes proper body alignment. Washcloth protects the eyes from soap and water. Friction aids in making the lather, which will cleanse the hair.

10. **ACTION** Rinse thoroughly by pouring warm water through the hair. Rinse until the soap is completely out of the hair. Apply one more soaping if the hair does not feel squeaky clean and if the patient can tolerate the procedure again.

    RATIONALE A squeaky sound when clean, rinsed hair strands are pulled through your fingers indicates hair is completely rinsed.

11. **ACTION** Apply a rinse or conditioner if requested or ordered. Rinse thoroughly.

    RATIONALE Decreases tangles and adds moisture.

12. **ACTION** Wrap head in towel, dry face and shoulders. Remove shampoo tray and basin.

RATIONALE Towel decreases chills. Removing tray and basin prevents spills.

13. **ACTION** Towel-dry hair and scalp, using more towels if needed. Comb hair; use a hair dryer if needed.

    RATIONALE Towel drying promotes quicker drying of the hair. Combing removes tangles and styles the hair.

14. **ACTION** Position patient for comfort and finish arranging the hair as desired by patient.

    RATIONALE Promotes comfort and demonstrates respect for patient's wishes.

15. **ACTION** Clean equipment and restore the unit, lowering the bed and raising the side rail.

    RATIONALE Cleaning readies equipment for next use. Restoring unit promotes safety.

■ Evaluation

16. **ACTION** Assess condition of hair and scalp. How does patient feel now?

    RATIONALE Promotes a sense of well-being and cleanliness as hair is left clean and groomed.

■ Documentation

17. **ACTION** Document the patient response and tolerance of the procedure. Note any abnormalities of the hair or scalp found during the procedure.

    RATIONALE Validates effectiveness and provides for consistency among personnel.

Documentation Example

8/2 1030 Bed shampoo given. Complained of being tired and weak. Stated it felt "very good to have clean hair again." No abnormalities of hair or scalp noted. Bed down and call bell within reach.

_____
(Nurse's signature)

?CRITICAL THINKING QUESTIONS

1. What needs to be done before deciding on what and how to give your patient a shampoo in bed?

2. Some cultures cover their hair, especially the women. What would you do if your patient is Muslim and a medicated hair shampoo is ordered?

Shaving may be done before, during, or after the bath. Many male patients confined to bed can shave themselves if you set up the equipment. A weak or otherwise debilitated man will need your assistance to care for his facial hair. Either a safety razor or an electric razor may be used. An electric razor must be checked before use for any possible electrical hazard.

Any razor should be used on only one patient to provide for infection control. The main considerations in shaving a patient are to be gentle and to use short strokes with the safety razor (Figure 19-10). Check the patient's chart to see if the patient has any bleeding tendencies or is receiving medication that would contraindicate the use of a safety razor. Steps 19-2 describe

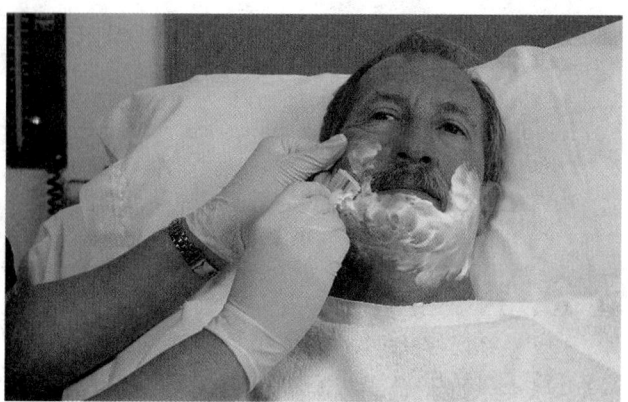

FIGURE **19-10** Shaving in the direction of hair growth.

how to shave a male patient. A safety razor should not be used when a patient has a low platelet count, is receiving an anticoagulant, is undergoing chemotherapy, or is on high-dose aspirin therapy.

Mustache and Beard Care. A patient with a mustache and/or beard needs daily care to these areas. The areas must be kept clean and free of food particles. Mustaches and beards may be cleansed with a warm damp washcloth or washed with soap or shampoo. **You may not shave off a beard or mustache without a written, informed consent.**

Nail Care

Most patients can perform nail care for themselves as part of their daily hygiene routine. You may need to provide care for those who are unconscious, blind, confused, unsteady, or in a cast or traction. Nail care includes regular trimming, cleaning under the nails, and cuticle care, and is usually done with the bath. Nails should be kept clean and trimmed according to the institution's policy and patient preference. The toenails of a diabetic patient or one with circulatory disease of the lower extremities should not be cut without a physician's order. You need to check your agency's policy to see if an order is needed to trim the fingernails of the diabetic patient.

Soak the nails in warm soapy water for 5 to 10 minutes, especially if they are dirty or thickened. Use an orangewood stick to clean under nails because a metal nail file can make the nails rough and trap dirt. Push cuticles back gently with the stick to prevent hangnails, which are pieces of skin that are partially de-

---

Steps 19-2 | Shaving a Male Patient

A shave can improve a man's appearance and give him a sense of well-being. Unless he has his own electric razor, a safety razor must be used. Practicing by shaving a family member or friend will increase your confidence in the procedure.

■ Shaving a Male Patient with a Safety Razor

1. *ACTION* Clean the face and neck with warm water. Place a warm washcloth on the patient's face for several minutes. Drape the patient and protect the bed linens from water.

   RATIONALE Cleaning reduces the surface bacteria should a cut occur. Application of warm washcloth reduces the chance of cuts because warm water softens the skin. Draping patient keeps linens dry and promotes patient comfort.

2. *ACTION* Apply shaving cream to face and neck or use lathered soap as a substitute.

   RATIONALE Lubricates skin so the razor glides more easily.

3. *ACTION* Hold a safety razor at a 30- to 45-degree angle in your dominant hand. Carefully pull the patient's skin taut with your other hand. Use firm, short motions in the direction of hair growth to shave the area.

   RATIONALE Decreases the chance of cutting or nicking the skin. Prevents pulling of the skin. Many patients, if able, will instruct the nurse on personal preference regarding shaving technique.

4. *ACTION* Rinse the razor every two or three strokes, changing the water as needed.

   RATIONALE Cleans razor of hair and ensures a closer, even shave. Clean water prevents contamination.

5. *ACTION* Short downward strokes are used for the upper lip area.

   RATIONALE Decreases chance of cuts or nicks.

6. *ACTION* Rinse area with a washcloth and clean, warm water. Dry area.

   RATIONALE Promotes comfort, removes shaved hair, and decreases surface bacteria.

7. *ACTION* Assess area for cuts, nicks, or hair. Apply lotion or aftershave if desired by patient.

   RATIONALE Lotion promotes comfort by moisturizing the skin. Aftershave closes the pores opened by the moist heat through astringent action.

■ Shaving a Male Patient with an Electric Razor

1. **ACTION** Apply preshave lotion or skin conditioner.

   RATIONALE Softens beard and skin.

2. **ACTION** Turn on razor; holding the skin taut, begin shaving one side of the face. Gently stroke the razor downward in the direction of hair growth.

RATIONALE Prevents pulling of the facial hairs and skin abrasion.

3. **ACTION** Offer lotion or aftershave when finished.

   RATIONALE Provides comfort.

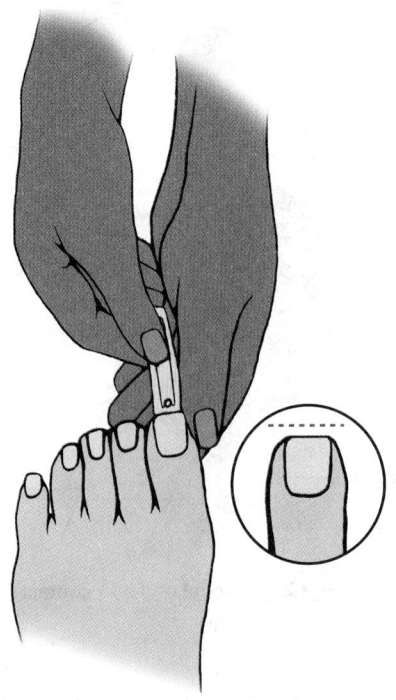

FIGURE **19-11** Cut toenails straight across and then smooth the corners.

Patient Teaching 19-1

Hygiene and Skin Care

Good hygiene practices and appropriate skin care techniques can be taught to patients during bath time. The following points should be covered:

* Hygiene care is important in maintaining health.
* Use warm, not hot, water and a mild soap when bathing to decrease irritation and prevent dry skin.
* For patients who will spend time outdoors, sunscreen with a minimum sun protection factor (SPF) of 15 should be used on all exposed areas to prevent skin cancer year round and not just in the summer; reapply sunscreen every 2 hours.
* Skin should be checked for any changes such as redness and rashes, changes in moles, or skin growths.
* Safety concerns need to be addressed, such as water temperature and preventing falls in the shower and tub.
* Prevent dry skin by avoiding cold or dry air and using creams or oils on the skin.
* Eat a balanced diet to promote skin health.
* Remove moisture from urine, stool, perspiration, or wound drainage to maintain skin integrity.
* Toenails should be clipped or filed straight across to preserve skin integrity; smooth any sharp edges.

tached at the base of the fingernail. Hangnails are painful and a possible source of infection.

Use nail clippers to cut the toenails straight across to prevent them from growing into the skin along the sides (Figure 19-11). This can cause pain or infection and leads to a condition called ingrown toenails. Ingrown toenails often require a surgical procedure to correct.

You may need to observe the color of the nail beds continually to monitor circulation in the extremities. Examples of when such monitoring is needed are after surgery, during traction, when the patient is in a cast, or to detect a failure in the general systemic circulation. Nail polish will need to be removed in these instances to allow monitoring. Patient Teaching 19-1 summarizes important points for hygiene and skin care.

Eye Care

Assess your patient's eyes for drainage, crusting, or redness. Notify the physician if any abnormalities are found. Routine eye care is described in Skill 19-1. If crusting is noted, soak the eyelid with a warm, damp washcloth for 2 to 3 minutes to soften the crust and ease its removal. Use a different part of the cloth for each eyelid. Unconscious patients may need more frequent eye care or the administration of lubricating drops as ordered. Older adults often develop dry eyes (Health Promotion Points 19-1).

Glasses and Contacts. Store glasses in a case when not in use. Most glasses today have plastic lenses that are easier to scratch than glass. To clean either type of lens, use clean warm water and a soft cloth to wipe dry. Do not use a paper towel on plastic lenses because it may scratch the lenses.

Contact lenses are classified as to whether they are hard or soft. Hard lenses feel like a firm plastic disk, whereas soft lenses have the consistency of a thick plastic food wrap. Before removing lenses, wash hands thoroughly and wear gloves. Many contact lenses today may be worn for an extended period of time.

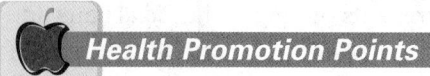

Health Promotion Points 19-1

Eye Care for Older Adults

- Adults should have glaucoma screening done every 2 to 3 years after age 40. Glaucoma is one of the leading causes of blindness.
- Older adults should be regularly checked for cataracts and macular degeneration.
- Encourage use of an Amsler grid at home to detect signs of macular degeneration.
- Wearing a brimmed hat and dark glasses when outdoors helps prevent cataracts.
- Encourage the use of artificial tears for those who experience dry eyes to help prevent infection.

Removal of Contact Lenses. To remove a hard lens, perform hand hygiene and cup your nondominant hand below the patient's eye. Move the lens directly over the cornea. Pull the upper eyelid up above the edge of the lens; pull the lower lid down to the lower edge of the lens. Press slightly on the lower lid at the edge of the lens; the lens should slide out between the eyelids.

To remove a soft lens, perform hand hygiene and place a drop of wetting solution or sterile saline in the eyes to moisten the contact surface. Using your nondominant hand, open the eye with your middle finger and thumb. Use the index finger of your dominant hand and place it gently on the lower edge of the lens and slide it down toward the lower lid. Gently pinch the lens between your index finger and thumb and lift it out (Figure 19-12).

Sometimes the techniques described do not work. In this case, get a lens suction cup to remove the contact lens. If a suction cup is not available, check with a colleague who wears such lenses and is familiar with the procedure for assistance.

Cleaning Contact Lenses. Lenses should be cleaned with commercially prepared cleaning solutions. Moisten the lens and rub it gently between the fingers to remove accumulated dirt and secretions while holding it over a basin of water or a stoppered sink with some water in the bottom. Rinse with the wetting solution, rinsing solution, or sterile saline. Replace the lens in the patient's eye or store in sterile saline in the case. **It is important to place the lens in the correct compartment of the case, either right or left.** If a case is not available, store the contact lenses in sterile cups filled with sterile saline and marked "right" or "left" and labeled with the patient's name.

Artificial Eye. Sometimes because of trauma, infection, or tumor, a patient has had an eye removed. The patient may have an artificial eye that is either permanently implanted or removable. An eye that is not implanted needs to be removed on a daily basis for clean-

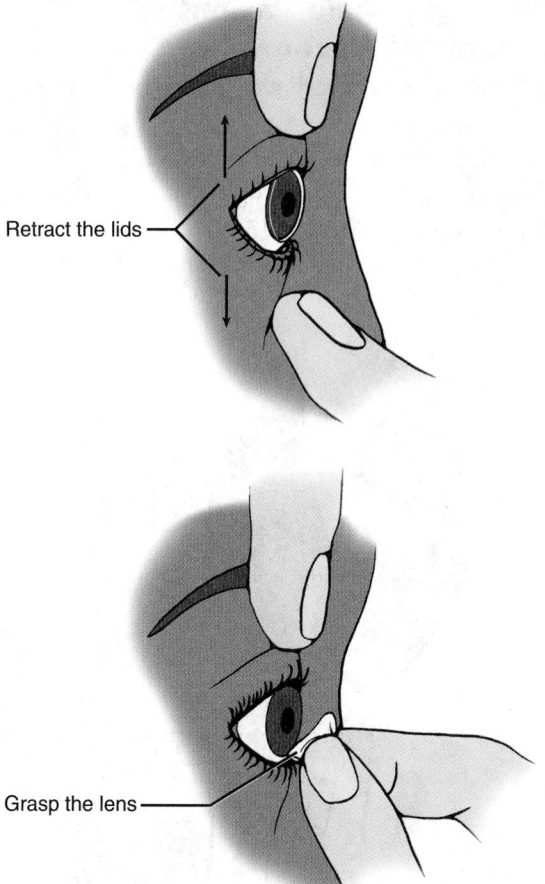

Retract the lids

Grasp the lens

FIGURE **19-12** Removal of a soft contact lens.

ing. Usually the patient will care for this independently, but some may need assistance.

To remove an artificial eye, pull down the lower eyelid and put a little pressure just below the eye. Cup your other hand below the eye to catch it as it moves out of the socket. Assess the socket for any signs of infection. Report any redness or drainage immediately. Cleanse the artificial eye with normal saline. The edges of the eye socket may be cleansed with warm tap water or saline. To replace the eye, pull down the lower lid and lift the upper lid. Place the eye in the socket and be sure the eyelids fit smoothly over the eye.

Ear Care

Hearing acuity may be affected if cerumen or foreign material collects in the external ear canal. Remove these materials by gently washing the external ear canal with a warm washcloth. **No object, including cotton-tipped applicators, should be inserted into the ear canal.** The applicators compact the cerumen, making it more difficult to clean the ear. You may need to irrigate the ear if the wax is dried or excessive (Home Care Considerations 19-1). Notify the physician if irrigation is needed.

Hearing Aids. Hearing aids amplify sound and must be cleaned daily (Figure 19-13). There are five types of

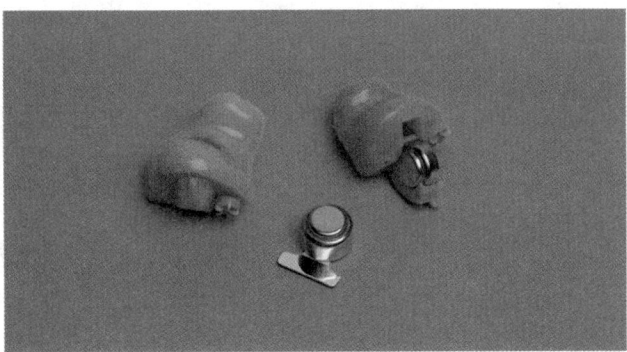

FIGURE **19-13** Hearing aids.

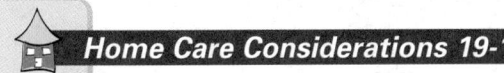

Removing Cerumen

A kit can be obtained at the drug store that provides drops that will soften cerumen so that it can be easily flushed out with the small ear syringe that comes with the kit. Patients who tend to build up considerable cerumen that interferes with hearing should be encouraged to use the kit on a periodic basis.

hearing aids: (1) body worn (rarely seen today), (2) behind the ear, (3) attached to the eyeglasses, (4) in the ear, and (5) in the ear canal. Do not drop or bump hearing aids because this can cause damage. Store the aid in its case to prevent damage and to avoid the accumulation of dust and dirt when not in use. Clean the earpiece with soap and water daily to prevent the buildup of wax and debris. Do not submerge the hearing aid in water. If the hearing aid is not working, check to make sure the unit is turned on, the battery is installed correctly (it may need to be replaced), and there are no cracks or breaks in the plastic housing or tubing.

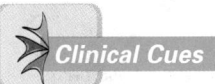

When the hearing aid is out of the ear and in its case, the battery cover should be opened so that the battery disengages.

Evaluation

During evaluation, you determine whether the expected outcomes set during the planning stage of the nursing process have been met. Evaluation statements indicating the expected outcomes for hygiene have been met are as follows:

- No evidence of redness, irritation, or breaks in skin integrity; skin integrity is maintained.
- Hair is clean and neatly styled each day per patient preference.
- The mucous membranes are pink and moist, without signs or symptoms of irritation or odor.

Feedback from the patient and other personnel should be obtained during evaluation.

Self-evaluation is important too. Did you encourage the patient to function independently? Did you use good body alignment when providing care? Were active measures taken to prevent pressure ulcers? The information gathered will indicate if any changes need to be made in the plan. If so, document the progress made and the changes for other staff.

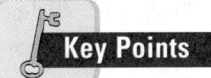

Key Points

- The skin is the largest organ of the body. The main functions of the skin are to protect, sense, regulate temperature, excrete, and secrete.
- Changes from aging may cause the skin to (1) wrinkle and sag, (2) become dry and itchy, (3) have altered temperature control, and (4) be more fragile and slower to heal.
- Hygiene is the practice of cleanliness that helps to preserve health. To determine self-care abilities, assess the patient's physical and cognitive ability.
- A pressure ulcer is an ulcer that forms from a local interference with circulation, and is graded according to four stages.
- The AHRQ lists five risk factors for developing pressure ulcers (see Box 19-1).
- Particular attention should be paid to assessing areas over bony prominences.
- Staging of ulcers may be inhibited in patients with darker skin, if eschar is present, or in patients with orthopedic devices in place.
- The purposes of bathing are to cleanse the skin, promote comfort, stimulate circulation, and remove waste products from the skin.
- When providing perineal care for a female, the area must be wiped from the pubic area down to the rectal area to prevent infection. When providing perineal care for an uncircumcised male, be sure to reposition the foreskin after cleansing.
- Maintaining oral hygiene prevents halitosis, feelings of uncleanliness, and dental caries.
- Hair care improves morale and body image. Hair and beards may not be cut without a written, informed consent.
- Shaving with a safety razor is contraindicated in patients who are on anticoagulants, chemotherapy, or high doses of aspirin or who are immunocompromised.
- Toenails must be trimmed straight across. An order is needed to trim the toenails of patients with diabetes or peripheral vascular disease.
- To provide eye care, wipe from the inner to the outer part of the eye using a different portion of the washcloth for each eye.

 Go to your **Companion CD-ROM** for an Audio Glossary, animations, video clips, and more.

evolve Be sure to visit the companion Evolve site at http://evolve.elsevier.com/deWit/fundamental/ for additional online resources.

NCLEX-PN® EXAMINATION-STYLE REVIEW QUESTIONS

*Choose the **best** answer(s) for each question.*

1. A healthy epidermis is important because it:
   1. contains elastic and collagen fibers.
   2. acts as a barrier to entry of pathogenic organisms.
   3. supplies nutrition to the underlying dermis.
   4. contains nerves that send messages to the brain.

2. A factor in skin problems common to elderly adults is: *(Select all that apply.)*
   1. skin tends to be dry because of increased gland activity.
   2. hair becomes thicker and grows more slowly.
   3. nails become thin and more brittle.
   4. fewer nutrients are available from the reduced diet.
   5. skin is less elastic and more fragile.

3. Your patient has an area at the left trochanter that is reddened with slightly abraded skin. You would stage this as a _____ pressure ulcer.
   1. stage I
   2. stage II
   3. stage III
   4. stage IV

4. The extremities are washed from distal to proximal because this:
   1. promotes safety.
   2. cleanses the skin better than proximal to distal.
   3. supplies vital skin oils.
   4. promotes venous return to the heart.

5. A stage III pressure ulcer is characterized by:
   1. a partial-thickness skin loss involving epidermis/dermis.
   2. a reddened area that does not blanch.
   3. an area of induration.
   4. a full-thickness skin loss that looks like a deep crater.

6. Special attention is given to skin over bony prominences because:
   1. pressure ulcers are more likely to develop.
   2. pressure ulcers develop only in these areas.
   3. these areas are often dirtier.
   4. the skin here tends to hold moisture.

7. A partial bath includes bathing the:
   1. face, hands, and feet.
   2. face, hands, perineum, axillae, and back.
   3. face, hands, perineum, and axillae.
   4. face, hands, back, perineum, and feet.

8. When providing foot care for the diabetic patient, you must remember to:
   1. cut the cuticles to prevent hangnails.
   2. never soak the feet.
   3. check for an order before trimming the nails straight across.
   4. check for an order before trimming the nails in a curved manner so there are not any sharp points to irritate the skin.

9. A back rub should be offered to every patient because it:
   1. is an active form of exercise.
   2. increases medication absorption.
   3. is an expected nursing service.
   4. is relaxing and decreases tension.

10. Prevention of pressure ulcers is promoted by: *(Select all that apply.)*
    1. changing the patient's position every 2 hours.
    2. directly massaging reddened areas.
    3. keeping the heels of the immobile patient off of the bed.
    4. using lift devices such as a trapeze bar to move patients.

CRITICAL THINKING ACTIVITIES *Read each clinical scenario and discuss the questions with your classmates*

Scenario A
While assisting a female patient during her bath, you notice that she cleanses herself from the rectum to the pubic area. You remember that she has a history of having recurrent vaginal infections. What will you do? How will you explain perineal care and proper toileting techniques to her?

Scenario B
Your postoperative patient has a history of a cerebrovascular accident (CVA) with weakness on his left side. In the hospital, he has performed most of his hygiene care independently and states that he "likes doing things for himself." What would you tell the family of your patient when they say they always do their father's complete bath at home so that he doesn't get tired?

Patient Environment and Safety

Objectives

Upon completing this chapter, you should be able to:

Theory

1. Discuss nursing responsibilities for environmental management.
2. Identify common noises in health care facilities and ways to minimize their effects on patients.
3. Explain the importance of neatness and order in the patient's environment.
4. Describe methods to prevent mechanical and thermal accidents and injury in health care facilities and the home.
5. Discuss the various forms of bioterrorism, safety measures to be taken, signs and symptoms of agents used, and measures to treat or contain the threat.
6. Demonstrate knowledge of the legal implications of using protective devices.
7. Discuss the principles for using protective devices.

Clinical Practice

1. Discuss how the health care facility's environment affects your patient.
2. Using correct technique, make an unoccupied and an occupied bed.
3. Explain, according to your facility's procedures, how to clean up a biohazard spill.
4. Discuss your clinical facility's response plan to a bioterrorism threat.
5. Given an emergency scenario, practice triaging the victims.
6. Correctly apply a vest protective device.

Skills

Skill 20-1	Making an Unoccupied Bed
Skill 20-2	Making an Occupied Bed
Skill 20-3	Applying a Protective Device

Key Terms

Be sure to check out the bonus material on the Companion CD-ROM, including selected audio pronunciations.

acute radiation sickness (ARS) (p. 327)
biohazard (BĪ-ō-hă-zărd, p. 326)
bioterrorism (p. 326)
environment (ĕn-VĪ-rŏn-mĕnt, p. 315)
humidity (hū-MĬ-dĭ-tē, p. 315)
poison (p. 328)
ventilation (p. 315)

The **environment** is the total of all elements and conditions that surround us and influence our development. Caring for the patient's environment is important in providing holistic care. The goal is to provide safety while making the patient as comfortable as possible. This chapter presents information on the factors that are controllable in a patient's environment, beds and bed making, how to provide a safe environment, and when and how to apply a protective device.

FACTORS AFFECTING THE ENVIRONMENT

The same environmental factors Florence Nightingale wrote about over a century and a half ago are still important today. Temperature, ventilation, humidity, lighting, odor, and noise all are items that must be controlled.

TEMPERATURE

Infants and older adults may need their rooms warmer than usual because of their poor temperature regulation. Keep room temperature between 68° and 74° F (20° and 23° C). Operating rooms and critical care areas are kept slightly cooler to reduce the patient's metabolic demands.

VENTILATION

Ventilation is the process or act of supplying a building or room continuously with fresh air. Most health care facilities have central air-conditioning units that regulate temperature, humidity, and air exchange. Fans are discouraged because air currents spread microorganisms. A table fan may be ordered if the patient has a respiratory condition because the patient may find it easier to breathe when air movement is felt. To maintain patient safety, do not open windows in the hospital. At home, windows may be opened at the top and bottom to encourage air circulation.

HUMIDITY

Humidity is the amount of moisture in the air. A range from 30% to 50% is normally comfortable. Very low humidity will dry respiratory passages and a person's skin. Most hospitals maintain a low humidity setting to discourage the growth of microorganisms. Vaporizers or humidifiers may be ordered for a patient with a respiratory condition who requires more humidity.

LIGHTING

A sunny, cheerful room can improve a patient's spirits. Areas must have adequate lighting for tasks and to prevent accidents and injury. The light should be bright enough to see without glare and to avoid eyestrain, and be soft and diffuse to prevent sharp shadows. Ideally, your patient will be able to control the lights independently. Appropriate interior and exterior lighting in the home helps protect it against crime.

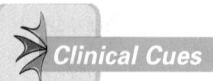

At night when the patient is sleeping, use a flashlight to provide very low diffuse light to check the patient without disturbing her. The flashlight is used to check fluid levels in drainage containers, amount of intravenous (IV) fluid remaining, and the like.

ODOR CONTROL

Illness changes sensory perceptions. Odors that ordinarily are pleasant may make the patient feel nauseated. Health care facilities may have unpleasant odors from bedpans, urinals, wounds, and so forth. Good ventilation and cleanliness will effectively control odors. Box 20-1 lists odor control measures.

| Box 20-1 | *Odor Control* |

- Reduce offensive odors by emptying and rinsing the bedpan, bedside commode, urinal, and emesis basin promptly. Change soiled linens as soon as possible.
- Dispose of used dressings, catheters, urine bags, tubing, intravenous bags, and other disposable equipment by placing in a closed plastic bag according to Standard Precautions guidelines and facility procedure. Dispose of them in the dirty or soiled utility room. **Nothing that could become odorous should be thrown in the patient's unit trash can.**
- Avoid being the source of odors yourself. Odors that linger include cigarette smoke; strong foods, such as onions or garlic; and perspiration or body odors. Eliminate these by bathing, using deodorant, and wearing clean clothes. **Perfumes, scented lotions, or scented cosmetics should not be worn in a patient care setting.**
- Remove old, disintegrating flowers and stagnant water promptly.
- Consult with your patient before using a room deodorizer or spray. These items can help control lingering odors, but your patient may be allergic or sensitive to the deodorizer itself. You might offend the patient if you spray a deodorizer throughout the room without asking permission first.

NOISE CONTROL

Noise is inevitable in health care facilities. The hospital should be a place for rest and quiet, yet a patient may experience sensory overload from all of the noise.

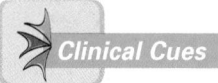

If not contraindicated, the patient who is disturbed by noise during sleep might try using foam earplugs to mask the noise. They will not prevent a patient from hearing a fire alarm and can be very helpful for a restful night's sleep.

Moving equipment in the halls, visitors, and health care personnel all combine to raise the sound level. Sound-absorbing flooring and ceiling materials, carpeting, and plastic equipment are used to reduce noise. The main cause of noise is people. To reduce noise, avoid long conversations on the intercom by going to the patient's room to talk. Encourage staff to limit conversations in the hallway and to speak in lowered voices. Tact is very important when dealing with patients, their visitors, and colleagues. Soft, pleasant background music may be played to mask other sounds and promote relaxation.

? *Think Critically About . . .* your patient's roommate has the television on very loud and your patient is unable to get any rest. What would you do to help your patient?

INTERIOR DESIGN

Patients' rooms and public areas often look more like a hotel now as opposed to the stark white of the past. Rooms have draperies and colorful bedspreads. These changes are to promote comfort by providing a homelike environment for the patient.

NEATNESS

It is important to provide a neat and tidy atmosphere for your patient. Keep the unit in enough order to be safe, but not so rigid that the patient may not have possessions from home. **Straighten the patient unit after making the bed. Old dishes and unused equipment should be removed promptly.** The over-the-bed table should be cleared, and wiped off if needed, before meals are served. Obtain the patient's permission before disposing of newspapers or magazines. Check and straighten the unit each time you enter and as time permits.

PRIVACY

Privacy is essential for a patient's well-being. Always knock gently and identify yourself before entering the room. In multiple-patient rooms, close the curtain around the patient for personal tasks such as using a bedpan and bathing. Post a sign on the door informing others of such tasks to discourage them from entering the room.

PATIENT UNIT

Each patient unit contains a bed, bedside cabinet, over-the-bed table, chair, call light, and closet (Figure 20-1). The unit usually has an over-the-bed light and a television and/or radio.

BEDS

A hospital mattress is usually firm and has a covering that can be cleansed easily between patients. An overlay (air or gel filled) may be used with a mattress to reduce the risk of pressure ulcers, but newer hospital mattresses are designed to reduce pressure areas. Beds used for health care are usually on wheels and equipped with side rails. The patient may use the rails to change position or to get out of bed. Side rails can be a safety hazard. You need to make sure that the mattress fits snugly to the rails and that the rails are close enough together so that the patient's head is not able to fit through the rails. **Always check to make sure the bed wheels are locked, unless you are moving the bed.**

BED POSITIONS

Most hospitals have electric beds, on which the position is changed with controls on the side rails. Other facilities use manual beds, on which the position is changed by the use of a crank (Home Care Considerations 20-1). The bed is usually kept in the "low position" (i.e., close to the floor). The bed can be placed in various positions (Figure 20-2).

BED MAKING

Bed rest may be an important part of the treatment for your patient. Most patients may be out of bed for short periods of time as they recover. An unoccupied bed is

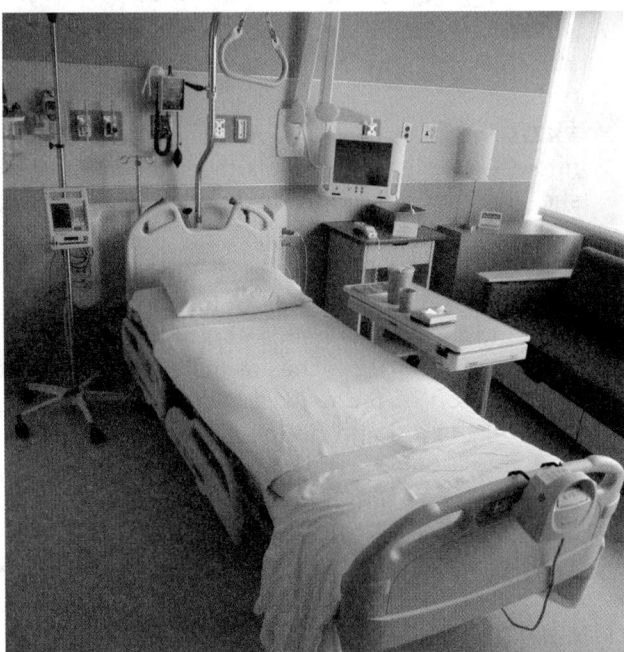

FIGURE **20-1** Common articles found in a patient unit: a hospital bed, bedside table, over-the-bed table, and chair.

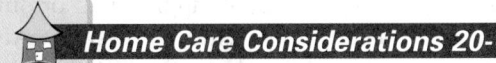

Home Care Considerations 20-1

Home Bed Safety Rail

A small-handle side rail or transfer rail may be purchased for a regular bed at home. This rail is attached to a large board that is placed under the mattress. The weight of the patient and mattress secures the rail, which the patient uses to adjust position or get in or out of bed.

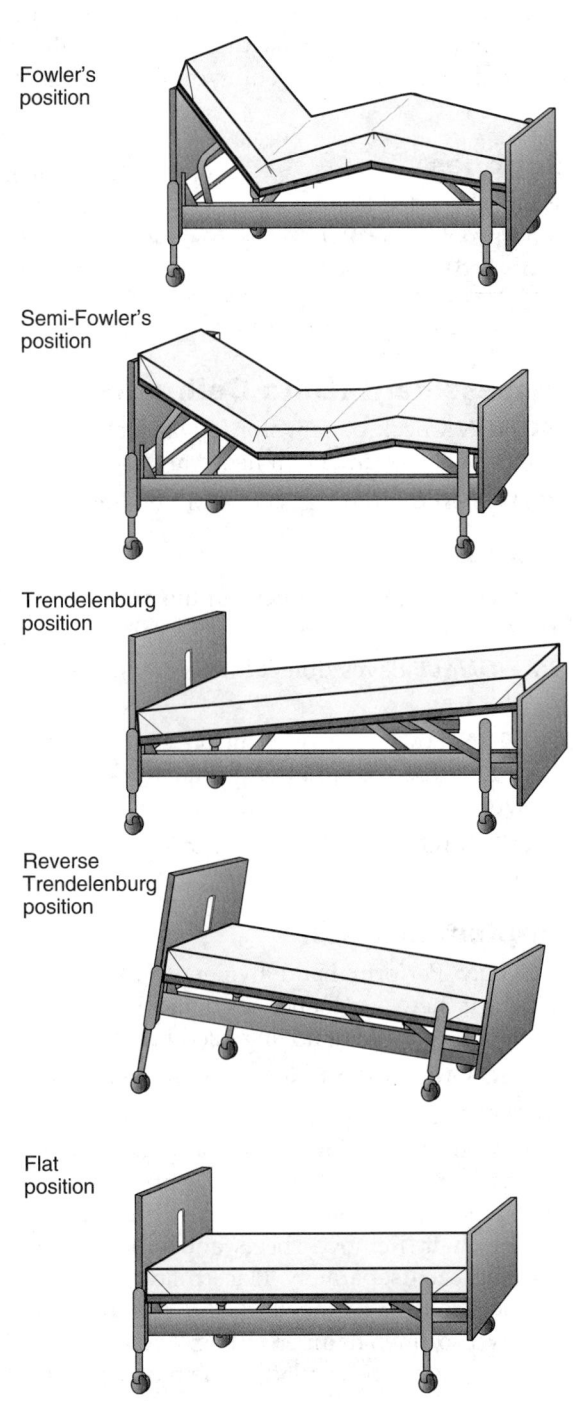

Fowler's position

Semi-Fowler's position

Trendelenburg position

Reverse Trendelenburg position

Flat position

FIGURE **20-2** Hospital beds can be adjusted to different positions.

made when the patient is out of bed in the chair or out of the room for a diagnostic procedure or therapy. **An occupied bed is made only if the patient absolutely cannot be out of bed.** For example, a patient whose activity order is bed rest with bathroom privileges would have the bed made while she is using the bathroom. Skill 20-1 and Skill 20-2 describe how to make an unoccupied and an occupied bed, respectively. Bed linens should be neat, orderly, and free of wrinkles. Linens that are rumpled may interfere with movement or cause the patient to fall when getting out of bed. Some important guidelines for making any bed are listed in Box 20-2 on p. 323.

Skill 20-1 | Making an Unoccupied Bed

Today, most beds are made when they are unoccupied. Many patients may be out of bed for the length of time it takes to make the bed. If the patient is allowed out of bed, make the bed at that time to reduce the work for both you and the patient.

■ Supplies
✓ Straight or fitted bottom sheet
✓ Waterproof underpad (if needed)
✓ Drawsheet or lift sheet (if needed)
✓ Top sheet
✓ Pillows (1 or more)
✓ Linen bag or hamper
✓ Spread and/or blanket
✓ Pillowcases (1 or more)

Review and carry out the Standard Steps in Appendix 3.

■ Assessment (Data Collection)
1. **ACTION** Check patient's orders and ability to be out of bed. Obtain help if necessary.

   RATIONALE Promotes safety for you and patient.

■ Planning
2. **ACTION** Arrange the linens in the order in which they will be used.

   RATIONALE Saves time if linens are in correct order for use.

3. **ACTION** Lower the side rail on your side of the bed. Raise bed to an appropriate working height for you.

   RATIONALE Provides easy access to materials. Prevents back strain and injury.

■ Implementation
4. **ACTION** Perform hand hygiene and don clean gloves if there is a chance of contact with blood or body fluids while removing used linen.

   RATIONALE Prevents spread of microorganisms.

5. **ACTION** Loosen all linens on your side of the bed. Go to other side, lower that rail, and loosen the linens from the head to the foot of the bed. Fold bedspread if not soiled; place over the back of patient's chair. Remove sheets and pillowcases, removing each separately. Place pillows on a clean surface, roll linens together, and put them in the pillowcase, linen hamper, or bag. Avoid shaking or fanning the linens or placing them on the floor.

   RATIONALE Loosening permits linens to be removed easily; bedspread and pillows are ready to be replaced. If a linen hamper or bag is not available, place the soiled linen in the pillowcase. Place on the foot of the bed or over-the-bed table to prevent spread of microorganisms.

Make the Bed on One Side
6. **ACTION** Check the mattress. Clean if soiled. Move mattress to the head of the bed if needed by grasping it in the center and at the bottom edge while facing the head of the bed and slide it up.

   RATIONALE Mattress is cleaned before making the bed. Mattresses tend to move to the foot of the bed when the head of the bed is raised.

7. **ACTION** Make the bed on one side at a time. Place all center folds in the linens at the center of the bed.

   RATIONALE Decreases the number of steps for the nurse. Centering linens puts the same amount of sheet on both sides of the bed.

8. **ACTION** Place and center the bottom sheet on the mattress. Unfold the sheet right side out so that the wide hem end is at the top of the mattress and the narrow hem end is at the foot of the bed. Tuck about 12 inches of the sheet smoothly over the top of the mattress. If a fitted sheet is used, fit the top and bottom corners of the mattress into it on your side.

   RATIONALE Secures sheet snugly to the head of the bed and evenly distributes linens.

9. **ACTION** Miter the corner at the head of the bed by picking up the side edge of the sheet so that it forms a triangle with the head of the bed, with the side edge perpendicular to the bed. Using the palm of your hand, hold the sheet against the side

of the mattress and tuck excess under mattress. Drop the sheet over your hand; then withdraw your hand and tuck the flap of the sheet under the mattress.

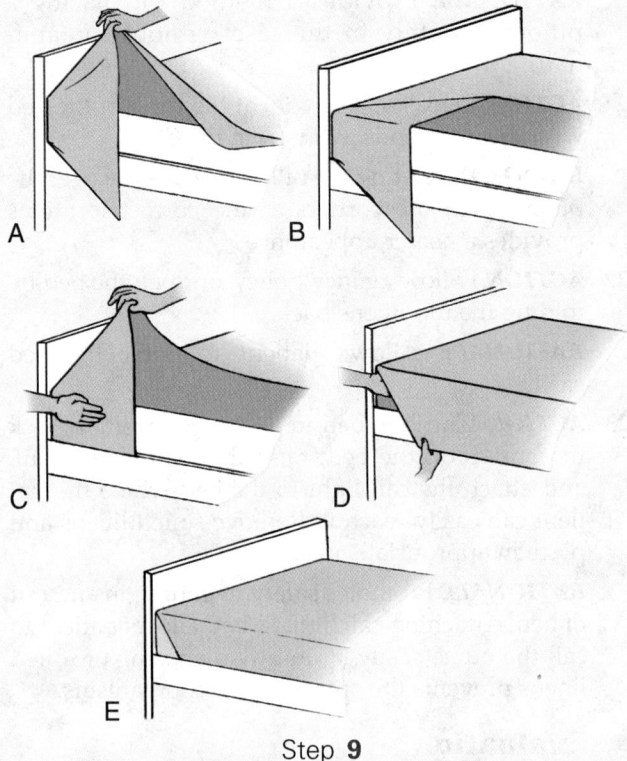

Step **9**

RATIONALE Holds the corners in place.

10. **ACTION** Position the drawsheet or lift sheet (if used) over the middle of the bed. Unfold and tuck both sheets in, on this side, from head to foot. If a lift sheet is used, do not tuck it under the mattress.

    RATIONALE Protects the bottom linens from soiling by placing the drawsheet from the patient's shoulders to below the hips. A lift sheet aids in repositioning the patient.

11. **ACTION** Place upper edge of the top sheet at the top of the mattress, seam (bottom) side up, and unfold it toward the foot of the bed.

    RATIONALE Placing top sheet seam side up avoids irritation from the seam when a cuff is formed over the spread.

12. **ACTION** Position the blanket or spread 4 inches from the top of the mattress, and unfold it toward the foot. Repeat for extra blankets.

    RATIONALE Allows sheet to be cuffed over top covers.

13. **ACTION** Tuck the sheet, blankets, and spread under the bottom of the mattress as one unit if a toe pleat is not needed. Miter the corner by lifting the top linens away from the mattress and up onto the bed about 18 inches from the bottom of the bed. A triangle should be formed. Tuck excess linens hanging below mattress level under it, bring down

the upper portion of the linens, and smooth them into a neat diagonal line.

RATIONALE Secures the linens under mattress. Top covers are not tucked under down the sides of the mattress to allow the patient to get in and out of bed easily.

Make the Bed on the Other Side

14. **ACTION** Fan-fold the top linen back toward the center of the bed while tucking in the bottom sheet and drawsheet. Miter the corner.

    RATIONALE Folding the top linen back allows you to see any wrinkles and remedy them. Mitering holds bottom sheet in place.

15. **ACTION** Grasp the edges of the bottom sheet tightly in both hands with the knuckles on top. Pull tightly down over the side; tuck under the mattress along the side, working down the side from head to foot. Pull the sheet diagonally at the bottom corner of the mattress to remove wrinkles.

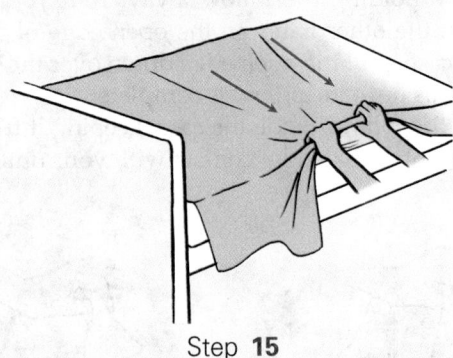

Step **15**

RATIONALE Provides a smooth bottom sheet without wrinkles that may cause pressure areas.

16. **ACTION** Grasp drawsheet (if used); pull tightly and tuck it in over the side of the mattress. If this is to be used as a lift sheet, do not tuck it under the mattress.

    RATIONALE Saves time because a lift sheet is used often.

17. **ACTION** Smooth top linens from the head to the foot of the bed if a toe pleat is not needed. Fold sheet, blanket, and spread under the mattress at the foot of the bed as one unit. Miter the corner of the top linens.

    RATIONALE Provides patient with a wrinkle-free bed.

18. **ACTION** Make toe pleats as indicated. Two examples of toe pleats:

    a. At the center of the top linens, at the foot of the bed, make a 6-inch lengthwise pleat in the top linens before tucking the covers under the mattress.

Continued

Skill 20-1 | Making an Unoccupied Bed—cont'd

b. Fold a 2-inch horizontal pleat, 6 to 8 inches from the foot of the bed, across the top linens before tucking the covers under the mattress.

RATIONALE Allows room for the patient's feet to move and prevents formation of pressure ulcers from the weight of the linens on the toes.

19. *ACTION* Move to the head of the bed and fold back the top sheet, forming a cuff 4 to 6 inches over the edge of the blanket and spread.

RATIONALE Provides a smooth edge under patient's chin and prevents soiling of blanket and spread.

20. *ACTION* Apply the pillowcase by grasping the closed end of the pillowcase and, with the other hand, gather one side of the open pillowcase up over the hand at the closed end. Grasp the pillow at the center of one end through the pillowcase while holding the pillow away from your body. With the other hand on the open edge of the pillowcase, pull the open edge down over the pillow. Do this until the pillow is completely covered. Adjust the pillow inside the case, keeping it from being contaminated by contact with your uniform.

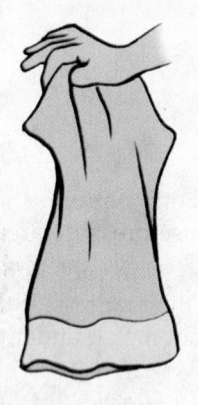
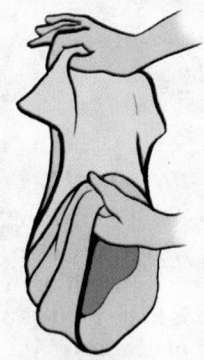
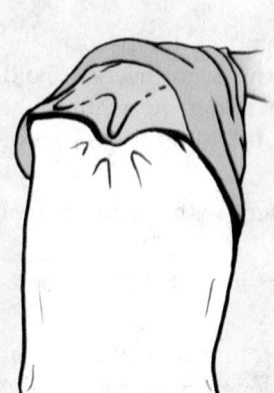
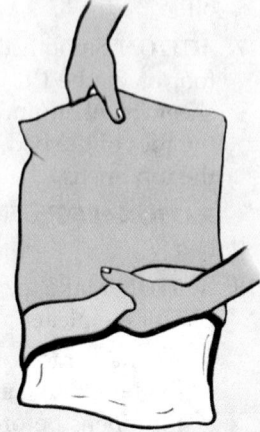

Step **20**

RATIONALE Provides a method for placing a pillow smoothly in the case without contaminating it.

21. *ACTION* Place the pillow(s) at the head of the bed with the open ends away from the door.

RATIONALE Fitting the pillowcase evenly over the pillow with the corners at the correct locations provides a neater appearance.

22. *ACTION* Follow agency policy, or open the bed by folding the top linens back.

RATIONALE Allows patient to enter the bed easily.

23. *ACTION* Place the bed in its lowest position, lock the brakes on the bed, raise the far top side rail, and attach the call light to the bed where the patient can easily reach it. Remove soiled linens and place in appropriate area.

RATIONALE Promotes safety in getting in and out of bed. Attaching call light to bed allows patient to call the nurse easily. Promptly disposing of soiled linens prevents the spread of microorganisms.

■ Evaluation

24. *ACTION* Assess the patient's area. Is the bed neat, smooth, and wrinkle-free? Is everything within easy reach of the patient? Is the unit straight and orderly? Is the bed in the lowest locked position?

RATIONALE Promotes safety. Patient does not have to reach for items.

■ Documentation

25. *ACTION* Document linen change if required by agency policy.

RATIONALE Validates that the procedure was performed.

Documentation Example

4/19 0800   Patient out of bed in chair. Linens changed, bed locked and in low position, call light within reach.

_____
(Nurse's signature)

?CRITICAL THINKING QUESTIONS

1. Why is it inadvisable to gather linen needed for two or three rooms and then carry it all around to deliver to the rooms at the beginning of the shift?

2. Why is it a good idea to pull the old linens apart and separate them if they are bunched up, before rolling them together to take off the bed and put into the linen hamper?

Skill 20-2 | Making an Occupied Bed

Linens are changed with the patient in bed if bed rest has been ordered. The procedure is easier and quicker when carried out by two people. Nursing research has shown that many patients experience greater benefit from getting out of bed than remaining on total bed rest. Hence, fewer beds are now made as occupied beds.

■ Supplies

✓ Bath blanket

✓ Bath supplies (if combining with a bed bath)

✓ Linens (as listed in Skill 20-1)

Review and carry out the Standard Steps in Appendix 3.

■ Assessment (Data Collection)

1. **ACTION** Check patient's orders to ensure patient is not allowed out of bed. Obtain help if necessary.

   RATIONALE Ensures medical plan will be followed. Promotes safety.

■ Planning

2. **ACTION** Arrange the linens in the order in which they will be used.

   RATIONALE Saves time.

3. **ACTION** Make sure the bed is locked and lower the side rail on your side. The other rail should be raised. Raise the bed to an appropriate working height.

   RATIONALE Prevents back strain and injury.

■ Implementation

4. **ACTION** Perform hand hygiene and don clean gloves if there is a chance of contact with blood or body fluids during procedure.

   RATIONALE Prevents spread of microorganisms.

5. **ACTION** Loosen the blanket and spread from the foot of the bed, and remove each piece separately. If unsoiled, fold and place item over the back of patient's chair. Place any soiled linens in the soiled linen or hamper bag.

   RATIONALE Placing unsoiled items over back chair saves time by readying linens to be replaced.

6. **ACTION** Place a bath blanket over the patient and the top sheet, unfold it, and ask the patient to hold the top, or tuck under the patient's shoulders. Remove the top sheet from beneath the bath blanket, and place in linen hamper or bag.

   RATIONALE Provides warmth and privacy.

7. **ACTION** Move the mattress to the head of the bed. Patient may help by grasping the headboard and pulling if able, or have another staff member help you.

RATIONALE Allows more room for the feet at the end of the bed.

8. **ACTION** Move the patient into a side-lying position at the far side of the bed, facing away from you. Assist the patient into proper alignment. Place a pillow under the head and at the patient's back to keep the patient in place if necessary.

   RATIONALE Provides safety. Allows near side of bed to be made.

9. **ACTION** Loosen the bottom linens from the top and side of the bed; roll each piece of linen as close to the patient as possible.

   a. Smooth the mattress cover (if present), and put the bottom sheet on the bed with the center fold at the center of the mattress. Fan-fold the portion of the sheet that is for the other side of the bed with the center fold at the center of the mattress.

   b. Push the folded linen under the rolled, soiled bottom sheets that are being removed. Tuck the near side of the bottom sheet under the head of the mattress, and miter the corner. Tuck the sheet under the mattress from the head to the foot of the bed.

   RATIONALE Allows soiled linens to be removed and clean linens to be placed when the patient rolls to the other side of the bed.

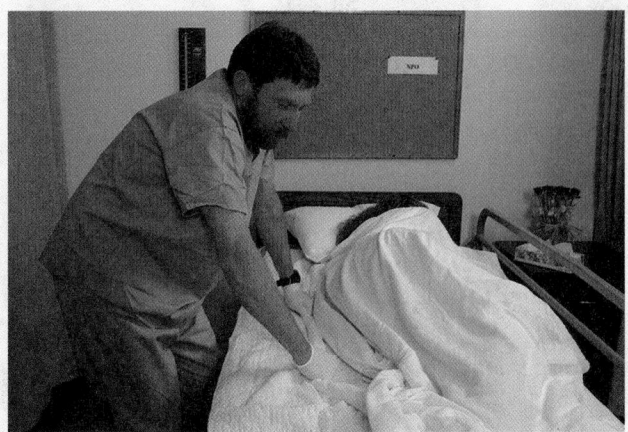

Step **9A**

Continued

Skill 20-2 | Making an Occupied Bed—cont'd

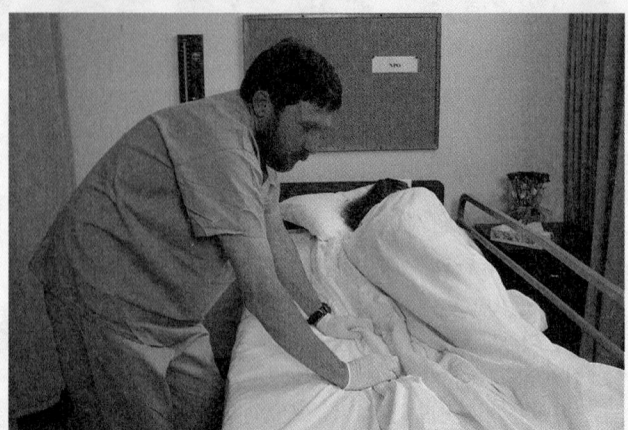

Step **9B**

10. **ACTION** Place the drawsheet on the bed (optional), centering it on the mattress so that it reaches from the patient's shoulders to below the hips. Fan-fold the far side of the sheet, and push it under the rolled bottom sheets. Tuck the near side under the mattress. Raise the side rail.

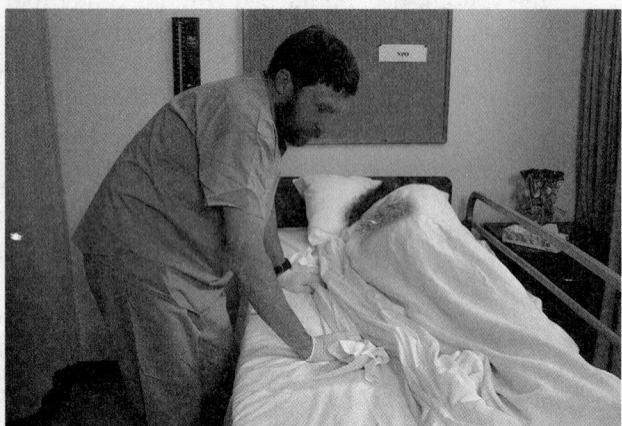

Step **10**

RATIONALE Allows removal of a soiled drawsheet when the patient is turned.

11. **ACTION** Go to the other side of the bed, lower that rail, and move the patient to the far side of the bed. If the patient can turn easily, ask the patient to roll to the opposite side. Adjust the patient's alignment, and reposition the bath blanket. Ask the patient to grab the raised side rail for support.

RATIONALE Allows removal of soiled linens and placement of clean linens. Raised rail provides safety.

12. **ACTION** Loosen the bottom linens and roll them up. Place in the linen hamper or bag, or in the used pillowcase.

RATIONALE Prevents the spread of microorganisms.

13. **ACTION** If a mattress cover is used, smooth out any wrinkles. Pull the bottom sheet across the mattress, fold over the top of the mattress and smooth, tighten, tuck the excess sheet under the mattress, and miter the corner.

RATIONALE Prevents wrinkles that may cause pressure ulcers.

14. **ACTION** Pull the drawsheet from the center of the bed; to pull tightly, place your knee against the mattress while pulling. Tighten, smooth, and tuck sheets under the side of the mattress from head to foot.

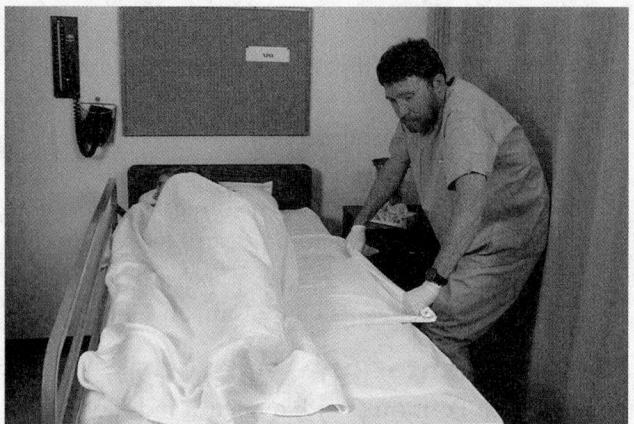

Step **14**

RATIONALE Protects the bottom sheet from soiling.

15. **ACTION** Allow the patient to roll onto back. Place the top sheet over the patient and the bath blanket with the top edge folded down a few inches beneath the chin. Have the patient hold the top of the sheet and remove the bath blanket. Position the blanket (if used) and spread in the same manner. Smooth the top linens and tuck the excess at the foot under the bottom of the mattress if a toe pleat is not needed. Miter the corner on the near side, then far side. Fold the top edge of the sheet over the blanket, and spread to form a cuff.

RATIONALE Keeps the patient warm and protects privacy while the top linens are placed.

16. **ACTION** Make a toe pleat in the top sheet and blanket if desired as described in Skill 20-1, Step 18.

RATIONALE Provides extra room for the feet.

17. **ACTION** Remove the used pillowcase and place in the linen hamper or bag. Apply the clean pillowcase

by grasping the closed end of the case in one hand and gathering one side from the open end up over the other hand. Grasp the pillow at the center of one end through the pillowcase while holding the pillow away from your body. Smooth the pillowcase down over the pillow. Place beneath the patient's head with the open end away from the door.

RATIONALE Places pillow in the case without contaminating it. Fitting the pillowcase evenly over the pillow with the corners at the correct locations provides a neater appearance.

18. *ACTION* Lower the bed, lock the brakes on the bed,, replace call light, and restore the unit. Remove the linen hamper or bag and place in appropriate area.

RATIONALE Provides safety for the patient and a method to call the nurse. Promptly disposing of soiled linens helps prevent the spread of microorganisms.

■ Evaluation

19. *ACTION* Assess the patient's area. Are the linens neat, smooth, and wrinkle-free? Is the unit restored?

RATIONALE Restoring the unit promotes safety because the patient does not have to reach for items.

■ Documentation

20. *ACTION* Document linen change on the flow sheet or in the nurse's notes, depending on agency policy.

RATIONALE Validates the completion of the procedure.

Documentation Example

10/15 0900   Linens changed on occupied bed, which is in a locked, low position.

_____
(Nurse's signature)

■ Special Considerations

✓ If the patient is in traction, the bed may have to be made from the top to the bottom (head of bed to foot of bed), instead of side to side. The same principles are applied from top to bottom. The patient may use the trapeze bar if able to help lift as you work the sheets down the bed.

✓ Linens should be smoothed, with wrinkles removed, whenever the patient is turned.

Home Care Considerations

• For the home care patient, a large plastic bag can be used crosswise under the hip area to protect the mattress from soiling. It is placed beneath the mattress pad to prevent any discomfort to the patient.

?CRITICAL THINKING QUESTIONS

1. For work efficiency, is it better to work with a colleague, helping him make occupied beds and then having him help you, or to make your occupied beds on your own?

2. When a patient is to be on bed rest, how can you sometimes make the bed when she is not in it?

Box 20-2 | *Guidelines for Bed Making*

• Use good body alignment, a wide base of support, and a proper working height when making the bed. Face the direction of movement and bend at the knees, not the back.

• Complete the linen change on one side before moving to the other side to save time and conserve energy.

• Avoid contaminating clean linen. Once linens enter a unit, they are exposed to that patient's microorganisms and must not be returned to the clean supply or used elsewhere.

• Unfold linens onto the bed. Do not flip or fan linens, to avoid stirring up air currents. Microorganisms travel on air currents and could be carried out of the unit.

• Remove linens one piece at a time to avoid wrapping dentures, eyeglasses, religious objects, or other patient belongings in soiled linens.

• Do not place used or soiled linen from one patient on the bed, table, or chairs belonging to another patient's unit.

• Carry used or soiled linens away from the body and place them in closed linen hampers or bags. Use a pillowcase if a linen bag is not available, and transport it to the linen hamper or chute. **Do not place soiled linens on the floor.**

SAFETY

Safety is a primary concern when caring for your patients. Safety is needed to prevent accidents and possible injuries to patients, visitors, and health care personnel. Methods of meeting the following 2009

National Patient Safety Goals from The Joint Commission are presented in the appropriate chapters of this text:

• Improve the accuracy of patient identification

• Improve the effectiveness of communication among caregivers.

- Standardize a list of abbreviations, acronyms, symbols and dose designations that are not to be used throughout the organization.
- Measure and assess, and if appropriate, take action to improve the timeline of reporting, and the timeliness of receipt by the responsible licensed caregiver, of critical test results and values.
- Reduce the risk of health care–associated infections.
- Accurately and completely reconcile medications across the continuum of care.
- Reduce the risk of patient harm resulting from falls Encourage patients' active involvement in their own care as a patient safety strategy.
- The organization identifies safety risks inherent in its patient population.

The most common accidents among patients are falls, burns, cuts, and bruises. Fights with others, loss of personal possessions, choking, and electrical shock also occur. Home safety is another issue you will need to discuss with your patients. You must be aware of possible safety hazards and correct them to prevent accidents. Box 20-3 describes nursing actions to promote patient safety.

HAZARDS
Falls

Falls are a safety hazard. The three most common factors that predispose a person to falls are impaired physical mobility, altered mental status, and sensory and/or motor deficits. The Joint Commission 2008 safety goals require that every patient be assessed and periodically reassessed for risk for falling, particularly correlating the patient's medications with increased risk for falls. Action must be taken to mitigate any identified risk. An example of a fall risk assessment tool is presented in Figure 20-3. Chapter 40 provides safety tips to prevent the elderly from falling in the home. Patients at risk for falls may have a leg or bed alarm placed. These alarms sense a change in position or pressure and

---

Box 20-3 | *Nursing Actions to Promote Patient Safety*

IN A HEALTH CARE FACILITY
- Orient the patient and family when admitted to the room with regard to operation of call bell system, bed, television, and radio. Check to be sure the patient can operate the controls.
- On admission, assess the patient's gait and risk for falling. If needed, have the patient call for help to get up.
- Evaluate the patient's drug regimen for side effects that may increase the risk of falling (i.e., those that affect the central nervous system or cause orthostatic hypotension, dizziness, or drowsiness).
- Keep the bed in the low position if not giving direct care.
- Put mattress onto the floor or a low platform, if there is a high risk for a fall and the patient does not ask for help.
- **Toilet the patient on a regular schedule to decrease the chance the patient will try to get out of bed unassisted.**
- Lock the bed wheels to prevent the bed from rolling when the patient attempts to get in or out.
- Provide a night-light to aid patients in going to the bathroom at night, to decrease disorientation, and to prevent bumping into furniture.
- Encourage the use of firm, nonskid slippers to prevent slipping while walking.
- Answer call lights quickly so that the patient learns to trust you and does not feel the need to get up without help.
- Tell the patient when you will next check in, and be prompt.
- Be sure the patient is comfortable and all desired items and call bell are in easy reach before you leave the room.
- Encourage use of grab bars for the toilet, tub, and shower.
- Place the high-risk or restless patient in a room close to the nurses' station so you may check on the patient often.

- Stay with the patient who is confused, agitated, or unsteady whenever the patient is up.
- Restrict fluids after 6 P.M. if a patient is up at night frequently to empty the bladder and has a history of injury when out of bed.
- Provide diversionary and social activities that confused and restless patients might enjoy. Seating patients confined to a wheelchair close to the nurses' station often provides enough stimulation to occupy their thoughts and reduce their need to wander.
- Be sure wheelchair brakes are locked before transferring a patient into or out of it.

IN THE HOME
- Place a nonskid bath mat in the tub and shower.
- Use night-lights for moving from the bedroom to the bathroom at night.
- Suggest the installation of grab bars for the bathroom by both the toilet and bathtub/shower.
- Install door buzzers or bed alarms that sound when the patient leaves the bed or opens an outside door.
- Keep the furniture arrangement and position of personal items constant to decrease confusion and eliminate the need to hunt for items.
- Maintain sufficient activity during the day to prevent too much napping, which can lead to nighttime wandering.
- Encourage removal of extension cords because these may cause a fall.
- Caution the patient that toys and animals may also cause falls. Removing an animal from the home because of risk of a fall must be carefully weighed against the social and emotional importance of the companionship a pet provides.
- Inform the patient and the family that hospital beds may be obtained or rented for home use. Provide appropriate community resources as indicated.

Fall Risk Assessment

Place a check mark in front of the items that apply to the patient.

General Information
____ Age over 70
____ History of falls*
____ Confusion at times
____ Confused most of the time*
____ Impaired memory or judgment
____ Unable to follow directions*
____ Needs assistance with elimination
____ Visual impairment
____ Feels physically weak*

Medications
____ Receiving central nervous system suppressants (narcotic, sedative, tranquilizer, hypnotic, antidepressant, psychotropic, anticonvulsant)
____ Receiving medication that causes orthostatic hypotension (antihypertensive, diuretic)*
____ Medication that may cause diarrhea (cathartic)
____ Medication that may alter blood glucose levels (insulin, hypoglycemics)

Gait and Balance
____ Poor balance when standing*
____ Balance problems when walking*
____ Swaying, lurching, or slapping gait*
____ Unstable when making turns*
____ Needs assistive device (walker, cane, holds on to furniture)*

Note: A check mark on any starred item indicates a risk for falls. A combination of four or more of the unstarred items indicates a risk for falls.

FIGURE **20-3** Fall risk assessment tool.

sound an alarm to alert health care workers or family members that patients are attempting to get out of bed or a chair (Figure 20-4) (Resnick, 2004).

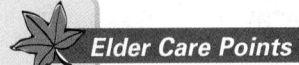
Elder Care Points

Falls are the most frequent cause of injury for the elderly patient in an acute care facility.

Burns

Burn prevention includes protecting the patient from accidental thermal injury and the threat of fire. Thermal injuries may be caused by either hot or cold materials. A person with diabetes or impaired circulation,

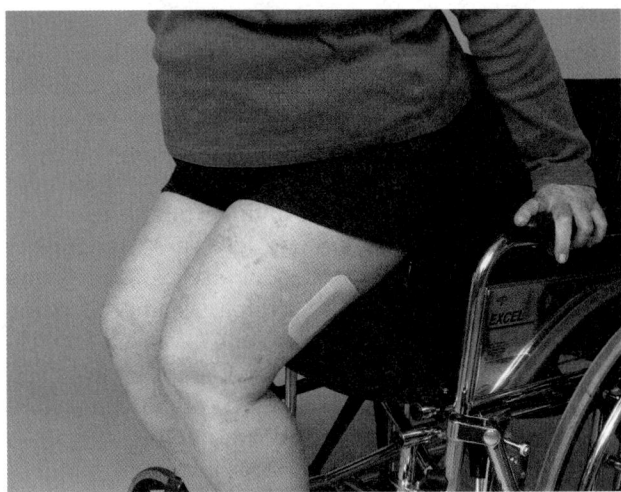
FIGURE **20-4** Leg alarm.

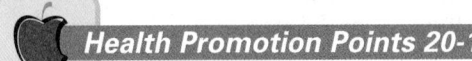
Health Promotion Points 20-1

Smoking Cessation

Patients and residents of long-term care facilities who smoke should be given information on how to quit smoking. Smoking causes damage to the lungs, blood vessels, etc., and decreases the oxygen-carrying capacity of the blood. Positive reinforcement for efforts to quit smoking is very important.

or who is paralyzed or on drugs that alter mental awareness, is more easily burned than a person in good health. To prevent these injuries, use a barrier between the patient's skin and the thermal application. Check the temperature of oral liquids before giving them to the patient. Warn the patient if a food or drink is hot. Caution the patient to avoid lying on, or sleeping with, heating pads or ice packs. Inspect electrical cords for frayed or broken areas that may cause sparks or fires. The engineering staff must check all electrical appliances brought into the hospital from home before use to ensure safety.

Smoking

Smoking is banned in most health care facilities; however, some long-term care agencies allow smoking in designated areas. Carefully supervise the patient who wants to smoke and is sedated, confused, or irrational. Warn your patient not to smoke in bed. **Smoking is never allowed when oxygen is in use because a spark could cause a fire.** Any equipment that might cause a spark is also prohibited near oxygen. Inform your patient who uses oxygen at home, and the family, of this risk.

Reducing tobacco use is one of the leading health indicators of *Healthy People 2010*. Second-hand smoke relates to another goal of *Healthy People 2010*, that of environmental air quality. Encourage your patients not to smoke (Health Promotion Points 20-1) (Duke Center for Nicotine and Smoking Cessation Research, 2007).

Fire

Fire is a possibility in any setting. **You must know and be familiar with your institution's fire regulations.** This includes knowing the location of the fire extinguishers, fire alarms, and escape routes, and how to notify the telephone operator of a fire in your area.

There are three basic types of fire extinguishers: A, B, and C. Type A is a water-under-pressure extinguisher that is used for paper, wood, or cloth fires. Type B contains carbon dioxide and is used for gasoline, oil, paint, fat, and flammable liquid fires. Type C is used for electrical fires and contains carbon dioxide. The most commonly seen extinguisher is an ABC combination extinguisher that can be used on any kind of fire.

Most agencies use the *RACE* acronym to respond to a fire because it is easy to remember. Should a fire occur, you must

- **R**escue any patients in immediate danger by removing them from the area.
- **A**ctivate the fire alarm system.
- **C**ontain the fire by closing doors and any open windows.
- **E**xtinguish the flames with an appropriate extinguisher.

Use proper body mechanics to evacuate patients to prevent injury. Protect against possible smoke inhalation by placing wet towels across the bottom of closed doors and have people hold wet washcloths over their noses and mouths. This traps most of the smoke in the washcloth during breathing. Box 20-4 lists home fire safety precautions.

? *Think Critically About* . . . Why do facilities schedule announced and unannounced fire drills?

HAZARDOUS MATERIALS
Biohazards

A biohazard is a biologic agent, chemical, or condition that can be harmful to a person's health. The Occupational Safety and Health Administration (OSHA) classifies materials in the work environment according to the degree of hazard to health that they impose. OSHA publishes specific guidelines for labeling, handling, cleaning spills, and disposing of these materials. Mercury is an example of a biohazard, as are blood and most body fluids. There should be a material safety data sheet (MSDS) for each biohazard substance stored or used on the nursing unit. These sheets are consulted for recommended methods of storage, labeling, handling spills, and disposal. Everyone must comply with these guidelines.

Bioterrorism and Other Terrorism Agents

Terrorist activities are designed to cause panic, fear, and chaos and disrupt an area's rescue and medical systems. Bioterrorism is the release of pathogenic

Box 20-4 *Fire Safety in the Home*

- Make sure there are two clear exits from each room and everyone knows and has practiced using the escape routes.
- Install smoke detectors on each level of your home.
- Never smoke in bed. Use sturdy, nonspill ashtrays. Check furniture for any smoldering cigarette butts after parties.
- Identify your house with large, easily seen address numbers for the fire department.
- Store matches, lighters, and flammable liquids out of the reach of children. Paints, thinners, and other flammable liquids should be stored in their original containers, away from heat, sparks, or flame. **Never store gasoline or propane inside the home.**
- Never leave cooking food unattended. Keep cooking areas clear of combustible materials.
- Keep your attic free from combustibles such as magazines and newspapers.
- Chimneys and central heating systems should be inspected at least once per year and cleaned if necessary.
- Never overload electrical circuits or bypass fuses or circuit breakers. Do not run extension cords under furniture or carpets, or across doorways.
- Use portable space heaters with care.
- Do not allow smoking in a home where oxygen is in use.

microorganisms into a community to achieve political and/or military goals. Common diseases, symptoms, and incubation periods for agents used in bioterrorism are listed in Table 20-1. It is important to know the early signs and symptoms of these agents because many of them initially present as vague or flulike symptoms.

Chemical terrorism is the use of certain compounds to cause destruction to achieve political and/or military goals. Health care agencies and institutions have developed plans and methods to handle these threats to safety. Chemical agents come in liquid, gas, and solid forms. Temperature and pressure can affect the form of the chemical agents. There are several types of chemical threats, including pulmonary agents, cyanide agents, nerve agents, vesicants, and incapacitating agents. Table 20-2 lists the agents used in the different kinds of chemical threats and the symptoms associated with each type.

Radiation is a form of energy that can come from man-made sources as well as the sun and outer space. Some elements that release radiation exist naturally in the soil, such as uranium. Plutonium, which is used in nuclear power plants, is also used to make nuclear bombs. Terrorists may use radioactive substances attached to an explosive device (a "dirty bomb") to disperse radiation. There are three basic ways to protect the body from radiation: time (decrease the amount of time near a source), distance (increase your distance from a source), and shielding (increase the barrier or shield between you and the source). Acute radiation sickness (ARS) develops when most or all of the body is exposed to a high dose of radiation usually over a short period of time. Initial symptoms of ARS are nausea, vomiting, and diarrhea. Loss of appetite, fatigue, fever, skin damage, hair loss, and potentially seizures, coma, and death are possible later effects.

You must be familiar with your institution's policies and procedures for handling victims of a terrorist attack. Knowing how to respond to terrorist attacks with various agents will help prepare you should a crisis happen in your area. Being prepared will help to alleviate your anxiety and increase your confidence in dealing with such unpredictable instances. In turn,

Table 20-1 | *Common Diseases Spread Through Bioterrorism*

BIOLOGIC AGENTS USED AS WEAPONS	SYMPTOMS	INCUBATION PERIOD (DAYS)
Anthrax	Flulike symptoms that improve, then respiratory and circulatory collapse occurs; chest x-ray shows widened mediastinum caused by thoracic edema; skin lesions involve vesicles with a black eschar center and enlarged adjacent lymph nodes.	1-45
Botulism	Difficulty speaking and swallowing, blurred or double vision; respiratory distress, descending muscular paralysis. *Note:* Inhaled form has no gastrointestinal symptoms.	1-5
Ebola virus *(Filovirus)*	Abrupt onset of fever, headache, muscle pain, gastrointestinal upset, maculopapular rash on the trunk, petechiae, and progressive bleeding.	4-10
Lassa fever (arenavirus)	Fever, retrosternal pain, tremor of tongue and hands; hearing loss.	7-16
Plague	Fever, mucopurulent sputum, chest pain, hemoptysis, purpura.	2-3
Ricin (cytotoxin from castor beans)	Acute onset of fever, chest tightness, cough, dyspnea, nausea, and arthralgias. Pulmonary edema occurs within 18-24 hr. Death occurs in 36-72 hr.	4-8 hr
Smallpox	Chickenpox-like lesions starting on the face and extremities, with progression from one stage of the lesions to the next *together.*	12 (average)
Tularemia	Fever, pneumonia, nonproductive cough, periorbital edema.	3-5

Modified from Leifer, G. (2007). *Introduction to Maternity & Pediatric Nursing* (5th ed., p. 723). Philadelphia: Elsevier Saunders, and *Medical Management of Biological Casualities Handbook* (2001). U.S. Army Medical Research Institute of Infectious Diseases.

Table 20-2 | *Types, Symptoms, and Effects of Chemical Weapons*

TYPE	EXAMPLES	SYMPTOMS	EFFECTS
Pulmonary agents	Phosgene (CG) Diphosgene (DP) Chloropicrin (PS) Chlorine (CL)	Irritate eyes and tracheobronchial tree. Tears, coughing, and chest discomfort. May appear minor at first but gets worse to include dyspnea and tachypnea.	Damages alveolar-capillary membranes during inhalation. Can result in pulmonary edema.
Cyanide agents	Hydrogen cyanide (AC) Cyanogen chloride (CK)	Odor of bitter almonds on the breath is a classic sign but may not be detected. Severe respiratory distress in an acyanotic person. Skin coloring may be cherry red, cyanotic, or normal. Irritation of eyes, nose, and airways.	Cyanide prevents intracellular oxygenation. Exposure to high concentrations can lead to death in 6-8 min. Severe exposure may result in asystole.
Nerve agents	Tabun (GA) Sarin (GB) Soman (GD) GF VX	Pupil constriction, red eyes, reduced vision, airway constriction, uncontrolled rhinorrhea, salivation, tearing, and sweating. Uncontrolled secretions in the gastrointestinal and respiratory tracts as well. May lead to convulsions, paralysis, and death.	Most toxic of the known chemical agents. Major effects seen in skeletal and smooth muscles.
Vesicants	Sulfur mustard (H, HD) Lewisite (L) Phosgene oxime (CX; not technically a vesicant but it causes skin lesions, so is included in this category because it has similar effects)	Irritate exposed skin and membranes. Mustard is the only one that does not cause immediate symptoms, but it can cause tissue damage within several minutes without burning or redness. Typical onset for all agents is 4-8 hr.	Cause blisters or vesicles, which is how this type gets its name. They also damage the eyes through direct contact and airways if inhaled. These agents are deadlier than pulmonary agents or cyanide.
Incapacitating agents	BZ	Range of usual onset is 30 min to 4 hr. May see paranoia to full-blown delirium and periods of deep sleep that have clawing or climbing movements. Person at risk of hyperthermia and injury from own random movements.	Designed to impair, not kill, victims through hallucinations, illusions, and nausea and vomiting. In most cases do not cause death.

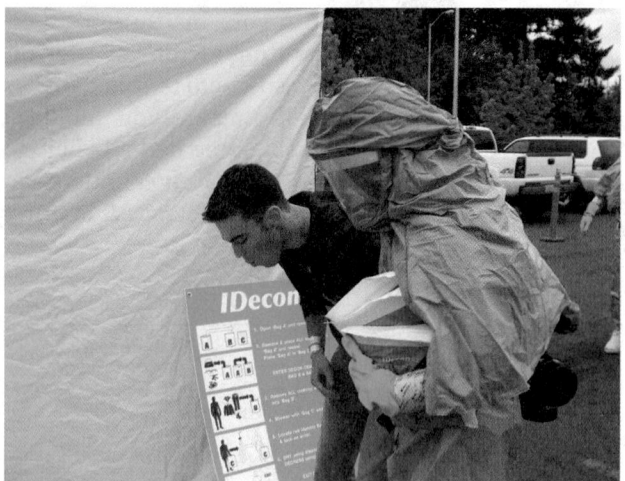

FIGURE **20-5** Biohazard suits worn by personnel assisting victims (drill at Southwestern Medical Center, Vancouver, WA.)

this will help you manage your patients' fears and give more effective care.

Decontamination. When a terrorist attack has occurred, such as the one with Sarin gas in the Tokyo subway, a portable decontamination unit with a specially trained staff is set up outside the emergency room (ER). The staff must wear masks and protective clothing that are impervious to chemicals and cover *all* skin surfaces (Figure 20-5). Military Mission-Oriented Protective Posture (MOPP) suits may be used that have a hooded pullover top, drawstring trousers, rubber boots, and gloves. A chemical mask with filtered respirator must be worn with the suit. There is an emergency protocol from the local health department's disaster response plan that is followed to decontaminate victims before they enter the hospital building. Thorough scrubbing of the all of the person's skin is often part of the protocol.

Triage and Treatment. Patients are triaged as they enter the ER. They are assessed and labeled according to the priority of care as "immediate," "delayed," "minimal," or "expectant." Patients who require lifesaving care are labeled "immediate"; care for those in need of major or prolonged care can be "delayed" briefly; those with minor injuries to be attended are labeled "minimal"; and "expectant" indicates those with severe life-threatening injuries who probably will not survive in spite of medical care. Triage priorities are based on the premise that limited medical resources should be used on those patients who will most likely live if they receive treatment.

Treatment is based on the type of agent to which the patient was exposed and the degree of exposure. Antibiotics are used for some of the biologic agents, and antidotes may be used for some of the chemicals and poisonous gases (Center for the Study of Bioterrorism & Emerging Infections, 2001). Otherwise, treatment is directed at supporting organ function while the body tries to recover. Life support measures using drugs, ventilators, and dialysis, if needed, are used.

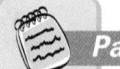 *Patient Teaching 20-1*

Poison Prevention

All patients should be taught the following safety precautions:

- Never call medicine "candy." Store all medicines in childproof containers.
- Keep toxic substances in a locked cabinet or closet out of the reach of children. Label with poison stickers.
- Always keep toxic substances in their original labeled container. Never put toxic substances in beverage or food containers.
- Obtain the poison control center number from your local operator. Keep it near the telephone so you do not need to search for it in an emergency.
- Never induce vomiting unless instructed by a professional. Depending upon the type of poison (e.g., lye, gasoline, grease, or some cleaning and petroleum products), vomiting may cause more damage.
- Keep syrup of ipecac on hand to induce vomiting if so directed. Vinegar or lemon juice may be recommended for use with alkaline substances. Milk may be suggested to counteract acid substances.
- It is important to note that older adults may obtain prescription medications in bottles that are not childproof. If they have young grandchildren or other visitors, these items should be kept out of reach or, safer still, in a locked cabinet.

Poison

A **poison** is a substance that when ingested, inhaled, absorbed, applied, injected, or developed within the body, may cause functional or structural disturbances. This is possible even if only a very small amount of the poison is encountered. Agents used in chemical terrorism fit into this category. Treatments and antidotes for poisoning can be obtained from a poison control center or are listed on some containers. **Some poisons do not have antidotes or treatments.** When reporting a known or suspected poisoning, have the label handy. Report the following:

- Name of the product
- Patient's age
- Amount you believe is involved
- Any symptoms and/or complaints you observe

Patient Teaching 20-1 lists information for patient teaching about poisons.

PROTECTIVE DEVICES

Protective devices, formerly called restraints, were overused in the past. Restricting movement on a long-term basis caused problems such as muscle weakness, atrophy, loss of bone mass, joint contractures, constipation, incontinence, pressure ulcers, depression, and cognitive impairment. The patient's self-concept and mood were negatively affected, and both the patient and family were affected emotionally. Some staff used these devices as a way to punish or discipline a patient. **This is an illegal and totally unacceptable practice that constitutes malpractice.**

Restraints are used in two types of situations, for behavioral or nonbehavioral indications. A protective device is used for a behavioral health reason if the patient is in a psychiatric setting or has demonstrated a sudden change in mental status/behavior. Nonbehavioral usage is for the continuation of medical treatments. An instance of a nonbehavioral use would be an elderly person with a history of dementia who needs to have her IV site protected from attempts to dislodge the catheter. Health care workers must check patients in a behavioral health protective device more frequently. The array and use of physical and chemical protective devices (i.e., medication) in psychiatric/behavioral health settings are not covered in this text. **It is your responsibility to be aware of and follow the regulations in your facility and area.**

LEGAL IMPLICATIONS OF USING PROTECTIVE DEVICES

Federal and local laws have been passed that protect the patient from physical and mental abuse and from physical and chemical restraints except those that are authorized by a physician, in writing, for a specified and limited period of time, or that are needed in an emergency situation. The devices must be applied by licensed, qualified personnel.

The Joint Commission supports the use of protective devices if clinically necessary, but only as a last resort. This text has described the use of side rails of a bed as a way to increase a patient's independence in changing position or getting in or out of bed. However, in some situations and facilities, especially long-term care, full side rails are considered restraints because they limit a patient's ability to move, whereas half-rails are not.

ALTERNATIVES TO PROTECTIVE DEVICES

The goal is to move to a less restrictive environment. Health care workers are encouraged to find alternatives to the use of protective devices (University of Iowa College of Nursing, 1996). Many of the actions described in Box 20-3 involve frequent observations of the patient, which helps prevent patient injury and decrease the use of the devices. Family and friends of a patient who is confused can be encouraged to sit with the patient to promote safety.

PRINCIPLES RELATED TO THE USE OF PROTECTIVE DEVICES

Box 20-5 lists five principles related to the use of protective devices. In general, the device must be of direct benefit to the patient.

Box 20-5 | ***Principles Related to the Use of Protective Devices***

- The use of protective devices must help the patient or be needed for the continuation of medical therapy.
- Use the least amount of immobilization needed for the situation.
- For all devices that limit movement or immobilize the patient, there must be a written order. As soon as the device is no longer needed, the physician must be notified.
- Apply the device snugly but not so tightly as to interfere with blood circulation or nerve function.
- The device must be removed and the patient's position changed at least every 2 hours. Active or passive exercises are performed for immobilized joints and muscles.

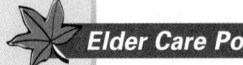 **Elder Care Points**

Older adults may be more confused in unfamiliar surroundings such as an acute care facility. Have family members bring in items from home that are familiar, such as photographs, a quilt, and so forth, to help older adults feel more comfortable. Frequently reorient them as to where they are and the time of day to reduce the need for a protective device.

For example, a patient who is confused may try to pull out a nasogastric tube. In order to continue medical treatment, it may be decided to place the patient's hand in a hand mitten. If this does not prevent the patient from pulling out the nasogastric tube, then a wrist or extremity device may be ordered. This situation illustrates the second principle. This patient did not require a vest or jacket device to prevent the dislodgement of the nasogastric tube.

Usually, the order must be written before applying a device. In an emergency, some agencies permit a device to be applied without a written order. You must obtain a written order as soon as possible (Communication Cues 20-1). When the protective device is no longer needed, obtain an order to discontinue it. The order usually specifies the type of device and how long it may be used (usually time-limited to no more than 24 hours depending on the patient's age).

When applying the protective device, make certain that the patient's movements or tugging will not impair circulation or nerve function. Padding the device with a soft washcloth or gauze pads will prevent skin irritation. The device should fit snugly when applied, but should not compromise the patient's neurovascular status. **You should be able to easily fit your index and middle fingers between the patient and the device.** A device that is secured too tightly may cause injury. Skill 20-3 describes how to apply different protective devices.

Communication Cues 20-1

Explaining the Need for a Protective Device

The situation below shows how a caregiver can explain the need for using a protective device to a family member.

Helen Klein is a 68-year-old patient in your unit. She was admitted for a right total hip replacement and has a history of Alzheimer's disease. Two hours ago, Mrs. Klein. returned to the unit postoperatively. Because of her diagnosis of Alzheimer's disease, you have placed her in a room near the nurses' station. Mrs. Klein is very confused, and only oriented to person. Shortly after she returned to the unit, her family went to dinner. You have tried repeatedly to orient her while her family is at dinner. You are now exiting the room after finding that Mrs. Klein was trying to get out of bed and has removed her dressing, drain, and IV line. You see her daughter coming down the hall. The daughter asks you, "How is my mother? Is she resting?"

NURSE: Your mother is fine, she is awake. May I talk with you for a minute?

MS. KLEIN: Sure.

(You should find a quiet, private place, out of Mrs. Klein's hearing, to talk with the daughter.)

NURSE: Ms. Klein, although your mother is stable, being in the hospital and changing her routine has added to your mother's confusion. While you were at dinner, she removed her dressing, drain, and IV line and was trying to get out of bed. We already have her in a room close to

the nurses' station so that we can check on her more frequently. Is it possible for you or another family member to spend the night with her?

MS. KLEIN: Why would you want me to do that? I did not think family members could stay with patients.

NURSE: For some patients, it is safer and they rest better if someone they are familiar with remains. This helps to keep the patient oriented and calm. If this is not possible, we may need to use a protective vest for your mother so that she does not get out of bed.

MS. KLEIN: You mean tie her down to the bed? That is cruel.

NURSE: A protective vest is secured to the bed, but it is not meant to be cruel. The purpose is to keep your mother safe. I do not want her to fall and endanger her new hip or suffer another injury.

MS. KLEIN: I see what you mean. I will talk with my brothers and sisters and see if one of us can spend the night with her. If we are with her, will she need to be tied down?

NURSE: It has been my experience that when a family member stays, the patient rests and remains in bed, so no, we would only use the vest if it is necessary to protect your mother.

Skill 20-3 | Applying a Protective Device

A protective device is used only after all alternative methods have been tried. Each type of device has its own purpose or main uses. A security or safety belt is used for the patient who is at a high risk for falls, or to secure a patient to a stretcher. A vest or jacket is used to assist a patient in maintaining proper body alignment when in a sitting position or to remind the patient not to get out of bed. An extremity immobilizer is used to prevent disruption to dressings, skin grafts, intravenous (IV) lines, urinary catheters, nasogastric tubes, and so forth. A mitten or hand mitt is used to keep the patient from scratching, to limit the ability to grasp tubes and catheters, or to prevent the patient from grasping the ties on a limb immobilizer.

■ Supplies
✓ Protective devices
✓ Belt
✓ Vest
✓ Extremity immobilizer
✓ Mitten or hand mitt
✓ Soap, washcloth, towel, and lotion

Review and carry out the Standard Steps in Appendix 3.

■ Assessment (Data Collection)

1. **ACTION** Assess whether all other possible measures have been used to resolve the safety problem and whether they have been effective.

   RATIONALE Ensures all possible methods of ensuring patient safety have been tried before using a protective device.

2. **ACTION** Check to see if there is an order for a protective device; if not, obtain one.

   RATIONALE Use of a protective device requires a written order.

3. **ACTION** Review your agency's policy and procedure for use.

   RATIONALE Keeps your practice within legal parameters.

4. **ACTION** Assess the skin and circulation in the area where the device will be applied.

   RATIONALE Provides baseline data prior to the application of the device.

■ Planning

5. *ACTION* Review manufacturer's instructions about the application of the device and obtain help if necessary.

RATIONALE Promotes correct usage and safety for you and patient.

■ Implementation

6. *ACTION* Explain the purpose and need for the device to the patient and family.

RATIONALE Decreases anxiety of patient and family.

7. *ACTION* Lock brakes on wheelchair or bed before proceeding.

RATIONALE Promotes safe application.

8. *ACTION* Apply the device and tie with a half-bow knot.

RATIONALE A half-bow knot fastens the device, yet can be easily and quickly untied by you in an emergency.

For Security or Safety Belt

9. *ACTION* With the patient sitting in a wheelchair, place the security belt around the waist or upper legs and slip one end of the tie through the slit on the opposite side.

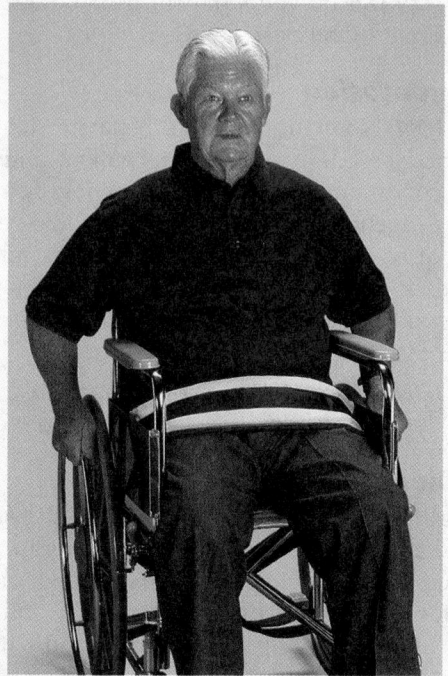

Step **9**

RATIONALE Secures belt to patient before it is attached to chair.

10. *ACTION* Bring both ends under the armrests and behind the chair (one on each side) and tie to the frame or fasten the buckle, if present.

RATIONALE Prevents patient from untying the protective device.

For Vest or Jacket Device

11. *ACTION* Place the vest on the patient, putting arms through the armholes, with the opening in the front (most are labeled for front and back).

RATIONALE Decreases the chance of choking if the patient slumps while wearing the vest. Promotes lung expansion.

12. *ACTION* Cross the straps in the front, slipping strap of underlapping side through the slit in the opposite overlapping side of the vest. Tie outside of the patient's reach, to the bed frame or the back of the chair.

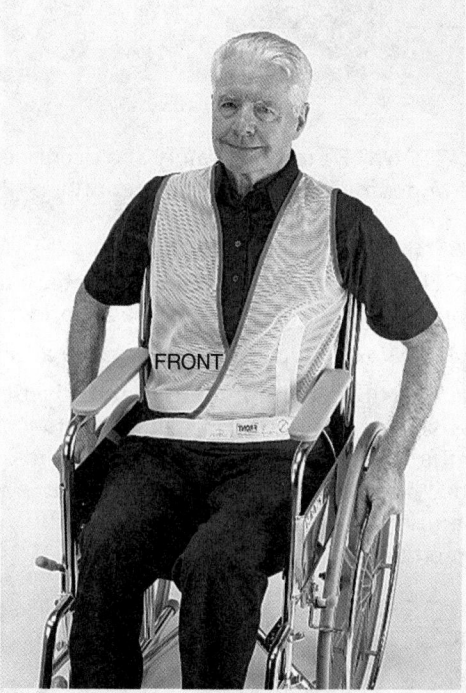

Step **12**

RATIONALE Promotes safety and prevents choking if patient slips down in bed or chair.

For Extremity Immobilizers

13. *ACTION* Wash and dry the patient's wrist(s) or ankle(s); apply lotion and massage areas.

RATIONALE Prepares patient for the application.

Continued

Skill 20-3 | Applying a Protective Device—cont'd

14. **ACTION** Apply immobilizer to the extremity needed—wrap the padded end around the wrist or ankle; pull the tie through the slit or buckle, or fasten with Velcro and attach to the bed frame.

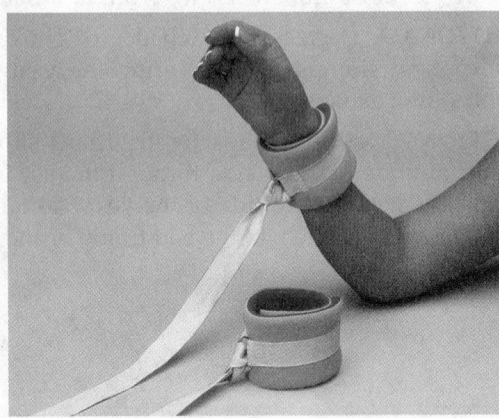

Step **14**

RATIONALE Promotes safety and decreases chance of impeding circulation of extremity.

For Mitten or Hand Mitt

15. **ACTION** Wash and dry the patient's hand thoroughly; apply lotion and massage hands.

    RATIONALE Prepares patient for the application.

16. **ACTION** Slip hand into mitt, and slip tie around wrist and secure. It is usually better to apply mitts to both hands so that the devices are not easily removed by patient. If patient is partially paralyzed, use only one mitt on the nonparalyzed hand.

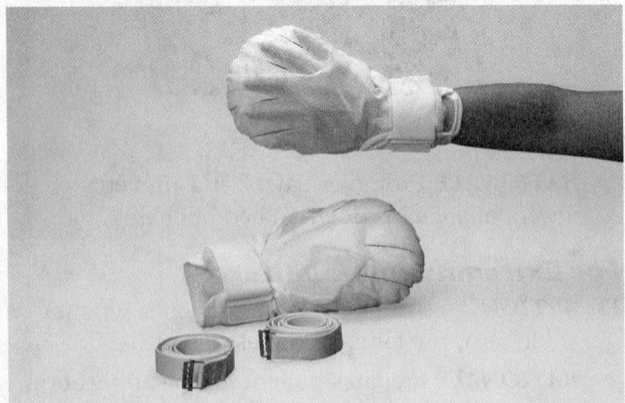

Step **16**

RATIONALE Promotes safety and prevents using fingers to pull out tubes and IV lines.

Evaluation

17. **ACTION** Check on the patient at least every 15 to 30 minutes or as directed by your agency and observe neurovascular function and patient's position and needs.

    RATIONALE Monitors patient for problems with the device and positioning and prevents patient's needs from going unmet.

18. **ACTION** At least every 2 hours (or according to agency policy), release the ties, change the patient's position, supervise active or provide passive range-of-motion (ROM) exercise, and assess the condition of the skin under the device. Remove only one device at a time.

    RATIONALE Provides safety while preventing joint stiffness and muscle aches.

19. **ACTION** Provide access to a call bell or other method to summon the nurse.

    RATIONALE Provides safety and makes patient feel less isolated.

20. **ACTION** Assess for the continued need for the device.

    RATIONALE Prevents patient from being in a device longer than necessary.

Documentation

21. **ACTION** Note the patient's behavior, alternative methods tried, explanation to patient and family, and condition of skin before applying device. Ongoing documentation includes periodic reevaluation of need for device, skin condition, pulses, patient's tolerance of device, times the restraints are removed and then reapplied, and the time when the device is removed and discontinued.

    RATIONALE Validates the need for the use of a device and that the device is being used correctly.

Documentation Examples

10/15 1400 Oriented to person only, thrashing in bed, and unable to understand directions to prevent dislodgement of IV line. Physician notified, order obtained for right wrist protective device, and device applied. Skin intact; fingers warm, dry, and with quick capillary refill. Call bell within reach.

_____
(Nurse's signature)

10/15 1600 Right wrist immobilizer removed and reapplied. Skin remains intact; passive ROM to R arm, wrist, and fingers. Sensation intact; no evidence of circulation impairment.

_____
(Nurse's signature)

■ Special Considerations

Home Care Considerations

You must consider the family or caregivers when
- Assessing their ability to stay with the patient attentively in effort to avoid the use of protective devices.
- Instructing them on interventions to try before using protective devices.
- Developing a written schedule for removal of the device, skin care, and exercise.
- Providing a documentation tool to track actual removal of the device and care given.
- Informing them of whom to notify should any abnormality be found.

?CRITICAL THINKING QUESTIONS

1. What would you do if your patient has wrist restraints ordered and there is an IV in the right wrist area?
2. What can happen if a restraint is too tight and circulation is impaired in an extremity?

Secure the ties of a protective device to an immovable part of the bed frame. Do not tie to the side rails because lowering the rails may cause the device to be pulled too tightly around the patient or cause strain on a joint of an immobilized extremity. Place the ties under the armrests of a chair and secure at the back to prevent the patient from sliding. This also prevents the patient from being able to slide the tie up and off the back of the chair.

Use a half-bow knot to secure the device to the bed frame or chair. It is a secure knot that will not slip, even if the patient tugs on the tie; however, it is easily undone by health care workers. A half-bow knot is similar to that used when tying shoes except only one loop is made (Figure 20-6).

Remove the device at least every 2 hours and perform active or passive range-of-motion exercises for immobilized joints and muscles. Moving joints, exercising muscles, and changing positions frequently help prevent complications. Use supportive pillows and pads to maintain position. Check the area distal to the device every 15 to 30 minutes. Observe for signs of adequate circulation, including pulses distal to the device. Signs that the circulation or nerve function has been impaired include coolness of the skin, change in color (particularly pallor or a bluish hue), numbness, pain, edema, and loss of sensation or movement. Remove the device immediately and contact the physician if any of these signs occurs.

?_Think Critically About . . ._ Your confused patient keeps getting out of her wheelchair. What would you try to keep her in the chair? If that does not work, what safety device do you think you would use?

DOCUMENTATION OF THE USE OF PROTECTIVE DEVICES

Objectively describe the behaviors you observed (i.e., the reason) that led you to believe there was a risk for injury. All alternative actions and methods that were tried before placing the device need to be documented. Document the time and from whom the order for the device was obtained, the type of device applied, the time of application, the name of the person applying the device, and the location of the device on the patient's body. Include the teaching done for the patient and family prior to the placement of the device. Obtain an informed consent as necessary. Document the periodic observations you make of the patient, including skin color, distal pulses, and so forth. Lastly, record the time when the device was discontinued and your name or the name of the person discontinuing the device. See Nursing Care Plan 20-1 for the care of a patient needing a protective device.

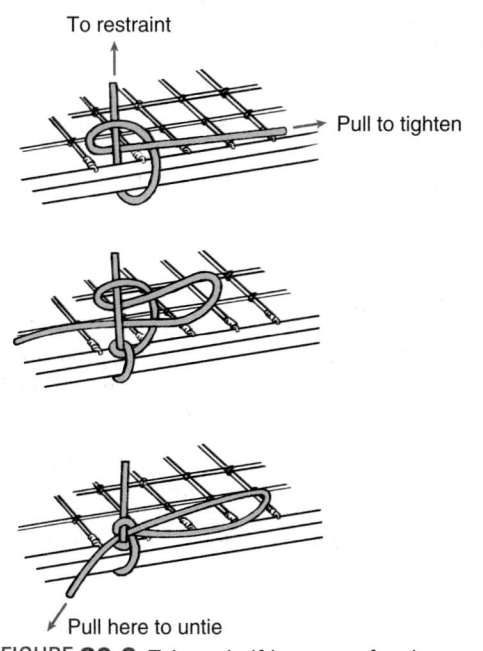

To restraint

Pull to tighten

Pull here to untie

FIGURE **20-6** Tying a half-bow or safety knot.

NURSING CARE PLAN 20-1

Care of the Patient Wearing a Protective Device

SCENARIO Hirosha Kumoto has Alzheimer's disease. She is in a room by the nurses' station. While her family was at dinner, you checked on her every 15 minutes. You tried to orient Ms. Kumoto to her surroundings. She is oriented ×1 only. Because Ms. Kumoto's family was not able to spend the night with her, it was decided to apply a safety vest.

PROBLEM/NURSING DIAGNOSIS *Patient is pulling out tubes and trying to get out of bed/Risk for injury related to* confusion and disorientation.
Supporting Assessment Data: Subjective: Asks over and over again: "Where am I? Why am I here?" *Objective*: Observed patient trying to get out of bed and climb over the side rails. Pt. removed postop dressing, drain, and IV.

Goals/Expected Outcomes	Nursing Interventions	Selected Rationales	Evaluation
No injury will be sustained during recovery period.	Assess patient's ability to follow medical regimen.	Assessment provides current information and data on patient condition.	*Has any injury been sustained?* No evidence of injury at this time.
	Try all alternative methods first, such as orienting patient, placing patient in a room by the nursing station, asking family to sit with patient PRN.	Protective devices are used only if alternative methods fail and are documented as failing.	Family member is with the patient intermittently.
	Obtain an order to apply protective device if above methods are not successful.	An order is required for any application of a protective device that restrains movements.	PRN order obtained from physician.
	Know your facility's policies and procedures before placing device.	Facilities differ on policies and procedures. You must follow your institution's rules.	
	Common practices are: • Assess skin condition before applying device.	Assessing skin condition prevents placing item over irritated uncovered area.	Skin intact without redness.
	• Assess patient every 15 to 30 min: check placement of device, patient positioning, and neurovascular status.	Frequent checks ensure patient has not untied device; device is in proper position with adequate neurovascular status.	Patient checked q 15 min. No problems noted.
	• At least every 2 hr, remove device and provide passive ROM exercises; reposition patient; reapply protective device as necessary.	Allows joint movement, helps to prevent contractures, prevents skin breakdown, and is refreshing for patient.	Repositioned and ROM provided q 2 hr.
	Continually reevaluate the need for the device. Get the order renewed q 24 hr as needed. Discontinue as soon as no longer necessary.	Devices are discontinued as soon as possible.	No fall or injury sustained. Meeting expected outcome.
Patient's family will verbalize understanding of need for the use of protective devices.	Explain to family the reasons for protective devices. Explain monitoring for safety.	When family understands that the goal is to keep family member safe, they are more likely to agree with use.	*Does the family understand?* Family verbalizes the need for using protective device when they are not present.
	Explain that all alternatives will be tried before placing protective device.	Communication helps prevent misunderstanding.	Full explanation given to family.
	Explain that the device will be removed as soon as is possible.	Reassures family that the patient will not always be restrained.	Expected outcome being met.

NURSING CARE PLAN 20-1

Care of the Patient Wearing a Protective Device—cont'd

Goals/Expected Outcomes	Nursing Interventions	Selected Rationales	Evaluation
Medically necessary devices will remain in place.	Use least restrictive protective device to ensure outcomes	Reassures family that the patient will not always be restrained.	Intravenous line and dressing remained in place. Expected outcome being met. Continue plan.

? CRITICAL THINKING QUESTIONS

1. The safety vest helps to prevent falls and maintain positioning. Would you use any other type of device for Ms. Kumoto? Why or why not? If so, what device would you consider using?

2. Does your facility offer any other alternatives to restraint use? Which policy do you feel is best? Why?

Key: *PRN*, As needed; *ROM*, range of motion.

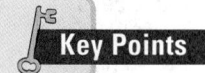

Key Points

- Many factors can be controlled in the patient's environment.
- Bright lighting is needed for performing procedures.
- Adequate night lighting is needed to prevent injury when going to the bathroom.
- The most common cause of noise pollution in a health care agency is people.
- Keep rooms neat and clean, while allowing patients to have personal items close to them.
- Privacy is important to a patient's well-being.
- A bed should be neat, clean, dry, and free from wrinkles.
- Bed making should be done, if possible, while the patient is out of bed.
- Safety is the primary concern when caring for patients.
- Falls are the most frequent cause of injury for the elderly patient in an acute care facility.

- *RACE* is the acronym for how to proceed in case of a fire.
- Know your agency's policy for cleaning up a biohazardous spill and handling bioterrorism or chemical terrorism occurrences.
- Protective devices are used only as a last resort.
- Use the least restrictive immobilizing device for the situation.
- A protective device should be applied snugly but should not impair neurovascular status.

 Go to your **Companion CD-ROM** for an Audio Glossary, animations, video clips, and more.

evolve Be sure to visit the companion Evolve site at http://evolve.elsevier.com/deWit/fundamental/ for additional online resources.

NCLEX-PN® EXAMINATION-STYLE REVIEW QUESTIONS

*Choose the **best** answer(s) for each question.*

1. Humidity in the hospital is kept between 30% and 50% for the purpose of:
   1. maintaining skin moisture.
   2. keeping the staff comfortable.
   3. humidifying the air.
   4. discouraging microbial growth.

2. In making a bed, it is important to remember: *(Select all that apply.)*
   1. to place soiled linens on the floor to avoid contaminating the bed.
   2. to unfold linens on the bed to avoid stirring up air currents.
   3. to return unused linens to the floor's clean linen area to prevent waste.
   4. to raise the bed during the linen change to prevent back strain.

3. Which of the following patients might be most likely to suffer a burn if left to tub bathe alone?
   1. An adult female who is to have abdominal surgery tomorrow
   2. An adult male who has been having back pain after a cystoscopy
   3. A patient taking drugs that alter mental awareness
   4. An alert elderly patient who prefers tub bathing

4. Which of the following would help prevent the most frequent cause of injury to the elderly patient? *(Select all that apply.)*

   1. Keeping pathways clear of papers and objects
   2. Grounding all electrical apparatuses in use
   3. Checking temperatures of fluids before serving them
   4. Providing a night-light in the bedroom and bathroom

5. If a biohazard spill occurs in the dirty utility room on your unit and you are unfamiliar with the product involved, you would first:

   1. dilute the spill with water.
   2. find the MSDS.
   3. don gloves.
   4. call a housekeeper.

6. The correct sequence of action in a fire is:

   1. call for help, activate the alarm, rescue a patient in danger, and extinguish the fire.
   2. rescue a patient in danger, activate the alarm, contain the fire, and extinguish the fire.
   3. call the hospital operator, race to close the fire doors, activate the alarm, and evacuate all patients.
   4. race to close the fire doors, activate the alarm, call the hospital operator, and evacuate all patients.

7. Which of the following findings **by itself** would indicate that a patient is at risk for falls?

   1. Age over 70
   2. Patient is receiving insulin
   3. Visual impairment
   4. Slapping gait or lurching

8. Your patient has a wrist restraint. Which of the following findings would you be concerned about?

   1. Quick capillary refill of the nail beds
   2. Skin that is warm and pink
   3. Ability to move fingers and toes
   4. Pallor of the nail beds

9. Terrorist attacks can occur from release of biologic or chemical agents or radiation. Bioterrorism is the release of _____ into a community to achieve political and/or military goals. *(Fill in the blank.)*

10. A patient immobilized by a protective device is at risk for:

    1. less attention from the staff.
    2. muscle weakness and increased bone density.
    3. constipation and impaired skin integrity.
    4. reduced capillary refill distal to the device.

CRITICAL THINKING ACTIVITIES *Read each clinical scenario and discuss the questions with your classmates.*

Scenario A
Two of your friends and fellow nursing students are talking and laughing rather loudly at the nursing station. What would you do?

Scenario B
While giving a bath to your bedridden patient, you notice smoke coming from the bathroom. What is your first action? That accomplished, how would you proceed?

Scenario C
If when, on a home care visit, you find several hazards to safety in the patient's home, how would you handle the situation?

Scenario: You notice a foul odor in your patient's room. How would you proceed?

evolve http://evolve.elsevier.com/deWit/fundamental/

Objectives

Upon completing this chapter, you should be able to:

Theory

1. Review the anatomic structures involved in the regulation of the vital signs and describe their functions.
2. Identify the physiologic mechanisms that regulate temperature, heart rate, blood pressure, and respiration.
3. List the factors that affect body temperature.
4. Discuss normal and abnormal characteristics of the pulse.
5. Describe the respiratory patterns considered to be normal and abnormal.
6. Explain the relationship of Korotkoff sounds to systolic and diastolic blood pressure.
7. State why pain is considered the fifth vital sign.

Clinical Practice

1. Measure and record the body temperature of an adult and a child at the oral, rectal, axillary, and tympanic (eardrum) sites using a glass, electronic, or tympanic thermometer.
2. Measure and record an apical pulse and a radial pulse.
3. Count and record respirations.
4. Measure and record blood pressure.
5. Use an automatic vital signs machine to monitor pulse and blood pressure.
6. Recognize deviations from normal vital sign patterns.
7. Determine factors that might be adversely affecting the patient's temperature, pulse, respiration, or blood pressure.

Skills

Skill 21-1 Measuring the Temperature with an Electronic Thermometer
Skill 21-2 Measuring the Temperature with a Tympanic or Temporal Artery Thermometer
Skill 21-3 Measuring the Radial Pulse
Skill 21-4 Measuring the Apical Pulse
Skill 21-5 Measuring Respirations
Skill 21-6 Measuring the Blood Pressure

Key Terms

Be sure to check out the bonus material on the Companion CD-ROM, including selected audio pronunciations.

apnea (ĂP-nē-ă, p. 358)
arrhythmia (ă-RĬTH-mē-ă, p. 355)
auscultation (ăw-skŭl-TĀ-shŭn, p. 359)
auscultatory gap (ăw-SKŬL-tă-tō-rē GĂP, p. 364)
axillary (ĂX-ĭ-lā-rē, p. 342)

basal metabolic rate (BMR) (BĀ-sĭl mĕ-tă-BŎ-lĭk RĀT, p. 338)
Biot's respirations (bē-ŌZ rĕ-spī-RĀ-shŭns, p. 358)
bradycardia (brăd-ē-KĂR-dē-ă, p. 353)
bradypnea (brăd-ē-PNĒ-ă, p. 358)
cardiac output (p. 339)
Cheyne-Stokes respirations (p. 358)
chills (p. 343)
core temperature (p. 342)
crackles (KRĂK-ŭlz, p. 358)
crisis (p. 344)
cyanosis (sī-ă-NŌ-sĭs, p. 357)
defervescence (dĕ-fĕr-VĔ-sĕns, p. 343)
diastolic pressure (dī-ă-STŎ-lĭk, p. 341)
dyspnea (DĬSP-nē-ă, p. 357)
eupnea (YĔWP-nē-ă, p. 357)
febrile (FĔB-rĭl, p. 343)
fever (p. 338)
hypertension (hī-pŭr-TĔN-shŭn, p. 364)
hyperthermia (hī-pŭr-THĔR-mē-ă, p. 343)
hyperventilation (p. 358)
hypotension (hī-pō-TĔN-shŭn, p. 365)
hypothermia (hī-pō-THĔR-mē-ă, p. 344)
hypoxemia (p. 358)
hypoxia (hī-PŎK-sē-ă, p. 339)
Korotkoff sounds (kŏ-RŌT-kŏf SOWNDS, p. 363)
Kussmaul's respirations (KŪS-măls rĕs-pī-RĀ-shŭnz, p. 358)
lysis (LĪ-sĭs, p. 344)
metabolism (mĕ-TĂ-bō-lĭ-sm, p. 338)
orthostatic hypotension (ŏr-thō-STĂT-ĭk hī-pō-TĔN-shŭn, p. 365)
overhydration (ō-vĕr-hī-DRĀ-shŭn, p. 341)
oximeter (ŏk-SĬM-ĕ-tĕr, p. 358)
oximetry (p. 358)
palpate (p. 351)
pulse deficit (p. 354)
pulse pressure (p. 359)
pyrexia (pī-RĔX-ē-ă, p. 339)
pyrogens (PĬ-rō-jĕnz, p. 339)
respiration (p. 340)
rhonchi (RŎNG-kī, p. 358)
shock (p. 364)
sphygmomanometer (sfĭg-mō-mă-NŎM-ĕ-tĕr, p. 359)
stertor (STĔR-tŏr, p. 358)
stethoscope (STĔTH-ō-skōp, p. 351)
stridor (STRĪ-dŏr, p. 358)
stroke volume (p. 339)
systolic pressure (sĭs-TŌL-ĭk, p. 341)
tachycardia (tăk-ē-KĂR-dē-ă, p. 353)
tachypnea (tăk-ĭp-NĒ-ă, p. 358)
tympanic membrane (tĭm-PĂN-ĭk, p. 342)
vital signs (p. 341)
wheeze (p. 358)

OVERVIEW OF STRUCTURE AND FUNCTION RELATED TO THE REGULATION OF VITAL SIGNS

How is body heat produced?

- Heat production is a by-product of metabolism (cellular chemical reactions in the body).

- When metabolism increases, more heat is produced. This is what causes fever (elevated temperature). When pathogens invade the body and the body attempts to destroy them, the increased activity (metabolism) causes fever. Pyrogens produced by some pathogens act on the body's thermostat and raise the body temperature.

- Basal metabolic rate (BMR) is the rate at which heat is produced when the body is at rest. The average BMR depends on the body surface area of the person.

What factors affect body heat production?

- Basal metabolic rate is affected by thyroid hormone. Excessive amounts of thyroid hormone cause an increase in the metabolic rate and the person feels warm; insufficient thyroid hormone results in a decreased metabolic rate and the person may feel cold.

- Other hormones that affect metabolic rate are epinephrine, norepinephrine, and testosterone. Because of their levels of testosterone, men have a higher BMR than women.

- Voluntary muscle movement of exercise increases the BMR and heat production.

- **The involuntary muscle action of shivering can increase heat production up to five times normal.**

How is body temperature regulated?

- The hypothalamus, located between the cerebral hemispheres, acts as a thermostat and controls body temperature by a feedback mechanism (Figure 21-1).

- The chemical reactions that occur in the body as it fights a pathogen cause the thermostat to reset to a higher level (a new *set point*).

- When the body heat rises above normal, the hypothalamus sends out a signal through the nervous system that causes vasodilation, sweating, and inhibition of heat production.

- If the body temperature drops below normal range, the hypothalamus sends messages for vasoconstriction of surface blood vessels to conserve heat and messages to induce shivering to increase heat production.

- Heat loss occurs through the skin's exposure to the environment. Heat loss occurs through (1) radiation, (2) conduction, (3) convection, and (4) evaporation.

- Blood flow from the internal organs carries heat to the skin. The heat is radiated to cooler objects in the vicinity of the person.

- When objects in the surroundings are warmer than the body, heat is radiated to the body and absorbed.

- When warm skin touches a cool object, heat is lost to the object by conduction. Ice bags applied to the skin increase conductive heat loss.

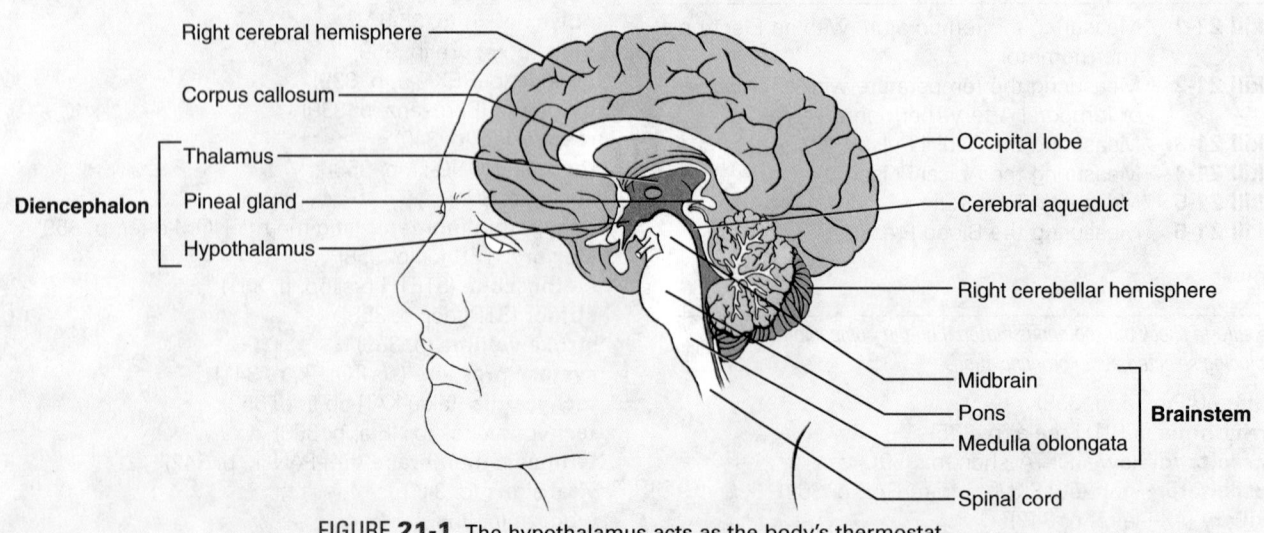

FIGURE **21-1** The hypothalamus acts as the body's thermostat.

- Air movement causes heat to be transferred from the skin to the air molecules by convection. Fast-moving air from an electric fan cools by convection. Heat loss increases when the skin is moistened and evaporation occurs.

- Sweat glands contribute to evaporative loss by secreting sweat in response to a message from the hypothalamus when the body temperature rises too high.

- As water evaporates from the skin, heat is transferred to the air. Heat is continually lost from the body by evaporation, resulting in a daily loss of 800 mL of water from the skin and lungs.

How does fever occur and what are its physiologic effects?

- Pyrexia (fever) occurs when normal mechanisms of the body cannot keep up with excessive heat production and body temperature rises. Pyrexia occurs when the body temperature rises above 100.4° F (38.0° C).

- When pyrogens (substances that cause fever) such as bacteria cause an immune response in the body, the hypothalamus is stimulated to raise the temperature set point.

- Altering the internal environment of the body and allowing the body to become hotter before triggering natural cooling mechanisms permit the body to become more hostile to the bacteria, and the immune system can more effectively destroy them. Fever also stimulates the immune system to produce substances to fight viruses.

- If the temperature rises above the new set point, the skin becomes flushed and moist.

- *Diaphoresis* is excessive sweat production, which attempts to cool the body by evaporation.

- When the metabolic rate rises and there is a greater demand for oxygen at the cellular level, fever occurs.

- Heart and respiratory rates rise in order to help the body meet the increased metabolic demand. If the oxygen demand cannot be met, *cellular* hypoxia (state of insufficient oxygen) occurs. Cerebral hypoxia may cause confusion in the individual.

What physiologic mechanisms control the pulse?

- Cardiac contractions produce the pulse. The surge of blood into the aorta causes a pressure wave that can be felt over a peripheral artery. Figure 21-2 shows the points on the body where the pulse may be felt.

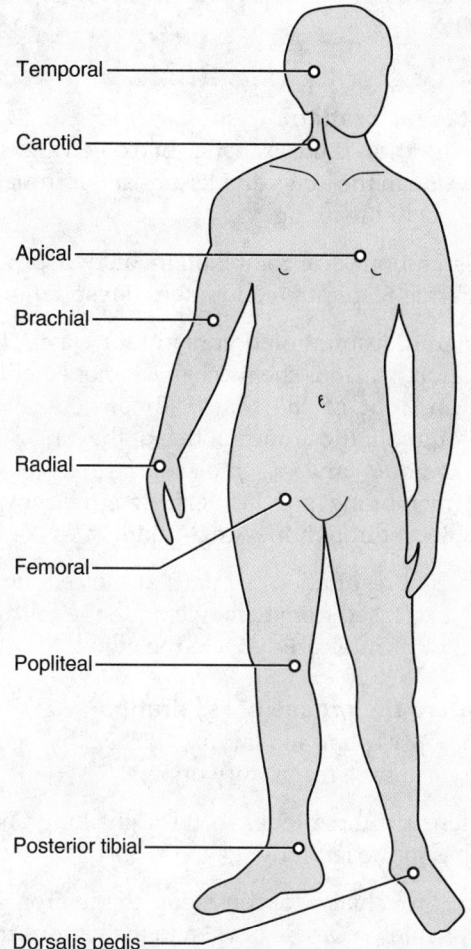

FIGURE **21-2** Pulse points.

- Cardiac contractions are normally initiated by the electrical impulse emerging from the sinoatrial (SA) node within the right atrium of the heart. If there is a problem with electrical conduction in the heart, the pulse rate is affected.

- When the heart contracts, an average of 60 to 70 mL of blood is propelled into the aorta. Stroke volume is the volume of blood pushed into the aorta per heartbeat. Stroke volume affects the character of the pulse. A weak pulse may indicate a fall in stroke volume.

- The amount of the blood circulating in the vascular system and the degree of vasodilation or vasoconstriction of the blood vessels can also affect stroke volume and the pulse.

- The pulse rate multiplied by the stroke volume equals the cardiac output. Cardiac output is the amount of blood pumped by the left ventricle in 1 minute. Average cardiac output in the adult is about 5 L of blood per minute.

Continued

OVERVIEW OF STRUCTURE AND FUNCTION RELATED TO THE REGULATION OF VITAL SIGNS—cont'd

What is respiration?

- **Respiration** is the exchange of oxygen and carbon dioxide in the lungs and tissues and is initiated by the act of breathing.

- Respiration is a combination of two processes: external respiration and internal respiration.

- External respiration occurs in four ways: (1) ventilation, which is the mechanical movement of air in and out of the lungs; (2) dispersion of air throughout the bronchial tree of the lungs; (3) diffusion of O_2 and CO_2 molecules across the alveolar membrane; and (4) perfusion, the movement of blood through the lungs and tissues.

- Internal respiration happens at the cellular level. O_2 is released from hemoglobin to the cell and the cell in turn releases CO_2 to the blood.

What are the organs of respiration?

- The nose, pharynx, larynx, trachea, bronchi, and lungs are the respiratory organs.

- There are three lobes in the right lung and two lobes in the left lung.

- The bronchial tree, consisting of the bronchi and bronchioles, carries oxygen to the various parts of the lungs (Figure 21-3).

- Movement of the diaphragm controls inhalation and exhalation. The slight negative pressure created in the chest during inspiration draws air into the lungs.

- Gas exchange with the blood occurs in the alveoli, tiny thin-walled sacs.

- Surfactant secreted by cells in the walls of the alveoli is necessary for alveoli to remain open; it reduces surface tension on the alveolar wall, allowing expansion.

How is respiration controlled?

- Breathing is an involuntary, automatic function controlled by the respiratory center located in the pons and medulla of the brainstem.

- The respiratory center works together with feedback mechanisms. The carotid body receptors in the common carotid arteries and the aortic body receptors lying adjacent to the aortic arch signal the respiratory centers to alter the rate or depth of respiration in response to decreased O_2 levels in the blood.

- Increasing levels of CO_2 and increasing hydrogen ion (H^+) concentration in the blood can activate these receptors also.

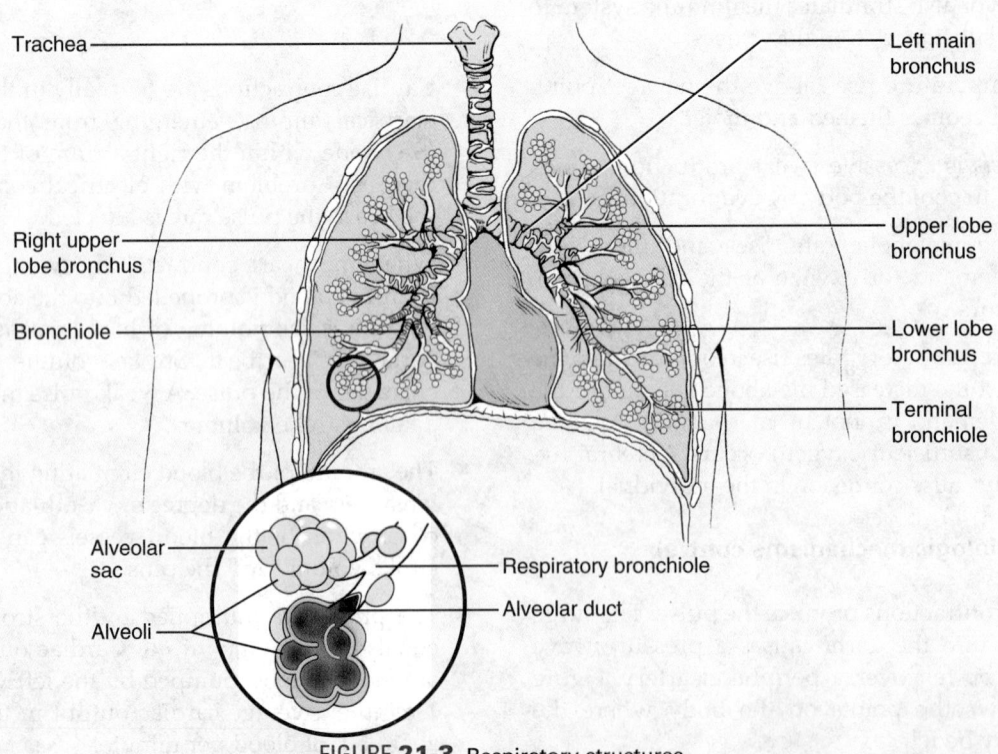

FIGURE **21-3** Respiratory structures.

- Messages are sent from the respiratory center to the respiratory muscles controlling the diaphragm and the intercostal muscles, thereby altering the respiratory rate or depth.

- The pumping action of the heart brings blood through the lung capillaries, where diffusion of O_2 and CO_2 can take place across the alveolar membrane.

- CO_2 is mainly carried as bicarbonate ion (HCO_3^-) in the blood until it reaches the lung. Carbon dioxide diffused into the lungs is released with exhalation.

What is blood pressure?

- Blood pressure is the pressure exerted on the arterial wall. The pressure changes depending on whether the heart is pumping or resting.

- Systolic pressure is the maximum pressure exerted on the artery during left ventricular contraction (systole).

- Diastolic pressure is the lower pressure exerted on the artery when the heart is at rest between contractions (diastole).

What physiologic factors directly affect the blood pressure?

- The amount of cardiac output (stroke volume × heart rate) affects the blood pressure. Blood pressure increases as stroke volume increases.

- If cardiac output falls, blood pressure falls.

- When vasoconstriction causes peripheral vascular resistance to rise, the pressure within the arterial system increases in order to push the blood along.

- When vasodilation occurs, vascular resistance drops and the pressure within the arterial system decreases.

- If blood volume increases, as in overhydration (excess fluid volume), blood pressure increases because there is more volume of blood in the same space (the vascular system).

- If blood volume decreases, as with bleeding or dehydration, blood pressure decreases.

- If the blood becomes thicker, as when excessive blood cells are manufactured, blood pressure increases because more pressure is needed to push the thicker fluid through the vascular system.

- When the vascular walls lose elasticity, as happens with arteriosclerosis and aging, blood pressure increases in order to push the blood through more rigid pathways.

What changes occur in vital signs with aging?

- Temperature is a less reliable indicator of health in the elderly. Fever is less likely to develop, but heat loss occurs more readily and can lead to hypothermia. The elderly person often has a lower normal temperature than the average adult. This may be due to a lower metabolic rate.

- The normal range for the heart rate does not change in the healthy elderly, but the rhythm may be slightly irregular.

- Respiratory rate may rise slightly as decreases in vital capacity and respiratory reserve occur.

- The systolic blood pressure rises slightly because the aorta and major arteries tend to harden with age. In many elderly, the diastolic pressure rises also.

The vital signs—temperature, pulse, respiration, blood pressure, and pain level—give some indication of the state of health of an individual. They represent interrelated physiologic systems of the body. Learning to measure vital signs is the beginning step in gathering assessment data for patients. Evaluation of vital sign data requires several readings so that a patient's status can be determined.

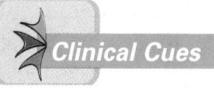
Clinical Cues

If another health care worker is assigned to take vital signs on your assigned patients, check the measurements to see how they fit in the overall picture of the patient's health status.

It is important to understand the physiologic mechanisms that regulate the vital signs and the factors that can affect each one.

MEASURING BODY TEMPERATURE

Normal body temperature ranges from 97.5° F to 99.5° F (36.4° C to 37.5° C), and varies considerably among individuals. Two scales are used to measure temperature: Fahrenheit and Celsius. Table 21-1 presents temperature correlations between the two scales. The temperature in a healthy young adult averages 98.6° F (37.0° C). It varies within the normal range as the body adjusts to changes in the amount of heat produced or the amount of heat lost. Some people run a low-normal or a

Table 21-1 *Comparison of Temperature Scales**

FAHRENHEIT	CELSIUS (CENTIGRADE)
95.0°	35.0°
95.9°	35.5°
96.8°	36.0°
97.7°	36.5°
98.6°	37.0°
99.5°	37.5°
100.4°	38.0°
101.3°	38.5°
102.2°	39.0°
103.1°	39.5°
104.0°	40.0°
104.9°	40.5°

*To change Celsius to Fahrenheit, multiply by 9/5 and add 32. To change Fahrenheit to Celsius, subtract 32 and multiply by 5/9.

high-normal temperature consistently; this represents the normal body temperature for them. **It is important to know the patient's usual temperature and then compare changes with that measurement.**

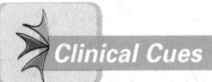
Clinical Cues

The patient's temperature usually does not indicate a fever unless it is over 100.2° F (37.8° C). Sometimes the temperature elevation is a body reaction to surgery or injury, rather than an indication of fever, and is expected to occur.

FACTORS INFLUENCING TEMPERATURE READINGS

The temperature reading obtained will vary according to the site used. Measurement sites are the mouth, rectum, axilla (armpit), ear, and on the skin. Most temperatures are measured orally, rectally, via the tympanic membrane (eardrum), or via the temporal artery. **Rectal temperatures are usually about 1° higher and axillary temperatures are about 1° lower than those measured orally.** The axillary temperature is the temperature taken in the armpit. The electronic thermometer is switched to the rectal setting and attached to a different probe before taking a rectal temperature, and the reading should be recorded as a rectal temperature. The rectal temperature is usually taken with the patient in the left Sims' position so that the rectum is positioned to accept the thermometer probe.

Sometimes the physician indicates the site of temperature to be taken; when it is not indicated, follow agency protocol.

The temporal artery thermometer is the most accurate noninvasive way to measure body temperature. It is passed over the temporal artery in the forehead. It captures the naturally emitted heat from the skin over the temporal artery, taking 1000 readings per second and selects the highest reading. It provides an accurate arterial temperature. The probe is gently stroked across the forehead to the far side (Figure 21-4). The arterial temperature is close to rectal temperature, but almost

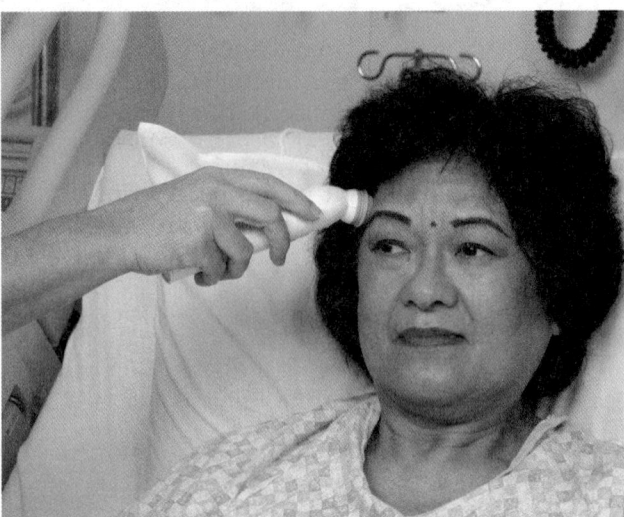
FIGURE **21-4** Slide the temporal artery thermometer across the forehead.

1° F (0.5° C) higher than an oral temperature. Ideally the temporal artery thermometer should be slid across the forehead above the brow ridges in a relatively straight line. Temporal artery temperature is unaffected by eating, drinking, smoking, or mouth breathing. If the person has been side-lying with part of the forehead into the pillow, allow the skin to cool to room temperature before using the thermometer.

Measuring tympanic temperature involves insertion of the thermometer probe into the auditory canal. The probe must be pointed at the tympanic membrane for the reading to be accurate. This is another easy and quick method of measuring the temperature. The graduated size of the probe prevents injury to the tympanic membrane. Tympanic membrane temperature is a good indicator of core body temperature. Core temperature is the temperature of the deep tissues of the body. The thermometer measures heat radiated as infrared energy from the tympanic membrane. The same blood vessels serve the hypothalamus and the membrane, so the temperature is close to core temperature at the hypothalamus. Temperatures taken with a tympanic thermometer are not subject to variations caused by eating hot or cold foods or liquids, smoking, or chewing gum. They can be affected by an ear infection or excessive wax that blocks the canal.

Think Critically About . . . Can you name three advantages of a tympanic thermometer over an oral thermometer? What is the advantage of a temporal artery thermometer?

Tympanic and temporal artery thermometers are more expensive than home electronic thermometers and are not universally used at home. Oral temperatures are convenient for older children and adults. The glass clinical thermometer must be left in place under the tongue for at least 3 minutes to register the temperature accurately, although newer types of electronic, chemical, and infrared thermometers register in much less time. If the patient has recently swallowed hot or cold foods or liquids or has been smoking or chewing gum, wait 15 to 30 minutes for these effects to pass for a more accurate measurement. **A glass thermometer is never used orally if the patient is uncooperative or at risk for biting on the thermometer.**

Rectal temperatures are taken when an accurate temperature cannot be obtained orally and a tympanic or temporal artery thermometer is not available. The rectal route may be used when there is nasal congestion or there has been nasal or oral surgery, the patient is unable to keep the mouth closed, or there is a risk for seizures. Rectal temperatures should not be used for cardiac patients or patients who have had rectal surgery.

Axillary temperatures are taken when oral or rectal temperatures are contraindicated and a tympanic or temporal artery thermometer is not available. They are a less reliable measure. Factors that may affect the body temperature are listed in Box 21-1.

? *Think Critically About . . .* Can you explain the physiologic process that causes a pregnant woman's temperature to be higher than that of the nonpregnant female?

PROBLEMS OF TEMPERATURE REGULATION
Hyperthermia

A condition in which the patient's temperature is above the normal range (100.4° F or 38.0° C) is called a fever, a febrile state, or pyrexia. However, fever is often not considered significant until the temperature reaches 101.3° F or 38.5° C. A fever is usually a common symptom of infection in which the heightened temperature helps to destroy invading bacteria. Very high fevers, such as those greater than 105.8° F or 41° C, cause damage to body cells, particularly those of the central nervous system. Hyperthermia (above-normal body temperature) may also occur after brain injury.

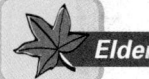
Elder Care Points

Very elderly patients tend to have a lower base body temperature, with frail elderly base temperature often being 96° F (35.6° C). If an elevation of 2° F. (1.1° C) occurs, fever is present (Yoshikawa & Norman, 1998).

In fever, the physiologic thermostat is reset at a higher level than normal and the heat-producing mechanisms of the body elevate the body temperature to the new setting. Because of chemical reactions in the body, chills (sensations of cold and shaking of the

---

Box 21-1 *Factors that Affect Body Temperature*

- **Time of Day (Circadian Rhythm).** The body temperature on awakening is generally in the low-normal range because of inactivity of the muscles. Conversely, the afternoon body temperature may be high-normal owing to the body's metabolic processes, the patient's activity, and the temperature of the atmosphere.
- **Environmental Temperature.** As might be expected, the body temperature is lower in cold weather and higher in hot weather.
- **Age of the Patient.** At birth, heat-regulating mechanisms are generally not fully developed, so there may be marked ups and downs in body temperature during the first year of life.
- **Physical Exercise.** Physical exercise uses large muscles, which create body heat by burning up the glucose and fat in the tissues. Muscle action generates heat, and core temperature rises.
- **Menstrual Cycle and Pregnancy.** Body temperature drops slightly just before female *ovulation* (the normal monthly ripening and release of the ovum) and then may rise 1° above normal during ovulation. Within a day or two preceding the onset of the next menstrual period, the temperature drops again. During pregnancy, the body temperature may consistently stay at high-normal because of an increase in the patient's metabolic rate.
- **Emotional Stress.** Highly emotional states cause an elevation in body temperature. The emotions increase hormone secretion, and the body activities required for this increase heat production.
- **Disease Conditions.** Bacteria, viruses, and toxins from some infective agents and the chemical reactions of the inflammatory response may produce fever. **Fever is a protective defense mechanism that the body uses to fight pathogens and their toxins.**
- **Drugs.** Certain drugs may cause temperature elevation because of the chemical action they have in the body.

body) may occur. The metabolic rate increases by about 7% for each degree Fahrenheit (10% for each degree Celsius) rise in temperature.

The course of a fever can be observed on the recorded graph in the patient's chart. There are three distinct stages in a fever: onset, febrile, and defervescence (abatement of fever). Onset may occur gradually or suddenly. The body responds to a pyrogen by trying to conserve and manufacture heat to raise the set point for core temperature. The person feels cold, and will add clothes or covers, curl up in a ball, and turn up the heat in order to feel warm. Chills, increased respiratory rate, and increased pulse rate mark this stage. During the febrile stage, the body temperature rises to the new set point established by the hypothalamus and remains there until there is resolution of the cause of the fever. **If the fever is very high, or if it lasts for an extended period, dehydration, delirium, and convulsions may occur.** Dehydration occurs as fluid is

Box 21-2 *Fever Patterns*

- **Constant:** The temperature is continuously elevated with less than 1° of variation within a 24-hour period.
- **Intermittent:** Alternating rise and fall of the temperature (e.g., low in the morning, high in the afternoon, or low for 2 to 3 days followed by a high temperature for 2 to 3 days).
- **Remittent:** A high temperature falls, usually in the morning, and again rises later in the day. The temperature never falls to normal in this type of fever until recovery occurs.
- **Relapsing:** The temperature falls to normal and then rises again in a repeating pattern.

lost with perspiration and more rapid breathing. Delirium and convulsions may occur because neurologic function is affected when the temperature in the brain rises. The stage of defervescence brings lowering of the body temperature to normal. The person feels warm and the skin may be moist.

A crisis (abrupt decline in fever) may occur when the body controls the infection, or a lysis (gradual return to a normal temperature) may mark the decline of the fever. Fevers are classified as constant, intermittent, remittent, or relapsing (Box 21-2).

Elder Care Points

The temperature in the elderly may not reflect the degree of seriousness of the illness because temperature may not rise significantly.

Hypothermia

Hypothermia (subnormal body temperature) refers to a lowering of the temperature of the entire body, not just a portion of it. The thermal regulating center in the hypothalamus is greatly impaired when the temperature of the body falls below 94° F (34.4° C). At this level, the activity of the cells is reduced, less heat is produced, and sleepiness and coma are apt to develop. Those at risk for hypothermia include postoperative patients who have been cooled during surgery, newborn infants whose skin is exposed to cool room temperatures, elderly or debilitated patients, and those exposed to cold temperatures for prolonged periods.

Elder Care Points

- The elderly, like infants, lose considerable body heat through the scalp. Wearing a hat, even indoors, helps prevent heat loss in cold weather.
- The elderly person with inadequate home heating is at risk for hypothermia during cold weather.

People exposed to extremely cold weather often suffer frostbite of the ears, nose, hands, and feet, where exposed tissue and feet and hands freeze. If the frozen part is thawed immediately, there is little effect on tissues. However, if frostbite is prolonged, it causes death of cells and loss of the frozen area.

Nursing activities for treating the patient with a below-normal body temperature should focus on reducing heat loss and supplying additional warmth. These activities may include (1) providing additional clothing or blankets for warmth (an electric blanket is most effective for raising temperature); (2) giving warm fluids, if permitted; (3) adjusting the temperature of the room to 72° F (22.2° C) or higher; (4) eliminating drafts; (5) increasing the patient's muscle activity; and (6) submerging frostbitten areas in a warm bath, with water temperature no warmer than 107° F or 41.8° C.

MEASURING BODY TEMPERATURE

Clinical thermometers are used to measure the body temperature, and there are a growing number of different types on the market. The thermometer made of glass with a mercury-filled bulb is not used anymore because if the thermometer gets broken, mercury and its vapor, which are toxic, are released. Glass thermometers are now filled with nonmercury material. Health facilities often use electronic digital thermometers, tympanic thermometers, temporal artery thermometers, and disposable, single-use thermometers.

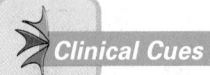

Clinical Cues

Be certain the patient has not eaten, drunk fluids, or smoked within the previous 15 minutes as this will cause an erroneous reading. A glass thermometer must remain in the sublingual pocket for 3 to 5 minutes to accurately reflect the body temperature.

Taking an Oral Temperature

The tip of the thermometer or probe should be placed in the sublingual pocket (Figure 21-5). The patient should keep the tongue down, close the mouth, and

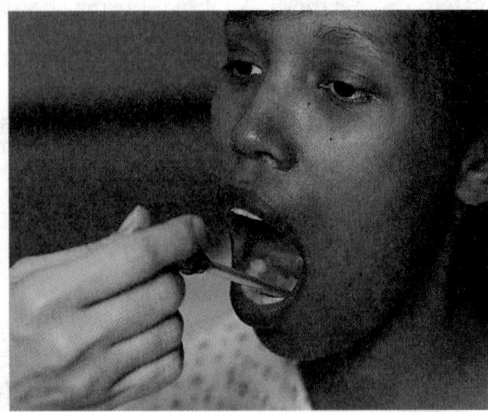

FIGURE **21-5** Measuring the temperature of the home care patient. Place the tip of the thermometer under the tongue in the sublingual pocket.

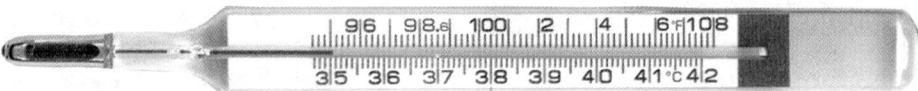

FIGURE **21-6** Nonmercury "Geratherm" glass thermometer.

keep the lips closed. A plastic sleeve or probe cover is used. Remove the plastic sleeve before reading a glass thermometer.

Taking a Rectal Temperature

Provide privacy and ask the patient to turn to the side facing away from you with the knees slightly flexed; drape the patient to reveal only the anal area. Don gloves and lubricate the tip of the rectal thermometer or probe, lift the upper buttock slightly so that the anus can be clearly seen. Insert the lubricated bulb into the rectum directed toward the umbilicus about 0.5 to 1.5 inches. Hold the thermometer in place for 3 to 5 minutes or until the correct temperature is indicated. Wipe the thermometer or probe from the stem toward the bulb or probe tip. Wipe the buttocks to remove lubricant or stool. Correctly dispose of tissues and gloves and perform hand hygiene.

Taking an Axillary Temperature

Place the thermometer in the center of the patient's dry axilla (armpit). A wet axilla will produce a false reading. Ask the patient to hold the arm tightly against the chest. The arm may rest on the chest. Leave the thermometer in place for 3 to 8 minutes or until the thermometer indicates the reading is complete. Remove and wipe the thermometer clean from the stem to the tip.

GLASS THERMOMETERS

The glass thermometer has a bulb containing an alloy of elements called Galinstan and a stem in which the substance can rise (Figure 21-6). On the stem, is a graduated scale representing degrees of temperature from 94° to 106.8° F. (The range on a Celsius thermometer scale is 34° to 43° C.) The alloy in the bulb expands when the bulb is in contact with body heat and registers on the scale in the stem. The bulb may be long and slender or blunt like the short, fat bulb used for rectal thermometers. Rectal thermometers often have a red tip or color on the stem to signify that they are for rectal use only and should not be used orally. Oral thermometers may also be used to take axillary temperatures. All glass thermometers must have the alloy below the normal range before using them, which is accomplished by shaking down the alloy. This is done by holding the thermometer firmly by the distal glass end and flicking the wrist in a quick motion several times to bring the alloy down to the bulb (Safety Alert 21-1).

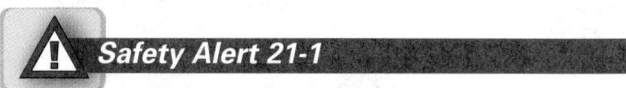

⚠ Safety Alert 21-1

Glass Thermometers

A glass thermometer should not be used orally if the patient is unconscious, subject to seizures, confused, or agitated because it might break if the patient bites on it. This thermometer should not be used orally on an infant or toddler who cannot hold it in the mouth properly or who might bite down on it.

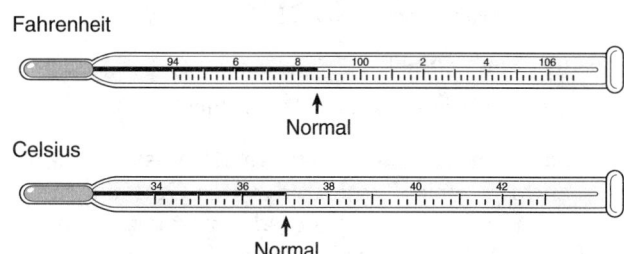

FIGURE **21-7** Reading the thermometer in Fahrenheit and Celsius.

Rectal and oral thermometers must be kept separated so they are not confused. Glass thermometers are very slippery when soapy; be especially careful when washing the thermometer. Glass thermometers may still be used in homes as not everyone has obtained a new type of thermometer. Nurses should be able to teach parents how to read a glass thermometer (Figure 21-7).

Reading the Glass Thermometer

Hold the thermometer horizontally at eye level and rotate it toward you until you can clearly see the column of alloy. Note where the end of the alloy is on the lined scale. The stem of the Galinstan alloy–in-glass thermometer contains the scale for measuring the temperature. The scale may be calibrated in either Fahrenheit or Celsius degrees, or it may have both scales. The Celsius scale has long lines indicating the degree and short lines for each one tenth of a degree. In contrast, the Fahrenheit scale has an arrow marking the normal temperature of 98.6° F. Long lines on the scale represent each degree, but only the even-numbered degrees are written as 96°, 98°, 100°, and so on. Short lines between the degree lines represent two tenths of a degree. All temperatures are recorded as ending in an even number when using this thermometer because it does not measure odd tenths of a degree. For example, one would read and record 99.2° F or 99.8° F but never

Home Care Considerations 21-1

Taking the Temperature at Home

- Teach the home care patient or family to cleanse the thermometer by using a clean tissue and wiping with a twisting motion from the tip toward the bulb, and then washing it in warm soapy water and rinsing with cold water.
- The thermometer should be disinfected in 70% to 90% isopropyl alcohol or a 1:10 solution of household bleach and water.
- The thermometer should be rinsed after disinfection, dried, and stored in a dry container.

99.3° F or 99.7° F. **To convert temperature from one scale to another, use these formulas:**
Fahrenheit to Celsius:

$$(\text{Fahrenheit} - 32) \times 5/9 = \text{Celsius}$$

Celsius to Fahrenheit:

$$(\text{Celsius} \times 9/5) + 32 = \text{Fahrenheit}$$

Lukewarm water is used to wash a glass thermometer, and it is rinsed with cold water. Oral and rectal thermometers should be stored separately to avoid confusing them (Home Care Considerations 21-1).

ELECTRONIC THERMOMETERS

The portable, battery-operated electronic thermometers register body temperature in 5 seconds to 1 minute. There may be an on-off button to activate

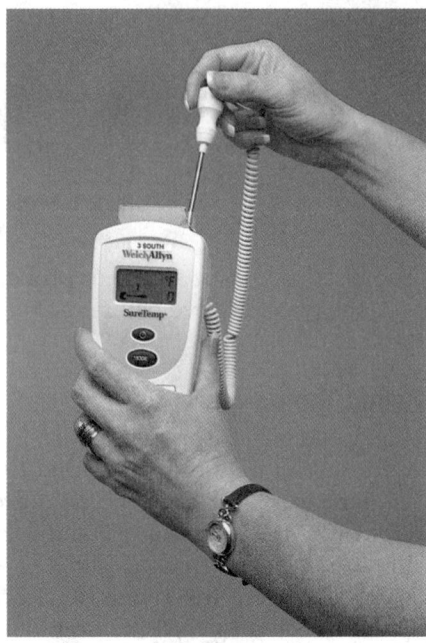

FIGURE **21-8** An electronic thermometer.

the battery, and a warm-up period may be required (Figure 21-8). The oral probe is placed in a plastic cover or sheath that is used one time and then discarded. The correct disposable probe cover and the correct setting should be used for the electronic thermometer when taking an oral or rectal temperature. The temperature is displayed digitally on a small screen on the hand-held unit. The reading is in tenths of a degree, so temperatures taken with this unit may end in odd numbers, such as 99.5° F (37.5° C). Skill 21-1 describes the use of an electronic thermometer.

Skill 21-1 | Measuring the Temperature with an Electronic Thermometer

An electronic thermometer may be used to measure temperature, without worry about injury, for patients who are at risk for seizure disorders. If a rectal temperature is desired, a special rectal probe is used along with a rectal probe cover.

■ Supplies
✓ Electronic thermometer
✓ Probe covers
✓ Pencil and paper

Review and carry out the Standard Steps in Appendix 3.

■ Assessment (Data Collection)

1. *ACTION* Perform hand hygiene, identify the patient, and explain the procedure. Ask whether the patient has had anything to eat or drink in the past 15 minutes.

RATIONALE Reduces the transfer of microorganisms, ensures that correct patient is undergoing the procedure, and puts the patient at ease. Eating, drinking, or smoking alters the temperature of the oral cavity.

■ Planning

2. *ACTION* Check to be certain there are probe covers in the container. Check the low battery light to ensure proper functioning of the thermometer.

RATIONALE Probe must not be used without a cover. A low battery must be replaced in order to obtain an accurate temperature measurement.

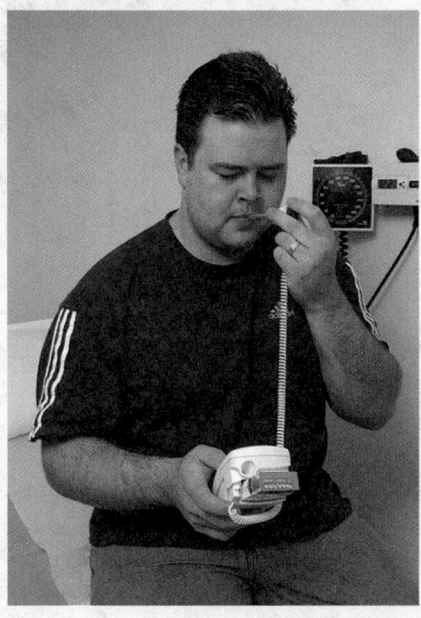

Step **2**

■ Implementation

3. *ACTION* Remove the probe from the unit, and push it down into a probe cover until a slight click is heard.

   RATIONALE The probe cover must be firmly in place for the unit to operate correctly.

4. *ACTION* Place the probe under the tongue in the side sublingual pocket. Ask the patient to close the lips and keep them closed.

   RATIONALE The probe must be in contact with tissue rich in blood supply to obtain an accurate temperature.

5. *ACTION* Hold the unit steady, or allow the patient to hold it, and read the temperature on the screen when the light stops flashing or the unit beeps.

Step **5**

RATIONALE Many units will beep when the correct temperature is recorded. If the probe is not positioned correctly, the unit will not beep or will refuse to register a temperature.

6. *ACTION* Remove the probe from the mouth, and discard the probe cover into the waste container by pressing the ejector button.

   RATIONALE Ejecting the probe cover directly into the waste can prevents handling its contaminated surface. Probe covers are *never* reused. Be careful not to accidentally leave a probe cover in the bed.

7. *ACTION* Note the temperature, and clear the register by returning the probe to its holder.

   RATIONALE Returning the probe to its holder turns off the thermometer and saves the battery.

8. *ACTION* Record the patient's temperature on your worksheet.

   RATIONALE Noting the time and temperature on your worksheet makes it readily available when charting.

■ Evaluation

9. *ACTION* Ask yourself: Is the temperature elevated? Is it higher or lower than the last reading?

   RATIONALE Provides data to determine trend of the temperature.

■ Documentation

10. *ACTION* Record the time and temperature on the graphic sheet. Record measures taken if the temperature was elevated in the nurse's notes.

    RATIONALE Verifies temperature was taken and makes measurement data available.

Documentation Example
T 99.8° F.

■ Special Considerations

✓ If thermometer does not function, the probe cover may be loose. Remove the cover, insert the probe back into its storage location to reset, pull it out, and replace the cover, being certain it is snapped into place.

✓ A rectal probe attachment and probe cover may be used to take a rectal temperature if this probe is available.

?CRITICAL THINKING QUESTIONS

1. If the temperature reading obtained does not fit with the clinical symptoms and history, what would you do?

2. Many physicians feel that using an electronic thermometer is more accurate than using a tympanic thermometer for an ill adult. What do you think would be the reason for this?

Tympanic Thermometers

These portable, battery-operated electronic thermometers register temperatures in 1 to 2 seconds. A switch on many units may be set for infant and toddler or for child and adult. The auditory canal probe is placed in a plastic cover that is used one time and then discarded. The temperature is displayed digitally on a small screen on the hand-held unit. The reading is in tenths of a degree and can be displayed in degrees Fahrenheit or Celsius (Figure 21-9). Using a tympanic thermometer is explained in Skill 21-2.

Temporal Artery Skin Thermometer

The temporal artery thermometer is placed on the skin of the forehead over the temporal artery. It is an electronic thermometer that is fast and accurate. It is less

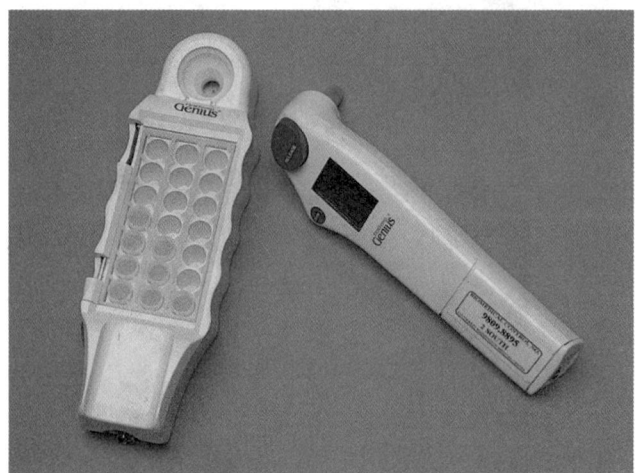

FIGURE **21-9** A tympanic thermometer.

Skill 21-2 | Measuring the Temperature with a Tympanic or Temporal Artery Thermometer

When placed into the auditory canal, a temporal thermometer produces a reading of core temperature. It is especially useful for measuring temperature in children.

■ Supplies
✓ Tympanic or temporal artery thermometer
✓ Probe covers
✓ Pencil and paper

Review and carry out the Standard Steps in Appendix 3.

■ Assessment (Data Collection)

1. **ACTION** Determine reason for measuring the temperature.

   RATIONALE Tells if measurement is routine or infection is suspected.

■ Planning

2. **ACTION** Check the low battery light. Set unit for the desired mode: infant-toddler or child-adult.

   RATIONALE If battery is low, the unit will not function. An inaccurate reading will be obtained if the wrong mode is used.

3. **ACTION** Check to see that there are probe covers in the container before going to the patient.

   RATIONALE Prevents an unnecessary trip to obtain the covers.

■ Implementation

4. **ACTION** Perform hand hygiene.

   RATIONALE Reduces transfer of microorganisms.

5. **ACTION** Remove the probe from the unit and attach a probe cover.

   RATIONALE The probe cover must be securely in place in order to obtain a reading. A disposable cover prevents transmission of microorganisms from one patient to another.

6. **ACTION** Gently place the probe in the ear canal until it seals the opening. Grasp the top of the pinna and gently pull up and back to straighten the ear canal of the adult if needed. Pull the lobe of the ear down or back to straighten the canal of a child under age 2 if needed. Point the probe slightly toward the face.

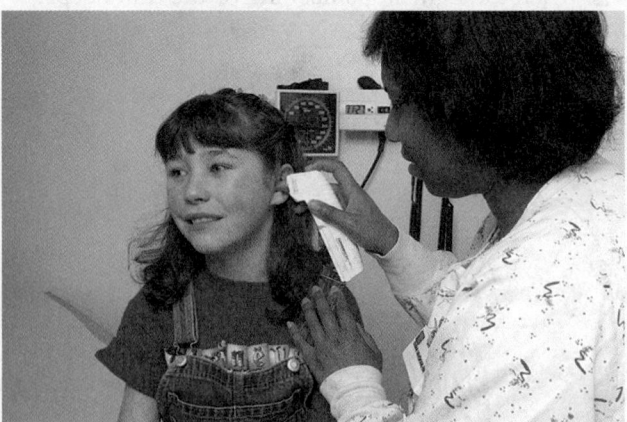

Step **6**

RATIONALE The probe must be pointed at the tympanic membrane and be sealed in the canal in order for the measurement to be taken. The auditory canal should be inspected for redness, swelling, discharge, or presence of cerumen or a foreign body before insertion of the probe.

7. *ACTION* Hold the unit steady. Steady the head with one hand if needed and press the button to take the reading.

   RATIONALE Head movement will break the seal of the probe in the canal.

8. *ACTION* Read the temperature and remove the probe. Praise a child for cooperating if appropriate.

   RATIONALE The temperature will be displayed on the small screen on the unit when it has been obtained.

9. *ACTION* Discard the probe cover in the waste receptacle.

   RATIONALE Probe covers are contaminated and are not designed to be reused.

10. *ACTION* Return the thermometer to the base unit for recharge.

    RATIONALE Returning the unit to the base prepares it for the next use.

11. *ACTION* Perform hand hygiene.

    RATIONALE Reduces transfer of microorganisms.

■ Evaluation

12. *ACTION* Ask yourself: Is the temperature elevated? Is it higher or lower than the previous reading?

    RATIONALE Provides data to determine temperature trend.

■ Documentation

13. *ACTION* Document the time and temperature on the graphic record or office chart. If more than one type of thermometer is used in the health care agency, designation of an aural temperature should be made.

    RATIONALE Notes that temperature was taken and makes measurement data available.

Documentation Example
T 100.3° F.

■ Special Considerations

✓ This thermometer should not be used if the patient has an inflammatory condition of the auditory canal or if there is discharge from the ear.

✓ Moving the probe laterally back and forth with small movements assists in positioning the probe so that it seals the canal.

✓ Having a parent hold the child's head against the body helps stabilize the head so that the probe can be placed in the ear.

✓ Approaching the small child or very elderly with a slow, smooth movement after explaining what you are going to do decreases reflex "ducking."

✓ A rectal probe attachment and probe cover may be used to take a rectal temperature if that probe is available.

? CRITICAL THINKING QUESTIONS

1. Will wax in an ear interfere with a tympanic thermometer reading? Why or why not?

2. If a 2-year-old child keeps turning his head away and squirming when you try to take a tympanic temperature, what would you do?

---

invasive than the tympanic thermometer and more reliable when used correctly (see Figure 21-4).

DISPOSABLE THERMOMETERS

Various types of single-use, disposable thermometers are available; among them are temperature-sensitive tapes that are placed on the forehead or abdomen to record the heat of the body. These are often used in newborn nurseries. Other types are the NexTemp thermometers (Figure 21-10). The sensor end of the shaft contains a series of dots arranged so that each one changes color at a different temperature from that of the preceding dot. Directions on the package explain how to use these thermometers. Most disposable thermometers will register the temperature within 2 minutes. They provide the least accurate readings of temperature.

APPLICATION of the NURSING PROCESS
Assessment (Data Collection)

Choose the appropriate site for temperature measurement based on the age and condition of the patient and the type of thermometer available. Determine if factors are present that might alter the temperature reading. The rectal method may be used when a tympanic or temporal artery thermometer is not available for patients who have wired jaws, who have a nasogastric tube in place and cannot breathe easily with the mouth closed, or who may have seizures.

Check the electronic thermometer battery before measuring the patient's temperature. A low battery may make the measurement inaccurate.

Choose the right mode (infant-toddler or child-adult) on the tympanic thermometer before measuring

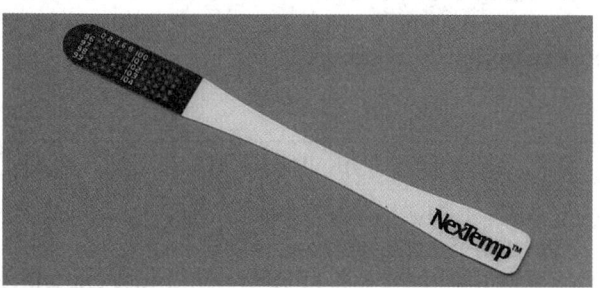

FIGURE **21-10** A disposable thermometer.

the patient's temperature. An inaccurate reading will result if the thermometer is not set properly.

Nursing Diagnosis

Nursing diagnoses for patients with alterations of normal temperature might be:

- Hyperthermia related to infection or excessive heat exposure
- Hypothermia related to prolonged exposure to cold
- Ineffective thermoregulation related to neurologic injury

Abnormalities found on assessment of the other vital signs (pulse, respiration, blood pressure) may indicate problems in various body systems. When such findings remain abnormal, nursing diagnoses would be written that address those problems.

Planning

Expected outcomes are written for each nursing diagnosis:

- Patient's temperature will return to normal after 3 days of antibiotic therapy.
- Normal body temperature will be regained within 6 hours.
- Temperature will be maintained below 102.5° F with use of hypothermia blanket.

Further expected outcomes would be written for nursing diagnoses established by abnormalities in other vital signs.

Implementation

Temperature is taken upon admission to the health care facility so that a baseline for comparison of future measurements is available. The physician orders the schedule for taking all the vital signs or the nurse takes them according to agency standards. Other times the temperature should be taken are as follows:

- Every 4 hours when a known infection is present
- Every 2 to 4 hours when a fever is present
- When the patient is "not feeling right"
- When the patient is receiving drugs that may affect the temperature
- Before surgery or an invasive procedure, then at regular intervals afterward as prescribed by hospital protocol

Measures to reduce fever are presented in Box 21-3. Other interventions are presented in Nursing Care Plan 21-1.

Evaluation

To evaluate success of the plan, determine whether expected outcomes have been met. Evaluation of measures to keep temperature within normal range is performed by analyzing the trend of the temperature

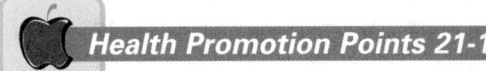

Box 21-3 | *Nursing Interventions to Reduce Fever*

- Encourage a large fluid intake unless contraindicated.
- Lower the room temperature by adjusting the thermostat or opening doors or windows.
- Increase the rate of circulating air with a fan.
- Remove items of clothing or bed covers.
- Control or reduce the amount of body activity.
- Carry out the physician's orders for cooling measures and supportive treatment: tepid sponge bath; cooling blanket; high-calorie diet and fluids; medication to lower temperature and combat the disease.

Health Promotion Points 21-1

Promoting Home Use of a Thermometer

When working with patients outside of the hospital setting, be certain that they own a thermometer and know how to use it. Many people do not own a thermometer. Teach the patient and family how to care for the thermometer.

on the graphic record. A fever that is decreasing when the patient is receiving antibiotics for an infection is one indication that the antibiotic therapy is effective. For the hypothermic patient, if the temperature returns to normal with the use of the warming blanket, the expected outcomes are met (Health Promotion Points 21-1).

Elder Care Points

- The average temperature in the older adult is 96.5° to 97.5° F. (35.8° to 36.4° C).
- Body temperature in the very elderly tends to be quite low in the morning upon awakening. This is because the metabolic rate slows during sleep and inactivity.
- The lack of subcutaneous fat allows the elder's body to cool more readily than bodies of younger people.

Evaluation to determine whether expected outcomes have been met for nursing diagnoses related to abnormalities in the other vital signs would include measurements indicating that those vital signs are now within normal limits.

MEASURING THE PULSE

Each time the heart contracts to force blood into an already full *aorta* (artery leading from the heart), the arterial walls in the vascular system must expand to

NURSING CARE PLAN 21-1

Care of the Patient with Elevated Body Temperature

SCENARIO Mr. Johnson, age 72, came to the clinic with malaise and temperature elevation. He has been ill for several days.

PROBLEM/NURSING DIAGNOSIS *Temperature 102.2° (39.0° C), chills*/Hyperthermia related to infectious process. *Supporting Assessment Data: Subjective:* "I feel terrible and I'm really wrung-out." *Objective:* Temperature 102.2°F (39.0° C), flushed skin, skin warm to touch; pulse 98, BP 132/84, respiratory rate 26.

Goals/Expected Outcomes	Nursing Interventions	Selected Rationales	Evaluation
Patient's temperature will decrease 1 degree within 8 hours.	Instruct to keep clothing and linen dry and to use only light clothing or linens.	Allows heat loss through conduction and convection.	*Is body covering kept to the minimum needed to prevent chilling?* Patient acknowledges instructions.
Patient's temperature will decrease to normal within 48 hours.	Advise to monitor temperature at home and to administer acetaminophen q 6 hr as ordered for temperature over 102.2° (39.0° C).	Tracks temperature trend; antipyretic will reduce temperature.	*Does patient have a thermometer at home and does he know how to use it?* States he will monitor his temperature with his thermometer.
	Instruct to limit activities and to increase frequency and length of rest periods until temperature is normal.	Activity increases metabolic rate, contributing to heat production.	*Does patient agree to limit his activities?* States he wants to go to church tomorrow, but will stay home and rest.
	Instruct to increase oral fluid intake with desired fluids.	Fluids will be insensibly lost and need to be replaced in order to lower temperature.	*Is patient willing to increase fluid intake?* States he has juice, tea, water, and soft drinks at home and will increase his intake.

? CRITICAL THINKING QUESTIONS

1. If the patient's temperature continues to rise, what interventions would you suggest?

2. How does using only light bed covers and sleepwear or light clothing assist specifically in lowering the body temperature?

---

accept the increase in pressure. The pressure wave causing this expansion is called the *pulse.* By counting each pulsation of the arterial wall, you can determine the pulse rate.

COMMON PULSE POINTS

The pulse can be felt wherever a superficial artery can be held against firm tissue, such as a bone (see Figure 21-2). The pulse is felt most strongly over the following areas:
- Radial artery in the wrist at the base of the thumb
- Temporal artery just in front of the ear
- Carotid artery on the front side of the neck
- Femoral artery in the groin
- Apical pulse over the apex of the heart (the actual beat of the heart)
- Popliteal pulse behind the knee
- Pedal pulse of the posterior tibial artery on the inside of the ankle behind the malleolus, in the groove between the malleolus and Achilles tendon and dorsalis pedis on the arch of the foot

The radial artery in the wrist is most often chosen to palpate (feel) the pulse when taking vital signs. It is best found by placing the flat part of the first two fingers against the tendon, or cord, on the thumb side of the inner wrist and then rolling the fingers slightly outward into the little trough on the thumb side of the wrist. Skill 21-3 describes measurement of the radial pulse. When it is difficult to find or to count the radial pulse, the apical beat of the heart is counted for a full minute with the use of a stethoscope (device that augments sounds from within the body). The apical pulse is counted when it is

Skill 21-3 | Measuring the Radial Pulse

The radial pulse is measured whenever vital signs are taken. The pulse quality and character should be noted while the pulse is being counted. When the radial pulse is irregular, the apical pulse should also be taken.

■ Supplies
✓ Digital watch or watch with second hand

✓ Pen and paper

Review and carry out the Standard Steps in Appendix 3.

■ Assessment (Data Collection)
1. *ACTION* Identify the patient.

   RATIONALE Ensures that the pulse will be recorded for the correct person.

■ Planning
2. *ACTION* Explain the procedure.

   RATIONALE Puts the patient at ease.

■ Implementation
3. *ACTION* Perform hand hygiene.

   RATIONALE Reduces transfer of microorganisms.

4. *ACTION* Place the pads of two or three fingers lightly over the radial artery with the patient's hand palm down.

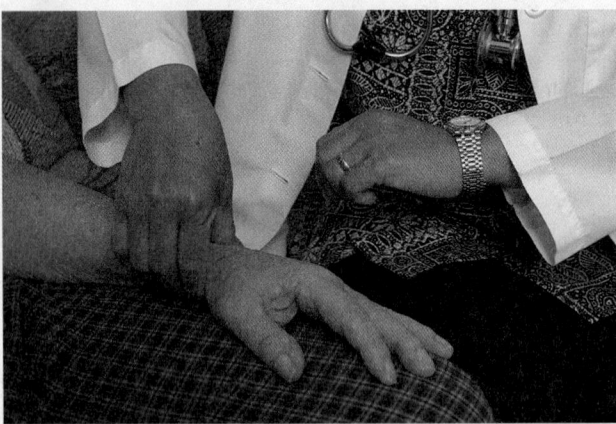

Step **4**

   RATIONALE Fingers are used rather than the thumb because the thumb has a strong pulse that could be confused with that of the patient.

5. *ACTION* Begin with a beat, and count the next beat as "1." Count the pulsations for 30 seconds and multiply by 2 to obtain the rate per minute. Note the regularity, strength, and character of the pulse.

   RATIONALE If the first beat is counted "1," the total count will be inaccurate because you should count only each full cardiac cycle. Counting for 30 seconds rather than 15 provides a more accurate measurement of the pulse. Whenever the pulse is irregular, very rapid, or very slow, count for a full minute.

6. *ACTION* Jot down the count.

   RATIONALE Prevents forgetting the result.

7. *ACTION* Perform hand hygiene.

   RATIONALE Reduces transfer of microorganisms.

■ Evaluation
8. *ACTION* Ask yourself: Is the result within normal range for the patient? Is the pulse slower or faster than previous readings? Has the patient ever had a pulse irregularity?

   RATIONALE Provides data regarding an alteration from normal for the patient.

■ Documentation
9. *ACTION* Record the time and pulse rate on the graphic sheet or on the office chart. Note any abnormalities in quality or rhythm in the nurse's notes. Report abnormalities as appropriate.

   RATIONALE Notes pulse measurement and any abnormality.

Documentation Example
P 92; irregular.

■ Special Considerations
✓ If the pulse is difficult to palpate, use lighter pressure. Change to the other wrist if there is still difficulty.

?CRITICAL THINKING QUESTIONS
1. If a radial pulse is difficult to feel or thready, how would you count the pulse?

2. If an adult patient's pulse rate is 105 bpm, what questions should you ask before assuming that this the patient has a heart problem?

important to have an accurate measure of the heart rate and may be ordered by the physician for patients with heart conditions. Nurses routinely take an apical pulse before administering digitalis and beta blocker medication. The apical, rather than the radial, pulse is also taken on children younger than 2 years. Locate the apical heart sound by placing the stethoscope on a point midway between the imaginary line running from the middle of the left clavicle through the left nipple in the fifth intercostal space (Figure 21-11, Skill 21-4).

PULSE RATE

The pulse rate varies widely and is influenced by a large number of factors (Table 21-2). The term tachycardia is used to refer to a pulse greater than 100 beats per minute (bpm); bradycardia indicates a slow pulse that is less than 60 bpm. The average pulse rate in an adult is 72 bpm. Tachycardia or bradycardia should be reported to the charge nurse or the physician. Medications may be prescribed to speed up the pulse when it

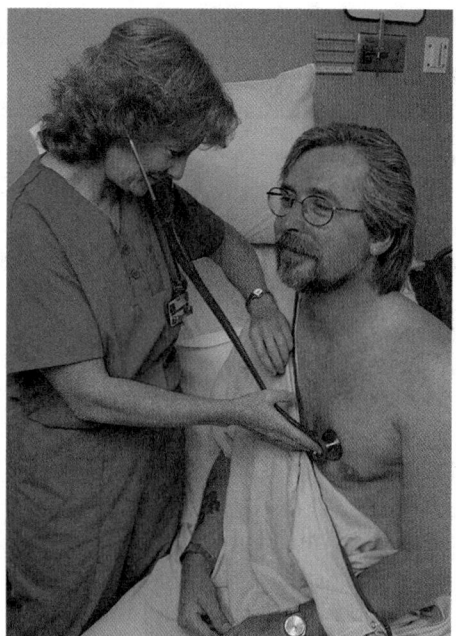

FIGURE **21-11** Counting the apical pulse.

Skill 21-4 | Measuring the Apical Pulse

The apical pulse is measured during a physical examination, whenever the radial pulse is irregular, or when the patient has congestive heart failure, has had heart surgery, or is recovering from a myocardial infarction. An apical pulse measurement is required before the patient is given digitalis or beta blocker–type heart medication.

■ Supplies
✓ Stethoscope
✓ Digital watch or watch with second hand

Review and carry out the Standard Steps in Appendix 3.

■ Assessment (Data Collection)

1. *ACTION* Determine if the patient has a known heart arrhythmia.

   RATIONALE Provides a baseline against which to compare the apical pulse.

■ Planning

2. *ACTION* Perform hand hygiene. Provide privacy; explain the procedure. Eliminate extraneous noise.

   RATIONALE Reduces transfer of microorganisms, protects the patient's right to privacy, and puts the patient at ease. Turning off the TV and closing the door provides a quieter environment.

■ Implementation

3. *ACTION* Expose the left chest. Warm the diaphragm of the stethoscope in the palm of your hand for a minute or two.

   RATIONALE Sounds are transmitted through the stethoscope best if it is placed on bare skin. A cold stethoscope is unpleasant for the patient.

4. *ACTION* Locate the apex of the heart by palpating for the fifth intercostal space at the midclavicular line.

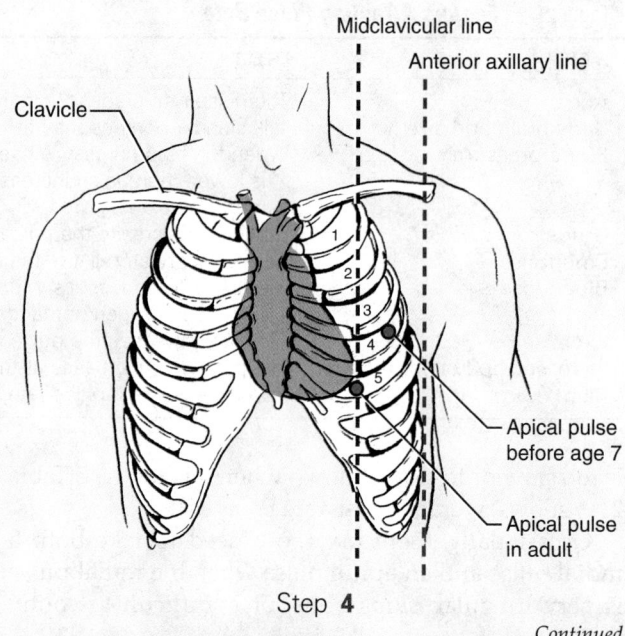

Step **4**

Continued

Skill 21-4 | Measuring the Apical Pulse—cont'd

RATIONALE The apex of the healthy heart is located at the fifth intercostal space on the midclavicular line.

5. *ACTION* Listen to the heart sounds with the diaphragm of the stethoscope.

RATIONALE The high-pitched heart sounds are heard best with the diaphragm. If the sounds are not heard clearly, move the stethoscope around slightly until sound is heard.

6. *ACTION* Count the number of beats for 1 minute.

RATIONALE While counting, note the rhythm and the strength of the beat.

7. *ACTION* Cover the chest, make the patient comfortable, and restore the unit. Jot down the apical pulse.

RATIONALE Prevents chilling and protects privacy. Restoring the patient's personal belongings to their former places, placing the call light at hand, and raising the side rails as needed protects safety.

8. *ACTION* Perform hand hygiene.

RATIONALE Reduces the transfer of microorganisms.

▪ Evaluation

9. *ACTION* Ask yourself: Was the apical pulse irregular? Has it been irregular before? Is this the same type of irregularity?

RATIONALE Answers to questions provide further data regarding heart status of the patient.

▪ Documentation

10. *ACTION* Note on the graphic record that the pulse was taken apically. If the apical pulse was irregular, note the finding in the nurse's notes.

RATIONALE Identifies the method by which the pulse was taken. Any abnormality should be documented in the nurse's notes.

▪ Special Considerations

✓ An apical pulse is the preferred method of measuring the pulse in children under 2 years of age.

✓ Care should be taken not to frighten a patient if the radial pulse is irregular and you then take the apical pulse. Explain to the patient that you could not obtain an accurate count radially and wish to listen to the heart directly.

✓ Do not start counting the apical pulse until you can hear it clearly. This sometimes takes a few beats in order to tune the ear to the soft beat.

✓ If the sound is difficult to hear, ask the patient to lean forward to bring the heart closer to the chest wall.

?CRITICAL THINKING QUESTIONS

1. If your patient has a very thick chest and it is difficult to hear the apical pulse, how would you verify the heart rate you measured as being accurate?

2. When a patient's vital signs are being taken by an electronic vital signs monitor, can you be sure the heart rate is accurate? How would you verify that it is?

Table 21-2 *Factors Affecting Pulse Rate*

FACTOR	EFFECT
Age	The pulse rate gradually diminishes from birth to adulthood.
Body build and size	Tall, slender persons may have a slower pulse rate than short, stout persons.
Blood pressure	When the blood pressure rises, it causes a decrease in the pulse rate. When the blood pressure is lower, there is an increase in the pulse rate because the heart is attempting to increase the output of blood.
Drugs	Stimulants increase the pulse rate. Depressants decrease the pulse rate.
Emotions	Acute anxiety stimulates the sympathetic nervous system, increasing the heart rate.
Blood loss	Excessive blood loss, as with hemorrhage, increases the heart rate as the body tries to meet the tissue oxygen demands.
Exercise	Exercise increases the pulse rate because the heart pumps faster to meet circulatory needs.
Increased body temperature	The pulse rate increases at the rate of 7-10 beats for each degree of temperature.
Pain	Pain increases the pulse rate.

is too slow or to slow it down when it is too fast. Table 21-3 shows average pulse rate by age.

Occasionally, there may be a need to take both a radial pulse and an apical pulse when the radial pulse is very irregular, skips beats, or is difficult to count. This requires two people to count the radial and apical pulses at the same time to determine whether there is a pulse deficit (difference between the apical and radial pulse). The nurses use one watch visible to both when counting the apical-radial pulse and begin and

Table 21-3 | *Average Pulse Rates*

AGE GROUP	AVERAGE PULSE RATE AT REST (BEATS PER MINUTE)
Normal pulse range	60-100
Some athletes	45-60
Adult male	72
Adult female	76-80
Child (age 5 yr)	95
Child (age 1 yr)	110
Newborn	120-160

end counting at the same time. One nurse counts the radial pulse and the other counts the apical pulse. The radial pulse subtracted from the apical pulse equals the pulse deficit.

As the blood travels farther away from the heart, the distinct wave of the pulse begins to fade, but the pulse can be palpated at the ankle or top of the foot. Pedal pulses are checked to determine whether there is any blockage in the circulation in the artery up to that point, especially in patients who have had cardiac catheterization using the femoral artery for the insertion of the catheter or those who have had surgery on the leg. Most nurses mark an "X" on the skin over the spot where the pedal pulse is felt so that all staff use the same location. When the pedal pulse is difficult to locate, a Doppler ultrasound stethoscope must be used (Figure 21-12).

PULSE CHARACTERISTICS

When the pulse is being counted, the rate, rhythm, and volume should be noted. **Timing is begun with a beat that is not counted; the next beat is "1."** An arrhythmia (irregular pulse) has a period of normal rhythm broken by periods of irregularity or skipped beats. This can occur as a temporary condition from emotional stress or fright. A continuing arrhythmia may be indicative of heart disease or a medication's side effects and should be reported to the charge nurse or physician and recorded. Figure 21-13 shows various pulse rates and rhythms.

The volume or strength of the pulse is just as important as the rate. With moderate pressure of the first two or three fingers on the vessel, a strong pulse will be felt regularly and with good force (Health Promotion Points 21-2). There are several terms to describe the strength of a pulse. The most common are

- Weak and regular (even beats with poor force), or 1+
- Strong and regular (even beats with moderate force), or 2+
- Full and bounding (even beats with strong force), or 3+
- Feeble (barely palpable)
- Irregular (both strong and weak beats occur within 1 minute)

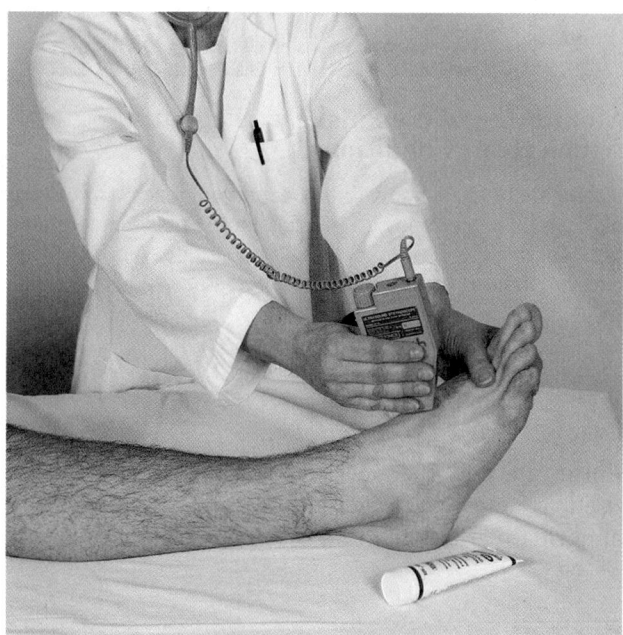

FIGURE **21-12** Checking a pedal pulse with a Doppler stethoscope.

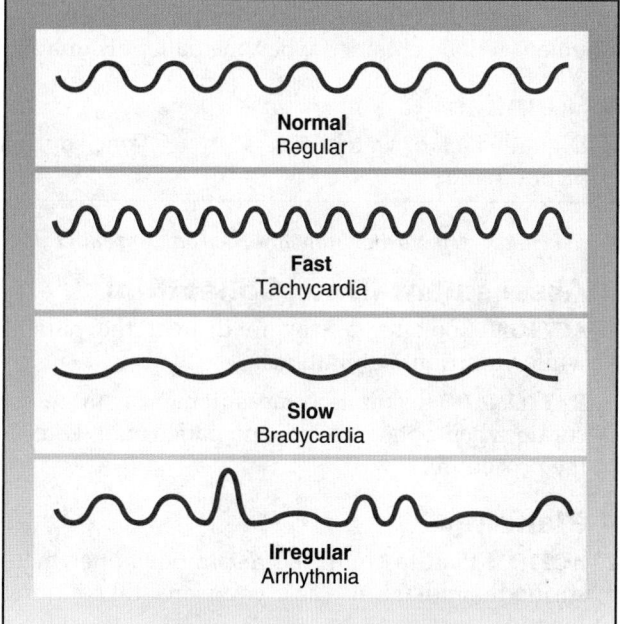

FIGURE **21-13** Pulse rhythms.

- Thready (generally indicates that it is weak and may be irregular)
- Absent (no pulse palpable or heard on auscultation)

Think Critically About . . . If an elderly patient who is receiving intravenous (IV) therapy had a pulse of 78, strong and regular, at 8 A.M. and at noon the pulse is 84, full, and bounding, what might account for the change?

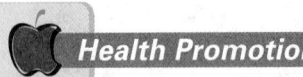

Health Promotion Points 21-2

Monitoring of the Pulse by a Patient with a Heart Condition

If the patient has a known heart condition, teach him to take his own pulse correctly and to assess the pulse characteristics. Ask him to keep a log of his pulse rates. Inquire if he knows when or what he should report to the physician.

APPLICATION of the NURSING PROCESS

Pulse rate and characteristics are assessment factors used to help determine cardiovascular health. Pulse abnormalities are defining characteristics for a variety of nursing diagnoses and are considered together with other assessment data. Changes in pulse rate are used for evaluation of the patient's response to different types of interventions, such as ambulation, bathing, dressing, or exercising.

MEASURING RESPIRATIONS

Measuring the respirations is done each time a full set of vital signs is taken. **A change in respiratory rate may indicate a change in a patient's condition, but is always considered along with the other vital signs and assessment data.** The respirations should be counted for 30 seconds and multiplied by 2. In someone who is known to be very ill or who has irregular respirations, count for a full minute (Skill 21-5).

Skill 21-5 | Measuring Respirations

Respirations are measured each time vital signs are obtained. The depth and character of respirations, as well as the number of breaths per minute, should be noted. The most accurate measurement will be obtained when the patient is unaware that you are counting respirations.

■ Supplies
✓ Digital watch or watch with second hand
✓ Pencil and paper

Review and carry out the Standard Steps in Appendix 3.

■ Assessment (Data Collection)
1. **ACTION** Look for a way to distract the patient while you count respirations.

   RATIONALE Respiration measurement is more accurate when obtained with the patient unaware of the procedure.

■ Planning
2. **ACTION** Plan to count the respirations after measuring the radial pulse as if you were still counting the pulse.

   RATIONALE May make the patient unaware that you are counting respirations.

■ Implementation
3. **ACTION** Perform hand hygiene and tell the patient you are going to take the vital signs.

   RATIONALE Reduces transfer of microorganisms and puts the patient at ease.

4. **ACTION** After taking the radial pulse with the wrist lying on the chest, continue holding the wrist while counting respirations or position your hand on the chest. Position the watch so that you can see both its dial and the rise and fall of the chest.

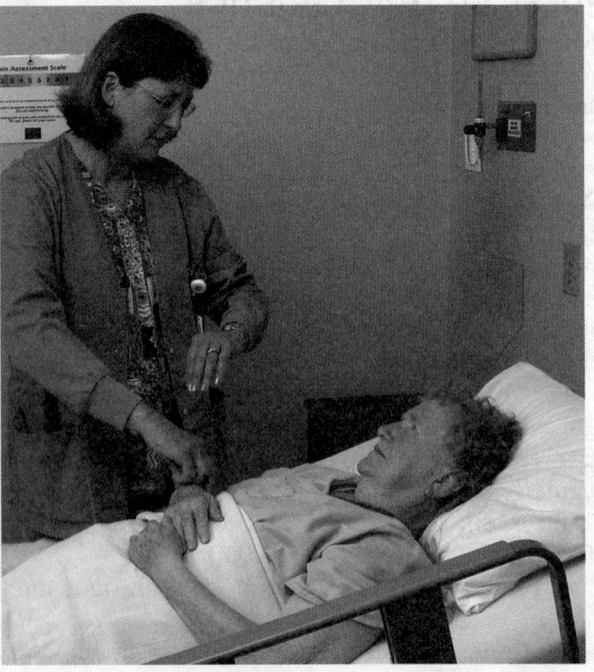

Step **4**

RATIONALE Looking like you are counting the pulse while watching the chest rise and fall helps distract the patient from his breathing. Alternately, having your hand on the patient's chest allows for the feeling of the rise and fall of the chest so you can count the respirations.

5. *ACTION* Count the respirations, noting rate, depth, pattern, and sounds. Count for 30 seconds by the watch and multiply by 2 to get the rate for 1 minute. If respirations are irregular, count for a full minute.

   RATIONALE Recall that a respiration includes both inspiration and expiration. Thirty seconds is sufficient for an accurate count if respirations are regular.

6. *ACTION* Jot down the measurement along with the pulse rate.

   RATIONALE Prevents forgetting the count.

7. *ACTION* Perform hand hygiene.

   RATIONALE Reduces transfer of microorganisms.

■ Evaluation

8. *ACTION* Ask yourself: Is the respiratory rate normal? Has it altered since the last measurement?

   RATIONALE Provides data to determine whether an alteration from normal is occurring.

■ Documentation

9. *ACTION* Record the time and respiratory rate on the graphic record, on the patient's office chart, or in the computer. If the character of respirations is abnormal or if the rate is irregular, document the findings in the nurse's notes.

   RATIONALE Notes respiratory rate and any abnormalities.

Documentation Example

R 36, shallow and moist sounding.

?CRITICAL THINKING QUESTIONS

1. If a patient is breathing very rapidly and shallowly, what is the best way to assess the number of respirations per minute?

2. What do you think is a better measure of a patient's respiratory status than counting respirations?

Table 21-4 *Normal Range of Respirations*

AGE GROUP	RESPIRATIONS PER MINUTE
Elderly	16-20
Healthy adult	12-20
Adolescent	16-20
Child (age 3 yr)	20-30
Infant (age 1 yr)	20-40
Newborn	30-80

Many of the factors that affect the pulse rate also affect the respiratory rate because the heart and lungs are closely connected in providing oxygen to sustain life. Although the rate and depth of respirations are controlled by the respiratory center in the brain, they are easily influenced by emotions, pain, degree of activity, age, fever, drugs, and disease conditions. The respiratory center is sensitive to changes in the carbon dioxide level in the blood and, to a lesser degree, in the oxygen level. Individuals can voluntarily control the rate and depth of respirations somewhat, as may happen when patients are aware that their respirations are being counted.

The respiratory rates vary according to age. Table 21-4 shows the normal range. The ratio of respirations to heartbeats is fairly constant at approximately 1 respiration to 4 heartbeats. **In addition, the rate of respirations increases during fever as the body attempts to remove excess heat.** Increased levels of carbon dioxide or lower levels of oxygen in the blood cause an increase in the respiratory rate to restore the chemical balance and expel the carbon dioxide.

Head injury or any increased intracranial pressure will depress the respiratory center and result in shallow or slow breathing.

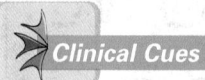
Clinical Cues

Certain drugs, such as narcotic analgesics and some sedatives, tend to depress the respiratory rate. Assess respiratory quality and count the rate each time before you administer one of these drugs.

If an adult does not breathe at a minimal rate of 12 respirations per minute and in sufficient depth, some of the following symptoms of hypoxia may be noted as a result of low oxygen supply in the blood:

- Apprehension and restlessness
- Confusion, dizziness, and change in the level of consciousness
- Cyanosis (bluish discoloration) or skin color changes, particularly around the mouth and in the nail beds

RESPIRATORY PATTERNS

As respirations are being counted, observe for variations in the pattern of breathing (Figure 21-14). Eupnea (a normal, relaxed breathing pattern) is effortless, quite evenly paced, regular, and automatic. The inspiratory phase is a bit shorter than the expiratory phase. Changes from this normal pattern are described in a variety of ways.

Dyspnea (difficult and labored breathing) is often accompanied by flared nostrils, anxious appearance, and statements such as "I can't get enough air." It is very important to know how much activity causes the dyspnea: Does it occur when walking down the hall, trying to eat a meal, or even when trying to talk?

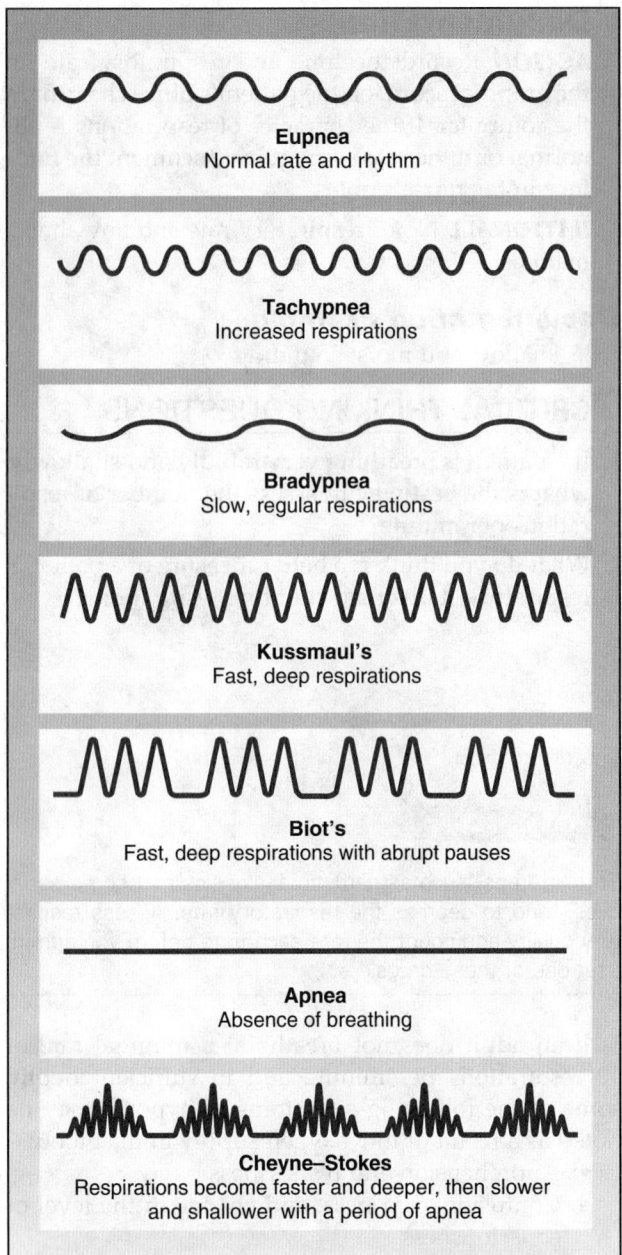

FIGURE **21-14** Respiratory patterns.

Tachypnea (increased or rapid breathing) results from the presence of fever and a number of diseases. **Breathing rate increases about four breaths for each 1° F or 0.5° C increase in temperature.**

Bradypnea (slow and shallow breathing) results when a limited amount of air is exchanged and less oxygen is taken in. This type of breathing often leads to hypoxemia (decreased levels of oxygen in the blood). It is often seen in patients who are under medical sedation, who are recovering from anesthesia or abdominal surgery, or who are in a weak or debilitated condition.

Hyperventilation is a pattern of breathing in which there is an increase in the rate and the depth of breaths and carbon dioxide is expelled, causing the blood level of carbon dioxide to fall. The condition is

seen after severe exertion, during high levels of anxiety or fear, and with fever and conditions such as diabetic acidosis.

Kussmaul's respirations have an increased rate and depth with panting and long, grunting exhalation. Kussmaul's respirations are seen in patients with diabetic acidosis and renal failure.

Biot's respirations are shallow for two or three breaths with a period of variable apnea. These respirations occur in patients with increased intracranial pressure. Such changes from the normal respiratory pattern of breathing should be reported to the charge nurse or physician so that appropriate treatment can be carried out.

Cheyne-Stokes respirations consist of a pattern of dyspnea followed by a short period of apnea (absence of breathing). Respirations are faster and deeper, then slower, and are followed by a period of no breathing, with continuation of this cycle. It is seen in critically ill patients with brain conditions, in patients with heart or kidney failure, and in cases of drug overdose.

Some of the terms used to describe noisy respirations are

- Crackles: Abnormal, nonmusical sound heard on auscultation of the lungs during inspiration; also called *rales*. Sound like hair rubbed between the fingers next to the ear.
- Rhonchi: Continuous dry, rattling sounds heard on auscultation of the lungs caused by partial obstruction.
- Stertor: Snoring sound produced when patients are unable to cough up secretions from the trachea or bronchi.
- Stridor: Crowing sound on inspiration caused by obstruction of the upper air passages, as occurs in croup or laryngitis.
- Wheeze: Whistling sound of air forced past a partial obstruction, as found in asthma or emphysema.

Abnormal patterns of respiration are covered more fully in Chapter 28.

Assessment of the respiratory rate and pattern must be analyzed together with other data such as breath sounds and arterial oxygen saturation in order to determine a patient's specific problem. Measurement of respirations may be performed to evaluate a patient's response to activity.

MEASURING OXYGEN SATURATION OF THE BLOOD

Another method of monitoring function of the respiratory system is pulse oximetry (measurement of oxygen). With a pulse oximeter (machine that measures oxygen in the blood), changes in arterial oxygen saturation can be tracked. Oxygen saturation may be spot checked or continuously monitored (Figure 21-15). The device measures oxygen saturation by determining the percentage of hemoglobin that is bound with

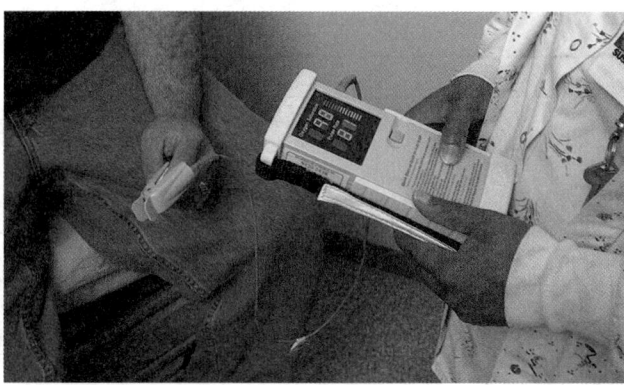

FIGURE **21-15** Measuring oxygen saturation with a portable pulse oximeter.

Table 21-5 *Classification of Blood Pressure (BP)*

BP CLASSIFICATION	SYSTOLIC BLOOD PRESSURE (mm Hg)	DIASTOLIC BLOOD PRESSURE (mm Hg)
Normal	<120	and <80
Prehypertension	120-139	or 80-89
Stage 1 hypertension	140-159	or 90-99
Stage 2 hypertension	≥160	or ≥100

oxygen. A sensor or probe is attached to an area of the patient through which infrared and red light can reach the capillary bed. Oxyhemoglobin absorbs more infrared than red light. A microprocessor in the monitor receives the information from the sensor-probe, computes the saturation value, and displays it on the monitor screen. A finger or toe clip-on probe is most commonly used, but adhesive sensors can be applied to the nose or the forehead. A clip-on probe is available for use on an earlobe or an infant's foot.

Many agencies are using a combination vital signs monitor and oximeter for scheduled vital sign measurements. The oxygen saturation is charted on the graphic sheet with the vital signs or on the electronic flow sheet in the computer. Further information about pulse oximetry can be found in Chapter 28.

MEASURING THE BLOOD PRESSURE

By measuring the blood pressure (BP), you obtain information about the effectiveness of the heart contractions, the adequacy of the blood volume in the system, and the presence of any obstruction or interference to flow through the blood vessels. Blood pressure is measured with the use of a sphygmomanometer and a stethoscope. The sphygmomanometer occludes the artery and then slowly allows blood flow through it. The stethoscope is used for auscultation (hearing) of the sounds made in the artery by the beats of the heart. The average blood pressure in a healthy young adult is 120/70 mm Hg: 120 is the systolic pressure, 70 is the diastolic pressure, and the difference between the two, or 40, is the pulse pressure. As a result of the many factors influencing it, the blood pressure is a dynamic force that can vary from minute to minute as the heart adjusts to demands and responses of the body and mind. Infants have very low blood pressure, and the blood pressure gradually but steadily increases with age. Normal blood pressure for any adult should be less than 120/80. The current guidelines of the National Heart, Lung, and Blood Institute, a division of the National Institutes of Health, indicate that the nor-

mal range for blood pressure should be much lower than previously thought (Table 21-5).

It is important to know the usual range of pressure of each patient and some of the factors that may be influencing it rather than to make judgments based on just one measurement (Table 21-6). Ask patients whether they have high or low pressure, or consult the chart for other readings that have been recorded. A reading of 110/60 may be normal for a 21-year-old man but low for a 70-year-old whose average pressure is 154/90. A noisy environment and crowded room conditions may cause a temporary elevation of blood pressure. Anxiety, fear, and stress elevate the blood pressure. Take a person's blood pressure in a quiet room with a relaxed environment.

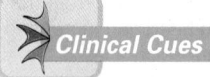
Clinical Cues

Patients should be allowed to sit in a chair, with their feet flat on the floor, and rest for at least 5 minutes before blood pressure measurements are taken. Crossing the legs at the knee causes an elevation in systolic and diastolic pressure. If taking a supine pressure, the patient should rest supine for at least 1 minute before the measurement is taken. The arm should be elevated in either position so that the brachial artery site for the reading is at the level of the right atrium. Prop the arm on a pillow when using the supine position.

EQUIPMENT USED FOR MEASURING BLOOD PRESSURE

Although direct measurement of blood pressure with an arterial catheter is the best method, the sphygmomanometer (device used to indirectly measure blood pressure) with an occlusive cuff and the stethoscope are the most commonly used pieces of equipment for measuring blood pressure (Figure 21-16). Two types of manometers were traditionally used in clinical settings: the mercury gauge, when greater accuracy is needed, and the aneroid gauge, which is a smaller unit and easy to carry but less accurate. Many hospitals have manometers attached to the wall in each patient's room. Mercury has been designated as a biohazard, and its use in medical equipment is being phased out. Although there is an effort to rid health care facilities of mercury-containing devices, many agencies and offices ha⌐ yet changed from mercury manometers becau⌐ are considered more accurate than the aneroid typ⌐ aneroid type is prone to mechanical alterations

Table 21-6 *Factors that Influence Blood Pressure*

FACTOR	INFLUENCE
Age	Newborns and infants have the lowest blood pressure. Blood pressure increases as age increases. It is highest in older adults because of a decrease in the elasticity of vessels, which causes an increase in resistance to blood flow. However, even in older adults a blood pressure above 140/90 mm Hg should not be considered normal.
Stress and emotions	Anxiety, pain, tension, worry, and stress raise blood pressure by stimulating the sympathetic nervous system, which causes vasoconstriction and a resulting increased heart rate.
Medication	Medications that lower blood pressure include narcotics, tranquilizers, hypnotics, diuretics, antihypertensives, and certain cardiac medications (particularly vasodilators). Medications that raise blood pressure include antihistamines, estrogen, and corticosteroids (glucocorticoids and mineralocorticoids).
Diurnal variation	Blood pressure is typically lowest in the early morning, with decreased activity, and highest in the afternoon or evening, with increased activity.
Sex	After puberty, males tend to have higher blood pressure than females. After menopause, women tend to have higher blood pressure than men of the same age.
Environment	A hot environment can lower blood pressure by causing vasodilation. A cold environment can raise it by causing vasoconstriction.
Exercise	Blood pressure increases with activity and exercise because the sympathetic nervous system responds to the body's increased need for oxygen.
Body position	Blood pressure is lowest in the recumbent position. It is slightly higher in the standing position because of sympathetic nervous system stimulation.
Right vs. left arm	About one fourth of the population has a difference of 10 (±5) mm Hg between the right and left arms.
Arm vs. leg	There is a difference of 10-40 mm Hg in systolic blood pressure between measurements taken using the arm and measurements taken using the leg.
Vasodilation	Parasympathetic nervous system stimulation causes blood vessels to increase in lumen diameter, thus lowering blood pressure. This may happen in response to warm temperatures, fever, and relaxation, for example.
Vasoconstriction	Sympathetic nervous system stimulation causes blood vessels to decrease in lumen diameter, thus raising blood pressure. This may happen in response to cold temperatures, for example.
Head injury	Injuries to the head and increased intracranial pressure result in increased blood pressure.
Reduced blood volume	Blood pressure decreases if the circulatory system contains an inadequate volume of blood, as from low cardiac output, hemorrhage, or shock.
Increased blood volume	Too much fluid in the cardiovascular system increases blood pressure.

From Harkreader, H., Hogan, M.A., & Thobaben, M. (2007). *Fundamentals of Nursing: Caring and Clinical Judgment* (3rd ed.). Philadelphia: Elsevier Saunders.

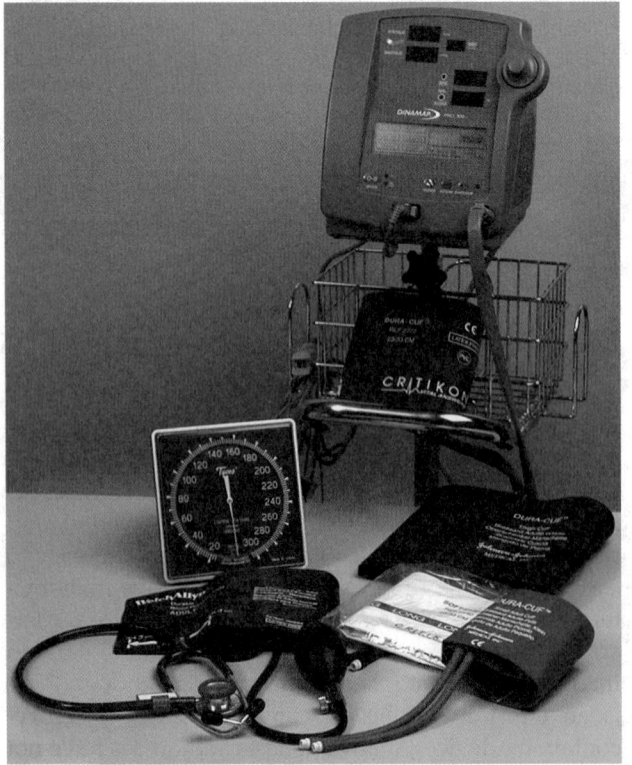

FIGURE **21-16** Equipment for measuring blood pressure. *Left,* Aneroid sphygmomanometer. *Right,* Electronic sphygmomanometer. *Front,* Stethoscope.

affect the accurate calibration of the device. Aneroid sphygmomanometers should be recalibrated every 6 to 12 months. Electronic vital signs monitors are replacing mercury manometers in hospitals.

An electronic sphygmomanometer takes the blood pressure almost automatically. The cuff is placed on the arm or wrist and pumped up. As the air is released, the systolic and diastolic pressures are displayed on a screen in the unit. This model does not require the use of a stethoscope for listening to pressure sounds, but it is much more expensive than the traditional manometer. The traditional manometer consists of a gauge for measuring the blood pressure; tubing running from the gauge to a cuff, which is wrapped around the arm or leg; and a control bulb that inflates and deflates the cuff. This sphygmomanometer is particularly useful for home monitoring.

The cuff must be the correct size to obtain an accurate blood pressure reading. A narrow cuff is used for small children and a wider cuff is needed for muscular or obese persons. **Using the wrong size produces errors as great as 25 mm Hg.** The proper width is 21% larger than the diameter of the arm, and the inflatable bladder should go around at least three fourths of the arm. A standard acoustic stethoscope with a "Y" tubing, soft ear tips, and diaphragm head is satisfactory for taking vital signs (Skill 21-6).

Skill 21-6 | Measuring the Blood Pressure

Blood pressure is measured each time vital signs are taken. Trends in blood pressure are monitored to detect early signs of complications from surgery, illness, or trauma.

■ Supplies
✓ Stethoscope

✓ Sphygmomanometer with correct-size cuff

✓ Pencil and paper

Review and carry out the Standard Steps in Appendix 3.

■ Assessment (Data Collection)

1. *ACTION* Identify the patient. Check to see what the patient's blood pressure is normally.

   RATIONALE Ensures that the blood pressure is recorded for the correct person. Knowing the usual pressure assists in knowing how high to inflate the cuff.

2. *ACTION* Assess the size of the patient's arm to determine the size of cuff needed.

   RATIONALE The bladder of the cuff should cover two thirds of the circumference of the upper arm.

3. *ACTION* Assess if there is a contraindication to taking the blood pressure on either arm.

   RATIONALE If a patient has had a mastectomy, a serious injury, a lymph node dissection, or has a dialysis shunt on the side of the arm chosen, use the other arm. If both arms are contraindicated, use a thigh cuff on a leg.

■ Planning

4. *ACTION* Provide privacy and reduce environmental noise. Explain the procedure and perform hand hygiene.

   RATIONALE Quieter environment allows you to hear the blood pressure sounds more accurately. Explaining procedure puts the patient at ease. Hand hygiene reduces transfer of microorganisms.

5. *ACTION* Place the patient in a comfortable position, sitting down or lying down, and allow the blood pressure to stabilize for 5 minutes before measuring it.

   RATIONALE Position changes alter hemodynamics within the body; blood pressure will stabilize within 5 minutes.

■ Implementation

6. *ACTION* Apply the cuff smoothly to the patient's arm, positioning the center of the bladder over the brachial artery and placing the cuff 1 to 2 inches above the antecubital space. Wrap the cuff firmly and smoothly around the arm and fasten it. Alternatively, position the cuff over the popliteal artery on the underside of the thigh.

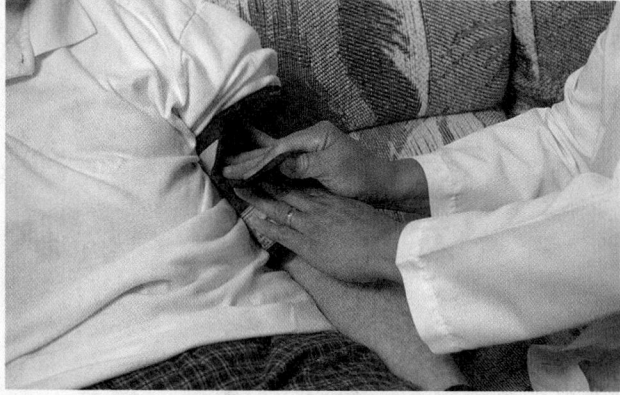

Step **6A**

RATIONALE The center of the bladder of the cuff must be over the brachial or popliteal artery for an accurate measurement to be taken.

7. *ACTION* Position the gauge so it can be easily visualized.

   RATIONALE Straining to see the lines on the gauge may cause an inaccurate reading.

8. *ACTION* Position and support the patient's arm or leg at the level of the heart.

   RATIONALE An arm or leg positioned above or below the level of the heart may cause an inaccurate reading.

9. *ACTION* Close the valve of the air pump by turning the screw valve clockwise until it is closed, but not so tightly that it cannot be easily released.

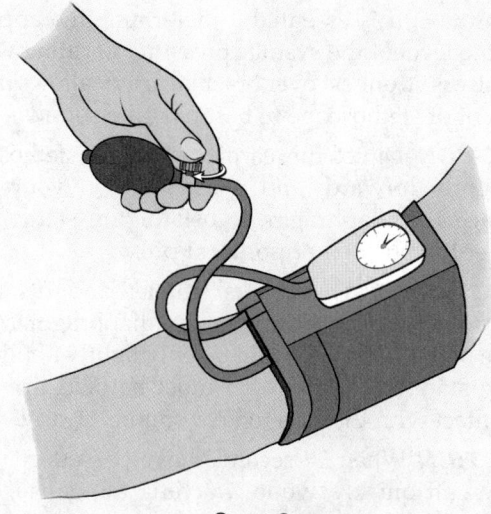

Step **9**

Continued

Skill 21-6 Measuring the Blood Pressure—cont'd

RATIONALE Closing the valve directs airflow into the cuff when the bulb is squeezed.

10. **ACTION** Palpate the brachial or popliteal artery for the strongest pulse area. Pump up the cuff until the artery is occluded, then release the valve and let the air out of the cuff. Radial artery may be palpated instead of brachial.

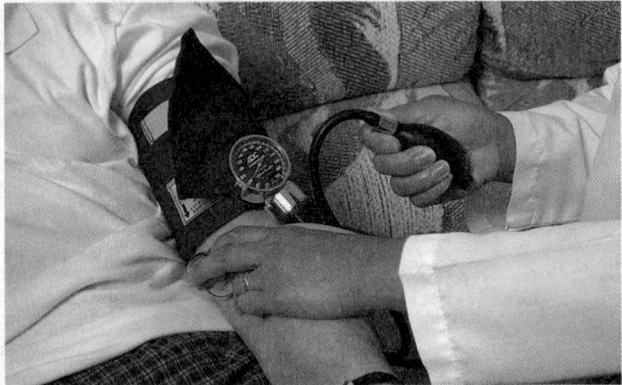

Step **10A**

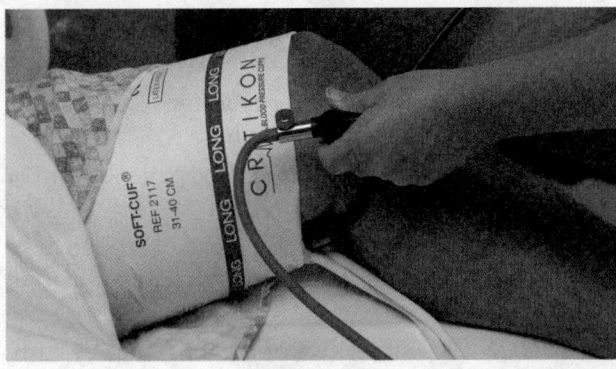

Step **10B**

RATIONALE Locating the pulse before pumping up the cuff is essential to determine the approximate level of the systolic pressure. Locating where pulse is strongest over brachial artery allows placement of stethoscope to best hear the sounds.

11. **ACTION** Direct the earpieces of the stethoscope slightly forward, and place them in your ears. Place the diaphragm or bell of the stethoscope over the brachial or popliteal pulse.

RATIONALE The bell is smaller and fits more closely over the skin than the diaphragm. When the bell is used, it should be only lightly applied to the skin. The diaphragm must be held firmly in contact with the skin to hear sounds clearly.

12. **ACTION** When 30 seconds have passed, reinflate the cuff quickly, while watching the gauge, to at

least 30 points higher than the point at which you no longer can feel the pulse.

RATIONALE Ensures that the cuff is inflated to a point above the patient's systolic blood pressure and prevents missing an auscultatory gap (period where sound disappears). Keeping the mercury column at eye level gives a more accurate reading. The aneroid gauge should be read with the eyes directly over or in line with it.

13. **ACTION** Deflate the cuff at a constant rate of 2 mm Hg/sec by unscrewing the valve on the bulb pump counterclockwise.

RATIONALE Deflating too rapidly or too slowly gives false readings. Avoiding contact of the stethoscope tubing with the clothing, cuff, or tubing of the sphygmomanometer will decrease the possibility of extraneous noise.

14. **ACTION** Listen for the first Korotkoff sound, and note this as the systolic blood pressure. Continue to listen and steadily deflate the cuff until muffling is heard; note this point. Continue deflating until the last Korotkoff sound is heard; note this point. Replace the patient's clothing if needed.

RATIONALE The point of muffling of Korotkoff sounds is considered the most accurate measurement of blood pressure in children; the point at which the last Korotkoff sound is heard is considered most accurate for adults. If sleeve was pushed up, replacing it shows courtesy to the patient.

15. **ACTION** Deflate the cuff completely. Jot down the blood pressure reading.

RATIONALE Deflating prepares the cuff for next use. Jotting the measurement on your worksheet makes it readily available when recording on the patient's chart.

16. **ACTION** Perform hand hygiene.

RATIONALE Reduces the transfer of microorganisms.

17. **ACTION** If you turned off the TV or radio, turn it back on. Restore the unit as it was.

RATIONALE Shows courtesy and caring to the patient. Replacing personal articles and the call light within reach prevents accidents.

■ **Evaluation**

18. **ACTION** Ask yourself: Is the blood pressure within normal range? Is it elevated? Is it dangerously low? Is there a considerable unexplained difference between this reading and the former reading?

RATIONALE Answers provide data regarding further assessments that may need to be made. Excessively high or low pressure should be reported to the physician.

■ Documentation

19. *ACTION* Document the time and pressure on the graphic sheet; record any new abnormality in the nurse's notes with your assessment. Blood pressure is recorded with the systolic pressure as the top number of a fraction and the diastolic pressure as the bottom number.

RATIONALE Demonstrates trend of blood pressure and communicates any abnormality.

Documentation Example

BP 136/84 (If muffling occurs, record as 136/92/84.) If thigh cuff is used, note that it is a thigh blood pressure.

■ Special Considerations

✓ Use appropriate cuff size with the bladder of the cuff covering two thirds of the arm circumference. Three sizes should be available: pediatric, adult, and large adult. A poorly fitting cuff provides inaccurate measurement.

✓ When using a thigh cuff, turn the patient onto the abdomen if possible and wrap the cuff about 2 inches above the knee. Place the stethoscope over the popliteal artery.

✓ To palpate a blood pressure when sound cannot be heard, locate the radial pulse, inflate the cuff per usual routine, and let the pressure fall; note the pressure at which the radial pulse is first felt. This is the systolic pressure; diastolic pressure cannot be determined by this method. This measure will be 2 to 5 mm Hg lower than that obtained by auscultation.

✓ If an ambulatory care patient has "white coat syndrome" (BP rises whenever the patient is approached by a medical person), retake the pressure before the patient leaves the office or clinic.

✓ Teach hypertensive patients the importance of monitoring their blood pressure frequently.

✓ Encourage the purchase of a home blood pressure unit.

✓ If a wrist BP monitor is used, advise that the wrist must be positioned at the level of the right atrium for accuracy.

✓ Digital blood pressure monitoring systems with large number readouts are available for the elderly with poor vision.

✓ An elderly hypertensive patient's blood pressure should regularly be checked with the patient standing and lying down and on both arms. *This method detects hypotensive reactions to blood pressure medication more accurately.*

✓ Whenever blood pressure is measured on a patient new to the office or health facility, take the blood pressure on both arms.

✓ If in doubt that an accurate pressure was obtained, ask another nurse to recheck the patient's blood pressure.

? CRITICAL THINKING QUESTIONS

1. When you have difficulty adequately hearing a patient's blood pressure sounds, what would you do to obtain an accurate measurement?

2. If a patient has fresh casts on both arms, how would you measure the blood pressure? Describe how you would do this.

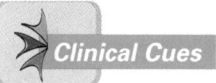
Clinical Cues

Always use the markings on the cuff to measure the arm-to-cuff width to verify that the cuff is the correct size. If in doubt, use a larger cuff as it will not alter the readings by being a bit too large.

If the sounds are very faint, try using the other arm, or use a Doppler stethoscope to amplify the sounds so that accurate readings occur.

KOROTKOFF SOUNDS

While measuring blood pressure, certain sounds may be heard that relate to the effect of the blood pressure cuff on the arterial wall. These sounds, called Korotkoff sounds, were identified by a Russian surgeon and are numbered as follows:

Phase I: Tapping—systolic pressure indicated by faint, clear tapping sounds that gradually grow louder

Auscultatory gap: No sound—silence as cuff deflates for 30 to 40 mm Hg; common with hypertension

Phase II: Swishing—murmur or swishing sounds that increase as the cuff is deflated

Phase III: Knocking—louder knocking sound that occurs with each heartbeat

Phase IV: Muffling—a sudden change or muffling of the sound (indicates diastolic pressure in children and some adults)

Phase V: Silence—disappearance of sound (marks diastolic pressure in adults)

It is important to continue to listen until the cuff is deflated so that you do not mistake an auscultatory gap for the last Korotkoff sound. Follow the guidelines in Box 21-4 when measuring the blood pressure.

When the blood pressure cannot be determined by auscultation, the palpation method is used to estimate systolic pressure. Diastolic pressure cannot be measured this way. With the blood pressure cuff in place on the upper arm, palpate the radial artery. Inflate the

Box 21-4 | *Guidelines for Measuring Blood Pressure*

To obtain an accurate reading and to avoid problems that lead to errors, use the following guidelines when measuring blood pressure:

- Have the patient lie down or sit and rest for 5 minutes. If sitting, have patient keep feet flat on the floor.
- Use the brachial artery in the elbow joint of either arm. The arm should be supported on a surface at the level of the heart.
- Check the condition of the equipment, and position the manometer gauge so it can be seen at eye level from a distance of 1 to 3 feet. The gauge indicator should be at zero when the cuff is deflated. Use the correct cuff size.
- Bare the arm, and place the cuff and stethoscope directly on the skin. Bunched or wrinkled clothing prevents the correct placement of the cuff.
- Palpate the brachial or radial artery before taking the blood pressure when the patient is new to you. Inflate the cuff while palpating the artery and note the level at which the pulse disappears. Deflate the cuff. Wait 30 to 60 seconds before reinflating for the auscultated readings. (For repeated measurements on familiar patients, you may forgo the palpated pressure, but inflate to 10 to 20 points above the person's usual systolic reading.)

- Make sure the diaphragm of the stethoscope is placed firmly but lightly over the artery. All surface edges of the diaphragm should be in contact with the skin. Do not place the thumb over the bell or top of the stethoscope to hold it in place.
- Inflate the cuff to 30 mm Hg above where the pulse disappeared on palpation with inflation to prevent missing an **auscultatory gap** (period when no sound is heard).
- Allow the cuff to deflate very slowly at 2 mm/sec. Any faster causes erroneous readings of both systolic and diastolic pressure.
- Once the cuff is starting to deflate, continue to deflate slowly all the way to zero. Do not stop midway and begin to inflate again, because this gives a false reading.
- Listen for the different sounds while steadily deflating the cuff, and identify the systolic and diastolic pressures. The phase I sound is the systolic pressure; the disappearance or phase V sound is the diastolic pressure. If the sound persists down to zero, then indicate the point at which the phase IV sound occurred and record both, as in this example: 130/62/0 (see Skill 21-6).

blood pressure cuff 30 mm Hg above the point at which the radial pulse disappears. Release the valve and allow mercury to fall 2 mm Hg per second, noting the point on the manometer when the radial pulse is again felt.

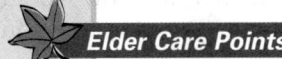 **Elder Care Points**

- It is wise to always first palpate the artery to detect at what level on the manometer no pulse is felt before taking the blood pressure of an elderly person.
- Many older adults with hypertension have an auscultatory gap in their Korotkoff sounds. If you simply pump up the cuff until you don't hear any sound and then let air out of the cuff, you may miss the upper point of the systolic blood pressure.

HYPERTENSION

Pressure consistently elevated above the normal range is called **hypertension**. Hypertension is most often found in people living in urban areas, and in those under considerable emotional stress; it affects more men than women and is twice as prevalent in blacks as in whites. Obesity is another factor contributing to hypertension. Some people may have hypertension without any risk factors. **Prolonged hypertension can cause permanent damage to the brain, the kidneys, the heart, and the retina of the eye. It is the cause of many cerebrovascular accidents (strokes).**

A systolic pressure above 140 and a diastolic pressure above 90 are regarded as being outside the normal range (hypertension). Prehypertension is a sys-

 Elder Care Points

- The pulse pressure of the elderly person is often widened because the systolic pressure tends to go up with age more quickly than the diastolic pressure.
- The elderly often experience orthostatic hypotension (drop in blood pressure when arising to a standing position) because the elasticity of the blood vessels decreases with old age. This predisposes to pooling of blood in the lower extremities upon standing and may cause dizziness. These patients are at risk for falls. Placing special elastic stockings on the lower extremities may lessen the problem.

tolic pressure above 120 and a diastolic pressure above 80. Pressures consistently higher than these should be reported to the charge nurse or physician if the patient usually has normal pressure, as should low pressures that indicate possible circulatory collapse or **shock** (condition of circulatory failure) (Health Promotion Points 21-3).

The *Healthy People 2010* goal of increasing quality and years of healthy life has an objective concerning elevated blood pressure. Objective 12.11 is directed at greater control of hypertension in the American population (Health Promotion Points 21-4).

?
Think Critically About . . . Why are several BP readings required before a diagnosis of hypertension can be made?

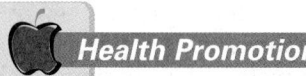

Health Promotion Points 21-3

Promoting Home Blood Pressure Monitoring

If the patient has been diagnosed with hypertension, encourage home monitoring of his blood pressure. Have him obtain a sphygmomanometer that is reliable and teach him to use it properly. Readings should be charted and tracked for changes.

Health Promotion Points 21-4

Healthy People 2010 Blood Pressure

Objective 12.11: Increase the proportion of adults with high blood pressure who are taking action to help control their blood pressure.

- Teach adults with high blood pressure the importance of controlling sodium intake, including reading food labels for sodium content and avoiding high-sodium foods, such as bacon, ham, and processed snacks.
- Refer overweight adults to a support group or weight reduction program.
- Teach about the importance of exercise and increased physical activity to reduce blood pressure.
- For the adult who smokes, teach about the relationship between cardiovascular disease and smoking; refer the individual to a smoking cessation program.
- Participate in community or health care agency health fairs to screen for hypertension and provide community education.
- Teach all adults to have their blood pressure taken at least once every 2 years; for those with hypertension, monitor blood pressure as recommended by the health care provider.

HYPOTENSION

Low blood pressure is called hypotension. Some people have a blood pressure that is normally below 90/60 mm Hg, but they are healthy with no other symptoms. However, hypotension with symptoms of shock or circulatory collapse is a dangerous condition that can rapidly progress to death unless treated. Shock is caused by hemorrhage, vomiting, diarrhea, burns, and myocardial infarction, among other conditions.

Signs and symptoms of shock are a decrease in blood pressure, an increase in pulse rate, cold and clammy skin, dizziness, blurred vision, and apprehension. Report such signs and symptoms to the charge nurse or physician without delay, and assist in treating the shock. See Chapter 37 for information about shock and its treatment.

Some patients experience postural or orthostatic hypotension (drop in blood pressure occurring with change from supine to standing or from sitting to standing position) from drug therapy, a neurologic problem, or dehydration. Blood pressure should be taken in both the standing and sitting positions for

Box 21-5 | *Technique for Determining Orthostatic Hypotension*

When the patient is experiencing fatigue, light-headedness, falls, visual blurring, or syncope, check for orthostatic hypotension.
- Measure the pulse rate. Then, with the patient supine and the brachial artery at the level of the right atrium, measure the blood pressure. Record the measurements.
- Assist the patient to a standing position. Immediately measure the pulse. Again with the brachial artery at the level of the right atrium, measure the blood pressure within 3 minutes of assisting the patient to stand.
- Determine the difference between the supine and standing systolic blood pressures. Determine the difference between the supine and standing diastolic blood pressures.

If there is a 20 mm Hg decrease in the systolic blood pressure or a 10 mm Hg decrease in the diastolic blood pressure when standing, the patient has orthostatic hypotension. Variations in heart rate are helpful in determining the cause of the orthostatic hypotension. A tachycardic response indicates dehydration or volume depletion.

these patients. A drop of 15 to 20 mm Hg from the patient's normal baseline pressure combined with symptoms of faintness, blurred vision, dizziness, or syncope signifies orthostatic hypotension. It is due to a failure of vasomotor compensatory mechanisms in response to position changes or to baroreceptor reflex impairment (Box 21-5).

APPLICATION of the NURSING PROCESS

Blood pressure measurements are considered along with the pulse rate in evaluating the general health of the cardiovascular system. Abnormalities such as hypotension, hypertension, and narrow or wide pulse pressure are defining characteristics for various nursing diagnoses and are considered along with other assessment data when choosing an appropriate diagnosis. Blood pressure is often assessed to determine how the patient is responding to a procedure or to drug treatment. This measurement is used to evaluate the patient's response to medication for hypertension. It is an important measurement in evaluating cardiovascular disease and in monitoring for shock.

PAIN, THE FIFTH VITAL SIGN

New standards of The Joint Commission state that pain is to be considered the "fifth" vital sign. The Joint Commission (2000) has recognized that "all patients have the right to pain relief." For this reason, pain is assessed and recorded along with the other vital signs. The assessment must include pain location, intensity,

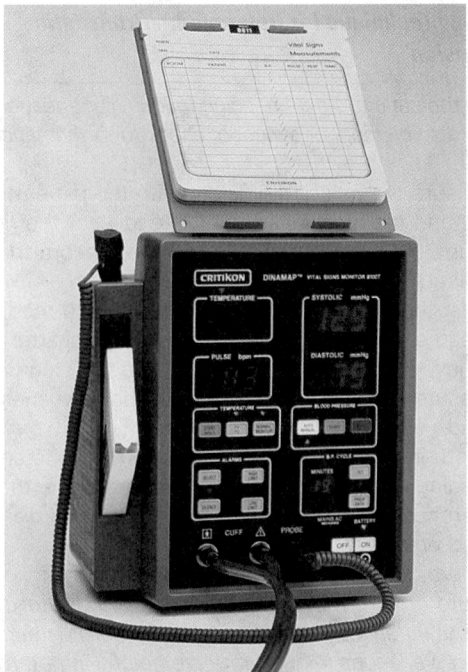

FIGURE **21-17** Automated vital signs monitor. (Courtesy of Critikon Inc., Tampa, Florida.)

character, frequency, and duration. A version of a standardized pain scale is used for the assessment. The assessment findings are often charted along with the vital signs on the graphic record. Follow-up on the assessment findings and treatment of pain is done according to agency policy. Chapter 31 presents further information on the assessment and treatment of pain.

AUTOMATED VITAL SIGN MONITORS

Lightweight, portable, automated units are available that measure blood pressure and heart rate simultaneously (Figure 21-17). Measurements can be obtained in 21 to 45 seconds. It is also possible to program most units to measure these vital signs at specified intervals. The vital signs are displayed digitally and may be retrieved using the unit's stored data capability. BioSign machines, newly introduced in the United States, can measure heart rate, respiration, blood oxygen level, temperature, and blood pressure and compare their relative status.

CHARTING VITAL SIGNS

The vital signs should be written down as soon as the measurements are obtained. It is easy to make errors or to forget the readings, especially when measuring vital signs for more than one patient. If computer entry is used, enter the vital signs before going to the next patient. Some nursing units record the vital signs on a jot board or worksheet used as a quick reference by nurses and physicians. Then the vital signs are recorded on the patient's chart by the unit secretary or the nurse. In ad-

dition, any unusual or abnormal findings may be written in the nurse's notes because of their importance to the patient's condition. The method for charting vital signs on a graphic record is shown in Figure 21-18.

RECORDING TEMPERATURE MEASUREMENTS

The bottom half of the graphic sheet in Figure 21-18 is for recording the temperature. Note that the range of degrees for temperature is 96° F to 105° F. Guidelines for charting on the graphic record are as follows:

- Record in even numbers. The graphic sheet is scored so that each line equals two tenths of a degree. Do not use odd numbers unless an electronic thermometer was used with measurements accurate to one tenth of a degree.
- Place a dot on the center of the appropriate line; the dot should be at the intersection of the appropriate hour and temperature reading.
- Connect the dots with a straight, accurate line.
- If the temperature is rectal, write ® above the dot.
- If the temperature is axillary, write @ above the dot.
- With computerized charting, the graphing is done automatically when the numbers are entered.

RECORDING PULSE MEASUREMENTS

The pulse is charted on the same page as the temperature in a table or on a graph. On a graph, each line between the bold lines represents 10 pulse beats.

Record the pulse on a graph in even numbers, such as 80, 86, and 102. Connect the dots with a straight, accurate line when a graph is used.

RECORDING RESPIRATION MEASUREMENTS

The lower portion of a graphic sheet sometimes may be used for recording the respiratory rate on the sheet or in a table. When the respiratory rate to be recorded on a graph is one of the numbers indicated on the sheet (such as 20 or 40), place the dot in the center of the appropriate line. Otherwise, the dot is centered at the correct vertical distance between two lines.

Record on a graph in even numbers, such as 22 and 46. Connect the dots with a straight, accurate line.

RECORDING BLOOD PRESSURE MEASUREMENTS

Many graphic sheets now contain a section labeled "blood pressure" and provide space for recording the readings. Write the systolic pressure above the slanted line and the diastolic pressure below the line.

Evaluating Vital Sign Trends

When vital signs are outside the expected norms, reflect a gradual trend, or have changed significantly compared with the previous vital signs, nursing ac-

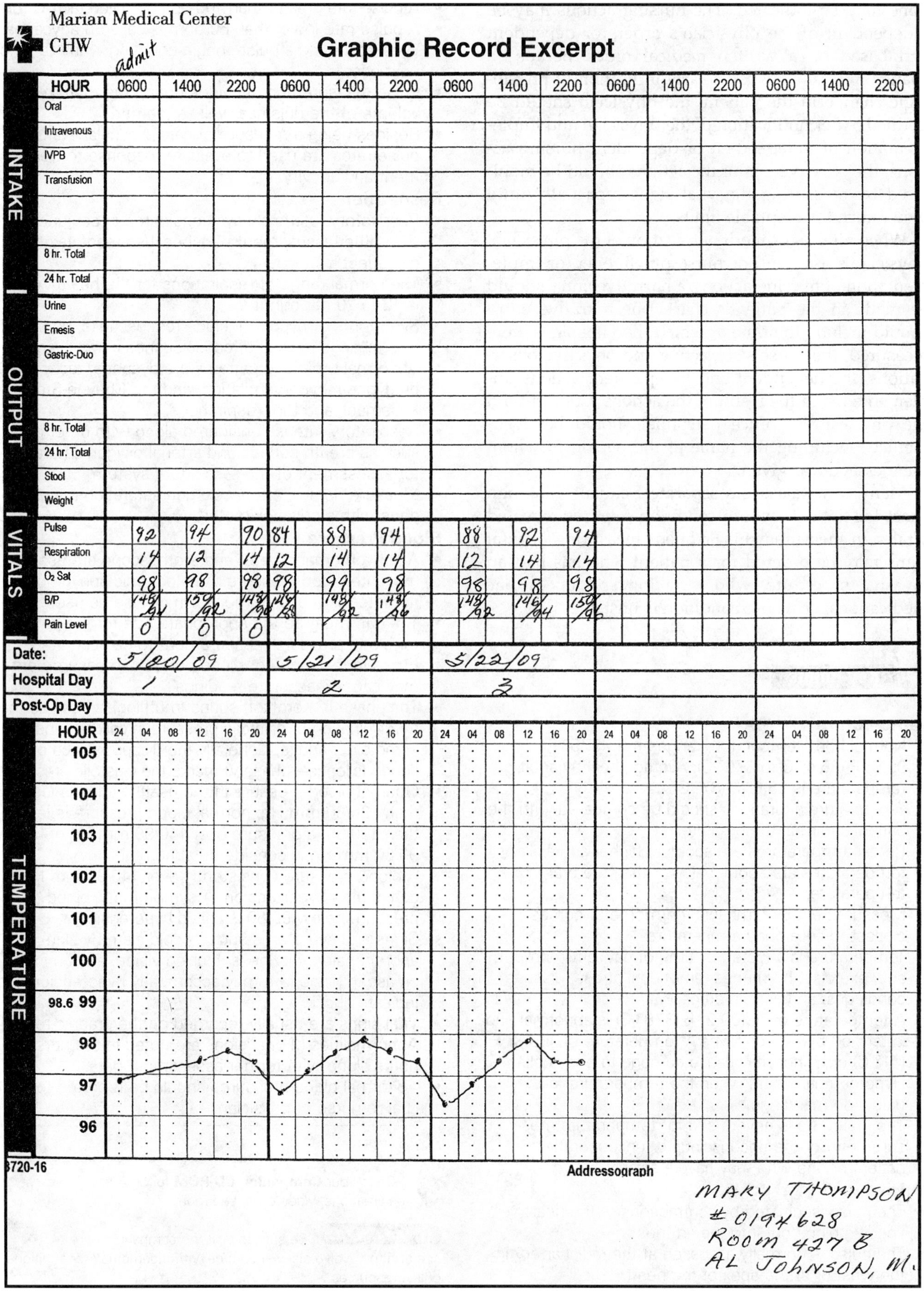

Marian Medical Center
CHW *admit*

Graphic Record Excerpt

HOUR	0600	1400	2200	0600	1400	2200	0600	1400	2200	0600	1400	2200	0600	1400	2200
INTAKE															
Oral															
Intravenous															
IVPB															
Transfusion															
8 hr. Total															
24 hr. Total															
OUTPUT															
Urine															
Emesis															
Gastric-Duo															
8 hr. Total															
24 hr. Total															
Stool															
Weight															
VITALS															
Pulse	92	94	90	84	88	94	88	92	94						
Respiration	14	12	14	12	14	14	12	14	14						
O₂ Sat	98	98	98	98	99	98	98	98	98						
B/P	148/94	159/92	148/90	148/88	148/92	148/96	148/92	146/94	159/96						
Pain Level	0	0	0												

Date:	5/20/09			5/21/09			5/22/09								
Hospital Day	1			2			3								
Post-Op Day															

HOUR	24	04	08	12	16	20	24	04	08	12	16	20	24	04	08	12	16	20	24	04	08	12	16	20	24	04	08	12	16	20
105																														
104																														
103																														
102																														
101																														
100																														
98.6 99																														
98																														
97																														
96																														

(TEMPERATURE)

3720-16

Addressograph

MARY THOMPSON
#0194628
ROOM 427 B
AL JOHNSON, M.

FIGURE **21-18** Graphic record of vital signs.

tions may be indicated. The nursing actions may be independent of the physician's orders or dependent and based on a written medical order. Because a change in vital signs is an early indication of physiologic change in the patient, the physician should be notified. After notification of the physician and implementation of independent or dependent nursing actions, the effectiveness of the actions should be monitored by measuring the vital signs repeatedly until they return to acceptable limits.

When vital signs merit notification of the physician, physician's assistant, or nurse practitioner, or implementation of nursing actions, a narrative entry should be made in the patient's chart. The narrative entry should include the time at which the vital signs were measured, the nurse's subjective and objective observations, the dependent and independent actions implemented, and the result of the actions. Contact with the physician or office personnel should be documented, including the name of the person to whom the message was given.

Many hospitals use a separate frequent vital sign sheet for patients whose condition requires repeated vital sign measurement. Frequent measuring of vital signs may be ordered for a patient who has had an invasive procedure, who is taking specific cardiac medications, or whose condition is unstable.

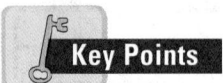
Key Points

Temperature
- Normal body temperature ranges from 97.5° F to 99.5° F (36.4° C to 37.5° C). Average healthy adult temperature is 98.6° F (37° C).
- Temperature alterations should be compared with the patient's normal temperature.
- Rectal temperatures are about 1° higher and axillary temperatures are about 1° lower than the oral temperature.
- Measurement by tympanic thermometer comes closest to core body temperature.
- Temperature is affected by time of day, environment, age, exercise, hormones, emotional stress, disease conditions, and certain drugs.
- A temperature over 100.2° F (37.8° C) is abnormal and is termed *pyrexia* or *fever*. A temperature of 105.8° F (41° C) or higher may cause damage to body cells.
- Hypothermia occurs when the temperature falls below normal range.
- The oral route is never used for temperature measurement for the unconscious or uncooperative patient or one who may have a seizure.

Pulse
- The pulse is initiated by contractions of the heart sending blood out into the arteries.
- The pulse is normally assessed at the radial artery in the wrist or at the apex of the heart.
- Normal pulse rate in the adult ranges from 60 to 100 bpm, with the average being 72 bpm.

- A pulse rate greater than 100 bpm is called tachycardia.
- A pulse rate lower than 60 bpm is called bradycardia.
- When counting a pulse, begin counting with "0"; the next beat is "1."
- Pulse measurement includes noting the rhythm and volume of the pulse as well as the rate.
- Besides being a measure of cardiovascular status, pulse rates are used to evaluate response to treatment and activity.

Respiration
- Respiratory rate is always considered in conjunction with other assessment data because many factors can affect it.
- The normal range of respirations for the healthy adult is 12 to 20 per minute.
- Symptoms of hypoxia include restlessness, confusion, change in level of consciousness, and cyanosis.
- Abnormal breathing patterns are dyspnea, tachypnea, bradypnea, hyperventilation, and the Cheyne-Stokes, Kussmaul, and Biot respirations.
- Respiratory rate is considered along with other data such as breath sounds and arterial oxygen saturation for assessment of the respiratory system.
- Measurement of arterial oxygen saturation may be done with a pulse oximeter.

Blood Pressure
- A sphygmomanometer and stethoscope are used to measure blood pressure. An electronic sphygmomanometer or vital sign monitor may also be used.
- The cuff must be the appropriate size for the patient for blood pressure measurement to be accurate.
- Errors in technique of blood pressure measurement may cause inaccurate readings.
- The phase IV Korotkoff sound (muffling) is used as the determination of diastolic pressure in children and in some older adults. Generally the disappearance of sound (silence—phase V) marks the diastolic pressure.
- Optimal blood pressure in the healthy adult is less than 120/80 mm Hg; normal blood pressure is less than 130/85; a pressure over 140/90 mm Hg or below 90/60 mm Hg is considered abnormal.
- A blood pressure consistently over 140/90 mm Hg constitutes hypertension. A symptomatic blood pressure below 90/60 is called hypotension.
- Signs and symptoms such as cold clammy skin, apprehension, dizziness, blurred vision, and an increase in pulse rate may accompany hypotension and indicate shock.
- Vital signs are usually recorded on the graphic record. Abnormalities of vital signs are noted in the nurse's notes along with further assessment data.
- Abnormal blood pressures should be reported to the charge nurse or physician.

Go to your **Companion CD-ROM** for an Audio Glossary, animations, video clips, and more.

evolve Be sure to visit the companion Evolve site at http://evolve.elsevier.com/deWit/fundamental/ for additional online resources.

NCLEX-PN® EXAMINATION-STYLE REVIEW QUESTIONS

*Choose the **best** answer(s) for each question.*

1. The nursing assistant reports to the nurse that the temperature of a patient who is first-day postoperative is 100.4° F. Which of the following actions should the nurse take first?
   1. Notify the surgeon of the temperature elevation.
   2. Check the preoperative temperature reading.
   3. Tell the nursing assistant to take the temperature again in 2 hours.
   4. Prepare to administer an acetaminophen PRN-ordered suppository.

2. Temperature greater than 105.8° F or 41° C should be treated promptly to reduce the fever because of:
   1. chemical reactions to oxygen in the bloodstream.
   2. potential damage to the cells of the central nervous system.
   3. heavy perspiration, reducing the amount of urine produced.
   4. the increased workload of the heart.

3. A newly admitted patient has a respiratory rate of 16 per minute. Which action should the nurse take?
   1. Recount the respirations in 5 minutes.
   2. Note the respiratory rate on the chart.
   3. Check the chart for signs of a respiratory disorder.
   4. Ask the patient to cough to clear the lungs.

4. The person who makes harsh high sounds upon inspiration has what kind of respiratory condition?
   1. Dyspnea
   2. Stridor
   3. Hyperventilation
   4. Cheyne-Stokes respirations

5. Pulse oximetry is used to:
   1. count the respiratory rate.
   2. determine the amount of oxygen taken into the lungs.
   3. measure carbon dioxide in the blood.
   4. determine the amount of oxygen carried in the blood.

6. A patient who has a blood pressure decrease from supine to standing of 20 mm Hg or more systolic, or 10 mm Hg or more diastolic, has _____ _____. *(Fill in the blank.)*

7. A patient whose blood pressure is consistently 136/80 is classified as having:
   1. normal blood pressure.
   2. hypotension.
   3. prehypertension.
   4. stage I hypertension.

8. Symptoms of shock that may be seen with hypotension are: *(Select all that apply.)*
   1. tachypnea.
   2. apprehension.
   3. tachycardia.
   4. cool, clammy skin.

9. When assigning vital sign measurement to the nursing assistant, the nurse says to take the apical pulse for the full 60 seconds. Which patient's condition would *most* warrant this instruction?
   1. A patient who is bradycardic
   2. A patient whose usual heart rate is 76
   3. A patient who is tachycardic
   4. A patient whose heart rate is irregular

10. Factors that may cause an inaccurate blood pressure reading are: *(Select all that apply.)*
    1. letting the manometer fall at 4 mm Hg per second.
    2. pumping the cuff up 20 points over the known systolic pressure.
    3. raising the arm with the BP cuff attached 4 inches above height of the heart.
    4. using a cuff that is 10% larger than the diameter of the arm.

CRITICAL THINKING ACTIVITIES *Read each clinical scenario and discuss the questions with your classmates.*

Scenario A
A mother brings her toddler into the clinic because he has been pulling at his ear and seems feverish. The child cried most of the night and is quite upset now.

1. How would you obtain accurate vital signs on this child?
2. Will a heart rate or respiratory rate be accurate if taken when a child is crying?

Scenario B
Richard Montez comes to the clinic for the first time because he has a sore throat. You find that his blood pressure measurement is 186/112 mm Hg.

1. Do you think this is an accurate measurement?
2. What would you do next?

3. What factors might be affecting Mr. Montez's blood pressure at this time?
4. What are the guidelines for determining if a patient has hypertension?

Scenario C
Mary Hartson comes to the clinic after pulling a back muscle. She is experiencing considerable pain. Her vital signs are usually BP 128/32, pulse 76, respirations 14, and temperature 97.8° F. What would you expect to find when you take her vital signs during this visit to the clinic?

Assessment is a vitally important nursing function. It is a continual process in which the nurse is constantly appraising the condition of patients. Nurses are expected to be able to assess lung sounds properly, identify abnormal heart sounds, determine when there might be something wrong in the abdomen, monitor circulatory status, detect neurologic changes, note skin problems, and recognize signs and symptoms of problems in any body system. When an illness occurs, it is likely to affect more than one body system. Although it is rare that a staff nurse will have the time to do a thorough physical examination of each patient assigned, the nurse must perform a quick focused assessment of each patient at the beginning of each shift and is responsible for assessing all body systems. The nurse is the person who is with the patient the most, and must monitor for subtle changes in condition. Good assessment skills can quickly identify new signs and symptoms that indicate complications of an illness or adverse side effects of medical therapy. This is especially important when working with home care or long-term care patients because the nurse is often the only health professional who sees the patient at regular intervals. The LPN/LVN charge nurse in the long-term care facility acts as the "eyes and ears" of the physician, as does the home care nurse.

The majority of people have had a physical examination at some time in their lives. Physical examinations are usually required for entry into schools, for the issuance of insurance policies, for employment, for particular types of driver's licenses, and for induction into military service. A complete physical examination is performed on patients who seek regular medical care every 1 to 5 years, depending on age and health condition. The nurse often assists with the physician's examination of the patient. This chapter introduces the methods used to obtain information about physiologic and psychosocial functioning and the ways to assist the examiner with the physical examination.

> **?**
> *Think Critically About . . .* Can you describe your last physical examination? What was done? What questions were you asked?

APPLICATION of the NURSING PROCESS

Assessment (Data Collection)

When a patient is admitted to the hospital, long-term care facility, home care service, or other agency, a nurse performs an initial assessment. This assessment usually includes gathering a history and demographic data and performing a brief physical examination. This type of assessment is covered in Chapter 5 along with interviewing (see Boxes 5-2 and 5-3).

Data Collection

Along with the physical examination, nurses are also expected to obtain some historical data concerning the patient's past and present state of health. The type of information required for the hospital nurse's admission history form is covered in Chapters 5 and 23. Students are often required to complete a history form to turn in with the nursing care plan. The information pertinent to daily care that you should know about the patient includes health history factors and psychosocial data. Certainly, knowledge of the current health problems is essential, and you should review the chart for these data or obtain them from the patient if the data are not yet on the chart.

Psychosocial and Cultural Assessment

To care for the whole patient rather than just tend to an area of physical need, nurses must be aware of how the illness is affecting the patient's life. Exploration of concerns regarding not only health but also all other areas of the patient's life is appropriate. If a mother is very worried about the care of her small children at home, energy will be focused on this area rather than on healing.

Assess for cultural preferences and health beliefs so that an individualized plan of care can be formulated. Cultural assessment is mainly a matter of asking the patient and family about preferences for food, bathing, and personal care, what they think about their illness and treatment, and who should be consulted about decisions. Phrase questions in a positive, nonthreatening way. Do not assume that just because a person is a member of a certain ethnic group, he or she has beliefs and practices common to that group. Box 22-1 provides a patient interview guide. Further information on cultural assessment is presented in Chapter 14.

Box 22-1 | *Patient Interview Guide*

SOCIAL DATA
- What is your marital status? Who is a significant person in your life?
- Do you have health insurance?
- What is/was your occupation?
- How has your admission affected things at home?
- Do you have any visual or hearing deficits?
- Do you wear dentures?
- Do you have any prosthesis, such as an artificial limb or joint?
- Are you an active member of any organization?
- Are you allergic to any medications? What happens when you take them?
- What prescription drugs do you take and how often? What over-the-counter medications do you take regularly or occasionally?
- Do you have any food allergies? Any allergies to any other substances? What happens when you eat or come into contact with any of these things?
- What do you like to eat? Are you presently on a special diet? Any special favorite foods? Do you have any food dislikes or intolerances?
- Do you or have you ever smoked? How much? For how long? When did you quit?
- Do you enjoy wine or other alcohol? When and about how much do you drink?

- Do you need assistance with your activities or with your personal care?
- Have you had previous surgeries or serious injuries?
- What health problems do you have?
- Do you routinely see other physicians? For what?
- What brought about your admission here?

PHYSICAL DATA
Review of Systems
Ask questions about the presence of the following:

Head and Neck
- Do you have frequent headaches or dizziness?
- Do you have problems with your ears? Are you hard of hearing, do have ringing in your ears, do you use a hearing aid?
- Do you have visual problems, wear contact lenses or glasses? Have you ever been told you have glaucoma or cataracts, any problems with your eyes in general? When was your last eye examination?
- Do you have frequent colds or nasal allergies, sinus infections, frequent sore throats, hoarseness, trouble swallowing, or swollen glands?
- When was your last dental examination? Any problem with gum disease or mouth sores?
- Do you have difficulty sleeping at night? Do you often take naps?

Continued

Box 22-1 *Patient Interview Guide—cont'd*

PHYSICAL DATA—cont'd
Review of Systems—cont'd

Chest

- Do you have a frequent cough? Is it a dry cough or do you bring up sputum? Can you describe the sputum for me?
- Do you have a history of lung problems such as pneumonia, asthma, wheezing, bronchitis, or emphysema?
- Have you had or ever been exposed to tuberculosis?
- Have you had any occupational exposure to any respiratory hazards?
- Have you ever had angina, chest pain, heart attack, or irregular heartbeats? Any palpitations, murmurs, or shortness of breath?
- Do you experience leg pains or cramps after walking a short distance?
- Do you have a pacemaker? Automatic defibrillator?
- Have you ever been told you have high blood pressure (hypertension)?
- Female: Do you routinely do breast self-exams? When was your last mammogram? Do you have any discharge from your nipples or any breast lumps?

Abdomen

- Do you have frequent indigestion, gas, bloating, heartburn, nausea, or vomiting?
- Do you experience excessive thirst or hunger?
- Do you have frequent bowel movements, a change in your bowel routine, or a change in the appearance of your bowel movements? Frequent diarrhea or constipation?
- Have you ever had rectal bleeding, black or tar-colored stools? Do you have excessive gas?
- Have you ever had hemorrhoids?
- Have you ever had problems with your gallbladder or liver?

Genitourinary

- Have you had problems urinating? Do you regularly have to get up during the night to urinate?
- Have you experienced urgency or frequency on a regular basis? Do you get the urge to urinate and then cannot void?
- Do you have problems with dribbling of urine or unexpectedly urinating when you laugh or cough?
- Have you ever had a urinary tract infection? Do you have them often?
- Any history of kidney stones?
- Female: Are you sexually active? Any vaginal problems or problems in the genital area? Any problems with your menstrual cycle? When was the last menstrual period? Any bleeding between periods or after menopause? When was your last Pap smear? Have you had any unusual vaginal discharge? Any history of herpes or other sexually transmitted disease?
- Male: Are you sexually active? Any genital problems or penile discharge? Any history of herpes or other sexually transmitted diseases? Any prostate problems?

Extremities and Musculoskeletal

- Do you have any joint pain or stiffness?
- Any muscle pain or back problems?
- Are you able to move your body in a full range of motion?
- Do you have any problems with circulation in your legs or arms?
- Do you bruise easily or have any skin lesions?
- Any history of phlebitis, thrombophlebitis, gout, or arthritis?
- Any fractures or injuries?
- Any artificial joints?

Endocrine

- Have you ever been diagnosed with thyroid problems? Hyper- or hypothyroid?
- Have you ever been told you have diabetes? Type 1 (insulin-dependent diabetes mellitus) or type 2 (non–insulin-dependent diabetes mellitus)? How long ago were you diagnosed? Do you take insulin or an oral agent to control your blood sugar?

 Elder Care Points

If the elderly person has difficulty with memory, data may be gathered from a family member or significant other.

? *Think Critically About* . . . What specific areas would you include in an overall assessment of a patient?

Physical Assessment

When patients are first encountered, observe their behavior and appearance and make a judgment about their health status. Some of these data may lead to the conclusion that a person is ill, has an elevated temperature, or is malnourished. In addition to observa-

tions, it is essential to ask the right questions and measure various body functions. The assessment thus provides a complete picture of physiologic functioning. When combined with a health and psychosocial history, it forms a health database for the individual. The information gathered from the physical assessment can be used for a variety of purposes. These include the following:

- Determining the patient's level of health and physiologic functioning
- Arriving at a tentative nursing diagnosis of a health problem
- Confirming a diagnosis of dysfunction, disease, or inability to carry out activities of daily living (ADLs)
- Indicating specific body areas or systems for additional testing or examination

Box 22-2 | *Taking a History of a New Illness or Problem*

When a patient presents with a new problem or illness, ask the following questions:
- What is the problem?
- When did it start? How did it start?
- Are the symptoms getting worse or remaining the same?
- Did anything seem to precipitate this illness or problem?
- How is it affecting you? Does it interfere with your usual activities?
- How often do the symptoms occur? Under what circumstances? Is there a relationship to meals? Is this a seasonal problem for you?
- If there is pain, where is it? Can you describe it? How would you rate it on a scale of 0 to 10?
- What, if anything, seems to relieve your symptoms?

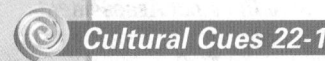
Cultural Cues 22-1

Ask Before Touching

Many cultures, including those of India, China, and the Arab countries, do not permit the touching of a female by a male outside of the family. Male nurses should seek permission from the female patient before touching her and should understand that it is not a personal issue if the female patient requests a female nurse or physician.

- Evaluating the effectiveness of prescribed treatment and therapy and observing for adverse side effects
- Monitoring for changes in body function

When the patient presents with a new illness or complaint, obtain a history of that illness or complaint with the questions in Box 22-2.

The physical assessment can be performed in a variety of settings, such as hospitals, health centers, clinics, schools, long-term care facilities, and physicians' or nurse practitioners' offices (Cultural Cues 22-1). The examination can be performed by a physician, nurse, physician's assistant, nurse practitioner, clinical nurse specialist, or other clinician, depending on the type of assessment, its purpose, and the policies of the particular agency. The assessment of physiologic functioning ranges from a comprehensive, in-depth examination that includes all systems of the body to a brief, scanning type of examination confined to a specific body part or system. Vocabulary specific to physical assessment is provided in Box 22-3.

Physical Examination Techniques

Because assessment is also a tool for nurses to use in planning nursing care, attention must be focused on methods of gathering information. In addition to using interviewing and communication skills, information is obtained by using the senses: sight, hearing, smell, and touch. The most helpful of these senses is sight, closely followed by touch.

Inspection and Observation. Through the sense of sight, nurses are able to inspect the various parts of the body and observe the behavioral responses of patients. When assessing the physiologic condition of a patient, the nurse or examiner uses inspection to make observations about the patient's general appearance, contours of the body, skin tone and color, rashes, scars and lesions (tissue damage or abnormality), deformities or

extremity weakness, characteristics of movements, and respirations.

Think Critically About . . . Can you think of other signs you might observe during physical examination?

Palpation. The sense of touch can be used to obtain a great deal of clinical information about patients. Palpation is performed with the hands and uses touch to feel various parts of the body. Palpation can be used to detect the size, shape, and position of parts of the body and the texture, temperature, and moisture of the skin. Palpation is used to ascertain the following:
- The presence of muscle spasm or rigidity
- Pain, swelling, or presence of a growth
- Any restriction in movement of a body part
- Skin temperature, turgor (elasticity), and presence of edema (fluid in the tissues)

Skillful palpation is based on knowing how to use the fingers and hands effectively. The backs of the hands and fingers are used to investigate differences in skin temperature over an inflamed joint or a foot with poor circulation. The skin is thinner on the back of the hand and more sensitive to changes in temperature. The pads of the fingers are used to palpate the size, position, and consistency of various structures, such as the lymph nodes and breast tissue. The palm of the hand is used to detect vibrations or tremors (involuntary fine movement of the body or limbs), and the thumb and index finger are used to check skin turgor, joint position, and the firmness of muscles and other tissues.

The abdomen is usually palpated lightly to identify painful or tender areas or to locate masses or abnormal collections of fluid. The pads of the fingers are used in light palpation, and pressure is exerted to indent the skin about 1 to 2 cm (½ to ¾ inch) (Figure 22-1). Deep palpation depresses the skin 4 to 5 cm (1½ to 2 inches) and can be done using one or both hands. When palpating, watch the patient's face for signs of discomfort and discontinue if it causes pain.

Percussion. Percussion is another method of obtaining information about structures of the body. It in-

Box 22-3 *Vocabulary Specific to Physical Assessment*

ADLs: Activities of daily living: bathing, dressing, grooming, cleansing teeth, shaving, toileting, etc.

Ascites: Abnormal accumulation of serous fluid within the peritoneal cavity.

Bruit: Abnormal sound heard on auscultation, a kind of swishing sound.

Cognitive: Relating to the mental process of knowing, remembering, relating; connected thinking.

Cyanosis: A bluish tinge to the skin, nail beds, or mucous membranes, indicating a significant decrease in oxygenation.

Ecchymosis: Blue or purplish patch on the skin or mucous membrane that is not elevated; bruising.

Erythema: Redness of the skin caused by congestion of the capillaries in the lower layers of the skin that occurs with any skin injury, infection, or inflammation.

Extension posture: Arms are stiffly extended, adducted, and hyperpronated with hyperextension of the legs and plantar flexion of the feet; indicates disruption of the motor fibers in the midbrain and brainstem; formerly called *decerebrate posture.*

Fissure: A narrow slit.

Flexion posture: Internal rotation and adduction of the arms with flexion of the elbows, wrists, and fingers, resulting from neurologic injury and interruption of voluntary motor tracts; extension of the legs may also be seen. Formerly called *decorticate posture.*

Guaiac: Test for blood in the stool.

Gurgles: Wet sounds heard when auscultating the lungs; newer term for rhonchi; gurgle sounds also occur in the bowel.

Inspection: Visual examination for detection of abnormal signs or qualities.

Integument: The skin covering the body.

Jaundice: Yellowness of the skin, sclera, mucous membranes, and excretions resulting from hyperbilirubinemia and deposition of bile pigments; also called *icterus.*

Jugular venous distention (JVD): Visible thickening of the jugular veins when the patient is positioned sitting in bed at a 15- to 35-degree angle; assessed as a sign of congestive heart failure or overhydration.

Lethargy: Abnormal drowsiness or stupor.

Murmur: A periodic sound of short duration of cardiac or vascular origin.

Ophthalmoscope: Lighted instrument used for viewing the interior of the eye.

Orientation: Awareness of one's environment with reference to place, time, and people.

Otoscope: Lighted instrument used to visualize the tympanic membrane and interior of the ear canal.

Pallor: Paleness of the skin.

Papanicolaou (Pap) smear: A microscopic laboratory examination used to determine the presence of malignant cells from body secretions (respiratory, genitourinary, or digestive tract).

Patent: Freely open (e.g., a patent drain).

Petechiae: Pinpoint, round, purplish red spots that are not raised, caused by intradermal or submucosal hemorrhage; a significant sign for various diseases.

Pigmentation: The deposition of coloring matter in the skin.

Proctoscopic examination: Examination of the rectum with a lighted instrument.

Rinne test: A test to compare bone and air conduction of sound, performed with a tuning fork.

Sanguineous: Bloody.

Scar: A mark remaining after the healing of a wound.

Serosanguineous: Composed of serum and blood.

Sigmoidoscopy: An examination of the sigmoid colon using a lighted instrument.

Sign: Any objective evidence of disease or dysfunction.

Sore: A term for a painful lesion of the skin or mucous membrane.

Speculum: A short, funnel-like tube for examining canals, such as the nasal canal and the vaginal canal.

Sputum: Mucous secretions of the lungs ejected through the mouth.

Symptom: Any indication of disease perceived by the patient; subjective information.

Tinnitus: A noise in the ears such as ringing, buzzing, or roaring.

Tuning fork: A forked metal instrument used to test hearing and the sense of vibration.

Vertigo: A sensation of rotation or whirling movement; dizziness.

Weber test: A test of bone conduction of sound performed with a tuning fork placed in the center of the forehead of the skull.

Wheeze: A high-pitched respiratory sound that often indicates narrowed airways; common in patients with asthma.

Wound: Bodily injury caused by physical means with disruption of the skin or other structure.

---

volves light, quick tapping on the body surface to produce sounds. Variations in the sounds reflect the characteristics of the organs or structures below the surface. Percussion is used primarily over the chest and abdomen to determine the size, location, and density of organs that lie within. The most common type of percussion consists of striking the middle finger of one hand with the index or middle finger of the other hand. When tapping, do not move the forearm; all the force is generated by a quick snap of the wrist (Figure 22-2). The tapping finger makes a quick contact with the other hand, and after two or three taps in one location, the hands are moved to another area. Different sounds are emitted as the examiner moves from one resonant area to a less or more resonant one. The sounds vary in their intensity, pitch, and duration. Sounds differ depending on the presence of underlying air, fluid, or a solid organ.

Auscultation. Auscultation is the process of listening to sounds produced in the body with the aid of the stethoscope. It is particularly valuable in hearing sounds produced in the heart, lungs, and abdomen. Nurses use

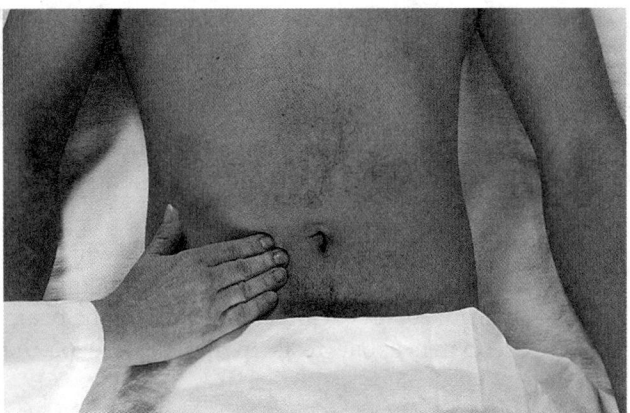

FIGURE **22-1** Palpate the abdomen for areas of tenderness.

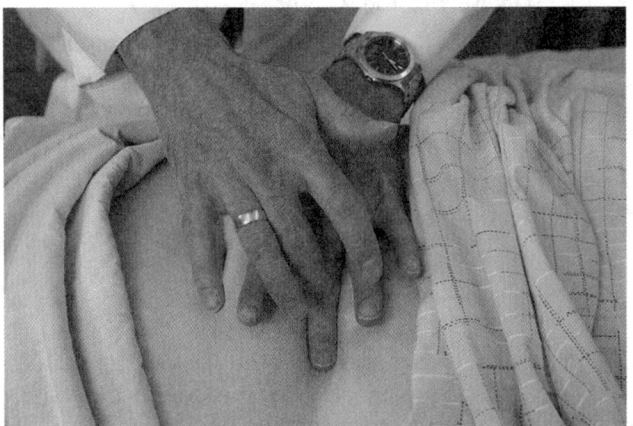

FIGURE **22-2** Technique for percussion.

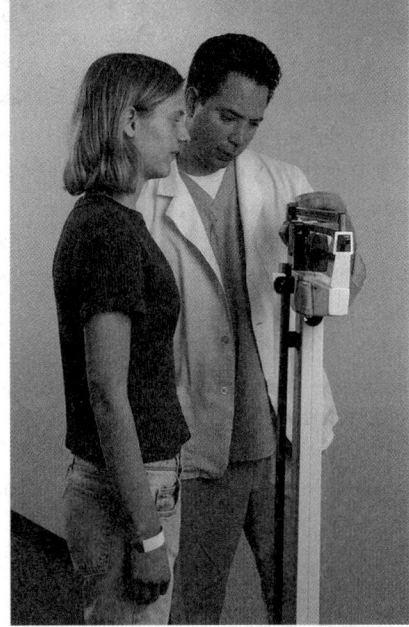

FIGURE **22-3** Weighing the adult.

the stethoscope to take blood pressure readings, to listen to the lungs, to assess heart sounds, and to check for the presence of bowel sounds. When listening to the lungs, the diaphragm of the stethoscope is used; heart valve sounds are best assessed through the bell of the stethoscope placed lightly on the chest wall. To properly use a stethoscope, place the earpieces in your ears so that they point forward toward your nose. The diaphragm is used to detect high-pitched sounds—breath, bowel, and normal heart sounds. The diaphragm (larger, flat surface) is held firmly against the skin and may leave a ring on the skin when lifted. The bell piece (smaller, cupped piece) is used to detect low-pitched sounds such as abnormal heart sounds made by the valves. It is held lightly against the skin; pressing harder obliterates the low-pitched sounds.

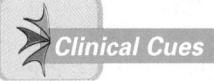

Do not place your thumb over the bell of the stethoscope when holding the diaphragm against the skin. If you do, you may only hear your own pulse transmitted via your thumb.

Olfaction. Olfaction refers to the sense of smell. The nose is used to identify characteristic smells associated with specific problems. A sweetish odor to the breath

can indicate diabetic acidosis; alcohol on the breath can provide a clue to the patient's lethargy or irrationality. Mouth odor that is foul may indicate periodontal disease or poor oral hygiene. A foul or sweet odor coming from under a cast or a wound indicates infection. A foul odor in the female genital area may indicate a vaginal infection.

Basic Physical Examination

The basics of physical examination are the foundation on which the nurse begins to build expertise. As medical-surgical conditions, pediatrics, and obstetric care are studied, further assessment skills will be learned.

Height and Weight. A basic nursing function is to weigh and measure the patient. Adult weight is most frequently measured on the standing scale (Figure 22-3). Weight can also be measured by using a built-in scale in a bed or a chair scale. Weight is measured consistently without or with shoes depending on the practice setting. Steps 22-1 provides the steps for weighing the adult. Infants are weighed in an infant scale (Figure 22-4). The infant is placed on a clean paper cover or the scale is cleansed after each weighing. The infant is weighed with one hand hovering closely to prevent a fall while adjusting the scale weights. **Never leave an infant unattended on the scale.**

Height is measured from the sole of the foot to the crown of the head. A vertical measuring rod is generally used with the patient standing erect and looking straight ahead. Shoes should not be worn when the patient is measured. The most common device used to measure adults and older children is the height rod attached to a standing scale. The rod is raised to a height greater than the person to be measured and the extension bar is raised. The person stands with the feet together centered under the rod with the back to the

Steps 22-1 | Weighing the Adult with a Standing Balance Scale

The adult is weighed on admission to the health care facility and periodically during clinic or office visits.

1. **ACTION** Check that the scale is properly calibrated and balanced by moving both weights to zero. The bar should rest in the middle of the space.

   RATIONALE Ensures that the patient's weight measurement will be accurate.

2. **ACTION** Move the large weight indicator on the lower part of the scale to the general range of the patient's weight (e.g., 50, 100, 150, 200, 250, or 300 lb).

   RATIONALE Prepares the scale by approximating the patient's weight.

3. **ACTION** Place a clean paper cover on the foot plate of the scale.

   RATIONALE Prevents transfer of microorganisms.

4. **ACTION** Assist the patient onto the scale, without shoes. Be certain that both feet are totally on the scale.

RATIONALE Shoes add to normal body weight. If a part of the foot is off the scale, the scale will not weigh accurately.

5. **ACTION** Ask the patient to remain still while adjusting the weights. Slide the other weight along the upper portion of the scale along the weight beam until the balance bar rests in the middle of the space.

   RATIONALE If the patient moves, the scale balance beam will swing wildly.

6. **ACTION** Record the weight.

   RATIONALE Recording the number immediately helps to prevent forgetting the exact number.

7. **ACTION** Assist the patient off of the scale and allow to put shoes on.

   RATIONALE Assisting the patient prevents falls when getting off the scale.

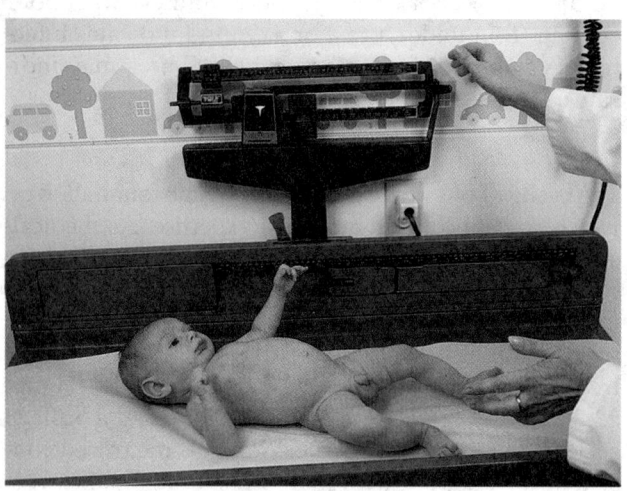

FIGURE **22-4** Weighing the infant.

rod and looks straight ahead. The extension rod is lowered while keeping it at a 90-degree angle until it rests level on the patient's head.

Infants and children younger than 3 years of age are measured in the supine position with the legs fully extended. In the physician's office, when an infant measurement board is not available, the length can be closely approximated by placing the infant on the paper covering an examining table, marking at the top of the head with the head in good alignment and the infant looking up, and then making another mark at the base of the heel with the leg fully extended. The distance between the marks is measured with a measuring tape. A second person is usually needed to help position the infant or toddler. Most measuring devices

are marked in inches and in centimeters, with fractions of these units to ensure an exact measurement. A standard for comparison of measured heights and weights that allows determination as to whether the patient's weight is within normal limits is the Metropolitan Height and Weight Chart (Table 22-1), or for children, standard growth charts. A body mass index chart is provided in Chapter 26 (see Table 26-8).

Children are weighed and measured frequently to track growth and determine if there is normal progression. Older patients should be measured yearly to track decreases in height that might indicate alterations in the spine such as those caused by osteoporosis.

Vital Signs Measurement. Vital signs should be measured at the time of the physical examination. If previous measurements are available, the present ones are compared with them. Blood pressure should be measured on both arms after the patient has been quietly sitting or lying down for at least 5 minutes.

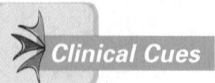
Clinical Cues

The blood pressure reading will be more accurate if the patient's feet are flat on the floor, the brachial artery is at the level of the right atrium, and neither you nor the patient talks during the procedure. (See Chapter 21 for guidelines for taking a blood pressure measurement.)

If it is abnormal, it should be measured on both arms and with the patient in a standing position as well. **Never take the blood pressure on the arm con-**

Table 22-1 *Metropolitan Height and Weight Tables for Men and Women According to Frame, Ages 25-59*

WOMEN*					MEN*			
HEIGHT (IN SHOES)† FEET	INCHES	SMALL FRAME	MEDIUM FRAME	LARGE FRAME	HEIGHT (IN SHOES)† FEET	INCHES	SMALL FRAME	MEDIUM FRAME	LARGE FRAME
4	10	102-111	109-121	118-131	5	2	128-134	131-141	138-150
4	11	103-113	111-123	120-134	5	3	130-136	133-143	140-153
5	0	104-115	113-126	122-137	5	4	132-138	135-145	142-156
5	1	106-118	115-129	125-140	5	5	134-140	137-148	144-160
5	2	108-121	118-132	128-143	5	6	136-142	139-151	146-164
5	3	111-124	121-135	131-147	5	7	138-145	142-154	149-168
5	4	114-127	124-138	134-151	5	8	140-148	145-157	152-172
5	5	117-130	127-141	137-155	5	9	142-151	148-160	155-176
5	6	120-133	130-144	140-159	5	10	144-154	151-163	158-180
5	7	123-136	133-147	143-163	5	11	146-157	154-166	161-184
5	8	126-139	136-150	146-167	6	0	149-160	157-170	164-188
5	9	129-142	139-153	149-170	6	1	152-164	160-174	168-192
5	10	132-145	142-156	152-173	6	2	155-168	164-178	172-197
5	11	135-148	145-159	155-176	6	3	158-172	167-182	176-202
6	0	138-151	148-162	158-179	6	4	162-176	171-187	181-207

Source of basic data: Build Study, 1979. Society of Actuaries and Association of Life Insurance Medical Directors of America, 1980. Copyright © 1996, 1999 Metropolitan Life Insurance Company. Courtesy of the Metropolitan Life Insurance Company.
*Weight in pounds in indoor clothing weighing 5 pounds for men and 3 pounds for women.
†Shoes with 1-inch heels.

taining a dialysis shunt or on the side where a mastectomy and lymph node dissection have occurred. If blood pressure is elevated during an office or clinic visit, the pressure should be taken again just before the patient leaves. Many patients become anxious when facing an examination or interview with a physician.

? *Think Critically About* . . . If you take a patient's blood pressure and it measures 148/94, what would you do?

The radial pulse is assessed and, if it is irregular, the apical pulse is counted. Respirations are also assessed, as is the temperature. Techniques for measuring vital signs are presented in Chapter 21. In office practice, the temperature is taken if the patient has a complaint that might alter the body temperature. Respirations are counted if there is a problem in the respiratory system. **In the hospital, the full set of vital signs is assessed.**

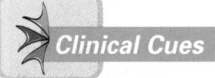
Clinical Cues

Whenever an illness is present that is affecting the respiratory system, you should count the respirations for a full minute. Note the character and depth of the respirations as well as the rate.

Review of Body Systems

Head and Neck. Assess the general appearance of the patient, the color and tone of the skin and its condition, appearance of the eyes, and condition of the hair. Does the nose seem stuffy? Is it drippy? Do the teeth appear clean? Does the patient seem to have difficulty hearing? Are the pupils equal in size? Do the eyes move in unison? Are there any extra movements of the eyes or lids? Are the cornea and lens clear or is there an opacity? When was the last eye examination? Is the patient alert and oriented? Does thinking seem logical? Does the neck appear normal? Are there complaints about swollen lymph nodes? Is the neck positioned midline to the head? Does neck movement seem normal and without stiffness? Perform a visual acuity exam as described in Steps 22-2 (Figure 22-5). Hearing can be quickly and easily tested using the audioscope (Figure 22-6). Directions for testing are included with the unit. Each ear is tested with four frequencies.

Chest, Heart, and Lungs. The chest should rise and fall with respiration symmetrically on both sides of the body. By placing the thumbs over the posterior vertebrae at the level of the tenth rib and noting whether the movement of each thumb is the same upon inspiration, chest excursion can be observed. The spine should be inspected from the rear and the side. It should be in midline with gentle concave and convex curves when viewed laterally. The shoulders should appear to be at equal height. Note whether lordosis (exaggerated lumbar curve), kyphosis (increased curve in the thoracic area), or scoliosis (pronounced lateral curvature of the spine) is present.

Inspect the anterior chest to see if there is a noticeable point of maximal impulse (PMI) of the heart. It will be located at or close to the fifth intercostal space at the midclavicular line. Place the diaphragm of the stethoscope over this area and listen for the heart sounds, S_1 and S_2. S_1 is the "lub" sound and S_2 is the "dub" sound. S_1 is loudest at the apex of the heart in the mitral area. S_2 is softer at this location and can be

Steps 22-2 Testing Visual Acuity

The Snellen eye chart is used to test visual acuity. This is performed by the nurse during a physical examination at an office or clinic and when there is a question of a problem with vision.

1. **ACTION** Position the patient 20 feet from the Snellen chart (see Figure 22-5).

   RATIONALE Accuracy of the test depends on maintaining the correct distance from the chart.

2. **ACTION** Ask the patient to leave on corrective lenses (except reading glasses) and cover one eye with an opaque card.

   RATIONALE Vision of each eye is tested individually.

3. **ACTION** Instruct the patient to read through the chart to the smallest line in print possible, reading from left to right.

   RATIONALE Identifies the person's visual acuity in that eye.

4. **ACTION** Record the fraction at the end of the last line read and indicate number of missed letters and whether corrective lenses were worn (i.e., 20/30, −2 with contact lenses).

   RATIONALE The number beside the smallest print read is the visual acuity score; other designations indicate how the test was performed.

5. **ACTION** Test the other eye and record the visual acuity.

   RATIONALE Vision must be tested in both eyes individually.

6. **ACTION** Perform the test with both eyes uncovered. Record the score.

   RATIONALE Tests acuity in both eyes together.

7. **ACTION** If the patient cannot read the top number even with glasses, position her closer to the chart.

   RATIONALE The score distance is altered according to how far the patient is from the chart.

8. **ACTION** Record the scores.

   RATIONALE Documents results of the test.

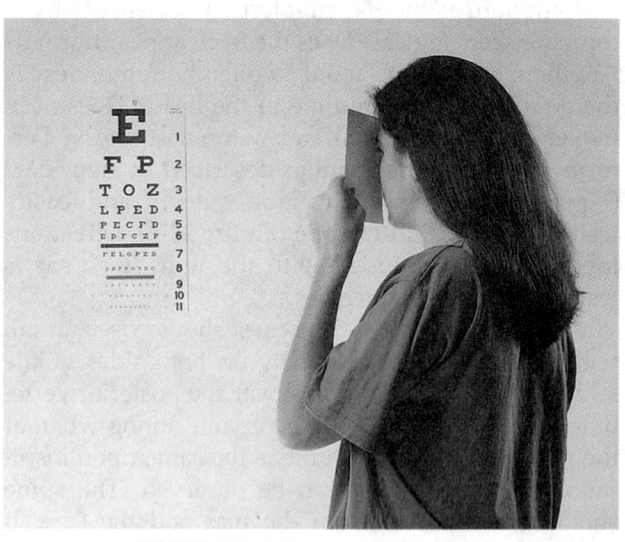

FIGURE **22-5** Testing visual acuity.

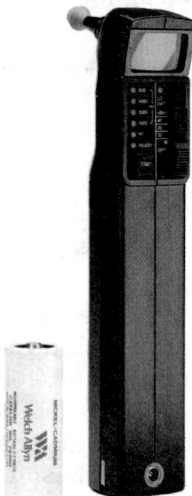

FIGURE **22-6** Audioscope instrument for testing hearing.

heard more loudly over the aortic area (Figure 22-7). The sounds are heard best if the stethoscope is placed against the skin rather than the cloth of the gown or shirt. (*Check the **Companion CD** for audio files of heart and lung sounds.*) Count the apical pulse and note whether it is regular. Determine if there are sounds present other than the two normal heart sounds, such as the swish of a murmur (Steps 22-3). After mastering basic heart sounds, you can practice listening to the valve sounds with the bell of the stethoscope placed lightly on the skin. The locations for listening to the valves are shown in Figure 22-7.

It takes considerable practice to hear all but the loudest heart murmurs and to determine the type. You will learn more about abnormal heart sound assessment and further techniques for assessing each body system in your medical-surgical nursing courses.

Lung sounds are auscultated using the diaphragm of the stethoscope. The sounds are created by air moving through passageways of varying diameter and length. The sounds vary in pitch and duration depending on the area of auscultation (Figure 22-8). Sounds over the trachea are loud and coarse. They are equal in length for inspiration and expiration and have

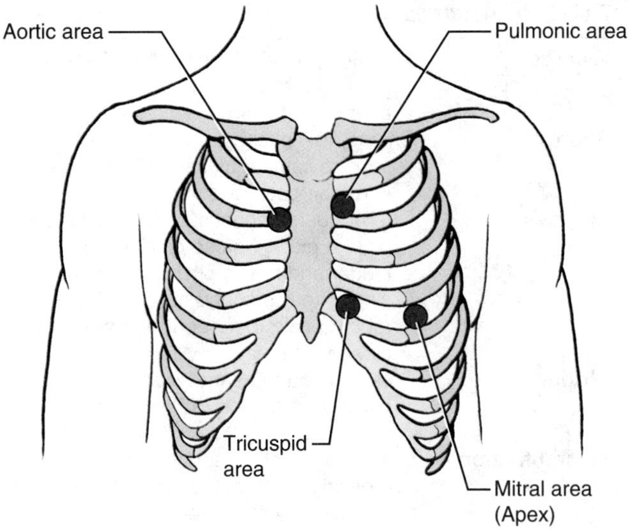

FIGURE **22-7** Auscultate the heart in each area.

no pause between them. They are medium in tonality and loudness. Vesicular sounds are the soft, rustling sounds heard in the periphery of the lung fields. They are longer on inspiration than expiration and there is no pause between them. Table 22-2 presents adventitious sounds (abnormal lung sounds). Auscultation is done in a systematic manner according to a set pattern (Figure 22-9). Steps 22-4 presents the steps for performing lung auscultation. Auscultation is performed on initial assessment, and once per shift for all bed rest patients and for patients who have a respiratory problem or who are at risk for a respiratory problem.

Skin and Extremities. The skin should be inspected for any rash or lesions (Table 22-3, p. 382). There should be no flaking or excessive dryness. Turgor is checked by gently pinching up a bit of skin on the arm or over the sternum. If the skin is slow to return to a flat position, the patient is most likely dehydrated. If the skin returns to the original position in less than 3 seconds, the turgor is "brisk." Ask about any changes in moles or other lesions. Check the nails for discoloration or abnormal appearance. Nail fungus may cause this. Abnormally shaped fingertips may indicate a cardiopulmonary problem.

Check capillary refill time by observing the color of the nail bed and then compressing the nail bed with the thumbnail or the distal end of a capped pen. Re-

a slight pause between them. When you are listening over the upper area of the chest over the bronchi, the sounds are harsh and loud and are shorter on inspiration than expiration. There is a pause between the two sounds. The bronchovesicular sounds are those heard over the central chest or back. Normally they are equal in length during inspiration and expiration and have

Steps 22-3   Basic Assessment of Heart Sounds

Heart sounds are assessed on admission to the health facility or agency's care and then once each shift in the hospital. A quiet room is needed to assess heart sounds; turn off the TV or radio.

1. **ACTION** Perform hand hygiene and explain the procedure. Provide privacy by closing the door or closing the curtains.

   RATIONALE Reduces transfer of microorganisms; explaining the procedure places the patient more at ease. Closing the door or curtains protects patient's right to privacy and prevents embarrassment.

2. **ACTION** Have the patient sit upright or elevate the head of the bed 45 to 90 degrees if not contraindicated.

   RATIONALE A sitting position brings the heart closer to the anterior chest wall.

3. **ACTION** Loosen or remove clothing.

   RATIONALE Allows anatomic landmarks to be identified and the stethoscope to be placed on the skin.

4. **ACTION** Place the diaphragm of the stethoscope at the apex of the heart (fifth intercostal space at the midclavicular line) and identify S_1 and S_2, the "lub" and "dub" sounds. Count the apical pulse rate.

   RATIONALE Heart sounds are normally the loudest at the apex of the heart. "Lub" and "dub" together make up one heartbeat.

5. **ACTION** Using the bell of the stethoscope, auscultate in the four valve areas for abnormal sounds (see Figure 22-7).

   RATIONALE The bell picks up lower-pitched sounds.

6. **ACTION** Replace clothing and make the patient comfortable. Lower the bed and raise the side rails if they were moved. Turn the TV or radio back on when finished.

   RATIONALE Prevents chilling, protects privacy, shows consideration and caring.

7. **ACTION** Report murmurs or any sound that is different from an S_1 or S_2.

   RATIONALE Abnormal sounds may indicate a change in condition.

8. **ACTION** Record the apical heart rate and presence of normal or abnormal sounds.

   RATIONALE Notes rate and any abnormal sounds: for example, "Apical rate 74, regular with normal S_1S_2."

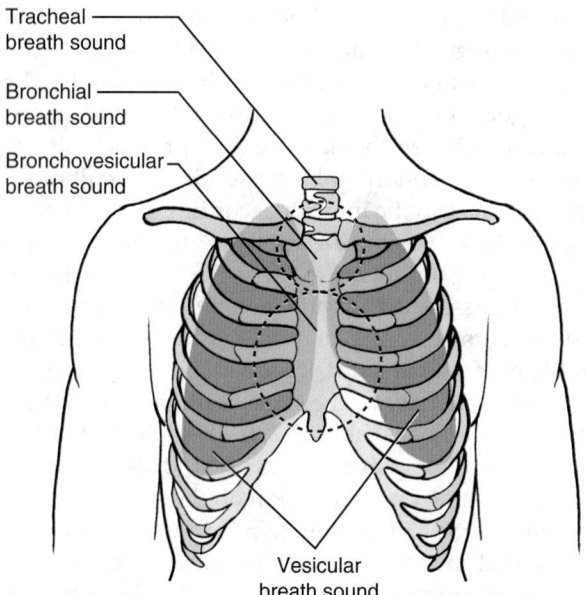

FIGURE **22-8** Locations of normal lung sounds.

Tracheal breath sound
Bronchial breath sound
Bronchovesicular breath sound
Vesicular breath sound

Table 22-2	*Abnormal Lung Sounds*
Wheeze	Whistling, musical, high-pitched sound produced by air being forced through a narrowed airway.
Rhonchi	Coarse, low-pitched, sonorous, rattling sounds caused by secretions in the larger air passages.
Crackles	Fine or coarse sounds. Fine crackles are high in pitch. Coarse crackles are louder and low in pitch. Crackles are similar to the sound produced by rubbing hairs between the fingers close to the ear.
Stridor	Croaking sound heard when there is partial obstruction of the upper air passages.
Pleural friction rub	Grating or scratchy sound similar to creaking shoe leather or opening a squeaky door. Caused when irritated pleural membranes rub over each other.

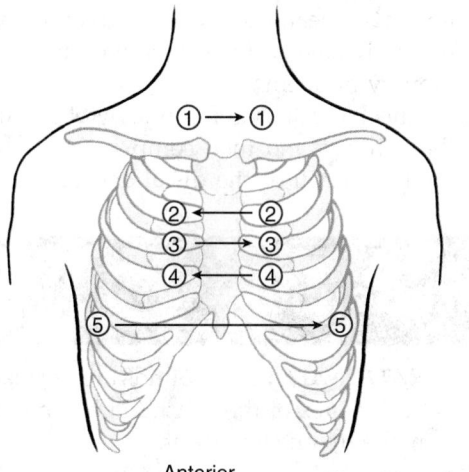

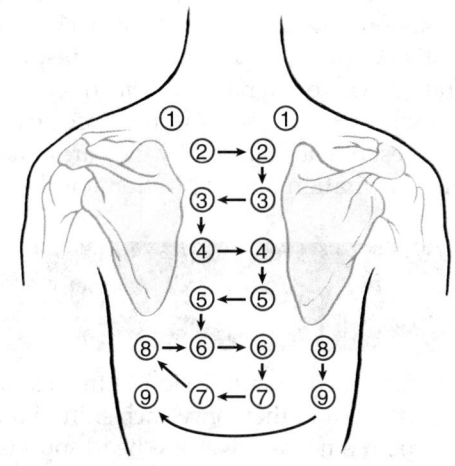

Anterior
Posterior

FIGURE **22-9** Sites for auscultation of the lung fields.

lease the pressure and note how quickly the color returns to the nail bed. If the color returns slowly, check again and count the seconds ("one–one thousand, two–one thousand," etc.) to estimate the number of seconds it takes for the color to return. **Normal refill time is less than 3 seconds.** This is not an accurate assessment of circulation, but it can be useful.

Peripheral pulses should be compared bilaterally. It is most important to check the dorsalis pedis pulse as this is an indication of the quality of circulation in the lower extremities.

Assess for generalized edema by checking for weight gain over a short period of time. Ask about shoe and ring tightness, and sock patterns left on the ankles when socks are removed. Look for eye and hand puffiness and abdominal fullness. To check for dependent edema, press the fingers into the tissue over the tibia just above the ankle. If an indentation remains, *pitting edema* is present (Figure 22-10). To describe edema, you can use the terms *taut, tight, puffy,* *indented,* or *pitting.* If pitting is present, it is classified according to its depth.

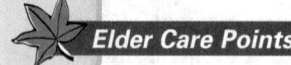

Elder Care Points

- The skin of the elderly is less elastic and drier than that of the younger person. Skin begins to sag. Skin turgor is not an accurate measure of hydration in the elderly. Checking the mucous membranes is a better assessment technique.
- The elderly are prone to develop lesions related to aging, such as brown spots (*lentigines*) and *actinic keratoses* (reddened, flaky areas that are precancerous).

Inquire about any abnormal sensations in the skin. Is there any tingling or twitching? Can the patient feel the difference between warmth and cold?

Inquire about any change in muscle strength. Does the patient ambulate normally? Is there weakness or

Steps 22-4 Auscultating the Lungs

1. **ACTION** Perform hand hygiene and explain what you are going to do.

   RATIONALE Prevents spread of microorganisms; explanation prepares the patient for the procedure.

2. **ACTION** Eliminate extraneous noise from the area; turn off the radio or TV, close the door as needed. Ask the patient not to talk.

   RATIONALE Lung sounds are heard more clearly without noise interference.

3. **ACTION** Provide privacy by drawing the curtain around the bed or closing the door to the room; adjust the blinds if the window faces a walkway or if others can see in easily.

   RATIONALE Protects the privacy of the patient; displays caring and courtesy.

4. **ACTION** Help the patient assume a sitting position with the back away from the bed or chair. Raise the bed to working height and lower the side rail.

   RATIONALE It is easier to auscultate the posterior of the lungs with the patient in a sitting position. If a sitting position is not possible, the patient can be turned to the side to auscultate over the back. Raising the bed and lowering the side rail makes it easier to auscultate without straining back muscles.

5. **ACTION** Remove or loosen clothing so that the stethoscope can be applied to the skin in the correct locations.

   RATIONALE It is easier to visualize anatomic landmarks if clothing is removed or loosened. Sounds are heard more clearly when the stethoscope is placed on the skin rather than on fabric.

6. **ACTION** Warm the diaphragm of the stethoscope with your hand.

   RATIONALE Reduces discomfort for the patient.

7. **ACTION** Ask the patient to breathe in and out slowly and deeply through an open mouth.

   RATIONALE Reduces air turbulence noise and helps prevent hyperventilation.

8. **ACTION** Apply the diaphragm of the stethoscope to the posterior of the chest and listen in each location (see Figure 22-9) for a full inspiration and expiration. Move the stethoscope from one side to the other. Do not listen over bone; place the stethoscope between the scapula, beside the vertebrae, and between the ribs.

   RATIONALE Ensures that all areas of the posterior lungs are auscultated. Helps pick up both inspiratory and expiratory abnormal sounds. Moving from side to side helps to compare sounds heard.

9. **ACTION** Move around to the front of the patient and auscultate the anterior and lateral areas of the lungs in a methodical side-to-side fashion.

   RATIONALE Provides a comprehensive assessment.

10. **ACTION** If noise from hair on the chest is heard, press the diaphragm more firmly onto the chest.

    RATIONALE Hair noise obscures lung sounds.

11. **ACTION** If rhonchi or crackles are heard, ask the patient to take a couple of deep breaths and to turn the head away and cough.

    RATIONALE Deep breathing and coughing may clear the passages.

12. **ACTION** Compare sounds heard on the right with those on the left for each area.

    RATIONALE Aids in the detection of abnormal sounds.

13. **ACTION** Rearrange the patient's clothing and turn the radio or TV back on. Lower the bed if it was raised; replace side rails if they were lowered, and make the patient comfortable.

    RATIONALE Restoring the unit protects privacy and promotes comfort and safety.

14. **ACTION** Perform hand hygiene.

    RATIONALE Reduces transfer of microorganisms.

15. **ACTION** Document findings.

    RATIONALE Provides data for future comparison.

paralysis of any extremity? Inquire about fatigue level. Is there any difficulty with bending and moving, as when getting in and out of a chair or a car?

The Abdomen. Bowel sounds are assessed on admission and once a shift for all patients. Bowel sounds are produced by the contractions of the small and large intestine. They are wavelike in character and are clicks and gurgles that occur from 5 to 30 times a minute. They are quite active after eating. Between meals it is normal to hear only a few sounds. Bowel sounds are judged to be *hyperactive* if they are very frequent, *hypoactive* if there are long periods of silence, and *absent* if no sound is heard for 2 to 5 minutes in any of the four quadrants. Auscultate for bowel sounds with the patient in a supine position. Lightly place the stethoscope over a quadrant (quarter) of the abdomen and listen; if no sound is heard, progress through the other quadrants until sounds are heard or listen for at least 2 minutes (Figure 22-11).

Table 22-3	*Types of Skin Lesions*				

LESION	DESCRIPTION	LESION	DESCRIPTION
Macule	Circumscribed, flat area with a change in skin color; less than 1 cm in diameter *Examples:* freckles, petechiae, measles, flat mole (nevus)	**Plaque**	Circumscribed, elevated, superficial, solid lesion; greater than 1 cm in diameter *Examples:* psoriasis, seborrheic and active keratoses
Papule	Elevated, solid lesion; less than 1 cm in diameter *Examples:* wart (verruca), elevated moles	**Wheal**	Firm, edematous, irregularly shaped area; diameter variable *Examples:* insect bite, urticaria
Vesicle	Circumscribed, superficial collection of serous fluid; less than 1 cm in diameter *Examples:* varicella (chickenpox), herpes zoster (shingles), second-degree burn	**Pustule**	Elevated, superficial lesion filled with purulent fluid *Examples:* acne, impetigo

From Lewis, S.L., Heitkemper, M.M., & Dirksen, S.R. (2007). *Medical-Surgical Nursing: Assessment and Management of Clinical Problems* (7th ed.). St. Louis: Mosby.

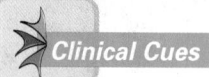

Clinical Cues

If you press when you palpate the abdomen before auscultating, or press too hard with the stethoscope, you may cause bowel sounds to occur that would not have normally been there.

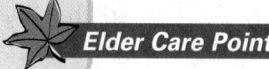

Elder Care Points

- Skin sensation and sensory function tend to diminish with aging.
- Muscle strength and joint flexibility may be decreased in the elderly.

Next, if the patient has a gastrointestinal problem, percuss over each quadrant of the abdomen. This is done by placing the hyperextended middle finger on the skin while the other fingers are raised off the skin and striking that finger with the curved middle finger of the other hand by flexing at the wrist in a tapping motion (see Figure 22-2). The sound will be dull over solid tissue and resonant over air-filled areas. If a lot of resonant areas are present, there is quite a bit of gas in the bowel.

After auscultating and percussing, gently palpate each quadrant of the abdomen looking for areas of tenderness, pain, and abnormal masses. When documenting the findings, a reference to the size of the abdomen establishes a baseline for future comparison.

Genitalia, Anus, and Rectum. Unless the patient has a specific complaint in these areas, the nurse does not visually assess them. They may be assessed, however, when bathing the patient, performing perineal care, or

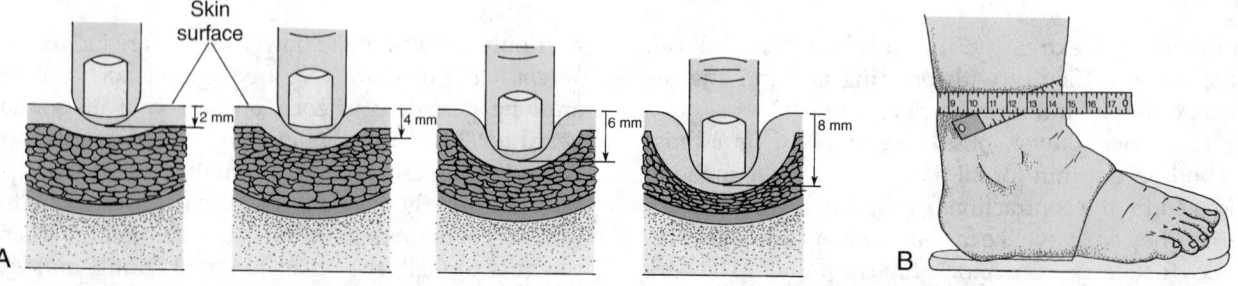

FIGURE **22-10** A, Measuring pitting edema. B, Measuring pedal edema.

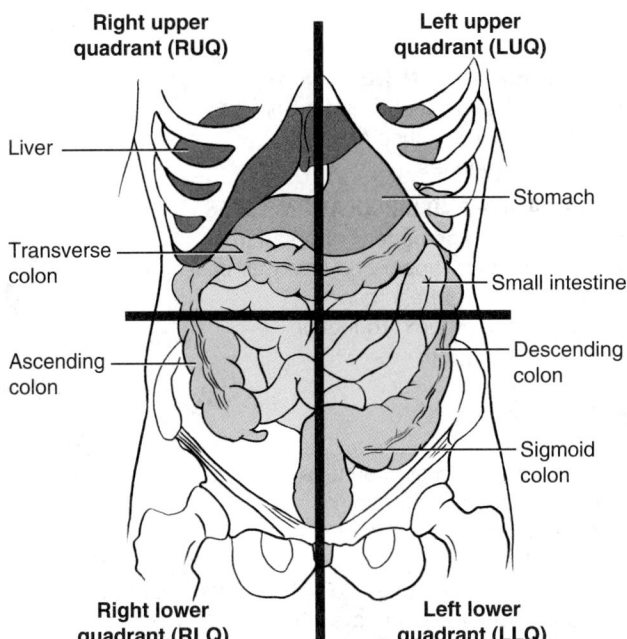

FIGURE **22-11** Auscultation of bowel sounds; listen in each quadrant.

assisting with toileting. Ask the patient if there are any problems with these areas.

Nursing Diagnosis

Nursing diagnoses are formulated or chosen depending on the problems found on assessment. The data are analyzed and the problems identified. The RN is often responsible for identifying the nursing diagnoses, but the LPN/LVN may need to choose the appropriate diagnoses from the North American Nursing Diagnosis Association–International (NANDA-I) list if no RN is present during the shift. This may be the case in long-term care facilities in the evening or on the night shift.

Planning

Appropriate goals or expected outcomes are written for each nursing diagnosis identified. The nurse sets priorities of care based on the most urgent needs of each assigned patient. A work organization plan is made incorporating all the tasks and assessments that need to be made during the shift.

Implementation

Assessment of patients involves interviewing and gathering a history, performing the physical examination, or assisting the physician while the physical examination is performed.

In many instances, a nursing assessment of the areas of basic need is more appropriate than a total physical assessment by the nurse. A systematic way to perform such an assessment is to use the acronym RNS HOPE. The acronym stands for
- **R**est and activity
- **N**utrition, fluids, and electrolytes
- **S**afety and security

- **H**ygiene and grooming
- **O**xygenation and circulation needs
- **P**sychosocial and learning
- **E**limination

The data to be covered for this assessment of psychosocial and physiologic functioning are listed in Box 22-4. Information gathered from this assessment is then analyzed, and a nursing care plan is prepared using the nursing process. After the initial assessment and development of the care plan, additional information is gathered in particularly pertinent areas to update the plan and evaluate progress. Skill 22-l describes the systematic performance of a physical examination.

Each patient should also be assessed at the beginning of each shift or shortly thereafter. This is a quick head-to-toe assessment on which the nurse establishes priorities of care and organizes the work for the shift (Box 22-5, p. 386).

Patient and Family Teaching

A good time to do teaching regarding preventive health care is while you are assessing the patient. Topics can include the following:
- The need for regular physical examinations
- Recommended periodic diagnostic tests
- The need for immunizations
- The necessity of regular dental examinations
- The warning signs of cancer (Patient Teaching 22-1, p. 386)
- The way to perform breast self-examination (Figure 22-12, p. 387) (Cultural Cues 22-2, p. 388)
- The method of performing testicular self-examination

Patients are also taught about the purpose of diagnostic tests ordered and what they will experience when undergoing them. Every patient should inquire about recommended diagnostic tests: digital rectal exam, stool for occult blood, sigmoidoscopy or colonoscopy, prostate-specific antigen (PSA) level (men), mammography and Papanicolaou (Pap) smear (women), blood glucose level, complete blood count (CBC) and metabolic panel of laboratory tests, urinalysis, full eye examination, and hearing test.

Assisting with a Physical Examination

Nurses often assist the examiner with various aspects of the physical examination. You may be asked to do the initial screening of the patient before the patient is seen by the examiner. A brief history of any complaints is obtained, vital signs are taken, and the patient is prepared for the examination. You should explain the examination procedure to the patient, answer any questions the patient has, and generally try to put the patient at ease. The examiner will explore each part of the body in considerable depth.

Positioning and Draping. You will prepare the patient for the particular type of examination the examiner is going to perform. Most examinations begin with the

Box 22-4 *Basic Needs Assessment*

Data to be gathered include:

REST AND ACTIVITY NEEDS

- Body proportion and appearance
- Range of motion in joints
- Muscular strength
- Balance and equilibrium
- Ability to perform ADLs (e.g., bathing, dressing, grooming, feeding, elimination, and ambulation)
- Sleep pattern, including interruptions and quality
- Hours of bed rest per day
- Pain

NUTRITIONAL, FLUID, AND ELECTROLYTE NEEDS

- Height and usual weight
- Unusual gain or loss of weight
- Caloric needs for level of activity
- Amount and type of food ingested daily
- Vitality level and amount of appetite
- Compliance with prescribed diet
- General body appearance
- Fluid intake and output during past 24 hours, even if intake and output records have not been kept. (Question patient and family to arrive at an estimated amount.)
- Abnormal loss of body fluid through suctioning, vomiting, diarrhea, hemorrhage, wound drainage, burns, and so forth
- Tubes used to instill or drain fluids (e.g., intravenous therapy, catheters, food supplements, and total parenteral nutrition)
- Fluid volume; edema; weight change
- Normal filling of neck veins
- Turgor of skin and moistness of mucous membranes
- Laboratory values of blood factors (e.g., hemoglobin, hematocrit, and electrolyte levels)

SAFETY AND SECURITY

- Potential risks for injury; skin condition; pressure areas
- Sensory deficits (e.g., deafness, blindness, or aphasia)
- Muscular weakness (e.g., paresis or paralysis)
- Speaks and understands English
- Need for side rails or safety devices

HYGIENE AND GROOMING

- Ability to bathe, dress, and groom self
- Amount of assistance needed
- Preferred routines

OXYGENATION AND CIRCULATION NEEDS

- Rate, depth, and pattern of breathing
- Breath sounds, upper and lower air passages, auscultated front and back
- Cough and sputum production
- Level of consciousness
- Orientation to reality
- Blood pressure
- Heart sounds
- Pulse rate and characteristics
- Jugular venous distention
- Peripheral pulses
- Skin color and temperature
- Laboratory values (e.g., complete blood count [CBC], arterial blood gases) (if available)
- Tolerance for usual ADLs

PSYCHOSOCIAL NEEDS

- Desire for spiritual assistance
- Support system
- Mental outlook
- Usual coping mechanisms
- Need for social service consult
- Financial worries
- Fears and concerns
- Knowledge deficits and learning needs

ELIMINATION

- Characteristics and amount of urinary output
- Characteristics and regularity of bowel movements
- Control of urinary and anal sphincters
- Alterations in elimination (e.g., use of laxatives or presence of catheter or ostomy)
- Bowel sounds and abdominal characteristics
- Presence of pain, burning, or other discomfort
- Signs of dehydration, temperature control

Skill 22-1 | Performing a Physical Examination

Nursing physical assessments are of various types and depth depending on the situation and the need. The assessment guide presented here is for a basic nursing physical examination. Further assessment would be indicated for areas where abnormalities are detected. With experience, you will add other assessment techniques to this basic examination.

■ Supplies
✓ Stethoscope
✓ Sphygmomanometer
✓ Thermometer
✓ Scale with measuring rod
✓ Patient gown

Review and carry out the Standard Steps in Appendix 3.

1. **ACTION** Interview the patient and obtain a thorough history.

RATIONALE Provides data regarding past medical problems, current complaints, and risk factors for various disorders.

2. **ACTION** Ask the patient to put on a patient gown.

RATIONALE Provides easy access to various parts of the body for examination.

3. **ACTION** Weigh and measure the patient. Record the measurements.

   RATIONALE Establishes baseline height and weight.

4. **ACTION** With the patient in a seated position, examine the head and neck.

   RATIONALE Allows the blood pressure to stabilize while performing another part of the examination.

5. **ACTION** Examine the skin and joints of the extremities. Check and compare the peripheral pulses bilaterally.

   RATIONALE Provides data about possible joint problems and skin lesions and possible circulatory problems. Detects presence and quality of peripheral pulses.

6. **ACTION** Measure the blood pressure, pulse, respirations, and temperature.

   RATIONALE Supplies information about vital functions of the body.

7. **ACTION** Auscultate the heart and listen in valve areas and count the apical heart rate.

   RATIONALE Determines abnormalities of heart rate and rhythm and presence of abnormal sounds.

8. **ACTION** Auscultate the lungs and check for bilateral equal chest movement with respiration.

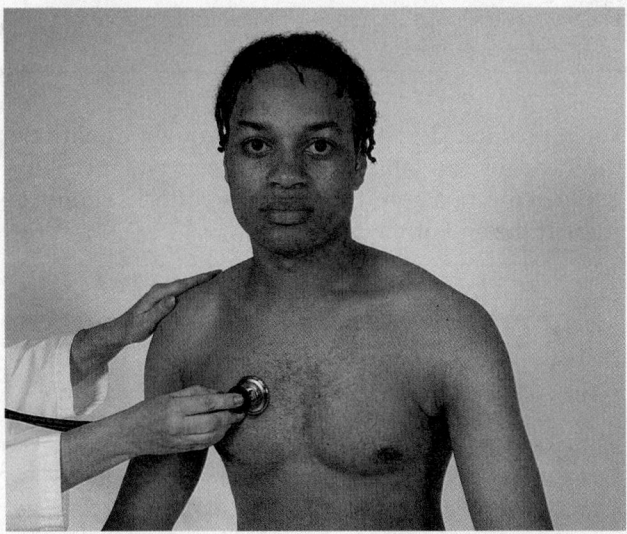

Step **7**

RATIONALE Noting rate, rhythm, and depth of respiration and comparing sounds from one side with the other helps determine if lung abnormalities are present.

9. **ACTION** Have the patient recline to a supine position on the examining table or bed and assess the abdomen. Auscultate for bowel sounds, percuss for areas of excessive gas, and palpate gently for tenderness.

   RATIONALE Determines if bowel sounds are present and normal, whether excess air is in the colon, and whether tenderness is present.

10. **ACTION** Obtain any needed specimens.

    RATIONALE Provides specimens for ordered diagnostic tests.

11. **ACTION** Direct further attention to any area in which a problem was discovered or in which the patient has a complaint.

    RATIONALE Gathers data to be brought to the attention of the physician, nurse practitioner, or physician's assistant.

12. **ACTION** If an eye examination is indicated, check visual acuity.

    RATIONALE Determines whether further eye examination is needed for visual correction.

13. **ACTION** If need indicates, check hearing using an audioscope.

    RATIONALE Screens for hearing abnormalities requiring referral for further testing.

14. **ACTION** Document the findings of the physical examination.

    RATIONALE Provides a written record of the findings. Provides baseline data with which future assessment can be compared.

15. **ACTION** Allow the patient to dress and ask if there are any questions.

    RATIONALE Shows courtesy and caring.

■ Special Considerations

✓ Review the physical changes of aging before deciding that a finding is "abnormal" in the elderly person.

✓ Allow the elderly patient time to adjust to position changes and assist the person to move slowly.

✓ If any neurologic abnormality is noted, perform a neurologic check (see Skill 22-2).

✓ During the assessment, question the patient about the latest dental and eye exams. Inquire as to status of diagnostic tests recommended periodically for preventive health care and cancer detection.

? CRITICAL THINKING QUESTIONS

1. If you have a patient who cannot communicate verbally with you and who seems confused, how would you go about obtaining the assessment data you need?

2. If you are doing an assessment on a patient who came in with a respiratory problem and you notice a suspicious-looking mole on the lower leg, how would you go about getting the physician to pay attention to that finding?

Box 22-5 | *Shift Head-to-Toe Assessment*

INITIAL OBSERVATION
- Skin color
- Appearance
- Affect
- Ease of respiration
- How the patient is feeling

HEAD
- Ability to respond to questions
- Appearance of eyes
- Ability to communicate
- Level of consciousness
- Presence of confusion
- Presence of jugular venous distention

VITAL SIGNS
- Temperature
- Pulse rate, rhythm, and quality
- Respiration, rate, depth, and pattern
- Blood pressure: compare with previous readings
- Oxygen saturation of the blood

PAIN
- Level of pain
- Frequency of use of medication
- Present status; need for medication
- Patient-controlled analgesia (PCA) pump functioning; medication left

CHEST: GENERAL HEART AND LUNG ASSESSMENT
- Auscultate lung fields
- Listen to heart rate at apex
- Inspect for equal bilateral movement of chest wall

ABDOMEN
- Appetite
- Shape
- Soft or hard
- Bowel sounds
- Time of last bowel movement
- Voiding status

EXTREMITIES
- Normal movement bilaterally
- Skin turgor and temperature
- Skin lesions or pressure areas
- Sensation
- Presence of edema
- Peripheral pulses; compare bilaterally

TUBES AND EQUIPMENT
- Intravenous catheter: condition of site, fluid in progress, rate, additives; time next fluid is to be hung
- Nasogastric tube: suction setting; amount and character of drainage; patency of tube, security of tube
- Urinary catheter: character and quantity of drainage; tube not under patient
- Dressings: location, drains in place, wound suction devices, amount and character of wound drainage
- Oxygen cannula: liter flow rate
- Pulse oximeter: intact probe; readings
- Traction: correct weight, body alignment weights hanging free
- Other equipment: applied properly, functioning as ordered

ASSESSMENT OF NEEDS
- Call bell in reach
- Tissues and waste container in reach
- TV control in reach
- Water and personal items positioned conveniently
- Room temperature suitable
- Room neat and tidy
- Determine what supplies will be needed in room for remainder of shift

Patient Teaching 22-1

The Warning Signs of Cancer

Patients should be taught to check with their physician if they find any of these warning signs of cancer:
- Change in bowel or bladder habits
- A sore that does not heal
- Unusual bleeding or discharge
- Thickening or a lump in the breast or elsewhere
- Indigestion or difficulty in swallowing
- Obvious change in a wart or mole
- Nagging cough or hoarseness

patient seated on the end of the examination table with a drape over the lap and legs. The patient will then assume a supine position and the drape is pulled up over the upper body so that the chest and/or abdomen can be exposed. For the lithotomy position used to examine the female genitalia and for the pelvic exam, stirrups are used to hold the patient's feet in an ele-

vated position. The pillow can be brought down from the head of the table to cushion the patient's head while in this position. The patient's buttocks should be right at the end of the table.

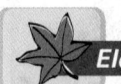

Elder Care Points

- The elderly person becomes chilled quickly because she has less subcutaneous tissue. Be certain draping is sufficient to prevent chilling.
- The elderly may become stiff when in a particular position on the examining table and should be slowly helped to a seated position for a couple of minutes and then assisted to stand and descend from the table.

The knee-chest position is sometimes used for a rectal examination. A lateral or Sims' position is used for a flexible sigmoidoscopy examination of the lower colon. A prone position may be needed for examination of lesions on the back or removal of lesions on the back of the legs or on the back (Figure 22-13).

1. POSITIONS

Visual Inspection: Standing in each position, look for changes in contour and shape of the breasts, color and texture of the skin and nipple and evidence of discharge from the nipples.

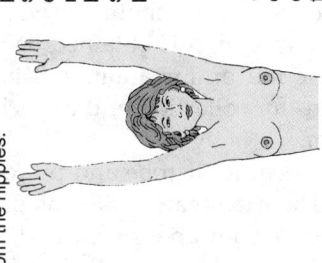

Arms raised above head

Hands on hips

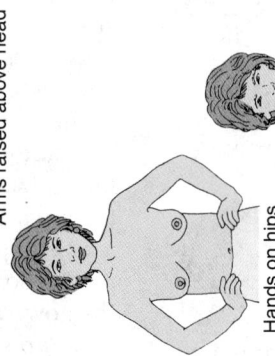

Bending forward

Arms relaxed at side

Palpation: Flat and Side-Lying:
Use your left hand to palpate the right breast, while holding your right arm at a right angle to the rib cage, with the elbow bent. Repeat the procedure on the other side. The side-lying position allows a woman, especially one with large breasts, to most effectively examine the outer half of the breast. A woman with small breasts may need only the flat position.

Side-lying Position: Lie on the opposite side of the breast to be examined. Rotate the shoulder (on the same side as the breast to be examined) back to the flat surface.

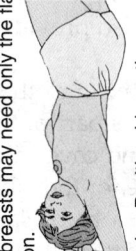

Flat Position: Lie flat on your back with a pillow or folded towel under the shoulder of the breast to be examined.

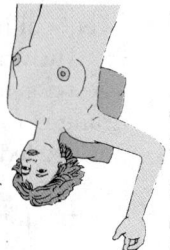

2. PERIMETER

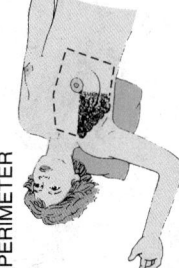

The examination area is bounded by a line that extends down from the middle of the armpit to just beneath the breast, continues across the underside of the breast to the middle of the breast bone, then moves up to and along the collarbone and back to the middle of the armpit. Most breast cancers occur in the upper outer area of the breast (shaded area).

3. PALPATION WITH PADS OF FINGERS

Use the pads of three or four fingers to examine every inch of your breast tissue. Move your fingers in circles about the size of a dime.

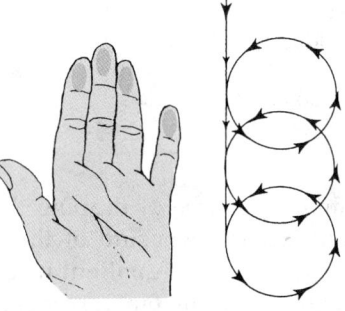

Do not lift your fingers from your breast between palpations. You can use powder or lotion to help your fingers glide from one spot to the next.

4. PRESSURE

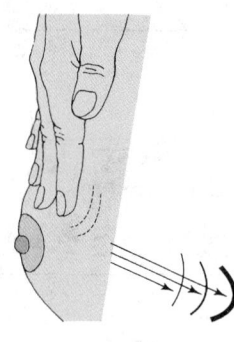

Use varying levels of pressure for each palpation, from light to deep, to examine the full thickness of your breast tissue. Using pressure will not injure the breast.

5. PATTERN OF SEARCH

Vertical Strip:

Using the following search pattern to examine all of your breast tissue, palpate carefully beneath the nipple. Any incision should also be carefully examined from end to end. Women who have had any breast surgery should examine the entire area and the incision.

Start in the armpit, proceed downward to the lower boundary. Move a finger's width toward the middle and continue palpating upward until you reach the collar bone. Repeat this until you have covered all the breast tissue. Make at least six strips before the nipple and four strips after the nipple. You may need between 10 and 16 strips.

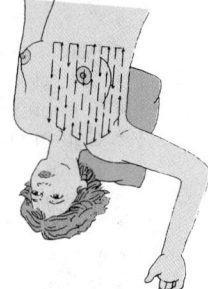

Nipple Discharge:
Squeeze your nipples to check for discharge. Many women have a normal discharge.

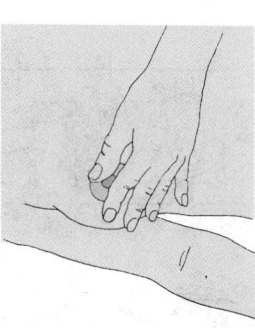

Axillary Examination:
Examine the breast tissue that extends into your armpit while your arm is relaxed at your side.

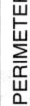

6. PRACTICE WITH FEEDBACK

It is important that you perform breast self-examination (BSE) while your instructor watches to be sure you are doing it correctly. Practice your skills until you feel comfortable and confident.

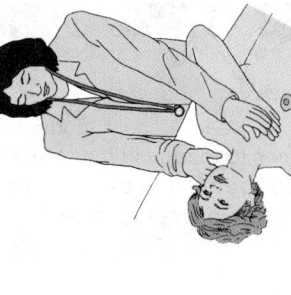

FIGURE **22-12** How to perform breast self-examination.

Cultural Cues 22-2

Modesty

Although Chinese women may not seem unduly modest, they are very modest when it comes to touch and tend to be uncomfortable touching their own bodies. It is essential to understand this reluctance when teaching breast self-exam. Stressing the benefits of the procedure may help overcome the problem.

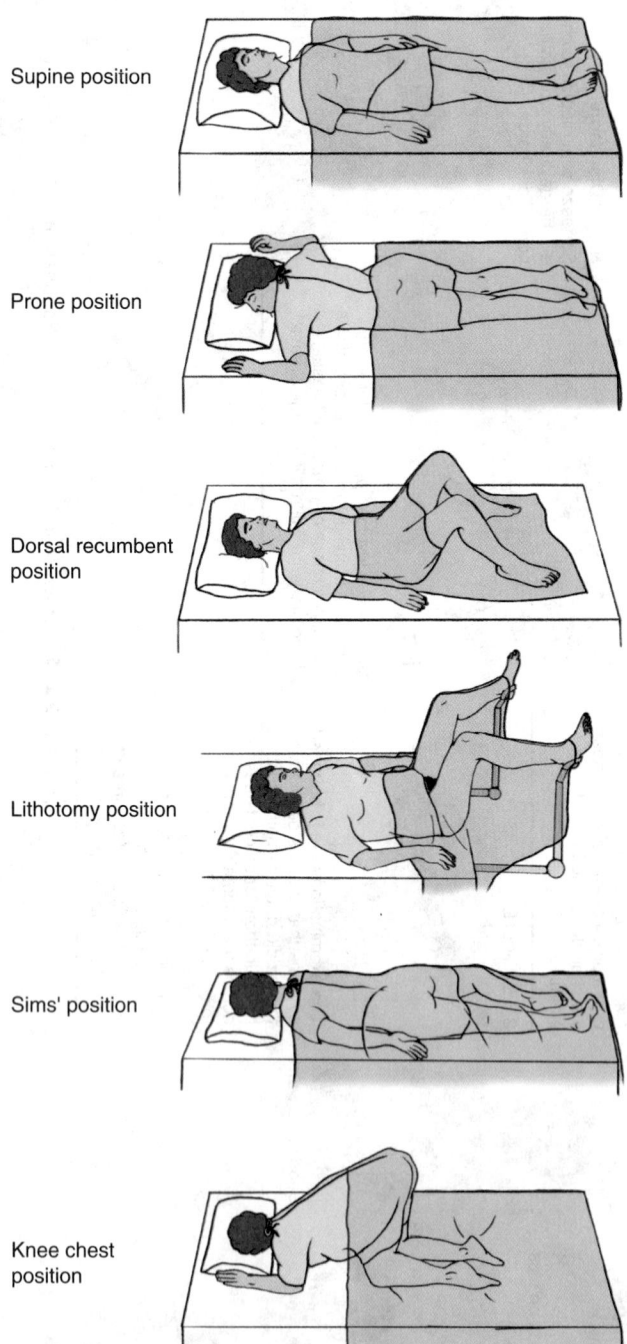

FIGURE **22-13** Positions for physical examination and procedures.

Box 22-6 **Equipment and Supplies for the Physical Examination**

The examiner should have the following items available to perform a physical examination:
- Examination gown
- Drape(s)
- Stethoscope
- Thermometer
- Sphygmomanometer
- Scale with height rod
- Tape measure
- Otoscope
- Ophthalmoscope
- Percussion hammer
- Tuning fork
- Tongue blades
- Cotton-tipped applicators
- Laboratory and x-ray request forms
- Examination lamp
- Flashlight
- Nasal speculum
- Vaginal speculum
- Rectal speculum
- Lubricant
- Snellen eye chart
- Tonometer
- Eye occluder or card
- Audioscope or ticking watch
- Papanicolaou smear supplies
- Test card for occult blood

The primary purpose of draping the patient is to prevent unnecessary exposure of the patient's body during the examination. **A patient who feels exposed and embarrassed will be tense, restless, and less able to cooperate.** Proper draping contributes to the patient's feeling of being cared for and promotes relaxation. The drapes also provide some warmth and prevent chilling.

The drapes may be of cloth or paper. The examining gown is also used as part of the drape as it can be arranged to expose and cover different parts of the body as needed. To drape for the lithotomy position, provide a draping sheet or a bath blanket turned so that one corner forms a triangle that falls between the legs.

Elements of the Physical Examination. Before a pelvic examination, the bladder should be emptied. If a urine specimen is required, it is obtained before the patient undresses for the examination. A labeled container and directions for collection of the specimen are given to the patient.

Ask the patient to disrobe and put on an examination gown. The examination table is prepared with a fresh paper cover, a drape is provided, and the necessary equipment for the physical examination is made ready (Box 22-6). Explain to the patient how to put on the gown and how to place the drape. If a pelvic exam and Pap smear are to be performed, a vaginal speculum, gloves, and lubricating jelly for the internal examination are placed conveniently. Fixative for the slide is placed within reach, or the ThinPrep jar is opened. Large cotton-tipped swabs should be within reach. The kit for the smear is opened and labeled and the patient's name and the date are placed on the end of the slide in pencil. The label is affixed to the Thin-Prep jar when that is used. The laboratory requisition slip is filled in. The examination light is positioned so that the examiner can adjust the light.

A female nurse must be present in the room any time a male health care provider performs a pelvic or breast examination of a patient. When the examiner is ready, the stirrups on the examination table are pulled out and the patient is helped to assume a lithotomy position. The drape is kept over the lower half of the patient's body during the positioning. The examiner takes specimens for the Pap smear and then performs the pelvic examination.

For the male patient, a glove, lubricant, and a test card for occult blood in the stool are placed adjacent to the examination table. The examiner will perform a rectal examination of the prostate for men over age 40.

Other common procedures that the nurse may be asked to perform are a urine dip, a hemoglobin measurement, a random blood sugar measurement, an electrocardiogram, and possibly a spirometry reading. Blood may need to be drawn for blood chemistry tests and a complete blood count. These procedures are covered in Chapter 24.

After the nurse has prepared the patient, the examiner will systematically assess every body system. The ophthalmoscope is used to check the interior of the eye (Figure 22-14). The light in the room is dimmed for this procedure. Pupil response is tested by shining the light into first one eye and then the other and watching the pupils contract.

The ears are examined with an otoscope after the outer ear is palpated for tenderness or nodules. With this instrument the physician can visualize the ear canal and the tympanic membrane (Figure 22-15). It is normal for cerumen to be in the ear. If there is an excessive amount, the ear may need to be lavaged.

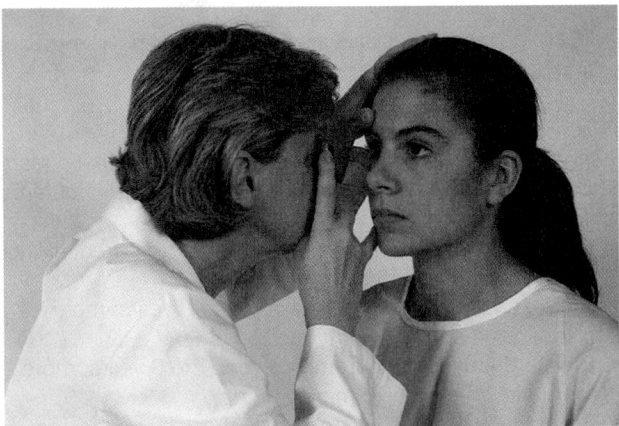
FIGURE **22-14** Checking the eye with an ophthalmoscope.

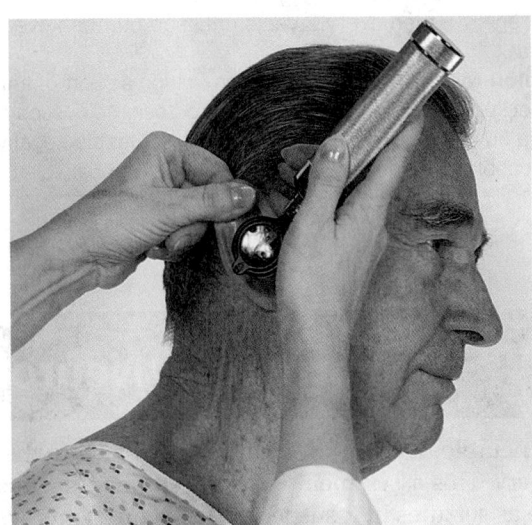
FIGURE **22-15** Checking the ear with an otoscope.

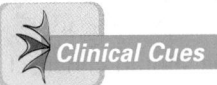
Clinical Cues

If the ear is to be lavaged, it is helpful to instill a wax dissolver into the ear and to let it sit for 10 to 30 minutes before lavaging. This makes the lavage procedure shorter and more comfortable for the patient.

Hearing may be initially tested with the use of a tuning fork. The Weber test is performed by striking the tuning fork and placing it in the middle of the patient's forehead or the skull. The patient says whether the sound is heard equally in both ears. The Rinne test compares air versus bone conduction of sound; sound is normally heard longer by air conduction. The tuning fork is struck and placed beside the ear. It is then struck and placed on the bone behind the ear. The patient says which sound lasted longer.

After the head and neck, chest, lungs, and heart have been examined, the patient will be asked to lie down supine on the examination table. The abdomen is assessed with the patient in this position. Further assessment of the extremities may be performed. When the examination is complete, the patient is often asked to dress and then the findings are discussed (Health Promotion Points 22-1).

Special Focused Examinations

At times you will need to perform a neurologic check, which is a brief form of a neurologic examination. The neurologic check is performed at regular intervals on patients who have experienced a head injury or who have had brain surgery. **It is done for any patient at risk of increasing intracranial pressure.** Skill 22-2 presents the steps of the neurologic check. The pupil size is measured under normal light conditions. Pupils are normally round and equal in size. A flashlight is used to make the pupils constrict. They should constrict briskly when stimulated by the light.

Health Promotion Points 22-1

Recommended Periodic Diagnostic Tests

Patients should be taught that the following diagnostic tests should be performed periodically to prevent health problems or detect cancer:

- **Blood pressure:** Annual measurement; more frequently if elevated above 140/90 mm Hg.
- **Cholesterol:** Measurement every 1 to 3 years; more frequently if above 200 mg/dL.
- **Blood glucose:** Measurement every 1 to 3 years; more frequently if above 110 mg/dL.
- **Breast:** Monthly self-examination; check by physician, nurse practitioner, or physician's assistant every 3 years until age 40, then every year. Mammogram beginning at age 40, then every 2 years until age 50, then every year.
- **Colon-rectum:** Digital rectal examination as part of annual checkup every year after age 40. Proctosigmoidoscopy at age 50 and 51, then every 3 to 5 years if test is negative. Stool blood test every year beginning at age 50.

- **Cervix and uterus:** If cervix and uterus are present, pelvic examination every year. Pap test for all adult women and sexually active adolescents. After three consecutive normal annual examinations, test may be performed every 3 years at discretion of physician.
- **Testicles and prostate:** Beginning at age 14, testicular self-examination (TSE) once a month. Beginning at age 40 for men, a digital rectal examination (DRE) annually. Beginning at age 50, prostate-specific antigen (PSA) blood test annually.
- **Skin:** Self-examination once a month with consultation with dermatologist for pale, waxlike, pearly nodules and asymmetric moles, abnormal pigmentation moles with an irregular border, or changes in moles.
- **Oral:** Yearly dental examination. Inspect sides and bottom of tongue every few months.
- **Eye:** Examination every 3 to 5 years; after age 40 every 2 to 3 years, particularly testing for glaucoma; more frequently for those with diabetes or eye disease.

Skill 22-2 | Performing a Neurologic Check

The neurologic check is done for any patient who has sustained a head injury or had cranial surgery. This assessment is also performed for those patients who have a neurologic problem such as seizures or a suspected central nervous system infection. This assessment is often performed every 2 hours to determine if there is neurologic deterioration.

■ Supplies
✓ Flashlight
✓ Pupil measuring guide
✓ Pen with the cap on

Review and carry out the Standard Steps in Appendix 3.

1. **ACTION** Ask the patient questions to test orientation to person, place, and time. Ask if patient remembers where she is, what month it is, who is president, when she was born, or other relevant questions. Do not ask the same questions each time the neurologic check is performed.

   RATIONALE Checks degree of mental orientation.

2. **ACTION** With the room lights subdued, examine the size of the pupils and determine if they are equal in size. Measure the size.

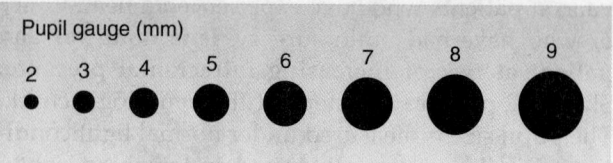

Step **2**

RATIONALE Increasing intracranial pressure, when extreme, causes one or both pupils to dilate.

3. **ACTION** Turn the flashlight on and position it lateral to the eye on the same plane. Slowly bring it over to shine directly on the pupil of the eye on that side and watch to see whether the pupil constricts. Quickly move the light back away to the side of the head.

   RATIONALE The pupil of that eye should constrict briskly and return to its former size after the light is averted.

4. **ACTION** Perform the same maneuver for the other eye. Briefly shine the light directly onto the pupil and watch for the pupillary reaction. Briefly shine the light directly onto the pupil again and watch the other eye for pupil constriction indicating a consensual reflex.

   RATIONALE If the pupil reacts sluggishly, it indicates that intracranial pressure is rising. This should be reported to the physician immediately.

5. **ACTION** Ask the patient to follow your finger, pen, or pencil with her eyes as you move it to the cardinal (primary) points. Test on one side and then the other.

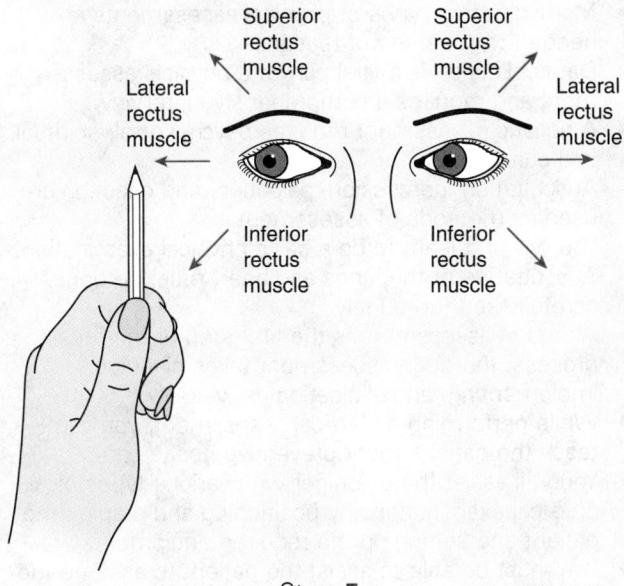

Superior rectus muscle

Superior rectus muscle

Lateral rectus muscle

Lateral rectus muscle

Inferior rectus muscle

Inferior rectus muscle

Step **5**

RATIONALE Watch the patient's eyes to see whether the patient tracks your finger without nystagmus (jerky movements). Checking these eye movements provides information about cranial nerves III, IV, and VI.

6. **ACTION** Ask the patient to follow your commands. Ask the patient to do specific things, such as rotate the left foot at the ankle or touch the nose with the right index finger.

RATIONALE The ability to follow commands indicates intact cognition and motor pathways.

7. **ACTION** Test extremity muscle strength by having the patient push against your hands with the sole of one foot and then with the other. Then have the patient grasp your crossed index and middle fingers on both hands with her hands. Check for the degree of strength and equality of strength on both sides.

RATIONALE Decreases in muscle strength can indicate pressure on certain areas within the brain or a problem within the spinal cord or muscles themselves. When weakness occurs on one side only, it can indicate a problem on the opposite side of the brain. Crossing the fingers prevents excessive pain.

For the Comatose Patient

8. **ACTION** Check the patient's response to a stimulus by pressing on the area near the base of a fingernail with a hard object or by applying pressure with two fingers in a grasp position on the trapezius muscle.

RATIONALE Note whether the patient grimaces, withdraws away from the stimulus, displays flexion posture, or displays extension posture. The Glasgow Coma Scale may be used to rank the patient's condition (see Table 22-4).

9. **ACTION** Make the patient comfortable. Document the findings, precisely charting any abnormalities found.

RATIONALE Making the patient comfortable shows caring and concern. Documentation notes result of the examination and provides data for future comparison.

?CRITICAL THINKING QUESTIONS

1. Can you explain why pupils might react sluggishly when intracranial pressure is rising?

2. What other questions could you ask the patient besides "Where are you?" "What day is it?" and "Who is president?" that would give you a good indication of the patient's orientation?

Both pupils should get smaller when either eye is stimulated by the light. This is called the *consensual reflex*. Pupils will also constrict when looking at a near object and then dilate when viewing a far object. This is called *accommodation*. Normal findings are often documented using the acronym PERRLA, meaning *Pupils Equal, Round,* and *Reactive to Light and Accommodation*. Eye muscles are tested by checking extraocular movements (EOMs). The patient is asked to track the nurse's finger or an object as it is moved to six different positions. The eyes normally move in a coordinated manner. Absence of movement or irregular movement may indicate cranial nerve damage or a neurologic problem. The Glasgow Coma Scale is used in most hospitals to score the neurologic exam (Table 22-4). It provides a baseline against which changes can be evaluated.

Vital signs are taken at the time of the neurologic check because diseases that increase intracranial pressure can affect the vital signs, although such changes often do not occur until quite late, when circulation to the brain has been impaired. The pulse and respiratory rates slow while the temperature and blood pressure rise.

Evaluation

Evaluating the techniques of physical assessment and the thoroughness of data collection is an individual responsibility. Questions to ask are as follows:
- Were all areas assessed adequately?
- Were there any pieces of data missing from the assessment form?
- Was the patient comfortable during the assessment?

Table 22-4 *Glasgow Coma Scale**

EYE OPENING

Spontaneous	4
To sound	3
To pain	2
Never	1

MOTOR RESPONSE

Obeys commands	6
Localizes pain	5
Normal flexion (withdrawal)	4
Abnormal flexion posturing	3
Extension posturing	2
None	1

VERBAL RESPONSE

Oriented	5
Confused conversation	4
Inappropriate words	3
Incomprehensible sounds	2
None	1

*The highest possible score is 15. A score of 7 or less indicates coma.

- Did the interaction remain focused on the assessment?
- Was all equipment available for the examination?
- Was the patient positioned and draped appropriately?
- Were procedures and their purpose explained to the patient?

A thorough, efficient assessment takes considerable practice. Assessment skills will improve with practice over time.

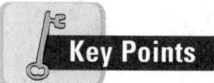

Key Points

- Nurses are expected to be able to perform a basic physical assessment.
- Assessment skill comes with practice over time.
- One of nursing's most important roles is to assess ill patients for signs of complications.

- Assessment of the home care patient is especially important because you are acting as the "eyes and ears" of the physician for the patient who cannot go to the office.
- Many different types of physical assessments are needed for a variety of reasons.
- Data collection is a vital part of a physical assessment and requires a comprehensive interview.
- A holistic assessment requires psychosocial, spiritual, and cultural data.
- Auscultation, percussion, palpation, and olfaction are used as methods of assessment.
- You will first learn to do a basic physical examination.
- Auscultation of the lungs and heart must be done carefully and thoroughly.
- Although assessment is the first step of the nursing process, thorough assessment takes planning, implementing, and evaluation as well.
- While performing a physical assessment, you can teach the patient about preventive health care.
- You will assist the examiner with various types of physical examinations by positioning and draping the patient and setting up the required equipment.
- You must be able to assist the patient to assume the supine, lithotomy, prone, Sims', and lateral positions.
- Draping protects the patient's privacy and modesty and helps prevent chilling.
- Laboratory requisitions must be filled out for all specimens to be sent for analysis.
- A neurologic check is often performed by nurses every few hours on patients at risk of increasing intracranial pressure.
- The Glasgow Coma Scale is used to score the neurologic check and to quantify the neurologic condition of the patient.

 Go to your **Companion CD-ROM** for an Audio Glossary, animations, video clips, and more.

evolve Be sure to visit the companion Evolve site at http://evolve.elsevier.com/deWit/fundamental/ for additional online resources.

NCLEX-PN® EXAMINATION-STYLE REVIEW QUESTIONS

*Choose the **best** answer(s) for each question.*

An assessment is assigned on a 66-year-old woman who has a history of congestive heart failure. She was hospitalized 3 days ago with pneumonia and is confused.

1. Detection of air within the intestinal system is assessed by _____. *(Fill in the blank.)*

2. Wet, crinkly sounds in the lungs heard on auscultation are referred to as:
   1. rubs.
   2. crackles.
   3. rhonchi.
   4. tinkles.

3. A holistic nursing assessment of a patient is necessary to:
   1. formulate an effective nursing care plan.
   2. establish patient trust in the nurse.
   3. determine the patient's physical problems.
   4. detect adverse effects of treatment.

4. When auscultating heart sounds (S_1 and S_2), listen at:
   1. the base of the heart with the bell.
   2. an area above the left nipple with the bell.
   3. 2 inches below the right nipple with the diaphragm.
   4. the fifth intercostal space at the midclavicular line with the diaphragm.

5. When listening to lung sounds, you should: *(Select all that apply.)*

   1. use the bell of the stethoscope.
   2. turn off the radio or TV.
   3. use the diaphragm of the stethoscope.
   4. listen in two or three places.
   5. follow a systematic pattern of stethoscope placement.

6. Neurologic assessments or neuro checks are performed for the patient who has experienced an intracranial injury to detect: *(Select all that apply.)*

   1. mentation.
   2. increasing intracranial pressure.
   3. coordination.
   4. pupil health.
   5. decreasing consciousness.

7. If the patient requires a pelvic examination, you would position the patient on the table in which position until the examiner is ready to perform the examination?

   1. Supine
   2. Sims'
   3. Knee-chest
   4. Lithotomy

8. When gathering data for a patient database for a patient with a respiratory complaint, which pieces of information are essential to obtain? *(Select all that apply.)*

   1. Location of pain or tenderness
   2. Ability to sleep
   3. Abnormal breath sounds
   4. Feelings of dyspnea

9. When a blood pressure (BP) reading is abnormal on initial assessment, it is best to check the BP:

   1. on the other arm.
   2. on both arms sitting and standing.
   3. with the patient standing.
   4. after a 5-minute wait.

10. When performing an initial assessment on a patient, which piece of information is most important to obtain?

   1. Where the patient is living
   2. Any allergies to medications
   3. Treatment for previous illnesses
   4. Date of previous diagnostic tests

CRITICAL THINKING ACTIVITIES *Read each clinical scenario and discuss the questions with your classmates.*

Scenario A
How could you obtain needed information for your initial assessment from a patient who is deaf?

Scenario B
If you are not certain that the blood pressure measurement you obtained is accurate, what would you do?

Scenario C
How would you handle the situation if your patient refuses to answer the questions you are asking during your assessment interview?

Scenario D
What would you do if you are to assess a patient of the opposite sex and the person does not want you to do the assessment?

23 Admitting, Transferring, and Discharging Patients

evolve http://evolve.elsevier.com/deWit/fundamental/

TYPES OF ADMISSIONS

Each day, thousands of people are admitted to hospitals. This is part of the daily routine for the nurse, but for the patient it is a major event. You must not lose sight of its impact on those admitted for care.

Illness, injury, and the need for surgery are highly stressful, particularly if associated with loss of function, chronic health problems, a change in body appearance, or a terminal diagnosis. The financial impact can be devastating, both because of the cost of care and due to the loss of income. These stresses extend to include the family and often close friends and associates as well.

? *Think Critically About . . .* How would the need to go into the hospital affect or alter your life right now?

ROUTINE ADMISSIONS

Routine admissions are those that are scheduled in advance. The physician and patient have agreed to the admission as the most appropriate way to address the medical need, and the patient has had at least a short period of time in which to make plans and arrangements for this interruption in the usual routine (Cultural Cues 23-1).

Many facilities have specific units that provide for day-stay or same-day surgeries. These patients will arrive a couple of hours before the procedure and, after a short recovery period in the day-stay unit, go home the same day. Although considered outpatients, day-stay patients must still meet the same admission criteria as routine admissions. If their condition is such that they cannot go home the same day, they are usually admitted to an inpatient nursing unit because most day-stay units do not remain open at night.

EMERGENCY ADMISSIONS

An emergency admission is one for which there was no prior planning. These occur when sudden illness, injury, or abrupt worsening of an existing condition requires immediate admission for treatment. Such admissions tend to be particularly stressful for both the

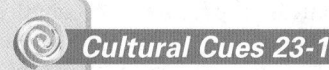

Cultural Cues 23-1

Family Care

In some cultures, it is expected that family members go with the patient and stay with them in the hospital. It is up to the nurse to ensure that the family is allowed to spend time with their loved one without causing disruption for the other patients. Providing a family room or a secluded corner and allowing one or two visitors at a time can meet this need.

---

patient and close family and friends. In addition to worry and fear about the medical problem, there may be prior commitments that now cannot be met or children who need care. These concerns can have a direct effect on the patient's response to treatment.

THE ADMISSION PROCESS

PREADMISSION PROCEDURES AND REQUIREMENTS

Routine admissions normally take place the day of the scheduled procedure. For this reason, most facilities require that the patient come in a day or two before admission to complete the administrative paperwork and have any admitting laboratory work or other studies completed.

Insurance companies and health care regulatory organizations mandate that specific criteria be met when an individual is admitted to the hospital. For routine admissions, these are completed in advance. However, in an emergency situation, they take place as the patient is being stabilized in the emergency department and prepared for admission. These are discussed below.

Authorization for Admission

Most third-party payers require prior authorization for hospital admission. There are a variety of third-party payers, including private or employer-provided coverage through major insurance companies, managed care plans (health care plans in which all medical care except emergency care is managed and must be preauthorized by the insuring group), and health maintenance organizations (HMOs) (organizations that provide most outpatient care at organization clinics, may provide inpatient care at organization hospitals, and must authorize usage of outside services). Government plans include Medicaid (state medical care coverage for low-income individuals and families), Medicare (medical care coverage provided through the Social Security Administration primarily for people age 65 and over), and TRICARE, previously called CHAMPUS (coverage in civilian facilities for military staff, family, and retirees).

In most cases it is the responsibility of the physician's office to obtain this authorization. If authorization is denied, it means that the patient's insurance carrier has refused to accept liability for payment. All payment programs and plans have criteria that define the services covered. For example, most plans do not cover procedures that are regarded as purely cosmetic, such as a face lift or breast augmentation, but these same plans may cover cosmetic procedures if they are to repair the effects of an injury or a necessary surgical procedure such as a mastectomy.

Admitting Department Function

The admitting department is responsible for making sure that all admission criteria are met. They collect the personal and insurance information and verify the authorization for admission. In many facilities, the admitting department is part of the business office and responsible for making payment arrangements on insurance deductibles and co-pays (the amounts the insurance carrier may require the patient to pay for care). They may also collect deposits and make payment arrangements for noncovered services.

For an emergency admission, this process may become the responsibility of the emergency department clerical staff.

Laboratory Work and X-Ray Examinations

As mentioned, lab work and examinations related to the planned course of treatment are commonly done before a routine admission. This includes procedures such as x-rays, computed tomography (CT) scans, and magnetic resonance imaging (MRI).

DAY OF ADMISSION

Patients are usually required to report to the hospital 1 or 2 hours before the scheduled procedure. For early procedures, this often means that they arrive near the end of the night shift rather than on the day shift. Day-stay units typically begin the day shift early, at 5 or 6 A.M., to accommodate the early arrivals.

Patient Orientation to Nursing Unit

Newly admitted patients, particularly those who have never been hospitalized before, may be nervous and very unsure of what to expect. You can do a great deal to alleviate their anxiety during the initial contact by orienting them to the nursing unit.

You should smile, make eye contact, and call the patient by name. A good example of the initial contact would be, "Hello, Mr. Jones. My name is Sandra Smith. I'm an LPN/LVN and I'll be one of your nurses today." It is important that the patient be given the names of all caregivers and their specific roles. **Never assume that a patient wishes to be called by his or her first name.** They are entitled to be addressed in the manner that is most comfortable for them.

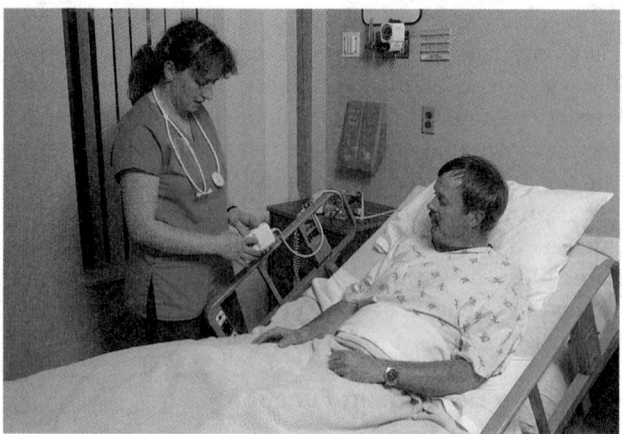

FIGURE **23-1** Nurse orienting patient to unit.

Proceed to orient the patient to the unit. Show the location of the call bell and demonstrate its use. Show the location of the bathroom and use of the emergency call bell next to the toilet. Also show the patient how to operate the television and the telephone (Figure 23-1). Explain about visiting hours and, if one is available, give the patient a printed orientation handout with this information. If the patient is to receive nothing by mouth (NPO), explain or reinforce this information. If the patient is not NPO and has no ordered fluid restriction, fill the water carafe and place it within the patient's reach.

Although this initial contact is frequently brief and may immediately precede hurried preparations for surgery or other procedures, the patient must be made to feel welcome and valued. **The patient must also be given ample opportunity to have questions answered and procedures explained.** If the patient is too ill at the time of admission for a full orientation, it should be done as soon as the patient's condition permits.

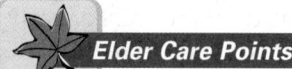

Elder Care Points

Age and failing health can decrease an older person's ability to cope with and understand change. These patients often need extra time and support in making the adjustment to a hospital stay.

Care of Patient Belongings. Hospitals provide very little space for personal belongings, but patients may find great comfort in wearing their own bathrobe or having a special picture on the bedside table or shelf. You can assist your patients to put belongings in the closet and encourage them to send home anything that will have no use during their stay. Valuables such as credit cards, money, or jewelry should be sent home with a family member. If this is not possible, obtain a valuables envelope and arrange for safe storage of these items following your facility's specific protocol. Document all other items, such as dentures, hearing aids, or bedside clock, on the patient belongings list. Items that plug into electrical outlets need to be

checked by the maintenance department to ensure they are properly grounded. During the patient's stay, this list should be updated to indicate things sent home or new items brought in for the patient's use.

Some patients will bring in their medications from home. Each facility will have a specific protocol regarding these medications. The medication reconciliation process should be used, comparing the patient's medication orders to all of the medications that the patient has been taking. Most facilities will ask that you make a list of the medications and then send them home with the family. **It is important to notify the physician of any medications the patient has been taking at home that are not included in the present orders.** Know the proper procedure for your facility and follow it at all times.

Initial Nursing Assessment (Data Collection)

The nursing assessment in an acute care facility is written by the RN, but the LPN/LVN can greatly assist in this process by data gathering during the initial contact. Vital signs, lists of medications (including all over-the-counter medications, supplements, and herbals the patient takes), and information about allergies, previous hospital stays, illnesses, and surgeries can all be obtained by the LPN/LVN and given to the RN for use in the actual assessment. In some facilities, the nursing assessment is done during a preadmission interview, which greatly reduces the tasks that must be accomplished before patients are sent for their scheduled procedures.

LPN/LVNs are frequently charge nurses in skilled nursing facilities and are responsible for completing the written assessment and care plan. When writing an assessment, it is important to accurately describe your findings. Most facilities use a check-off system, but a narrative description is still required. Table 23-1 shows the items to be assessed and gives examples of descriptive terms.

Figure 23-2 shows an example of the typical assessment form. Chapter 5 gives specific information on assessment data collection and use of nursing diagnoses. Chapter 6 discusses the writing of care plans.

Preparing the Chart

Most care facilities have unit secretaries who assist in the admission process by preparing the actual chart, transcribing orders, preparing lab slips and x-ray requests, and filling out consent forms. It is the responsibility of the nurse to check that everything has been accurately transcribed by the secretary. If the orders have been correctly transcribed, the nurse then signs immediately below them and also writes the date and time signed. The nurse must be able to set up a chart and do the transcription if there is no unit secretary available. Regardless of who does the actual transcription of orders and completion of request forms and consents, the nurse who checks and signs the orders is directly responsible for their accuracy. In most acute

Table 23-1 *Admission Assessment Data Gathering*

ASSESSMENT CATEGORY	EXAMPLES OF DATA
Level of consciousness	Alert, lethargic, drowsy, difficult to arouse, unresponsive to unpleasant stimuli, comatose
Vital signs	Temperature (include how taken [e.g., oral, tympanic, rectal, or axillary], and whether Fahrenheit or centigrade)
	Pulse rate
	Pulse quality (e.g., bounding, thready, regular, or irregular)
	Respiratory rate
	Respiratory quality (e.g., labored, shallow)
	Respiratory status (e.g. unlabored, labored, wheezing, cough [productive or nonproductive], shortness of breath, use of accessory muscles, or abnormal breath sounds on auscultation [name or describe abnormal sounds])
	Blood pressure (systolic and diastolic)
	Height and weight (the patient should be weighed and measured rather than accepting the stated height and weight, unless the medical condition prevents this)
Ability to communicate	Language spoken, speech impediment or impairment, or decreased ability to understand verbal communication
Vision and hearing	Visual impairment, including type and degree; hearing impairment, including degree; ability to read Braille, use sign language, or read lips
Condition of skin	Skin breaks or tears, bruises, abrasions, pressure areas, excessive dryness, birthmarks, rashes, surgical incisions, wounds
Prosthetic and assistive devices	Hearing aid, glasses, contact lenses, dentures, braces, walker, wheelchair, cane, artificial limbs, wigs
Other health problems and concerns	Pain or discomfort, loss of function or loss of normal control of function, restricted movement, alteration in sensation, additional diagnoses other than that for which admission is occurring (e.g., diabetes mellitus, heart disease)

care facilities orders are verified by the RN, but in some acute facilities and in most skilled nursing facilities, this duty is performed by the LPN/LVN.

Admission orders are often long and complex. For safety, the individual transcribing the orders should make a checkmark by each order as it is processed. The nurse who reviews the orders must verify that each order has been processed and that the transcription is accurate. **This means the nurse must read every lab slip, procedure request, and consent form, correcting as necessary.** If there has been an error on a document to be signed, any changes must be clear and must be initialed. Any deletions must be crossed out with a single line, with the word "error" and the nurse's initials written above. If a consent form has been transcribed inaccurately, or if the physician orders a change in the wording, it should be destroyed and a new form written for the patient's signature.

Once transcription of the orders has been verified, the orders are signed. A line is drawn along the left margin of the orders being verified and then the nurse signs with the date and time immediately below the last order and the physician's signature. The facility may require that this be done in red ink, or have some other specific protocol. Know and follow the policy of your facility.

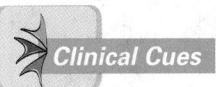
Clinical Cues

Avoiding conversing with co-workers while signing off orders helps ensure that mistakes are not made due to interruption and distraction.

Hospitals and other facilities have specific protocols for noting allergies. In most institutions they are not only written on the plan of care, but are also displayed on the front of the chart. In addition, patients often are given a colored armband with the allergies clearly listed.

PLAN OF CARE

Preparation of the written plan of care is part of the assessment and is done by the nurse with input from all the members of the health care team. The basis of the plan of care is the nursing process and nursing diagnosis, both of which are covered in detail in Chapters 4, 5, and 6.

PATIENT TRANSFER TO ANOTHER HOSPITAL UNIT

Changes in condition may require that a patient be transferred from one nursing unit to another. As patients in the intensive care unit (ICU) or cardiac care unit (CCU) become stable, they are often transferred to a definitive observation unit (DOU), also sometimes called a step-down unit, or to the med-surg unit. A patient who was originally admitted to the medical or surgical unit may become less stable and be transferred to the DOU, ICU, or CCU.

When a patient is to be transferred, the patient's physician must be notified and approve the transfer. In situations of sudden deterioration of condition, the patient may be moved immediately per established hospital protocols, but in general transfers from one

Text continued on p. 401

ADMISSION ASSESSMENT

GENERAL ADMISSION INFORMATION

Date of admission: _____ **Time:** _____

From: ☐ Home ☐ Hospital _____ ☐ Other _____ ☐ W/C ☐ Gurney ☐ Ambulated

Language spoken: ☐ English ☐ Other _____ **Able to read:** ☐ Yes ☐ No

Diagnosis: _____

Vital signs: T _____ P _____ R _____ B/P _____ **Pain level:** _____

Height: _____ **Weight:** _____ Recent gain or loss? ☐ No ☐ Yes Amount: _____

ALLERGIES

Medication allergies: _____ Reaction: _____

_____ Reaction: _____

_____ Reaction: _____

Food allergies: _____ Reaction: _____

Other allergies: _____ Reaction: _____

COMMUNICATION

Speech ☐ Clear ☐ Mild to Moderately aphasic ☐ Severely aphasic ☐ Needs speech assessment

MENTAL STATUS

		Score
ORIENTATION	☐ Able to state name ☐ Able to state birth date (1 point each, 2 possible)	
	Able to state: ☐ Year ☐ Season ☐ Month ☐ Day of week ☐ Today's date (1 point each, 5 possible)	
REGISTRATION	☐ Able to repeat series of three words: table, apple, horse (6 points, decrease by 1 point for each try)	
CALCULATION	☐ Able to count backward from 100 by 7 (100-93-86-79-72) (5 points. Stop at fifth number, 1 point for each successful number. Resident may do as subtraction, e.g., 100 – 7 is 93, 93 – 7 is 86, etc.)	
RECALL	☐ Able to repeat the three words from Registration question (3 points, 1 point for each correct word)	
LANGUAGE	☐ Able to name objects: pencil, watch (1 point each) ☐ Able to repeat "No ifs, ands, or buts." (1 point) ☐ Able to follow three-stage command: "Pick up the paper, fold it, and lay it on the table." (3 points) ☐ Able to compose and write a simple sentence. (1 point)	
Total score (highest possible is 27)		

MOOD/BEHAVIOR

☐ Quite ☐ Passive ☐ Friendly ☐ Depressed ☐ Elated ☐ Cooperative ☐ Combative ☐ Secure ☐ Homesick ☐ Questioning
☐ Fearful ☐ Noisy ☐ Talkative ☐ Lethargic ☐ Hyperactive

FUNCTIONAL/NEUROMUSCULAR

PUPILS: ☐ Equally round and reactive **Right:** Size _____ Reactive _____ **Left:** Size _____ Reactive _____

VISION:

Right: ☐ Adequate ☐ Adequate w/glasses ☐ Poor ☐ Blind **Left:** ☐ Adequate ☐ Adequate w/glasses ☐ Poor ☐ Blind

HEARING:

Right: ☐ Adequate ☐ Adequate w/aid ☐ Poor ☐ Deaf **Left:** ☐ Adequate ☐ Adequate w/aid ☐ Poor ☐ Deaf

STRENGTH:

Grip: ☐ Equal ☐ Weak right ☐ Absent right ☐ Weak left ☐ Absent left

Legs (push): ☐ Equal ☐ Weak right ☐ Absent right ☐ Weak left ☐ Absent left

SKIN CONDITION

☐ **No problems identified** (skin intact, moist mucous membranes)

Color: ☐ Normal ☐ Pale ☐ Jaundiced ☐ Cyanotic ☐ Ashen

Condition: ☐ Warm ☐ Cool ☐ Dry ☐ Clammy ☐ Diaphoretic ☐ Mottled

Turgor: ☐ Elastic ☐ Decreased ☐ Tenting

Indicate marks or lesions on the figures to the right using the following codes:

B = bruising

P = pressure ulcer: Stage I, II, III, IV

L = laceration

S = scar

R = rash (describe in notes)

A = abrasion

BU = burn

E = edema

C = cyanosis

U = ulceration other than pressure ulcer

SI = surgical incision (recent)

L FRONT BACK R R L

Stamp lower right corner with patient identification information

FIGURE **23-2** Admission record for skilled nursing. The entire form (three pages) is included on your companion CD-ROM.

nursing area to another require a specific order by the attending physician. The admissions office, or in some facilities the business office, must be notified of any transfers.

It is also important that the patient's family or significant other be notified, preferably prior to the actual transfer. In emergency situations, notification should be made as soon as possible.

Each facility has specific guidelines as to documentation, but it is always necessary that the transfer be recorded in the nursing notes, by both the nurse transferring the patient and the nurse receiving the patient. The care plan must be reviewed and revised and a full report given to the receiving nurse when the patient arrives on the new unit.

Failure to pass on necessary information in the process of transferring a patient has been cited as a major factor in patient care errors. The major accrediting body in the United States, The Joint Commission, has added "improving the effectiveness of communication among caregivers" to their patient safety goals. Their guidelines state that every facility is to have procedures in place that provide for accurate communication of patient information at the time of any transfer, whether to another nursing unit, to an ancillary department for tests or procedures, or to another facility. This information will include a complete listing of the patient's current medications. They further state that this should include the opportunity for the person receiving the patient to ask questions regarding the patient and the plan of treatment.

Loss of patient belongings is most likely to happen during a transfer from one unit to another. This is particularly true of durable medical equipment, such as walkers, canes, and wheelchairs, because they are often overlooked on the assumption that they belong to the facility rather than the patient. **For this reason, all equipment brought to the hospital by the patient should be clearly labeled, usually with a wide piece of tape on which the patient's name is written in large letters.**

Glasses, dentures, hearing aids, and jewelry are the other most frequently lost items, and replacement can be very expensive for the facility. Check the drawers, shelves, patient bathroom, and bed linens carefully to ensure that such things are not accidentally thrown away or sent to the laundry.

DISCHARGING THE PATIENT

Discharge planning begins at admission, particularly when the diagnosis indicates the patient will need rehabilitation or long-term assistance. Members of the health care team must document needs to be addressed so the patient can be discharged from acute care. The discharge planner (an RN who implements and organizes the plan for patient discharge) will use

this information, as well as information gathered from the patient, the family, and the physician, to make appropriate discharge arrangements for the patient.

The actual discharge orders are written by the physician. When discharge orders are received, you should assist as needed with notifying the family or significant other, collecting patient belongings, and preparing the patient for the ride home or to a new facility. Just prior to discharge, retrieve any valuables stored in the hospital safe, and have the patient sign for them in accordance with hospital protocol.

DISCHARGE TO AN EXTENDED CARE OR REHABILITATION FACILITY

Acute hospital stays are often short, and patients may not be well enough to go directly home at the time of discharge. A growing number of patients are being discharged to rehabilitation or extended-care facilities.

To ensure that information regarding necessary treatments, medications, and special needs is clearly communicated, the RN completes a detailed patient information sheet for the receiving facility (Figure 23-3). Information recorded includes primary and secondary diagnoses; current orders; medications (including over-the-counter medications, dietary supplements, and any herbals the patient takes), noting dosage, route, frequency, and time of last dose given; physician names and phone numbers; and a brief synopsis of the hospital stay. It is preferable but not always possible for the discharging nurse to call the admitting nurse at the new facility and give a verbal report prior to sending the patient.

If the patient is to be transferred by ambulance, arrangements for this service are made by the hospital's discharge planner. If the patient is able to go by private car and the physician is in agreement, the patient is taken to the car via wheelchair by a staff member.

Any records to be transferred with the patient must be ready in an envelope before the transporting vehicle arrives. Often a copy of the discharge summary and instructions has also been faxed to the receiving facility to allow them to make advanced arrangements for the patient's arrival.

Just prior to the time of discharge, assist the patient with packing of personal belongings. You should also assist the patient as necessary to dress in a manner appropriate to the mode of transport and the weather conditions.

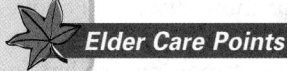
Elder Care Points

The need to be transferred from the hospital to a rehabilitation or long-term care facility can be confusing and frightening for elderly patients. Whenever possible, have a family member or a close friend either travel with patients or meet them when they arrive at the new facility to smooth this transition.

INTERFACILITY TRANSFER AND ORDER FORM

PATIENT			BIRTHDATE	AGE	SEX	MARITAL STATUS S M W D SEP	RELIGION	HOSPITAL #

ADDRESS	CITY	PHONE	ADM. DATE	DISCHARGE DATE

NEAREST RELATIVE OR FRIEND	RELATIONSHIP	PHONE	PHYSICIAN IN CHARGE AT TIME OF TRANSFER	PHONE

TRANSFERRED TO	ADDRESS	PHONE	TRANSFERRED FROM	DISCHARGE COORD.

DISCHARGE DIAGNOSIS	SURGERY/DATE

Rehab Potential ❑ Good ❑ Fair ❑ Poor
Patient informed of condition ❑ Yes ❑ No If No/Why not?_____
Date of Chest X-ray or PPd _____ Results_____
Durable Power of Attorney: ❑ Yes ❑ No
Durable Power of Attorney For Health Care: ❑ Yes ❑ No
CPR Status ❑ Yes ❑ No
    Discussed with Family ❑ Yes ❑ No   Discussed with Patient ❑ Yes ❑ No

Foley Catheter: ❑ Yes ❑ No   Catheter Size_____ Balloon Size_____
Reason for Catheter: ❑ Neurogenic ❑ Postoperative
❑ Other____
Replace Foley Cath. Every 30 days and/or PRN non-patency ❑ Yes ❑ No

Diet:_____.
NG or G Tube: ❑ Yes ❑ No   Give _____ Cal _____ cc
House Formula: or_____ every 24 Hrs.
Flush tube with _____ cc of water every _____ Hrs. and post medication administration.
Replace NG tube when plugged, PRN. ❑ Yes ❑ No Routine Dental Care: ❑ Yes
Podiatry Care: q .3 mon. PRN (For mycotic/hypertrophic nails) ❑ Yes ❑ No
May participate in activity plan not in conflict with treatment plan.

"I certify that post-hospital ECF services are required on inpatient basis, because of individual need for skilled nursing care on a continuous basis for condition(s) for which patient was receiving inpatient hospital care."

REHABILITATIVE THERAPY
P.T. Evaluation ❑ Yes ❑ No Rx Plan:
Speech Evaluation ❑ Yes ❑ No Rx Plan:
OT Evaluation ❑ Yes ❑ No Rx Plan:

MOBILITY LEVEL: ❑ UP IN CHAIR ❑ UP AD LIB ❑ BED REST ❑ OTHER:

TREATMENT/WOUND AND SKIN CARE (SPECIFIC AREA TREATED): ISOLATION ❑ YES ❑ NO

RA ABGs (COPY)	O₂ (ROUTE) LPM	CONT.	PRN	CHANGE CANNULA, TUBING, HUMIDIFIER Q 5 DAYS
DIABETIC MONITORING:		DIALYSIS ❑		RADIATION THERAPY ❑

ALLERGIES:

MEDICATIONS	DOSAGE & FREQUENCY	DIAGNOSES (Every medication must have a diagnosis)

HISTORY AND PHYSICAL UPDATE ❑ YES ❑ NO   IF YES: PLEASE COMMENT.

PERIODIC LABS: (Any required to monitor meds)	FREQUENCY:

SIGNATURE_____ M.D. DATE_____

FIGURE **23-3** Interfacility transfer form.

DISCHARGE HOME

Patients being discharged directly home require essentially the same preparations as those discussed above. Most patients discharged directly home will travel by private car, but special transport may be needed for patients with severe mobility restrictions. It is the nurse's responsibility to verify that necessary arrangements have been made so the discharge goes smoothly for the patient and family.

Written discharge instructions are prepared by the RN and reviewed with the patient and often with family members as well. Both the patient and the nurse sign the form, a copy is given to the patient, and one is placed in the chart. The discharge form lists medications, activity restrictions, special diet instructions, and ordered follow-up appointments. The name and phone number of the physician are also listed. This is particularly important if the patient is being cared for by a new physician. For example, an accident victim may have been assigned an orthopedic surgeon during admission through the emergency department and will need to know how to contact this physician for care following discharge.

Home Health Care

Many patients, particularly the elderly, receive home health care following discharge. Home health services may include skilled nursing, such as wound care, diabetic care and teaching, and intravenous medication administration. Physical, occupational, or speech therapy and respiratory care are also often part of home care services, as is personal care performed by a home health aide. Counseling and information regarding long-term planning, financial assistance, or community services available can be provided by a medical social worker (MSW). Many services that were once available only to hospital patients are now routinely provided in the home setting.

There are many advantages to home health care. These include reduced cost, decreased exposure to potentially serious infections, and most important, being in a familiar, comfortable environment. Medicare, Medicaid, and some insurance and managed care plans provide for payment of portions or all of these services when ordered by a physician.

Discharge Against Medical Advice

Occasionally a patient will insist on leaving the hospital against the advice of the physician. The patient has the right to make this choice. It is the responsibility of the health care team to help patients understand how the decision to leave the hospital may impact their health. Listen to what the patient has to say, answer questions, and offer to ask the physician or supervising nurse to talk with the patient.

If the patient's ultimate decision is to leave, notify the physician immediately. If the physician feels it is inappropriate for a discharge order to be written, the patient is asked to sign a form stating that he is leaving against medical advice (AMA). Sometimes a patient will refuse to sign. You must document this, and then date and sign the form in the space provided. The patient's stated reasons for leaving are written in the nursing notes.

When patients choose to leave against medical advice, they also need to be informed that insurance carriers will sometimes refuse to pay the hospital bill and that they would then become liable. Document this information in the chart.

DEATH OF A PATIENT

Although there is a growing trend toward remaining at home to die, most deaths still occur in hospitals and long-term care facilities. It is often a difficult time for family, friends, and at times even the hospital staff. Death after a long, good life or at the end of lingering illness or pain may be seen as a kind and welcome release. Death of a vigorous, active adult or a child, however, is often viewed as unfair and even unthinkable. Death may also bring great disruption to family life, especially if the individual was the primary wage earner or provider of care for the family children. See Chapter 15 for more about care of the dying patient.

PROVIDING SUPPORT FOR SIGNIFICANT OTHERS

Often the most important gift we can give the bereaved is just being there. Simply sit and listen while they talk of their loss and the fears about the changes it will bring. People need to grieve; it is an important step in healing.

Many people derive significant comfort from spiritual or religious beliefs and practices. Offer to call their priest, minister, rabbi, or spiritual advisor. If death is anticipated, doing this while the patient still lives can be particularly helpful, especially if the religious beliefs include specific predeath rituals.

You can also offer to make phone calls or arrangements for someone to come and take the significant other's home if this seems appropriate. An elderly widow or widower alone at the bedside of the just-deceased spouse, for example, may have difficulty making such a decision without some guidance or assistance.

Allow the family and friends adequate time at the bedside to say their good-byes. Crying, touching their loved one, and hugging each other are all part of a necessary human process in dealing with grief.

It is important to note that you must have dealt with your own feelings about death before you can be a good support person for someone else. Young nurses should not feel personally rejected if the family looks to older staff members for comfort and assistance. Older individuals have usually had more opportunity to experience loss through death, and family members frequently feel they will have a deeper understanding of the impact.

Think Critically About . . . How do you feel about caring for a patient who is dying?

PRONOUNCEMENT OF DEATH

In most states it is still required that a physician pronounce death. You must be familiar with the policy and procedure for your facility and adhere to it. The time life signs ceased, the time death was pronounced, and the name of the person making the official pronouncement must be documented in the nursing notes.

AUTOPSIES

Most deaths are not followed by an autopsy (examination of the remains by a pathologist to determine cause of death). Autopsy is usually performed when the patient has died of unknown causes, has died at the hands of another, or has not been seen within a specific period of time by a physician. In such cases the death becomes a coroner's case, and it is the coroner (city/county medical officer responsible for investigating unexplained death) who orders and authorizes the autopsy. The laws governing autopsy in these instances vary, and facility guidelines will follow local state law.

Autopsy may also be performed when it is felt that information valuable to medical research may be obtained, or when the family has questions about the cause of death. In such cases, the next of kin must authorize the autopsy.

ORGAN DONATION

The need for donor organs grows continually. Thousands of people each year owe their opportunity for a longer, healthier life to an organ donation. Requests to the family for organ donation are usually done by a physician or a nurse specially trained to do this. When handled in a sensitive, caring manner, requests for organ donation can be an opportunity for the family to allow something good to come out of a personal tragedy.

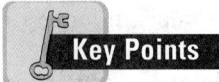

Key Points

- Admissions may be planned or occur in response to a medical emergency, but it is always a stressful event for the patient.
- Many procedures, including surgery, are now done as outpatient services, with the patient being cared for in a day-stay unit.
- The majority of health care payment plans require that authorization be obtained by the physician's office prior to a routine or elective admission.
- The admission department is responsible for determining that all admission criteria have been met and payment arrangements have been made.
- Because patients are often admitted only 1 or 2 hours prior to a procedure, lab work and x-rays are frequently done a day or two prior to admission.
- You must make patients feel welcome and orient them to the unit and hospital routine.
- Patients should be asked to send all valuables, unnecessary items, and medicines home if possible.
- Patient belongings, particularly those that are necessary for their care, such as wheelchairs, walkers, and canes, should be clearly labeled with the patient's name.

- In an acute care facility, the admission assessment and care plan are written by an RN, with the LPN/LVN providing data for this purpose.
- LPNs/LVNs may be charge nurses in some skilled nursing facilities and assume full responsibility for the initial assessment and writing of the care plan.
- Transfer of a patient from one unit to another requires a physician order, and care must be taken that the family is notified and all patient belongings are moved with the patient.
- The RN discharge planner begins discharge plans at the time of admission to ensure that patient needs will be adequately met after leaving the facility.
- The length of stay in an acute facility is often short, and the patient may need to spend some time in a skilled nursing facility or rehabilitation unit before going home.
- Written discharge instructions, complete with medications, treatments, and copies of necessary medical records, must accompany the patient being transferred to another facility.
- Patients discharged to their homes must be provided with written instructions regarding medications, treatments, and follow-up care.
- Home health care may be ordered before discharge, particularly for elderly patients. This may include skilled nursing, personal care assistance, therapy, and assessment by a social worker.
- If a patient chooses to leave the hospital against the advice of the physician, the nurse must notify the physician and ask the patient to sign a form acknowledging that the physician advises against leaving.
- When a patient dies, the nurse can frequently be of great assistance to the family and friends simply by being available to listen and providing them with privacy.
- Death is usually pronounced by the physician and must be accurately noted in the medical record, including the time life signs ceased, the time death was officially pronounced, and by whom.
- Autopsy is only performed for specific reasons and must be ordered by the coroner or authorized by the next of kin.

Go to your **Companion CD-ROM** for an Audio Glossary, animations, video clips, and more.

 evolve Be sure to visit the companion Evolve site at http://evolve.elsevier.com/deWit/fundamental/ for additional online resources.

NCLEX-PN® EXAMINATION-STYLE REVIEW QUESTIONS

*Choose the **best** answer(s) for each question.*

1. Obtaining authorization for an emergency admission is often the responsibility of:
   1. the physician's office.
   2. the patient.
   3. the emergency department clerical staff.
   4. the admissions office.

2. When instructing a patient scheduled for same-day surgery, you tell would him to: *(Select all that apply.)*
   1. report to the same-day surgery unit 3 to 4 hours before the scheduled procedure.
   2. bring only essential items to the hospital.
   3. have someone available to take him home after the procedure.
   4. report to the same-day surgery unit 1 to 2 hours before the scheduled procedure.

3. When making the first contact with a patient, it is most important to:
   1. verify the payment source.
   2. send all personal belongings home.
   3. make the patient feel welcome.
   4. have the patient remove all jewelry.

4. In an acute care facility, the person responsible for the initial nursing assessment is:
   1. the admissions staff.
   2. the RN.
   3. the RN or LVN.
   4. the physician.

5. In a skilled nursing facility, the person responsible for the initial nursing assessment may be: *(Select all that apply.)*
   1. the LPN/LVN.
   2. the admissions staff.
   3. the RN.
   4. the physician.

6. Orders are verified and signed off by:
   1. the unit secretary.
   2. the licensed nurse.
   3. the physician.
   4. the nursing supervisor.

7. If a patient brings credit cards, money, and jewelry to the hospital, you can provide for their security by: *(Select all that apply.)*
   1. sending all of the items home with the family.
   2. placing the contents in a valuables envelope and storing it in the bedside drawer.
   3. placing the contents in a valuables envelope to be stored in a safe.
   4. making a list of all the items on a "belongings list" and placing it in the chart.

8. When transferring a patient to another facility, copies of pertinent medical records:
   1. are the responsibility of the family to deliver.
   2. must accompany the patient.
   3. are mailed at the time of transfer.
   4. must be delivered by hospital messenger because they are confidential.

9. Discharge instructions for patients who go directly home from the hospital should include: *(Select all that apply.)*
   1. physician's phone number for follow-up appointment.
   2. instructions on how and when to take medications.
   3. instructions for activity restrictions and exercises to be performed.
   4. signs and symptoms of complications to report to the physician.

10. If a patient decides to leave against medical advice:
    1. he must be detained until the physician can come in and talk with him.
    2. he must sign a release or he may not leave the facility.
    3. a court order should be obtained to force him to remain for treatment.
    4. he has the legal right to do so.

11. An autopsy may be required when: *(Select all that apply.)*
    1. a patient dies after a 4-day hospitalization.
    2. a patient dies within 24 hours of admission.
    3. a patient dies without being under a physician's care outside the hospital.
    4. the cause of death is uncertain.

CRITICAL THINKING ACTIVITIES *Read each clinical scenario and discuss the questions with your classmates.*

Scenario A
What might you say to make a nervous patient and family feel more relaxed during the admission process?

Scenario B
What would you do if a family wanted to discuss organ donation?

Diagnostic Tests and Specimen Collection

Objectives

Upon completing this chapter, you should be able to:

Theory

1. Describe each of the seven categories of tests that are commonly performed.
2. Discuss appropriate psychosocial care and teaching for patients undergoing diagnostic tests or procedures.
3. Prepare to perform a capillary hemoglobin test, a venipuncture, a throat culture, an electrocardiogram, a urine dipstick test, and a stool for occult blood test.
4. Explain factors to be considered when an older adult is to undergo diagnostic testing.

Clinical Practice

1. Provide pre- and post-test nursing care, including appropriate teaching, for patients undergoing diagnostic tests and procedures.
2. Attend to psychosocial concerns of patients undergoing various diagnostic tests.
3. Perform a random blood glucose test using capillary blood and a glucometer.
4. Perform patient teaching for a magnetic resonance imaging (MRI) test.
5. Describe how to prepare a patient for and assist with aspiration procedures such as lumbar puncture, thoracentesis, paracentesis, bone marrow aspiration, and liver biopsy.
6. Correctly use Standard Precautions whenever obtaining or handling specimens for diagnostic tests.
7. List the steps for assisting with a pelvic exam and Pap test.
8. Correctly fill out laboratory and test requisition forms.

Skills & Steps

Skills

Skill 24-1 Phlebotomy and Obtaining Blood Samples with a Vacutainer System
Skill 24-2 Performing a Capillary Blood Test: Blood Glucose or Hemoglobin
Skill 24-3 Performing a Urine Dipstick Test
Skill 24-4 Obtaining a Stool Specimen for Occult Blood, Culture, or Ova and Parasites
Skill 24-5 Obtaining Culture Specimens: Throat and Wound
Skill 24-6 Assisting with a Pelvic Examination and Pap Test (Smear)

Steps

Steps 24-1 Obtaining an ECG Tracing (Electrocardiogram)
Steps 24-2 Assisting with a Flexible Sigmoidoscopy

Key Terms

 Be sure to check out the bonus material on the Companion CD-ROM, including selected audio pronunciations.

anemias (p. 406)
aspiration (p. 415)
biopsy (p. 415)
colonoscopy (KŌ-lŏn-Ŏ-skō-pē, p. 423)
culture (p. 405)
cystoscopy (sĭst-Ŏ-skō-pē, p. 424)
electroencephalogram (EEG) (ē-LĔK-trō-ĕn-SĔ-fă-lō-grăm, p. 425)
endoscope (ĔN-dō-skōp, p. 423)
gastroscopy (găs-TRŎ-skō-pē, p. 423)
hematoma (hē-mă-TŌ-mă, p. 422)
jaundice (JĂWN-dĭs, p. 425)
panel (p. 410)
polyps (PŎL-ĭps, p. 423)
smears (p. 425)
transducer (trăns-DŪ-sĕr, p. 418)
venipuncture (VĔN-ĭ-pŭnk-chŭr, p. 407)

Diagnostic tests and procedures provide important information about complex chemical reactions that affect physiologic functioning of the body. Laboratory examinations of blood, urine, and other body fluids and tissues provide accurate information about the function of various organs and physiologic mechanisms. The information is helpful in making or confirming a diagnosis or in evaluating the effectiveness of a treatment. This chapter introduces basic information about common diagnostic tests and procedures. It is necessary to check the instructions from the particular department of the facility in which the test is to be performed for the specifics of patient preparation because this may vary somewhat from facility to facility. Box 24-1 provides terms with definitions specific to diagnostic testing.

APPLICATION of the NURSING PROCESS

Assessment (Data Collection)

When a diagnostic test or procedure is ordered, assess what the patient knows about the test. This will establish what teaching is needed. Inquire about concerns the patient may have about the test. Determine if there

Box 24-1 | *Terminology for Diagnostic Testing*

Angiography: Method of injecting a dye into an artery and obtaining an x-ray of blood vessels, tumors, and lesions

Arteriography: Radiography of an artery or arterial system after injection of a contrast medium into the bloodstream.

Bronchoscopy: Inspection of the interior of the tracheobronchial tree through a bronchoscope.

Cardiac catheterization: Introduction of a catheter into the heart chambers to confirm a diagnosis or to evaluate the extent of the disease process.

Colposcopy: Gynecologic examination that uses the colposcope to examine the walls of the vagina and the cervix.

Complete blood count (CBC): Includes type and number of red blood cells, white blood cells, platelets, and hemoglobin.

Computed tomography scan (CT scan): Through use of a computer, cathode ray tubes emit radiation at different depths to show density of tissues and organs, indicating malformations, tumors, and so on. Also called *computed axial tomography (CAT) scan.*

Conization: Coring or removal of the mucous lining of the cervical canal and its glands by means of cutting with a high-frequency current; performed when a Pap smear indicates abnormal cells.

Cytology: The study of the structure, function, and pathology of cells.

Endoscopic retrograde cholangiopancreatography (ERCP): Examination of the biliary system done through a flexible endoscope and instillation of contrast medium into the ampulla of Vater of the pancreas.

Esophagogastroduodenoscopy (EGD): Endoscopic examination of the esophagus, stomach, and duodenum.

Fluoroscopy: Examination by means of fluoroscope using x-rays displayed on a fluorescent screen.

Glucometer: Small machine used to measure glucose content of capillary blood.

Hematology: Study of blood and its components.

Histology: Branch of anatomy dealing with the structure, composition, and function of tissues.

Intravenous pyelography (IVP): Injection of a dye into a vein to show urine flow through the renal pelvis, ureters, and bladder on x-ray.

KUB x-ray: X-ray of the kidneys, ureters, and bladder.

Lumbar puncture: Insertion of a hollow needle into the subarachnoid space between the third and fourth lumbar vertebrae to withdraw samples of cerebrospinal fluid for analysis and to measure the pressure; also called *spinal puncture* and *spinal tap.*

Magnetic resonance imaging (MRI): Noninvasive method, based on magnetic fields, of visualizing soft tissue without the use of contrast media or ionizing radiation.

Papanicolaou (Pap) smear: A laboratory test to determine cancer, especially cervical, vaginal, or uterine cancer.

Paracentesis: A needle puncture of the abdomen to remove ascites fluid, perform a lavage, or initiate peritoneal dialysis.

Proctosigmoidoscopy: Examination of the rectum and sigmoid colon with a sigmoidoscope.

Radiography: The making of film records of internal structures of the body by exposure of film sensitized to x-rays.

Radioimmunoassay (RIA): Use of radionuclides, following principles of immunology, to measure materials present in blood in minute amounts.

Radionuclides: Radioactive substances that disintegrate with the emission of electromagnetic radiation.

Radiopharmaceutical: A radioactive pharmaceutical substance used for diagnostic or therapeutic purposes.

Sequential multiple assay (SMA): A series of assay tests for a variety of chemical substances performed one after another on one blood or serum sample by a chemical analyzer.

Thoracentesis: Insertion of a needle through the chest wall to the pleural space to drain fluid or air or to instill medication.

Treadmill stress test: A test that measures heart rate and blood pressure response to clinically controlled active exercise on a treadmill (a machine with a moving belt on which one walks while staying in one place).

Ultrasonography: A technique in which deep structures of the body are visualized by recording the reflections (echoes) of ultrasonic waves directed into the tissues.

---

will be any special nursing measures needed to protect the safety of the patient. Assess wounds each shift for signs of infection so that the physician can be alerted to the need for a culture (the growing of microorganisms in or on a medium designed for their growth). Assess the patient for allergies to medication and to iodine and other procedure skin prep solutions used for diagnostic testing.

Nursing Diagnosis

Nursing diagnoses will be those pertinent to the problems for which a diagnostic test or procedure is ordered. "Deficient knowledge" related to the type of diagnostic test is appropriate if the patient is unfamiliar with the test. A few examples of nursing diagnoses for which diagnostic tests might be part of the treatment plan include the following:

- Impaired urinary elimination related to dysuria and foul-smelling urine
- Pain related to raw, sore throat
- Pain related to inflammation and swelling at wound site

Planning

Verify that any items needed for patient preparation for the ordered test are on hand. Check to see that pretest medications have arrived on the unit 1 to 2 hours before the scheduled test time. Plan when to do any teaching

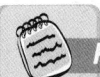

Patient Teaching 24-1

Diagnostic Tests

The following guidelines should be considered when preparing to teach patients about the diagnostic tests they are to undergo. You should also consider the instructions for the specific preparation for the test available from the department performing the test. Teach the patient:

• What the test is for
• What will be experienced during the test
• Whether or not it is necessary to refrain from eating or drinking before the test and for how many hours
• Whether there is special preparation for the test (medications to be taken, special diet, laxatives, enemas, need to drink a lot of water)
• Whether routine medications may be taken before the test
• When the result will probably be available
• Any post-test measures such as drinking more water, taking a laxative, or remaining on bed rest for a certain number of hours
• Whether it is necessary to arrange for someone to drive her home after the test
• About how long the test usually takes
• Any aftereffects of the test or procedure

about the test or procedure. Review information about the procedure to prepare for teaching. Include the pre- and post-test care in your work schedule. A test involving the colon will require the administration of enemas, which can be time consuming. Many diagnostic tests require measuring vital signs frequently when the patient returns to the nursing unit. Expected outcomes are written for the particular nursing diagnosis associated with the problem for which the test is being performed.

Implementation

One of the most important nursing measures is to make certain that the patient has received adequate teaching about the test or procedure to be performed and that concerns have been addressed (Patient Teaching 24-1). Carry out the pre- and post-test actions for the particular test or procedure ordered (Assignment Considerations 24-1). Obtain a signed consent for any invasive procedure requiring one.

Laboratory Tests

Tests can be performed on any body fluid or tissue to detect changes from the normal state. Because blood bathes and nourishes all body tissues and collects waste products to be eliminated, chemical changes in the blood can be signs of disease. Analysis of urine also provides a rich source of information about cellular activity.

Hematology Tests. *Hematology* is the study of blood and its components. The complete blood count (CBC) provides information about the state of health or presence of illness (Table 24-1). Changes in the number,

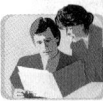

Assignment Considerations 24-1

Post-Test Assessments

Thoughtful consideration should occur before assigning vital sign measurements to UAPs after invasive diagnostic tests. Vital signs are not the only parameters that usually need to be assessed. The patient may need to be monitored for bleeding, neurologic abnormalities, decreases in sensation or function, increasing pain, and general changes in condition. The licensed nurse needs to check the patient personally frequently.

Table 24-1 | *Example of a Complete Blood Count (CBC) (Adult)*

COMPONENT	TEST VALUE	NORMAL RANGE
WBC	6.8 K/μL	4.5-11.0 mm^3
RBC	4.59 M/μL	4.6-5.4 mm^3
Hgb	14.0 g/dL	12.0-18.0 g/dL
HCT	40.8 mL/dL	37.0-54.0 mL/dL
MCV	89.0 μm^3	80.0-96.0 μm^3
MCH	30.6 pg/cell	26.0-34.0 pg/cell
RDW	11.3%	11.4%-16.2%
PLT	252,000/mm^3	150,000-400,000/mm^3
Neutrophil (band)	50%	54%-62%
Lymphocyte	36%	25%-33%
Monocyte	12%	3%-13%
Eosinophil	2%	1%-3%
Basophil	0%	0%-1%
RBC morphology	Normal	Normal

Key: *HCT,* Hematocrit; *Hgb,* hemoglobin; *MCH,* mean corpuscular hemoglobin; *MCV,* mean corpuscular volume; μL, microliter; μm, micrometer; *PLT,* platelets; *RBC,* red blood cell; *RDW,* red cell distribution width; *WBC,* white blood cell.

size, or appearance of red blood cells (erythrocytes) occur in diseases associated with types of anemia. The *hematocrit* refers to the separation of blood and is the amount of blood cells in relation to the amount of plasma. It is decreased in severe anemias (low red blood cell count) and massive blood losses but is higher than normal in dehydration and shock.

During infections, the type and number of white blood cells (*leukocytes*) increase (*leukocytosis*). The neutrophil count, in particular, can be significant. When infection is severe, the bone marrow releases more granulocytes as a compensatory measure. Many young, immature polymorphonuclear neutrophils called "bands" are released into the bloodstream.

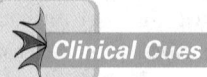

Clinical Cues

Most labs used to report the cells on the differential white blood cell (WBC) count by order of maturity, with the less mature cell forms being on the left side of the report. Therefore, a "shift to the left" in the number of cells, or an increase in bands, may indicate infection.

Certain drugs may cause such a sharp fall in leukocytes (*leukopenia*) that the individual is unable to fight

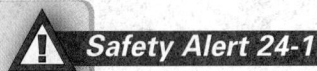

Safety Alert 24-1

Bleeding Danger

Spontaneous bleeding is a serious danger when the platelet count falls below 20,000/mm³ of blood. Observe for bleeding gums, blood in the urine, and oozing from needlesticks.

off infection. Hemoglobin testing shows the capacity of the blood to transport oxygen from the lungs to the tissues. Hemoglobin levels drop when there is bleeding within the body. A normal platelet count is 150 to 400/mm³ of blood. Platelet activity is essential to blood clotting (Safety Alert 24-1).

In addition to the CBC, tests of bleeding and clotting time of the blood may be done. Knowledge about the length of bleeding time is essential before most surgeries or extensive dental extractions are performed. Common tests for clotting time are the prothrombin time (PT) and activated partial thromboplastin time (APTT). The prothrombin time is prolonged in certain diseases of the liver and in certain blood disorders. **Prothrombin time is widely used to adjust dosages of anticoagulant drugs such as sodium warfarin (Coumadin).** This test is reported using International Normalized Ratio (INR) numbers. The partial thromboplastin time is used for monitoring clotting time during heparin therapy.

The erythrocyte sedimentation rate (ESR) measures the rate at which the red blood cells settle out of unclotted blood in 1 hour. Inflammatory conditions cause the cells to settle more rapidly. The more rapid the settling, the higher the ESR.

Think Critically About . . . The patient's hemoglobin when she was admitted was 13.8 g/dL. Two days later it is 13.2 g/dL. Is this significant? What could it mean?

Blood Chemistry Tests. Chemical laboratory tests are performed on whole blood, plasma, serum, and other body fluids such as urine, spinal fluid, and gastric contents. Blood chemistries are commonly obtained to detect changes in biochemical reactions in the body and to determine a diagnosis. They provide information about the electrolyte balance, the ability of the body to metabolize nutrients, the function of organs, and the presence or accumulation of toxic substances. Most laboratory forms list the normal values for each test with the results of the test.

Food and drink are usually withheld for 8 to 12 hours prior to blood chemistry tests. The blood specimen for a complete blood count, chemistry, or serology test is obtained by venipuncture (puncture of the vein with a needle). Hemoglobin may be determined from a fingerstick for capillary blood. **Gloves must be worn and Standard Precautions are required, as are steps to prevent continued bleeding from the puncture site.** The blood specimens are collected in tubes with color-coded stoppers, which indicate the type of anticoagulant, if any, the tubes contain (Skill 24-1).

Skill 24-1 | Phlebotomy and Obtaining Blood Samples with a Vacutainer System

Blood tests are the most commonly ordered diagnostic procedure. **Every time a venipuncture is performed for blood sampling, two patient identifiers must be used to verify that the procedure is being performed on the correct patient. The room number cannot be one of the identifiers. Patient name and patient number or birth date are valid identifiers.** When there is not a laboratory with a phlebotomist on the premises, the nurse is usually responsible for obtaining the needed blood samples. The Vacutainer system is the most common method used to obtain blood samples. Blood can be drawn using a syringe and needle with the same venipuncture technique. The correct tube, indicated by the color of its top, must be used for the test ordered.

■ Supplies

✓ Tube labels
✓ Pen
✓ Tape
✓ Latex gloves
✓ Vacutainer tubes

✓ Vacutainer holder
✓ Vacutainer needle with needle guard
✓ Towel, paper towel, or underpad
✓ Tourniquet
✓ Alcohol swabs

✓ 2 × 2 Gauze squares
✓ Bandage
✓ Cotton balls
✓ Biohazard sharps container
✓ Biohazard plastic bag
✓ Requisition slip

Review and carry out the Standard Steps in Appendix 3.

■ Assessment (Data Collection)

1. **ACTION** Check the physician's order for tests to be done.

RATIONALE Determines type of tube to be used.

2. **ACTION** Ask the patient's name or check the wristband.

Continued

Skill 24-1 | Phlebotomy and Obtaining Blood Samples with a Vacutainer System—cont'd

RATIONALE Verifies that the right patient will have blood drawn.

■ Planning

3. *ACTION* Check to see that the needed tubes and materials are on hand.

   RATIONALE Prevents having to stop and obtain supplies.

■ Implementation

4. *ACTION* Fill out a label for each tube.

   RATIONALE Ensures that tubes will be correctly labeled.

5. *ACTION* Explain the procedure to the patient and have her sit with the arm on a table or lie down with the arm stretched out at the side.

   RATIONALE Explaining procedure decreases fear of the unknown. Positioning provides stable access to the venipuncture site.

6. *ACTION* Perform hand hygiene and put on latex gloves.

   RATIONALE Reduces transfer of microorganisms.

7. *ACTION* Select an appropriate venipuncture site, avoiding scars, lesions, or a vessel in which IV fluids are infusing.

   RATIONALE Scar tissue is difficult to puncture; a puncture over a lesion may introduce microorganisms into the blood; IV fluids may alter the test results.

8. *ACTION* Place the Vacutainer tube inside the holder, but do not push it onto the needle; position the Vacutainer holder and tubes within easy reach.

   RATIONALE Preparing the system for use allows you to pick up the equipment with one hand after you have stabilized the vessel.

9. *ACTION* Lower the extremity so the site is below the heart.

   RATIONALE A dependent position enhances blood flow to the site.

10. *ACTION* Apply a tourniquet to the extremity 2 to 4 inches above the venipuncture site. It should be moderately tight. Ask the patient to make a fist (unless a potassium level specimen is being drawn).

    RATIONALE The tourniquet obstructs blood flow out of the vessel and causes the vein to fill with blood. A distended vein is easier to palpate and puncture. Making a fist aids in vein distention, but will elevate the reading for potassium by forcing potassium out of cells.

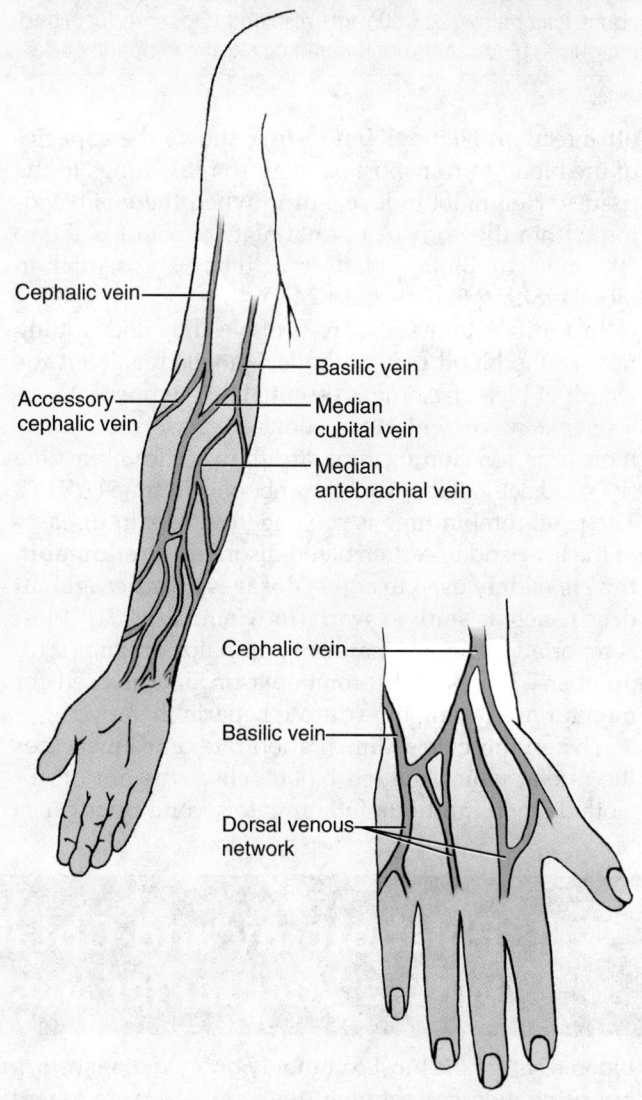

Cephalic vein
Basilic vein
Accessory cephalic vein
Median cubital vein
Median antebrachial vein
Cephalic vein
Basilic vein
Dorsal venous network

Step **7**

11. *ACTION* Cleanse the site with 70% alcohol in a circular motion outward; allow the area to dry.

    RATIONALE Alcohol decreases the number of microorganisms on the skin, preventing their transfer to the blood.

12. *ACTION* Pick up the Vacutainer holder and tube in your dominant hand and remove the needle cover.

    RATIONALE Prepares the unit for venipuncture.

13. *ACTION* Anchor the vein with the thumb of your nondominant hand far enough below the site so that the needle will not touch the thumb as it enters the vessel.

    RATIONALE Stabilizes the vein so that it does not roll when venipuncture is performed.

14. **ACTION** Hold the Vacutainer unit with the needle bevel facing up and position it at a 30-degree angle over the desired venipuncture site.

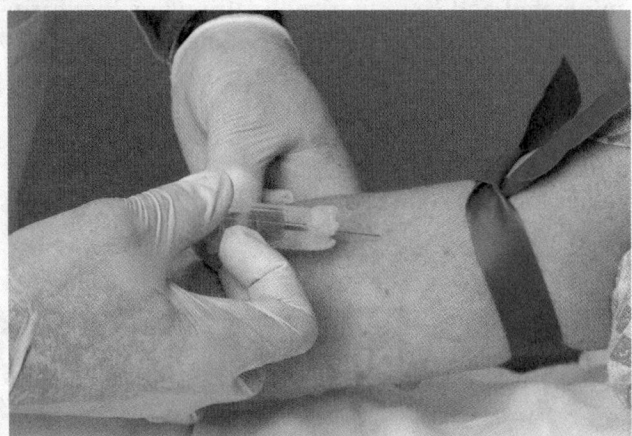

Step **14**

RATIONALE Positions needle for entry into the vessel.

15. **ACTION** Puncture the site, and, while stabilizing the Vacutainer unit, press the tube stopper onto the needle; blood running into the tube indicates successful venipuncture.

RATIONALE Stabilizing the unit prevents pushing the needle through the vein when pressing the tube stopper onto the Vacutainer needle.

16. **ACTION** Allow the tube to fill completely.

RATIONALE Ensures a sufficient quantity of blood to perform the test.

17. **ACTION** If further specimens are needed, stabilize holder and remove filled tube and set safely aside. Place next tube carefully on needle and allow to fill. Repeat until all required tubes are filled. Remove final tube.

RATIONALE Obtains sufficient blood for all ordered tests. Stabilized holder prevents pushing needle through vessel wall. Removing last tube before removing needle prevents introducing air into the tube.

18. **ACTION** Loosen the tourniquet, and withdraw the needle from the vein and secure the needle guard.

RATIONALE Loosening the tourniquet before withdrawing the needle will decrease the amount of bleeding that occurs.

19. **ACTION** Immediately apply a dry gauze pad with pressure to the vein to stop the bleeding.

RATIONALE A dry pad aids coagulation of the blood, and pressure constricts the vessel, decreasing bleeding.

20. **ACTION** Apply a small adhesive bandage over the puncture site.

RATIONALE Decreases entrance of microorganisms at the site and helps prevent further bleeding.

21. **ACTION** Carefully remove and dispose of the Vacutainer needle in a biohazard sharps container.

RATIONALE Prevents accidental needlesticks.

22. **ACTION** Remove and label the tube(s) of blood, and place in a biohazard bag.

RATIONALE Labeling the tube(s) correctly identifies the patient's blood. A biohazard bag prevents blood contamination should the tube(s) become broken.

23. **ACTION** Fill out the laboratory requisition slip, and attach it to the blood samples; send it to the laboratory.

RATIONALE Identifies the correct test to be done for the right patient.

24. **ACTION** Remove gloves and perform hand hygiene.

RATIONALE Reduces transfer of microorganisms and removes powder from hands.

■ Evaluation

25. **ACTION** Check to be certain the correct tubes were used and all the samples have been obtained with adequate blood in each tube.

RATIONALE Ensures that patient will not have to return for another venipuncture.

■ Documentation

26. **ACTION** Note the procedure and samples obtained on the patient's medical record; include how they were sent to the laboratory.

RATIONALE Verifies that the ordered blood samples were drawn and sent to the laboratory.

Documentation Example

1/8 0700 Successful venipuncture; 3 tubes drawn and sent to lab for CBC, SMA-12, and VDRL. No hematoma at site; bleeding stopped and bandage applied. Patient tolerated procedure without problems.

_____
(Nurse's signature)

?CRITICAL THINKING QUESTIONS

1. An elderly woman tells you technicians and nurses always have difficulty drawing her blood samples because she has tiny veins. What would you do to ensure a successful venipuncture?

2. If you have done three "sticks" on a patient for blood samples and have not been successful, what would you do?

Blood glucose tests are essential in the diagnosis and control of diabetes. Testing the amount of blood glucose can be done outside the laboratory using capillary blood from a fingerstick, test strips, and a machine called a glucometer (Skill 24-2). The tests of bilirubin, alanine aminotransferase (ALT), and alkaline phosphatase (ALP) are used to measure liver function. Blood urea nitrogen (BUN) and creatinine levels are important indicators of kidney dysfunction. Damage to striated and heart muscle can be detected by testing for blood levels of lactate dehydrogenase (LDH), creatine kinase (CK), and aspartate aminotransferase (AST). Other tests are used to determine toxic levels of substances such as barbiturates, lead, arsenic, and medications. **Most laboratories are equipped with automated and computerized instruments that carry out multiple tests on a single specimen.** One model is the sequential multiple assay (SMA, SMAC) unit, which can be programmed to run a battery of screening tests on one blood sample. Table 24-2 shows a typical SMA-12 panel (group of tests) with normal values for each component.

Skill 24-2 | Performing a Capillary Blood Test: Blood Glucose or Hemoglobin

Random blood sugar tests are performed for known diabetic patients and for patients who are showing signs and symptoms of hyperglycemia or hypoglycemia. A quick screening test for anemia is done by measuring hemoglobin. Both of these tests are done with capillary blood taken from a fingertip and are frequently done by the nurse in the physician's office or clinic.

■ Supplies
✓ Gloves
✓ Cotton ball
✓ Fingerstick device holder
✓ Bandage

✓ Lancet
✓ Alcohol swabs

For Random Blood Sugar
✓ Glucometer (Accu-Chek)
✓ Glucometer strips

For Hemoglobin Test
✓ Hemoglobin capillary flow collector
✓ Clean gauze pad
✓ HemoCue machine

Review and carry out the Standard Steps in Appendix 3.

■ Assessment (Data Collection)

1. *ACTION* Gather equipment and assess whether all supplies are on hand.

   RATIONALE Prevents having to stop procedure to fetch needed items.

2. *ACTION* Identify the patient and determine what is known about the procedure.

   RATIONALE Identifies what information needs to be given to patient.

■ Planning

3. *ACTION* Plan which finger to use and ask patient to allow hand to hang downward. If hand is cold, have patient warm it under running warm water, or warm it with your hands.

   RATIONALE Holding hand down and warming it brings blood to the fingertips.

■ Implementation

4. *ACTION* Perform hand hygiene and put on gloves. Cleanse the chosen fingertip thoroughly with an alcohol swab. Ask the patient to hold the finger separated from the others and not to touch anything as the alcohol dries.

   RATIONALE Removes bacteria from the finger, preparing it for the puncture. Alcohol will dry while machine is set up, saving time.

A: For Blood Glucose Test

5. *ACTION* Turn on the machine, place the lancet in the holder, and remove the lancet cover. Cock the lancet device. Check the control number that appears on the screen with the control number on the bottle of test strips.

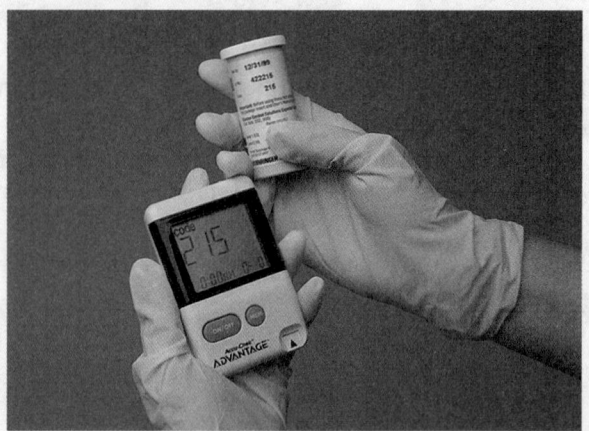

Step **5**

RATIONALE Prepares the equipment to puncture the skin. Checking control number ensures that the correct setting is used for the machine because it must match the strip number.

6. *ACTION* Remove a test strip from the bottle and insert the end with the metal strips into the machine. (For machines that have intervening steps, check the manufacturer's directions. Some machines require that the specimen be obtained and a certain time period elapse before the strip is placed in the machine.)

RATIONALE Prepares the machine to read the amount of glucose in the blood.

7. *ACTION* Place the fingerstick device firmly on the skin and push the release button, causing the lancet to pierce the skin.

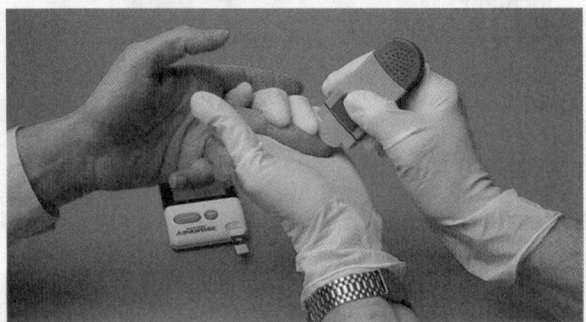
Step 7

RATIONALE With the device at a right angle to the fingerprint lines, the needle should pierce the skin deeply enough to provide free blood flow with little pressure.

8. *ACTION* If machine directions indicate need, wipe away the first drop of blood with a clean cotton ball.

RATIONALE First drop often contains a large portion of serous fluid that dilutes the specimen, causing false result.

9. *ACTION* Lightly squeeze the finger, gently milking down the finger toward the tip until a large drop of blood has formed on the tip.

RATIONALE Provides an adequate amount of blood for the specimen.

10. *ACTION* Lightly apply the drop of blood to the pad on the test strip and apply a clean cotton ball to the puncture wound with pressure. Ask patient to hold the cotton ball tightly in place.

RATIONALE Applying blood to test strip begins the test. Pad must be completely covered with blood for accurate result. Pressure and dry cotton ball stop bleeding.

11. *ACTION* For alternate type of glucometer, start the timer and place the test strip on a paper towel beside the timer. At 60 seconds, place the test strip into the machine. See the manufacturer's directions.

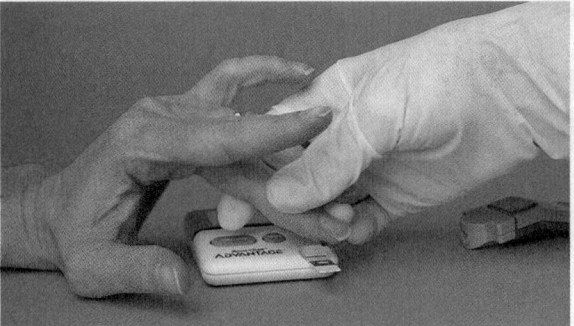
Step 10

RATIONALE Some machines require different procedures for an accurate result.

■ Evaluation: Blood Glucose Test

12. *ACTION* Note the reading on the screen of the machine and record it. Turn the machine off. Share the result with the patient.

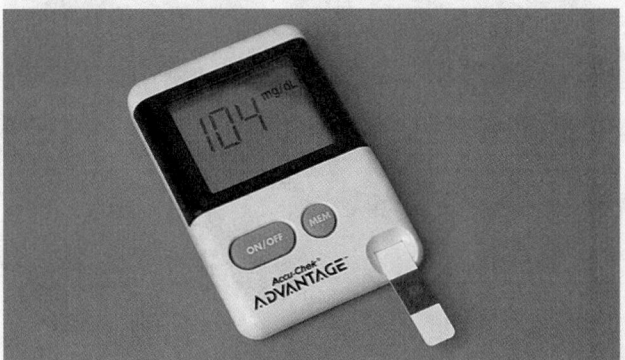
Step 12

RATIONALE Machine will provide a reading. If "error" appears, turn off the machine and start the procedure over from the beginning. Too much or too little blood on the test strip may cause an error. It is necessary for the patient to know the reading in order to participate in care.

13. *ACTION* Assess whether the patient's finger is still bleeding. Stop the bleeding and apply an adhesive bandage if patient desires one.

RATIONALE Prevents blood continuing to flow; prevents transmission of possible blood-borne pathogens.

14. *ACTION* Dispose of the test strip, lancet, and blood-tinged supplies in the appropriate hazardous materials waste receptacles. Remove the gloves and perform hand hygiene.

RATIONALE Prevents the transmission of blood-borne pathogens.

15. *ACTION* Document the procedure and the reading on the patient's medical record. In the inpatient facility, record the reading on the appropriate flow sheets.

Continued

Skill 24-2 | Performing a Capillary Blood Test: Blood Glucose or Hemoglobin—cont'd

RATIONALE Provides a record of the reading; patients on insulin have a place on the medication administration record (MAR) for the recording of the blood glucose reading.

B: For Hemoglobin Test

After Step 4:

5. **ACTION** Perform the fingerstick as in Step 7 for *Blood Glucose Test*. Wipe away the first drop of blood and obtain a large drop of blood. Hold the capillary collection device with the point in the drop of blood to draw up the blood.

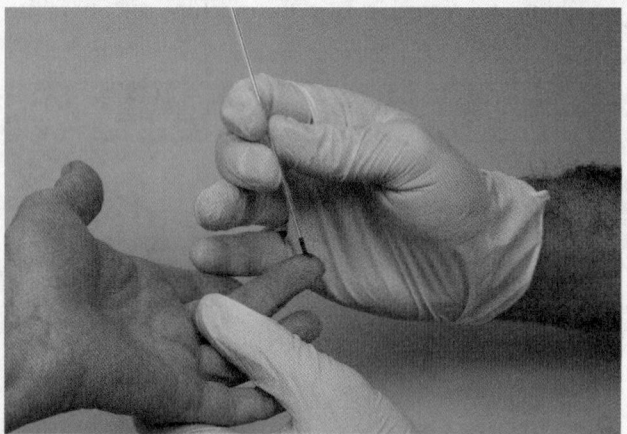

Step **5**

RATIONALE Blood will flow into the test stick.

6. **ACTION** Gently wipe the flat back side of the test stick on the clean gauze pad.

   RATIONALE Removes excess blood.

7. **ACTION** Place a clean cotton ball tightly against the puncture wound.

   RATIONALE Stops the bleeding.

8. **ACTION** Remove used supplies from the area. Turn on the hemoglobin machine and place the test stick into the proper slot according to the manufacturer's directions.

   RATIONALE Disposes of used supplies. Prepares machine to take the reading.

9. **ACTION** Note the reading and write it down.

   RATIONALE Obtains the result and prevents forgetting the number read.

10. **ACTION** Turn off the machine and dispose of the used capillary blood stick in the sharps container. Remove the gloves and perform hand hygiene.

RATIONALE Reduces chance of transfer of blood-borne pathogens.

11. **ACTION** Share the result with the patient; apply an adhesive bandage to the puncture wound if desired.

    RATIONALE Sharing result keeps patient informed. Bandaging prevents further bleeding and protects wound.

■ Evaluation: Hemoglobin Test

12. **ACTION** Determine if hemoglobin level is within normal range.

    RATIONALE Teaching may be needed regarding iron-rich foods and/or iron medication if level is low.

■ Documentation

Documentation Example

1/6 1030   Capillary Hgb 11.8 g/dL.

_____

(Nurse's signature)

■ Special Considerations

✓ Warming the hand before attempting the fingerstick provides a greater chance of a successful specimen on the first attempt.

✓ Small children will need to be held by the parent or another nurse.

✓ Children should be told that it will "be a tiny sting" and that they will see blood. Do not lie to the child.

✓ Having children use a finger puppet on the other hand sometimes will distract them sufficiently from the procedure that they will hold still.

✓ The elderly bleed more easily than younger persons and may not need as deep a puncture.

✓ The puncture depth of the lancet needle can be adjusted by pushing the lancet further in or pulling it out a little from the holder.

This procedure should never be performed without the use of gloves due to the risk of contamination with blood.

?CRITICAL THINKING QUESTIONS

1. If you get an error message when performing a fingerstick for blood glucose, what would you do?

2. If the result of the fingerstick Hgb on a pregnant patient is 10.6 g/dL, is this a normal value? (You may need to consult an obstetric nursing text or a laboratory manual for the answer.)

Table 24-2 | *Sequential Multiple Assay (SMA) Panel (SMA-12)*

TESTS INCLUDED	NORMAL RANGE*
Albumin	3.5-5.2 g/dL
Alkaline phosphatase (ALT)	35-150 Units/L
Aspartate aminotransferase (AST)	1-36 Units/L
Bilirubin, total	8.4-10.4 mg/dL
Calcium, serum	8.4-10.6 mg/dL
Cholesterol	60-180 mg/dL
Glucose	70-100 mg/dL
Lactate dehydrogenase (LDH)	110-220 Units/L
Phosphate	3.0-4.5 mg/dL
Total protein	6.0-8.0 g/dL
Urea nitrogen (BUN)	11-23 mg/dL
Uric acid	2.2-8.0 mg/dL

*Normal range may vary among laboratories depending on the type of test performed and the reagents used. (The SMA-6, SMA-7, and SMA-20 are different panels containing tests for 6, 7, and 20 substances.)

Think Critically About . . . The patient was admitted with malaise and fever. The ESR was 27 mm/hr upon admission. Today it is 34 mm/hr. What does this indicate?

Serology Tests. Serology tests are based on the analysis of blood serum. They are important in diagnosing many diseases stemming from bacterial and viral infections. Diseases such as dysentery, rheumatic fever, typhoid, influenza, rubella, and syphilis produce positive reactions related to antigen antibodies. Radioimmunoassays, which are based on principles of immunity, use radionuclides (radioactive material; formerly called radioisotopes), such as iodine-125 and iodine-131, to detect minute particles of protein in the blood. Blood typing and identification of blood factors may also be carried out in the serology section of the laboratory. Examples of common serology tests are listed in Box 24-2. Most serology tests can be done without restricting the patient's food or fluid intake. However, some of the radioimmunoassays may require the administration of the radionuclide drug at a certain time before drawing blood for the test. For viral infections, two separate specimens are needed to show a rise in titer during the illness.

Urinalysis. Analysis of urine provides valuable information about the function of the kidneys and other biologic processes within the body. Organic compounds found in the urine include urea, uric acid, creatinine, and hippuric acid. Inorganic substances found are sodium, chloride, phosphate, potassium, and ammonia. Urine composition varies according to fluid intake and diet; therefore, the time the specimen is obtained may influence the results.

Box 24-2 | *Examples of Serology Tests*

There are many different types of serology tests that may be ordered. Common examples are
- Agglutination tests for specific organisms
- Antistreptolysin-O titer
- Blood typing: ABO groups and Rh
- Carcinoembryonic antigen (CEA) assay
- Coombs' test
- C-reactive protein antiserum
- Heterophil antibody titer
- Immunoelectrophoresis
- Immunoglobulin (Ig) types: IgG, IgA, IgM, IgE, and IgD
- Radioimmunoassays
- Tests for syphilis
  - *Treponema pallidum*–microhemagglutination (TP-MHA)
  - Venereal Disease Research Laboratory (VDRL)
  - Fluorescent treponemal antibody (FTA)
- Enzyme-linked immunosorbent assay (ELISA) antibody test for human immunodeficiency virus (HIV)
- Western blot

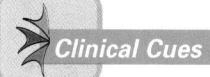 **Clinical Cues**

Urine deteriorates quite rapidly, so specimens should be analyzed soon after collection. Send the specimen to the laboratory quickly or refrigerate it.

Urine specimens can be classified as
- Single, catheterized, or random specimens that can be collected at any time, with no special preparation required (a specimen of the first voiding in the morning is preferred because it is more concentrated)
- Midstream specimens, in which the external genitalia are cleansed, a small amount of urine is passed, and then a midportion of the voiding is collected in a sterile container and used for a culture. The procedure for obtaining a midstream specimen is located in Chapter 29.
- Timed, long-period specimens, in which all urine is collected over a 12- or 24-hour period and placed in a container containing some type of preservative.

Generally, no special instructions are required for the single, random specimen. Often a urine dipstick test is performed to screen the specimen for abnormalities. Urine dips are performed using test strips or sticks that have various chemicals impregnated in them (Skill 24-3). Patient Teaching 29-1 in Chapter 29 provides instructions for the midstream specimen. The method for obtaining a specimen from an indwelling urinary catheter is listed in Steps 29-1 in Chapter 29. A laboratory manual must be consulted for instructions on carrying out special types of urine tests. Some tests require restriction of fluid intake; others require that

Skill 24-3 Performing a Urine Dipstick Test

Urine dipsticks are manufactured to test for several substances in the urine. They provide a quick and easy way to screen for abnormalities in the urine in the physician's office, at home, in the clinic, in the long-term care facility, or on the hospital nursing unit. A random or mid-stream urine specimen is used for the test.

■ Supplies

✓ Multistix for urine testing ✓ Timer/watch
✓ Gloves ✓ Urine specimen

Review and carry out the Standard Steps in Appendix 3.

■ Assessment (Data Collection)

1. **ACTION** Assess whether patient can produce urine specimen.

   RATIONALE If patient has recently emptied the bladder, it may be necessary for her to drink some water and wait a while before producing specimen.

■ Planning

2. **ACTION** Determine that Multistix and gloves are on hand.

   RATIONALE Prevents hunting for supplies when ready to test specimen.

■ Implementation

3. **ACTION** Fill in a lab report form with the patient's name, physician's name, date, and your initials.

   RATIONALE Sheet is ready for recording of the test results.

4. **ACTION** Obtain the specimen, put on gloves, and wet the dipstick with urine, making certain that each colored square is moistened. Remove the stick from the urine quickly and gently tap it on the side of the container to remove excess urine.

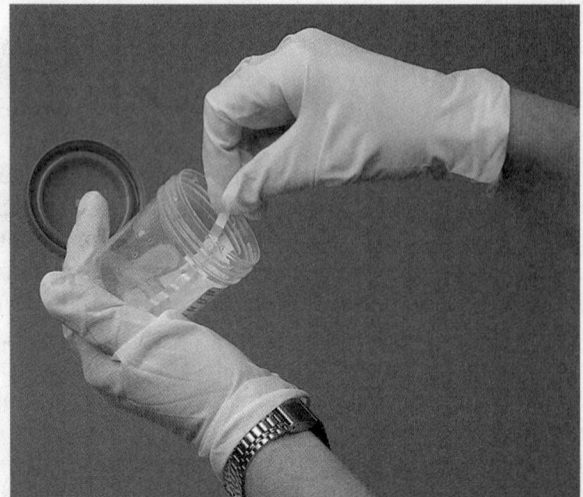

Step **4**

RATIONALE The stick can be dipped into the urine or a small amount of urine can be poured down the stick while holding it over the toilet or a work-room sink.

5. **ACTION** Start timing the tests immediately after wetting the stick.

   RATIONALE Exact timing is necessary for accuracy of the test results. Some portions of the test require 30 seconds before reading; others are read at 40 seconds, 45 seconds, or 60 seconds.

■ Evaluation

6. **ACTION** Hold the stick horizontally and compare the color chart on the side of the Multistix bottle with the color on the strip at the correct time interval.

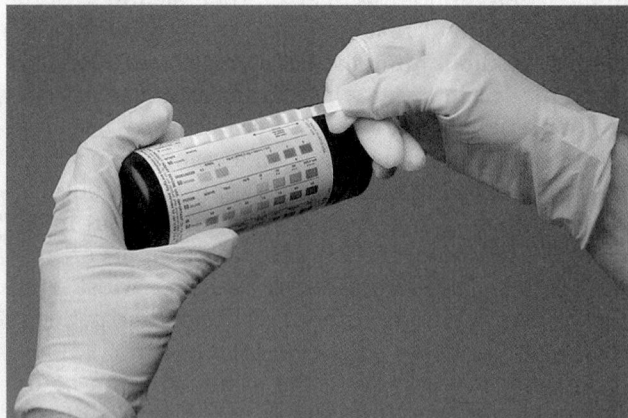

Step **6**

RATIONALE Allows for close comparison of the colors for each square on the stick with the color chart on the bottle.

7. **ACTION** Write down the result for each component of the test on the lab report form.

   RATIONALE Records the test results.

8. **ACTION** Dispose of urine, container, and used Multistix correctly in biohazard waste receptacle. Remove gloves and perform hand hygiene.

   RATIONALE Reduces transfer of microorganisms.

9. *ACTION* Share results with patient or give the report to the physician.

RATIONALE Participation of patient in testing and care improves understanding of treatment. Documentation is the completed laboratory slip.

■ Special Considerations

✓ Certain medications and vitamins may discolor the urine and interfere with accurate reading of the test results.

✓ Urine specimens must be tested while they are fresh for the result to be accurate.

Patient Teaching 24-2

Collection of a 24-Hour Urine Specimen

Give the patient a 24-hour urine collection container. Provide the following instructions:

* Empty the bladder into the toilet and begin timing the collection of the specimen.
* For the next 24 hours, add all urine to the collection container.
* Keep the container on ice or refrigerated if instructed to do so (depends on the laboratory and the type of test ordered).
* At the time the 24 hours is up, empty the bladder and add the urine to the collection container.
* Seal the collection container and return it to the laboratory or the physician's office as directed.

set amounts of fluids be given and urine specimens be obtained at specified times (Patient Teaching 24-2). A normal urinalysis is presented in Table 24-3.

Other Laboratory Tests. Among the other laboratory tests performed are bacteriology, histology, and cytology tests. Specimens of blood, urine, feces, and wound drainage, and samples of other body fluids or tissues, may be cultured to identify the disease-causing organism. To obtain a stool specimen, ask the patient to catch some stool in a container suspended in the toilet bowl, in a bedpan, or in plastic wrap draped on the rim of the toilet bowl. A small amount of stool is transferred to the appropriate container for a culture or a test for ova and parasites (O & P), or onto cards for the occult blood test (Skill 24-4). Aseptic technique must be maintained when collecting specimens for culture and sensitivity. In sensitivity tests, the identified organism is subjected to various antibiotic drugs to see which ones are most effective in killing it. With new culture media that contain chromogens that interact with bacterial and fungal enzymes, organisms can be identified after only 24 hours of incubation.

Histology and cytology tests involve the study of tissues and cells. Confirmation of a diagnosis often depends on viewing tissues under a microscope to see the effects of the disease. Organs and tissues removed

✓ If the patient produces the specimen at home, ask that it be refrigerated until it can be brought in for testing.

?CRITICAL THINKING QUESTIONS

1. If some of the test strip squares turn an odd color after exposure to urine, what would you do?
2. If a patient's specimen was obtained 2 hours ago and brought to the office, will the test results of a urine dip be accurate?

Table 24-3 | *Normal Urinalysis*

CHARACTERISTIC	NORMAL VALUE
Color	Yellow, straw, dark yellow, amber
Character	Clear
Specific gravity (sp gr)	1.010-1.030
Acetone, ketones	Negative
Glucose (gluc)	Negative
Protein (Alb)	Negative
Nitrite	Negative
Occult blood	Negative
pH	4.6-8.0
Odor	Faint (not fruity, musty, fishy, or fetid)
Urobilinogen	Negative or 0.1-1 Ehrlich Units/dL
Cells	
Erythrocytes	2 or fewer per high-power field
Leukocytes	4 or fewer per high-power field
Casts	None
Crystals	Small amount
Bacteria or fungi	None
Parasites	None
Epithelium	10 or fewer cells per high-power field

at biopsy (surgical excision of a small amount of tissue) are studied closely and a pathology report is prepared. Studies of tissues and cells are performed to detect carcinogenic, metabolic, vascular, and other changes.

A variety of procedures may be used to obtain specimens for bacteriologic or cytologic examinations. Venipuncture and bone marrow aspiration (withdrawal of fluid or cells) yield specimens for culture or cytologic studies; urine specimens can be obtained from catheters and by clean-catch procedures. Lumbar puncture is used to obtain spinal fluid for culture. Standard Precautions must be employed and aseptic technique followed to guard against infection or contamination of specimens.

Ultrasonography

Ultrasonography (sonography) is a noninvasive method of visualizing soft tissue structures of the body. **The sonogram is a recording of the reflection of the ultrasonic waves directed into the tissues.** The procedure is used to diagnose many pathologic

Skill 24-4 | Obtaining a Stool Specimen for Occult Blood, Culture, or Ova and Parasites

Nurses frequently need to obtain a stool specimen from a patient and test it for occult blood. Specimens may also be sent for culture or for tests for ova and parasites or other substances. Stool for ova and parasites must be sent to the laboratory immediately. In some states, stool testing is only permitted in the laboratory.

■ Supplies

✓ "Hat" collection container to place in the toilet
✓ Bedpan
✓ Toilet tissue

✓ Gloves
✓ Container with culture preservative
✓ Sterile swab(s)
✓ Specimen container for ova and parasites

✓ Test cards for stool for occult blood
✓ Wooden sticks
✓ Tongue blades

Review and carry out the Standard Steps in Appendix 3.

■ Assessment (Data Collection)

1. *ACTION* Determine if patient understands why specimen is needed.

   RATIONALE Understanding helps patient accept need for specimen.

2. *ACTION* Determine if patient will need to use a bedpan or can use the toilet to deposit the specimen.

   RATIONALE Identifies equipment needed.

■ Planning

3. *ACTION* Determine when patient usually has a bowel movement.

   RATIONALE Allows nurse to be available to collect the specimen.

4. *ACTION* Instruct patient about need for stool specimen.

   RATIONALE Understanding makes patient more cooperative.

■ Implementation

5. *ACTION* Place collection container by toilet or position patient on bedpan. Ask patient to use call button when specimen is ready.

   RATIONALE Container will be at hand when needed. Alerts nurse to collect specimen.

6. *ACTION* Instruct patient to void and use tissue before placing stool collection container in toilet to catch stool specimen; or clean and replace bedpan after voiding.

   RATIONALE Stool specimen should be free of urine or tissue.

7. *ACTION* Assist patient with cleansing of rectal area as needed. Assist to perform hand hygiene.

   RATIONALE Keeps patient clean and prevents spread of microorganisms.

8. *ACTION* Perform hand hygiene and put on gloves.

   RATIONALE Protects hands from fecal contamination.

9. *ACTION* Take specimen in covered bedpan to bathroom or utility room if bedpan was used.

   RATIONALE Provides private area in which to transfer the specimen to the lab container or onto the stool cards.

Stool Culture

10. *ACTION* Open specimen jar containing culture medium, placing lid upside down on counter. Withdraw sterile swab from culture tube or package and place it into stool to obtain stool sample the size of a bean. Place stool into the stool culture container with the culture medium. Taking care not to contaminate the inside of the jar lid, replace it on the container.

    RATIONALE Placing lid upside down prevents contamination of the lid. Prepares stool for laboratory culture.

Test for Ova and Parasites

11. *ACTION* Using wooden tongue blades, transfer a portion (1 inch or 2.5 cm) from the middle of the stool to the container for the ova and parasite specimen. If the stool is liquid, transfer about 15 mL of liquid stool to the container.

    RATIONALE Readies the specimen for the lab.

12. *ACTION* Send to the laboratory immediately with a filled-out requisition slip. Be certain specimen container is properly labeled with the patient's name, date, and room number, and physician's name.

    RATIONALE Identifies specimen as belonging to the patient; routes laboratory result to the correct physician.

Test for Occult Blood

13. ACTION Open the front window(s) of the specimen card.

RATIONALE Readies the card for receipt of the specimen.

14. ACTION With wooden stick, obtain a small amount of stool from the middle, interior portion of the specimen. Smear it on the area within the window of the stool card. Repeat if more than one window is to be filled for the test.

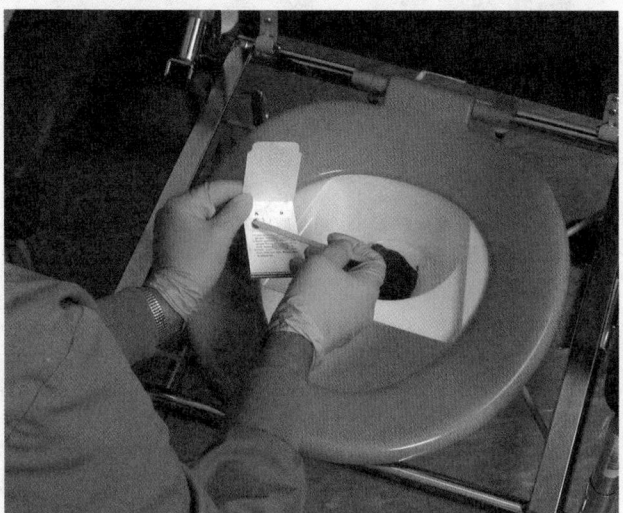

Step **14**

RATIONALE Places specimen within the testing area of the card. Only a very small amount of stool is required.

15. ACTION Open occult blood specimen card back window.

RATIONALE Provides access to the specimen for testing.

16. ACTION Place two drops of the occult blood specimen reagent on the stool smear and one drop on the control; repeat for each window on the card. (Check test instructions for number of drops of the reagent; some test instructions differ.)

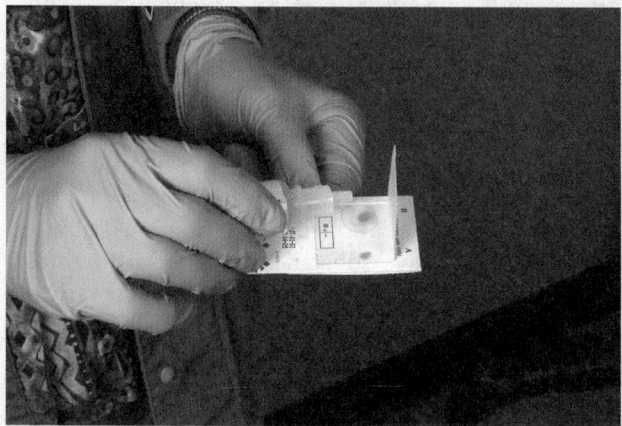

Step **16**

RATIONALE Begins the test.

17. ACTION Wait 30 seconds. Read the test, looking for blue discoloration in or around the stool smear. Check that the control turned blue.

RATIONALE Blue color within 30 seconds indicates that blood is present in the stool. Careful timing is essential to accuracy of the test.

18. ACTION Dispose of the test card in a biohazard waste container. Cleanse the bedpan or "hat" stool collection container. Remove gloves and perform hand hygiene.

RATIONALE Reduces transfer of microorganisms.

■ Evaluation

19. ACTION If test result is positive, be certain that patient adhered to the diet restrictions prior to testing. Ascertain if there were medications taken that could have produced a false-positive test result.

RATIONALE Ensures accuracy of test result.

■ Documentation

20. ACTION Fill in the lab test form with the patient's name, date, physician's name, type of test, and the result, or enter the result in the patient's chart.

RATIONALE Ensures that the test result is recorded.

Documentation Example

1/04 0915   Stool for occult blood negative ×2.

_____

(Nurse's signature)

■ Special Considerations

✓ False-positive and false-negative results for occult blood tests are prevented by the patient following the recommendations for diet and medication cessation for several days prior to the test. See particular test manufacturer's recommendation sheet.

✓ Stool cultures are often done in a series of three on specimens taken from different bowel movements.

❓CRITICAL THINKING QUESTIONS

1. Why do you think a stool specimen for ova and parasites needs to be fresh when it reaches the lab?

2. Why is it contraindicated to take aspirin for 5 days prior to obtaining a stool sample for an occult blood test?

conditions of the female reproductive organs, prostate, heart, kidney, pancreas, gallbladder, lymph nodes, liver, spleen, thyroid, eye, and peripheral blood vessels. It is often used in conjunction with radiography or nuclear medicine scans. The procedure is quick and does not usually produce much discomfort. Sonograms are produced with high-frequency sound waves that pass through the body. Echoes vary with tissue density, and the tracing produced is an echo-reflection map.

Patient preparation depends on the type of sonogram desired. For an abdominal sonogram, the patient is asked to drink a liter of water before the procedure. A gel or lubricant is applied to the skin over the area to be examined. The technician moves the transducer (wand emitting the sound waves) over the area with slight pressure. The echo-reflection pattern is displayed on a monitor, and pictures may be recorded or printed. The test takes approximately 35 to 45 minutes. There is no particular aftercare needed.

Radiology Procedures

X-Rays, Fluoroscopy, and Cineradiography. The radiology department uses radiography, fluoroscopy, and cineradiography to produce data to be used in diagnosis. Different types of radiation are used for diagnosis and treatment of disease: alpha rays, beta rays, gamma rays, and x-rays. The most widely used radiologic diagnostic technique, irradiation by x-ray, produces an image of the denser tissues of the body by passing rays through the part to expose a film. The denser tissues block the x-rays and prevent them from exposing the film; therefore, tissues appear as black, gray, or white images depending on the degree of density. X-rays of the bony skeleton are examples of this process. Radiopaque solutions and materials can be used in various organs to form shadows on the film that show size, location, and structure of less dense tissues (Figure 24-1).

Fluoroscopy is used to examine movement. X-rays are passed through the body part and are projected on a fluorescent screen. The dense tissues produce dark shadows on the film, whereas soft tissues appear whiter. To examine movement through organs or soft tissues, the room is made dark and a radiopaque substance is introduced into the body. For example, to observe movement and structure of the throat, esophagus, and stomach, barium is swallowed. Cineradiography is the method of adding a video camera to the fluoroscope equipment and making a photographic record of the procedure. It produces a videotape; therefore, the results can be viewed and examined in more detail.

The low intensities of diagnostic x-rays make them quite safe to use, because the exposure is of short duration and the rays do not penetrate deeply into the tissues. Higher intensity doses of radiation are harmful to the cells and are used therapeutically to bombard

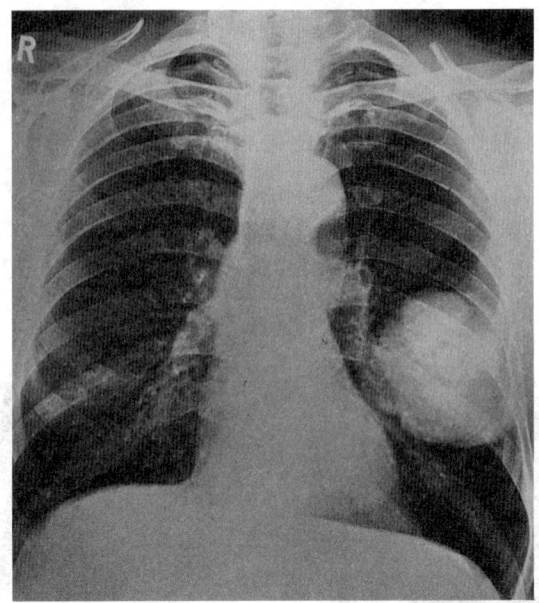

FIGURE **24-1** Chest x-ray showing a tumor.

and kill cancer cells in the body. Commonly performed radiologic procedures include the following:

- Chest x-ray
- Barium swallow and upper gastrointestinal (GI) series
- Barium enema and small bowel series
- Kidneys, ureters, and bladder (KUB) x-ray
- Gallbladder series and cholangiogram
- Intravenous pyelogram (IVP)
- X-rays of the bony skeleton, arthrogram, and myelogram
- Radionuclide scans
- Computed tomography scans (CT, CAT scans)

?Think Critically About . . . The patient asks how a sonogram works; can you explain the process in easy-to-understand terms?

Radionuclide Scans. Radionuclide scans are based on the fact that various organs and soft tissues of the body attract and concentrate certain radionuclides. These studies are carried out in the nuclear medicine department, which is often a division of the radiology department. A radioactive substance is injected into a vein and then, after a period of time to allow the organ being scanned to absorb the substance, a radioactivity scanner (scintillator) is passed over the area where the organ is located. Serial pictures are produced at intervals. The radioactive substance is passed in the urine fairly quickly. The patient is not considered radioactive. Radionuclides are used in scanning the thyroid gland, kidneys, brain, liver, lungs, bones, and pericardium and in determining blood volume. The time required for the scan depends on the organ being scanned (Safety Alert 24-2).

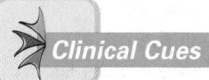

Safety Alert 24-2

Nuclear Scans and Pregnancy

Radionuclide tests are contraindicated for pregnant or nursing women. Always verify whether a woman is pregnant, could be pregnant, or is nursing before sending her for a nuclear scan.

Nursing care involves proper disposal of linens, waste materials, and body secretions that have been made radioactive. The patient is asked to empty the bladder when imaging is complete to reduce radiation exposure time. Assure patients that they are not radioactive or a danger to others in the vicinity.

Computed Tomography. Computed tomography (CT) x-rays of various organs and parts of the body are used to confirm a diagnosis, plan treatment, evaluate the effects of treatment, and guide needle placement in biopsy or aspiration. A computer enhances x-rays and allows examination of horizontal sections of the body at various angles to define tissue density.

Blood flow is assessed with CT angiography. A contrast medium in used for the procedure. The test is used for suspected pulmonary embolism and arteriovenous malformation, to determine patency of coronary arteries, and to detect blood flow patterns to tumors.

Clinical Cues

If a patient who has diabetes is to have a CT scan with an iodine-based contrast medium and is taking a drug containing metformin, the drug must be discontinued before the test and another means used to control blood sugar. Metformin can significantly alter renal function.

Most CT scans are noninvasive, but consent may be required for scans using a contrast medium. The preparation of the patient depends on the organ or part to be examined. The CT scan requires that the patient be in one position for 10 to 45 minutes. The patient is positioned on a table inside the scanner. The scanning machinery revolves around the body part being scanned. Data are fed into the computer, which produces images in shades of gray that indicate the different densities of the organ.

? *Think Critically About . . .* If your patient expresses fear at receiving a radionuclide for a particular diagnostic test, how could you reassure her?

Magnetic Resonance Imaging. Magnetic resonance imaging (MRI) is a noninvasive method of differentiating normal from abnormal tissue in the body. MRI is com-

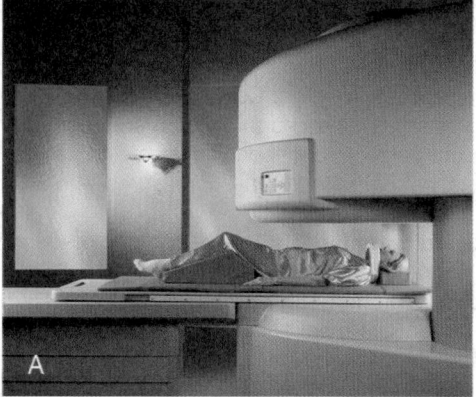

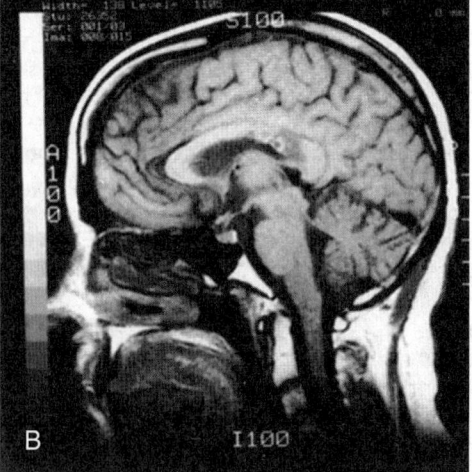

FIGURE **24-2** **A,** Magnetic resonance imaging (MRI) machine. **B,** Midline sagittal view of the brain using MRI.

monly used for the brain, knee joint, spine and spinal cord, and abdominal organs. The patient must lie flat and very still. The patient is placed on a table and then slid inside the large cylinder-shaped machine; the cylinder may be of open or closed design (Figure 24-2). As scanning takes place, loud clicks can be heard. The procedure takes up to 1½ hours. The patient can talk through an intercom system to the MRI staff. This may help relieve feelings of claustrophobia. Patients with metal devices implanted in the body, such as cardiac pacemakers, automatic implantable cardiac defibrillators, metal hip prostheses, artificial cardiac valves, vascular clips, or staples from recent surgery, cannot undergo this procedure because the machine emits a strong magnetic field.

Clinical Cues

For patients undergoing MRI, remove any transdermal medication patch, including a nicotine patch, as the metal backing may cause a burn from this procedure. Inquire about any internal prosthetic device that contains metal. Many patients become very anxious about being placed in an MRI scanner. Obtain an order for sedation, if needed, before the procedure.

| Box 24-3 | *Common Tests and Procedures for the Heart and Lungs*

EXAMINATIONS OF THE HEART

Cardiac catheterization: Complex procedure in which a long catheter is passed through an artery or vein to the heart to obtain information about defects, valves, patency of coronary arteries, pressures, and blood specimens.

Angiocardiography, left: Use of contrast medium to visualize the left side of the heart.

Digital subtraction angiography (DSA): Procedure in which contrast medium is injected into the arteries and the computer performs "digital subtraction" to reveal structures that block clear view of arteries.

Ventriculography, left: Use of contrast medium to define the formation of the left ventricle.

Electrocardiogram (ECG, EKG): Record of the electrical activity of the heart, which normally produces P, Q, R, S, and T waves.

Echocardiogram: Record of the position and motion of the heart produced by ultrasound waves; used to picture structure of the valves.

Electron beam computed tomography (EBCT): Computerized tomography of the heart, a noninvasive procedure, that shows calcified plaque in the coronary arteries.

Master two-step test: ECG made of heart response to the exercise of stepping up and down two steps that are 9 inches high.

Mixed venous oxygen saturation (SvO_2): A pulmonary artery catheter measures the oxygen saturation of venous blood as it returns to the right side of the heart.

Phonocardiogram: Graphic record of heart sounds.

Treadmill test: Test of the heart's response to graded levels of exercise or stress on a treadmill.

Vectorcardiography: Record of the direction and magnitude of the forces of the heart during one heartbeat.

Nuclear cardiography: Process in which radioisotopes are injected intravenously and the radioactive uptake is counted over the heart by a scintillation camera; tests provide information about myocardial contractility, myocardial perfusion, and cellular injury from infarction.

EXAMINATIONS OF PULMONARY FUNCTION

Oximetry: Test that monitors arterial or venous oxygen saturation; venous measurements are noninvasive because probe is attached to fingertip, earlobe, nose, or forehead (venous oxygen saturation); arterial readings are done by pulmonary artery catheter (arterial oxygen saturation).

Bronchospirometry: Method of measuring the air entering and leaving each lung separately; a double-lumen catheter with two balloons is passed into the bronchus under fluoroscopy.

Capnography: Method of monitoring the partial pressure of carbon dioxide in respiratory gases. Assists in detecting beginning hypoxia during anesthesia and in critically ill patients. Shows a pattern on a monitor screen with parameters for normal and abnormal.

Plethysmography: Method of measuring blood flow through the pulmonary capillaries, using an airtight "body box."

Radioactive gas perfusion tests: Use of radioactive tracers given intravenously to measure blood flow through the lungs; radionuclides are given for lung scans.

Spirometer: Instrument that measures the amount of air taken into the lungs and expelled.

Ventilation tests: Measurement of air volume moved in and out of the lungs; includes tidal volume, residual volume, minute respiratory volume, inspiratory reserve volume, expiratory reserve volume, etc.

Describe the machine and procedure to the patient. The underlying concept is one of changing magnetic fields, and information is translated into images of different densities of tissue in the body.

Nursing care involves obtaining consent and making certain that all surface metal (e.g., rings, watch) is removed from the patient's body. Instruct the patient to lie very still during the procedure and to keep the eyes closed to decrease feelings of claustrophobia. Music of the patient's choice may be provided. Teach the patient deep-breathing and rhythmic-breathing relaxation techniques.

? *Think Critically About . . .* The patient scheduled for an abdominal MRI says she doesn't think she can stand to hold still in a restricted position for more than 10 minutes. What would you do?

Cardiopulmonary Studies and Procedures

A battery of tests that range from simple to complex is used to diagnose heart or lung disease (Box 24-3).

Cardiac Studies

Electrocardiogram. The electrocardiogram (ECG, EKG) was one of the first diagnostic tests of heart activity and is still important because it is quick and easy and provides an immediate visual record. **The ECG consists of waves and lines that represent the electrical activity during the cardiac cycle** (Figure 24-3). There are P waves, the QRS complex, and the T wave. Sometimes a U wave is present. The person trained in interpreting the tracing can determine if the waves are normal or abnormal. Nurses in medical offices or clinics often are responsible for obtaining the ECG tracing. Clothing is removed from the upper body in order to apply the electrodes to the skin (Figure 24-4). Female patients are given a gown positioned with the ties in the front. Necklaces, bracelets, and watches are removed because

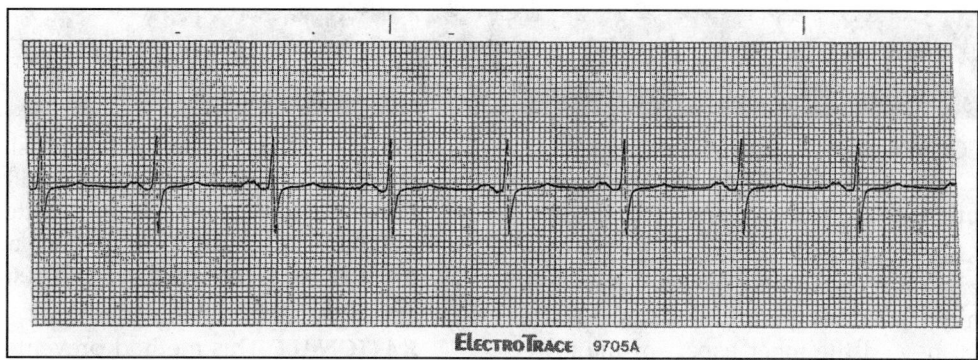

Criteria

1. Rate between 60–100 bpm and regular.
2. P wave precedes each QRS complex; PR interval between 0.12–0.20 second (3–5 small squares).
3. QRS duration between 0.04–0.12 second (1–3 small squares).
4. QRS complexes have essentially the same shape.

FIGURE **24-3** Normal electrocardiogram (ECG) tracing.

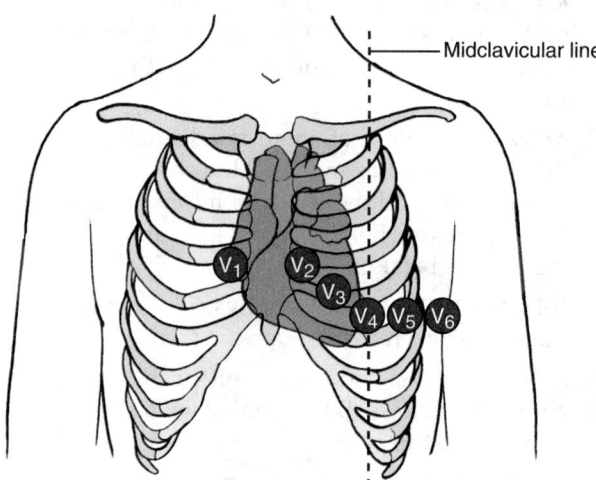

FIGURE **24-4** Positions for placing electrodes.

they sometimes interfere with the electrical tracing (Steps 24-1).

Cardiac Catheterization. Cardiac catheterization is a procedure used to determine the function of the heart, valves, and coronary circulation. During catheterization, readings can be taken of oxygen concentration at different sites, of pressure in the different heart chambers, and of cardiac output. Abnormal blood flow through the heart and the coronary vessels can be detected. Cardiac catheterization is of great value in diagnosing coronary artery disease and valvular dysfunction.

The patient signs a consent form and must have a complete history and physical examination before the procedure. Nothing is given by mouth for at least 6 hours, and a sedative-narcotic may be given to allay apprehension and anxiety.

Cardiac catheterization is a surgical procedure using surgical aseptic techniques. It is carried out in a special cardiac catheterization laboratory, radiology department, or surgical suite. A catheter is inserted into a vein

Legal & Ethical Considerations 24-1

Assessments after Cardiac Catheterization

It is a legal responsibility to check neurologic signs and distal pulses below the site of entry for a cardiac catheterization. Should a hematoma form at the entry site and pressure on the nerves be so great that function is lost in the leg or foot, the nurse would be legally liable if the pulses and sensation had not been regularly assessed. Document the assessment findings to protect against legal ramifications.

or artery and threaded into the heart for injection of contrast media and pressure readings. Heart action is observed by fluoroscopy and is continuously monitored by ECG until the tests are completed. A videotape is made to provide records of heart function. Postcatheterization nursing care includes ensuring the patient has bed rest for 2 to 12 hours, frequent checking of the pressure dressing over the insertion point, and measuring vital signs and the distal pulse every 10 to 15 minutes for the first hour and the temperature every 6 hours. When the femoral approach has been used, the patient's leg may be immobilized for several hours. This lessens the chance of bleeding. Unless a new self-sealing type of catheter was used, immobilization is often done by the placement of a special pressure device or by small sandbags. Observe closely for chest pain, dyspnea, bleeding from the wound, quality of pulses distal to the catheter entry point, abnormal neurologic signs, and any signs of infection (Legal & Ethical Considerations 24-1).

When a noninvasive procedure is desired and advisable, an electron beam tomography test may be performed on the heart. This will show the percentage of calcification present in the coronary arteries. Calcium deposits are part of the atherosclerosis process

Steps 24-1 Obtaining an ECG Tracing (Electrocardiogram)

Each type of ECG machine has its own set of operating instructions. Consult the manual for the machine on hand for variations in the operating procedure.

1. *ACTION* After the patient is positioned comfortably, shave hair as needed for electrode placement. The extremity electrodes go on the inner aspect of the upper arms and the inner aspect of the lower legs. The chest electrodes are placed on the chest in the correct sequence.

   RATIONALE Excessive hair interferes with good adherence of the electrodes. Electrode placement must be correct to obtain a readable tracing.

2. *ACTION* Hook the wires (leads) from the machine to the electrodes, matching up the correct lead with the correct electrode.

   RATIONALE There are labels indicating which wire goes to which electrode. If the wires are not attached to the correct electrode, the tracing will not be correct.

3. *ACTION* Turn the machine on; ask the patient to hold still. Press the auto-run button.

   RATIONALE The machine will begin the tracing and automatically stop after recording the beginning leads.

4. *ACTION* Press the manual-run button and immediately press the "1-2-3" button. Allow the machine to run through two full sheets of recording paper and press "stop."

   RATIONALE This sets the machine to record the other required leads.

5. *ACTION* Press "manual run" again and allow enough paper to run through the machine so that the patient's tracing can be torn off cleanly. Check the tracing for a correct appearance. Roll or fold up the tracing and place it to one side. The tracing should be on an even line and without tiny vibration lines indicating electrical interference. If the tracing is not clear, troubleshoot according to the manual with the machine and retake the tracing. Turn off the machine.

   RATIONALE This method prevents losing some of the patient's tracing. The machine should not be left on between uses.

6. *ACTION* Remove the lead wires from the electrodes. Stabilizing the skin, remove the adhesive-backed electrodes from the patient. Check to be certain that all electrodes have been removed.

   RATIONALE Stabilization prevents undue pulling on the patient's skin. Checking for electrodes prevents sending the patient away with an electrode still attached.

7. *ACTION* Check that there is adequate tracing for the required leads and label the sheets with the patient's name and the required information: age, sex, blood pressure, height and weight, and medications the patient is taking.

   RATIONALE Assists the physician in interpreting the tracing correctly.

8. *ACTION* Assist the patient off of the table. Allow patient to redress. Be certain all jewelry removed is returned to the patient.

   RATIONALE Shows caring; prevents jewelry from getting misplaced.

9. *ACTION* Document the procedure in the patient record. Route the tracing for interpretation.

   RATIONALE Provides information that the procedure was carried out. Allows the physician to interpret the tracing.

and can help predict the degree of risk for coronary occlusion or myocardial infarction.

Angiography and Arteriography. Angiography and arteriography are used to locate lesions, occluded vessels, tumors, and malformed blood vessels. A contrast medium is injected into an artery and x-rays are taken of the dye spreading through the vessels. The procedure may be used to diagnose problems in arteries anywhere in the body: heart, neck, brain, or extremities.

A consent form is signed and baseline vital signs are obtained. Usually the patient is given nothing by mouth for at least 6 hours, and a mild sedative or tranquilizer is given before the procedure. After the procedure, the patient is kept on bed rest for a number of hours, an ice pack is applied to the insertion point, and vital signs are measured periodically. The contrast medium insertion point is also checked for bleeding or formation of a hematoma (collection of clotted blood). Be alert for any reaction to the dye.

Treadmill Stress Test. The treadmill stress test measures the cardiac heart rate and blood pressure response to clinically controlled active exercise. It is used to diagnose heart capacity, to guide convalescence from a myocardial infarction (heart attack), and to determine response to medical treatment. While having heart action continuously monitored by ECG, the patient walks on a treadmill, pedals a stationary bicycle, or climbs a set of stairs (Figure 24-5). The speed and degree of the incline of the treadmill can be changed to increase the amount of work or stress on the heart. The speed and resistance of the exercise bicycle can also be

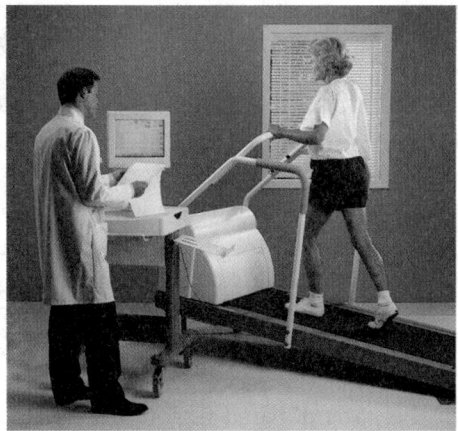

FIGURE **24-5** Cardiac treadmill stress test.

changed to meet the established standards for the test. The test is terminated when the desired heart rate is reached, the patient shows signs of fatigue, or the ECG shows signs of cardiac ischemia. Often thallium-201, a radioisotope, is used to show myocardial perfusion while exercising during the stress test. A consent form is signed, and the patient may have a light meal 4 to 6 hours before the test and must avoid caffeine and smoking for 4 hours prior to the test. The patient is told to discontinue taking medications when the test is for diagnostic purposes; medications may be taken when the test is to determine response to treatment. After a period of rest, the patient is able to resume usual activities.

Pulmonary Function Tests. Pulmonary function tests provide information about respiratory function, lung capacity, and diffusion of gases. Appointments are made for the tests to be performed in the pulmonary laboratory. Spirometers and other breathing devices may be used. No special preparation is required.

Endoscopic Examinations

There are many procedures based on the use of an endoscope (an instrument used to view inside a body cavity). Endoscopes are small metal or plastic devices or flexible tubes equipped with fiberoptics that provide direct light to the tissues being examined. Preparation of the patient depends on the test to be performed.

Gastroscopy. Gastroscopy is the visual inspection of the upper digestive tract and the stomach to obtain specimens of gastric contents and perform a biopsy on the stomach tissues. A signed consent form is required. The patient is instructed to take nothing by mouth for 8 hours before the examination. About 30 minutes before the procedure, an injection of an atropine-like drug and a sedative is given.

The test is conducted in the GI laboratory. A local anesthetic is sprayed on the pharynx, and a gastroscope is passed to the stomach. The scope has a fiberoptic system for its lens. The gastroscope may be equipped with a camera to take color photographs.

Washings are done to obtain specimens for cytology studies or a biopsy specimen is taken.

The patient should take nothing by mouth until the effects of the local anesthetic have worn off and the gag reflex has returned. After resting for a period of time, the patient can resume usual activities. Observe for signs of bleeding or unexplained pain, which might be due to perforation of an ulcer.

Proctosigmoidoscopy. Proctosigmoidoscopy is the visual inspection of the lower bowel and is used to check the lining for ulceration, polyps (growths protruding from a mucous membrane), tumors, inflammation, and other abnormalities. Consent is required for the procedure. The bowel should be clear of fecal material; therefore, a cathartic is given the night before the procedure and an enema may be ordered. The patient may be restricted to a liquid diet the day before the test. The patient should empty the bladder before the test and then assume a side-lying or Sims' position on a table. The sigmoidoscope is inserted. The fiberoptic lens enables the examiner to see the structures, and suction can be used to remove secretions. Air may be introduced to inflate the lower bowel to better view the wall, and biopsy forceps may be used to remove a specimen of tissue. Some abdominal cramping is usually experienced. No special aftercare is required. The nurse assists the physician with this procedure (Steps 24-2).

Colonoscopy. Colonoscopy is the inspection of the entire large intestine for polyps, areas of inflammation, and malignant lesions. It confirms suspicious findings of x-rays and is used to take biopsy specimens or remove polyps found on other studies or in patients with a known history of polyps.

The patient is placed on a clear liquid diet for 24 to 48 hours before the procedure, avoiding liquids that contain red or purple dye, and given nothing by mouth for at least 8 hours. Sometimes a particular diet is ordered for the 3 days before the test. Bowel cleansing with laxatives, cathartics, and enemas is performed in the 24 hours before the test. Bowel fluid must return clear before colonoscopy can be successfully performed. Sedation is given to promote relaxation and decrease awareness. The procedure takes 30 to 90 minutes.

A long, flexible fiberoptic endoscope is inserted anally and slowly advanced through the large intestine. The patient is generally well sedated throughout the procedure. A signed consent is required. Check the patient's laboratory values for CBC and clotting times to see that they are within normal limits. **Any iron medication, aspirin, and most anti-inflammatory drugs must be withheld for 3 days.** See that the patient is instructed in the clear liquid diet regimen and bowel-cleansing program. Administer the bowel preparation components as ordered. Give any ordered pretest medications. Teach the patient about the procedure and what to expect. Colonoscopy should not be done sooner than 10 to 14 days after barium GI studies. Obtain baseline vital signs. After the test, monitor

Steps 24-2 Assisting with a Flexible Sigmoidoscopy

Assisting with a sigmoidoscopy is often a duty of the nurse employed in a physician's office or clinic.

1. *ACTION* Set up the sigmoidoscopy equipment and check that the light is functioning and that the suction functions. Place gloves and lubricant on a prepared field.

   RATIONALE Checking prevents an equipment problem during the procedure.

2. *ACTION* Inquire if the patient completed the bowel preparation as instructed.

   RATIONALE Bowel must be clean for visualization of the mucosal walls.

3. *ACTION* Have the patient empty the bladder before the procedure.

   RATIONALE Prevents added discomfort during the procedure.

4. *ACTION* Ask the patient to remove all clothing from the waist down and put on a gown so that it ties in the back.

   RATIONALE Allows the examiner to access the anus.

5. *ACTION* Assist the patient onto the examining table and into the left lateral or Sims' position.

   RATIONALE Positions the rectum for entry of the sigmoidoscope.

6. *ACTION* Drape the patient so that only the anus is exposed.

   RATIONALE Protects the patient's modesty and privacy. Draping prevents unnecessary chilling.

7. *ACTION* Ask the patient to breathe slowly and deeply through the mouth during the procedure and to try to relax the lower abdominal and rectal muscles. Explain that discomfort is often due to air instilled to improve visualization.

   RATIONALE Breathing through the mouth slowly helps the patient to relax and to maintain relaxed muscles. Relaxing the muscles aids in the insertion and progression of the sigmoidoscope.

8. *ACTION* After the procedure, put on gloves and clean the patient's anal region of excess lubricant using tissue wipes. Allow the patient to rest before arising from the table.

   RATIONALE Cleaning prevents lubricant from getting on the table or the patient's clothes.

9. *ACTION* Remove gloves and perform hand hygiene.

   RATIONALE Reduces transfer of microorganisms.

10. *ACTION* Assist the patient off of the table and allow privacy to dress.

    RATIONALE Shows consideration for the patient.

11. *ACTION* Place biopsy specimens in fixative and label the containers; fill out a requisition slip. Send the biopsy specimens to the laboratory.

    RATIONALE Ensures that the specimen is labeled correctly and is sent to the laboratory.

12. *ACTION* After patient has left the room, clean up the room and cleanse the equipment.

    RATIONALE Prepares the room for the next patient. Equipment must be disinfected before next use.

the vital signs every half-hour for 2 hours and then according to facility protocol. Monitor rectal bleeding. Slight bleeding is expected if polyps were biopsied or removed. Keep the patient on bed rest for the time ordered. Someone must drive the patient home.

Cystoscopy. Cystoscopy is the visual inspection of the interior of the bladder for the collection of biopsy specimens, collection of urine separately from each ureter, and treatment of various conditions. It is valuable in diagnosing urologic ailments. Aseptic technique is used throughout the procedure to avoid introducing microorganisms and causing infections in the urinary tract. With the patient in the lithotomy position, the cystoscope is passed through the urethra and the bladder is visually inspected. Cystoscopy is often carried out in conjunction with the intravenous pyelogram (IVP) and is used for surgical procedures involved in transurethral resection of the prostate, removal of bladder tumors or polyps, and various other bladder treatments. Local or general anesthetics are used when cystoscopy will cause discomfort or pain.

A signed consent form is needed, and the patient is to be given nothing by mouth after midnight. Usually a cathartic is given the evening before the test to empty the colon of feces. Afterward the patient should be on bed rest for 3 to 4 hours or until recovered from the effects of anesthesia. Fluid intake should be increased, and it is common for the urine to be pink tinged after the procedure, but red urine and clots should be reported to the physician. Mild analgesics may be given for complaints of backache. Vital signs are checked, and temperature should be taken every 6 hours because some patients experience a fever a day or so af-

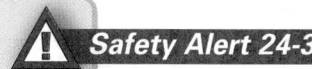

Safety Alert 24-3

Allergy

Allergy to iodine or shellfish must be assessed because an iodine-based contrast medium is used during the ERCP test.

ter the procedure resulting from the spread of an infection already present in the urinary tract.

Endoscopic Retrograde Cholangiopancreatography. Endoscopic retrograde cholangiopancreatography (ERCP) is used to identify a cause of biliary obstruction such as stricture, cyst, stones, or tumor. The procedure is usually done because jaundice (yellowness of the skin, mucous membranes, and sclera caused by presence of bile pigments) is present. The patient is placed on the x-ray or endoscopy table, and a local anesthetic is sprayed on the pharynx to help prevent gagging during insertion of the endoscope. The endoscope is inserted through the mouth and down into the duodenum after intravenous sedation, usually diazepam (Valium) or midazolam (Versed), is given. Atropine may be given to decrease secretions in the oropharynx. Secretin may also be given when the duodenum is reached to stop peristalsis. A catheter is inserted into the pancreatic duct via the endoscope and a contrast medium is injected. X-rays are taken. The procedure takes about an hour. The patient is monitored during the procedure for complications from medications or from perforation by the endoscope.

The patient is given nothing by mouth for 8 hours before the test. A sedative-narcotic and atropine are given in preparation for the insertion of the endoscope (Safety Alert 24-3). The patient must be in a fasting state, and a signed consent is required.

After the test, vital signs are monitored every half-hour for 2 hours and then hourly for 4 hours or until stable. The gag reflex must return before foods and fluid are offered.

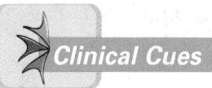

Clinical Cues

Offer a warm saline gargle or throat lozenges to reduce throat soreness.

Observe skin color for increasing jaundice after the test because irritation from the endoscope may make a stricture worse until inflammation subsides.

Aspirations

Aspirations are performed to obtain bone marrow, liver cells, spinal fluid, abdominal fluid, or fluid in the chest cavity. These procedures are usually performed at the bedside or in a procedure room by the physician, who is attended by a nurse. Most of these procedures are uncomfortable for the patient. Generally the nurse

obtains the equipment needed, opens sterile supplies as requested, positions and drapes the patient, and assists the physician. Pretest analgesia or sedation is administered if ordered. It is essential that the patient remain still during the procedure. Baseline vital signs are taken before the procedure begins. Table 24-4 provides information on positioning and care of patients undergoing an aspiration.

Electroencephalography

The neurologic and physiologic activity of the brain produces electrical charges that can be measured as brain waves. The tracing of the brain waves is an electroencephalogram (EEG). The EEG is done to localize and diagnose brain lesions, scars, epilepsy, infections, blood clots, and abscesses. It is also performed to determine brain death in comatose patients on life support systems.

Patients scheduled for an EEG are to have no stimulants, no sedatives, and no anticonvulsant drugs, such as phenytoin (Dilantin), for 48 hours before the test unless necessary to control seizures. It is not necessary to shave any hair, and generally there is no special preparation. Some electroencephalography laboratories require that the hair be shampooed and dried before the test.

The patient sits in a chair, or remains on a stretcher, in a quiet room, and electrodes are attached to the scalp with skin glue or paste, or a mesh cap containing the 19 to 25 electrodes is placed on the head (Figure 24-6, p. 428). The equipment detects the electrical energy generated by the brain and produces a graphic record of the brain waves. The patient should close the eyes and relax. A request to hyperventilate for some of the tracings may be made because abnormalities may then be more noticeable. Rapid shallow breathing causes alkalosis, which in turn produces vasoconstriction in the brain and may activate seizure activity. A flashing light may be held over the face in order to induce abnormal activity. The patient may be sleep deprived before the test or a sedative may be given when a sleeping electroencephalogram is desired. Sleep is helpful in producing abnormal brain activity, particularly that associated with epilepsy. The test may take up to 1 hour and 15 minutes. Any paste or gel used is washed away after the test.

Other Diagnostic Tests

Many other diagnostic tests are performed each day. They will be encountered in the units of study for the medical-surgical and obstetric nursing courses.

Nurses employed in physicians' offices, medical clinics, and in the hospital are required to obtain blood specimens and to perform certain diagnostic tests such as wound or throat culture (Skill 24-5), random blood sugars, hemoglobin levels, and urine dips. They also assist with Papanicolaou smears (application of secretions and cells on a slide) (Skill 24-6, p. 430) and sigmoidoscopies. It should be noted that there are many models of glucometers and hemoglobin machines. If

Table 24-4 *Aspiration Procedures*

PROCEDURE	EXPLANATION	IMPLEMENTATION
Lumbar puncture (spinal tap)	Insertion of a needle into the subarachnoid space in the spinal canal to obtain specimens of spinal fluid, measure the pressure, or instill dye, anesthetic, or medication	Take baseline vital signs. Patient is assisted to assume a side-lying flexed position.
Bone marrow aspiration	Insertion of a needle into the bone to extract bone marrow cells for laboratory analysis	Take baseline vital signs. Premedicate as ordered. Set up sterile tray and supplies; help patient assume correct position (depends on aspiration site). Warn patient when pressure and discomfort will be felt. Monitor patient's status during the procedure. Note characteristics of aspirate and document the procedure and patient response.
Liver biopsy (aspiration)	Insertion of a needle into the liver for the aspiration of liver cells	Take baseline vital signs. Have the patient empty the bladder. Premedicate as ordered. Set up the sterile tray and supplies. Assist the patient to a supine position at the far right side of the bed with the right arm over the head and the head turned to the left. Have patient practice taking a deep breath, blowing it all out, and holding the breath, then breathing normally. Explain that this will need to be done for the procedure. Warn patient when puncture is about to occur. After the procedure, assist to move to the center of the bed and turn onto the right side. Instruct to maintain position for 2 hr. Label specimen and send to laboratory with proper requisition. Keep patient on bed rest for 6 hr. Assess vital signs q 15 min × 4, then q 30 min × 4; then q 1 hr × 4; then q 4 hr.

Site of needle puncture

Third lumbar vertebra

Distal end of spinal cord

Dura mater

Subarachnoid space

Cauda equina

Sterile tray and supplies are set up for the physician. Tell patient not to cough and to breathe slowly and deeply. Hold patient's arms and legs in flexed position. Warn patient when discomfort will occur. When procedure is finished, label tubes with correct information. Be certain pressure dressing is intact over the puncture site. Instruct patient to maintain a dorsal recumbent position for 4-12 hr; turning side to side is permitted. Medicate for pain as needed. Document the procedure and patient's response.

Table 24-4 | *Aspiration Procedures—cont'd*

PROCEDURE	EXPLANATION	IMPLEMENTATION
Thoracentesis	Insertion of a needle through the chest wall into the pleural space to remove air, fluid, or blood collected there	Take baseline vital signs. Set up the sterile tray and supplies. Assist patient to sit leaning over an over-the-bed table padded with pillows. Support the patient's body in this position during the procedure. If the patient is unable to sit up, a side-lying position is used.

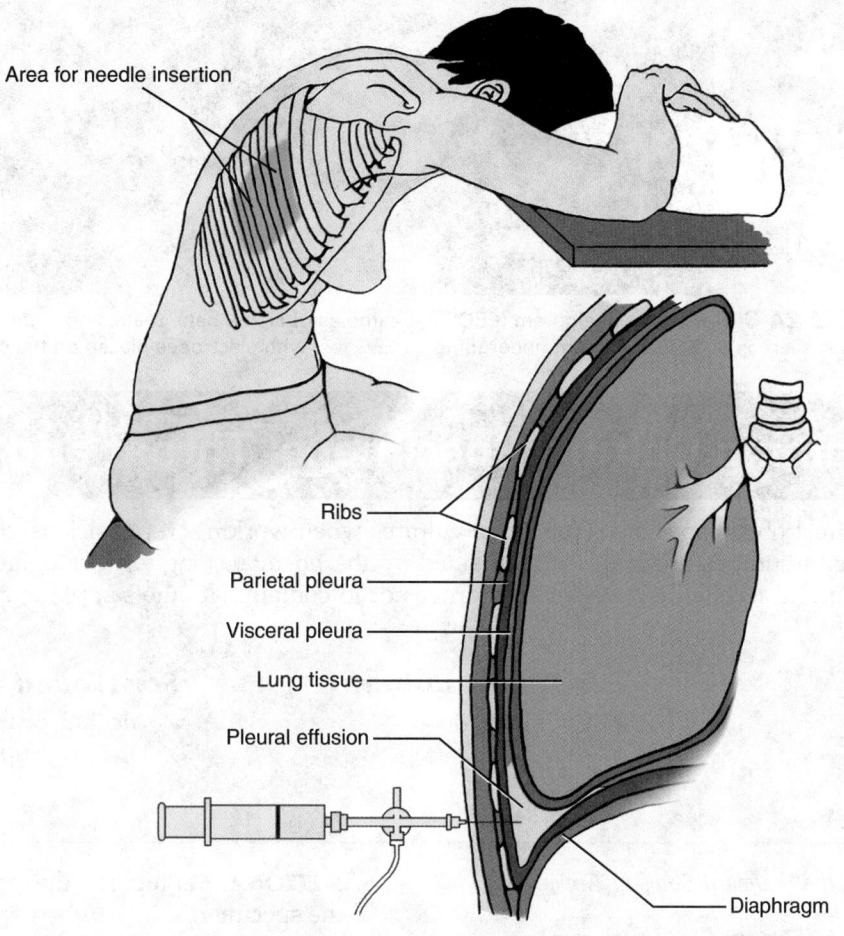

Area for needle insertion

Ribs

Parietal pleura

Visceral pleura

Lung tissue

Pleural effusion

Diaphragm

		Assess respiratory status during the procedure. Assist patient to a comfortable position in bed after procedure is finished. Label any specimens. Document the procedure and the patient's response.
Paracentesis	A needle puncture of the abdomen to remove ascites fluid, obtain fluid for analysis, or carry out peritoneal dialysis	Take baseline vital signs. Position the patient upright on the side of the bed or sitting backward on a straight chair with the feet supported. Set up the sterile tray and supplies. Sit in front of the patient and notify when puncture is to be made. Assess respiratory status continuously; assess vital signs after 15 min Explain to patient what the physician is doing. After the procedure, be certain the pressure dressing is intact. Assist the patient to a comfortable position in bed. Label specimens. Document the procedure and the patient's response. Monitor vital signs per agency protocol.

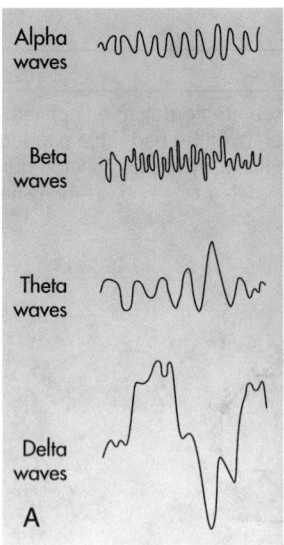
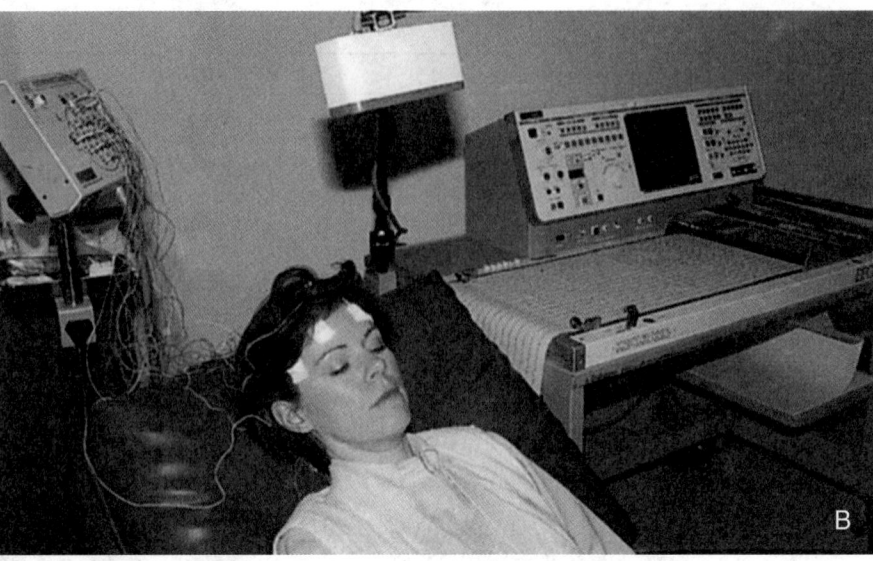

FIGURE **24-6** Electroencephalogram (EEG). **A,** Examples of alpha, beta, theta, and delta waves seen on an EEG. **B,** Patient undergoing an EEG test with electrodes placed on the scalp.

Skill 24-5 | Obtaining Culture Specimens: Throat and Wound

Nurses frequently must obtain specimens for throat cultures when working in physicians' offices or clinics. Wound cultures are frequently obtained by the hospital, long-term care, and home care nurse. Careful technique is essential in order not to contaminate the sample to be cultured.

■ Supplies
✓ Culture tube
✓ Label
✓ Requisition slip
✓ Biohazard plastic bag

For Throat Culture
✓ Tongue blade

For Wound Culture
✓ Alcohol swabs
✓ Dressing supplies

Review and carry out the Standard Steps in Appendix 3.

■ Assessment (Data Collection)

1. *ACTION* Check the physician's order for the specific culture.

   RATIONALE Determines type of tube to be used.

2. *ACTION* Identify the patient by asking her name, or check the ID armband.

   RATIONALE Verifies that the right patient will have the culture specimen obtained.

■ Planning

3. *ACTION* Verify that all supplies are on hand and that there is good lighting for the area to be cultured.

   RATIONALE Prevents having to stop and obtain supplies. Good lighting provides good visual field for obtaining the needed specimen.

■ Implementation

4. *ACTION* Explain the procedure to the patient and label the culture tube.

RATIONALE Prepares the patient and identifies the specimen.

5. *ACTION* Perform hand hygiene and put on gloves.

   RATIONALE Prevents contamination of the hands.

A: Throat

6. *ACTION* Position a light so that the pharynx may be viewed. Withdraw the sterile swab from the tube or package.

   RATIONALE The light from an otoscope works well; otherwise use an examining light. Pharynx must be visible to obtain the specimen.

7. *ACTION* Ask the patient to tip the head back slightly and open the mouth wide. Instruct the patient to sing a low note ("ah").

   RATIONALE Allows visualization of the pharynx and keeps the tongue out of the way.

8. *ACTION* Depressing the tongue with a tongue blade and, without touching the teeth, tongue, cheek, or gums, insert the sterile swab into the throat and rotate it slightly around the tonsil area

and the back wall, only touching areas of exudate (fluid with cellular debris from inflammation) or areas of inflammation. Withdraw the swab without touching other structures.

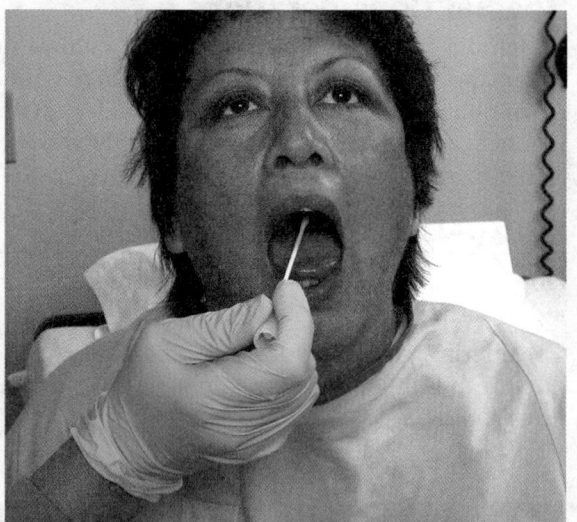

Step **8**

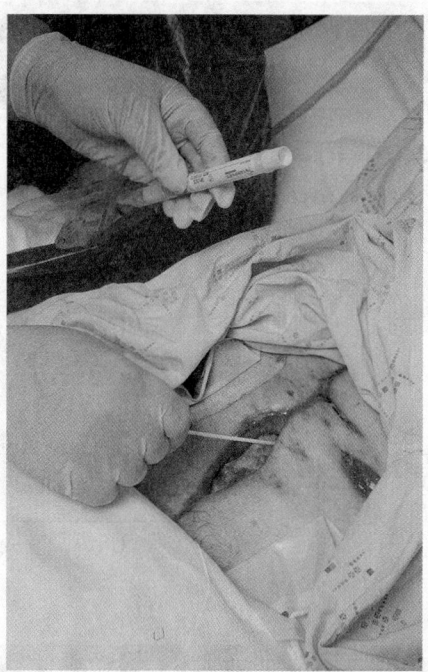

Step **10**

RATIONALE Obtains secretions that may contain microorganisms from the throat area only.

9. *ACTION* Place the swab into the culture tube without touching any other surface.

RATIONALE Prevents contamination of the specimen.

B: Wound (Aerobic Culture)

6. *ACTION* Remove dressing, folding soiled side together, and dispose of it in a biohazard waste container.

RATIONALE Prevents spread of microorganisms.

7. *ACTION* Cleanse the area around the wound edges with an antiseptic swab.

RATIONALE Removes old exudate and skin bacteria.

8. *ACTION* Remove and dispose of gloves properly.

RATIONALE Prevents transfer of microorganisms.

9. *ACTION* Open sterile gloves and dressing supplies.

RATIONALE Prepares equipment to take specimen and redress the wound.

10. *ACTION* Put on the gloves. Take the sterile swab(s) from the culture tube and insert the tip(s) into the wound where drainage is occurring; rotate the swab gently. Remove the swab(s) and replace them carefully in the culture tube without touching any other surface.

RATIONALE Obtains specimen from area most likely to contain microorganisms. Prevents contamination of the specimen.

11. *ACTION* Redress wound using sterile technique.

RATIONALE Prevents contamination of wound with microorganisms.

For Both Throat and Wound Cultures

12. *ACTION* Squeeze the ampule in the bottom of the culture tube to release the preservative solution. Press the swab into the solution to wet it thoroughly.

RATIONALE Preserves the specimen.

13. *ACTION* Remove the gloves and perform hand hygiene.

RATIONALE Reduces transfer of microorganisms.

14. *ACTION* Label the tube and fill out the laboratory requisition; send the culture to the lab.

RATIONALE Prevents the culture from being lost or mislabeled.

■ Evaluation

15. *ACTION* Review report when returned from lab to see what organism(s) have grown.

RATIONALE Type of organism will dictate the correct therapy.

16. *ACTION* Check orders to see if physician has ordered the appropriate therapy to treat the infection according to the laboratory sensitivity report. If not, call the physician.

RATIONALE Provides a check to see that treatment has been ordered for the infection.

Continued

Skill 24-5 Obtaining Culture Specimens: Throat and Wound—cont'd

■ Documentation

Documentation Example: Throat

12/22 1100 Throat culture obtained and sent to lab.

_____
(Nurse's signature)

Documentation Example: Wound

12/22 1300 Wound culture obtained from wound on right upper thigh. Wound redressed using sterile technique. Culture sent to lab.

_____
(Nurse's signature)

■ Special Considerations

✓ Anaerobic cultures require a different culture medium and procedure. Check the facility manual. Anaerobic cultures are performed from deep within wounds for organisms that cannot grow when exposed to air.

?CRITICAL THINKING QUESTIONS

1. How would you obtain a throat culture from a crying, squirming 5-year-old child?
2. Considering your daily tasks for the patient, when do you think the best time to obtain a wound culture would be?

Skill 24-6 Assisting with a Pelvic Examination and Pap Test (Smear)

Papanicolaou (Pap) smears are a frequent diagnostic test for cervical, vaginal, or endometrial cancer ordered in a medical office or a clinic. Occasionally a Pap smear may be obtained in the procedure room at the hospital. The Pap smear is done in conjunction with a pelvic exam on the female patient. Patients should not douche for 24 hours prior to the test. The specimens are either placed on slides or swished into a special solution in a container (ThinPrep type of Pap smear).

■ Supplies

✓ Disposable gloves
✓ Saline solution
✓ Examination table with stirrups
✓ Examination light
✓ Vaginal speculum
✓ Biohazard waste container
✓ Cotton-tipped applicator or cytology brush
✓ Cervical scraper
✓ Patient gown and drape
✓ Lubricant
✓ Examination stool
✓ Glass slide with a frosted edge or ThinPrep specimen container
✓ Pencil
✓ Pathology requisition slip
✓ Cytology fixative

Review and carry out the Standard Steps in Appendix 3.

■ Assessment (Data Collection)

1. **ACTION** Assess whether patient is familiar with the procedure.

   RATIONALE Determines patient's knowledge base.

2. **ACTION** Assess equipment and supplies on hand.

   RATIONALE Aids in determining what if any supplies are missing before starting the procedure.

■ Planning

3. **ACTION** Plan ahead and label the frosted end of the slide with the patient's name and date or label the ThinPrep container.

   RATIONALE Identifies the slide as belonging to the patient; prevents report error.

4. **ACTION** Fill out the requisition slip with the required information.

   RATIONALE Ensures that requisition is ready after smear is taken.

■ Implementation

5. **ACTION** Explain the procedure if patient is unfamiliar with it; answer questions.

   RATIONALE Decreases fear of the unknown and helps patient relax.

6. **ACTION** Set up the table and equipment as the examiner prefers.

   RATIONALE Prepares the equipment for the patient and the examiner.

7. **ACTION** Give the patient a gown, and ask that all clothing below the waist be removed and the gown put on so that it ties in the back; provide privacy.

   RATIONALE Allows the examiner to access the perineal area. If the examiner wishes to do a breast check, ask the patient to remove all clothing.

8. **ACTION** When patient is ready, assist onto the table with the lower half of the body covered with a drape. Assist into a lithotomy position with the feet in the stirrups and the buttocks right at the end of the table. The knees should be apart. The drape can be left free or positioned so that the corners can be wrapped around the lower legs and feet with the third corner hanging over the perineum.

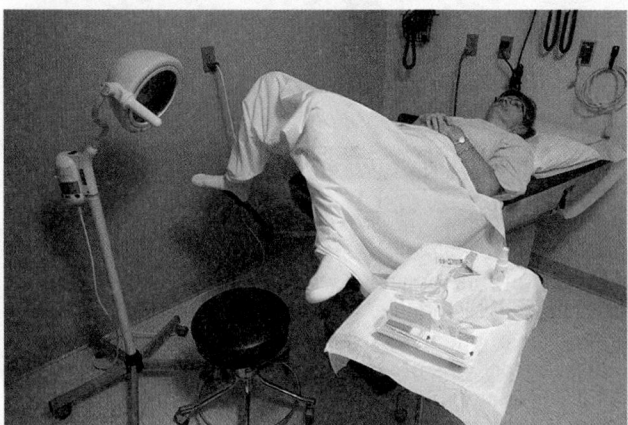

Step **8**

RATIONALE The lithotomy position allows the examiner to visualize the vagina and cervix with the speculum. The drape protects the patient's modesty and provides privacy. The third corner of the drape can be folded back when the examiner is ready to begin.

9. **ACTION** Reassure the patient and help her relax during the procedure by telling her to take deep, slow breaths through the mouth and to try to relax the abdominal muscles.

RATIONALE The procedure will go more smoothly if the patient is relaxed. The examiner will perform the pelvic examination after the smear has been taken.

10. **ACTION** Assist the examiner by passing equipment as requested.

RATIONALE Helps the procedure go quickly and smoothly.

11. **ACTION** Apply gloves and fix the slide(s) by flooding them with 95% ethyl alcohol or spraying them with cytology fixative according to the directions on the spray container. If ThinPrep container and solution was used, just close the container.

RATIONALE Smears on slides must be fixed within 10 seconds after collection to maintain the normal appearance of the cells and to prevent the smears from being exposed to contaminants in the air. Spray lightly from left to right and then from right to left.

12. **ACTION** When the procedure is finished, assist the patient to slide back, pull out the table extension and remove the feet simultaneously from the stirrups and lay them straight on the table. Ask pa-

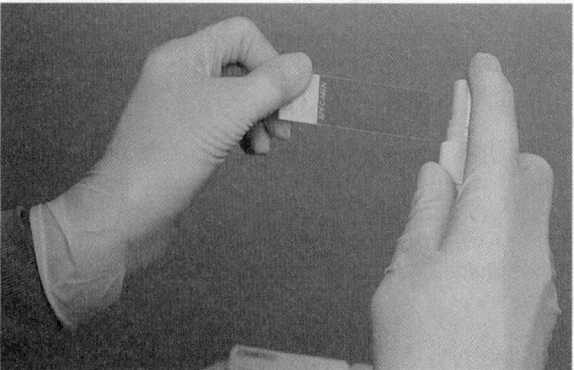

Step **11**

tient to slide back slightly onto table. When the patient is ready to sit up, assist to a sitting position as you slide the table extension into the table.

RATIONALE Shows consideration for the patient. Positions patient to sit up.

13. **ACTION** Allow the slide(s), if used, to dry for at least 5 minutes before packaging them in a slide container to send to the laboratory.

RATIONALE Prevents contamination or disruption of the smear.

14. **ACTION** Send the labeled container and the requisition slip to the laboratory.

RATIONALE Ensures that smear reaches laboratory.

■ Evaluation

15. **ACTION** Evaluate whether the procedure went smoothly. If not, consider what should be changed for the next time you assist with the procedure.

RATIONALE Assists in perfecting technique and helpfulness to patient and examiner.

■ Documentation

16. **ACTION** If examiner does not document the procedure on the patient's medical record, note that the procedure was done and the specimen sent to the laboratory.

RATIONALE Notes date procedure was performed.

Documentation Example

6/19 1015   Pap smear and pelvic examination done by Dr. Smith; tolerated without problems. Smear fixed and sent to pathology lab with requisition.

_____

(Nurse's signature)

?CRITICAL THINKING QUESTIONS

1. What would you say and do to help a young woman relax during her first pelvic examination and Pap smear?

2. If a patient's knees and legs are visibly shaking during a Pap smear and the examiner is having trouble seeing into the vagina, what would you do?

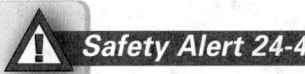

Safety Alert 24-4

Critical Laboratory Values

In 2005, The Joint Commission instituted Safety Goals requiring that the nurse notify the physician immediately of any laboratory test result considered "critical" when such a result arrives on the unit. Note in the chart that the phone call was made and to whom the laboratory result, and the importance of it, was given.

the machine to be used is different than the one indicated in Skill 24-2, the procedure may vary slightly. The correct steps for the procedure will be in the instruction manual accompanying the machine.

An important step is to fill out the laboratory or test requisition slip properly. Information generally required is the patient's name, physician's name, date, and type of test requested. For some tests, names of medications that the patient is taking will be requested. All specimens should be labeled on the container (not lid) with the patient's name, the date, and the physician's name.

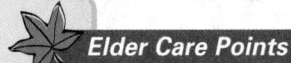

Elder Care Points

When elderly persons are taken to another department for a diagnostic test, it is important to send an extra blanket with them in case they have to wait in a holding area for an extended period. Too often these areas are cool and the cover sheet is not sufficient to keep elderly persons warm. An attendant should be with the patients or personnel should check on them frequently.

Evaluation

Evaluation involves determining whether the expected outcomes written for each nursing diagnosis have been met. The patient is assessed for potential adverse effects of the diagnostic procedure. One way to continually improve patient preparation is to ask patients after the procedure if there was anything they wish they had known in advance that had not been told to them. Information obtained in this way is often helpful for future patient teaching regarding a particular procedure.

Evaluation is also performed by comparing the results of tests performed from one day to another. For example, the WBC reading on a CBC indicates whether an infection is improving or worsening. If the treatment is effective against the infection, the WBC should be falling. When a serum potassium is low, the nurse checks the laboratory values to determine if the administration of extra potassium has corrected the problem (Safety Alert 24-4). The nurse is usually responsible for giving the home care patient appropriate instructions and patient teaching before scheduled tests and procedures. After the test is scheduled, a visit or telephone call allows for assessment of what the patient knows about the test. The nurse can provide explanation and teaching,

explain the pretest preparation, and determine that the patient can carry out the necessary preparation. If the patient needs assistance, then a family member may be enlisted to help or the nurse must schedule a visit at the appropriate time to help the patient with the preparation for the procedure. It should also be determined ahead of time that the patient has transportation available to the facility where the procedure is to be performed. When samples of blood or urine are needed for laboratory testing, the nurse can obtain the samples and deliver them to the laboratory. Check to see that the consent form is signed if one is required.

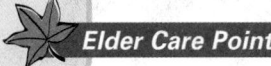

Elder Care Points

- Elderly patients who are repeatedly kept NPO (nothing by mouth) for various tests and procedures are susceptible to dehydration and electrolyte imbalances. Frequent assessment is needed to determine hydration status.
- A series of enemas can also upset electrolyte balance. Assess for signs of potassium and sodium imbalance after administering enemas.

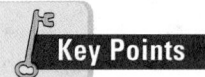

Key Points

- Diagnostic tests and procedures assist in making diagnoses and provide information about physiologic functioning.
- The nurse assesses what patients know about the test or procedure they are about to undergo. Teaching is based on current knowledge.
- Nursing diagnoses relate to the underlying problems for which the testing is being performed. *Deficient knowledge* is a nursing diagnosis used when the patient needs teaching.
- The nurse must plan time for diagnostic test preparation and post-test care into the daily work plan. Expected outcomes are written for the specific nursing diagnoses.
- The nurse implements teaching, pretest preparation, and post-test care for all patients undergoing diagnostic testing.
- Hematology tests are studies of the blood and its components. The CBC is the most commonly ordered hematology test.
- The erythrocyte sedimentation rate (ESR) is an indirect measure of inflammatory action in the body.
- Blood chemistry tests provide information about electrolyte balance; the ability of the body to metabolize nutrients; the function of the liver, kidney, muscles, and heart; and the accumulation of toxic substances. Chemistry tests are often ordered by SMA panel.
- Serology tests are helpful in diagnosing or confirming bacterial or viral infection.
- The urinalysis provides valuable information about the function of the kidneys and other biologic processes within the body.
- Cytologic studies of tissue and cells are performed to detect carcinogenic, metabolic, vascular, and other changes.

- Culture and sensitivity tests of body fluids are done in the bacteriology laboratory to determine organisms responsible for infection and the drugs that will kill them.
- Sonography uses sound waves and their echoes to picture structures within the body.
- Radiology uses x-rays to obtain pictures of bones and tissues within the body. An opaque contrast medium can be used to outline hollow organs.
- Radionuclide scans help determine abnormalities in structure or function of different organs.
- CT scans use a computer to enhance x-rays and allow visualization of structures within the body.
- Magnetic resonance imaging is based on electromagnetic fields and can produce clearer images of internal structures than CT scans.
- The ECG is a tracing of the electrical activity in the heart; the EEG traces the activity of the electrical pattern produced by brain waves.
- Cardiac catheterization is an invasive procedure to determine abnormalities of structure and function of the heart; it is combined with coronary angiography.
- All invasive tests or tests requiring injection of a contrast material or radionuclide require a signed consent form from the patient.

- Endoscopic examinations are performed by using a flexible fiberoptic instrument. A large portion of the gastrointestinal system can be visualized endoscopically.
- Aspirations are performed to extract fluid or tissue for study.
- Evaluation is based on whether the expected outcomes have been met. Laboratory values are compared to see if there is improvement in the patient's condition.
- The home care nurse sets up appointments for diagnostic testing for the home care patient, assists with test preparation, performs necessary teaching, and supervises post-test care.

 Go to your **Companion CD-ROM** for an Audio Glossary, animations, video clips, and more.

evolve Be sure to visit the companion Evolve site at http://evolve.elsevier.com/deWit/fundamental/ for additional online resources.

NCLEX-PN® EXAMINATION-STYLE REVIEW QUESTIONS

*Choose the **best** answer(s) for each question.*

1. A culture is obtained when a patient has a bladder infection for the purpose of:
   1. selecting the correct dose of medication.
   2. determining the prognosis of the disease.
   3. ruling out an infectious process.
   4. growing and identifying causative organisms.

2. The sensitivity part of a culture and sensitivity test is for the purpose of:
   1. identifying the causative organism of the infection.
   2. determining which medications are ineffective against the causative organism.
   3. testing anti-infectives to see which ones are most effective against the causative organism.
   4. growing colonies of the causative organism on a culture medium.

3. Tests for syphilis are considered _____ tests. *(Which type of test?) (Fill in the blank.)*

4. When taking a culture sample from an infected wound, the nurse should: *(Select all that apply.)*
   1. don sterile gloves to obtain the sample.
   2. swab the skin around the wound.
   3. swab into the center of the drainage area.
   4. cleanse the area around the wound.

5. Correct technique for obtaining a specimen for a throat culture is to use a sterile applicator and swab: *(Select all that apply.)*
   1. gum areas.
   2. exudate areas on tonsils.
   3. medial tongue and throat.
   4. inflamed areas in back of throat.

6. When instructing a patient about a magnetic resonance imaging test, you would explain that: *(Select all that apply.)*
   1. it is necessary to hold very still during the test.
   2. heavy sedation is usually provided prior to the test.
   3. loud noise will be heard during the test.
   4. communication with the technician is possible.

7. When instructing the patient about a colonoscopy, you would include that: *(Select all that apply.)*
   1. the prep for the procedure begins 24 to 48 hours beforehand.
   2. sedation will be given prior to the procedure.
   3. it is OK to drive home afterward.
   4. there is often some rectal bleeding afterward.

8. A lumbar puncture is a(n) _____ procedure. *(What type of procedure?) (Fill in the blank.)*

9. When caring for the patient who has just undergone a liver biopsy, you must:
   1. keep the patient positioned on the right side for 2 hours.
   2. apply pressure to the aspiration site by hand for 30 minutes.
   3. keep the patient on bed rest for 24 hours.
   4. turn the patient to the left side afterward.

10. When collecting a blood sample with a Vacutainer system, it is very important to:
    1. replace the tube stopper firmly for each sample.
    2. release the tourniquet after successful venipuncture.
    3. withdraw the holder and tube at the same time.
    4. stabilize the holder when changing tubes.

CRITICAL THINKING ACTIVITIES *Read each clinical scenario and discuss the questions with your classmates.*

Scenario A
The patient underwent a cardiac catheterization this morning.

1. What assessments would you need to make regularly afterward?

2. If you have difficulty finding the dorsalis pedis pulse in the leg where the catheter was inserted, what would you do?

3. What might it mean if the leg in which the catheter was introduced begins to swell?

Scenario B
The patient has blood chemistries ordered every morning. On the third day, she complains that she doesn't want this done because she is sick and becoming sicker because they are taking all her blood. How would you respond to the patient?

25 Fluid, Electrolyte, and Acid–Base Balance

evolve http://evolve.elsevier.com/deWit/fundamental/

Objectives

Upon completing this chapter, you should be able to:

Theory

1. List the various functions water performs in the body.
2. List the major electrolytes and the function of each.
3. Describe three ways in which body fluids are continually being distributed among the fluid compartments.
4. Identify the signs and symptoms of the common fluid and electrolyte imbalances.
5. State the main signs and symptoms of acid–base imbalances.

Clinical Practice

1. Assess an assigned patient for signs of fluid and electrolyte imbalance.
2. From patient laboratory results, identify electrolyte values that are abnormal.
3. Implement teaching for the patient with hypokalemia.
4. Develop a plan of care for a patient who has a fluid and electrolyte imbalance.
5. Identify patients who might be at risk for an acid–base imbalance.

Skills & Steps

Skill
Skill 25-1   Measuring Intake and Output

Key Terms

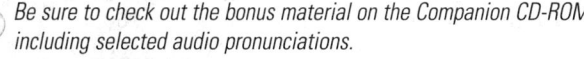

Be sure to check out the bonus material on the Companion CD-ROM, including selected audio pronunciations.

acidosis (ă-sĭ-DŌ-sĭs, p. 441)
active transport (p. 439)
alkalosis (ăl-kă-LŌ-sĭs, p. 444)
ascites (ă-SĪ-tēz, p. 441)
dehydration (dē-hī-DRĀ-shŭn, p. 437)
diffusion (dĭ-FŪ-zhŭn, p. 438)
edema (p. 441)
electrolytes (ĕ-LĔK-trō-līts, p. 436)
extracellular (ĕks-tră-SĔL-ū-lăr, p. 437)
filtration (fĭl-TRĀ-shŭn, p. 439)
hydrostatic pressure (hī-drō-STĂ-tĭk PRĔ-shŭr, p. 439)
hypercalcemia (hī-pĕr-kăl-SĒ-mē-ă, p. 444)
hyperchloremia (hī-pĕr-klōr-Ē-mē-ă, p. 445)
hyperkalemia (hī-pĕr-kă-LĒ-mē-ă, p. 442)
hypermagnesemia (hī-pĕr-măg-nĕ-SĒ-mē-ă, p. 445)
hypernatremia (hī-pĕr-nă-TRĒ-mē-ă, p. 441)

hyperphosphatemia (hī-pĕr-fŏs-fă-TĒ-mē-ă, p. 445)
hypertonic (hī-pĕr-TŎN-ĭk, p. 439)
hyperventilation (p. 447)
hypervolemia (hī-pĕr-vō-LĒ-mē-ă, p. 441)
hypocalcemia (hī-pō-kăl-SĒ-mē-ă, p. 444)
hypochloremia (hī-pō-klōr-Ē-mē-ă, p. 445)
hypokalemia (hī-pō-kă-LĒ-mē-ă, p. 442)
hypomagnesemia (hī-pō-măg-nĕ-SĒ-mē-ă, p. 444)
hyponatremia (hī-pō-nă-TRĒ-mē-ă, p. 441)
hypophosphatemia (hī-pō-fŏs-faw-TĒ-mē-ă, p. 445)
hypotonic (hī-pō-TŎN-ĭk, p. 439)
hypovolemia (hī-pō-vō-LĒ-mē-ă, p. 437)
interstitial (ĭn-tĕr-STĬSH-ăl, p. 437)
intracellular (ĭn-tră-SĔL-ū-lăr, p. 437)
intravascular (ĭn-tră-văs-kū-lăr, p. 437)
isotonic (ī-sō-TŎN-ĭk, p. 439)
osmosis (ŏz-MŌ-sĭs, p. 438)
tetany (TĔT-ă-nē, p. 447)
transcellular (trăns-SĒ-lū-lăr, p. 437)
turgor (p. 440)

COMPOSITION OF BODY FLUIDS

WATER

The two largest constituents of the body fluids are water and electrolytes. Water is present in greater proportion than electrolytes. Water serves many functions, but the four main functions of water in the body are (1) as a vehicle for the transportation of substances to and from the cells; (2) to aid heat regulation by providing perspiration, which evaporates; (3) to assist maintenance of hydrogen (H^+) balance in the body; and (4) to serve as a medium for the enzymatic action of digestion.

Over half of the body's weight is water. The amount varies by age, sex, and health status. The adult male body contains about 60% water; the adult female body, because of more fat tissue, contains about 50% water. The greater the amount of fat the body contains, the less the percentage of water it has because fat contains less water than other tissue. **The infant and the elderly person are more quickly and seriously affected by minor changes in their fluid balance and can become rapidly dehydrated.** The infant, because of its large body surface compared with body weight, loses more fluid through the skin than the adult. The

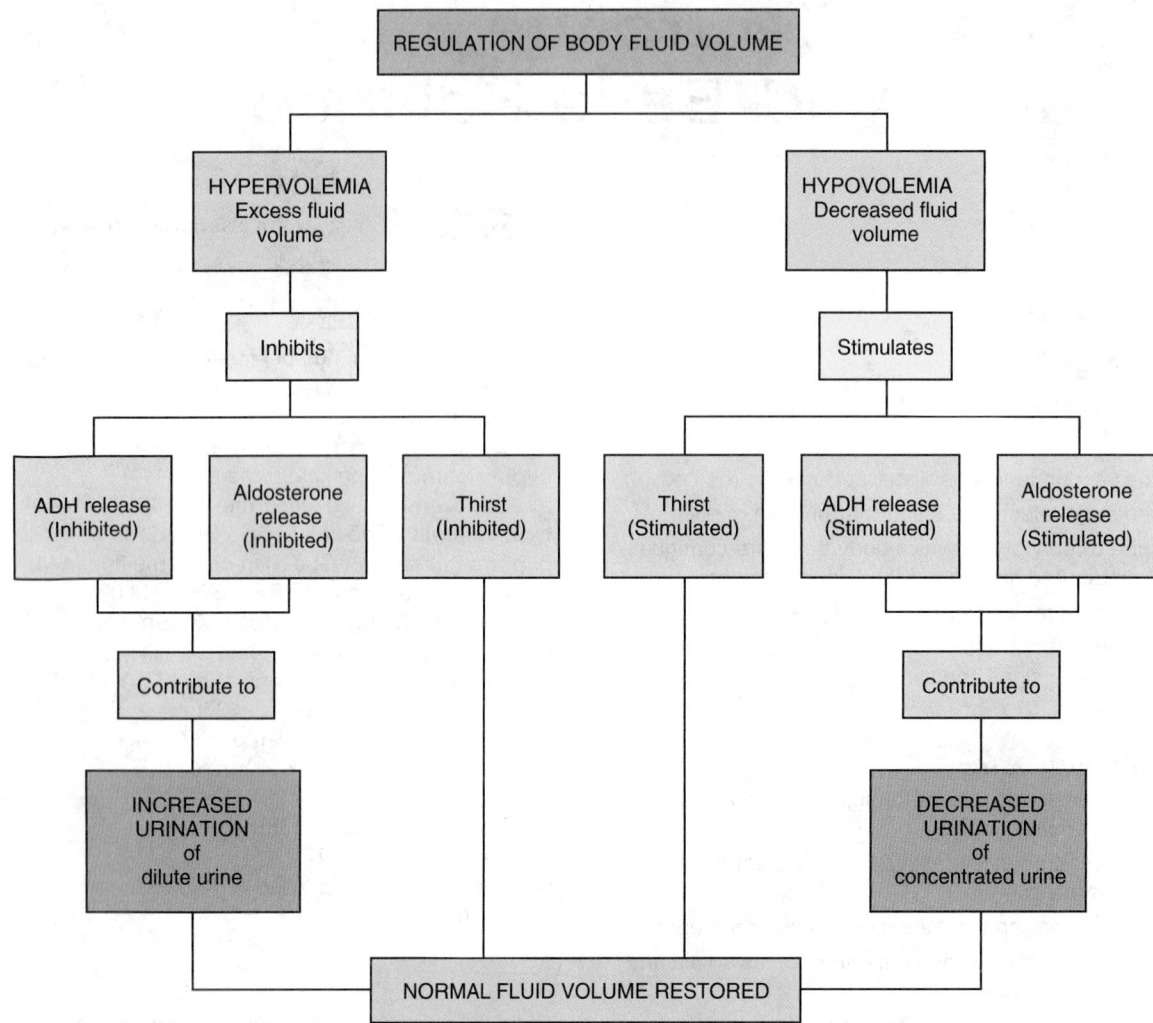

CONCEPT MAP **25-1** Regulation of body fluid volume.

kidneys of the infant are not as efficient as the adult's and less fluid is reabsorbed. The elderly person has an age-related decline in total body water, diminished thirst sensation, a decrease in urine-concentrating ability of the kidney, and a decrease in effectiveness of antidiuretic hormone. These factors cause dehydration to occur more quickly than in the younger adult. Dehydration may cause hypovolemia (Concept Map 25-1). If an excess of fluid volume is present in the body, hypervolemia occurs.

Water is critical to maintaining a state of homeostasis because water is the medium in which most metabolic and chemical reactions in the body take place. Without sufficient water, cells cannot function and death results.

Water is the avenue for transportation within the body. It carries nutrients to the cells and transports wastes for excretion. Body water continually moves in and out of the blood, through the lymph vessels, between the cells, and in and out of the cells. Table shows sources of water and avenues of water

Table 25-1 | *Sources of Water and Avenues of Loss*

SOURCES	24 HOURS	AVENUES OF LOSS	
Oral fluids	1500 mL	Urine	1500 mL
Food	800 mL	Perspiration	400 mL
Metabolism	200 mL	Feces	200 mL
		Expired air	400 mL
Total	2500 mL		2500 mL

? *Think Critically About . . .* How might NPO (nothing by mouth) status before tests or surgery affect a person's water balance?

ELECTROLYTES

Electrolytes are minerals or salts that are dissolved in body fluid. When in solution, they break up into particles known as *ions* that have a tiny electrical charge. The ions develop a positive electrical charge and are then known as *cations,* or they develop a negative electrical charge and are *anions.* **For each positively**

Table 25-2 | *The Major Electrolytes: Normal Range and Function*

ELECTROLYTE	NORMAL RANGE	FUNCTION
Sodium (Na^+)	135-145 mEq/L	Major cation of the extracellular fluid. Major role in regulation of water balance. Regulates extracellular fluid volume through osmotic pressure. Water follows sodium concentration in the body. Essential to the transmission of nerve impulses and helps maintain neuromuscular irritability. Important in controlling contractility of the heart. Helps maintain acid–base balance. Aids in maintenance of electroneutrality.
Potassium (K^+)	3.5-5.0 mEq/L	Major intracellular cation. Important to nerve transmission and muscle contraction. Helps maintain normal heart rhythm. Helps maintain plasma acid–base balance.
Calcium (Ca^{2+})	8.4-10.6 mg/dL	Involved in formation of bone and teeth. Necessary for blood coagulation. Essential for normal nerve and muscle activity.
Magnesium (Mg^{2+})	1.3-2.1 mg/dL	Necessary for building bones and teeth. Necessary for nerve transmission and is involved in muscle contraction. Plays an important role in many metabolic reactions, where it acts as a cofactor to cellular enzymes.
Phosphate (PO_4^{3-})	2.7-4.5 mg/dL	Necessary for formation of adenosine triphosphate (ATP). Cofactor in carbohydrate, protein, and lipid metabolism. Activates B-complex vitamins.
Chloride (Cl^-)	96-106 mEq/L	Helps maintain acid–base balance. Important to formation of hydrochloric acid for secretion to the stomach. Aids in maintaining plasma electroneutrality.
Bicarbonate (HCO_3^-)	22-26 mEq/L	A buffer that neutralizes excess acids in the body. Helps regulate acid–base balance.

charged cation in a fluid compartment, there must be a negatively charged anion so that a balance is maintained. As fluids move from compartment to compartment, the body works to maintain homeostasis in each compartment by balancing the anions and cations so that there is electrical neutrality. Electrolytes move within the body freely, but each has a primary location. Because disturbances in homeostasis upset the normal balance of electrolytes, the location and function of each electrolyte become important in understanding what is occurring in the body. **The major source of electrolytes is from the diet.** Table 25-2 presents the electrolytes, their normal ranges, and functions.

NONELECTROLYTES

The intermediate products of metabolism—amino acids (proteins), glucose, and fatty acids—are nonelectrolytes. They remain bound together when dissolved in body fluid. In the healthy individual who is eating normally, the nonelectrolytes circulating in the body fluid remain stable.

BLOOD

There are 4 to 6 L of circulating blood volume in the body, depending on body size and sex. Erythrocytes (red cells), leukocytes (white cells), and platelets (thrombocytes) are the blood cells that are carried in the plasma. **Any condition that alters body fluid volume also alters the plasma volume of the blood, and can affect blood pressure and circulation.** The plasma proteins and colloids contribute to plasma colloid osmotic pressure, which helps keep fluid in the vascular compartment.

Table 25-3 | *Body Fluid Distribution*

BODY FLUID	DISTRIBUTION
Extracellular fluid	Approximately ⅓ of total body water. Transports water, nutrients, oxygen, waste, etc., to and from the cells. Regulated by renal, metabolic, and neurologic factors. **High in sodium (Na^+) content.**
Intravascular fluid	Fluid within the blood vessels. Consists of plasma and fluid within blood cells. Contains large amounts of protein and electrolytes.
Interstitial fluid	Fluid in the spaces surrounding the cells. **High in sodium (Na^+) content.**
Transcellular fluid	Includes aqueous humor; saliva; cerebrospinal, pleural, peritoneal, synovial, and pericardial fluids; gastrointestinal secretions; and fluid in urinary system and lymphatics.
Intracellular fluid	About ⅔ of total body fluid. Fluid contained within the cell walls. Most cell walls are permeable to water. **High in potassium (K^+) content.**

DISTRIBUTION OF BODY FLUIDS

Body fluids are either intracellular (within the cell) or extracellular (outside of the cell). Extracellular fluid (ECF) is of three types: intravascular, interstitial, and transcellular. Table 25-3 describes these fluids. When fluid shifts from the plasma in the vascular space out to the interstitial space, blood volume drops and dehydration (removal of water from a tissue) and hypovolemia (decreased volume of plasma) may occur.

MOVEMENT OF FLUID AND ELECTROLYTES

The amount of fluid leaving the body should be balanced by water entering it. Water is taken in through the ingestion of fluids and food and is produced by cell metabolism. The thirst mechanism located in the hypothalamus helps control fluid balance in the body. It monitors fluid volume and concentration. Hypothalamic receptors sense when fluid is more concentrated and stimulate nerve impulses that are interpreted in the brain as thirst, which motivates the person to drink. Intake of sufficient water lowers the concentration and the receptors are no longer stimulated.

Fluid is lost in the urine and feces and through *insensible* (invisible) losses via exhaled air and through the skin as perspiration. **The kidney is the main organ through which fluid excretion is achieved.** Several hormones affect urine output, particularly antidiuretic hormone (ADH), aldosterone, and atrial natriuretic peptide (ANP). ADH is secreted by the posterior pituitary. More ADH is released when the blood becomes more concentrated or there is decreased circulating blood volume, and during times of pain, nausea, and stress. When this occurs, the renal tubules reabsorb more water, and urine output decreases. Aldosterone is released by the adrenal cortex when ECF volume is low or when sodium concentration is elevated, causing reabsorption of sodium from kidney tubules. This creates an osmotic gradient by which more water is retained. The release of aldosterone is stimulated by the renin-angiotensin-aldosterone system. ANP acts to protect the body from fluid overload and is released from sites in the myocardium and the brain. Blood volume and pressure also affect the glomerular filtration rate and urine output.

Water and the substances suspended or dissolved in it must move from compartment to compartment so that they are normally distributed within the body. They must pass through the semipermeable membranes of the body's cells to do this. The heart circulates blood throughout the body. As the blood flows through the capillaries, fluid and solutes can move into the interstitial spaces, where substances in every cell of the body can be exchanged. Several processes move fluids, electrolytes, nutrients, and waste products back and forth across the cell membranes (Figure 25-1).

Passive Transport

Diffusion. Diffusion is the process by which substances move back and forth across the membrane until they are evenly distributed throughout the available space. Substances will move from a high to a low concentration until the concentration on both sides of the membrane is equal. This is called movement down a concentration gradient. Glucose, oxygen, carbon dioxide, water, and other small ions and molecules move by diffusion. It is a process of equalization.

Diffusion may occur by movement along an electrical gradient as well. The attraction between particles of opposite charge and the repellent action between particles of like charge comprise an electrical gradient. Many intracellular proteins have a negative charge that tends to attract the positively charged sodium and potassium ions from the ECF.

Osmosis. Osmosis refers to the movement of pure solvent (liquid) across a membrane. Water diffuses by osmosis. When there are differences in concentration of fluids in the various compartments, water will be moved from the area of less solute concentration to the area of greater concentration until the solutions in the compartments are of equal concentration. The process takes place via a semipermeable membrane—a membrane that allows some substances to pass through but prevents the passage of other substances. Fluid moves between the interstitial and intracellular and the interstitial and intravascular compartments by osmosis. Cell wall membranes are semipermeable, as are the walls of blood vessels.

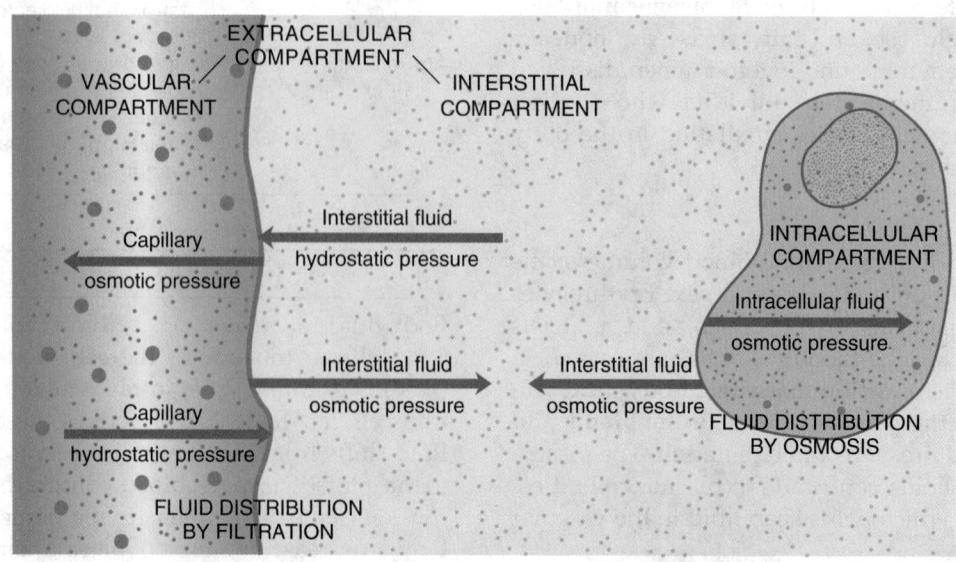

FIGURE **25-1** Factors that influence body fluid distribution.

When living cells are surrounded by a solution that has the same concentration of particles, the water concentration of the intracellular and extracellular fluids will be equal. Such a solution is termed isotonic (of equal solute concentration). If cells are surrounded by a solution that has a greater concentration of solute than the cells, the water in the cells will move to the more concentrated solution and the cells will dehydrate and shrink. The solution is hypertonic (of greater concentration) in relation to the cells. If the cells are surrounded by a solution that has less solute than the cells, the solution is hypotonic (of less concentration) in relation to the cells. The particles within the cells exert an osmotic pressure, drawing water inward through the semipermeable membrane. The cells swell from the extra fluid (overhydrate). These concepts are important to the administration of intravenous fluids (see Chapter 36). Solutions are classified as isotonic, hypertonic, or hypotonic according to their concentration of electrolytes and other solutes. **So, by osmosis water passes rather freely across cell membranes.** The process of osmosis is essential to the life of the cells and to the balance of water and electrolytes in the body. Osmotic pressure within vessels helps to keep fluid from leaking out into the interstitial spaces (Figure 25-2).

Filtration. Filtration is the movement of water and suspended substances outward through a semipermeable membrane. The pumping action of the heart creates hydrostatic pressure (pressure exerted by fluid) within the capillaries. Hydrostatic pressure causes fluid to press outward on the vessel. That force promotes filtration, forcing movement of water and electrolytes through the capillary wall to the interstitial fluid.

Active Transport

Active transport, contrary to diffusion, osmosis, and filtration, requires cellular energy. This force can move molecules into cells regardless of their electrical charge or the concentrations already in the cell. **Active transport may move substances from an area of lower concentration to an area of higher concentration.** The energy source for the process is adenosine triphosphate (ATP). ATP is produced during the complex metabolic processes in the body's cells. Enzyme reactions metabolize carbon chains of sugars, fatty acids, and amino acids, yielding carbon dioxide, water, and high-energy phosphate bonds. Active transport can

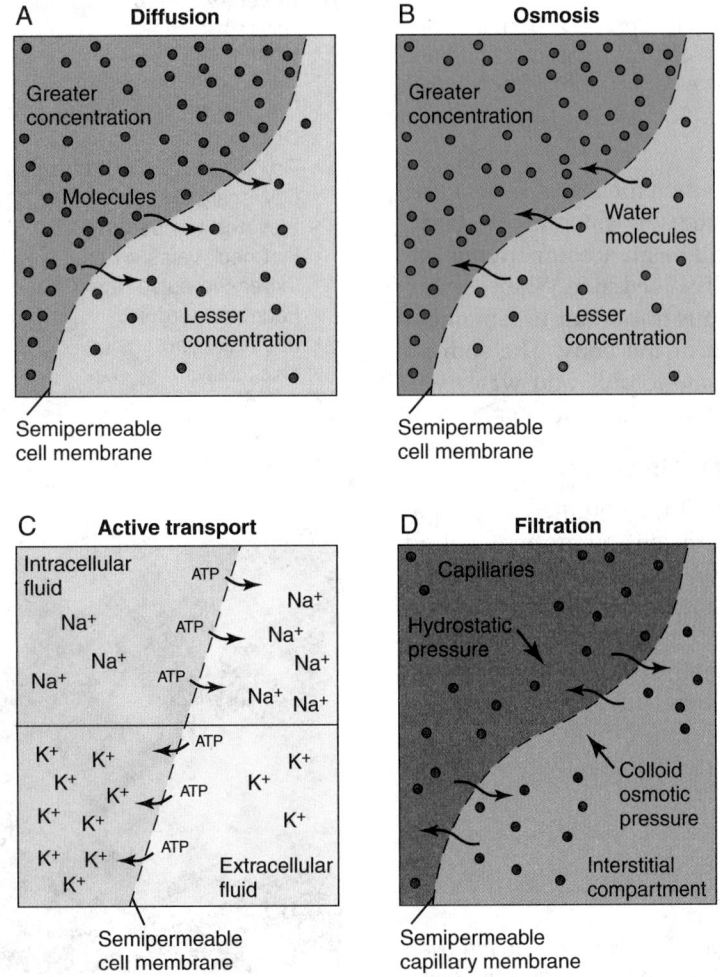

FIGURE **25-2** Movement of water and electrolytes by **A,** diffusion; **B,** osmosis; **C,** active transport; and **D,** filtration.

move amino acids, glucose, iron, hydrogen, sodium, potassium, and calcium through the cell membrane.

FLUID AND ELECTROLYTE IMBALANCES

Healthy people maintain intake and output balance by drinking sufficient fluids and eating a balanced diet each day. **The healthy kidney regulates fluid and electrolyte balance by regulating the volume and composition of extracellular fluid.** Illness affects fluid balance in many ways. The patient may be unable to ingest food or liquids, there may be a problem with absorption from the intestinal tract, or there may be a kidney impairment that affects excretion or reabsorption of water and electrolytes. Any disease that affects circulation (e.g., congestive heart failure) will ultimately affect the distribution and composition of body fluids. Burns, in which large amounts of body fluid may be lost through open wounds, also present problems of fluid balance. **In fact, any seriously ill patient is at risk for a fluid and electrolyte imbalance.**

 Elder Care Points

Any patient over age 65 is at risk for confusion from fluid and electrolyte imbalance. Always look for signs of a fluid and electrolyte imbalance when an elderly patient becomes confused.

A fluid imbalance exists when there is an excess (too much) or a deficit (too little) of water in the body. When this occurs, there will be an accompanying imbalance in the substances dissolved in it. When considering sodium imbalances, it is important to remember that water follows sodium in the body. The sodium concentration causes an osmotic pull, and water will go to where that concentration is highest.

DEFICIENT FLUID VOLUME

Those at risk for deficient fluid volume are (1) patients unable to take in sufficient quantities of fluid because of impaired swallowing, extreme weakness, disorientation or coma, or the unavailability of water; and (2) patients who lose excessive amounts of fluid through prolonged vomiting, diarrhea, hemorrhage, diaphoresis (sweating), or excessive wound drainage. Treatments that can cause a fluid deficit are diuretic therapy and gastrointestinal suction without fluid replacement.

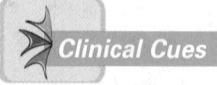 **Clinical Cues**

Keep an accurate record of the amount of drainage removed by suction so that adequate fluid can be replaced and dehydration can be avoided.

Burns and drainage from large wounds or fistulas can deplete the fluid volume. Treatment of fluid volume deficit involves remedying the underlying cause and replacing fluids.

Dehydration

When a fluid deficit occurs, it causes loss of water from the cells (dehydration); when there is too little water in the plasma, water is drawn out of the cells by osmosis to equalize the concentration, and the cells shrivel. Dehydration is treated by fluid administration, either orally or intravenously.

Signs and symptoms of dehydration are listed in Box 25-1. Tissue turgor (degree of elasticity) is checked by gently pinching up the skin over the abdomen, forearm, sternum, forehead, or thigh (Figure 25-3). In a person with normal fluid balance, the skin when pinched will immediately fall back to normal when released. If a fluid deficit is present, the skin may remain elevated or tented for several seconds after the pinch. This test measures skin elasticity as well and is not a valid indicator of fluid status in the elderly. Weight loss is another sign of dehydration. In the in-

Box 25-1 *Signs and Symptoms of Dehydration (Fluid Volume Deficit)*

- Complaints of dizziness
- Dark, concentrated urine
- Decreased urine production
- Dry mucous membrane
- Dry, cracked lips and tongue
- Dry, scaly skin
- Elevated temperature
- Flat neck veins when lying down
- Increased pulse rate
- Poor skin turgor
- Postural hypotension
- Thick saliva
- Thirst
- Weak, thready pulse
- Weakness

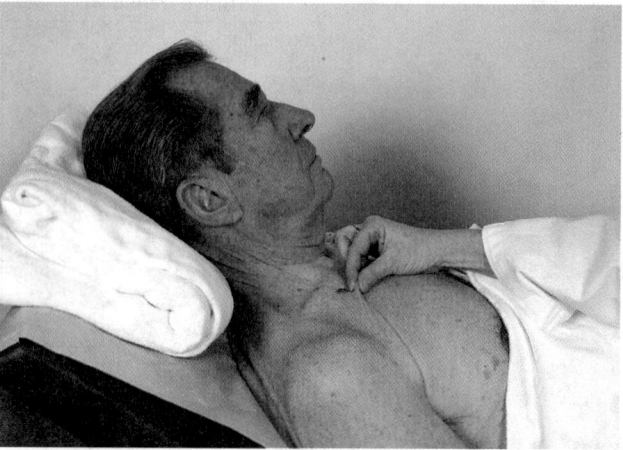

FIGURE **25-3** Testing for tissue turgor and signs of dehydration.

fant, severe fluid deficit is evident by sunken eyeballs and depression of the anterior fontanel.

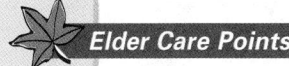
Elder Care Points

The elderly person who suffers from nausea, vomiting, or diarrhea is especially prone to dehydration. If the person has fever, this adds to the fluid loss. Because of the fluid and accompanying electrolyte losses, the person may become confused. Offering the patient small amounts of liquid frequently, if it can be kept down, or an electrolyte solution such as Gatorade, helps prevent additional problems.

EXCESS FLUID VOLUME

Healthy people do not ordinarily drink too much water. When people become ill they may take in more water than they excrete. This can happen if they receive intravenous fluid too quickly, are given tap water enemas, or are persuaded to drink more fluids than they can eliminate. If these events happen, the patient will suffer a fluid volume excess. Impaired elimination, such as occurs in renal failure, is an important cause of fluid volume excess. **Signs of overhydration are weight gain, crackles in the lungs, slow bounding pulse, elevated blood pressure, and possibly edema.** When fluid volume excess occurs, hypervolemia (excessive blood volume) may also occur. Hypervolemia causes an elevation of blood pressure.

Edema

Edema is an excessive accumulation of interstitial (tissue) fluid. It is often a sign of fluid overload, but may be from other causes. In ambulatory patients, the excessive fluid tends to accumulate in the lower extremities (Figure 25-4). In the bedridden patient, the fluid accumulates in the sacral region. These types of fluid accumulations are termed *dependent edema*. Generalized edema occurs when excess interstitial fluid is spread throughout the body. It is most visible in the hands and face, where swelling is detectable. Causes of generalized edema are (1) kidney failure, (2) heart failure, (3) liver failure, and (4) hormonal disorders involving the overproduction of aldosterone and ADH (Figure 25-5). Local edema may be caused by infection or injury and the resulting inflammation.

Treatment involves correcting the underlying cause and assisting the body to rebalance fluid content. Fluid intake may be restricted or diuretic drugs may be administered to cause excretion of the excess fluid. A diuretic is a drug that causes the kidneys to increase the excretion of fluid.

Think Critically About . . . Why should you auscultate the lungs of elderly patients who are receiving intravenous fluids even if they have no current lung problems?

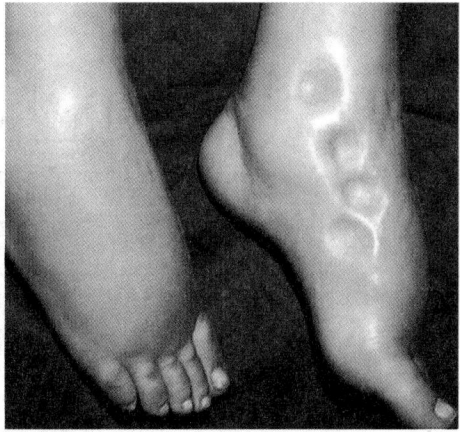
FIGURE 25-4 Example of pitting edema from fluid excess. The finger depressions do not refill quickly after pressure has been exerted.

ELECTROLYTE IMBALANCES

A summary of the normal ranges of the major electrolytes, the causes of imbalances, the signs and symptoms of imbalances, and nursing interventions is provided in Table 25-4.

Sodium Imbalances

Hyponatremia. **A deficit of sodium in the blood is called** hyponatremia (Na^+ <135 mEq/L). This can occur from a sodium loss or an excess of water. **This is the most common electrolyte imbalance patients experience.** Sodium loss may occur from excessive vomiting or diarrhea, in which fluid loss is replaced with plain water. Decreased secretion of aldosterone can result in sodium loss. Congestive heart failure, liver disease with ascites (abnormal accumulation of fluid within the peritoneal cavity), and sometimes chronic renal failure result in excessive water retention without concurrent sodium retention. This results in a hypervolemia combined with hyponatremia. The average intake of sodium is 6 to 12 g/day. If there is a problem with water balance, sodium may be restricted in the diet.

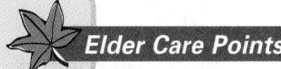
Elder Care Points

Elderly patients are more susceptible to hyponatremia than younger ones. Those taking thiazide diuretics or selective serotonin reuptake inhibitors (SSRIs) are particularly at risk for hyponatremia. The problem is especially prevalent in long-term care residents.

Hypernatremia. **When the serum sodium concentration rises above 145 mEq/L, a state of** hypernatremia **exists.** This occurs when there is an excess of sodium or a loss of body water. Excessive administration of sodium bicarbonate for the treatment of acidosis (excess of acid or depletion of alkaline substances in the blood and body tissues) is one cause. More commonly,

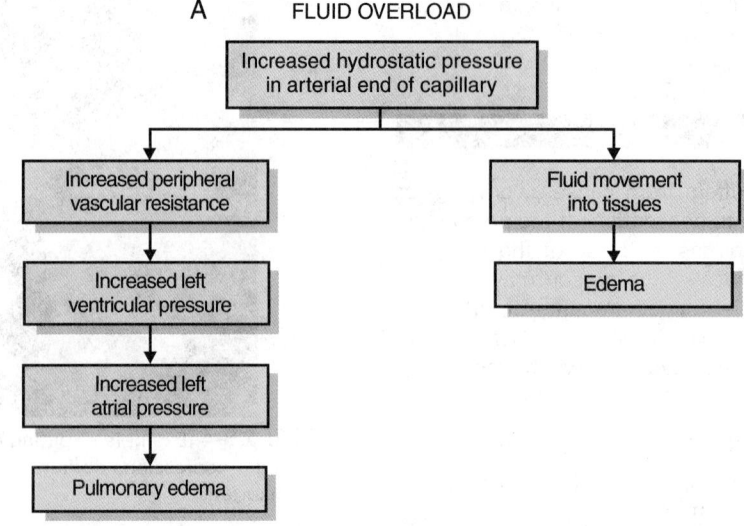

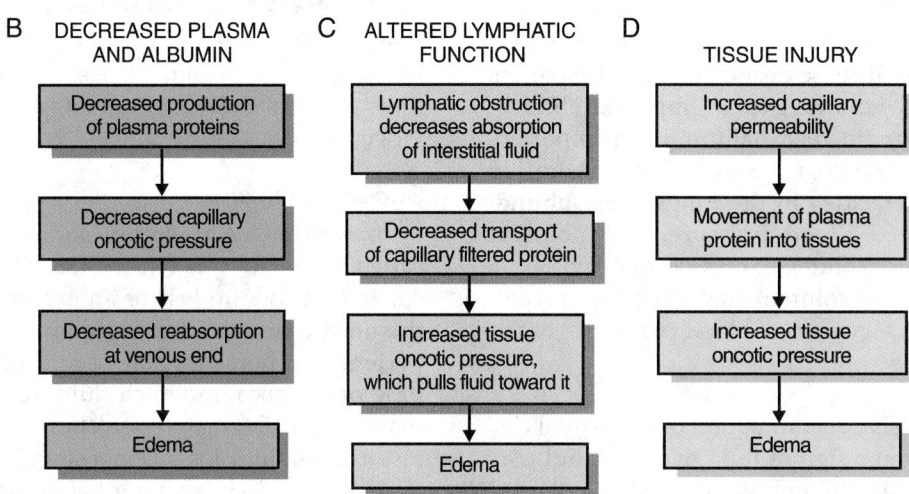

FIGURE **25-5** Mechanisms of edema formation. **A,** Fluid overload; **B,** decreased plasma and albumin; **C,** altered lymphatic function; and **D,** tissue injury.

water loss from fever, respiratory infection, or watery diarrhea is the cause.

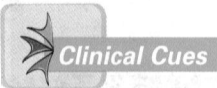

Patients on long-term corticosteroids that cause potassium depletion may develop hypernatremia. Observe for signs of edema in these patients.

Decreased water intake may occur in immobile, confused, or dependent patients or in those who have sustained damage to the thirst center in the hypothalamus. The body tries to correct the situation by conserving water through reabsorption in the renal tubules. Hypernatremia causes an osmotic shift of fluid from the cells to the interstitial spaces, causing a cellular dehydration and interruption of normal cell processes. Sodium intake is restricted for the patient with hypernatremia (Patient Teaching 25-1, p. 445).

Potassium Imbalances

Hypokalemia. **When the potassium level falls below 3.5 mEq/L,** hypokalemia **exists.** Extra potassium must be given to help correct the imbalance. Hypokalemia may occur due to poor diet, illness causing a shift of potassium from ECF to intracellular fluid (ICF), or increased potassium loss. Vomiting, diarrhea, gastrointestinal (GI) suction, excessive sweating, and diuretic therapy may deplete potassium levels. The patient is encouraged to eat foods high in potassium (Patient Teaching 25-2, p. 445), and intravenous replacement may be necessary (Safety Alert 25-1, p. 445).

Hyperkalemia. **When serum potassium level rises above 5.0 mEq/L, a state of** hyperkalemia **exists.** Patients with severe burns or crush injuries and those undergoing major surgery are at risk for hyperkalemia. The mechanical disruption of cell membranes causes a shift of potassium from the ICF to the ECF. Hyperkalemia occurs in renal failure, overuse of potassium-sparing diuretics, digitalis toxicity, overuse

Table 25-4 | *Electrolyte Imbalances*

SERUM VALUE	SIGNS AND SYMPTOMS	CAUSES/RISK FACTORS	NURSING INTERVENTIONS
SODIUM: NORMAL RANGE: 135-145 mEq/L			
<135 mEq/L	Central nervous system and neuromuscular changes resulting from failure of swollen cells to transmit electrical impulses. Mental confusion, altered level of consciousness, anxiety, coma, anorexia, nausea, vomiting, muscle cramps, seizures, decreased sensation.	Inadequate sodium intake, as in patients on low-sodium diets. Excessive intake or retention of water (kidney failure and heart failure). Loss of bile, which is rich in sodium, as a result of fistulas, drainage, gastrointestinal surgery, nausea and vomiting, and suction. Loss of sodium through burn wounds. Administration of IV fluids that do not contain electrolytes.	Restrict water intake as ordered for patients with congestive heart failure, kidney failure, and inadequate antidiuretic hormone production. Liberalize diet of patient on low-sodium diet. Closely monitor patient receiving IV solutions to correct hyponatremia. Replace water loss with fluids containing sodium.
>145 mEq/L	Dry mucous membranes, loss of skin turgor, intense thirst, flushed skin, oliguria, and possibly elevated temperature; weakness, lethargy, irritability, twitching, seizures, coma, intracranial bleeding.	High-sodium diet, inadequate water intake as in comatose, mentally confused, or debilitated patient. Excessive sweating, diarrhea, failure of kidney to reabsorb water from urine. Administration of high-protein, hyperosmotic tube feedings and osmotic diuretics.	Encourage increased fluid intake; measure I & O; give water between tube feedings; restrict sodium intake; monitor temperature.
POTASSIUM: NORMAL RANGE: 3.5-5.0 mEq/L			
<3.5 mEq/L	Abdominal pain, gaseous distention of intestines; cardiac dysrhythmias, muscle weakness, decreased reflexes, paralysis, paralytic ileus, urinary retention, lethargy, confusion, electrocardiogram (ECG) changes, increased urinary pH.	Inadequate intake of potassium-rich foods. Loss of potassium in urine when kidneys do not reabsorb the mineral. Loss of potassium from intestinal tract as a result of diarrhea or vomiting, drainage from fistulas, overuse of gastric suction. Improper use of diuretics.	Instruct patients (especially those taking diuretics) about foods high in potassium content; encourage intake. Observe closely for signs of digitalis toxicity in patients taking this drug. Teach patients to watch for signs of hypokalemia. Administer potassium chloride supplement as ordered. Monitor I & O and cardiac rhythm.
>5.0 mEq/L	Muscle weakness, hypotension, paresthesias, paralysis, cardiac dysrhythmias, ECG changes.	Conditions that alter kidney function or decrease kidney's ability to excrete potassium. Intestinal obstruction that prevents elimination of potassium in the feces. Addison's disease, digitalis toxicity, uncontrolled diabetes mellitus, insulin deficit, crushing injuries, and burns.	Decrease intake of foods high in potassium. Increase fluid intake to enhance urinary excretion of potassium; provide adequate carbohydrate intake to prevent use of body proteins for energy. Carefully administer proper dose of insulin to diabetic patients. Instruct patient in proper use of salt substitutes containing potassium.
CALCIUM: NORMAL RANGE: 8.4-10.6 mg/dL			
<8.4 mg/dL	Paresthesias, seizures, muscle spasms, tetany, hand spasm, positive Chvostek's sign, positive Trousseau's sign, cardiac dysrhythmia, wheezing, dyspnea, difficulty swallowing, colic, cardiac failure.	Inadequate dietary intake of calcium and vitamin D. Impaired absorption of calcium from intestinal tract, as in diarrhea, sprue, overuse of laxatives and enemas containing phosphates (phosphorus tends to be more readily absorbed from the intestinal tract than calcium and suppresses calcium retention in the body). The parathyroid regulates calcium and phosphorus levels. Hyposecretion of parathyroid hormone can result in hypocalcemia.	Encourage adults to consume sufficient calcium from cheese, broccoli, shrimp, and other dietary sources. Have 10% calcium gluconate solution at bedside of patient having thyroidectomy in case of surgical damage to the parathyroid glands. Give all oral medicines containing calcium ½ hour before meals to facilitate absorption.

Key: *ECG,* Electrocardiogram; *I & O,* intake and output; *IV,* intravenous.

Continued

Table 25-4 *Electrolyte Imbalances—cont'd*

SERUM VALUE	SIGNS AND SYMPTOMS	CAUSES/RISK FACTORS	NURSING INTERVENTIONS
CALCIUM: NORMAL RANGE: 8.4-10.6 mg/dL—cont'd			
>10.6 gm/dL	Anorexia, abdominal pain, constipation, polyuria, confusion, renal calculi, pathologic fractures, cardiac arrest.	Excess intake of calcium, as in patient taking antacids indiscriminately. Excess intake of vitamin D. Conditions that cause movement of calcium out of bones and into extracellular fluid (e.g., bone tumor, multiple fractures). Tumors of the lung, stomach, and kidney, and multiple myeloma. Immobility and osteoporosis.	Administer diuretics as prescribed to increase urinary output and calcium excretion. Monitor I & O; encourage high fluid intake (3000-4000 mL/day).
MAGNESIUM: NORMAL RANGE: 1.3-2.1 mEq/L			
<1.3 mEq/L	Insomnia, hyperactive reflexes, leg and foot cramps, twitching, tremors, seizures, cardiac arrhythmias, positive Chvostek's sign, positive Trousseau's sign, vertigo, hypocalcemia and hypokalemia.	Chronic malnutrition; chronic diarrhea. Bowel resection with ileostomy or colostomy; chronic alcoholism; prolonged gastric suction; acute pancreatitis; biliary or intestinal fistula; osmotic diuretic therapy; diabetic ketoacidosis.	Diet counseling to help patients at risk increase level of magnesium (e.g., milk and cereals). Monitor closely IV infusions of magnesium. Monitor I & O.
>2.1 mEq/L	Hypotension; sweating and flushing, nausea and vomiting; muscle weakness, paralysis, respiratory depression; cardiac dysrhythmias.	Overuse of antacids and cathartics containing magnesium; aspiration of sea water, as in near drowning. Chronic kidney failure.	Teach patients to avoid abuse of laxatives and antacids; instruct patients with renal problems to avoid over-the-counter drugs that contain magnesium. Encourage fluid intake to increase urinary excretion of magnesium if not contraindicated. Monitor I & O. Administer diuretics as ordered.
PHOSPHATE: NORMAL RANGE: 2.7-4.5 mg/dL			
<2.7 mg/dL	Confusion, seizures, numbness, weakness, possible coma. Chronic state may cause rickets and osteomalacia.	Vitamin D deficiency or hyperparathyroidism; use of aluminum-containing antacids.	Assess for vitamin D deficiency, hyperparathyroidism, or overuse of aluminum-containing antacids.
>4.5 mg/dL	Anorexia, nausea, vomiting.	Renal insufficiency.	Assess for restlessness, confusion, chest pain, and cyanosis. Monitor respirations. Check all electrolyte levels.

of potassium-containing salt substitutes, uncontrolled diabetes mellitus, and a variety of other illnesses.

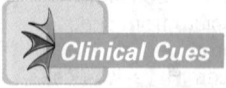
Clinical Cues

Hyperkalemia can cause life-threatening cardiac arrhythmia. Tall or peaked T waves may be seen on ECG. P waves may be small.

Calcium Imbalances

Hypocalcemia. **When the calcium level drops below 8.4 mg/dL,** hypocalcemia **occurs.** This can occur from nutritional deficiency of calcium or vitamin D. Hypocalcemia occurs in disorders in which there is a shift of calcium into the bone. Metastatic cancer invading bone is one such cause. Removal or injury of the parathyroid glands during thyroidectomy causes parathyroid hormone deficiency and consequent hypocalcemia. Excessive infusion of bicarbonate solution, alkalosis (excess of alkaline or decrease of acid substances in the blood and body fluids), blood transfusions, and hypoparathyroidism may cause hypocalcemia.

Hypercalcemia. Hypercalcemia, **a serum calcium level above 10.6 mg/dL,** can occur during periods of lengthy immobilization when calcium is mobilized from the bone or when an excess of calcium or vitamin D is taken into the body. Most cases are related to hyperparathyroidism or malignancy in which there is metastasis with bone resorption. Such malignancies include multiple myeloma and lung or renal cancers.

Magnesium Imbalances

Hypomagnesemia. Hypomagnesemia, **a serum level below 1.3 mEq/L,** results from malabsorption, malnutrition, or increased loss from renal tubular dysfunction

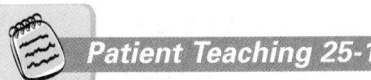

Foods High in Sodium

The patient experiencing a fluid volume excess or who is to decrease sodium intake should avoid the foods listed below. The patient who is low in sodium may add some of these foods to the diet.

- Buttermilk
- Canned meats or fish
- Canned soups (regular)
- Canned vegetables (regular)
- Casserole and pasta mixes
- Catsup
- Cheese (all kinds)
- Lunch meats
- Dried fruits
- Dried soup mixes
- Foods containing monosodium glutamate (MSG)
- Frozen vegetables with sauces
- Gravy mixes
- Ham
- Hot dogs
- Olives
- Pickles
- Prepared mustard
- Preserved meats
- Processed foods
- Salted nuts
- Salted popcorn
- Salted snack foods
- Softened water high in sodium
- Regular soy sauce
- Tomato or vegetable juice

Foods High in Potassium

The patient with hypokalemia should be encouraged to add the foods listed below to the daily diet. Patients in renal failure may need to restrict their intake of these foods.

- Apricots
- Avocados
- Bananas
- Cantaloupe
- Codfish
- Dates
- Meats
- Milk
- Orange juice
- Oranges
- Potatoes
- Raisins
- Salmon
- Tuna

or thiazide diuretic use. Extensive gastric suction or diarrhea can also cause it. Hypomagnesemia usually is present when hypokalemia and hypocalcemia occur.

Hypermagnesemia. Hypermagnesemia, **a serum level above 2.1 mEq/L,** occurs rarely and usually in the presence of renal failure, although magnesium-containing laxatives or antacids or severe dehydration can cause it.

Anion Imbalances

Imbalances of chloride, phosphate, and bicarbonate accompany cation imbalances because of the principle of electroneutrality. Hypochloremia, **a chloride level below 96 mEq/L, is associated with hyponatremia.** It can also occur with severe vomiting and is seen as a compensatory decrease in acid–base disorders. Hyperchloremia, **a chloride level above 106 mEq/L, occurs along**

Hypokalemia

Severe hypokalemia (K$^+$ < 2.5 mEq/L) may cause cardiac arrest. Potassium-wasting diuretics used without potassium replacement can cause hypokalemia. Premature ventricular contractions and changes in the ECG pattern such as ST segment depression, a prolonged Q-T interval, and U wave occurrence may be seen.

with hypernatremia and a form of metabolic acidosis. Hypophosphatemia **occurs when the level of phosphate falls below 3.0 mg/dL.** It may result from use of aluminum-containing antacids that bind phosphate, from vitamin D deficiency, or from hyperparathyroidism. Hyperphosphatemia, **a phosphate level above 4.5 mg/dL, commonly occurs in renal failure.**

? *Think Critically About . . .*

- Why may some elderly people have a low serum calcium even though they take in sufficient calcium in the diet?
- What type of fluid and electrolyte imbalances can occur in the patient who is undergoing diuretic therapy? Why?

ACID–BASE BALANCE

Acid–base balance is very important to maintaining homeostasis in the body because cell enzymes can function only within a very narrow range of pH.

pH

pH is a measure of the degree to which a solution is acidic or alkaline. Cell metabolism constantly produces carbon dioxide, which combines with water to form carbonic acid (H_2CO_3), which immediately breaks down into hydrogen ions and bicarbonate ions. The concentration of hydrogen ions (H$^+$) determines the pH reading. **The normal serum pH is 7.35 to 7.45.** Death may occur at a serum pH below 6.8 or above 7.8. Because of the production of acids by the body's metabolic systems, there is a tendency for the body to become acidic if homeostasis is upset.

BICARBONATE

Bicarbonate is a very important substance in maintaining acid–base balance. **The normal range of bicarbonate (HCO$_3^-$) is 22 to 26 mEq/L.** The major function of this alkaline electrolyte is the regulation of the acid–base balance in the body. Bicarbonate acts as a buffer to neutralize the excess acids in the body and maintain the bicarbonate-to–carbonic acid ratio at 20:1, which is needed for homeostasis. The kidneys selectively reabsorb or excrete bicarbonate to regulate serum levels and help maintain acid–base balance.

CONTROL MECHANISMS

For the serum pH to remain within the normal range of 7.35 to 7.45, the ratio of bicarbonate ion to carbonic acid must be 20:1. If one component of the ratio changes, the other must change proportionately to maintain the proper balance for serum pH to be within the normal range. There are three control mechanisms for pH. The first is the blood buffer system. The blood buffer system consists of weak acids and weak bases. These buffer pairs can act quickly to stabilize the serum pH. The buffer pair that is monitored in clinical settings is the sodium bicarbonate–carbonic acid buffer system. When an acid is added to the blood, it combines with the base (bicarbonate) component of the buffer, forming a weaker acid. Because weak acids do not readily release free H^+, changes in serum pH are minimized. When a base is added to the blood, it combines with the acid component of the buffer to form a weaker base. The other blood buffer systems are protein buffers and phosphate buffers. They mini-

mize pH changes but do not remove acid or base from the body.

The second control mechanism for pH is the lungs. In the lungs, the H^+ ion and the HCO_3^- ion dissociation reaction can be reversed, and water and carbon dioxide (CO_2) are reformed. The carbon dioxide and water are expired from the lungs, decreasing the amount of acid in the body. The lungs can either expel more CO_2 or conserve it to help balance the pH. The respiratory system can readjust quickly to help control serum pH.

The third control mechanism for pH is the urinary system. In the kidney, enzymes promote the dissociation of carbonic acid to free hydrogen ions, which can be excreted in the urine. The bicarbonate ions are returned to the blood to restore the levels of buffer. The kidneys reduce the acid content of the serum by exchanging hydrogen for sodium with the help of aldosterone, and can neutralize acids by combining them with ammonia and other chemicals. When there is excess alkali (base), the kidney can also excrete excess bicarbonate. This compensatory ability of the kidney takes more time to work than the compensatory action in the lungs. Figure 25-6 shows the interaction of these control mechanisms.

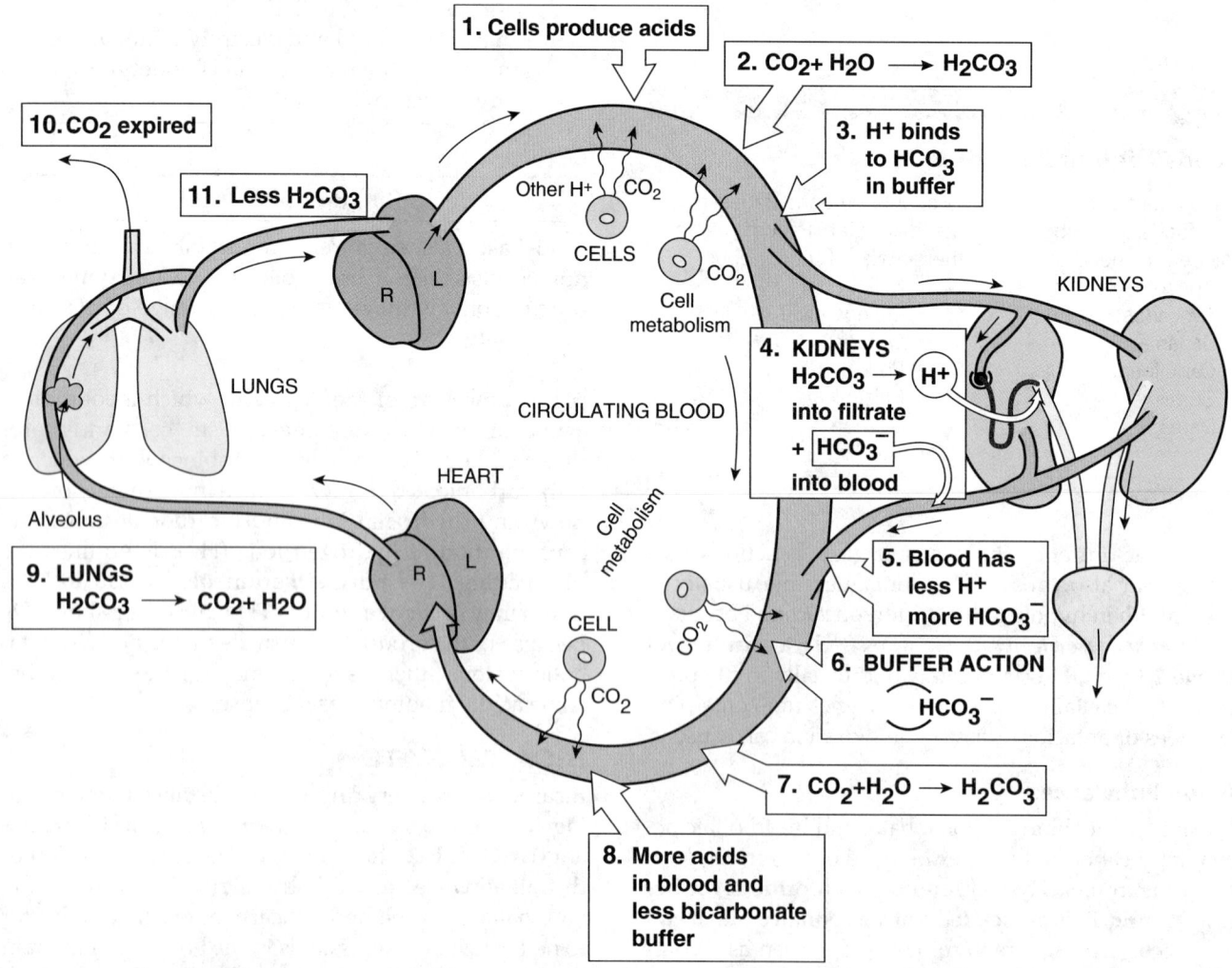

FIGURE **25-6** Regulation of acid–base balance by chemical buffers, respiratory system, and renal system.

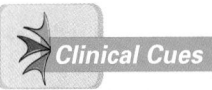

Clinical Cues

Usually about 3 days are needed for the kidneys to stabilize pH within normal range.

? *Think Critically About* . . . If the blood flow to the kidneys is reduced for a considerable period of time, what effect might it have on serum pH?

ACID–BASE IMBALANCES

There are four types of acid–base imbalances, as shown in Table 25-5. To determine if an acid–base imbalance exists, the pH, arterial CO_2 partial pressure ($Paco_2$), and HCO_3^- are measured by arterial blood gas analysis performed on a sample of arterial blood. **An increase in hydrogen ions results in acidosis (decrease in pH). A decrease in hydrogen ions results in alkalosis (increase in pH).** Imbalances may be acute or chronic. An initial change in carbon dioxide is nearly always due to a respiratory disorder. Disorders that show an initial change in bicarbonate ions are metabolic. The three control mechanisms continually work together to maintain acid–base balance. When an imbalance occurs, the lungs and kidneys try to *compensate* by working to bring the pH back toward normal limits.

RESPIRATORY ACIDOSIS

An increase in carbon dioxide levels occurs in a variety of disorders. It is seen in patients with acute problems such as airway obstruction, pneumonia, asthma, or chest injuries. It is also seen in patients taking opiates, which depress the respiratory rate. Chronic respiratory acidosis is prevalent among people with chronic obstructive pulmonary disease (COPD), also called chronic airflow limitation (CAL).

Table 25-5 *Four Acid–Base Imbalances*

IMBALANCE	CAUSES	BLOOD GAS VALUES*
Respiratory acidosis	Slow, shallow respirations	pH < 7.35
	Respiratory congestion/ obstruction	$Paco_2$ > 45 mm Hg
Metabolic acidosis	Shock (poor circulation)	pH < 7.35
	Diabetic ketoacidosis Renal failure Diarrhea	HCO_3^- < 22 mEq/L
Respiratory alkalosis	Hyperventilation	pH > 7.45 $Paco_2$ < 35 mm Hg
Metabolic alkalosis	Vomiting	pH > 7.45
	Excessive antacid intake Hypokalemia	HCO_3^- > 26 mEq/L

*Normal blood gas values: pH: 7.35-7.45; Pao_2: 80-100 mm Hg; $Paco_2$: 3-45 mm Hg; HCO_3^-: 22-26 mEq/L.

METABOLIC ACIDOSIS

An excessive loss of bicarbonate ions or an increased production or retention of hydrogen ions leads to metabolic acidosis. The loss of bicarbonate ions with diarrhea is one cause of metabolic acidosis. Metabolic acidosis also occurs when large amounts of acid are produced within the body. This happens when more energy than usual is expended and lactic acid builds up in the body, as occurs when oxygenation of tissue falls. The faulty metabolism of a diabetic patient causes a build up of ketoacids, resulting in metabolic acidosis. The other major cause of metabolic acidosis is kidney disease, in which there is decreased excretion of acids and decreased production of bicarbonate (Concept Map 25-2). In this instance, dialysis is required to maintain the pH within life-permitting limits.

Effects of Acidosis

Acidosis depresses the nervous system, causing headache, lethargy, weakness, and confusion. If the acidosis is unrelieved, coma and death will ensue. Evidence that the compensatory mechanisms are at work in metabolic acidosis is deep rapid breathing (Kussmaul's respirations) and secretion of urine with a low pH.

RESPIRATORY ALKALOSIS

Hyperventilation (a rapid respiratory rate) results in respiratory alkalosis. It is usually caused by anxiety, high fever, or an overdose of aspirin. Head injuries may also lead to hyperventilation. Treatment for hyperventilation is to treat the underlying disorder. The person may breathe through a re-breather mask temporarily, mixing the excessively exhaled carbon dioxide with oxygen so that carbon dioxide is inhaled.

METABOLIC ALKALOSIS

Vomiting resulting in loss of hydrochloric acid from the stomach may cause metabolic alkalosis; gastrointestinal suction can occasionally cause it also.

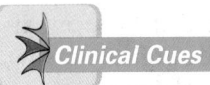

Clinical Cues

Hypokalemia (low serum potassium) is another cause of metabolic alkalosis as the kidney then retains K^+ while excreting H^+. Excessive consumption of antacids with bicarbonate can also upset the acid–base balance and cause alkalosis.

Effects of Alkalosis

Irritability of the nervous system occurs when the pH balance shifts to alkalosis. The patient may display restlessness, muscle twitching, and tingling and numbness of the fingers. If the alkalosis progresses, tetany will occur and seizures and coma result. Tetany is characterized by severe muscle cramps, carpopedal spasms, laryngeal spasms, and **stridor** (shrill harsh sound upon inspiration).

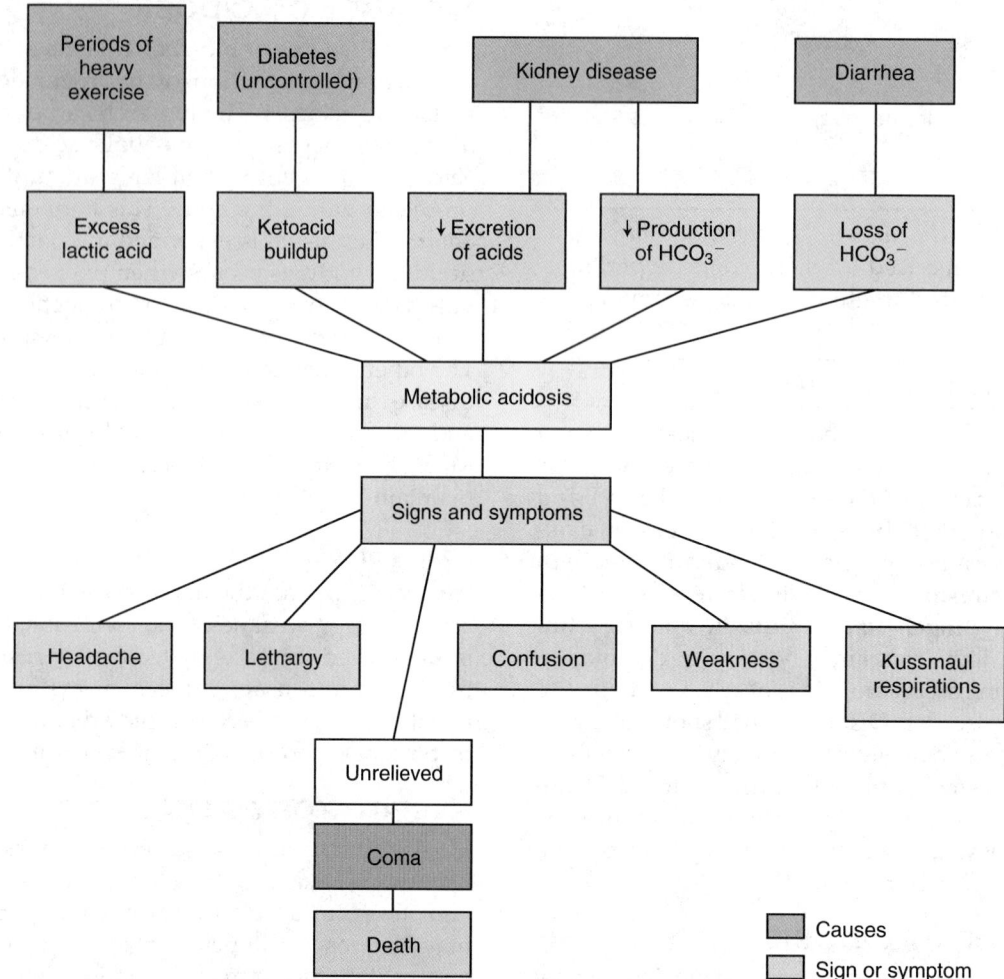

CONCEPT MAP **25-2** Causes, signs, and symptoms of metabolic acidosis.

Think Critically About . . . Can you identify the type of imbalance that might result from (1) rapid respiratory rate; (2) out-of-control diabetes; (3) renal failure; and (4) eating antacids for a nervous stomach?

More in-depth information about acid–base imbalances will be covered in your medical-surgical nursing courses and can be found in a medical-surgical nursing textbook.

APPLICATION of the NURSING PROCESS

Assessment (Data Collection)

First, assess the patient for risk of fluid, electrolyte, or acid–base imbalance. Then assess for physical signs and symptoms of alterations in normal balance. Examine laboratory test results for electrolyte levels that are outside the normal range. Evaluate blood gas determinations to determine if an acid–base imbalance exists and, if so, what type of imbalance is present. Evaluate intake and output (I & O) records to determine if there is a fluid imbalance. The urine volume the adult usually excretes in 24 hours is approximately 1500 mL. In

stressful situations, it may decrease slightly from the effects of increased aldosterone and ADH. Urine concentration provides another clue to the fluid status. Urine concentration is commonly measured by the specific gravity. The concentration of urine is compared with the specific gravity of distilled water, which is 1.000. Urine contains urea, electrolytes, and other substances, so its specific gravity will exceed 1.000. Urine specific gravity normally ranges between 1.003 and 1.030. The average range is 1.010 to 1.025. The urine specific gravity is measured with a urinometer, a refractometer, or a dipstick that contains a reagent for specific gravity.

Tracking daily weight is another way to assess for alterations in fluid balance (Assignment Considerations 25-1).

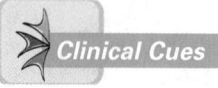 *Clinical Cues*

A weight gain or loss of 2.2 lb (1 kg) in 24 hours indicates a gain or loss of 1 L of fluid.

Skin turgor (elastic condition) is partially dependent on the amount of tissue fluid supporting the skin.

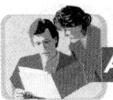

Daily Weight

When assigning the measurement of daily weight, remind the UAP that the weight needs to be measured at the same time every morning, with the patient in the same clothing, on the same scale, after the patient has voided and before eating. Otherwise accuracy in weight gain or loss is impossible. Ask the UAP to report to you any change of more than 2.2 lb (1 kg) immediately.

Checking skin turgor is useful when assessing fluid balance (see Figure 25-3). The sternum is one of the most reliable places to check skin turgor, particularly in the elderly.

Edema may be an indicator of fluid volume overload. Look for puffy eyelids and swollen hands. Edema may be sometimes evidenced by a pit developing when a fingertip is pressed into the tissue over a bony prominence, such as the malleolus or tibia, and held for 5 seconds. After the finger is removed, the pit slowly disappears. A better method of assessing the course of peripheral edema is to measure the circumference of the extremity in the same location each day.

Changes in vital signs are pertinent when assessing fluid, electrolyte, and acid–base balance. Fever increases fluid loss and predisposes the patient to fluid volume deficit. A pulse rate greater than 100 beats per minute (bpm) may be an early sign of decreased vascular volume from fluid volume deficit. A weak, thready pulse accompanies fluid volume deficit, and a bounding pulse is associated with fluid volume overload. Potassium and magnesium deficits may cause an irregular pulse rate. Rapid breathing may cause an alkaline blood pH by expelling large amounts of carbon dioxide, or it may be the body's way to compensate for an acidic blood pH. Moist respiratory sounds in the absence of cardiac or respiratory disease are a sign of excess fluid in the lungs from fluid overload. Fluid overload will cause a rise in systolic blood pressure.

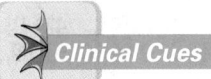

To assess for a fluid deficit, measure the blood pressure and pulse in the lying, sitting, and standing positions. If there is a systolic blood pressure drop of 20 mm Hg accompanied by a pulse rate increase of 10 bpm at 1 minute after the position change, deficient fluid volume is suggested.

Severe fluid volume deficit will decrease blood flow to the brain and result in decreased sensorium and confusion. Imbalances in sodium have direct effects on the brain volume and mental function as well.

Neuromuscular irritability is assessed when imbalances in calcium and magnesium are suspected.

Deep tendon reflexes may be tested to monitor neuromuscular irritability. Check for Chvostek's sign and Trousseau's sign when calcium or magnesium deficit is a possibility. Chvostek's sign is assessed by tapping the facial nerve about an inch in front of the earlobe. A unilateral twitching of the face is a positive response. A blood pressure cuff is placed on the arm and inflated above systolic pressure for 3 minutes to test for Trousseau's sign. If a spasm of the hand occurs, the reaction is positive. Deep tendon reflexes are tested by tapping a partially stretched muscle tendon with a percussion hammer. The extent of the reflex is scored from 0 to 4+, with 0 representing no response, 2+ a normal response, and 4+ a hyperactive response.

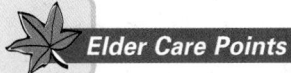

Elder Care Points

Checking for tenting is not an accurate way to assess dehydration in the elderly because their skin loses elasticity with aging and will tent with normal hydration. It is better to check for dry mucous membranes, concentrated urine, and other signs and symptoms in these patients.

Nursing Diagnosis

Using critical thinking, the assessment database is analyzed, problem areas are identified, and nursing diagnoses are chosen. Nursing diagnoses commonly used for patients with fluid, electrolyte, or acid–base imbalances are as follows:

- Deficient fluid volume
- Excess fluid volume
- Risk for imbalanced fluid volume
- Ineffective tissue perfusion
- Decreased cardiac output
- Impaired gas exchange
- Ineffective breathing pattern

Other nursing diagnoses may be appropriate as a result of the fluid, electrolyte, or acid–base imbalance or may be related to the cause of the imbalance, for example, diarrhea.

Planning

Collaboration with the patient and family or caregiver allows the best plan to be devised. Priorities of care are set. The goal is to restore the patient's fluid, electrolyte, or acid–base balance. Individual expected outcomes are written as appropriate. Expected outcomes might be as follows:

- Patient will exhibit normal skin turgor.
- Patient's weight will stabilize at normal baseline.
- Intake and output will be balanced.
- Blood gases will return to normal.
- Breath sounds will be clear to auscultation.
- There will be no evidence of edema.
- Electrolyte values will be within normal limits.

NURSING CARE PLAN 25-1

Care of the Patient with Dehydration

SCENARIO Nina Hiaji, age 76, is placed in the skilled care section of her retirement home. She has been ill for several days with the flu and fever. Her daughter found her confused and lethargic when she came to visit her this morning. Her temperature is 100.8° F (38.2° C), and her blood pressure is 132/72 (her normal pressure is 142/88). Her pulse is 96 and her skin is warm and dry. She is complaining of thirst. Her urine is dark and concentrated. Her oral mucous membranes appear dry and her saliva is thick and stringy. She is dehydrated and hypernatremic.

PROBLEM/NURSING DIAGNOSIS Very thirsty with fever and dehydration/**Deficient fluid volume** related to fever and lack of intake.
Supporting Assessment Data: Subjective: Thick saliva. *Objective:* Poor skin turgor at sternum. Has had flu for several days and has not been eating or drinking much.

Goals/Expected Outcomes	Nursing Interventions	Selected Rationale	Evaluation
Fluid balance will be normal within 24 hr.	Encourage intake of 8 oz of fluid every hour.	Fluid intake promotes rehydration.	*Is patient taking fluids?* Yes, took 32 oz by noon. Progressing toward goals.
	Provide mouth care every 4 hr and before meals.	Mouth care provides comfort and promotes appetite.	Provided q 4 hr and ac.
Patient will not be confused in 32 hr.	Reorient to person, place, and time frequently.	Reorientation decreases confusion.	*Is patient confused?* Yes, still confused.
	Monitor fluid intake and output and record it. Assess intake related to output.	Monitoring shows progress toward rehydration.	Intake 2645 mL. Output 2480 mL. Is rehydrating.
	Monitor laboratory values of electrolytes for signs of electrolyte imbalance.	Monitoring laboratory values indicates success or failure of interventions.	Laboratory values not available yet.
	Monitor for increasing signs of dehydration; notify physician if they appear.		
	Monitor IV therapy; prevent fluid volume excess. Fluid intake promotes rehydration.	Monitoring helps keep fluid therapy on track as ordered. Progressing toward goals.	IV flowing on time. Continue plan.

? CRITICAL THINKING QUESTIONS

1. Can you explain the physiologic process of how the flu and fever cause dehydration and hypernatremia?

2. Can you explain the physiologic mechanism of why postural hypotension may occur when a person is dehydrated? What causes the dizziness?

A specific time frame would be incorporated into the expected outcome. Nursing interventions are chosen to help the patient achieve the outcomes. Nursing Care Plan 25-1 presents examples of expected outcomes and nursing interventions.

Implementation

When patients are unable to take in sufficient fluids on their own, work with the physician to provide an adequate intake of fluid and electrolytes. If patients can swallow and retain fluid, assist them frequently with taking small amounts of fluid. Establish a plan for assisting with both hot and cold liquid consumption. With conscientious care, the need for intravenous feeding can be avoided. Assessment of what the patient prefers is helpful. In addition to water, fruit juices, bouillon, Popsicles, soft drinks, or gelatin can be offered. For patients who cannot drink and will need only short-term assistance, intravenous therapy is ordered (Table 25-6). See Chapter 36 for more discussion on intravenous therapies. For those who will be unable to take in fluids or food on their own for an extended period, a feeding tube must be placed or total parenteral nutrition (TPN) is started. Care of the patient with a feeding tube and TPN is discussed in Chapter 27. It is important to track the patient's intake and output whether there is a risk of fluid volume imbalance, actual deficit, or actual overhydration (fluid volume excess).

Table 25-6 | *Why Use This Intravenous Fluid?*

CATEGORY OF FLUID	TYPE OF FLUID AND EXAMPLES	ACTION	USE
Crystalloids	**Isotonic Fluids** 0.9% sodium chloride D₅W solution Ringer's solution Lactated Ringer's solution	Raise intravascular volume without causing cellular fluid shifts or changing the electrolyte concentrations in the plasma.	Used for fluid loss from vomiting and diarrhea, for those waiting for blood products, and for fluid loss during surgery.
	Hypertonic Fluids Concentrated dextrose in water: 20%, 30%, 40%, 50%, 60%, or 70% 3% or 5% sodium chloride solution	Draw fluid from the intracellular to the extracellular compartment, thereby relieving cellular edema.	Concentrated dextrose solution is often used to lower cerebral edema.
Colloids	**Albumin**	Draws fluid from the interstitial and intracellular spaces, replenishing intravascular volume.	Diminish ascites (intraperitoneal fluid), maintain blood pressure, and used in shock when crystalloid solutions are insufficient to maintain vascular volume.

Key: D_5W, 5% Dextrose in water.

Table 25-7 | *Measurement Equivalents*

HOUSEHOLD OR APOTHECARY MEASUREMENT	METRIC EQUIVALENT
15 drops; 15 minims	1 mL
1 teaspoon	5 mL
1 tablespoon	15 mL
1 ounce	30 mL
1 cup (8 ounces)	240 mL
1 pint	500 mL
1 quart	1000 mL
5 ice chips to 1 ice cube (1 ice chip = 1 teaspoon)	25 mL (about ½ volume of chips)

Table 25-8 | *Common Equivalents of Food Containers**

CONTAINER	VOLUME
Coffee cup	240 mL
Iced tea glass	320 mL
Juice glass	120 mL
Wax drinking cup	180 mL
Styrofoam cup	210 mL
Large glass	230 mL
Cream package	15 mL
Sherbet	90 mL
Soup, clear	120 mL
Soup, thick	180 mL
Gelatin	80 mL
Milk carton	240 mL

*May vary from one facility to another.

Think Critically About . . . What type of fluid and electrolyte imbalances is the patient who has intestinal flu and suffers from both vomiting and diarrhea likely to have?

Recording Intake and Output

To check oral intake at mealtimes, look at the tray before it is removed from the room and record the intake on the shift intake and output record. Fluids that must be measured include anything that is liquid or will become liquid if left at room temperature. Foods such as ice cream, sherbet, milk shakes, gelatin, and gruel or thinned baby cereals are counted as liquids. Amounts should be converted from household measures to milliliters or cubic centimeters (Table 25-7). Most facilities provide a list of the equivalent amounts contained in the type or size of dish used by the dietary department (Table 25-8). If this information is not available, and for the home care patient, use a graduated container to measure the capacity of various dishes and glasses. The amounts the patient drinks between meals are also recorded.

Intravenous (IV) fluid infused is added as intake. At the beginning of the shift during the report, note how much is left in an IV container that is in progress. Another IV container may be started during the shift when the old one is totally infused. By adding and subtracting, the total amount of IV intake can be calculated. For example, suppose a patient has 350 mL remaining in the IV bag at the beginning of the shift, it infuses, and a new bag is hung at 1:00 P.M. At the end of the shift, 200 mL has infused from the new bag. Add the 350 mL and the 200 mL for a total of 550 mL of IV intake for the shift. This amount is entered on the I & O record as intake under the IV column (Figure 25-7). Most fluids entering the patient's body are recorded as intake; blood and blood products administered are recorded separately.

Fluid output is also counted and recorded. The average urinary output in a 24-hour period is 1000 to 1500 mL; an output of less than 600 mL in a 24-hour period, or less than 30 mL/hr, should be reported to the charge nurse or physician. To measure urinary output, pour the urine from the bedpan or urinal into

	DATE	10/15/09			10/16/09											
	HOUR	0600	1400	2200	0600	1400	2200	0600	1400	2200	0600	1400	2200	0600	1400	2200
INTAKE	Oral	180	560	380	120	620	380									
	Intravenous	475	550	550	350	350	350									
	IVPB Piggyback															
	Transfusion															
	8 hr. Total															
	24 hr. Total			2695			2170									
OUTPUT	Urine	650	980	850	500	850	820									
	Emesis															
	Gastric-Duo															
	8 hr. Total															
	24 hr. Total			2480			2170									
	Stool															
	Weight															

FIGURE 25-7 Intake and output record.

a graduated container. (Gloves are always worn when handling urine containers.) The container is placed on a flat surface and the level of fluid is read at eye level. The amount is recorded on the I & O record under output. For the ambulatory patient, give instructions about saving urine and provide a collection container for the toilet. Ask the patient to call when the container needs emptying or show the patient how to measure and record the urine before disposing of it. Urine drainage bags are emptied before they become full or at least once a shift. The amount is measured and recorded on the I & O record.

Output from all other sources is measured, including drainage from nasogastric tubes, chest tubes, and wound drainage suction devices. If the patient has diarrhea, the liquid stool can be measured in the same manner as urine. Profuse perspiration that requires a change of dampened linen is noted on the I & O record according to agency protocol. Emesis is also measured and recorded as output. At the end of each shift, the total intake and total output are tallied and entered on the 24-hour I & O record in the chart. You do not need a physician's order for instituting the recording of I & O; this is a nursing responsibility (Skill 25-1).

The patient with a fluid volume excess may have an order for fluid restriction. This means that the patient may have only a certain amount of fluid over a 24-hour period. Work out a schedule of fluid intake so that liquids are spaced evenly and the patient does not receive all the allotted liquids in a short time. A typical schedule would be day: 600 mL; evening: 400 mL; night: 200 mL. If not prohibited, hard candies and chewing gum can help relieve thirst. Frequent oral care is essential.

Diuretics are often prescribed, particularly when there is a potential for congestive heart failure or pulmonary edema. Daily weight and electrolyte status must be monitored along with intake and output for these patients.

Skin care is particularly important in preventing a breakdown over an edematous area. The stretched skin is extremely fragile, has a decreased blood supply, and is no longer flexible. Keep bed linens dry and smooth and turn the patient frequently to relieve pressure over bony prominences. **Be very gentle in repositioning and turning the patient to avoid friction on the skin; use a lift sheet. A break in edematous skin can quickly form a pressure ulcer.**

The patient with a fluid volume excess may be placed on sodium restriction because sodium usually is retained along with water. Table salt is prohibited, and special attention must be paid to the foods and fluids allowed the patient. Items that should be particularly avoided are listed in Patient Teaching 25-1.

Laboratory values for electrolytes and acid–base balance are monitored to determine if treatment is effective, and imbalances are being corrected. When potassium is ordered, the level is checked before administering the next dose (Safety Alert 25-2). Urine output is assessed to ensure adequate flow. Orders for fluids are carefully checked before a new intravenous infusion is begun. Assessment for fluid imbalance is ongoing.

For the home care patient, thorough teaching is performed so that the patient can meet the requirements for fluid intake or restriction. Adherence to sodium restriction is monitored by checking the food intake of the patient periodically. Obtaining feedback regarding comprehension of instructions is a vital part of the

Skill 25-1 | Measuring Intake and Output

Intake and output (I & O) are measured and recorded whenever a patient has a potential or an actual fluid balance problem. The physician may order I & O monitoring, or the nurse may independently decide to monitor the patient's I & O. Usually, I & O are measured and recorded for every patient who is receiving IV therapy or has a nasogastric (NG) tube attached to suction, a Foley catheter, or other drainage tube.

■ Supplies

✓ I & O record sheet
✓ Bedpan or urinal
✓ Graduated measuring container
✓ "Hat" toilet collection device
✓ Gloves
✓ Pen or pencil

Review and carry out the Standard Steps in Appendix 3.

■ Assessment (Data Collection)

1. *ACTION* Determine need for recording I & O.

   RATIONALE There may be an order or a need to perform this nursing function.

2. *ACTION* Assess what equipment will be needed in the room to measure and record the I & O.

   RATIONALE Ensures that measuring container and I & O sheet are in the room when needed.

■ Planning

3. *ACTION* Note on I & O sheet all items that need to be recorded.

   RATIONALE Reminds everyone caring for patient that IV medications, NG tube irrigations, and wound drainage all need to be recorded.

4. *ACTION* Place a sign above the toilet stating that I & O is to be recorded. Tell personnel to record all intake.

   RATIONALE Sign above toilet alerts personnel to measure all urine before disposal. Intake will be recorded.

5. *ACTION* Ask the patient to use the call light when urine has been collected.

   RATIONALE Alerts personnel to measure the urine.

■ Implementation

6. *ACTION* Explain the procedure to the patient and ask that each amount of fluid taken between meals be recorded.

   RATIONALE The patient must understand the procedure in order to comply with the recording of I & O.

7. *ACTION* Calculate fluid intake before removing a food tray from the room.

   RATIONALE A more accurate count is obtained than when relying on memory.

8. *ACTION* Assess fluid intake each time you are in the room.

   RATIONALE It is easier for patients to remember what they drank if questioned soon afterward.

9. *ACTION* Put on gloves and measure and record all output.

   RATIONALE Gloves reduce the transfer of microorganisms. Output includes urine, diarrheal stool, emesis, gastric drainage, wound drainage, and excessive perspiration. A graduated container measures all liquid output accurately.

10. *ACTION* Dispose of the output in the commode and clean the equipment; remove gloves and perform hand hygiene.

    RATIONALE Removes a medium for growth of pathogens; reduces the transfer of microorganisms.

11. *ACTION* Note the amount of output in the correct column on the I & O sheet.

    RATIONALE Writing down the amount immediately helps provide an accurate record.

12. *ACTION* Note additional types of intake on the I & O sheet as they occur.

    RATIONALE Jotting down the amount of an IV infusion or the amount of gastric irrigant instilled helps maintain an accurate record of intake.

13. *ACTION* At the end of the shift, mark and record the amount of gastric suction secretions, wound drainage in collection devices, and chest drainage. Empty the urine collection bag and measure and record the output. If the suction collection container is full, dispose of the canister according to agency protocol and install a new one. Total the amount of output for the shift.

    RATIONALE For accuracy, all output must be recorded on the I & O sheet. Collection containers are emptied, the level at the end of the shift is marked with the date and time, or containers are replaced if they are full and disposable. All types of output are added together for the shift total.

Continued

Skill 25-1 | Measuring Intake and Output—cont'd

14. **ACTION** At the end of the shift, calculate the amount of IV fluid intake and add it to the intake side of the I & O sheet.

    RATIONALE All IV fluid infused is included as intake.

15. **ACTION** After the shift totals have been calculated, enter the amounts on the I & O flow sheet. At the end of a 24-hour period, total the amounts for all shifts for both intake and output.

    RATIONALE The total I & O amount over 24 hours presents the most accurate picture of the patient's fluid balance. What constitutes a normal intake and output depends on the condition of the patient and on any restrictions imposed.

16. **ACTION** Place a new shift I & O sheet in the patient's room; make certain the name and room number are on the sheet.

    RATIONALE A record form must be available for the recording of the I & O (see Figure 25-7).

■ Evaluation

17. **ACTION** Determine if the I & O are within normal limits. Compare the amounts to see if there is any indication of a fluid imbalance. Compare the total

with the totals from the previous 2 days to see if either intake or output is increasing.

RATIONALE If the output is greater or less than the intake, the patient may have a fluid imbalance. Comparison of the totals shows whether there is an increase in intake or output.

Documentation is done on the I & O sheet (see Figure 25-7) or on the computer flow sheet.

❓CRITICAL THINKING QUESTIONS

1. What would you do if you recorded the patient's intake for breakfast and 30 minutes later she vomits into the toilet?

2. Your patient is on a full liquid diet, has an IV running at 100 mL/hr, and receives an IV piggyback medication of 50 mL at 2 P.M. He has a Foley catheter. What would you include as output on your shift record? What would you include as intake?

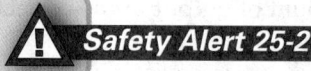

⚠ Safety Alert 25-2

Administering Potassium IV

If urine output is less than 30 mL/hr, potassium should not be given. Check IV fluids for added potassium before initiating IV therapy. Check the IV fluid that is in progress. Giving potassium when urine flow is inadequate may cause kidney damage.

---

teaching. Collaboration with the patient on the plan of care is essential to obtain patient compliance.

When acid–base imbalance occurs, control of the underlying disorder is instituted. Blood gases are monitored, and oxygen and electrolytes are administered as needed. Nursing measures to improve pulmonary function are instituted as appropriate.

❓ *Think Critically About . . .* What characteristics would you expect to find in a urine specimen from a patient who is dehydrated? How would it differ from a urine specimen from a patient who has a fluid volume excess?

Evaluation

Every 24 hours, evaluation is performed to see if the nursing interventions are assisting the patient to meet expected outcomes. If the patient is not progressing toward achievement of the outcomes, problem solving and critical thinking are used to determine why. The plan of care is altered appropriately. When outcomes are met, that portion of the plan is discontinued.

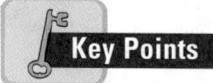

Key Points

- Water is essential to life.
- Body fluids are intracellular or extracellular and shift from one compartment to another.
- Fluid moves from compartment to compartment by diffusion, osmosis, filtration, and active transport (see Figure 25-2).
- Fluids are lost from the body through urine, feces, expired air, and perspiration; 24-hour output is approximately 2500 mL.
- Fluid is taken in or produced from liquids, digestion of food, or cell metabolism; this should total 2500 mL/day.
- The kidney is the major organ regulating fluid and electrolyte balance.

- Intake and output are balanced in the healthy individual.
- Daily fluid intake in the adult must be at least 1500 mL/day to maintain homeostasis.
- Illness affects fluid and electrolyte balance in many ways.
- Common causes of fluid volume deficit are vomiting, diarrhea, gastric suction, wound and fistula drainage, and burn injuries.
- A fluid volume deficit results in dehydration (see Box 25-1).
- The elderly and the very young can become dehydrated very quickly.
- Signs of fluid volume excess are weight gain; edema; elevated blood pressure; slow, bounding pulse; and crackles in the lungs.
- Causes of edema include kidney failure, heart failure, liver failure, and hormonal disorders.
- Tracking daily weight is a method of determining fluid volume excess or deficit.
- The body works to maintain a balance of anions and cations in each fluid compartment.
- Sodium is the predominant electrolyte in the extracellular fluid; potassium is the predominant electrolyte in the intracellular fluid.
- Whenever a water imbalance exists, there will be an accompanying sodium imbalance.
- Hyponatremia is a frequent cause of hospitalization of the elderly.
- It is important to know the causes of electrolyte imbalance, the normal range for the major electrolytes, and the signs and symptoms of imbalance (see Table 25-4).
- Acid–base balance is necessary to maintain homeostasis in the body.
- Normal serum pH is 7.35 to 7.45.
- Three mechanisms control pH in the body: the blood buffer system, lungs, and kidneys.

- An increase in hydrogen ions results in acidosis, as evidenced by a decrease in pH. There are two types of acidosis: respiratory and metabolic (see Table 25-5).
- Acidosis depresses the nervous system, causing headache, lethargy, weakness, and confusion, and can progress to coma and death.
- A decrease in hydrogen ions results in alkalosis, as evidenced by an increase in pH. There are two types of alkalosis: respiratory and metabolic (see Table 25-5).
- Alkalosis causes irritability of the nervous system with restlessness, muscle twitching, and tingling and numbness of the fingers; it can progress to tetany, seizures, and coma.
- Tissue turgor is not a reliable indicator of hydration status in the elderly; the mucous membranes should be checked for dryness.
- The conscientious nurse can keep the patient at risk of deficient fluid volume from developing it.
- Dependent edema is assessed by checking for pitting by pressing a fingertip against the tissue at a bony prominence.
- A physician's order is not necessary to institute recording of intake and output (I & O).
- Fluid restriction is often necessary for the patient who has excess fluid volume.
- Accurately recording I & O is essential in caring for a patient with a fluid imbalance.

 Go to your **Companion CD-ROM** for an Audio Glossary, animations, video clips, and more.

evolve   Be sure to visit the companion Evolve site at http://evolve.elsevier.com/deWit/fundamental/ for additional online resources.

NCLEX-PN® EXAMINATION-STYLE REVIEW QUESTIONS

*Choose the **best** answer(s) for each question.*

1. Which of the following patients would be at risk for a fluid imbalance? The patient: *(Select all that apply.)*
   1. with a history of congestive heart failure.
   2. who has severe burns.
   3. who is 5 days postoperative after abdominal surgery.
   4. suffering with influenza who has nausea and vomiting.
   5. with diabetes and early kidney failure.

2. The elderly individual is at greater risk for dehydration than the middle-aged adult because: *(Select all that apply.)*
   1. the elderly have a diminished sense of thirst.
   2. the elderly have less muscle mass as years advance.
   3. the elderly person's body is almost 80% water.
   4. compensatory mechanisms work less efficiently.

3. Your patient has been ordered to receive nothing by mouth today because of scheduled diagnostic tests. Even without fluid intake, what amount of fluids would be lost, if any?
   1. The 200 mL normally produced by metabolism of food
   2. None
   3. Only the minimum amount of urine needed to excrete wastes
   4. Urine and obligatory losses, totaling 1500 mL

4. The patient who ate a serving of soup (120 mL), a container of gelatin (80 mL), a glass of iced tea (320 mL), and a serving of sherbet (90 mL) had an intake of _____ mL.

5. An 82-year-old patient is admitted with vomiting and diarrhea. On assessment, you note that he is apprehensive and his skin is cool and pale. His pulse is rapid and his blood pressure is lower. These symptoms are indicative of:

   1. fluid overload.
   2. electrolyte imbalance.
   3. dehydration.
   4. intestinal flu.

6. Your patient has been ill with pneumonia and was admitted yesterday to start IV antibiotic therapy. He has a history of congestive heart failure and is taking digitalis and furosemide. He has not been eating well the past 3 days because he was feeling so bad. The physician ordered fluids and daily lab work yesterday. The patient seems more confused this morning and is very weak, and his urinary output has fallen. In order to determine what is causing these symptoms, you would first:

   1. check the morning electrolyte levels.
   2. call his physician.
   3. check yesterday's lab results.
   4. ask for an order for extra potassium.

7. A patient has food poisoning and has been vomiting frequently for the past 8 hours. If this continues, he will likely develop:

   1. metabolic acidosis.
   2. metabolic alkalosis.
   3. respiratory acidosis.
   4. respiratory alkalosis.

8. Patients who are undergoing diuretic therapy to decrease excess body fluid tend to lose potassium. If too much potassium is lost, the patient will have which of the following electrolyte and acid–base imbalances?

   1. Hyperkalemia; metabolic acidosis
   2. Hypokalemia; metabolic alkalosis
   3. Hyponatremia; metabolic acidosis
   4. Hypernatremia; metabolic alkalosis

9. One of the best methods to assess whether peripheral edema is increasing or decreasing is to:

   1. compare intake with output over several days.
   2. weigh the patient daily and compare weights.
   3. use a fingertip to assess for pitting edema of the tissue.
   4. measure the circumference of the affected extremity in the same location each day.

10. Signs and symptoms of hyponatremia include:

    1. confusion, muscle cramps, and anorexia.
    2. flushed skin and decreased urine output.
    3. bounding pulse and bradycardia.
    4. diarrhea and hyperactive bowel sounds.

CRITICAL THINKING ACTIVITIES *Read each clinical scenario and discuss the questions with your classmates.*

Scenario A
George Torres is admitted with a head injury. He is comatose and is breathing rapidly. His blood gases show a pH of 7.37, $Paco_2$ of 32, and HCO_3^- of 26. Compare these gases to normal values. What type of acid–base imbalance does this patient have?

Scenario B
Lena Mason, who has diabetes, is admitted in a stuporous condition. Her blood gases show a pH of 7.33, $Paco_2$ of 40, and HCO_3^- of 20. What type of acid–base imbalance does this patient have?

Scenario C
Douglas Byrd is on fluid restrictions and is to have no more than 1200 mL of fluid per day. This is his third day on restrictions and he is complaining bitterly of being thirsty. What creative ways can you think of to decrease his thirst while staying within his fluid allotment?

Scenario D
Ramon Hernandez is admitted in a very confused state from his home. His neighbor says he has been ill for several days. What would you do to assess him for dehydration and electrolyte imbalance?

Concepts of Basic Nutrition and Cultural Considerations

evolve http://evolve.elsevier.com/deWit/fundamental/

Objectives

Upon completing this chapter, you should be able to:

Theory

1. Review the structure and function of the gastrointestinal system.
2. Utilize the components of the USDA MyPyramid website to assist patients to plan their diets.
3. Discuss the function of proteins, carbohydrates, fats, vitamins, minerals, and water in the human body.
4. Identify food sources of proteins, carbohydrates, fats, vitamins, and minerals.
5. List medical conditions that may occur as a result of protein, calorie, vitamin, or mineral deficiency or excess.
6. Identify a variety of factors that influence nutrition.
7. Describe cultural influences on nutritional practices.
8. Identify nutritional needs throughout the life span.
9. Discuss components of a basic nutritional assessment.

Clinical Practice

1. Identify patients at risk for nutritional deficits.
2. Complete a nutritional assessment on an assigned patient.
3. Use therapeutic communication with a patient while discussing needed diet modification.
4. Develop a teaching plan for the patient for whom a therapeutic diet is prescribed.

Key Terms

Be sure to check out the bonus material on the Companion CD-ROM, including selected audio pronunciations.

amino acids (ă-MĒ-nō, p. 460)
body mass index (BMI) (p. 475)
carbohydrates (kăr-bō-HĪ-drātz, p. 463)
carotenoids (p. 466)
cholesterol (kō-LĔS-tĕr-ŏl) (p. 466)
colostrum (kō-LŎ-strŭm, p. 473)
complementary proteins (kŏm-plĕ-MĔN-tă-rē, p. 463)
complete proteins (p. 461)
digestion (p. 457)
essential amino acids (p. 460)
fat (p. 465)
fiber (p. 465)
fructose (FRŬK-tōs, p. 464)
glucose (p. 464)
incomplete proteins (p. 461)
kosher (p. 471)

kwashiorkor (kwăsh-ē-ŌR-kōr, p. 463)
lacto-ovo-vegetarian (LĂK-tō-Ō-vō-vĕ-jĭ-TĀ-rē-ăn, p. 463)
lactose (p. 464)
lactovegetarian (p. 463)
malnutrition (p. 463)
marasmus (mă-RĂZ-mŭs, p. 463)
metabolism (p. 457)
minerals (p. 467)
MyPyramid (p. 459)
nonessential amino acids (p. 460)
nutrients (p. 460)
nutrition (p. 457)
obesity (p. 473)
protein (p. 460)
saturated fats (p. 466)
sucrose (p. 464)
toxicity (p. 466)
unsaturated fats (p. 466)
vegan (VĒ-găn, p. 463)
vegetarians (vĕ-jĕ-TĀ-rē-ănz, p. 463)
vitamins (VĪ-tĭ-mĭnz, p. 466)

Health promotion and prevention of disease are major roles of the nurse: Adequate nutrition is an essential component of attaining and maintaining good health. Nutrition is the sum of processes involved in taking in nutrients and absorbing and using them. Nutrition is concerned with those properties of food that build sound bodies and promote health. To achieve adequate nutrition, individuals should consume a balanced diet containing adequate amounts of the essential nutrients for proper body function. The functions of nutrition include providing energy, regulating body processes, and building, maintaining, and repairing tissue.

The gastrointestinal (GI) system includes the mouth (with tongue and teeth), pharynx, esophagus, stomach, small intestine, and large intestine. The salivary glands, liver, gallbladder, and pancreas are accessory organs for the gastrointestinal system. Foods are digested and absorbed, and the nutrients in these foods are made available to all body cells through the process of metabolism (process by which large molecules are broken down into smaller molecules to make energy available to the organism). Metabolism enables the absorbed nutrients to enter the blood following digestion (process of converting food into chemical substances that can be ab-

OVERVIEW OF STRUCTURE AND FUNCTION OF THE GASTROINTESTINAL SYSTEM

Which structures are involved in the gastrointestinal (digestive) system?

- The gastrointestinal system is composed of the mouth, tongue, teeth, pharynx, esophagus, stomach, small intestine, large intestine, and anus (Figure 26-1).

- Accessory organs include the salivary glands, liver, gallbladder, and pancreas.

- The mouth is the first part of the digestive tract. It contains the teeth and tongue and receives secretions from the salivary glands.

- The tongue is composed mostly of skeletal muscle. It is the largest, most movable organ of the mouth.

- Adults have 32 permanent teeth. Teeth are categorized as incisors, cuspids, bicuspids, and molars.

- The parotid glands are the largest of the salivary glands. One is located on each side of the body anterior and inferior to the ear.

- The pharynx is a fibromuscular passageway that connects the nasal and oral cavities to the larynx and esophagus. Food is forced into the pharynx by the tongue.

- The esophagus is a collapsible muscular tube about 20 cm long. It is the passageway for movement of food to the stomach.

- The stomach is located in the upper left quadrant of the abdomen. The adult stomach has an average capacity of 1.5 L.

- The small intestine includes the duodenum, jejunum, and ileum. It is 2.5 cm in diameter and 6 meters long.

- The large intestine includes the cecum, ascending colon, transverse colon, descending colon, sigmoid colon, rectum, and anus. It is about 1.5 meters long.

- The liver is a large, reddish brown organ located in the upper right quadrant of the abdomen.

- The gallbladder is a pear-shaped sac that is attached to the surface of the liver by the cystic duct.

- The pancreas is a flat, elongated organ located along the posterior abdominal wall. The head of the pancreas is on the right side in the curve of the duodenum. The tail is on the left side, next to the spleen.

What are the functions of the organs of the gastrointestinal system?

- The mouth receives food and breaks it into small particles by chewing and mixing it with saliva.

- The tongue allows food to be manipulated in the mouth for chewing and mixing with saliva.

- The tongue helps position food for swallowing. Taste buds are also located on the tongue.

- The teeth are used for grasping, tearing, crushing, and grinding of food.

- The salivary glands secrete saliva into the mouth for mixing with food during chewing. Saliva breaks down food for tasting. Saliva plays a role in the chemical digestion of starches.

- The pharynx serves as a passageway for food to enter the esophagus through swallowing.

- The esophagus is the passageway for food to enter the stomach. The lining of the esophagus secretes mucus to ease the passage of food.

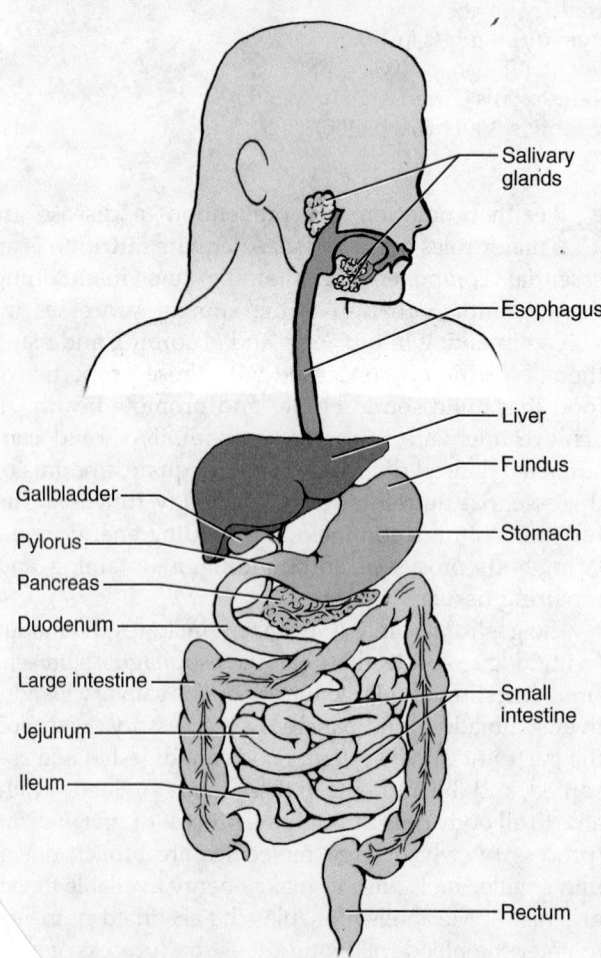

FIGURE **26-1** The gastrointestinal system.

- The stomach is a temporary storage place for food. The churning action of muscles of the stomach mixes food with gastric juices. Food is changed to a semiliquid state for passage to the small intestine. Gastric acids begin digestion of proteins. Vitamin B_{12} is absorbed in the stomach through the action of intrinsic factor secreted from the stomach wall.

- The small intestine receives food from the stomach, and secretions from the liver and pancreas. The process of digestion is finished in the small intestine. Nutrients are absorbed and residue is passed to the large intestine.

- The large intestine is the site of absorption of fluid and electrolytes and the elimination of waste products.

- The liver produces and secretes bile into the small intestine for digestion of fats. The liver plays a major role in digestion of fats, carbohydrates, and proteins through its metabolic functions.

- The gallbladder stores and concentrates bile. Fatty foods in the duodenum stimulate the flow of bile from the gallbladder to the duodenum.

- The pancreas secretes digestive juices into the small intestine for digestion of carbohydrates, proteins, and fats. The pancreas also secretes insulin for utilization of glucose.

What changes in the digestive system occur with aging?

- Increased dental caries and tooth loss may lead to decreased ability to chew food normally.

- Decreased sense of taste may lead to loss of appetite.

- Decreased gag reflex may increase the risk of choking and aspiration.

- Decreased muscle tone at sphincters may increase heartburn or risk of esophageal reflux.

- Decreased gastric secretions may interfere with digestion of food.

- Decreased peristalsis may increase the risk of constipation or bowel impaction.

sorbed into the blood and utilized by the body tissue), for the use of all body cells.

DIETARY GUIDELINES

USDA MyPYRAMID

The MyPyramid food guidance system developed by the U.S. Department of Agriculture (USDA) (Figure 26-2) shows the six food groups necessary for good nutrition and explains the use of each component. The pyramid is developed based on the 2005 USDA Dietary Guidelines for Americans. The guidelines describe a healthy diet as one that

- Emphasizes fruits, vegetables, whole grains, and fat-free or low-fat milk and milk products
- Includes lean meats, poultry, fish, beans, eggs, and nuts
- Is low in saturated fats, *trans* fats, cholesterol, sodium, and added sugars

The pyramid emphasizes a personalized approach to nutrition and is designed for individuals ages 2 and above. A variety of foods from each group is needed to achieve a healthy diet. See Figure 26-3 for the USDA's Food Guide Recommendations for a 2000-Calorie Diet.

The bread group consists of breads, cereals, rice, and pasta products, such as spaghetti and macaroni. The greatest number of servings per day should come from this group, and at least half should be whole-grain products. Three to five servings are recommended from the vegetable group. These servings are usually divided between lunch and dinner. The fruit group, which includes juices, is allocated two to four servings per day. Milk, yogurt, and cheese comprise the milk group, and intake should be three servings per day. The meat group includes meat, poultry, fish, dry beans, eggs, and nuts. Most Americans exceed the recommended two to three servings a day from the meat group. It is recommended that extra portions of grains and vegetables replace excess protein in the diet. This would decrease the amount of protein and fat that is now consumed in the usual adult diet. Fats, oils, and sweets are included in the MyPyramid dietary recommendations; however, they should be consumed sparingly. People of all ages are encouraged to adjust their exercise level and food intake to maintain body weight within the recommended limits. The American Heart Association released new recommendations in 2006 for diet and lifestyle. The American Heart Association 2006 Diet and Lifestyle Recommendations are presented in Box 26-1.

An alliance of federal and state agencies, the Healthy People Consortium, has contributed to the development of national health objectives. These objectives were revised in December 2005 and released by the Secretary's Council on National Health Promotion and Disease Prevention as Objectives for 2010 (Box 26-2, p. 462). *Healthy People 2010* also addressed the issue of disparities in risk for nutrition-related disease among ethnic minorities and low-income groups. Issues such as obesity and food insecurity (limited access to safe, nutritious food) was evident in the low-income, Hispanic, African American, Native American, and

Anatomy of MyPyramid

One size doesn't fit all

USDA's new MyPyramid symbolizes a personalized approach to healthy eating and physical activity. The symbol has been designed to be simple. It has been developed to remind consumers to make healthy food choices and to be active every day. The different parts of the symbol are described below.

Activity
Activity is represented by the steps and the person climbing them, as a reminder of the importance of daily physical activity.

Moderation
Moderation is represented by the narrowing of each food group from bottom to top. The wider base stands for foods with little or no solid fats or added sugars. These should be selected more often. The narrower top area stands for foods containing more added sugars and solid fats. The more active you are, the more of these foods can fit into your diet.

Personalization
Personalization is shown by the person on the steps, the slogan, and the URL. Find the kinds of amounts of food to eat each day at MyPyramid.gov

Proportionality
Proportionality is shown by the different widths of the food group bands. The widths suggest how much food a person should choose from each group. The widths are just a general guide, not exact proportions. Check the website for how much is right for you.

Variety
Variety is symbolized by the 6 color bands representing the 5 food groups of the Pyramid and oils. This illustrates that foods from all groups are needed each day for good health.

Gradual Improvement
Gradual improvement is encouraged by the slogan. It suggests that individuals can benefit from taking small steps to improve their diet and lifestyle each day.

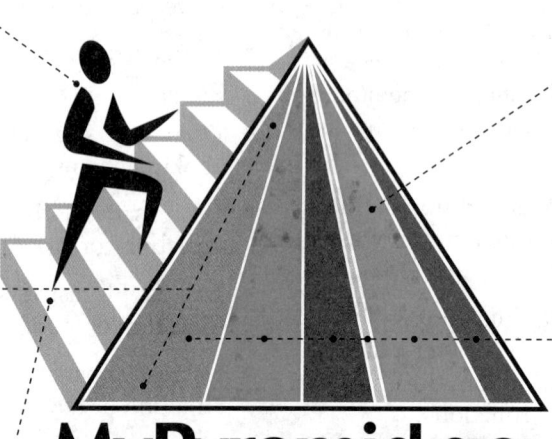

MyPyramid.gov
STEPS TO A HEALTHIER YOU

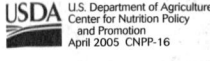 U.S. Department of Agriculture
Center for Nutrition Policy
and Promotion
April 2005 CNPP-16

USDA is an equal opportunity provider and employer.

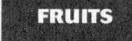

GRAINS VEGETABLES FRUITS OILS MILK MEAT & BEANS

FIGURE 26-2 The USDA MyPyramid. (From U.S. Department of Agriculture, April 2006.)

Asian/Pacific Islander American communities, especially among females. A major focus on meeting the objectives of this area of *Healthy People 2010* included improving accessibility of nutritional information, nutritional education, nutritional counseling and related services, and healthful foods in a variety of settings and for all population groups (*Healthy People 2010*, 2005).

Six nutrients (biochemical substances used by the body that must be supplied in adequate amounts from foods consumed) are essential to normal functioning: proteins, carbohydrates, fats, vitamins, minerals, and water.

PROTEIN

FUNCTIONS OF PROTEIN

~~constant~~ supply of protein is essential to meet the ~~~~ need to build and replace tissue and cells. Dur~~~~mes~~ of illness and after surgery, injuries, burns, or

blood loss, we require more protein production to help in rebuilding cells and tissues. Protein plays a role in maintaining fluid balance, acid–base balance, transportation of nutrients, and antibody, enzyme, and hormone production. Protein is also a source of energy for the body. **Protein supplies 4 calories per gram.** The body does not store protein except in body tissues and fluids, collectively referred to as the "amino acid" pool. The body will protect its protein stores by first using carbohydrates, then fat, for energy. If these are low or absent, the body will use dietary protein, then tissue protein, for energy.

Proteins are composed of amino acids (organic compounds that are the chief components of proteins). The body can produce some amino acids to build its own proteins. Nine amino acids are considered essential amino acids because they must be consumed through food sources. The liver can manufacture 11 amino acids; these are considered nonessential amino acids. For body cells to build proteins, they must have all amino acids.

GRAINS Make half your grains whole	VEGETABLES Vary your veggies	FRUITS Focus on fruits	MILK Get your calcium-rich foods	MEAT & BEANS Go lean with protein
Eat at least 3 oz of whole-grain cereals, breads, crackers, rice, or pasta every day 1 oz is about 1 slice of bread, about 1 cup of breakfast cereal, or ½ cup of cooked rice, cereal, or pasta	Eat more dark-green veggies like broccoli, spinach, and other dark leafy greens Eat more orange vegetables like carrots and sweet potatoes Eat more dry beans and peas like pinto beans, kidney beans, and lentils	Eat a variety of fruit Choose fresh, frozen, canned, or dried fruit Go easy on fruit juices	Go low-fat or fat-free when you choose milk, yogurt, and other milk products If you don't or can't consume milk, choose lactose-free products or other calcium sources such as fortified foods and beverages	Choose low-fat or lean meats and poultry Bake it, broil it, or grill it Vary your protein routine—choose more fish, beans, peas, nuts, and seeds

For a 2000-calorie diet, you need the amounts below from each food group. To find the amounts that are right for you, go to MyPyramid.gov.

Eat 6 oz every day	Eat 2½ cups every day	Eat 2 cups every day	Get 3 cups every day; for kids aged 2 to 8, it's 2	Eat 5½ oz. every day

Find your balance between food and physical activity
- Be sure to stay within your daily calorie needs.
- Be physically active for at least 30 minutes most days of the week.
- About 60 minutes a day of physical activity may be needed to prevent weight gain.
- For sustaining weight loss, at least 60 to 90 minutes a day of physical activity may be required.
- Children and teenagers should be physically active for 60 minutes every day, or most days.

Know the limits on fats, sugars, and salt (sodium)
- Make most of your fat sources from fish, nuts, and vegetable oils.
- Limit solid fats like butter, stick margarine, shortening, and lard, as well as foods that contain these.
- Check the Nutrition Facts label to keep saturated fats, *trans* fats, and sodium low.
- Choose food and beverages low in added sugars. Added sugars contribute calories with few, if any, nutrients.

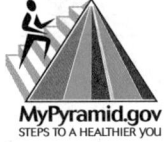
MyPyramid.gov
STEPS TO A HEALTHIER YOU

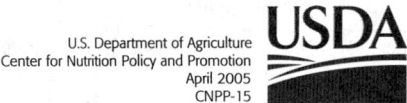
U.S. Department of Agriculture
Center for Nutrition Policy and Promotion
April 2005
CNPP-15
USDA is an equal opportunity provider and employer.

FIGURE 26-3 MyPyramid recommendations for 2000-calorie diet. (From U.S. Department of Agriculture, April 2006.)

Box 26-1 *American Heart Association 2006 Diet and Lifestyle Recommendations*

1. Use up at least as many calories as you take in.
   - Know how many calories you are eating
   - Increase physical activity as needed to match number of calories consumed
   - Plan at least 30 minutes of moderated physical activity each day
2. Eat a variety of nutritious foods from all the food groups. Choose foods such as vegetables, fruits, whole-grain products and fat-free or low-fat dairy products. Eat fish at least twice a week, especially fish high in omega-3 fatty acids (salmon, trout, herring) to reduce risk of coronary artery disease.
3. Eat less of the nutrient-poor foods and limit how much saturated fat, *trans* fat, cholesterol, and sodium you eat.
   - Choose lean meat and poultry without skin and prepare them without added saturated and *trans* fat.

- Cut back on foods containing hydrogenated vegetable oils to reduce *trans* fat in your diet.
- Reduce foods high in dietary cholesterol. Aim to eat less than 300 mg of cholesterol each day
- Reduce consumption of beverages and foods with added sugars.
- Aim to eat less than 2300 mg of sodium per day.
- If you drink alcohol, drink in moderation. That means 1 drink per day for females and 2 drinks per day for males.
- Follow the American Heart Association recommendations when you eat out, and keep an eye on your portion sizes.

Reprinted with permission www.americanheart.org. Copyright © 2008 American Heart Association.

FOOD SOURCES OF PROTEIN

Food sources of protein include meats, poultry, fish, eggs, dairy products, cereals, grains, legumes, and most vegetables. Animal sources (red meat, eggs, milk and milk products, poultry, fish) are complete (or high-quality) proteins because they contain all nine essential amino acids. Plant sources of protein are incomplete (or low-quality) proteins because they do not contain all essential amino acids. The only plant source of all nine essential amino acids is soybeans. Soybeans and soy

Box 26-2 | *Healthy People 2010: Objectives for Nutrition and Overweight*

19-1 Increase the proportion of adults who are at a healthy weight.

19-2 Reduce the proportion of adults who are obese.

19-3 Reduce the proportion of children and adolescents who are overweight or obese.

19-4 Reduce growth retardation among low-income children under age 5.

19-5 Increase the proportion of persons ages 2 years and older who consume at least two daily servings of fruit.

19-6 Increase the proportion of persons ages 2 years and older who consume at least three daily servings of vegetables with at least one third being dark green or orange vegetables.

19-7 Increase the proportion of persons ages 2 years and older who consume at least six daily servings of grain products, with at least three being whole grains.

19-8 Increase the proportion of persons ages 2 years and older who consume less than 10% of calories from saturated fat.

19-9 Increase the proportion of persons ages 2 years and older who consume no more than 30% of calories from total fat.

19-10 Increase the proportion of persons ages 2 years and older who consume 2400 mg or less of sodium daily.

19-11 Increase the proportion of persons ages 2 years and older who meet daily recommendations for calcium.

19-12 Reduce iron deficiency among young children and females of childbearing age.

19-13 Reduce anemia among low-income pregnant females in their third trimester.

19-14 (Developmental) Reduce iron deficiency among pregnant females.

19-15 (Developmental) Increase the proportion of children and adolescents ages 6 to 19 years whose intake of meals and snacks at schools contributes to good overall dietary quality.

19-16 Increase the proportion of worksites that offer nutrition or weight management classes or counseling.

19-17 Increase the proportion of physician office visits made by patients with a diagnosis of cardiovascular disease, diabetes, or hyperlipidemia that includes counseling or education related to diet and nutrition.

19-18 Increase food security among U.S. households and in so doing reduce hunger.

Courtesy of www.healthypeople.gov/Document/html/pdf/Volume2/Nutrition.pdf.

products can be a less expensive substitute for meat in the diet while supplying high-quality protein. Combining plant sources of foods can provide "complementary" complete protein intake in the diet (e.g., cereal with milk, beans with rice, peanut butter sandwiches).

DIETARY REFERENCE INTAKES OF PROTEIN

Dietary Reference Intakes (DRIs) have been developed by the U.S. National Academy of Sciences to eventually replace Recommended Daily Allowances. DRIs provide guidelines for estimating nutrient intake for planning and evaluating diets of healthy people. DRIs are a combination of four separate recommendations: Recommended Dietary Allowance (RDA, used by individuals to reduce disease risk); Adequate Intake (AI, used by individuals to set dietary goals); Estimated Average Requirement (EAR, used to plan diets for large groups); and Tolerable Upper Intake Level (UL, maximum amount a person can consume without health risk). Healthy adults require 0.8 g of protein per kilogram of body weight. **The average DRI is 46 to 56 g of protein per day for the healthy adult.** This can be achieved through a combination of meat and plant sources. Protein intake should be approximately 10% to 15% of the total daily calories. The typical American diet is high in protein (~75 g/day). A serving of protein is, for example, a 3-oz portion of meat or a serving

of beans equivalent to one-half cup of dry beans. A 3-oz serving is about the size of a deck of cards.

? Think Critically About . . . What size portion of meat is typical in your diet? Do you limit beans to one-half cup dry? Do you eat larger than a 3-oz portion of meat?

The DRI for protein may vary depending on activity level, state of health, and availability of protein food sources. Very active adults such as athletes and bodybuilders may raise their DRI to 1.2 to 1.4 g/kg, or up to a maximum of 1.7 to 1.8 g/kg. **The body requires more protein (1) during times of illness or injury, for such processes as cell repair and antibody production; and (2) during times of rapid tissue growth, such as pregnancy and lactation.** Individuals who are vegetarians or live in areas where meat sources of protein are scarce may need to consume up to 1.6 g/kg of complementary proteins to meet complete protein needs through combining foods.

To determine the protein requirement per day for a healthy adult, calculate as follows:

Weight in pounds ÷ 2.2 = _____ kg (1 kg = 2.2 lb)

_____ kg × 0.8 = _____ g of protein

PROTEIN DEFICIENCY

In many nations throughout the world, the availability of protein-rich food is limited. Millions of children under age 5 are affected by lack of protein intake. Lack of protein in young children can lead to permanent disabilities because of the fast rate of brain growth that occurs during this period. Extreme protein deficiency results in the conditions of marasmus and kwashiorkor. Marasmus is a form of protein–energy and nutrient malnutrition (a disorder of nutrition related to unbalanced diet, malabsorption, or lack of assimilation of nutrients) occurring chiefly in the first year of life, characterized by growth retardation and wasting of subcutaneous fat and muscle. Marasmus is the result of severe starvation. The body uses its carbohydrate and fat sources for energy. When these are depleted, protein muscle mass is used for energy. Use of muscle mass for energy will result in heart, lung, and kidney damage if the condition continues. Uncorrected, marasmus can lead to death.

Kwashiorkor is a condition occurring in infants and young children soon after weaning from breast milk. It is due to severe protein deficiency. **Kwashiorkor differs from marasmus in that adequate energy from other nutrients may be consumed; however, the diet is deficient in protein.** Symptoms of kwashiorkor include edema, pigment changes in the hair and skin, impaired growth and development, distention of the abdomen, and liver changes. These symptoms occur because low protein intake leads to changes in water balance, which leads to edema. Protein is the main component of hair. Therefore, deficiency results in changes in color and texture. The liver becomes fatty and loses it ability to function. Fatty enlargement of the liver results in an enlarged abdomen.

PROTEIN EXCESS

The average American diet supplies 1½ to 2 times the DRI for protein. Athletes and very active individuals may consume higher levels. High-protein diets for people who do not require a protein increase are stressful to the liver and kidneys. The kidneys must rid the body of excess waste products resulting from an increased protein intake. This increased stress on the kidneys can contribute to kidney damage. Protein is metabolized by the liver. Liver function is strained with the excess load of protein to metabolize, which could contribute to decreased liver function. High-protein diets, especially from meat sources, can lead to excess fat in the diet. High-fat diets are associated with increased risk of obesity, heart disease, and certain types of cancer (colon, breast, pancreas, and prostate).

VEGETARIAN DIETS

Many people have become vegetarians as a means to maintain desired weight and decrease the amount of animal fat in the diet. Cultural, religious, and personal factors (e.g., objection to the killing of animals for food) also influence a person's choice of a vegetarian diet. The primary types of vegetarian diets are as follows:

- Lacto-ovo-vegetarian: Dairy products, eggs, and plant foods are included in the diet.
- Lactovegetarian: Eggs are excluded. Dairy products and plant foods are included.
- Vegan: All animal food sources are excluded, including honey.

A vegetarian diet must be planned to include essential nutrients. Individuals choosing this dietary practice should engage in research and consult a nutrition specialist to ensure nutritional needs are met. The well-planned vegetarian diet is believed to offer health benefits such as reduced risk of heart disease, hypertension, diabetes, and obesity. The challenge is to plan meals that provide adequate levels of complete proteins, vitamins, and minerals. Vegans, in particular, may have a diet deficient in vitamin B_6, vitamin B_{12}, iron, zinc, calcium, riboflavin, and vitamin D. The more limited the vegetarian diet, the greater the risk of nutritional deficiencies.

Nutrient requirements can be met by combining categories of food to meet protein needs by following a modified version of the MyPyramid. Some combinations that provide a good protein source are whole grains plus legumes, legumes plus nuts or seeds, or whole grains, legumes, nuts, or seeds plus dairy products. Soybeans are a legume high in protein and contain all nine essential amino acids. Soy products are available in many sources, including tofu, legumes, protein powders, and soy milk. Mineral deficits can be avoided by eating dark green leafy vegetables, adding fruits with high levels of vitamin C to meals to aid in absorption of iron, or taking dietary supplements of calcium and vitamin B_{12} because these may be difficult to obtain in the absence of animal food sources.

Individuals who follow vegetarian diets meet their protein needs without consuming meat products. This is accomplished by combining plant sources of food to achieve a complete protein intake. These are called complementary proteins. Examples include red beans and rice, peanut butter on whole-wheat bread, bean soup with cornbread, or stir-fried vegetables with tofu.

Think Critically About . . . What nonmeat foods from a dinner you like could be combined to provide complete and adequate protein?

CARBOHYDRATES

Carbohydrates are the body's main source of energy. Carbohydrates should make up about 50% to 60% of the daily caloric intake. **Each gram of carbohydrate supplies 4 calories.** The three major forms of carbohydrates are simple carbohydrates, complex carbohydrates, and fiber. Complex carbohydrates should comprise about 90% of the total proportion of carbohydrates consumed. This category of carbohydrates contains fiber and other nutrients. Simple carbohydrates tend to be nutrient poor.

FUNCTIONS OF CARBOHYDRATES

Carbohydrates are a quick source of energy. They are easily converted to glucose, the fuel for the body's cells. Carbohydrates are important to the function of internal organs, the nervous system, and muscles. Carbohydrates are also needed to regulate protein and fat metabolism. They help to fight infection and promote growth of body tissues. Many carbohydrates are also high in dietary fiber, which is essential to the bulk in stool, aiding in regular waste elimination. High fiber intake is helpful in treating certain gastrointestinal disorders (e.g., constipation, hemorrhoids) and reducing blood cholesterol levels and synthesis.

SIMPLE CARBOHYDRATES

Glucose is the metabolized form of sugar in the body. It is found in table sugar (sucrose), fruit sugar (fruc-

tose), and milk sugar (lactose). These are quickly absorbed into the bloodstream as a ready source of energy for the cells. Sucrose is the major sweetener found in foods such as candy, ice cream, cookies, and cakes. The typical American diet is high in simple carbohydrates. Although simple sugars cause a quick rise in blood sugar, the level falls rapidly and can result in a return to a hunger state.

Think Critically About . . . Can you identify hidden sugar content of foods by reading the food label (Figure 26-4)? Sugar is added to many foods in the form of corn syrup, sucrose, lactose, maltose, and dextrin.

COMPLEX CARBOHYDRATES (STARCHES)

Complex carbohydrates are foods such as breads, pasta, cereal, potatoes, and rice. They are broken down into simple sugars for digestion, absorption, and use by the body. Starches provide a more consistent blood sugar level than simple sugars. Experts recommend

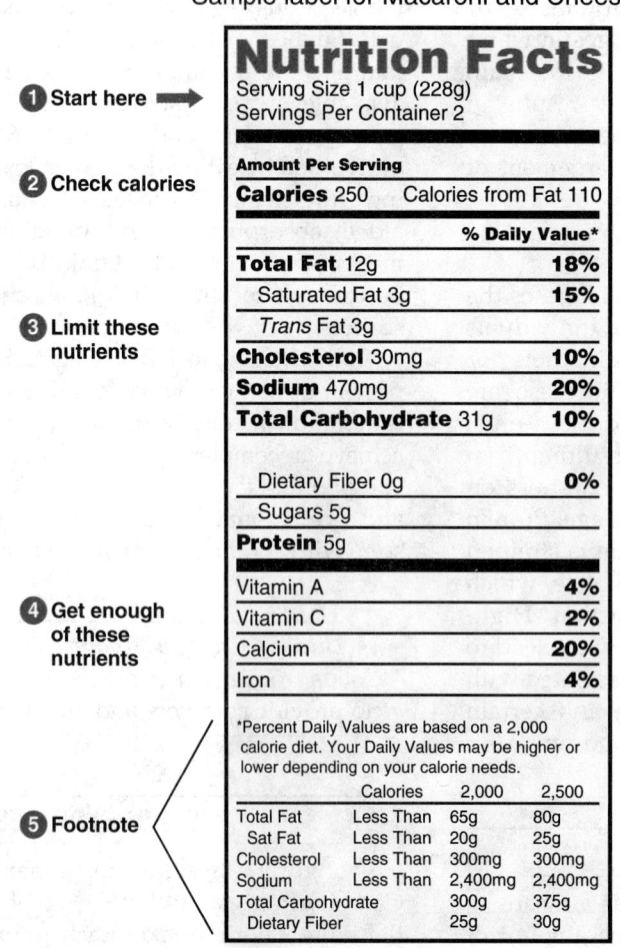

Sample label for Macaroni and Cheese

FIGURE **26-4** Food label.

Table 26-1 | *Carbohydrate Content of Selected Foods*

FOOD	QUANTITY	GRAMS OF CARBOHYDRATES
JUICE		
Apple	¾ cup	22
Grapefruit	¾ cup	17
Orange	¾ cup	20
FRUIT		
Banana	Medium	19
Apple	Medium	19
Grapefruit	½	11
Orange	Medium	15
Peach	Medium	10
Strawberries	½ cup	5
BREAD AND GRAINS		
Bagel	1	38
Cornbread	1 slice	28
Bread (white or wheat)	1 slice	12
VEGETABLES		
Corn	½ cup	15
Carrots	½ cup	6
Green beans	½ cup	4
Black beans	½ cup	20
Sweet potato	½ cup	32
Cauliflower	½ cup	2
DESSERTS		
Apple pie	1 slice	58
Cake with frosting	1 slice	35
Pecan pie	1 slice	65
Sorbet	½ cup	25
Ice cream	1 cup	32
Yogurt, plain	1 cup	16
MISCELLANEOUS		
Honey	1 tablespoon	17
Popcorn	1 cup	6
Red beans and rice	½ cup	40
Colas	12 ounces	38
Cashews	½ cup	22
Cream of Wheat	½ cup	32
Cornflakes	1 cup	20
Granola	1 cup	67
Grape Nuts	1 cup	93
Cheerios	1 cup	16

that 85% to 95% of carbohydrates consumed should be complex, and 5% to 15% should be simple sugars. The carbohydrate content of some common foods is listed in Table 26-1.

RECOMMENDATIONS FOR INTAKE

Dietary Reference Intakes (DRIs) were developed for carbohydrates in 2002. Children and adults need a minimum of 130 g of carbohydrates per day. Approximately 50% to 60% of total calories should be carbohydrates. Diet crazes, including both the Atkins diet and the South Beach diet, stresses low carbohydrate consumption. Several research studies conducted since 2002 suggest there may be benefits to low-carbohydrate diets as a means for weight loss. Compared to other meal plans, these diets may be effective for weight loss, maintaining weight loss, and improvement of high-density lipo-

protein (HDL) and triglyceride levels. Research is being conducted on the long-term effects of low-carbohydrate intake and, although the data are not in, there are questions about the nutritional effects and safety of long-term use of a low-carbohydrate diet. Some concerns include promotion of heart disease and increased risk of complications of liver and renal disease because of the high protein content of the diets. Most Americans need to increase complex carbohydrates and decrease consumption of simple sugar. It is suggested that the maximum intake of added sugars be limited to providing no more than 25% of energy.

> **?** *Think Critically About . . .* Can you determine your carbohydrate intake? Write down your food intake for the past 24 hours. Calculate total calories. What was the percentage of simple and complex carbohydrates? Divide carbohydrate calories by total calories.

FIBER

Dietary fiber is the portion of carbohydrates that cannot be broken down by intestinal enzymes and juices. Fiber passes through the small intestine and colon undigested. Food sources of fiber include whole-grain cereals and skins of fruits, vegetables, and legumes.

Fiber increases bulk in the stool, leading to good intestinal function and elimination. The presence of fiber in the colon also is beneficial in delaying absorption of carbohydrates and cholesterol from the intestine. This delay may be beneficial to diabetic patients by decreasing blood glucose levels. Some properties of fiber may also decrease absorption of fat. **Health experts recommend 21 to 38 g of fiber per day.** Fiber content in the diet can be increased by such practices as replacing white bread with whole-wheat bread and white rice with brown rice, or eating whole-grain cereals and pasta. Increasing intake of fresh fruit and vegetables, as well as beans and peas, will also increase fiber intake. Fiber content of selected foods is listed in Table 26-2.

FATS (LIPIDS)

Americans are becoming more aware of fats in their diets. Health promotion strategies emphasize the negative impact of fat on health. High fat intake has been linked to obesity, breast and colon cancer, hypertension and other cardiovascular diseases, and stroke. Triglycerides are the major lipid found in both foods and the body.

FUNCTIONS OF FAT

Fat is an essential nutrient. Fat supplies a concentrated form of energy. It also spares protein from being

Table 26-2 *Fiber Content of Selected Foods*

FOOD	QUANTITY	GRAMS OF FIBER
FRUITS		
Apple, unpeeled	1 small	3.0
Apple, peeled	1 small	2.0
Banana	1 medium	2.0
Orange	1 medium	1.7
Cantaloupe	½	3.0
Grapefruit	1 cup	3.0
Strawberries	1 cup	4.0
VEGETABLES		
Green beans	1 cup	1.9
Broccoli, raw	1 cup	3.5
Cauliflower, raw	1 cup	2.3
Celery, raw	1 cup	1.8
Corn, whole kernel	½ cup	3.0
Potato, with skin	1 medium	2.5
Sweet potato, baked	1 medium	3.0
GRAINS AND CEREALS		
Biscuit	1	1.0
Bread, white	1 slice	1.0
Bread, wheat	1 slice	2.0
All Bran	½ cup	9.0
Oatmeal, cooked	½ cup	4.0
Shredded Wheat	¾ cup	4.0
LEGUMES, COOKED		
Kidney beans	1 cup	19.0
Pinto beans	1 cup	20.0
Black-eyed peas	1 cup	16.0
Lima beans	1 cup	16.0
Black beans	1 cup	21.0

burned for energy. **Fat supplies 9 calories/g consumed.** Other functions of fat include the following:

- Provides a source of fatty acids
- Adds flavor to foods and contributes to texture
- Dissolves and transports fat-soluble vitamins and fat-soluble phytonutrients (carotenoids)
- Insulates and controls body temperature
- Makes food smell appetizing
- Cushions and protects body organs
- Facilitates transmission of nerve impulses
- Gives feeling of fullness after eating

Fats are made up of fatty acids and glycerol called triglycerides. Fatty acids are classified as either saturated fats or unsaturated fats. Fats can be of liquid or solid consistency. Fats that are liquid at room temperature are called *oils*. Most oils are unsaturated fat and include corn oil, safflower oil, and canola oil. *Omega-3 fatty acid* (found in salmon, trout, halibut, sardines, tuna, canola oil, soybean oil, omega-3–rich chicken eggs, and walnuts) is the most unsaturated form of fatty acid. These foods should be added to the diet as sources of unsaturated fat. Solid fats include shortening and lard and are saturated fats.

? *Think Critically About . . .* How much saturated and unsaturated fat is used in your home per day?

FOOD SOURCES OF FAT

Animal food sources provide the most saturated fatty acids, and vegetables, nuts, or seeds supply unsaturated fatty acids. Two saturated vegetable fats are coconut oil and palm oil. **There are three essential fatty acids: linoleic acid (found in corn oil, safflower oil, and sunflower oil), oleic acid (found in olive oil and beef), and linolenic acid (found in green leafy vegetables, walnuts, pecans, soybean oil, and soybean products).** These fatty acids are necessary for the production of healthy blood cells, healthy arteries, nerve function, and skin maintenance. Deficiencies of these three fatty acids may lead to illness or skin problems.

Most Americans consume more fat in the diet than is needed to maintain health. The recommended daily allowance of fat is 25% to 30% of total calories. Saturated fats should be limited to 10% of total fat intake, or 2.5% to 3% of total calories. Some cardiologists recommend diets of 20% fat for individuals at risk for heart disease and as low as 10% fat for individuals with a history of heart disease. Research has shown a marked reduction of risk for further complications of heart disease and in some instances reversal of cardiac pathology.

A component of fat, cholesterol, is linked to heart disease and hardening of the arteries. Cholesterol is only found in animal products and oils such as palm and coconut. Increased cholesterol level places the individual at risk for heart disease and stroke. Cholesterol, however, has an important role in the structure of essential hormones and in the conversion of vitamin D by the action of sunlight on the skin. Cholesterol is also essential to the production of bile in the liver. Table 26-3 lists fat content of selected foods.

VITAMINS

Vitamins are present in small amounts in a wide variety of food sources. They are essential nutrients that must be taken in through food sources or supplements. It is best to consume vitamins through food sources; however, vitamin supplements can provide the nutrients needed. Vitamins are classified as *fat soluble* or *water soluble*. Water-soluble vitamins are easily absorbed into the bloodstream for use by the body. Fat-soluble vitamins are absorbed in the small intestine the same as other fats by action of bile in the duodenum, and are stored in the liver.

The fat-soluble vitamins are vitamins A, D, E, and K. These vitamins, because they are stored in the body, can cause toxicity (poisoning) if ingested in excessive quantities. Vitamin A can be produced in the body by carotenoids (e.g., beta-carotene) Carotenoids act as antioxidants, protecting the cells and tissues from damage from free radicals, and have been shown to increase immunity, improve vision, and have a role in cancer prevention.

The water-soluble vitamins include the B-complex vitamins (thiamine, riboflavin, niacin, vitamin B_6, folic

Table 26-3 | *Fat Content of Selected Foods*

FOOD	QUANTITY	GRAMS OF FAT
DAIRY PRODUCTS/EGGS		
Milk, whole	1 cup	8
Milk, 2%	1 cup	5
Milk, 1%	1 cup	3
Ice cream	1 cup	14
Yogurt, plain	1 cup	3
Egg, whole	1	5
Egg white	1	0
Butter	1 tablespoon	12
Margarine	1 tablespoon	11
FISH		
Catfish, fried	3 ounces	11
Salmon, canned	3 ounces	2
Tuna, canned in oil	3 ounces	7
Tuna, canned in water	3 ounces	2
MEAT AND POULTRY		
Beef	3 ounces	26
Bacon	3 ounces	9
Ham	3 ounces	14
Pork chop	3 ounces	19
Frankfurter	1	13
Chicken breast, with skin	½	18
Chicken breast, without skin	½	3
Chicken leg, with skin	1	11
Chicken leg, without skin	1	2
FAST FOODS		
Whopper with cheese	1	48
Quarter-Pounder with cheese	1	29
Big Mac	1	32
French fries, small	1 serving	12
Wendy's Single	1	16
Wendy's Small Chili	1 serving	9
MISCELLANEOUS		
Mayonnaise	1 tablespoon	11
Avocado	1	30
Cashews	½ cup	32

acid, vitamin B_{12}, pantothenic acid, and biotin) and vitamin C. Some of these vitamins (especially niacin, vitamin B_6, and folate) accumulate in toxic amounts only if a person is taking large quantities of them as supplements or is suffering from kidney failure. Although vitamins do not have caloric value, they are essential to the body for the building of tissue and for proper cellular function and to facilitate the reactions that release energy from carbohydrates, proteins, and fats. Table 26-4 summarizes the function, common food sources, signs of deficiency, and signs of toxicity of fat-soluble and water-soluble vitamins.

MINERALS

Minerals are inorganic substances contained in animals and plants. They are essential for metabolism and cellular function. Minerals are categorized as major minerals (macro minerals) or trace minerals (micro minerals). The major minerals are calcium, magnesium, sodium, potassium, phosphorus, sulfur, and chlorine. Selected foods with high sodium content are listed in Table 26-5. Trace minerals are iron, copper, iodine, manganese, cobalt, zinc, molybdenum, selenium, fluoride, and chromium. **Minerals are necessary for proper muscle and nerve function and act as catalysts for many cellular functions.** They combine to form salts and are largely responsible for the acid–base balance of the body. Because mineral actions are interrelated, a deficiency of one mineral will affect the action of another mineral in the body. Other functions of minerals include the following:

- Maintaining rigidity and strength in teeth and bones
- Facilitating contraction and relaxation of muscles
- Assisting in blood clotting, and tissue repair and growth

Dietary Reference Intakes have been created for every mineral. Generally, sufficient minerals can be supplied by a balanced diet. Extra iron is needed when blood loss from surgery or trauma has occurred. The body does not manufacture its own minerals; therefore, all must be provided through food sources. Table 26-6 lists minerals, their function, food sources, signs of deficiency, and signs of toxicity.

WATER

Water is the most essential of all nutrients. The adult body is 50% to 60% water by weight. The proportion of water is dependent upon body composition, age, bone density, body weight, and hormone status. As the body ages, the percentage of body water decreases. **The water requirement for adults is approximately 1 mL/calorie of intake** (or 35 mL/kg in adults, 30 mL/kg in the elderly). Water requirements are increased for patients who are immobile, have a fever, or have diarrhea.

Water is used in every body process from digestion to absorption to elimination or secretion. Most foods contain water, and the body obtains a substantial amount of the water needed directly from food. Water is not stored in the body, and what is lost during 24 hours must be replaced. **A general rule is that the patient should take in an amount equal to the recorded fluid output plus 500 mL.**

FACTORS THAT INFLUENCE NUTRITION

To assist patients to reach their optimum nutritional state, you must consider a variety of factors that may influence an individual's ability to meet nutritional needs. A dietitian should be consulted if malnutrition or risk of malnutrition is suspected.

Table 26-4 *Vitamins*

VITAMIN	MAJOR FUNCTION	FOOD SOURCE	DEFICIENCY	TOXICITY
FAT-SOLUBLE VITAMINS				
Vitamin A (retinol)	Maintenance of epithelial cells and mucous membranes. Important for night vision. Necessary for adequate immune response	Liver, dark green leafy vegetables, deep orange vegetables and fruit	Night blindness; rough, dry skin; dry mucous membranes; xerophthalmia (an eye disease)	Appetite loss, hair loss, dry skin, bone and joint pain, enlarged liver and spleen, fetal malformations
Vitamin E	Protects red blood cells from rupture. Prevents destruction of vitamin A in the intestine. Helps maintain normal cell membranes	Vegetable oils, wheat germ, legumes, nuts, fish, green leafy vegetables	Breakdown of red blood cells	Decreased thyroid hormone level, increase in triglycerides
Vitamin K	Necessary for blood clotting	Dark green leafy vegetables, cauliflower, soybean oil, green tea, synthesis of intestinal bacteria	Hemorrhage	None known
Vitamin D	Aids in absorption of calcium and phosphorus, regulates blood levels of calcium. Promotes bone and teeth mineralization	Fortified milk, fish with bones, cod liver oil	Rickets (children) Osteomalacia (adults)	Calcification of soft tissues, hypercalcemia, renal stones, growth failure in children
WATER-SOLUBLE VITAMINS				
Vitamin B$_1$ (thiamine)	Carbohydrate metabolism; assists function of the heart, muscles, and nervous system. Promotes appetite and good function of the digestive tract	Whole grains, wheat germ, organ meats, pork, legumes, brewer's yeast	Polyneuritis, beriberi, fatigue, depression, poor appetite, edema, nervous instability, Wernicke's encephalopathy, Korsakoff's psychosis, spastic muscle contractions	None known
Vitamin B$_2$ (riboflavin)	Essential for certain enzyme systems that aid in the metabolism of carbohydrate, proteins, and fats	Milk and milk products, eggs, green leafy vegetables, organ meats, peanuts, whole grains	Tongue inflammation, scaling and burning skin, sensitive eyes, cataracts	None known
Vitamin B$_3$ (niacin)	Part of the enzymes that regulate energy metabolism. Promotes good physical and mental health and helps maintain the health of the skin, tongue, and digestive system. May be used as an anticoagulant	Meats and organ meats, whole-grain flour, enriched white flour, legumes, brewer's yeast	Pellagra, gastrointestinal disturbances, photosensitive dermatitis, depressive psychosis	Flushing caused by vasodilation; nausea and vomiting; abnormal glucose metabolism; abnormal plasma uric acid levels; abnormal liver function; gastric ulceration
Vitamin B$_6$ (pyridoxine)	Metabolism of proteins, amino acids, carbohydrates, and fats. Essential for proper growth and maintenance of body functions	Liver and red meats, whole grains, potatoes, green vegetables, corn	Believed to lead to convulsions, peripheral neuropathy, secondary pellagra, possible depression, oral lesions	Sensory nerve damage, numbness of extremities, ataxia, bone pain, muscle weakness

Adapted from Peckenpaugh, N.J., & Poleman, C.M. (2007). *Nutrition Essentials and Diet Therapy* (10th ed.). Philadelphia: Elsevier Saunders.

Table 26-4 | *Vitamins—cont'd*

VITAMIN	MAJOR FUNCTION	FOOD SOURCE	DEFICIENCY	TOXICITY
WATER-SOLUBLE VITAMINS—cont'd				
Vitamin B$_{12}$ (cobalamin)	Aids in hemoglobin synthesis, normal functioning of all cells, folic acid metabolism. Important in energy metabolism	Meats, organ meats, dry milk and milk products, eggs	Pernicious anemia, anorexia, degeneration of the spinal cord, various psychiatric disorders	None known
Folic acid	Formation of red blood cells and normal functioning of gastrointestinal tract. Aids in metabolism of proteins	Glandular meats, yeast, dark green leafy vegetables, legumes, whole grains	Impaired cell division, megaloblastic anemia, possible neural tube defect, various psychiatric disorders	None known
Vitamin C (ascorbic acid)	Helps protect the body against infections. Aids in wound healing	Citrus fruits, tomatoes, strawberries, cantaloupe, currants, broccoli, cabbage, potatoes, green peppers, green leafy vegetables	Scurvy, anemia, swollen and bleeding gums, loose teeth, poor wound healing, easy bruising from ruptured small blood vessels	Urinary stones, diarrhea, hypoglycemia

Table 26-5 | *Selected Foods with High Sodium Content*

FOOD	QUANTITY	MILLIGRAMS OF SODIUM
PREPARED FOODS		
Cream of potato soup	1 cup	1422
Tomato soup	1 cup	1022
Chili, no beans	1 cup	1024
Cheese ravioli	1 cup	1280
Cream of chicken soup	1 cup	1047
Chicken noodle soup	1 cup	1000
FAST FOOD		
Burger King Whopper	1	1105
Arby's Beef and Cheddar	1	1801
Subway Cold Cut Sub	6 inch	1651
Supreme pizza	1 slice	1313
MISCELLANEOUS FOODS		
Pickle	1 slice	56
Olive	1	75
Table salt	1 teaspoon	2300
Sausage link	1	643
Cheese	1 ounce	264
Soy sauce	1 tablespoon	1000
Taco seasoning	2 teaspoon	480

cious appetites, leading to concerns about weight management. Eating disorders are a concern during this growth period, especially among adolescent girls, but the prevalence in adolescent boys is increasing.

Physiologic changes and physical limitations may influence the eating habits of the elderly. The elderly may be at risk for inadequate nutrition because of income limits, loneliness, and difficulty obtaining and/or preparing food. Nutritional deficiencies can often mimic the dementia of aging, and elderly patients showing signs of dementia should be evaluated for deficiencies.

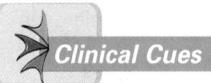

Clinical Cues

The elderly may also be overweight related to decreased activity and high fat intake. A method of accurately accessing overweight is to determine the waist-to-hip ratio. Measure the waist at the narrowest point, and the hips at the widest point. Divide the waist measurement by the hip measurement to determine the ratio. A ratio of 0.7 for women and 0.9 for men is considered healthy. The higher the ratio, the greater the risk for heart disease and other conditions related to overweight and obesity.

AGE

Infants are dependent upon others to meet their nutritional needs. Nutrition may be provided by breast milk or formula. As the child grows, nutritional needs change based on the stage of development. Parents and caregivers face the challenge of experimenting with a variety of foods and meal strategies to meet the needs of growing children.

Adolescents are strongly influenced by their peers. Food choices are often of the fast-food and pizza variety. Growth spurts during this time may result in vora-

ILLNESS

Nutritional needs usually increase during illness. Patients with diseases such as cancer and human immunodeficiency virus/acquired immunodeficiency syndrome (HIV/AIDS) experience loss of muscle mass, resulting in the need for more calories and protein. A loss of appetite may occur due to pain, nausea, vomiting, and stomatitis. These patients are a special challenge to health care workers.

Table 26-6 | *Minerals*

MINERAL	FUNCTION	FOOD SOURCE	DEFICIENCY	TOXICITY
Calcium	Muscle contraction and relaxation, coagulation, building of strong bones and teeth, plays role in nervous system function, aids in blood coagulation	Milk and milk products, dark green leafy vegetables, sardines, salmon with bones, tofu and other soy products, and hard water	Poor bone growth and tooth development, poor blood clotting, osteoporosis, rickets in children, osteomalacia in adults; possible hypertension	Kidney stones in predisposed individuals
Chloride	Maintenance of fluid and acid–base balance, aids in activation of gastric enzymes	Table salt, fish, vegetables	Disturbances in acid–base balance; possible growth retardation, psychomotor defects, and memory loss	None known
Magnesium	Builds strong teeth and bones, protein synthesis, regulation of heartbeat	Raw dark green leafy vegetables, nuts and soybeans, whole grains, bananas, apricots, seafood, coffee, tea, cocoa, hard water	Rare, but in disease states may lead to confusion, poor memory, cardiac arrhythmia	Increased calcium excretion
Phosphorus	Helps build strong bones and teeth, present in the nuclei of all cells, acid–base balance, factor in energy metabolism	Milk and milk products, eggs, meats, legumes, whole grains, soft drinks	With malabsorption can cause anorexia, weakness, stiff joints, and fragile bones	Hypocalcemia, tetany
Potassium	Acid–base balance, transmits nerve impulses and helps control muscle contractions and regulation of heartbeat; necessary for enzyme reactions	Apricots, bananas, oranges, grapefruit, green beans, broccoli, carrots, potatoes, meat, milk, peanut butter, legumes, molasses, coffee, tea, cocoa	May cause impaired growth, hypertension, bone fragility, diminished heart rate, arrhythmias, and death	Hyperkalemia, with cardiac disturbances
Sodium	Acid–base balance, fluid balance, transmits nerve impulses and helps control muscle contractions	Salt (major source), milk, milk products, and several vegetables	Hyponatremia, edema of lower extremities	May cause hypertension, can lead to renal disease and cardiovascular disease
Chromium	Activates enzymes, enhances the removal of glucose from the blood	Liver and other meats, whole grains, cheese, legumes, brewer's yeast	Weight loss, abnormalities of the central nervous system, possible aggravation of diabetes mellitus	Liver damage
Fluoride	Aids in formation of bones and teeth, decreases cavities	Fluoridated water, fish, tea, gelatin	Increased risk of dental caries	Mottling of teeth
Iodine	Helps regulate metabolism as a part of thyroid hormones; helps to keep skin, hair, and nails healthy	Iodized salt, saltwater fish, seaweed products	Goiter; cretinism in children born to iodine-deficient mothers	Goiter
Iron	Formation of hemoglobin	Liver, red meats, dark green leafy vegetables, fortified cereals, legumes, whole grains	Iron deficiency anemia	Idiopathic excess hemoglobin, which can lead to cirrhosis, diabetes mellitus, and cardiac enlargement
Zinc	Protein synthesis, normal growth and sexual development, wound healing, immune function, smell acuity	Whole grains, wheat germ, crabmeat, liver, brewer's yeast	Depressed immune function, poor growth, delayed sexual maturation	Severe anemia, nausea, vomiting, cramps, diarrhea, malaise, fatigue, renal damage

Adapted from Peckenpaugh, N.J., & Poleman, C.M. (2007). *Nutrition Essentials and Diet Therapy* (10th ed.). Philadelphia: Elsevier Saunders.

EMOTIONAL STATUS

An individual's emotional state has a strong influence on eating habits. Some persons tend to overeat during times of emotional distress, whereas others will lose their appetite. You should be aware of the patient's response to stress and take opportunities to intervene if nutrition is compromised.

ECONOMIC STATUS

Sufficient income does not guarantee optimum nutrition. However, it does provide the opportunity to make healthy choices. Individuals with limited income can benefit from patient education related to good nutritional choices because a balanced diet is affordable even with low income. In addition, patients should be referred to community and government programs (e.g., Women, Infants, and Children [WIC]; Supplemental Food Program) for assistance in meeting nutritional needs. Social workers and dietitians can be helpful in recommending community resources providing nutritional interventions and programs.

RELIGION

Religious practices and affiliations influence nutrition by dictating food preparation, foods allowed, and those to avoid. You must develop an awareness of and respect for patients' religious beliefs related to food to promote good nutrition effectively. Some common religious food practices include the following:

- *Islam:* No pork or pork products. No alcohol.
- *Judaism:* Foods prepared in kosher manner (prepared for use according to Jewish law). Separate dishes, pans, and silverware must be used to prepare and serve meat and dairy food. Meat and milk may not be eaten at the same meal. Pork, shellfish, crustaceans, and birds of prey are not allowed. Orthodox Jews follow stricter guidelines than others.
- *Seventh-Day Adventist:* No stimulants (coffee, tea). Shellfish, pork, and alcohol must be avoided. Many are lacto-ovo-vegetarians with emphasis on whole-grain foods.

CULTURE

Cultural influences, both ethnic and environmental, have an important impact on nutrition. Individuals are more likely to consume foods with which they are familiar. Most traditional ethnic diets can be modified to meet required nutritional needs. Many rely on combining incomplete proteins (rice and beans, etc.) to make complete proteins.

CULTURAL INFLUENCES ON NUTRITION

American society is composed of multiple cultures. Ethnicity, culture, and region of residence have a strong influence on nutrition. Awareness of nutritional preferences of different ethnic groups can enhance your ability to provide effective nutritional counseling.

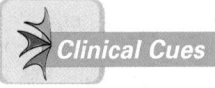
Clinical Cues

Consult with or refer patients to the dietitian/nutritionist to provide foods the patient will find acceptable to eat. Allowing family to prepare and provide food for the patient may be a means to ensure proper nutrition. Family members can be advised of any restrictions required because of specific medical needs.

AFRICAN AMERICAN

The African American diet closely resembles food preferences of the southern region of the United States. African and West Indian influences are also prevalent in the African American diet, as evidenced by inclusion of foods such as okra, black-eyed peas, and peanuts and peanut products in the diet.

Typical foods in the traditional African American diet include a variety of greens (collard, mustard, turnip, kale), dry beans, cornbread, sweet potatoes, pork, catfish, and chicken. Most meats and fish are prepared by frying. Seasonings for vegetables include smoked bacon, ham, and salted pork. Desserts may include sweet potato pie, peach cobbler, and fried pies. These preferences often contributed to high fat, sugar, and salt content in the traditional African American diet. Dietary counseling should include modification of the diet to accomplish a more healthy composition while maintaining the basic components of the diet.

HISPANIC AMERICAN

The Hispanic population is one of the fastest growing in the United States. Several groups are represented, including Mexican, Puerto Rican, and Cuban. Nutrition preferences have a Spanish and American Indian influence. The Hispanic diet is high in carbohydrates such as beans, rice, corn, and tortillas. Meats and meat dishes are heavily seasoned and spicy. The diet can be high in fat because of the use of lard in the preparation of fried foods. Desserts are very sweet and may be prepared with syrup-like sauces. Preferences for fried foods lead to high fat in the diet.

ASIAN AMERICAN

The popularity of Asian American cuisine is evident throughout the United States. The traditional Asian diet is high in carbohydrates and vegetables, and low in meat and fish. Mung beans and soybeans and products such as sprouts are also used. Vegetables are rarely eaten raw. They are stir-fried and added to meat, rice, or noodle dishes. The practice of adding monosodium glutamate (MSG) to enhance flavor has decreased. However, dishes may still have a high sodium and high fat content.

Table 26-7 *Culturally Diverse Food Patterns of Americans*

CULTURE	HISTORICAL DIETARY PATTERN*
African American	All meats, fish, and chicken; pork often consumed (spareribs, bacon, and sausage); vegetables cooked in salt pork for long periods of time; grits and cornbread muffins; some lactose intolerance. Popular vegetables include collard greens, beet greens, and sweet potatoes.
Chinese American	Rich in vegetables (bean sprouts, broccoli, bamboo shoots, and mushrooms). Vegetables cooked until crisp; meat consumed in small portions with other food. Soy sauce, tofu, peanut butter; limited milk and cheese; fish baked with native spices; soups with egg, meat, and vegetables. Tea is China's national beverage. Rice is staple of diet.
Jewish American	Diet varies according to whether family is Orthodox, Reform, or Conservative. For Orthodox family, food must be kosher (clean); meat is soaked in salt water to remove blood; only meat eaten is that of divided hoofed animals that chew a cud; fish without scales (shellfish) and pork are prohibited; milk and meat cannot be combined. Favorites are gefilte fish, lox (smoked salmon), herring, eggs, bagels, cream cheese, and matzo.
Laotian American	Numerous varieties of freshwater fish and shellfish (eaten fresh, dried, or salted); pork, beef, chicken, rabbit, often mixed with vegetables and spices; eggs, peanuts, black-eyed peas; vegetables eaten raw, as juice, or cooked with meat or fish and preserved by drying or pickling; sticky rice, rice or bean thread noodles, and legumes often used in desserts; soybean drink, sugar cane drink, tea, and coconut juice. Popular seasonings include padek, chilies, curry, tamarind, and red and black pepper.
Italian American	All meats, fish, and chicken, including cold cuts (salami, mortadella) and Italian pork sausage; pasta (staple of diet), breads, olive oil, wine, cheese, and all varieties of fruits and vegetables.
Japanese American	Fish and seafood (fresh, smoked, and raw) and beef. Food is cut into small portions. Principal fruit is nasi, which tastes much like a pear. Many vegetables are eaten, such as seaweed, bamboo shoots, onions, beans, and dried mushrooms (shitake); enjoy pickled vegetables. Rice is national staple. Beverages include tea and sake. Little cheese, milk, butter, or cream is consumed. Chief cooking fat is soybean oil or rice oil.
Mexican American	Chicken, pork chops, wieners, cold cuts, hamburger, eggs (used frequently), beans (eaten mashed or refried with lard), potatoes (basic item, usually fried), chilies, fresh tomatoes, corn (maize—often used as basic grain), tortillas, packaged cereals; little milk because of lactose intolerance.
American Indian	Acorn flour, a staple food made into mush or bread; salmon, fresh or dried; other varieties of fish, deer, duck, geese, and other small game; nuts such as buckeye and hazel; wild berries, seeds, and roots.
Puerto Rican American	Meat cooked in stews; poultry, pork, fish, dried beans or peas mixed with rice; milk in combination with coffee (cafe con leche), variety of fruits, starchy vegetables (plantains, cassava, sweet potatoes), salad, soft drinks.
Vietnamese American	Pork—most common meat; meats cut into small pieces and fried, boiled, or steamed; fish—all types of freshwater and saltwater fish and shellfish, often fried and dipped in fish sauce; eggs, soybeans, legumes, and wide variety of fruits and vegetables; rice often eaten with every meal; seasonings including oyster sauce, soy sauce, monosodium glutamate, ginger, garlic, nuoc mam sauce; tea, coffee, soft drinks, soybean milk.
Middle Eastern American	Lamb is the most commonly eaten meat. Pork is prohibited if the individual is of the Muslim or Jewish faith. Legumes such as black beans, chick peas, and lentils may be used for food preparation. Feta cheese is a favorite dairy product. Breads and cereals may include unleavened bread, and pita bread is commonly eaten. Eggplant is very common in the Middle Eastern diet. Fruits and vegetables are preferred raw. Preferred spices and herbs include dill, garlic, mint, cinnamon, oregano, parsley, pepper, and olive oil.

Adapted from Leifer, G. (2003). *Introduction to Maternity & Pediatric Nursing* (5th ed., p. 36). Philadelphia: Saunders; and data from Mahan, L.K., & Escott-Stump, S. (2008). *Krause's Food, Nutrition and Diet Therapy* (12th ed.). Philadelphia: Elsevier Saunders; and other sources.
*More diverse eating patterns occur as future generations of a culture become assimilated.

MIDDLE EASTERN AMERICAN

Food preferences among Middle Eastern cultures include fermented dairy products such as yogurt, meats, grains in the form or wheat or rice at each meal, fresh fruits, and vegetables. Some foods are specially prepared if the individual practices the Muslim religion. Food preparation includes grilling, frying, grinding, and stewing.

The nurse and dietitian can assist patients to modify diets to meet nutritional requirements. Meals can be made healthier by teaching patients to prepare food with less fat and sodium. Use of herbal, low-sodium seasoning can maintain the desired flavor. A summary of food patterns of American cultural groups can be found in Table 26-7.

NUTRITIONAL NEEDS THROUGHOUT THE LIFE SPAN

INFANTS

The first year of life marks the fastest growth period of human development. **By 6 months of age, the birth weight of the normal newborn should double. By the end of the first year, the birth weight should**

triple. The American Academy of Pediatrics recommends that infants be breast-fed or receive breast milk for the first full year of life. Emphasis on the importance of breast-feeding is a major component of prenatal education programs. In addition to providing complete nutrition, breast milk also provides immunity to most childhood diseases through the first few months of life. The first breast fluid, colostrum, is available at delivery. Colostrum also contributes to passage of meconium stool and growth of normal bacterial flora in the bowel. Within 7 to 10 days of delivery, the composition of breast milk changes. Protein and fat-soluble vitamin content decreases, and water-soluble vitamins, fat, and calories increase. By the 14th day, mature milk is produced. Breast milk rarely causes allergic responses in the infant.

Infant formulas are similar in composition to breast milk; however, nutrients in human milk are more easily digested and absorbed. Formulas are a modified form of cow's milk, made more digestible and with added carbohydrate and fat content. Infants with allergy to modified cow's milk may use soy-based formulas (unless soy allergy is a concern) or special hypoallergenic formulas. An advantage of bottle feeding is the opportunity to share the feeding responsibility with other caregivers. Feeding can be a time to build an emotional bond with the infant. Fathers, grandparents, and older siblings can also establish this bond. Breast-feeding mothers can pump their breasts so that the infant can be bottle-fed by other caregivers.

A milestone for infants is the introduction of solid foods. Pediatricians prefer adding solid foods to the diet at 4 to 6 months of age; however, some health care professionals encourage later introduction of solid foods (starting at 9 to 12 months) to further decrease the risk of food allergy or sensitivity. Many parents add solid foods earlier in the belief that solid foods will satisfy the infant and result in the infant sleeping through the night. This practice should be discouraged because the infant's GI system is still immature and is unable to digest cereals before 3 months of age. **Introducing solid foods before 4 to 6 months of age also increases the risk of the infant developing food allergies as the immune system matures.**

Solid foods should be introduced gradually, one item at a time. This provides the opportunity to identify allergic responses. A cereal such as rice is a good initial choice. Rice is easily tolerated and provides additional iron and calories. Another new food can be introduced in about 1 week. Each new food should be a single item. Introduction of combination foods decreases the ability to identify foods that may be responsible for an allergic response should one occur. As the child shows evidence of tolerating solid foods, weaning from the bottle or breast should be considered. Parents and caregivers should allow children to develop their own food preferences and to decide when and how much to eat.

TODDLERS AND PRESCHOOL CHILDREN

During the toddler and preschool years (ages 2 to 5), the growth rate tends to level off. The child consumes less milk and increases intake of solid foods. Toddlers' food choices may change frequently. They seem to have a hearty appetite at times, then show lack of appetite at other times. Specific food preferences may be evidenced (e.g., mashed potatoes and gravy); then the child suddenly refuses these items. Parents and caregivers become very frustrated with these reactions and are often concerned that the child is not obtaining adequate nutrition. Parents can use some of the following guidelines to assist toddlers to eat:

- Provide a pleasant environment at mealtimes.
- Avoid combination foods. Toddlers prefer single-item foods that do not touch each other on the plate.
- Provide plates and utensils in a size that can be easily handled by the small child.
- Provide small servings.
- Use dishes that are colorful and/or contain pictures of favorite characters.
- Avoid forcing a child to eat.
- Offer foods that are easy to chew.
- Try colorful foods (e.g., peas, carrots).

SCHOOL-AGE CHILDREN

School-age children may be influenced by their peer group when making food choices. They are very susceptible to commercial ads for fast food that show toys as prizes and show children in play areas when eating. Children at this age may desire sweet, non-nutritive foods such as soda, candy, cake, and ice cream. Parents and caregivers should serve as role models by eating nutritious meals and snacks and providing healthy meals and snacks for school time. Children should be served a well-balanced breakfast before leaving for school. Studies have shown that a healthy breakfast increases a child's ability to concentrate and achieve in school. Lunches could be taken from home or selected from the school cafeteria menu. Children should be taught to make wise choices from the school menu. Children from lower income families may be able to take advantage of government-sponsored school breakfast and lunch programs.

An increasing number of children come home after school to an environment without adult supervision. Parents can provide nutritious after-school snacks such as fruit and raw vegetables. Snacks high in sodium and sugar should be minimized or avoided. Because of the high calorie and high sodium preferences of many young children, obesity (excessive accumulation of body fat) can be a health issue during the school-age years.

ADOLESCENTS

Many physiologic changes occur during the adolescent years. Of these changes, the growth spurt and social and emotional changes related to puberty have great impact on nutrition and eating habits. Adolescents tend to consume many fast foods, either from fast-food restaurants or vending machines. Fast-food restaurants also serve as a social gathering place for many adolescents.

During the growth spurt (girls ages 10.5 to 14, and boys ages 12.5 to 14), the body requires more calories as well as nutrients such as B vitamins, calcium, vitamin D, and iron. Adolescent females require increased levels of iron after the menstrual cycle begins. Adolescent girls are very aware of their appearance. Concern about weight may lead to eating disorders, resulting in inadequate calories and nutrients for growth. Parental supervision and intervention may be critical to assisting the adolescent to meet appropriate nutritional needs. Parents can assist by

- Providing snacks high in calcium, iron, and protein
- Decreasing preparation of high-fat foods
- Teaching how to select more healthful choices from fast-food restaurants and preparing healthier versions at home with friends
- Keeping fruit juice and low-fat milk available instead of high-calorie sodas
- Keeping vegetable sticks and fresh fruit available as snack choices

ADULTS

Child-rearing, work, and family responsibilities have an influence on the eating habits of most adults. Many adults rely on fast food or convenience foods to meet their nutritional needs. Studies have shown that adults eat many of their meals, especially breakfast and lunch, from fast-food restaurants. Oftentimes the only meal consumed at home is the evening meal, and even that may not be prepared at home. Medical problems such as obesity and hypertension are prevalent during early and middle adulthood. This can be attributed to stress, poor eating habits, and lack of exercise. Lifestyle and dietary recommendations for adults include

- Decrease fat and sodium intake.
- Decrease intake of simple sugars.
- Increase fruit, fresh vegetables, and whole grains in the diet.
- Prepare more meals at home, where fat and sodium content can be controlled.
- Increase exercise.

Patient teaching about good nutrition and making healthy choices is very important. Many want to change habits, but may not have the needed information (Communication Cues 26-1).

OLDER ADULTS

Older adults are the group most at risk for inadequate nutrition. Many factors influence eating habits of

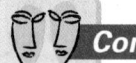 **Communication Cues 26-1**

The Patient with Hypertension

Mrs. Hernandez is readmitted to the hospital with a blood pressure of 190/120. She is sitting in a chair looking out the window. You notice she has been crying.

NURSE: "Good morning, Mrs. Hernandez. I'm Lisa, your nurse today."

MRS. HERNANDEZ: *(Continues to look out the window. Sobs quietly.)*

NURSE: "You seem upset, Mrs. Hernandez. How can I help you?"

MRS. HERNANDEZ: "This disease is going to kill me!" *(Continues to cry. Grasps arms of chair tightly.)*

NURSE: "Your disease is going to kill you?"

MRS. HERNANDEZ: "Yes! My blood pressure has gotten so high, and it's all my fault!"

NURSE: "Tell me more." *(Places hand on patient's shoulder, pulls up a chair, and sits next to her.)*

MRS. HERNANDEZ: "I take my medicine, but I just can't stop eating and lose weight. Look at my hands and feet. They are so swollen." *(Points at hands and feet.)*

NURSE: "Yes, I see they are swollen. Tell me about your diet at home."

MRS. HERNANDEZ: "I like a lot of salt in my food. My favorite foods are cheese, enchiladas, burritos, and chips. They don't taste good without lots of salt."

NURSE: "Seasoning is very important to making food taste good. Let's discuss ways to season the foods you like without using too much salt. The excess salt in your diet may be the cause of the swelling in your hands and feet."

MRS. HERNANDEZ: *(Looks up at nurse.)* "You can do that? I really want to learn to do this. I'm not ready to die!"

NURSE: "I hear you are afraid you will die from this disease. Uncontrolled blood pressure can put you at risk for serious complications, including death; however, managing your diet and taking your medications are ways to reduce those risks."

MRS. HERNANDEZ: *(Smiles at nurse.)* "Thanks for talking to me. Let's start talking about the things I need to know."

older adults. Economic status, physical disabilities, chronic disease, access to food sources, and physiologic changes must be considered when planning nutrition for this group. **Nutrient requirements do not change with aging except in the presence of disease and/or illness.** Older adults may need to decrease calories if activity level is decreased; however, increasing physical activity by including strength training and flexibility activities should be encouraged to promote appetite and a sense of well-being. Physiologic changes such as a decrease in taste and smell may decrease the appetite of many older adults. The taste of sweets remains strongest and may contribute to elderly people consuming more sweets than is advisable. Physical limitations such as chronic lung disease and arthritis make food preparation

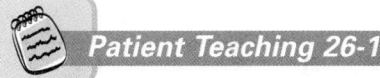

Patient Teaching 26-1

Improving Nutrition of Elderly Adults

Mrs. Lewis, a 76-year-old, has lived alone since her daughter and grandchildren moved away 3 months ago. She chose not to move and live with her daughter's family. For the past month, Mrs. Lewis has experienced a progressive decrease in appetite. She states she does not enjoy eating alone. She states it is too much trouble to cook for one person. Mrs. Lewis should be taught to

- Prepare several portions of favorite foods at one time, and place in freezer containers for easy access and preparation.
- Keep nutritious snacks available, including fruit, vegetable slices, and soft desserts such as puddings.
- Participate in church and/or community senior citizen social activities to increase socialization.
- Serve food in an attractive setting, even when eating alone.
- Listen to favorite music during mealtimes to serve as a stimulant when eating alone.
- Add flavorful, low-sodium seasoning to food.
- Maintain adequate fluid intake.
- Engage in exercise such as gardening or walking to stimulate appetite and provide a feeling of general well-being.

more difficult and may result in reliance on convenience foods that may not be nutritious. Many older adults have lost spouses and friends through death. Eating alone is not pleasant for many individuals. If possible, arrange for companionship during meals, such as sitters or attendance at senior day services centers. At least two meals a day are served at most centers. Some older adults have limited incomes and must limit food choices. Programs such as Meals on Wheels, the Food Stamp Program, and community food banks, as well as family intervention, can help older adults to meet nutritional needs. Social workers and dietitians can assist in making these referrals. Families can prepare meals that can be frozen and easily heated by the elderly person. Patient Teaching 26-1 gives strategies to assist older patients to meet nutritional needs.

Another concern for older adults living alone is senility. Many elders with memory loss may not remember eating and may not eat for long periods of time. Family intervention to provide supervision of meal preparation and eating can help to ensure the person is eating nutritionally and preparing foods safely.

APPLICATION of the NURSING PROCESS

Assessment (Data Collection)

The nurse should be aware of factors that may have a negative impact on the patient's nutritional status. The admission physical assessment is a good time to observe the patient for potential nutritional problems. Admission diagnoses such as cancer, kidney disease, liver disease, gastrointestinal disease, HIV/AIDS, obesity, diabetes mellitus, or hypertension indicate a need to address nutritional issues. Surgical procedures such as gastrectomy or colon resection also indicate the need to address nutrition. Dietitians should be consulted for any of these diagnoses.

The nutritional assessment begins with a complete medical, family, and social history. Information can be obtained from the family if the patient is unable to respond. The patient's income level, education, activity, and family status should be considered.

Physical examination should begin with observation of the patient's general appearance. Is the patient obese? Is there muscle wasting? Notation should be made of the patient's skin, hair, nails, eyes, mouth, and extremities. Neurologic function should be assessed as well. Height and weight should be measured. Weight gain or loss should be noted. Determination of the patient's thinness or excessive fatness should also be determined. A common technique used is to determine the patient's body mass index (BMI). The BMI uses height and weight to estimate fat values at which the risk for disease increases. The BMI may provide more useful information than body weight alone because ideal body weight formulas do not take into consideration individuals with large muscle mass. A simple way to determine the BMI is to multiply the weight in pounds by 705, then divide this figure by the square of the height in inches. For example, for a person who weighs 165 lb and is 5'8" tall:

$$165 \times 705 = 116,325$$
$$5'8" = 68 \text{ inches}$$
$$(68)^2 = 4624$$
$$116,325 \div 4624 = 25.16 \text{ (BMI of 25)}$$

A BMI chart with most calculations completed may also be used (Table 26-8). The chart is not all-inclusive. Use of a more extensive chart or calculations are required for those patients whose weight is outside the limits of the chart.

The recommended range for BMI is 18.5 to 24.9. A BMI below 18.5 is considered underweight, between 25 and 29.9 overweight, above 30 obese, and above 40 morbidly obese and at severe risk for disease. Waist circumference may also be a determining factor for risk of disease. A waist size greater than 35 inches for women and 40 inches for men is associated with increased risk for disease. The BMI serves as a screen only. Results should be evaluated with other assessment information to determine the patient's risk for disease.

You must also review results of laboratory studies as part of the nutritional assessment. Serum albumin (protein), hemoglobin, and hematocrit will indicate if the patient is at risk for malnutrition, anemic, or dehy-

Table 26-8 | Body Mass Index (BMI) Table

BMI	19	20	21	22	23	24	25	26	27	28	29	30	31	32	33	34	35
HEIGHT								WEIGHT (IN POUNDS)									
4'10" (58")	91	96	100	105	110	115	119	124	129	134	138	143	148	153	158	162	167
4'11" (59")	94	99	104	109	114	119	124	128	133	138	143	148	153	158	163	168	173
5' (60")	97	102	107	112	118	123	128	133	138	143	148	153	158	163	168	174	179
5'1" (61")	100	106	111	116	122	127	132	137	143	148	153	158	164	169	174	180	185
5'2" (62")	104	109	115	120	126	131	136	142	147	153	158	164	169	175	180	186	191
5'3" (63")	107	113	118	124	130	135	141	146	152	158	163	169	175	180	186	191	197
5'4" (64")	110	116	122	128	134	140	145	151	157	163	169	174	180	186	192	197	204
5'5" (65")	114	120	126	132	138	144	150	156	162	168	174	180	186	192	198	204	210
5'6" (66")	118	124	130	136	142	148	155	161	167	173	179	186	192	198	204	210	216
5'7" (67")	121	127	134	140	146	153	159	166	172	178	185	191	198	204	211	217	223
5'8" (68")	125	131	138	144	151	158	164	171	177	184	190	197	203	210	216	223	230
5'9" (69")	128	135	142	149	155	162	169	176	182	189	196	203	209	216	223	230	236
5'10" (70")	132	139	146	153	160	167	174	181	188	195	202	209	216	222	229	236	243
5'11" (71")	136	143	150	157	165	172	179	186	193	200	208	215	222	229	236	243	250
6' (72")	140	147	154	162	169	177	184	191	199	206	213	221	228	235	242	250	258
6'1" (73")	144	151	159	166	174	182	189	197	204	212	219	227	235	242	250	257	265
6'2" (74")	148	155	163	171	179	186	194	202	210	218	225	233	241	249	256	264	272
6'3" (75")	152	160	168	176	184	192	200	208	216	224	232	240	248	256	264	272	279

From National Heart, Lung, and Blood Institute. (2007). Obesity Education Initiative. U.S. Department of Health and Human Services, National Institutes of Health. Available at: www.nhlbisupport.com/bmi.

drated. Table 26-9 summarizes physical signs of malnutrition. Further assessment of the patient's nutritional status can be completed by asking the questions in Focused Assessment 26-1.

After completion of the nutritional assessment, determine if a nutritional problem is present. Document the findings and conclusions. Documentation should include a summary of the findings and indicate any problem identified and the course of action taken. Make a nutritional referral to the dietitian, with the physician's permission, if malnutrition or other nutritional problems are identified so that early intervention can be started.

Nursing Diagnosis

After data collection, nursing diagnoses and goals/expected outcomes should be formulated. Some nursing diagnoses related to nutrition include the following:

- Imbalanced nutrition: less than body requirements
- Imbalanced nutrition: more than body requirements
- Ineffective coping
- Deficient fluid volume
- Excess fluid volume
- Delayed growth and development

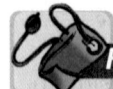

Focused Assessment 26-1

Assessment of Nutrition

The health care facility may have a nutritional assessment tool. If not, questions may be asked to assess the patient's nutritional patterns.

- What foods do you like/dislike?
- Are there foods that cause you discomfort? Examples: indigestion, diarrhea, constipation, or stuffy nose?
- What types of snacks do you eat? How often do you snack?
- What types and amount of fluids do you drink?
- What milk products do you use? How often?
- Do you eat bread at each meal? What type?
- How much fruit do you eat each day?
- Do you add salt to your food? How much?
- How often do you eat desserts?

- Do you use sugar or salt substitutes? What types?
- Do you drink alcohol? How much? How often? What type(s)?
- What types of meat do you eat? Chicken, red meat? How much do you eat each day?
- Do you eat fish? How often? How is it prepared?
- How much sugar do you add to foods and fluids?
- Have any members of your family been told they have diabetes?
- Are any immediate family members overweight?
- Is food prepared by anyone other than you? If so, do you make suggestions concerning meal planning?
- Do you read labels of prepared foods to determine fat and sodium content?

Table 26-9 *Physical Signs Indicating Possible Malnutrition*

NORMAL APPEARANCE	SIGNS ASSOCIATED WITH MALNUTRITION	DISORDERS, NUTRITIONAL DEFICITS	NON-NUTRITIONAL PROBLEMS
HAIR Shiny, firm, well rooted	Lack of natural shine: dull and dry, thin and sparse, dyspigmented, easily plucked (no pain)	Kwashiorkor and, less commonly, marasmus Protein deficiency	Excessive bleaching of hair Alopecia
FACE Skin color uniform, smooth, healthy appearance, not swollen	Scaling of skin around nostrils; swollen face (moon face)	Riboflavin	Acne vulgaris
EYES Bright, clear and shiny; no sores at corners of eyelids; membranes healthy pink and moist; no prominent blood vessels or mound of tissue or sclera	Pale conjunctiva Conjunctival xerosis (dullness), corneal xerosis (dullness); keratomalacia (softening of cornea) Redness and fissuring of eyelid corners Corneal arcus (white ring around eye); xanthelasma (small yellowish bumps around eyes)	Anemia (e.g., iron deficiency) Vitamin A Riboflavin, pyridoxine Hyperlipidemia	Bloodshot eyes from exposure to weather, lack of sleep, smoke, or excessive alcohol consumption
LIPS Smooth, not chapped or swollen	Angular cheilosis (white or pink lesions at corners of mouth	Riboflavin	Excessive salivation from improper-fitting dentures
TONGUE Deep red in appearance; not swollen or smooth	Magenta tongue (purplish); filiform papillae atrophy or hypertrophy (red tongue)	Riboflavin Folic acid Niacin	Leukoplakia
TEETH No cavities; no pain; bright	Mottled enamel, caries (cavities), missing teeth	Fluoride excess; excessive sugar	Malocclusion Periodontal disease Poor dental hygiene
GUMS Healthy; red; do not bleed; not swollen	Spongy, bleeding Receding gums	Vitamin C Scurvy	Periodontal disease
GLANDS Not swollen	Thyroid enlargement (front of neck swollen) Parotid enlargement (cheeks become swollen)	Iodine Starvation Bulimia	Allergic or inflammatory enlargement of thyroid
NERVOUS SYSTEM Psychological stability; normal reflexes	Psychomotor changes Mental confusion Sensory loss, motor weakness, loss of position sense, loss of vibration, loss of ankle and knee jerks, burning and tingling of hands and feet (paresthesia) Dementia	Kwashiorkor Protein deficiency Thiamine Niacin, vitamin B_{12}	

Adapted from Mahan, C.K., & Arlin, M. (2008). *Krause's Food, Nutrition and Diet Therapy* (10th ed., p. 375). Philadelphia: Elsevier Saunders; and Peckenpaugh, N.J. (2007). *Nutrition: Essentials and Diet Therapy* (12th ed., pp. 469-470). Philadelphia: Elsevier Saunders.

- Deficient knowledge
- Impaired swallowing
- Risk for aspiration

Planning

Some examples of goals and expected outcomes for the above nursing diagnoses are as follows:

- Patient will consume 2200 calories per day.
- Patient will restrict caloric intake to 1800 calories per day.
- Patient will verbalize methods to manage stress, such as relaxation exercises.
- Patient will consume 1500 mL of fluid per day.
- Patient with edema in upper and lower extremities will experience its decrease by day of discharge.
- Infant will gain 5 oz by day of discharge.
- Patient will choose appropriate foods from the hospital menu for a low-fat, low-cholesterol diet.
- Patient will consume at least 50% of a pureed diet.
- Patient will have breath sounds that remain clear with no evidence of aspiration on repeat swallow studies.

Implementation

Interventions for nutritional care include assisting patients with the meal tray, feeding when necessary, providing enteral nutrition or total parenteral nutrition when needed, teaching about proper diet, encouraging adherence to a therapeutic diet, and monitoring the patient's nutritional status.

Before serving a meal, provide for elimination by offering the bedpan or urinal or assisting the patient to the bathroom. Assist the patient to wash the hands and face as needed. Provide oral hygiene if desired. Create an attractive and pleasant environment for eating. Remove distracting articles, such as an emesis basin or a urinal, and use a spray or deodorizer to remove unpleasant odors in the room if not contraindicated. Position the patient comfortably for the meal, with the head of the bed elevated (if allowed), or assist the patient to sit up in a chair and clear the over-the-bed table for the diet tray.

When serving prepared trays from the dietary kitchen, serve those patients first who are able to feed themselves. Each tray should be checked against the unit dietary order list to verify that the correct diet tray has been prepared for each patient. Deliver the trays as quickly as possible to prevent food from cooling.

When dietary personnel deliver meal trays, the nurse is responsible for positioning the patient and setting up the tray to promote food and fluid intake (Assignment Considerations 26-1). Many people have difficulty opening the sealed packages of eating utensils and condiments. For the patient with an intravenous cannula in the hand, milk cartons and other sealed food items should be opened and prepared for

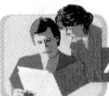

Assignment Considerations 26-1

Assigning of Feeding Responsibilities

Feeding patients may be delegated to unlicensed assistive personnel (UAP) such as certified nursing assistants or patient care technicians. Knowledge of the skill level of the UAP is essential to providing a pleasant and safe environment for the feeding experience.

---

eating. Attending to these details quickly after the trays are served helps the patient enjoy a warm meal.

Patient and Family Teaching

Depending on the patient's nutritional problem and type of diet prescribed, the following points may be included in the patient's teaching plan:

- Normal weight for body height and build
- Caloric intake needed to maintain normal weight
- Need for added calories, proteins, and vitamins to promote healing
- Foods high in iron and vitamin C that are used to build iron stores
- Use of "low-salt" or "no-salt" canned vegetables
- How to read food labels to determine the content and caloric value of various foods
- Use of a variety of herbs and spices to enhance the taste of food when salt is restricted
- Use of frequent small meals, which may be more appealing when appetite is diminished
- Ways to increase the amount of vegetables and fruit in the diet
- Methods of shopping wisely for prepared frozen foods when there is limited time available for food preparation
- Resources such as community food banks, Food Stamp Program, and WIC for patients with limited financial resources

Evaluation

Evaluation is based on the achievement of the expected outcomes. Review the goals/expected outcomes. Did the patients achieve them? Did they partially achieve them? If problems were not resolved, why not? While evaluating a patient's achievement of outcomes, you may need to work with the patient to change, modify, or eliminate some expectations (Nursing Care Plan 26-1).

Sample evaluation statements include the following:

- Patient gained 1 lb in 1 week.
- Patient lost 1 lb in 1 week.
- Patient consumed 90% of food and fluids at each meal.
- Patient made appropriate food choices from an 1800-calorie menu.

NURSING CARE PLAN 26-1

Care of the Patient with Malnutrition

SCENARIO Emily Montgomery is a 55-year-old female admitted with a diagnosis of pneumonia and malnutrition. Mrs. Montgomery was brought to the emergency room by a friend. She lives alone and does not work outside the home. Her husband of 30 years died about 1 year ago. She has a son and daughter; both are married and live about 100 miles away. Physical examination reveals a thin, frail-appearing woman in mild respiratory distress. She is receiving oxygen at 2 L/min and intravenous fluids of 5% dextrose and water with 40 mEq of potassium added. She is on a full liquid diet with orders to push oral fluids. She is 5′6″ tall and weighs 103 lb. She states she has had a poor appetite for the past year and usually eats one small meal daily. Mrs. Montgomery reports a 40-lb weight loss. Lab values: Hgb. 9.7, Hct. 30.1, Albumin 2.8.

PROBLEM/NURSING DIAGNOSIS *Considerable weight loss with malnutrition*/Imbalanced nutrition: less than body requirements related to loss of appetite.
Supporting Assessment Data: Subjective: States "I haven't had much of an appetite since my husband died. I usually eat one meal a day." ***Objective:*** Height 5′6″, weight 103 lb. Hemoglobin 9.7, hematocrit 30.1, albumin 2.8. Muscle wasting in the abdomen and all extremities, 40-lb weight loss.

Goals/Expected Outcomes	Nursing Interventions	Selected Rationale	Evaluation
Weight gain of at least 2 lb by date of discharge.	Obtain daily weights. Teach proper weight for height.	Provides information on patient progress and potential need for more interventions.	*Did patient gain at least 2 lb by discharge?* Gained 3 lb by date of discharge. Outcome met.
Consumes at least 85% of each meal by date of discharge.	Assess food likes and dislikes Refer to nutritionist	Adequate nutrition needed to return to optimal level of health.	*Did patient consume at least 85% of each meal?* Consumed 90% of each meal. Outcome met.
Hemoglobin, hematocrit, and albumin levels within normal limits by time of discharge.	Assess energy level. Provide rest periods Monitor lab studies for hemoglobin, hematocrit, and albumin levels.	Levels within normal limits help provide proper oxygenation to tissues, and evidence of adequate protein, resulting in an increase in energy level.	*Were lab values within normal limits?* Hemoglobin 11.3, hematocrit 40.9, albumin 3.2 at time of discharge Progressing toward expected outcome.

PROBLEM/NURSING DIAGNOSIS Husband of 30 years died 1 year ago/*Depression, isolation*/Ineffectual individual coping related to death of husband.
Supporting Assessment Data: Subjective: States loss of appetite since death of husband, eats one meal daily. ***Objective:*** Thin, frail appearing, depressed, withdrawn appearance.

Goals/Expected Outcomes	Nursing Interventions	Selected Rationale	Evaluation
Verbalizes feeling of well-being by time of discharge.	Assess economic and social factors that may hinder achievement of optimal nutrition. Refer to social services for follow-through on social needs.	Provides subjective data concerning patient progress.	*Did patient express improvement in well-being?* States "I feel better, but I still get tired sometimes." Progressing toward outcome.
Energy level increased to perform activities of daily living with assistance by date of discharge.	Assess level of activity tolerance.	Promotes patient's self-care abilities.	*Did patient complete activities of daily living with limited assistance by time of discharge?* Completes daily hygiene with minimal assistance. Requires occasional rest periods. Progressing toward expected outcome.

Continued

NURSING CARE PLAN 26-1
Care of the Patient with Malnutrition—cont'd

PROBLEM/NURSING DIAGNOSIS Eats only one small meal each day/*Lack of understanding of appropriate food choices*/Deficient knowledge related to choosing diet with adequate calories and nutrients.
Supporting Assessment Data: Subjective: States poor appetite, eats one meal per day. ***Objective:*** 40-lb weight loss, muscle wasting.

Goals/Expected Outcomes	Nursing Interventions	Selected Rationale	Evaluation
Demonstrates the ability to choose balanced diet from a hospital menu by date of discharge.	Teach components of nutritious diet. Provide daily menus to choose appropriate foods. Involve family in discussion concerning nutritional needs.	Provides information concerning patient's ability to care for self and level of compliance.	*Did patient choose appropriate food items from menus?* Chose appropriate foods from menu for 2 days prior to discharge. Outcome met.

? CRITICAL THINKING QUESTIONS

1. The patient is ready for discharge. What strategies could the family use to ensure the plan of care is followed?

2. What are some signs and symptoms the patient should be taught to report to the health care provider?

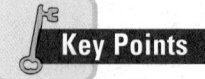
Key Points

- To achieve good nutrition, individuals should consume a balanced diet containing all essential nutrients: proteins, carbohydrates, fats, vitamins, minerals, and water.
- USDA MyPyramid divides foods into six groups and contains recommendations for daily servings of each group.
- General dietary recommendations include
  - Increase total complex carbohydrates.
  - Decrease saturated fats and *trans*-fatty acids.
  - Decrease sugar intake.
  - Eat more fiber, especially soluble fiber.
  - Decrease sodium intake.
  - Consume alcohol in moderation or not at all.
- Dietary Reference Intakes (DRIs) were developed by the U.S. National Academy of Sciences and are taking the place of Recommended Daily Allowances.
- Protein is needed for building tissues, regeneration of cells, tissue healing, and energy, and supplies 4 calories/g.
- Carbohydrates are the main source of energy for the body and supply 4 calories/g.
- Functions of carbohydrates include a quick source of energy and regulation of protein and fat metabolism.
- Dietary fiber is the portion of carbohydrates that cannot be broken down by intestinal enzymes and juices. Food sources include whole-grain cereals and skins of fruit, vegetables, and legumes.
- Fiber increases bulk in the stool, leading to good intestinal function and elimination.
- High fat intake has been linked to obesity, breast and colon cancer, hypertension and other cardiovascular diseases, and stroke.
- Fats are classified as saturated (solid at room temperature) and unsaturated (liquid at room temperature). Fat provides a concentrated source of energy, supplying 9 calories/g.
- Functions of fat include absorption of fatty acid, adding flavor to foods, absorption of fat-soluble vitamins, and insulation and control of body temperature.
- Vitamins are classified as fat soluble or water soluble. Fat-soluble vitamins are vitamins A, D, E, and K. Water-soluble vitamins are the B-complex vitamins and vitamin C.
- Minerals are essential for metabolism and cellular function. Major minerals (dietary needs are more than 100 mg/day) include calcium, magnesium, sodium, potassium, phosphorus, sulfur, and chlorine. Iron, zinc, fluoride, chromium, selenium, iodine, and copper are called trace minerals because the body requires less than 100 mg/day of each.
- Minerals also play a role in maintaining strong teeth and bones, and blood clotting.
- Water is involved in all the body's chemical processes and is the most essential of all nutrients.
- Awareness of a patient's economic status can help the nurse individualize patient care.
- Awareness of and respect for patients' religious and cultural preferences is important to meeting their nutritional needs.
- The first year of life marks the fastest growth period of human development. Birth weight should double by the end of 6 months and triple by the end of 1 year.
- Infant nutrition usually consists of breast milk or formula for the first year with solid foods introduced gradually, one food at a time, so that symptoms of allergy or sensitivity can be noted.
- Toddlers and preschool children tend to be finicky eaters. Providing child-size, colorful dishes and serving small portions may motivate eating in small children.

- School-age children are influenced by their peers and are at risk for obesity because of preference for fast foods, and sweet desserts and snacks.
- Children at risk for poor nutrition should be referred to school breakfast and lunch programs.
- Puberty and the adolescent growth spurt increase nutritional requirements of protein, calcium, and iron.
- Teaching adolescents how to make wise choices at fast-food establishments can be very important.
- Eating disorders, especially among adolescent girls, are prevalent during this developmental stage.
- Adults should be taught to make wise choices in food selection to help avoid conditions such as obesity, hypertension, diabetes mellitus, and cardiovascular disease.
- Elderly adults may be at risk for malnutrition. Chronic disease and physical disability may interfere with the elderly meeting nutritional needs.
- Elderly adults with limited incomes should be referred to community and/or government agencies for assistance.

- A nutritional assessment should be completed on every patient who is at risk for nutritional deficit or who shows subjective or objective signs of malnutrition.
- Patients with gastrointestinal disorders, cancer, HIV/AIDS, abdominal surgery, and immobility are types of patients who are at risk for malnutrition and should be evaluated by the dietitian.
- The recommended BMI range is 18.5 to 24.9 for an adult.
- Patients should be referred to the dietitian for determination of nutritional needs.
- The nursing process is a tool for determining the patient's nutritional risks and providing care.

 Go to your **Companion CD-ROM** for an Audio Glossary, animations, video clips, and more.

evolve   Be sure to visit the companion Evolve site at http://evolve.elsevier.com/deWit/fundamental/ for additional online resources.

NCLEX-PN® EXAMINATION-STYLE REVIEW QUESTIONS

*Choose the **best** answer(s) for each question.*

1. When teaching a patient about essential nutrients, which of the following will the nurse explain provides energy to the body? *(Select all that apply.)*
   1. Proteins
   2. Vitamin C
   3. Potassium
   4. Fats
   5. Iron
   6. Carbohydrates

2. The major nutrient(s) involved in fluid balance are: *(Select all that apply.)*
   1. fat.
   2. potassium.
   3. niacin
   4. carbohydrates.
   5. sodium.
   6. chloride.

3. The patient's potassium level is reported as 2.5 mEq/L. The nurse recognizes this as a critically low value. The patient is at high risk for _____. *(Fill in the blank.)*

4. Carbohydrate digestion begins when:
   1. food is mixed with fluid.
   2. pancreatic enzymes are present in the small intestine.
   3. the teeth break up the food and mix it with saliva.
   4. food reaches the stomach and is mixed with gastric acid.

5. The major component necessary for metabolism of carbohydrate is:
   1. pancreatic enzymes.
   2. insulin secreted by the pancreas.
   3. bile secreted by the liver.
   4. mucus secreted from the duodenum.

6. A woman's BMI is measured as 26. This BMI level is classified as:
   1. underweight.
   2. within normal limits.
   3. overweight.
   4. obese.

7. A patient who weighs 185 lb is placed on a 2200-calorie diet. How many grams of protein should the diet contain to meet the maximum recommended daily requirement of this nutrient?
   1. 56 g
   2. 67 g
   3. 75 g
   4. 82 g

8. The dietitian recommends an increase of fiber in the diet. Which of the following foods is a good source of fiber?
   1. Celery
   2. Chicken breast
   3. Milk
   4. Beans

9. The nurse teaches the patient that which of the following has the least saturated fat in the diet?
   1. Ground beef
   2. Salmon
   3. Shrimp
   4. Chicken

10. During a physical examination of a patient, which of the following is NOT indicative of malnutrition?
    1. Dry, brittle hair
    2. Absence of gray hair
    3. Brittle nails
    4. Dull-appearing eyes

CRITICAL THINKING ACTIVITIES *Read each clinical scenario and discuss the questions with your classmates.*

Scenario A

Ray Brown, age 28, is 6'1" and weighs 250 lb. He states he has had difficulty remaining on the 2500-calorie diet prescribed by the dietitian. History reveals Mr. Brown's diet is mainly a traditional African American diet, including many high-fat and high-sodium foods.

1. Calculate Mr. Brown's BMI.
2. What medical conditions is Mr. Brown at risk for because of his present weight and eating habits?
3. How can Mr. Brown's diet be modified to help him meet his weight loss goal and dietary needs?

Scenario B

Tina Aquirre, age 19, is a student at a local community college. She frequently skips breakfast and lunch or grabs a sweet roll and soda midmorning and a candy bar and soda midafternoon. She is experiencing fatigue and inability to concentrate during late afternoon classes.

1. How do you explain Tina's fatigue in the late afternoon?
2. What nutritional strategies would you suggest to help Tina meet her nutritional needs and provide needed energy for her classes?

Scenario C

Sam Minor, a 56-year-old accountant, is diagnosed with hypertension. His blood pressure is 164/100 when he comes to the physician's office for a checkup.

1. What additional assessment data do you need to develop a teaching plan for Mr. Minor to meet his nutritional needs?
2. Develop a teaching care plan for Mr. Minor.

Scenario D

Marian Chou, age 50, is undergoing chemotherapy for liver cancer. She is experiencing loss of appetite, nausea, and abdominal pain.

1. What nursing diagnoses are appropriate for Mrs. Chou?
2. What nursing interventions would you implement to assist Mrs. Chou to stimulate her desire to eat and take fluids?

27 Diet Therapy and Assisted Feeding

Objectives

Upon completing this chapter, you should be able to:

Theory

1. Identify the role of the nurse related to diet therapy and special diet.
2. Compare and contrast a full liquid diet with a clear liquid diet.
3. Describe health issues related to nutrition.
4. List disease processes that may benefit from diet therapy.
5. Verbalize the rationale for tube feedings.
6. List the steps for the procedure to insert, irrigate, and remove a nasogastric tube.
7. Discuss the procedure for tube feeding.
8. Identify the medical rationale and nursing care for a patient receiving total parenteral nutrition (TPN).

Clinical Practice

1. Develop a teaching plan for nutritional therapy.
2. Utilize therapeutic communication with a patient who needs a special diet.
3. Demonstrate insertion, irrigation, and removal of a nasogastric tube.
4. Demonstrate feeding a patient through a nasogastric tube or percutaneous endoscopic gastrostomy (PEG) tube.

Skills & Steps

Skills

Skill 27-1	Assisting a Patient with Feeding
Skill 27-2	Inserting a Nasogastric Tube
Skill 27-3	Using a Feeding Pump
Skill 27-4	Administering a Nasogastric/Duodenal Tube Feeding or Feeding via a PEG Tube

Steps

Steps 27-1	Nasogastric Tube Irrigation
Steps 27-2	Nasogastric Tube Removal

Key Terms

Be sure to check out the bonus material on the Companion CD-ROM, including selected audio pronunciations.

anorexia nervosa (ăn-ō-RĔK-sē-a nĕr-VŌ-sa, p. 486)
atherosclerosis (ăth-ĕr-ō-sklē-RŌ-sĭs, p. 489)
bulimia (bū-LĒ-mē-a, p. 487)
congestive heart failure (CHF) (cŏn-JĔS-tĭv HĂRT FĀL-yŭr, p. 489)

diabetes mellitus (dī-ă-BĒ-tēz MĔL-ĭ-tĭs, p. 489)
dysphagia (dĭs-FĀ-jē-a, p. 492)
feeding pump (p. 498)
gastrostomy tubes (găs-TRŎS-to-mē, p. 492)
glycosuria (glī-kōs-ŪR-ē-a, p. 498)
hyperosmolality (HĪ-pĕr-ŎS-mō-LĂ-lĭ-tē, p. 502)
hypertension (p. 487)
jejunostomy or duodenal tubes (jē-jūn-AW-stō-mē, p. 493)
myocardial infarction (MI) (p. 489)
nasogastric tubes (nā-zō-GĂS-trĭk, p. 492)
NPO (p. 486)
percutaneous endoscopic gastrostomy (PEG) tubes (pĕr-kū-TĀ-nē-ŭs găs-TRŎS-to-mē, p. 492)
postoperative (p. 486)
preoperatively (prē-Ŏ-pĕr-ă-tĭv-lē, p. 486)
residue (p. 486)
total parenteral nutrition (TPN) (pă-RĔN-tĕr-ăl, p. 502)

THE GOALS OF DIET THERAPY

The goals of diet therapy are to treat and manage disease, prevent complications, and restore health through appropriate diet. Patients in hospitals and other health care facilities have multiple dietary needs due to disease processes, surgical procedures, physical health, and cultural, religious, and individual preferences. The specific diet for each patient is prescribed on the physician's order sheet. Some patients may have diets without restrictions that are similar to meals eaten at home. For other patients, diet therapy is a significant factor in their medical treatment. **You can assist patients to meet their nutritional goals by completing a thorough nutritional assessment.** The patient's food and fluid intake should be monitored and the response to therapy documented. Weight gain or loss, percentage of meals eaten, and ability to tolerate the diet should be included in the documentation. Modification of the diet to increase effectiveness of therapy can be accomplished through discussion with the patient, physician, and dietitian.

Patients who may need assistance with food and fluid intake are those who have paralysis of the arms, are visually impaired, have an intravenous line in their hand or arm, or are severely impaired or weak (Figure 27-1). You may delegate this task to the nursing assistant or a family member if appropriate (Skill 27-1).

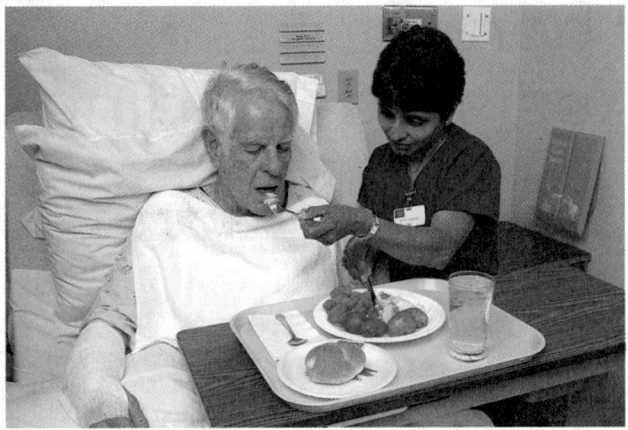

FIGURE **27-1** Assisting with feeding.

Skill 27-1 | Assisting a Patient with Feeding

Assisting a patient with feeding is a nursing responsibility. Patients with physical or mental impairment may require the expertise of a nurse to ensure safe feeding procedure is followed.

■ Supplies
✓ Tray with dishes of food
✓ Over-the-bed or tray table
✓ Utensils
✓ Napkin
✓ Straw
✓ Small towel or extra napkin

Review and carry out the Standard Steps in Appendix 3.

■ Assessment (Data Collection)
1. **ACTION** Assess the patient's need for assistance with feeding.

   RATIONALE Guides type of assistance to be given.

■ Planning
2. **ACTION** Check the diet on the tray with the diet sheet.

   RATIONALE Ensures that the patient receives the correct diet.

3. **ACTION** Clear the over-the-bed table, and place the diet tray on it. Position the patient in as high a Fowler's position as is comfortable and permitted. Or assist the patient to a chair. Position the over-the-bed table with the diet tray on it in front of the patient.

   RATIONALE Swallowing is enhanced by an upright position.

4. **ACTION** Protect the patient's clothing and bed linens with a towel or napkin.

   RATIONALE Protects clothing or bed linens from soiling if food is spilled.

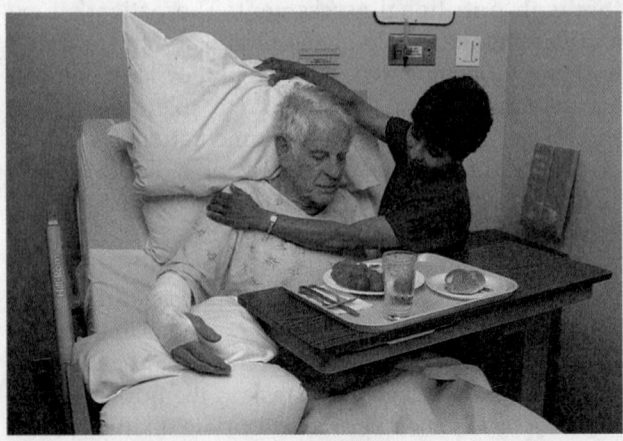

Step **3**

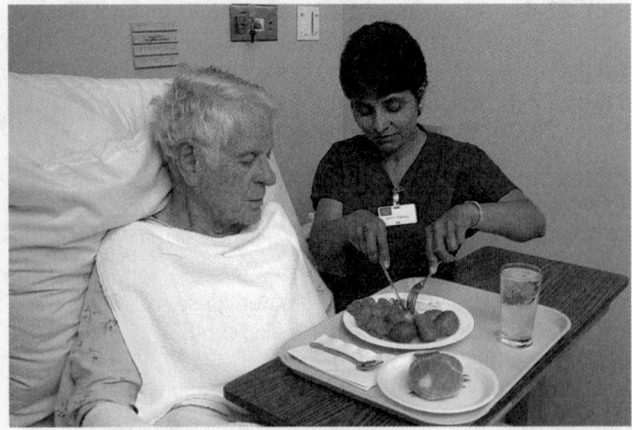

Step **4**

5. ACTION Open the containers of food, fluids, condiments, and eating utensils.

RATIONALE Prepares the food for feeding the patient.

■ Implementation

6. ACTION Ask which foods the patient prefers to begin with. Add condiments as desired by the patient. Alternate foods as the patient desires. Offer small bites, and wait until the patient has chewed and swallowed before offering the next bite.

RATIONALE A relaxed, unhurried manner will encourage the patient to eat more of the meal.

7. ACTION Offer fluids when the patient indicates they are desired. Place a flexible straw in the fluid container and grasp it a few inches from the mouth end when steadying it for the patient to grasp with the lips. Be certain the liquid is not too hot.

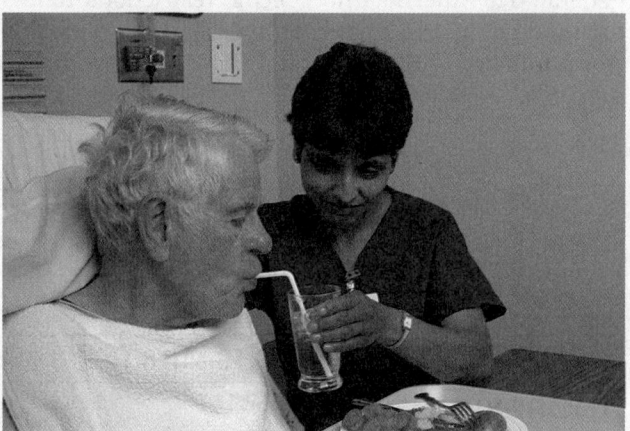

Step **7**

RATIONALE Liquids help wash down food. Do not add too much liquid as this will interfere with digestion. A straw masks the degree of heat in the fluid, and patients may burn their mouths if the liquid is too hot.

8. ACTION Wipe the mouth at intervals as needed. Talk with the patient during the meal. Try not to appear rushed.

RATIONALE Removal of food particles from the sides of the mouth preserves the patient's dignity. Conversation adds to the social atmosphere and can improve food intake.

9. ACTION Encourage patients who are physically capable to feed themselves as much as possible.

RATIONALE Self-feeding increases self-esteem.

10. ACTION Refrain from insisting that the patient finish all the meal.

RATIONALE Gentle persuasion to take just another bite is appropriate for the patient who is taking a smaller amount of nutrients than required, but the patient's wishes must be respected.

11. ACTION When the meal is finished, remove the tray, and offer an opportunity to perform hand hygiene and brush the teeth.

RATIONALE The patient's hands may have become soiled if the patient participated in feeding. Oral hygiene refreshes the mouth and removes retained food particles.

The Visually Impaired Patient

12. ACTION For the patient who is visually impaired but is able to self-feed, describe what foods are on the plate and tray. Orient the patient to the position of the foods on the plate by describing the plate as if it is a clock face with particular foods positioned at, for example, 12:00, 3:00, 6:00, and 9:00.

RATIONALE Many patients who have their eyes bandaged or who are blind are still able to feed themselves if given adequate orientation to the plate and tray.

13. ACTION Complete procedure as listed for the patient who needs assistance.

RATIONALE Patients with additional impairment may need nursing assistance for feeding.

■ Evaluation

14. ACTION Assess patient's tolerance of the meal, the amount consumed, and any difficulty experienced.

RATIONALE Provides information for modification of diet if necessary.

■ Documentation

15. ACTION Document the feeding and the patient's response.

RATIONALE Documents nutritional intake and how it is tolerated. Communicates progress to the health care team.

Documentation Example

2/16 1200   Fed lunch; ate 50% of meal. Had difficulty chewing and swallowing meats. Occasional coughing when swallowing. Discussed with physician. Diet changed to pureed meats.

_____

(Nurse's signature)

?CRITICAL THINKING QUESTIONS

1. The patient requires assistance with feeding, but is reluctant to allow the nurse to help. Identify strategies the nurse might use to make the procedure more acceptable.

2. The patient is recovering from a cerebrovascular accident (CVA). Right-sided weakness is noted on assessment. What safety measures might the nurse use to reduce the risk of complications during assisted feeding?

THE POSTOPERATIVE PATIENT

Patients scheduled for surgical procedures may have special dietary needs. Ideally, the surgical patient should be well nourished preoperatively (before surgery) to facilitate postoperative (after surgery) healing and recovery.

Preoperative patients are usually NPO (no food or fluids by mouth) 6 to 8 hours before the procedure. This practice decreases the risk of vomiting while under anesthesia, which could lead to aspiration of stomach contents. Aspiration can result in serious respiratory complications.

? *Think Critically About . . .* How does the anatomy of the gastrointestinal tract relate to the risk of aspiration when a patient is under anesthesia?

Postoperative patients progress from a clear liquid diet to a full liquid diet. Solid foods are added when the patient can tolerate them without nausea, vomiting, or other abdominal discomfort.

Clear liquids are started when the patient has a return of bowel sounds detected by auscultation. The goal is to introduce fluids that have low residue (remains after digestion), are easily digested, and have low risk of causing abdominal discomfort. Abdominal distress, such as vomiting and distention, can cause injury to surgical incisions.

Foods that are clear fluids at room temperature (e.g., gelatin, Popsicles) and liquids that are clear are on the clear liquid diet. Some physicians will restrict use of cola drinks on a clear liquid diet, but will allow carbonated drinks that are clear, such as white lemon-lime soda or ginger ale. Clear liquid diets are used short term because the diet is deficient in most nutrients. Bouillon (broth) added to the diet adds small amounts of protein and some electrolytes.

The patient progresses to full liquids when clear liquids are tolerated. Full liquid diets include all fluids, custards, ice cream, sherbet, puddings, and strained cereals. Full liquids can be used for long-term dietary management because protein and other essential nutrients, vitamins, and minerals are available from the foods allowed. Foods allowed in clear liquid diets and full liquid diets are compared in Table 27-1.

Patients recovering from surgical procedures that involved manipulation of or surgical incision into the stomach or bowel may progress to a soft diet before attempting a general or regular diet. Soft diets are low in fiber, and foods have a soft consistency. Foods allowed on a soft diet include eggs, breads without seeds, boiled or mashed potatoes, soups, fruit, juices, tender cooked vegetables, ground or softly cooked meats, cooked cereals, and milk products (see Summary of Basic Hospital Diets in Appendix 5). As the patient's condition progresses, the diet is advanced to general. This diet has no specific restrictions unless required because of a patient's specific disease process (see Summary of Basic Hospital Diets in Appendix 5).

? *Think Critically About . . .* Your patient is scheduled for a bowel resection. How would you discuss dietary goals with your preoperative patient? Can you explain expected dietary progression and rationale to your patient?

HEALTH ISSUES RELATED TO NUTRITION

ANOREXIA NERVOSA

Anorexia nervosa is a mental disorder characterized by refusal to maintain a normal minimum body weight, intense fear of becoming obese, and a severe disturbance in body image. It is prevalent among adolescent and young women who become obsessed with being thin; however, adolescent and young men may also be affected. They view themselves as obese despite being

Table 27-1 *Full Liquid and Clear Liquid Diets*

FOOD ALLOWED ON A CLEAR LIQUID DIET	FOOD ALLOWED ON A FULL LIQUID DIET
Grape, apple, and cranberry juice	Milk and milk beverages
Strained fruit juices	Yogurt, eggnog, pudding
Vegetable broth	Custard and ice cream
Carbonated water (preferably clear)	Pureed meats and vegetables in cream soups
Clear fruit-flavored drinks	Strained fruit juices
Sweetened gelatin and ices	Vegetable juices
Clear candies	Sweetened plain gelatin
Popsicles	Cooked refined cereals
Tea, coffee	Strained or blended gruel
Clear broth	All other beverages
	Cream, margarine, butter
	Sherbet
	Popsicles

extremely underweight. Patients with anorexia nervosa may refuse to eat, or food intake is dangerously low. **If not corrected, anorexia nervosa can be fatal.** Treatment is a combination of nutritional intervention and psychological counseling (Rader Clinics, 2007).

Collaboration among the patient, family, physician, mental health professional, nurse, and dietitian is crucial. A nutritional plan that is acceptable to the patient should be initiated. The treatment goals are to plan and achieve a nutritious, healthy eating pattern and to attain a body weight that is acceptable to the patient. The patient must have a willingness to remain in psychological therapy and follow nutritional recommendations to achieve treatment success (Communication Cues 27-1).

BULIMIA

Bulimia is an eating disorder characterized by episodic binge eating, followed by behaviors designed to prevent weight gain, including purging, fasting, use of laxatives, and excessive exercise. Women with bulimia are aware of their problem and often feel ashamed of the behavior. Treatment of bulimia is usually easier because of this awareness. Psychological as well as nutritional counseling is necessary. Addition of nutri-

tional supplements, and monitoring patients after eating to ensure purging does not occur may be included in the treatment plan. Medical conditions such as esophageal and peptic ulcers may accompany bulimia because of the gastric acid exposure during frequently induced vomiting. This condition must be treated along with providing the psychological counseling needed to stop these practices.

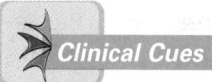

Clinical Cues

The patient with an eating disorder requires careful observation and skilled therapeutic communication. You should observe the patient for evidence of "hoarding" food, and structure communication to achieve compliance with the treatment regimen.

Nursing interventions for patients with anorexia nervosa and bulimia include diet management, patient teaching, and monitoring progress. Teaching should include principles of healthy weight maintenance, components of a healthy diet, the dangers of fasting and purging, and availability of community support groups. Nurses should document the patient's weight, compliance with nutritional recommendations, and eating behaviors; the effectiveness of the diet; and need for modification of any aspect of the treatment plan (Bond, 2005).

OBESITY

The incidence of obesity is rapidly increasing in the United States. Research by the Centers for Disease Control and Prevention (Centers for Disease Control, 2008) estimates that about 62% of Americans are overweight; of those, about 32.5% are obese. Obesity is defined as excessive accumulation of fat, not merely being overweight according to height and weight standards. Many factors contribute to obesity, including genetics, environment, poor eating habits, lack of knowledge about good nutrition, body physiology, age, and gender. Diet therapy to manage obesity must be individualized and incorporate all factors relevant to the patient.

The fact that obesity increases the risk of cardiovascular disease, diabetes, hypertension (abnormally elevated blood pressure), gallbladder disease, and joint disease is well documented. The goal of diet therapy is to improve health and quality of life. Long-term success of weight loss programs is low. **Approximately 5% of obese persons who reach their desired weight maintain the weight loss over a 2- to 5-year period.** Therefore, reaching a specific weight should not be the only measure of success.

To accomplish weight loss, the individual must expend more energy than is consumed through intake of calories. Exercise designed to match the ability of the patient is usually a component of weight loss programs. Diet therapy is dependent on the patient's

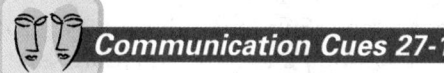

Communication Cues 27-1

The Patient with Anorexia Nervosa

Terri Mashburn is a 16-year-old high school junior admitted with a diagnosis of anorexia nervosa. Terri has lost 30 lb over the past 3 months as a result of refusing to eat and excessive exercise. She is observed during all meals. You are assigned to sit with Terri during her lunch.

NURSE: "Hello, Terri. Your lunch is here. I'm going to sit with you while you eat."

TERRI: *(Moves from chair to bed.)* "You can take that away. I can't eat that stuff! I'm not hungry anyway." *(Curls up in bed; hides face in pillow.)*

NURSE: *(Places tray on table. Sits on bed next to Terri.)* "You seem upset, Terri. Tell me what's bothering you." *(Places hand on Terri's shoulder.)*

TERRI: "Nothing is bothering me. I just don't want to eat."

NURSE: "Tell me about that."

TERRI: "The nurse weighed me this morning. I've gained 2 lb since I've been here. This food is making me fat!"

NURSE: "I know you are concerned about your weight. Let's talk about the medical plan concerning your weight."

TERRI: *(Sits up in bed.)* "OK, but you are not going to make me eat all that food."

NURSE: *(Brings tray to beside.)* "Tell me which foods you will eat. If you do not like any of them, I can get whatever you want from the dietary department."

TERRI: *(Raises cover on food.)* "None of that will do. It will make me fat. I'll eat a salad and an apple. Sprite to drink will be all right."

NURSE: "I will call dietary now." *(Calls dietary department to order food.)* "Now, let's review your medical plan while we wait."

degree of obesity. Obesity is characterized as mild to morbid. A mildly obese person is about 20% to 30% above ideal body weight. Morbidly obese people are at least 100 lb above their ideal body weight. Excessive body fat is present in all instances of obesity. Very-low-calorie diets (500 calories/day or less), appetite suppressants, or surgical intervention may be used to treat obesity. Surgical procedures such as stomach stapling, jaw wiring, and gastric bypass are usually a last resort for individuals who are morbidly obese and have severe medical conditions. Diet therapy to treat obesity should include the following:

- Consultation and continued follow-up with a physician
- Referral and continued follow-up with a dietitian for nutritional assessment and assistance with meal planning
- Development of a meal plan that is realistic and acceptable to the patient
- An exercise program that takes the patient's interests and physical limitations into consideration
- Foods from all groups of the MyPyramid
- Recommended dietary allowances of all nutrients

Current approaches to treatment of obesity include bariatric surgical procedures. These procedures include gastric bypass and laparoscopic elastic banding (lap band). These procedures have been successful for many individuals who have been unsuccessful at weight loss by other methods; however, there are many potential complications of which the patient must be fully informed (Mayo Clinic, 2007b).

PREGNANCY

Nutritional status prior to and during pregnancy can influence the health of the mother and the fetus. Nutritional assessment and counseling are important throughout the pregnancy to reduce the risk of complications such as low-birth-weight infants and pregnancy-induced hypertension. Factors to consider when counseling a pregnant woman include her nutritional status prior to pregnancy, her age, and the number of pregnancies. An increase in nutrients is needed for healthy growth of fetal and maternal tissues. Counseling should include emphasis on maternal weight gain. Weight gain during pregnancy should consist of a gain of 2 to 4 lb during the first trimester and 1 lb per week during the second and third trimesters. The recommendation for calorie consumption is no increase during the first trimester and an increase of 300 calories/day during the second and third trimesters. These serve as guidelines only. Factors to consider include the patient's prepregnancy weight and body mass index (BMI), and the general health of the mother and baby (Mayo Clinic, 2007a). Table 27-2 summarizes dietary needs during pregnancy and lactation.

SUBSTANCE ABUSE

Individuals who abuse alcohol and other drugs often present to health care facilities with nutritional deficits. Substance abuse interferes with food intake by decreasing appetite, decreasing the amount of financial resources for food, and substituting calories in alcohol for calories in food. Substance abuse may also lead to impaired absorption and reduced storage and use of nutrients, as well as increased metabolic needs. **Thiamine deficiency is often present with alcohol abuse.** Patients seen in a health care facility with a history of substance abuse should be assessed for nutritional deficits. Medical treatment will usually include fluid and electrolyte supplements; vitamin and mineral supplements, especially thiamine; and a high-calorie, high-carbohydrate diet. Liver damage is com-

---

Table 27-2 *Changes in Nutrient Requirements During Pregnancy*

FOOD GROUP	NONPREGNANT WOMEN	PREGNANT WOMEN
Milk		
Adult	2 cups or more	3 cups or more
Adolescent	4 cups or more	5 cups or more
Vegetables and fruits	1 serving	2 servings
Citrus or alternate	1 serving at least every other day	1 serving daily
Dark green or deep orange vegetable		
Other fruits or vegetables, including potatoes	3 or 4 servings	2 servings
Meat or protein alternative	2 servings or more	3 servings or more (6 oz cooked or more)
		Include serving with high iron content once per week (e.g., 3 oz red meat)
Cereal and bread	6 servings or more	6 servings or more
Other		Use iodized salt
		Drink water or other beverages—at least 6-8 cups daily

Modified from Peckenpaugh, N.J., & Poleman, C. M. (2007). *Nutrition Essentials and Diet Therapy* (10th ed.). Philadelphia: Saunders.

mon in substance abuse because of the increased stress of metabolizing excessive alcohol and drugs. Dietary fat may be restricted if liver function is impaired. The nurse plays a vital role in assessment of nutritional status and evaluation of the progress of treatment.

DISEASE PROCESSES THAT BENEFIT FROM DIET THERAPY

CARDIOVASCULAR DISEASE

Cardiovascular disease includes diseases of blood vessels, hypertension, myocardial infarction (MI) (loss of blood supply to the heart muscle), and congestive heart failure (CHF) (pump failure of the right or left ventricle). Diet therapy is focused on reduction of fat and sodium intake. Excessive fat intake, especially saturated fat, leads to development of atherosclerosis. Atherosclerosis is the accumulation of fatty deposits on the walls of blood vessels. This process leads to narrowing of the vessel diameter, resulting in decreased blood supply to major organs. Narrow blood vessels increase the workload of the heart, resulting in hypertension as the heart attempts to circulate blood. Dietary management includes reduction of fat intake (30% or less of total calories) and reduction of cholesterol. There are three types of cholesterol in the blood. *High-density lipoprotein* (HDL) is referred to as "good cholesterol" because high blood levels tend to cleanse vessels of fatty deposits. Elevated blood levels of *low-density lipoprotein* (LDL) increase deposits of fat on vessel walls. *Very-low-density lipoprotein* (VLDL) serves as a carrier for *triglycerides* in the blood; therefore, levels should be kept low. Triglycerides are a type of fat that contributes to atherosclerosis and coronary artery disease. Increased levels may also indicate poor management of diseases such as diabetes. Red meats, eggs, and high-fat dairy products contain large amounts of saturated fat. Consumption of low-fat dairy products, vegetable oils, poultry, and fish is desirable to lower cholesterol levels (see Low-Fat Diets in Appendix 5).

Control of sodium in the diet is therapeutic in prevention and management of cardiovascular disease. Large amounts of sodium cause fluid retention. Increased fluid volume in patients with CHF increases the workload of the heart and results in increased respiratory distress and edema in the legs and feet. Increased fluid volume and edema can also lead to hypertension. New research shows that Dietary Approaches to Stop Hypertension (DASH)—diets low in sodium and high in fruits, vegetables, nuts, seeds, legumes, and low-fat dairy products—can lower blood pressure even in healthy people. This might prevent hypertension later in life. The health care provider may prescribe a regular diet with no added salt, or sodium restriction from 250 mg to 4 g. **One teaspoon of salt contains 2300 mg of sodium.** Sodium content is very concentrated in many foods, and exceeding limits can occur easily. Patients should be taught to read food and beverage labels for sodium content and avoid adding salt to foods during cooking. Salt substitutes and no-salt seasonings may be used in cooking. Patients should consult with the physician or dietitian before using salt substitutes because many contain ingredients that should be avoided by some people (see Sodium-Restricted Diets in Appendix 5).

Think Critically About . . . Are you aware of the amount of sodium you consume? Read the labels for sodium content of your favorite snack foods. Develop an awareness of the amount of salt you add to foods at the table or during meal preparation.

DIABETES MELLITUS

Diabetes mellitus is a disturbance of the metabolism of carbohydrates and the use of glucose by the body. There are two main types of diabetes. *Type 1 diabetes* (insulin-dependent diabetes mellitus [IDDM]) occurs when the beta cells of the pancreas stop secreting insulin. Insulin is needed to transport glucose across the cell wall. Type 1 diabetes usually develops at an early age and was previously referred to as *juvenile diabetes*.

Type 2 diabetes (non–insulin-dependent [NIDDM]) occurs when glucose receptors on the cell membrane lose their sensitivity to insulin. Insulin is secreted in normal or excessive amounts; however, the receptor sites will not allow most glucose to enter the cell. Type 2 diabetes usually develops after age 40 and was previously referred to as *adult-onset diabetes*; however, an increased incidence of type 2 diabetes among young adults has been identified.

The incidence of diabetes is increasing at an alarming rate in the United States. Of particular concern is the prevalence of type 2 diabetes among late adolescent and young adult individuals. **Americans of African American and Hispanic ethnic background are at greatest risk of development of diabetes.** The goal of diet therapy for patients with diabetes is to control the amount of carbohydrates in the diet to maintain the blood glucose level at 70 to 100 mg/dL. Generally patients should distribute carbohydrate intake throughout the day and avoid ingestion of large amounts of carbohydrates at one meal. Dietary recommendations are a daily meal plan of 45% to 60% carbohydrates, 20% to 25% protein, and 20% to 25% fat. Calorie restriction will be included if the patient is overweight. Patients with type 2 diabetes are typically overweight. The majority of carbohydrates should be complex (brown rice, pasta, whole-grain foods, legumes). All carbohydrates are converted to glucose for energy. Complex carbohydrates usually contain more nutrients and higher fiber content. Research suggests that fiber delays the absorption of glucose, resulting in

Table 27-3	Dietary Strategies for the Two Main Types of Diabetes Mellitus	
DIETARY STRATEGY	**TYPE 1 (NONOBESE)**	**TYPE 2 (USUALLY OBESE)**
Decrease energy intake (kilocalories)	No	Yes
Increase frequency and number of feedings	Yes	May be necessary to balance carbohydrate intake
Plan consistent daily ratio of protein, carbohydrate, and fat for each feeding	Desirable	May be desirable to avoid excessive carbohydrate content in a meal
Use extra or planned food to treat or prevent hypoglycemia	Very important	Important if patient uses insulin as adjunct to oral medications
Plan regular times for meals and snacks	Very important	May be important, especially if insulin is used
Use extra food for unusual exercise	Yes	Usually not necessary; develop strategy based on individual patient need
During illness, use small, frequent feedings of carbohydrate to prevent starvation ketoacidosis	Important	Usually not necessary because of resistance to ketoacidosis; develop strategy based on individual patient need

Adapted from Williams, S.R. & Schlenker, E. (2003). *Essentials of Nutrition and Diet Therapy* (8th ed., p. 385.). St. Louis: Mosby.

lower blood glucose levels. A summary of general dietary strategies for patients with diabetes is provided in Table 27-3.

Patients with diabetes are at higher risk for cardiovascular disease, hypertension, kidney disease, blindness, and stroke. The nurse should encourage diabetic patients to monitor their blood glucose closely, especially the effect of carbohydrate intake on blood levels, and to consult with and follow the dietary recommendations of a dietitian or nutritionist. The American Diabetes Association recommends a diet of moderate complex carbohydrates, including pasta, beans, whole grains, rice, and fruit. The remainder of the dietary recommendations consists of decreasing the amount of protein to about 25% of total calories, and limiting fat intake to no more than 30% of total calories. Because of the increased incidence of heart disease in diabetic patients, the fat intake should be 20% to 25%. Foods high in saturated fats should be limited or avoided. Patients should be advised to limit the amount of salt added to the diet.

Patients should be instructed in ways to include favorite foods into the diet and remain within their individual dietary plan. The plan should be developed taking into consideration the type of diabetes, the patient's activity level, and whether or not the patient is overweight. Every diabetic patient responds differently to carbohydrate intake. A serving of carbohydrates is 15 g regardless of the type of food. A patient can monitor his response to particular carbohydrates by measuring the blood glucose 1½ to 2 hours after eating. A blood glucose level of 180 mg/dL or below usually indicates an acceptable level following meals. Patients should be taught to read food labels to determine the amount of carbohydrates in a specific food and include that food in the diet as part of the overall meal plan. A patient may consume simple carbohydrates such as ice cream or candy if they are part of the daily allowance of carbohydrates and not additional. Inclusion of these foods should be dependent on good diabetes control as determined by the health care provider. Dietary counseling related to reducing fat and

sodium in the diet should be a part of the meal plan (Nursing Care Plan 27-1).

? *Think Critically About* . . . Do you have a close family member with diabetes? Genetics play an important role in the development of type 2 diabetes. What steps can you take to prevent the onset of type 2 diabetes?

HIV/AIDS

HIV (human immunodeficiency virus) and AIDS (acquired immunodeficiency syndrome) are associated with severe diarrhea, profound weight loss, and muscle wasting. Some patients lose as much as 50% of their body weight as a result of treatment, multiple infections, loss of appetite, malignancies, and gastrointestinal disorders. Diet therapy is directed toward replacement of fluids and electrolytes, weight gain, replacement of muscle mass through protein intake, and maintaining the strength of the immune system. Patients should be referred to the dietitian as soon as they are diagnosed as HIV positive. Developing good nutritional practices is important in maintaining function of the immune system. **Research suggests that diet therapy can be a factor in delaying the onset of full-blown AIDS.**

Calorie intake should be increased for patients with HIV/AIDS. Emphasis should be placed on protein intake. Infections, an impaired immune system, and medical treatment may result in painful lesions in the mouth and ulcerations in the esophagus and stomach. Solid food may be difficult to eat. Milkshakes with added calories and supplements such as Ensure or Sustacal can be used to provide calories and protein. Fluids and electrolytes may be replaced intravenously (see High-Calorie/Protein Diets in Appendix 5). Dietary considerations include the following:

- Maintaining high calorie intake
- Increasing protein intake to maintain or increase muscle mass

NURSING CARE PLAN 27-1

Diet Therapy for a Patient with Type 2 Diabetes

SCENARIO Teresa James is a 46-year-old African American diagnosed with type 2 diabetes 3 months prior to admission. T.J. is an attorney in a busy law firm. She states she rarely has time to plan and prepare meals. "I just grab something on the run or eat out." Mrs. James' blood glucose is 413 mg/dL on admission. She is 5'3" and weighs 187 lb.

PROBLEM/NURSING DIAGNOSIS *Hyperglycemia (uncontrolled blood sugar)*/Noncompliance related to unwillingness/inability to make lifestyle adjustments.

Supporting Assessment Data Subjective: Patient states, "I don't have time for meal planning and preparation. I just grab something on the go or eat out." **Objective:** Blood glucose 413 mg/dL. Weight 187 lb.

Goals/Expected Outcomes	Nursing Interventions	Selected Rationale	Evaluation
Weight loss of 2 lb by discharge date.	Assess knowledge of disease process. Assess willingness to make lifestyle changes. Referral to dietitian for diet planning.	Establishes knowledge base about disease process Provides baseline data for patient compliance. Provides resource for component of needed lifestyle changes.	*Has weight loss occurred?* Weight loss of 2 lb by discharge date. Goal met.
Blood glucose level below 130 mg/dL by second day of admission.	Assess patient skill of measuring blood glucose. Provide instruction as needed.	Establishes patient's ability to complete skill. Patient must monitor blood glucose to assess diabetes control and patient response to carbohydrates in diet.	*Has blood glucose dropped?* Blood glucose 128 mg/dL by second day of admission. Outcome achieved.
Verbalizes understanding of relationship of medications to diet.	Teach about medications, their use, administration, and side effects. Teach signs and symptoms of hypoglycemia and hyperglycemia. Teach interventions for episodes of hypoglycemia and hyperglycemia.	Encourages patient compliance with dietary and pharmacotherapeutic management of disease process.	*Does patient understand about medication and diet?* Verbalizes relationship of medications to diet. Outcome achieved.

PROBLEM/NURSING DIAGNOSIS *Acknowledges inability to make appropriate food choices*/Deficient knowledge related to meal planning for diabetes, relationship of diet to management of disease.

Supporting Assessment Data Subjective: Patient states, "I don't have time for meal planning and preparation. I just grab something on the go or eat out." **Objective:** Blood glucose 413 mg/dL. Weight 187 lb.

Goals/Expected Outcomes	Nursing Interventions	Selected Rationale	Evaluation
Demonstrates the ability to choose appropriately from a variety of fast-food and restaurant menus.	Provide variety of fast-food and restaurant menus.	Provides patient with flexibility in meal planning. Promotes understanding of dietary exchanges.	*Does patient choose appropriate foods?* Demonstrates ability to choose appropriate foods from fast-food and restaurant menus. Outcome achieved.
Demonstrates the ability to develop a 24-hr meal plan.	Provide a variety of foods to compile menu.	Demonstrates patient's understanding of meal plan.	*Can patient develop a 24-hr meal plan?* Demonstrates development of 24-hr meal plan. Outcome achieved.
Verbalizes a weight management plan.	Advise of proper weight.	Weight management is critical component of control of disease process.	*Has patient developed a weight-loss plan?* Verbalizes she will begin an exercise program to assist with weight management. Progressing toward outcome.

Continued

NURSING CARE PLAN 27-1

Diet Therapy for a Patient with Type 2 Diabetes—cont'd

? CRITICAL THINKING QUESTIONS

1. You are asked to provide a list of dietary recommendations to a patient with diabetes. What will you include in the list?

2. Your patient states he does not understand how to use the American Diabetes Association (ADA) Exchange List. Briefly describe the use of the Exchange List and its implications for the diabetic patient.

- Offering bland, soft, or pureed foods when the mouth is painful
- Adding thickening agents to liquids if swallowing is difficult
- Adding seasonings to help food taste more appealing
- Encouraging small, frequent meals

Complete assessment of health and nutritional status is important for patients diagnosed with HIV/AIDS. Typical nursing diagnoses for HIV/AIDS patients are as follows:

- Impaired oral mucous membrane related to impaired immune system
- Imbalanced nutrition: less than body requirements related to anorexia, and/or oral lesions
- Fluid volume deficit related to prolonged diarrhea and decreased fluid intake

Table 27-4 provides a summary of nutritional recommendations for diseases/disorders of various body systems.

ASSISTED FEEDING

Patients with acute illness and neurologic disorders may be unable to tolerate oral fluid intake. Patients may experience dysphagia (difficulty swallowing) following a stroke or develop an increased risk for malnutrition from the effects of inflammatory bowel disease, HIV/AIDS, and cancer treatment. There are several types of enteral tubes. Tubes may be placed through the nose into the stomach (nasogastric tubes), placed directly into the stomach (gastrostomy tubes or percutaneous endoscopic gastrostomy [PEG] tubes),

Table 27-4 *Diet Therapy for Specific Diseases and Disorders*

CONDITION	DIET THERAPY
Gastroesophageal reflux disease (GERD): reflux of gastric contents into the esophagus, causing irritation	Assess foods that are best or least tolerated. Decrease alcohol, chocolate, and fat intake. Avoid cigarette smoking. Increase protein intake for healing. Lose weight if appropriate.
Peptic ulcer: loss of tissues lining the esophagus, stomach, and duodenum	Increase iron in diet because of blood loss from ulcers. Increase protein and vitamin C. Avoid eating snacks that stimulate gastric acid. Eat small, frequent meals. Avoid medications that irritate the mucosa (e.g., aspirin, ibuprofen).
Dumping syndrome: nausea, weakness, sweating, palpitations, diarrhea, occurring after a patient has had a gastrectomy	Eat small, frequent meals. Decrease intake of simple carbohydrates. Drink fluids 45-60 minutes before or after meals. Lie down from 15-20 minutes after meals to decrease dumping.
Inflammatory bowel disease: inflammation of the bowel causing malabsorption of nutrients (e.g., Crohn's disease, ulcerative colitis)	Avoid foods that cause symptoms. May be NPO for bowel rest. TPN in severe cases. High-calorie, high-protein, low-fat, low-fiber, lactose-restricted diet.
Diverticulosis/diverticulitis: formation of small sacs protruding through the bowel wall	Clear liquid diet during acute phase. Progression to high-fiber diet. (See Clear Liquid Diet and Guidelines for High-Fiber Diets in Appendix 5.)
Liver disease: cirrhosis, hepatitis	Intake and output. High-protein diet to increase lean mass. Restrict protein in advanced stages. High-calorie diet for energy. Fat-restricted diet. Nutritional supplements. Avoid foods that irritate the esophagus because of esophageal varices. NPO during the acute phase.
Nausea and vomiting	Avoid food during the acute phases of nausea and vomiting. Limit foods to bland, low-fat choices when they can be tolerated (e.g., dry toast and crackers). Clear liquids in small amounts. Eat small frequent meals.
Renal failure	High-calorie, high-carbohydrate, low-protein diet. Control of sodium, potassium, and phosphorus in the diet.
Renal calculi	Calcium- or oxalate-restricted diets may be ordered (restrict legumes, nuts, dark green leafy vegetables, citrus fruits). Modified calcium restriction may be ordered. High fluid intake is usually indicated.

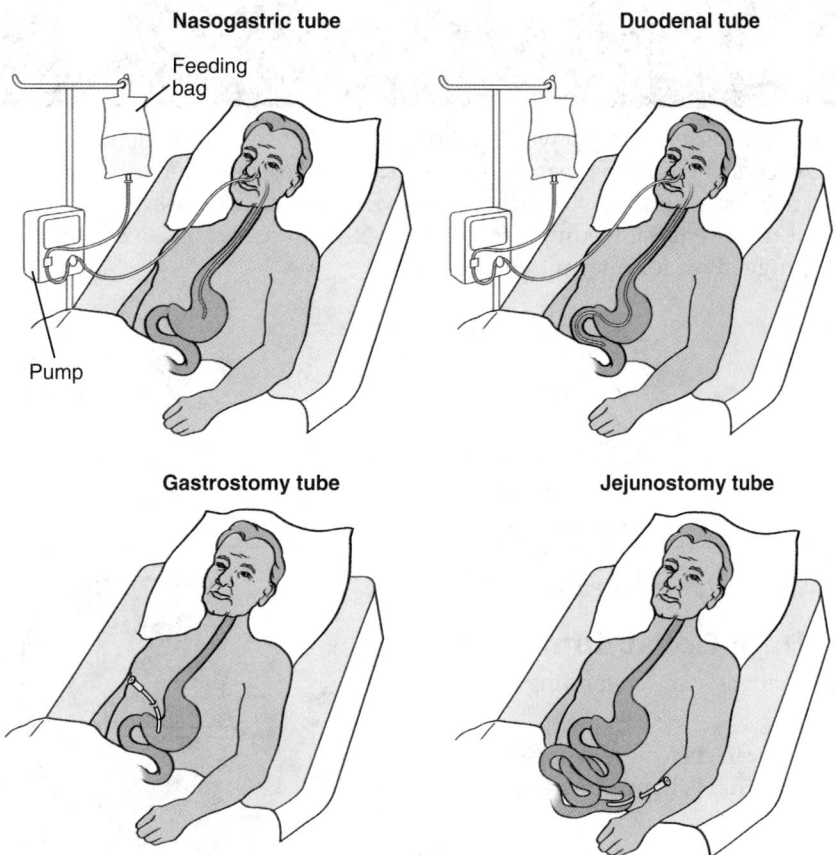

Nasogastric tube

Feeding bag

Pump

Duodenal tube

Gastrostomy tube

Jejunostomy tube

FIGURE **27-2** Anatomic locations for nasogastric, duodenal, gastrostomy, and jejunostomy tubes.

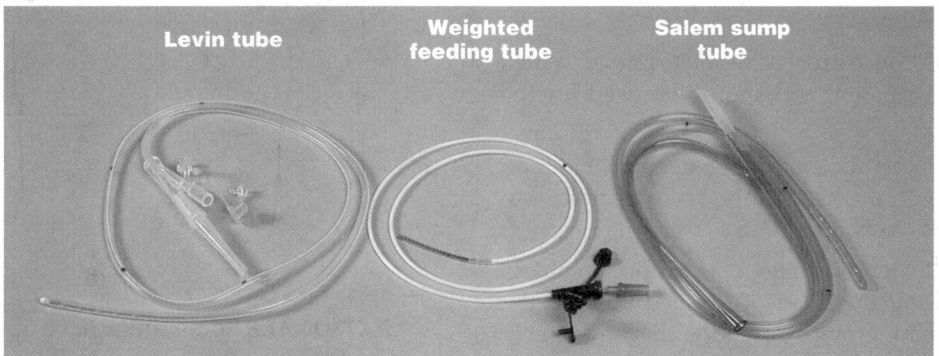

Levin tube   **Weighted feeding tube**   **Salem sump tube**

FIGURE **27-3** Nasogastric and enteral feeding tubes.

or placed into the intestine (jejunostomy or duodenal tubes) (Figure 27-2).

NASOGASTRIC AND ENTERAL TUBES

Nasogastric (NG) tube placement is usually a temporary measure to provide nutritional support. The tube is placed through the nose and esophagus into the stomach. The nasogastric tube may be used for other purposes, such as the following (Figure 27-3):

- Decompression of the stomach, such as removing stomach contents prior to or after surgery
- Obtaining specimen for lab analysis
- Gastric lavage for patients with gastrointestinal bleeding or for removal of ingested toxins
- Administration of medications (see Chapter 34, Skill 34-4)

When enteral nutrition is anticipated over an extended period of time, small-bore feeding tubes (8 to 10 Fr.) may be inserted. Small-bore tubes are soft, flexible tubes that must be inserted by a skilled person using a guidewire or stylet. Patients who are active may find the tube restrictive and inconvenient. Nursing care of patients with NG tubes involves insertion, irrigation, administration of tube feeding, checking for placement, and removal of the tube.

Success in inserting the tube is more likely if the confidence of the patient is gained first. Tube insertion is more difficult if the patient is unable to cooperate, such as unconscious patients or patients with impaired mental function (Skill 27-2). Explain the procedure and its benefit to the patient prior to beginning insertion. Proper placement of small-bore tubes should be verified by x-ray.

Skill 27-2 | Inserting a Nasogastric Tube

A nasogastric (NG) tube is inserted per a physician's order and is used with suction when a patient is experiencing excessive vomiting, needs stomach decompression after surgery on the intestinal tract, or is at risk for aspirating stomach contents because of decreased level of consciousness. If the patient needs enteral feedings, the tube is either attached to a feeding pump or left unattached and plugged off for intermittent feedings.

■ Supplies

✓ Stethoscope
✓ Gloves
✓ Drape or towel
✓ Tongue blade
✓ NG tube
✓ Flashlight

✓ Glass of water, straw
✓ Tape
✓ Water-soluble lubricant
✓ Plug for tube
✓ Irrigation syringe and solution container
✓ Safety pin

✓ Tissues
✓ Normal saline solution
✓ Suction machine and connecting tubing, or feeding pump and tubing

---

Review and carry out Standard Steps in Appendix 3.

■ Assessment (Data Collection)

1. *ACTION* Assess the patient's understanding of the procedure.

   RATIONALE Patients can be more cooperative when they understand what is happening to them.

■ Planning

2. *ACTION* Check the airflow through the nostrils: Close one side of the nose, and check the airflow through the other.

   RATIONALE This procedure determines which nostril is most patent and should be used for the tube's passageway.

3. *ACTION* Gather all equipment needed. Position the patient with the head of the bed elevated 30 to 90 degrees. Raise head of bed to working height.

   RATIONALE Demonstrates good time management. Elevating the head of the bed enables the tube to move by gravity down the digestive tract.

4. *ACTION* Hand the emesis basin and the tissues to the patient. Otherwise, place the emesis basin close beside the patient's face with the tissues near the pillow. Agree on a hand signal that will instruct you to stop if the patient experiences too much discomfort.

   RATIONALE The basin will catch emesis if the patient vomits. The signal allows the patient some control of the procedure.

5. *ACTION* Put on gloves.

   RATIONALE Barrier protection is needed in case the patient vomits or there is spillage of gastric contents.

6. *ACTION* Measure the distance the tube is to be inserted by measuring from the tip of the nose to the tip of the ear and then to the xiphoid process. Mark it with a piece of tape.

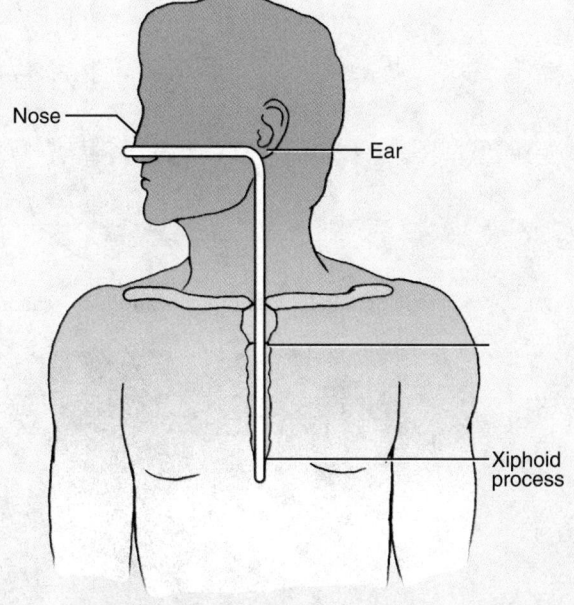

Step **6**

RATIONALE Some tubes have approximate target markings on them: one black band indicating the length of the tubing needed to reach the stomach, two bands for the pylorus, and three bands for the duodenum. Marking the tube after measurement individualizes the tube length.

7. *ACTION* Chill or warm the tube to the desired stiffness for insertion.

   RATIONALE A too limp or too stiff tube is difficult to insert. Placing a soft rubber tube in a basin of ice will stiffen it; placing a stiff plastic tube in a basin of warm water will soften it.

■ Implementation

8. *ACTION* Lubricate the tip of the tube and insert it through the nostril with the best airflow. If changing the NG tube, insert it in the nostril other than the one previously used to avoid further irritation of the tissue. With the patient's head hyperex-

tended, aim the tube down and toward the ear. Twist the tube slightly as you advance it. If you encounter severe resistance, withdraw the tube and insert it in the other nostril. Do not forcibly push it because you could injure tissue and cause bleeding.

RATIONALE Using the largest passageway for insertion of the tube decreases tissue trauma. For easier insertion, use water or a water-based lubricant to moisten the tip of the tube. Do not use an oil-based lubricant because of the possibility of lipid aspiration.

9. **ACTION** As the tube reaches the back of the throat, have the patient take sips of water through the straw, drop the head forward, and begin to swallow.

RATIONALE Encouragement is offered by saying "swallow," "swallow," when advancing the tube.

10. **ACTION** Check the position of the tube as it passes down the back of the patient's throat by having the patient open his mouth and hold down the tongue with a tongue depressor. If the tube is coiled up in the mouth, withdraw it into the nose and begin again by having the patient bend head forward and swallow. The patient can signal you to stop for a moment to rest, if necessary, but avoid waiting too long.

RATIONALE Difficulty with the tube entering the esophagus opening sometimes occurs.

11. **ACTION** Advance the tube each time the patient swallows.

RATIONALE The tube advances more easily with the assistance of esophageal peristalsis.

12. **ACTION** Check the placement of the tube:

   A. Use the irrigating syringe to pull back, using gentle suction, and aspirate stomach contents. If none are obtained, turn the patient onto the left side and insert the tube another 1 to 2 inches. Test the fluid pH; instill 30 mL of air and obtain a sample of fluid. Fluid can be tested using pH strips.

   B. When tube placement has been properly established and the tube is secured to the patient, thereafter some facilities will allow checking by injecting 10 to 20 mL of air into the tube with the irrigating syringe and listening with the stethoscope placed to the left of the tip of the xiphoid. The air makes a "swooshing" sound as it enters the stomach, but the patient may belch if the tube is in the esophagus. However, this is not recommended as "best practice."

RATIONALE When the target point on the tube has reached the nose, the tube should be in the stomach; this must be verified with a pH check of the aspirated fluid. Gastric pH is 1 to 4, intestinal and

respiratory pH is greater than 6. A pH greater than 6 indicates the tube is in the trachea. If there is a question about placement, contact the physician.

13. **ACTION** Tape the tube securely to the face. Clean the bridge of the nose with a prep pad or apply tincture of benzoin to it. Cut a 4-inch long piece of 1-inch tape; split it up the middle for 3 inches. Place the solid piece of tape on the bridge of the nose, and spiral the split ends down the tube. Secure the tape with one more piece across the bridge of the nose. Be certain the tube is not rubbing the side of the naris because it can cause necrosis.

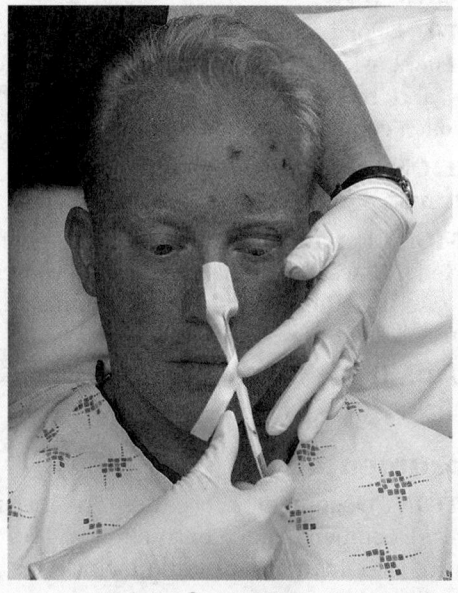

Step **13**

RATIONALE The tube must be secured so that it is not easily dislodged. Commercially made NG tube holders are available and may be used in your facility.

14. **ACTION** Attach the free end of the tube to the connecting tubing attached to the suction machine or feeding tube. Turn the suction machine or wall unit to low intermittent suction for a patient who needs stomach decompression. If using a feeding pump, adjust the drip rate to the rate prescribed by the physician, connect the tubing, and turn on the pump. When the patient is up and not attached to the suction machine or feeding pump, loosely loop the tube in a circle, secure the loop with adhesive tape, and pin the tube to the gown.

RATIONALE Low, intermittent suction is usually ordered to prevent damage to the stomach mucosa. Securing the tube to the gown helps prevent pulling the tube, which is uncomfortable for the patient and can dislodge the tube.

15. **ACTION** Remove gloves. Position the tube by looping it above the stomach level, placing a piece of tape around it to make a tab, and fastening the tab to the gown with a safety pin.

Continued

Skill 27-2 | Inserting a Nasogastric Tube—cont'd

RATIONALE Prevents the tube from becoming dislodged.

16. *ACTION* Perform hand hygiene before leaving the room.

    RATIONALE Hand hygiene is necessary even after wearing gloves to prevent transmission of organisms to others.

■ Evaluation

17. *ACTION* For patient who needs stomach decompression, ask the patient if nausea is relieved. Assess abdomen for distention. Note the flow of stomach contents into the suction canister.

    RATIONALE Determines effectiveness of procedure.

18. *ACTION* If feeding tube is inserted and feeding started, assess residual stomach contents in 4 hours. If patient is able to communicate, ask if there is any abdominal discomfort.

    RATIONALE Evaluates patient's tolerance of tube feeding.

■ Documentation

19. *ACTION* Document procedure on the nurse's notes. Document intake on the intake and output record. Documentation should include

    - Reason for tube insertion
    - Time of procedure
    - Type of procedure
    - Type and size of tube
    - Patient's tolerance of procedure
    - Amount and characteristics of stomach contents

    RATIONALE Provides members of the health care team with description of the procedure and the patient's response.

Documentation Example

2/13 1300 Number 16 Levin tube inserted in right nostril. 500 mL dark green fluid returned. Vomited 200 mL dark green fluid during tube insertion. Tube taped to nose. States nausea and abdominal pain relieved after tube insertion. Tube connected to low, intermittent suction.

_____

(Nurse's signature)

■ Special Considerations

✓ Insertion of NG tube in patients who are unconscious or have endotracheal tubes in place may require assistance. Seek the help of another nurse to ensure patient safety.

✓ Consult with the physician before inserting an NG tube into the nostril of a patient who has had nasal or throat surgery or trauma to the nose. Special care is usually required.

✓ Patients with mental impairment may attempt to pull out the feeding tube. Protective mittens may be applied to prevent pulling out the tube.

✓ Keeping the suction connecting tubing above the entrance to a portable suction unit helps the suction to work more efficiently.

?CRITICAL THINKING QUESTIONS

1. The nurse inserts a nasogastric tube and checks for placement. When 20 mL of air is instilled, the nurse hears a "swoosh" over the stomach. The nurse aspirates 10 mL of fluid from the tube. The pH strip test 7.0. What action should the nurse take?

2. The patient has a nasogastric tube inserted postoperatively. The nurse notes that there has been no drainage from the tube in the past hour. List appropriate nursing actions.

Nasogastric tubes should be monitored frequently. **Check tube placement prior to feeding or administering medications.** Patients with decreased level of consciousness and decreased cough or gag reflex may not exhibit expected symptoms if the tube is displaced into the respiratory tract. Placement of the tube in the respiratory tract can lead to severe respiratory complications if the tube enters the pleural space or if misplacement is not detected prior to feeding or medication administration.

The nasogastric tube is irrigated to ensure it is patent. Usually 30 to 60 mL of normal saline solution is sufficient to flush the tube. The amount used for irrigation must be counted as part of the recorded intake (Steps 27-1). When therapy is completed or the patient is able to tolerate oral feedings, the nasogastric tube can be removed (Steps 27-2).

PERCUTANEOUS ENDOSCOPIC GASTROSTOMY TUBES

A PEG tube is generally used when a patient requires long-term nutritional support. The PEG tube has replaced surgical gastrostomy tube placement in most situations. The PEG tube has several advantages over surgical gastrostomy, including reduced procedure time, cost, and recovery time, and no need for general anesthesia. The tube is placed via endoscopy either in the day surgery unit or gastrointestinal (GI) lab. The PEG tube allows patients more freedom of ambulation and allows the patient the opportunity to administer his own feeding easily. A PEG tube can be removed easily when it is no longer indicated.

Care of the PEG tube is similar to that of the NG tube. **Tube placement should be checked at least every shift**

Steps 27-1 | Nasogastric Tube Irrigation

Nasogastric tubes are irrigated to verify patency and keep them from clogging. They may be irrigated every few hours or once a day depending on the situation and the physician's orders.

Review and carry out the Standard Steps in Appendix 3.

1. **ACTION** Check physician's order for frequency of irrigation, and amount and type of solution.

   RATIONALE Ensures following procedure as ordered.

2. **ACTION** Assess the color, amount, and characteristics of gastric secretions.

   RATIONALE Provides baseline information.

3. **ACTION** Assess bowel sounds.

   RATIONALE Bowel sounds are evidence of return or improvement of bowel function.

4. **ACTION** Assess patient for complaints of discomfort.

   RATIONALE Information may indicate potential complications.

5. **ACTION** Position the patient in semi-Fowler's position at 30 to 60 degrees.

   RATIONALE A slightly upright position helps prevent reflux.

6. **ACTION** Perform hand hygiene and put on gloves.

   RATIONALE Possible contact with body fluids requires the use of gloves.

7. **ACTION** Verify proper placement of the tube.

   RATIONALE Prevents instilling irrigation fluid into the lungs.

8. **ACTION** Fill the syringe with the irrigating solution, usually normal saline, by holding the syringe between your index finger and thumb. Place the tip of the syringe in the solution, and pull the plunger up to obtain at least 30 mL of solution.

   RATIONALE Normal saline is isotonic and will not upset electrolyte balance. Cola has shown to be an effective irrigation solution following tube feedings.

9. **ACTION** Disconnect the gastric tube from the suction tubing on the machine; hold the connecting tubing between the last two fingers of your nondominant hand; hold the gastric tube in a fistlike grasp with the other fingers of that hand.

   RATIONALE The tube may be irrigated only if disconnected from suction.

10. **ACTION** Attach the filled syringe to the free end of the gastric tube and instill the solution.

    RATIONALE Assists in clearing the tube.

11. **ACTION** When irrigation is completed, attach the gastric tube to the suction tubing; restart the suction.

    RATIONALE Checking that the suction machine or unit is turned on will ensure correct function.

12. **ACTION** Remove gloves and perform hand hygiene; make the patient comfortable.

    RATIONALE Performing hand hygiene prevents spread of microorganisms.

13. **ACTION** Add amount of irrigating solution to intake record.

    RATIONALE Documents intake.

---

and prior to feeding or administration of medication. Check the patient's chart for the placement measurements. Measure the tube length from skin level to the end of the placement adapter. Compare the measurements. Higher measurements indicate the tube has migrated outward. If the tube becomes dislodged, the nurse should notify the charge nurse and the physician. Follow the facility policy and licensure regulations regarding reinsertion of the tube. The tube may be reinserted by an LPN/LVN if permitted by the scope of practice. Document your findings and report them to the physician if discrepancies are present.

Daily care of the tube involves washing the tube insertion site with soap and water. Use a cotton swab moistened with saline or half-strength peroxide to remove encrustation. Assess the skin for evidence of irritation, maceration, or signs of infection. Dry the site and reposition the external disk to prevent sticking to the skin. Document your assessment and treatment of the site. Observe the patient for abdominal distention or aspiration. Abdominal pain, vomiting, or respiratory distress may be signs of complication. Prior to feeding or administration of medications, the amount of residual fluid in the stomach should be assessed. If a continuous feeding is in progress, stop the infusion prior to checking for residual. Use an irrigation syringe to withdraw stomach contents. If the residual volume is greater than 150 mL, replace the withdrawn fluids and delay further feeding for 1 to 2 hours. (Facility policies vary. Follow the policy in your facility of practice.) **Keep the patient's bed elevated at least 30 degrees at all times if the patient is on continuous feeding to facilitate stomach emptying and prevent aspiration.** Further discussion of various tubes for medical conditions can be found in your medical-surgical textbook.

Steps 27-2 Nasogastric Tube Removal

When the condition for which the NG tube was inserted has resolved, the tube is discontinued.

Review and carry out the Standard Steps in Appendix 3.

1. **ACTION** Check physician's order sheet for order to remove NG tube.

   RATIONALE Prevents removal of the tube while still needed.

2. **ACTION** Assess amount, color, and character of drainage in suction canister.

   RATIONALE Amount, color, and character of drainage must be documented on the chart.

3. **ACTION** Explain procedure to patient.

   RATIONALE Helps gain patient's confidence and cooperation.

4. **ACTION** Elevate head of bed to 30 degrees.

   RATIONALE Position is more comfortable for patient.

5. **ACTION** Perform hand hygiene and put on gloves.

   RATIONALE Protection against exposure to body fluids.

6. **ACTION** Turn off suction or tube feeding pump if present. Place the towel or basin where the withdrawn tube can be placed into it quickly. Flush the tube with 20 mL of water followed by 20 mL of air. Pinch off the tube and pull out gently but quickly.

   RATIONALE Flushing the tube clears gastric content from the tube that may leak into the esophagus and cause irritation. Instillation of air pushes tube away from stomach lining and reduces the risk of trauma during removal. Pinching off the tube prevents spillage of any residual fluid.

7. **ACTION** Offer mouth care.

   RATIONALE Mouth care removes unpleasant taste from the mouth.

8. **ACTION** Measure and record the gastric drainage. Rinse or dispose of the drainage container and tube following facility policy.

   RATIONALE Gastric drainage is recorded as part of output for the shift.

9. **ACTION** Remove gloves and perform hand hygiene.

   RATIONALE Prevents spread of microorganisms.

10. **ACTION** Assess every 2 hours for signs of nausea, vomiting, or abdominal distention. Assess bowel sounds.

    RATIONALE Provides for early recognition of intolerance to removal of NG tube.

11. **ACTION** Document the time the tube was removed and the patient's response to the procedure. If the tube was used for suction, record amount and characteristics of drainage.

    RATIONALE Documentation provides communication to other health care personnel concerning the care provided to the patient.

FEEDING TUBES AND PUMPS

Tube feedings can be continuous or intermittent. Continuous feeding is effective for patients who cannot tolerate large amounts of fluids at one time. Intermittent feeding is beneficial for patients who are able to feed themselves or when beginning to reintroduce oral feeding. Intermittent feeding more closely resembles regular meals. Feelings of hunger stimulate appetite and aid in the transition from tube to oral feeding.

The amount of tube feeding is prescribed by the physician and usually ranges from 8 to 12 oz per feeding. It may be necessary to start with smaller amounts and increase the feeding as the patient is able to tolerate the formula. A daily amount of 2000 mL is generally sufficient to meet the patient's nutritional requirements. High concentrations of carbohydrates are needed to increase the caloric content of the formula above this amount, but this often leads to diarrhea. If a syringe is used, it should be 30 mL or larger, and the formula should flow in by gravity; **it should not be pushed in** as a bolus or in large amounts. Allow about 10 minutes for an intermittent feeding to flow into the tube. Flush the tube with 30 mL of water after each feeding to prevent clogging. Facility policy may include use of carbonated sodas such as cola or ginger ale to flush tubing.

Continuous feedings are instilled into the tube drop by drop in much the same manner as an intravenous feeding. For this purpose, a feeding pump and a tube feeding set similar to an intravenous administration set is used (Skill 27-3). The rate is set on the pump, or the drops are regulated through the drip chamber to control the amount given; this device can be used with NG tubes, PEG tubes, or jejunostomy tubes (Skill 27-4). Tube feedings contain a high level of glucose to provide the necessary calories. They should be given slowly to prevent diarrhea and glycosuria (sugar in the urine). The preferred method is to give the feedings slowly over a 24-hour period. When feedings are

Skill 27-3 | Using a Feeding Pump

Continuous feeding via feeding pump is usually prescribed when a patient requires long-term nutritional support or cannot tolerate large volumes of feeding formula at one time.

■ **Supplies**

✓ Feeding formula
✓ Irrigating syringe
✓ Feeding pump
✓ Stethoscope
✓ Tubing for pump
✓ Gloves
✓ Feeding tube bag
✓ Glass of water

Review and carry out Standard Steps in Appendix 3.

■ **Assessment (Data Collection)**

1. *ACTION* Check the physician's order for type, amount, and flow rate of feeding.

   RATIONALE Ensures correct feeding formula is administered.

2. *ACTION* Put on gloves. Assess tube placement or residual if PEG tube is in place.

   RATIONALE Possibility of coming in contact with body fluids requires wearing gloves. Assessing placement determines NG tube is in the stomach, and prevents infusion of feeding into respiratory tract. Check residual to determine if stomach is emptying effectively.

■ **Planning**

3. *ACTION* Elevate head of bed at least 30 degrees. Keep bed elevated at all times.

   RATIONALE Assists in preventing gastric reflux and/or aspiration of feeding.

4. *ACTION* Open tubing and feeding bag and connect to feeding pump with tubing clamp closed. Open formula and pour enough to infuse over a 4- to 6-hour period. If using commercially prepared feeding container, close the roller clamp on the tubing, spike the infusion port and fill the drip chamber.

   RATIONALE Small amount of feeding formula in bag prevents spoilage of formula. Some formulas are prepared in an administration container. These formulas are prepared to hang for up to 24 hours.

5. *ACTION* Open the clamp and prime the tubing by allowing the formula to fill the length of the tubing.

   RATIONALE Prevents air from entering the stomach and causing abdominal distention and discomfort.

■ **Implementation**

6. *ACTION* Attach the tubing to the NG tube or PEG tube. Set the flow rate and turn on the pump.

   RATIONALE Begins administration of feeding formula.

7. *ACTION* Observe the infusion for 2 to 3 minutes before leaving patient.

   RATIONALE Determines if formula is infusing properly.

8. *ACTION* Remove gloves and perform hand hygiene.

   RATIONALE Prevents spread of microorganisms.

■ **Evaluation**

9. *ACTION* Assess patient for signs of complications, including abdominal distention, abdominal pain, nausea, or vomiting.

   RATIONALE Determines patient's tolerance of tube feeding.

10. *ACTION* Assess stomach residual every 4 hours by aspirating contents.

    RATIONALE Determines if stomach is emptying properly.

■ **Documentation**

11. *ACTION* Document the time the infusion was started, type of formula, amount, and flow rate. Include checking for tube placement or check for residual. Document patient's response to the infusion.

    RATIONALE Verifies nutritional intake and patient response.

Documentation Example

2/14 1000   Feeding via pump initiated with 200 mL formula at 50 mL/hr. Tube patent and in place with return of gastric secretions. Positioned ↑ 30 degrees. Bowel sounds present all 4 quads.

(Nurse's signature)

? CRITICAL THINKING QUESTIONS

1. The nurse discovers the feeding solution bag empty and the pump continuing to infuse. Identify nursing interventions.

2. The home care nurse discovers the patient resting on the left side with the head on a pillow and the head of the bed flat. A continuous tube feeding is infusing at 30 mL/hr. What action, if any, should the nurse take?

Skill 27-4 | Administering a Nasogastric/Duodenal Tube Feeding or Feeding via a PEG Tube

Tube feedings are administered to patients who cannot ingest food orally but do not have a problem with absorption of nutrients from the intestinal tract. They may be used for short-term or long-term nutritional support. Intermittent feedings should only be used with stomach tubes.

■ Supplies
✓ Large syringe or feeding bag and feeding formula
✓ Tubing
✓ Feeding pump (if needed)
✓ Stethoscope
✓ Gloves
✓ Adaptor for syringe for small-bore tubes
✓ Glass of water

Review and carry out the Standard Steps in Appendix 3.

■ Assessment (Data Collection)

1. **ACTION** Check the physician's order for type of feeding, amount, and strength of solution.

   RATIONALE Ensures feeding is given according to physician's order.

2. **ACTION** Assess abdomen for distention or tenderness.

   RATIONALE Identifies discomfort prior to feeding to avoid complication.

■ Planning

3. **ACTION** Elevate the head of the bed 30 degrees.

   RATIONALE Elevation allows gravity to help flow of the formula into the stomach and thus helps prevent reflux. The position should be maintained at least 30 to 60 minutes after the feeding.

4. **ACTION** Perform hand hygiene. Put on gloves.

   RATIONALE Possible contact with body fluids requires the use of gloves.

■ Implementation

5. **ACTION** Pinch off the tube and remove the plug, cap, or clamp.

   RATIONALE Pinching the tube prevents fluid leaking from the tube.

6. **ACTION** Check placement of the tube. For NG tube, attach syringe and aspirate small amount of stomach contents (5 to 10 mL); if no fluid is obtained, check the tube placement by introducing air through the tube and listening to the left of the xiphoid process with the stethoscope for a "swoosh"; for a small-bore feeding tube, verify that placement has been checked by x-ray. Reinstill aspirated fluid.

   RATIONALE Obtaining gastric or intestinal contents is the best evidence of proper tube placement. Small-bore feeding tubes frequently will collapse when aspiration is attempted and nothing can be obtained. Stomach or intestinal contents are high in electrolytes, and removal depletes electro-

lytes. When more than 150 mL of residual formula are obtained, the physician should be notified because it is an indication that the feeding is not well tolerated.

For Intermittent Feedings

7. **ACTION** Pinch off the tube and pour the formula into a gavage bag or the barrel of the syringe, keeping it no more than 18 inches above the level of entry into the stomach or intestine. If a gavage bag is used, fill it with the prescribed amount of formula and regulate it to run in slowly over 30 minutes.

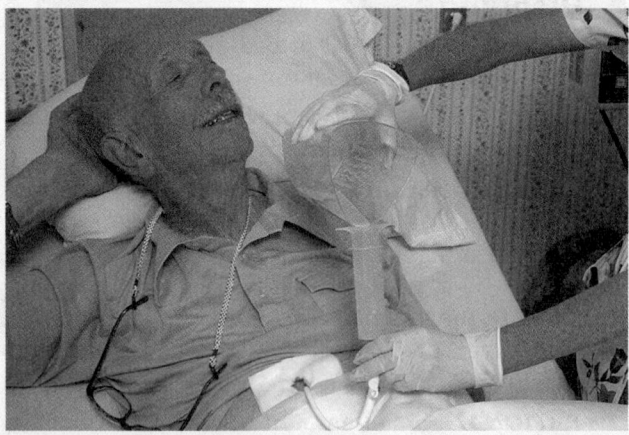

Step **7**

   RATIONALE The formula should be given over 10 minutes or longer; gravity pull will draw it in. Flow can be regulated by raising and lowering the container.

8. **ACTION** Add formula to keep the neck of the syringe filled. Continue adding formula to the syringe until the prescribed amount is given. Flush the tube with 30 to 60 mL of water.

   RATIONALE If the formula level falls below the neck of the syringe, air will enter the tubing and the intestinal tract, causing discomfort as a result of distention. Flushing the tube helps to prevent clogging.

For Continuous Tube Feeding

9. ***ACTION*** Fill the feeding bag with the prescribed amount of formula, clear the tubing of air, and attach it to an intravenous pole or infusion pump. Set the rate according to the physician order.

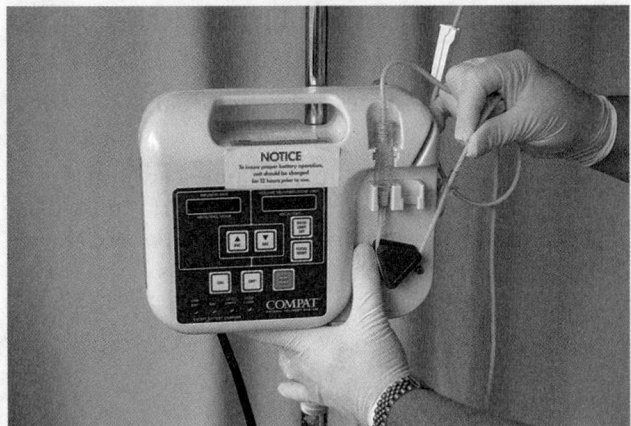

Step **9**

RATIONALE Feeding bag can be hung at room temperature for 4 hours within the hospital environment. A feeding pump delivers a controlled flow of formula. Some gavage bags have a pocket in which to place ice; this type of bag can allow the formula to hang up to 6 hours when ice is present.

10. ***ACTION*** Verify enteral, gastrostomy, or jejunostomy tube placement.

RATIONALE Jejunostomy tube sutures must be secure. Aspirating usually will not produce fluid from the jejunum; air cannot be easily detected when instilled into the jejunum. If the tube is not in place, the feeding could spill into the abdominal cavity, causing a chemical peritonitis.

11. ***ACTION*** Check the amount of residual from the previous feeding for gastrostomy tube by aspirating with a syringe; reinstill the fluid.

RATIONALE Residual should be checked every 4 hours for continuous gastrostomy tube feedings.

12. ***ACTION*** Attach the tubing from the feeding bag to the enteral, gastrostomy, or jejunostomy tube using an adaptor as needed. Turn on the pump and check the drip rate; begin feeding.

RATIONALE Drip rate should be checked frequently. Patient tolerance of the feeding should be assessed every hour while the patient is awake. Increasing abdominal distention or pain indicates a problem.

13. ***ACTION*** Follow the formula with 1 to 2 oz of water to clear the tube. Keep the liquid level above the neck of the syringe or bag to prevent air bub-

bles from collecting in the system or in the patient's intestinal tract.

RATIONALE Water helps clear the tubing and prevents clogging.

For Both Intermittent and Continuous Tube Feeding

14. ***ACTION*** Remove the syringe or connecting tubing, and clamp the tube by inserting the plug and covering with a cap protector or with a gauze 2 × 2 secured with a rubber band; a clamp may also be used (for intermittent feedings).

RATIONALE This prevents backflow of the formula or stomach fluid.

15. ***ACTION*** In the home, wash the bag and tubing or other equipment with soap and water every 8 hours; change the bag and tubing or syringe every 24 hours.

RATIONALE In home setting, equipment is washed with soap and water every 8 hours but may be reused for 3 to 7 days. Equipment is rinsed thoroughly after each feeding in the hospital and in the home.

16. ***ACTION*** Remove gloves and perform hand hygiene.

RATIONALE Prevents spread of microorganisms.

▪ Evaluation

17. ***ACTION*** Assess patient for evidence of discomfort or complications such as nausea, vomiting, and respiratory distress.

RATIONALE Provides evidence of patient's tolerance of tube feedings.

18. ***ACTION*** Monitor lab values, weight daily.

RATIONALE Assesses evidence of resolution of malnutrition.

▪ Documentation

19. ***ACTION*** Documentation should contain type of formula given, amount, verification of tube placement or securing sutures, amount of residual if obtained, and any signs of intolerance of the feeding.

RATIONALE Documents nutritional intake and any problems.

Documentation Example

5/16 1300 240 mL Jevity given via PEG tube. Checked for residual prior to feeding. 25 mL gastric contents aspirated and reinstilled. Abdomen soft, bowel sounds present in all quadrants. Tolerated feeding without evidence of discomfort. Head of bed remains at 30 degrees.

(Nurse's signature)

Continued

Skill 27-4   Administering a Nasogastric/Duodenal Tube Feeding or Feeding via a PEG Tube—cont'd

 Home Care Considerations

Nursing support for patient and family is essential. Teaching should involve patient and family if possible. Teaching plan should include

- Type of feeding
- Amount of feeding
- Operation of the feeding pump if used
- Checking for tube placement
- Signs and symptoms of complications
- Positioning the patient
- Procedure for manual feeding
- Safety factors during feeding
- Signs of problems to report

? CRITICAL THINKING QUESTIONS

1. The patient is receiving continuous tube feeding at 70 mL/hr. The nurse checks residual and returns 500 mL. What action(s) should the nurse take?

2. The caregiver reports to the home care nurse that the patient has been coughing and "milk-like" drainage has been noted around the patient's nose. List appropriate nursing interventions.

---

ordered for four or more times a day, the patient is usually given 150 to 240 mL per feeding and advanced at a rate of 50 mL/day until the desired volume is tolerated. Principles to observe when administering tube feedings are summarized in Box 27-1.

Box 27-1   *Principles of Tube Feeding*

Principles to follow when giving patients tube feedings:
- Elevate the head of the bed 30 to 90 degrees before feeding and leave it up for 30 to 60 minutes after the feeding.
- Keep the head of the bed elevated at least 30 degrees at all times if the patient is receiving continuous feeding.
- Assess bowel sounds at least once every 8 hours.
- Assess abdomen for distention.
- Check the tube position within the gastrointestinal (GI) tract before each feeding is started or at least once each shift.
- Check for gastric residual by aspirating via the gastric tube before each intermittent feeding or at least every 4 hours if the patient is receiving continuous feeding. If the gastric residual is greater than one half the volume given in the last feeding or greater than 150 mL when continuous feeding is in progress, replace the residual and delay the next feeding for 1 to 2 hours.
- Perform a fingerstick blood glucose every 4 to 6 hours as ordered for hyperglycemia until the patient demonstrates a normal blood glucose level.
- If nausea occurs, stop the feeding and notify the physician.
- Record an accurate intake and output record. Dehydration can occur because of diarrhea or the high glucose content of the formula.
- If persistent diarrhea occurs, notify the physician.

TOTAL PARENTERAL NUTRITION

Total parenteral nutrition (TPN) is a method of delivering total nutrition through a catheter placed in a large central vein (e.g., subclavian vein). A large vein with high blood flow is needed to dilute the solution rapidly. The solution may also be infused through a port implanted in the patient's chest wall, or a **peripherally inserted central catheter (PICC).** These options are used for patients receiving long-term therapy, such as victims of massive burns, intestinal obstruction, inflammatory bowel disease, AIDS, or cancer chemotherapy.

TPN is composed of high concentrations of carbohydrates as the main source of energy. Protein is provided through solutions of all amino acids. Solutions of other essential nutrients are also added to the infusion. Fatty acids are administered through lipid solutions that are infused daily or several times per week. TPN solutions are started slowly to allow the body to adjust to the high level of glucose concentration and the hyperosmolality (increased concentration of solutes within the fluid) of the solution. Usually 1000 to 2000 mL is administered the first 24 hours. After the first 24 hours, the infusion is increased until the desired volume is met. Monitoring of TPN should be ongoing. The infusion rate should be assessed through-

Elder Care Points

Elderly patients are at risk for fluid overload when receiving large volumes of intravenous fluids. Patients should be assessed for symptoms of fluid overload, including increased pulse rate, cough, respiratory distress, crackles on auscultation of the lungs, and imbalance in intake and output.

Table 27-5 *Monitoring Total Parenteral Nutrition**

ITEM TO ASSESS	WHEN TO ASSESS
IV site (PICC, central line, MediPort)	Every 4 hours. Observe for redness, swelling, or drainage from site.
Patient response	Every shift. Observe for signs of restlessness or discomfort.
Blood glucose	Every 6-8 hours. Report abnormal levels to the physician.
Vital signs	Every 4-8 hours. Abnormal vital signs may signal development of complications.
Weight	Daily or weekly as ordered. Evaluates patient's response.
Intake and output	Every shift. Abnormal urinary output may signal hyperglycemia or altered kidney function.
Flow rate	Every 4 hours. Prescribed flow rates should be followed to prevent hyperglycemic intolerance to TPN.
Electrolytes, CBC, BUN	Daily or as ordered. Evaluates patient's response.
Nutritional status	Ongoing. Includes weight, albumin levels, status of muscle mass.

*Baseline levels of blood chemistry, vital signs, weight, and nutritional status should be completed prior to beginning total parenteral nutrition (TPN) infusion. Compare ongoing monitoring to baseline results.
Key: *BUN,* Blood urea nitrogen; *CBC,* complete blood count; *IV,* intravenous; *PICC,* a peripherally inserted central catheter.

out the shift. If the rate is lower or higher than the prescribed rate, you should adjust the infusion to the correct flow rate. **Attempts should not be made to catch up if the rate has slowed. The rapid infusion of glucose can be harmful to the patient.** Table 27-5 summarizes the steps for monitoring TPN.

APPLICATION of the NURSING PROCESS

The steps of the nursing process are applied when caring for patients with NG or intestinal tubes.

Assessment (Data Collection)

- Assess reason for the tube. This information is necessary for evaluating the tube's effectiveness.
- Assess patient's understanding of the procedure.
- Assess function of the tube at least every 4 hours.
- Assess for signs of complications (i.e., nausea, vomiting, abdominal distention, abdominal pain, respiratory distress).

Nursing Diagnosis

Nursing diagnoses appropriate for patients requiring nutritional assistance are as follows:
- Risk for deficient fluid volume related to diarrhea or excessive vomiting
- Imbalanced nutrition: less than body requirements related to anorexia or NPO status
- Risk for injury related to aspiration of stomach contents into the respiratory tract from difficulty swallowing

Planning

Establish goals/expected outcomes based on the nursing diagnoses chosen. Examples of goals/expected outcomes are as follows:
- The patient will tolerate food and fluids without vomiting.
- The patient will consume at least 90% of all meals.
- The patient's breath sounds will remain clear without evidence of aspiration of food or fluids.

- The patient will gain 2 lb by time of discharge.
- The patient's stools will be formed.

Implementation

Nursing measures include frequent mouth care to prevent drying and cracking of the mucous membranes. To keep the mouth and lips moist, swab the oral cavity with a gauze pad or cotton swab that has been moistened with normal saline or water.

The nostrils often become dry and tender. If not contraindicated, a room humidifier can be helpful for the patient who is experiencing nose and throat discomfort. The nares should be cleansed with a swab and warm water daily or as needed. Water-soluble lubricant can be used on the nares. Other nursing actions include the following:
- Provide freedom of movement by securing the tubing to the patient's clothing to permit maximum activity without pulling on the nares.
- Do not permit the tubing to be kinked, as the flow of tube feeding will be cut off.
- Keep the environment clean, quiet, and well ventilated.

Patient Teaching 27-1 provides information to discuss with patients or caregivers of patients with NG or intestinal tubes.

Evaluation

Determine whether goals were met, partially met, or unmet. Retain, revise, or terminate nursing diagnoses, goals, or nursing interventions as appropriate. Evaluate the patient's ability to take food by mouth without nausea or vomiting. Evaluate nutritional parameters to ascertain success of tube feeding. Reassess abdominal peristalsis, signs of intestinal bleeding, or their absence.

Examples of evaluation statements are as follows:
- The patient takes food by mouth without nausea or vomiting.
- The patient gained ½ lb per week while receiving tube feedings.

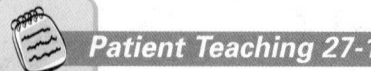

Patient Teaching 27-1

Patient with a Nasogastric or Intestinal Feeding Tube

Discuss the need for and advantages of having a nasogastric (NG) or intestinal tube in place. Teach the patient or primary caregiver the following:

- Perform oral care every 2 hours while awake to decrease mouth dryness; keep lips moistened.
- Be aware of the possible side effects from tube feeding, such as nausea, diarrhea, constipation, vomiting, or hyperglycemia.
- Keep the tube taped to the nose or face and attached to gown or clothing so that it does not hang lower than the stomach or point of entry into the patient's body.
- Keep the patient sitting up at an angle of at least 30 degrees for 1 hour after feedings to prevent reflux and possible aspiration of formula.
- Administer tube feedings at room temperature. Keep open formula refrigerated between feedings.
- Discard prepared or open refrigerated formula after 24 to 48 hours.
- Aspirate gastric fluid from the tube to check placement before giving each feeding (for nasogastric tube).
- Irrigate the tube with a small amount of water before and after each feeding.
- Clear the tube with water between each medication and after the last medication is given. Use 30 mL of water first, then give one medication, instill 5 mL of water, give next medication, instill 5 mL of water, and so on. When all medications are given, instill 30 mL of water to clear the tube.
- **Never** mix medications together because this causes clumping, which clogs tubes.
- Keep tubing clamped when not in use.
- Keep the area around the gastrostomy or jejunostomy tube clean with half-strength hydrogen peroxide or warm water.

- The patient takes food by mouth without aspiration of stomach contents into the airway.
- The patient has solid stools by time of discharge.

Documentation

Document the following:

- Size of tube inserted and how the patient tolerated the procedure
- Amount of formula given; result of tube feeding
- How placement of the tube is checked and amount of and character of gastric residual at each feeding
- Presence or absence of bowel sounds each shift
- Problems with nausea, constipation, or diarrhea
- Date and time of tube removal

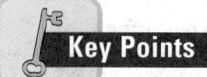

Key Points

- Nursing knowledge and understanding of diet therapy are important to assist patients to meet their nutritional needs.
- Diet therapy may involve progressive introduction of foods, such as clear liquid to full liquids, following surgery.
- Patients with eating disorders (anorexia nervosa, bulimia) pose a special challenge to nurses and other medical professionals.
- Dietary management of eating disorders must include psychological and nutritional counseling.
- Obesity is an increasing health care problem. Success of nutritional therapy for obese patients is low. Interventions include behavior modification, calorie control, appetite depressants, surgery, and psychological counseling.
- Maintaining optimum nutrition during pregnancy is critical to maternal health and healthy development of fetal tissues.
- Nutritional deficits are often found in patients with substance abuse. Nutritional assessment must be completed to determine nutritional status and to develop a plan to correct deficits.
- Diet therapy can be beneficial in the management of many disease processes, including gastrointestinal disorders, cardiovascular diseases, diabetes, nausea and vomiting, urinary disorders, cancer, and HIV/AIDS.
- Enteral tubes are sometimes prescribed when patients are unable to eat, or when food in the digestive tract aggravates a disease process. Enteral tubes may be used short or long term.
- NG tubes may be used to decompress the bowel, analyze gastric contents, or remove toxins.
- Nursing responsibilities when tubes are in place include patient teaching, tube insertion and removal, verification of placement, irrigation of tube, administration and management of tube feedings, and assessment for the development of complications.
- Patients experiencing severe malnutrition related to disease or treatment may require long-term and extensive nutritional support. Total parenteral nutrition (TPN) may be prescribed to meet those needs. TPN is composed of all amino acids and essential nutrients. Fatty acids are administered through lipid infusions. Calories are added through highly concentrated glucose solutions.
- Nursing knowledge concerning management of TPN is essential for success of treatment. Nurses are responsible for assessing the patient for potential complications and ensuring that the fluids are administered as ordered. Evaluation of the patient's response to treatment should be documented in the medical record.

  Go to your **Companion CD-ROM** for an Audio Glossary, animations, video clips, and more.

evolve Be sure to visit the companion Evolve site at http://evolve.elsevier.com/deWit/fundamental/ for additional online resources.

NCLEX-PN® EXAMINATION-STYLE REVIEW QUESTIONS

*Choose the **best** answer(s) for each question.*

1. When teaching the patient about a clear liquid diet, which of the following would the nurse instruct to include in the meal plan? *(Select all that apply.)*

    1. Milk
    2. Ginger ale
    3. Custard
    4. Cream of chicken soup
    5. Jell-O
    6. Popsicles
    7. Cream of Wheat
    8. Chicken broth

2. A patient is 5'6" tall and weighs 92 lb. Which of the following may be indicators of an eating disorder? *(Select all that apply.)*

    1. Makes a milkshake prior to bedtime
    2. Skips breakfast on a regular basis
    3. Exercises 3 hours daily
    4. Takes a laxative after each meal
    5. Eats large salads daily
    6. Purges meals

3. A patient asks how her diet should be changed during her pregnancy. The best response by the nurse would be:

    1. "Eat as much as you wish since you are 'eating for two.'"
    2. "Decrease calories by 100 per day to avoid weight gain."
    3. "A change in calorie intake is not necessary if prenatal vitamins are taken daily."
    4. "Increase calories by 300 per day during the second and third trimesters."

4. The major factor responsible for malnutrition in alcoholics is:

    1. substitution of alcohol calories for food calories.
    2. thiamine deficit.
    3. lack of access to food.
    4. malabsorption of nutrients.

5. A patient is admitted to the hospital with a diagnosis of congestive heart failure (CHF). Teaching related to diet therapy for CHF should include:

    1. reduction of fat and protein.
    2. increasing calories and fluids.
    3. reduction of sodium intake.
    4. increasing simple carbohydrates.

6. A diabetic patient asks if a slice of cake can be added to the meal for dessert. The best response by the nurse would be:

    1. "Diabetic patients should not eat cake."
    2. "Yes, but you must omit other carbohydrates of equal value from the meal."
    3. "You will have to check with your physician."
    4. "Yes, but don't do this too often."

7. After administration of an enteral feeding or during continuous feeding, how should the nurse position the patient? _____
   (Fill in the blank.)

8. A patient is receiving TPN. The night nurse reported that the infusion rate had been increased to 75 mL/hr. When you make your rounds at 8 A.M., you discover the rate is still infusing at 50 mL/hr. The appropriate nursing action is to:

    1. increase the rate to 75 mL/hr now.
    2. notify the physician immediately.
    3. change the rate to 125 mL/hr for 4 hours to catch up.
    4. leave the rate at 50 mL/hr because the patient is tolerating oral fluids.

9. The nurse teaches a diabetic patient to limit saturated fat and sodium intake because:

    1. all diabetic patients are at risk for obesity.
    2. these foods contribute to higher glucose levels.
    3. these nutrients are nonessential.
    4. diabetic patients are at risk for cardiovascular disease.

10. The nurse teaches a patient who will receive TPN at home to report symptoms of excessive thirst, voiding, and hunger to the health care provider. These symptoms are indicative of which complication of TPN?

    1. Fluid overload
    2. Protein excess
    3. Hyperglycemia
    4. Malnutrition

CRITICAL THINKING ACTIVITIES *Read each clinical scenario and discuss the questions with your classmates.*

Scenario A

Martin Stevens is admitted with exacerbation of symptoms of inflammatory bowel disease. He is placed NPO. Lab studies reveal severe electrolyte imbalance and malnutrition. TPN is ordered.

1. What are indications for TPN?
2. What is the composition of TPN?
3. Describe nursing interventions for patients receiving TPN.

Scenario B

Flora Smith, age 87, is cared for in her home following a stroke. She is unable to swallow and has a PEG tube in place. Her daughter administers continuous tube feeding using a feeding pump.

1. What parameters will you assess when you visit Mrs. Smith?
2. What factors will indicate tolerance of the feeding?
3. What complications may occur?
4. What teaching points will you review with Mrs. Smith's daughter?

Scenario C

James Kelly, age 42, is newly diagnosed with type 2 diabetes.

1. Differentiate between the types of diabetes.
2. What is the goal of dietary management of diabetes?
3. What are the recommendations for distribution of calories for a patient with diabetes?

Scenario D

Maria Torres, age 32, visits a health clinic for advice concerning weight loss. She is 5'9" tall and weighs 288 lb. She states she has been walking for 30 minutes three times a week for the past 2 weeks.

1. Ms. Torres is at high risk for which medical conditions?
2. How would you determine her dietary needs?
3. What diagnostic tests would be appropriate?
4. Develop a teaching plan for Ms. Torres.

CHAPTER 28

Assisting with Respiration and Oxygen Delivery

evolve http://evolve.elsevier.com/deWit/fundamental/

Objectives

Upon completing this chapter, you should be able to:

Theory

1. Explain how the respiratory system functions.
2. Name three causes of hypoxia.
3. Identify procedures to be followed in the event of respiratory or cardiac arrest.
4. Describe the various methods used for oxygen delivery.
5. List safety precautions to be observed when patients are receiving oxygen therapy.

Clinical Practice

1. Prepare to assist patients to clear the airway via coughing, postural drainage, suctioning, abdominal thrusts (Heimlich maneuver), and inhalation therapy.
2. Regulate oxygen flow and correctly apply an oxygen delivery device.
3. Prepare to provide care for the tracheostomy patient.
4. Prepare to care for the patient who has a chest tube and drainage system.

Skills & Steps

Skills

Skill 28-1   Using a Pulse Oximeter
Skill 28-2   Administering Abdominal Thrusts (Heimlich Maneuver)
Skill 28-3   Cardiopulmonary Resuscitation
Skill 28-4   Administering Oxygen
Skill 28-5   Nasopharyngeal Suctioning
Skill 28-6   Endotracheal and Tracheostomy Suctioning
Skill 28-7   Providing Tracheostomy Care

Steps

Steps 28-1   Maintaining a Disposable Water-Seal Chest Drainage System

Key Terms

Be sure to check out the bonus material on the Companion CD-ROM, including selected audio pronunciations.

anoxia (ă-NŎX-ē-a, p. 507)
apnea (p. 526)
atelectasis (ă-tě-LĔK-tă-sĭs, p. 529)
cannula (KĂN-ū-la, p. 518)
cyanosis (p. 510)
dyspnea (p. 509)
endotracheal (ĔN-dō-TRĀ-kē-ăl, p. 526)
expectorate (ĕk-SPĔK-tō-rāt, p. 518)

expiration (p. 508)
humidifier (hū-MĬ-dĭ-fī-ĕr, p. 519)
hypercapnia (hī-pĕr-KĂP-nē-a, p. 509)
hypoxemia (hī-pŏx-SĒ-mē-a, p. 507)
hypoxia (p. 507)
inspiration (p. 508)
nebulizer (NĚ-bū-lī-zĕr, p. 518)
obturator (ŎB-tŭ-rā-tŏr, p. 532)
retractions (p. 510)
stridor (p. 510)
tachypnea (p. 510)
tenacious (tě-NĀ-shŭs, p. 524)
tracheostomy (trā-kē-ŎS-tō-mē, p. 526)

Maintaining an open airway and providing adequate ventilation for every patient are primary nursing responsibilities. Oxygen is needed by all cells of the body to metabolize nutrients and produce the energy needed to function. When anoxia (condition of being without oxygen) occurs, cell metabolism slows down, and some cells begin to die. Through the act of breathing, we take in air that contains about 21% oxygen. An exchange of gases takes place in the lungs as oxygen is absorbed into the bloodstream and carbon dioxide, a waste product of cell metabolism, is released in the exhaled air. **The most common cause of respiratory insufficiency is obstruction of the airway.** Fortunately, obstruction is often easily reversed through the use of positioning and suctioning techniques.

Nurses must identify patients with breathing problems, take appropriate nursing actions to help relieve airway obstructions, and initiate or maintain oxygen therapy competently when it is used in the patient's treatment.

HYPOXEMIA

The foremost problem of the respiratory system is the disturbance of the levels of the gases oxygen and carbon dioxide in the bloodstream. This disturbance causes *respiratory insufficiency,* the inability of the body to meet its oxygen needs and remove excess amounts of carbon dioxide. The decreased amount of oxygen in the bloodstream is called hypoxemia and leads to a reduced amount of oxygen available to meet cellular needs, or the condition of hypoxia. Increased levels of

OVERVIEW OF STRUCTURE AND FUNCTION OF THE RESPIRATORY SYSTEM

Which structures are involved in respiration?

- The nose, mouth, pharynx, larynx, and trachea comprise the upper respiratory system (Figure 28-1).

- The trachea divides into the right and left main bronchi, which lead to the right and left lung.

- The right lung has three lobes, and the left lung has two lobes.

- Within each lung, the bronchi divide into smaller and smaller branches and then divide into bronchioles attaching to the alveoli.

- The *alveoli* (air sacs) are the terminal respiratory units of the lung and are lined with mucous membrane. There are between 300 million and 1 billion alveoli in the lungs.

- The diaphragm beneath the lungs moves, causing enlargement of the thoracic cavity. Because of negative pressure within the cavity, air flows in and inspiration (movement of air into the lungs) occurs. When the diaphragm muscle relaxes, the thoracic cavity space is decreased and air is forced out of the lungs in expiration (movement of air out of the lungs).

- The chest muscles combine with diaphragm action to move air in and out of the lungs.

- The respiratory muscles depend on nerve impulses from the spinal cord.

- The thoracic cage allows the respiratory muscles to function correctly.

What are the functions of the respiratory structures?

- The upper respiratory pathways carry air to and from the lungs.

- Air is warmed and humidified as it passes through the upper airway passages.

- The bronchi channel air to and from the lungs. The mucous membrane lining the bronchial tree contains tiny hairlike projections, or *cilia*, that trap and help remove small foreign particles that are inhaled.

- The mucous membrane secretes mucus that assists cilia in cleansing foreign substances from the respiratory tract.

- The alveoli contain macrophages that quickly phagocytize inhaled bacteria and other foreign particles.

- The mucus and cilia propel the foreign substances toward the entrance of the respiratory tract; the cough reflex works to expel the secretions.

- The central nervous system controls respiration.

- Chemoreceptors located in the aorta and carotid arteries sense changes in oxygen or carbon dioxide and send signals to the brainstem.

- The signals of changing levels of hydrogen ions in the blood (indicated by pH), carbon dioxide, and

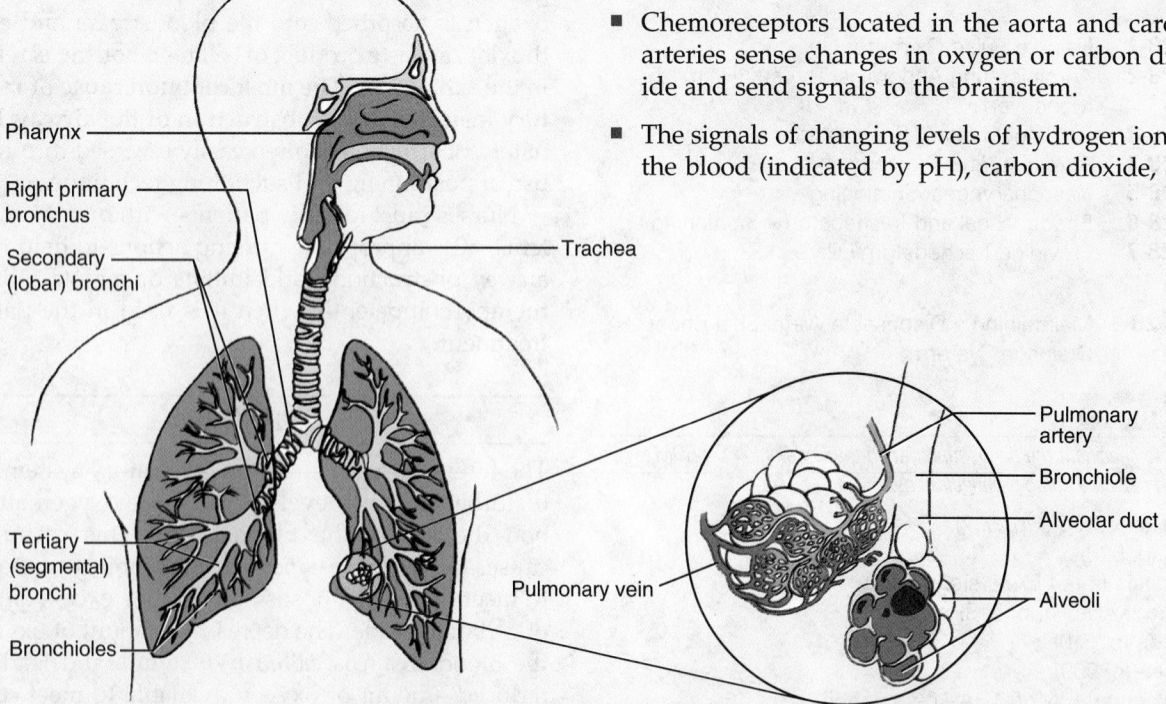

FIGURE **28-1** The respiratory system.

oxygen trigger the respiratory center in the medulla to send signals through the spinal cord to the nerves that control the respiratory muscles, causing an increased or decreased rate of respiration.

- Chemoreceptors send signals in response to changes in arterial blood gases.

- During normal breathing, about 500 mL of air moves in and out of the lungs with each breath.

- Oxygen diffuses across the alveolar membrane into the blood; carbon dioxide diffuses across the alveolar membrane from the blood to the alveoli.

- The blood transports oxygen to the cells and carries carbon dioxide from the cells to the lungs. Most of the oxygen is transported attached to the hemoglobin molecule in the red blood cells. The largest portion of carbon dioxide is transported to the lungs in the plasma portion of the blood.

What changes occur with aging that affect respiration?

- Alterations in connective tissue after age 70 cause decreased elasticity of the thorax and respiratory tissues.

- Total body water decreases 50% after age 70 and consequently respiratory membranes are drier, leading to thickened mucus.

- There is some degree of impairment of the cilia in the airways, decreasing their efficiency in removing mucus and foreign material.

- There is a loss of elastic recoil during expiration, and respiratory muscles must be used to complete expiration.

- Tissue changes cause thickening of the alveolar membrane, decreasing the ease of gas diffusion across the membrane. Oxygen saturation decreases, with partial pressure of oxygen (Po_2) dropping to 75 to 80 mm Hg from the usual 80 to 100 mm Hg.

- The elderly patient therefore has less respiratory reserve, making it more difficult for the body to meet demands for increased oxygenation.

carbon dioxide are described as **hypercapnia** (too much carbon dioxide in the blood).

Hypoxemia poses a dangerous threat to patients. The onset may be rapid and obvious or it may be insidious and gradual, with no clear-cut symptoms of **dyspnea** (difficulty breathing) or shortness of breath. Prompt recognition of the problem and swift action are needed when airways become obstructed. Box 28-1 lists common causes of hypoxia. Persistent hypoxic states require the combined efforts of a team consisting of a physician, respiratory therapist, laboratory technologist, and nurse.

SYMPTOMS OF HYPOXIA

The symptoms of hypoxia are those resulting from decreased oxygenation of various organs. The tissues of the body differ in their ability to survive by means of anaerobic metabolism—without oxygen. Brain cells,

---

Box 28-1 | *Common Causes of Hypoxia*

OBSTRUCTION OF THE AIRWAY
- Occlusion by tongue or mucous secretions
- Inflammation from croup, asthma, tracheobronchitis, laryngitis
- Occlusion by foreign body: aspiration, vomitus
- Chemical and heat burns with resultant inflammation
- Chronic obstructive pulmonary disease (chronic airflow limitation) causing collapse of airways
- Near drowning: occlusion by water

RESTRICTED MOVEMENT OF THE THORACIC CAGE OR THE PLEURA
- Abdominal surgery (incisional pain restricts movement)
- Chest injuries (flail chest, penetrating wounds)
- Pneumothorax (spontaneous or traumatic)
- Extreme obesity (restricts thoracic movement)
- Diseases (spinal arthritis, peritonitis, ascites, kyphoscoliosis)

DECREASED NEUROMUSCULAR FUNCTION
- Depressed central nervous system: drugs including sedatives and anesthesia agents, brain trauma, cerebrovascular accident
- Coma (diabetic, uremic, and from brain injuries)
- Diseases (multiple sclerosis, myasthenia gravis, poliomyelitis, Guillain-Barré syndrome)

DISTURBANCES IN DIFFUSION OF GASES
- Diseases (pulmonary fibrosis, emphysema)
- Trauma (contusion)
- Emboli, fat embolus
- Tumors, benign or malignant
- Respiratory distress syndrome

ENVIRONMENTAL CAUSES
- High altitude (decreased oxygen in the atmosphere)

Table 28-1 *Signs of Hypoxia and Respiratory Insufficiency*

EARLY SIGNS	INITIALLY	LATER	LATEST
Sits up to breathe	Blood pressure up	Blood pressure down	Cyanosis
Complains "I can't catch my breath"	Pulse up	Pulse down	Muscle retractions
Memory lapse	Respirations up	Dysrhythmia	
Mental dullness		Use of accessory muscles	
Restlessness		Stridor	

however, cannot withstand deprivation of oxygen and very quickly show the effects of hypoxia. The areas of memory, judgment, and intellectual ability are most readily affected. The heart and the retina of the eye are also highly vulnerable to reductions in oxygen. Other organs are also affected, such as the kidney, which retains more sodium when hypoxic.

Because the brain, retina, and heart are most susceptible to slight changes in oxygenation, the earliest signs of hypoxia involve these organs. Patients just do not seem right even though the vital signs are within normal limits. There may be signs of confusion. Patients who have difficulty breathing often become very anxious, and their anxiety increases the respiratory rate, although the higher rate may not increase the oxygenation. Tachypnea or stridor may be present. Dysrhythmias develop as the amount of oxygen supplied to the heart muscle is reduced. Patients with labored breathing, such as seen in obstructive pulmonary disease, use 30% to 50% of their energy just to breathe. Cyanosis (blue tinge to skin or mucous membrane) and retractions (muscles move inward on inspiration) of accessory muscles of the neck, chest, and abdomen are late signs of respiratory insufficiency (Table 28-1 and Concept Map 28-1). Hypoxia depresses body functions and disturbs the acid–base balance of the body. Less oxygen in the bloodstream leads to respiratory acidosis (see Chapter 25). Hypoxia is treated by administering oxygen and correcting the cause. Blood gases are a valuable tool for determining the degree and possible cause of hypoxia.

Patients suffering from hypoxia are highly susceptible to respiratory infection. Inadequate inflation of the lungs results in pooling of secretions and provides a medium for growth of microorganisms. It is essential that the respiratory patient be protected from hospital-acquired infections. Personnel with a respiratory infection should be kept out of the patient's environment.

? *Think Critically About . . .* How would you know that a patient is in respiratory distress? What signs and symptoms might be present?

PULSE OXIMETRY

Pulse oximetry is used for any patient thought to be at risk of hypoxia. With the pulse oximeter, changes in arterial oxygen saturation can be continuously

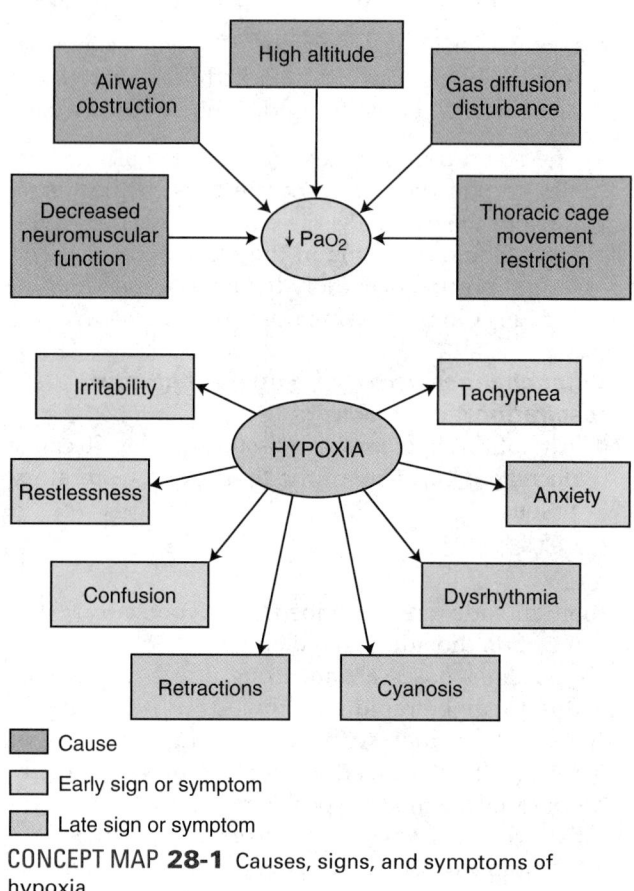

CONCEPT MAP **28-1** Causes, signs, and symptoms of hypoxia.

tracked. Because pulse oximetry is a form of continuous monitoring, in some ways it is more valuable than arterial blood gases for monitoring hypoxemia. The device measures oxygen saturation by determining the percentage of hemoglobin that is bound with oxygen. A sensor or probe is attached to an appendage of the patient through which infrared and red light can reach the capillary vascular bed (Skill 28-1, Figure 28-2). Oxyhemoglobin absorbs more infrared than red light. A microprocessor in the monitor receives the information from the sensor/probe, computes the saturation value, and displays it on the monitor screen.

Adhesive sensors can be applied to the nose or the forehead. Clip-on probes are used on the earlobe, fingertip, toe, or infant's foot. Adhesive sensors are generally disposable, whereas clip-on probes may be reusable.

Skill 28-1 | Using a Pulse Oximeter

Pulse oximetry provides the pulse oxygen saturation level (SpO_2), which is a reliable measure of oxygen saturation of the blood. It is a noninvasive measurement of the amount of oxygen carried by hemoglobin. In this manner, intermittent or continuous monitoring of oxygen saturation can be obtained. This is a painless procedure that allows the patient's response to treatment for hypoxia to be immediately evaluated. The procedure may not be accurate if the patient has had recent tests using intravenous dye or is jaundiced. The oximeter sensor contains both red and infrared light-emitting diodes (LEDs) and a photodetector. The photodetector registers light passing through the vascular bed, and the microprocessor determines oxygen saturation from the data received. It is most accurate when there is no direct sunlight or fluorescent light on the patient. The normal SpO_2 is greater than 90%. The sensor should be placed on a site that is free of moisture and has good local circulation.

■ Supplies
✓ Pulse oximeter
✓ Probe (clip-on or adhesive)

Review and carry out the Standard Steps in Appendix 3.

■ Assessment (Data Collection)

1. **ACTION** Assess for an appropriate site for placement of the sensor.

   RATIONALE The fingertip is the most common site, because light is easily passed through the tissue.

■ Planning

2. **ACTION** Set up the oximeter; plug in machine and turn on the power and check for proper function.

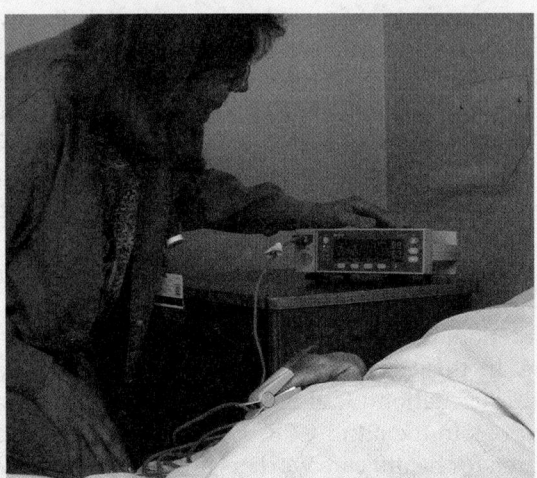

Step **2**

   RATIONALE Prepares machine to measure oxygen saturation. Check the manufacturer's instruction book.

■ Implementation

3. **ACTION** Remove dark nail polish or artificial nail if using a fingertip sensor.

   RATIONALE Dark nail polish or artificial nails distort readings.

4. **ACTION** Attach the correct sensor for the site flush to the skin and secure it.

   RATIONALE Different sensor probes are used for the fingertip, toe, or earlobe. Probe must be in contact with the skin to produce accurate readings.

5. **ACTION** Turn on machine and set alarms to predetermined saturation levels if monitoring is to be continuous. Tell patient alarm will sound if probe falls off or is moved. Correlate oximeter pulse rate with patient's radial pulse.

   RATIONALE Alarm will sound if saturation falls below set level or if probe is loosened or dislodged. Patient will know what to expect.

6. **ACTION** Read oxygen saturation level on screen and record it.

   RATIONALE Provides baseline data for beginning of monitoring; 10 seconds to 2 minutes are required for stabilization of unit.

■ Evaluation

7. **ACTION** Note and record the oximeter readings every hour.

   RATIONALE Normal SpO_2 saturation is 90% to 100%. When levels fall below 90%, action should be initiated immediately because the patient is on the brink of hypoxia, since as PaO_2 falls, a more rapid decrease occurs in oxygen saturation of the blood due to the oxyhemoglobin dissociation curve.

8. **ACTION** Rotate site of clip-on probes every 4 hours and disposable probes at least every 24 hours.

   RATIONALE Skin breakdown can occur with prolonged use of a probe. Apply skin cream to previously used area if skin dryness occurs.

Continued

Skill 28-1 | Using a Pulse Oximeter—cont'd

9. *ACTION* Adjust oxygen flow according to readings and physician's orders.

   RATIONALE Oxygen flow rate may be increased or decreased per physician's orders depending on the Spo_2 level.

10. *ACTION* Check the oximeter's calibration per manufacturer's directions at least once a day.

    RATIONALE Ensures that saturation readings are accurate.

11. *ACTION* When the order for pulse oximetry is discontinued, take a final reading, remove the probe, disconnect the machine, and clean the sensor site and the equipment.

    RATIONALE Prepares equipment for next use.

12. *ACTION* Record time of discontinuation of procedure and the final oximetry reading.

    RATIONALE Verifies testing has been discontinued.

■ Documentation

Documentation Example

10/12 1400 Spo_2 92%; O_2 by nasal cannula at 4 L/min.

———————————————

(Nurse's signature)

■ Special Considerations

✓ A small portable oximeter can be used to spot-check a patient's oxygen saturation. The probe is applied in the same manner as in this skill.

? CRITICAL THINKING QUESTIONS

1. What might be two nursing actions you could take if your patient, who has had trauma to the ribs as well as a leg fracture, develops a Pao_2 of 86%?

2. What simple measures can you have a patient take that might increase the Pao_2 when it begins to decrease?

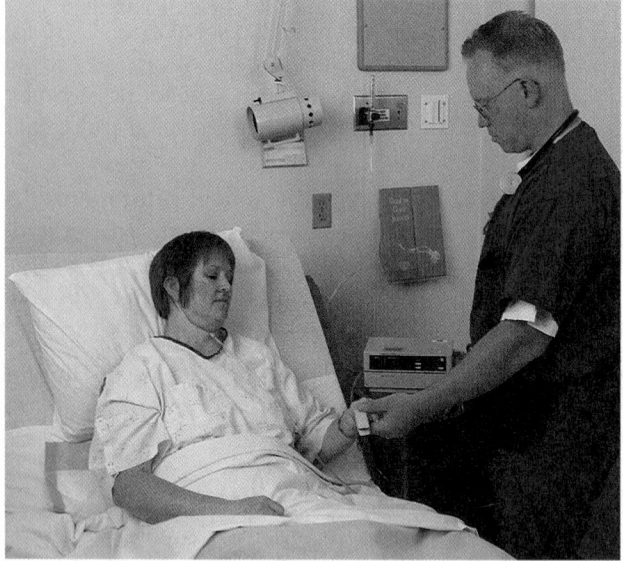

FIGURE **28-2** Monitoring oxygen saturation with the pulse oximeter.

AIRWAY OBSTRUCTION AND RESPIRATORY ARREST

Sometimes the airway becomes obstructed with a foreign object or food that goes down the throat the wrong way. If a person seems to be choking and cannot breathe, there is a set pattern of responses you should make. It is hoped that the person will exhibit the universal signal for choking, signaling for help (Figure 28-3). In this event you should perform abdominal thrusts (Heimlich maneuver) (Skill 28-2). The steps are the same for adults and children older than 1 year of age, but different for infants. For an infant, the ability to cry is the best sign that the airway is unobstructed. **In the unconscious person, the most common cause of airway obstruction is the tongue.**

If the airway is obstructed for an extended period, the heart may stop due to hypoxia. Sometimes the obstruction may be cleared, but the victim has no pulse. In this instance, you must start cardiopulmonary resuscitation (Skill 28-3). Current guidelines and variations in the adult CPR procedure for infants and children for health care workers are listed in Table 28-2 on p. 517. New guidelines for public bystanders state that giving 30 chest compressions—instead of 15—for every two rescue breaths is adequate. Fast, hard chest compressions can be used rather than being combined with rescue breathing if the bystander is reluctant to give mouth-to-mouth breaths.

> **Clinical Cues**
>
> If the patient has on colored nail polish, the sensor will function best if the polish is removed or the sensor is positioned on the sides of the finger.
>
> Another way to measure oxygenation is by determining oxygen saturation. This is an invasive procedure usually done in the critical care unit. Chapter 24 contains a description.

? • *Think Critically About . . .* What are two advantages of pulse oximetry over arterial blood gases for monitoring oxygenation?

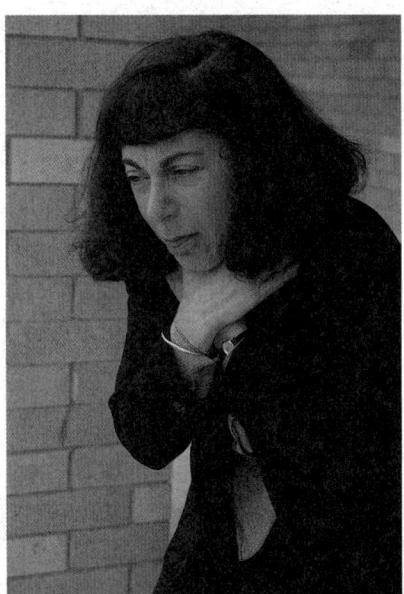

FIGURE **28-3** The hand grasping the throat is the universal signal for choking.

CLEARING RESPIRATORY SECRETIONS

THE EFFECTIVE COUGH

Mucus and secretions of the respiratory tract are typical causes of obstruction of the free passage of air. **The simplest method of clearing the air passages is to cough effectively.** Deep breathing and coughing are two standard measures used to clear secretions and prevent hypoxia. Deep breathing increases oxygenation, opens alveoli, and may precipitate coughing. Many patients with lung disease or the inability to forcibly expel a volume of air need to be taught how to cough effectively (Patient Teaching 28-1, p. 518). They must learn to make the most of their air volume to remove the obstructing materials. Ineffective coughing spasms may produce additional hypoxia, lead to the rupture of the alveoli, or even precipitate the collapse of air passages. Although forceful exhalation can be used with patients who are lying down, it is more effective for patients in the sitting position. For forceful exhalation coughing, the patient takes two deep

---

Skill 28-2 | Administering Abdominal Thrusts (Heimlich Maneuver)

Abdominal thrusts below the diaphragm, also called the Heimlich maneuver, is administered to either a conscious or an unconscious victim with airway obstruction. The purpose of the maneuver is to dislodge whatever is obstructing the airway and reestablish normal respiration.

■ For a Conscious Person

1. *ACTION* Ask person if she can speak.

   RATIONALE Establishes if person can get air into and out of the lungs.

2. *ACTION* If unable to talk or coughing is proving ineffective, position herself to deliver abdominal thrusts.

   RATIONALE Person needs assistance to dislodge obstruction.

3. *ACTION* Stand behind the person and place arms around the person's waist.

   RATIONALE Places hands at the correct height to deliver the thrusts.

4. *ACTION* Make a fist with one hand and place the other hand over the fist.

   RATIONALE Prepares the hands to deliver a solid thrust.

5. *ACTION* Place the hands halfway between the xiphoid process and the umbilicus with the thumb of the fist inward.

   RATIONALE Locates correct position for thrust delivery.

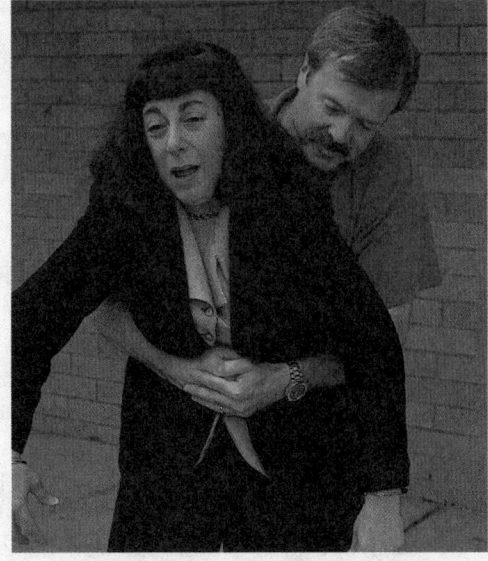

Step **6**

6. *ACTION* Using an upward rotating motion of the fist, forcefully thrust the hands into the abdomen at an upward angle.

   RATIONALE Creates an artificial cough, making the diaphragm move and forcing air out of the lungs.

Continued

Skill 28-2 | Administering Abdominal Thrusts (Heimlich Maneuver)—cont'd

7. **ACTION** Repeat the thrusts until the foreign body is expelled or the person becomes unconscious.

   RATIONALE The person cannot get air into the lungs until the obstruction is removed.

■ For an Unconscious Person

8. **ACTION** Call for help and/or activate emergency medical system (EMS) and slide the victim to the floor and place on back.

   RATIONALE Positions victim for airway opening maneuver and finger sweeps.

9. **ACTION** Tilt the victim's head back, grasp tongue and lower jaw between thumb and forefinger, and lift the jaw. If some foreign matter can be seen, use the index finger of the other hand to perform a finger sweep with a hook motion, being careful not to force the object farther down the throat.

   RATIONALE Allows rescuer to see into the mouth and pulls tongue away from back of throat.

10. **ACTION** Open airway and attempt to ventilate; if unsuccessful, reposition head and try again.

    RATIONALE Airway must be open for air to enter the lungs. Repositioning will often open the airway.

11. **ACTION** If ventilation is not successful, kneel straddling the victim's thighs and facing the head.

    RATIONALE Positions your body to deliver abdominal thrusts.

12. **ACTION** Locate the xiphoid process and the umbilicus, and place the heel of one hand over the back of the other slightly above the umbilicus.

    RATIONALE Positions hands for effective thrusts. Ensures you are not thrusting over the xiphoid.

13. **ACTION** Press heel of hand toward head with five quick abdominal thrusts or until foreign object dislodges.

    RATIONALE Causes artificial cough, forcing air from the lungs, which may dislodge an obstruction.

14. **ACTION** Use head tilt–jaw lift (or jaw-/chin thrust if patient is unconscious), to open mouth and, if a foreign body can be seen, sweep with a curved finger down inside of the cheek toward base of tongue, sweeping the debris out the other side of the mouth.

    RATIONALE Removes any dislodged object.

15. **ACTION** Open the airway and attempt to ventilate by pinching off the nose and placing the mouth over the patient's mouth.

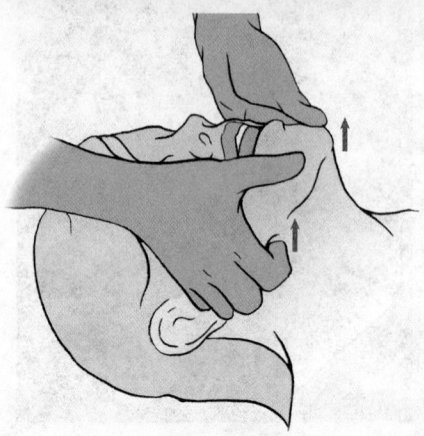

Step **14**

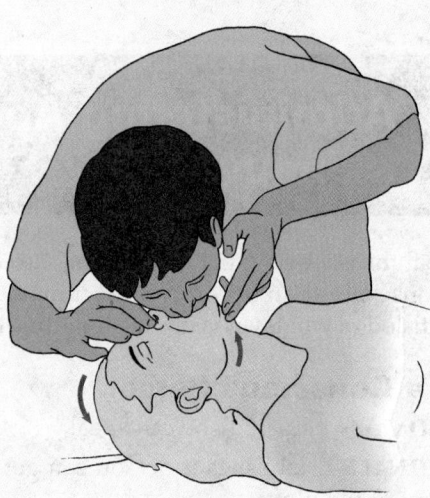

Step **15**

RATIONALE If airway is open, breaths will go into victim's lungs. If airway is still obstructed, attempt to ventilate will be unsuccessful.

16. **ACTION** If ventilation is not successful, repeat steps 12 through 14. Repeat sequence until foreign body is dislodged. If person resumes breathing, turn to side with arms in front of the body.

    RATIONALE Person cannot breathe if obstruction is present. Side-lying recovery position aids continued respiration and prevents aspiration if person vomits.

■ For the Conscious Infant

17. **ACTION** Place the infant face down straddling your arm, keeping the head lower than the trunk. Place your hand under the chest and around the jaw for support.

RATIONALE Positions the infant for effective back blows; position assists object to move up into or out of mouth.

18. **ACTION** Deliver five blows between the shoulder blades.

    RATIONALE Force of the blows should dislodge foreign body.

19. **ACTION** Sandwich the infant between your arms and turn her over. With the head down, deliver five chest thrusts using two fingers over the lower half of the sternum.

    RATIONALE Helps dislodge object.

20. **ACTION** Repeat steps 17 through 19 until object is dislodged.

    RATIONALE Infant cannot breathe when object is in airway.

■ For the Unconscious Infant

21. **ACTION** Turn the infant over, place on your thigh or hard surface, and open the airway. Perform tongue-jaw lift. If you can see the object, carefully perform a finger sweep to remove it.

    RATIONALE Position allows visualization of object in the mouth; finger sweep removes object.

22. **ACTION** Open the airway and attempt to ventilate with your mouth over the infant's mouth and nose.

    RATIONALE If the airway is unobstructed, the chest will rise.

23. **ACTION** If the chest does not rise, reposition the head and attempt to ventilate again.

RATIONALE Airway is obstructed; repositioning may open it.

24. **ACTION** If unable to ventilate, reposition the infant straddling your arm and repeat the back blows and chest thrust sequences.

    RATIONALE No air can reach the lungs if the airway is obstructed.

25. **ACTION** Perform tongue-jaw lift and, if you can see object, finger sweep it out.

    RATIONALE Removes the obstructing object.

26. **ACTION** If unable to see anything, repeat back blows and chest thrust sequences. Activate EMS if the obstruction is not relieved within 1 minute.

    RATIONALE Repeating sequences will dislodge object. EMS activation will bring help.

■ Special Considerations

✓ If victim is pregnant, use chest thrusts rather than abdominal thrusts to dislodge the obstruction; place the heel of one hand over the lower third of the sternum and the other hand on top of it. Give five quick thrusts.

✓ If the victim is obese, chest thrusts may be more effective.

?CRITICAL THINKING QUESTIONS

1. What do you think are the most common causes of choking in adults?

2. What should you teach parents of young children regarding types of foods to avoid serving and supervision when they are eating?

Skill 28-3 | Cardiopulmonary Resuscitation

Cardiopulmonary resuscitation (CPR) must be started whenever someone is found in respiratory or cardiac arrest, meaning without breathing or without a heartbeat. It is vitally important to call for help while beginning to assess the victim. The following method is appropriate for adults. See Table 28-2 for differences for the child or infant.

1. **ACTION** Shake victim and shout name or "Are you OK?"

   RATIONALE Arouses victim if she is not unconscious.

2. **ACTION** Call for help: activate the emergency medical system.

   RATIONALE Emergency assistance and supplies for advanced life support should arrive within minutes.

3. **ACTION** Place the victim supine on a firm surface, kneel beside the person, and open the airway by placing the heel of one hand on the forehead and two fingers of your other hand on the bony prominence of the chin; lift the chin to open the airway.

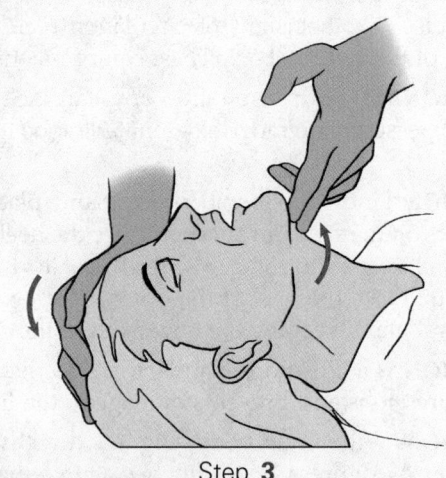

Step **3**

Continued

Skill 28-3 | Cardiopulmonary Resuscitation—cont'd

RATIONALE Opens airway, allowing airflow to occur if victim is breathing.

4. *ACTION* Look, listen, and feel for air movement by turning your face toward the victim's chest and your ear and cheek toward the victim's mouth.

   RATIONALE Allows you to observe the chest for rise and fall of respiration, feel airflow on your cheek from the mouth, and hear the sound of airflow with your ear.

5. *ACTION* If mask is available, place it over the victim's nose and mouth with the bridge of the nose as a guide. If no mask is available, maintain the head tilt and seal the nose with your fingers. Take a deep breath and, forming a seal around the victim's mouth with your own, give two 1-second breaths that make the chest rise. If the first breath does not go in, the airway may have become obstructed; reposition with head tilt–chin lift and try to deliver the breaths again, watching to see that the chest rises and falls. If the airway is obstructed, perform the Heimlich maneuver.

   RATIONALE A rescue breathing mask protects the rescuer from the victim's secretions. Slow, long breaths help prevent air from entering the stomach. Rising and falling of the chest indicates that the airway is unobstructed. If the airway becomes obstructed, air will not enter. The Heimlich maneuver assists in dislodging an obstruction.

6. *ACTION* Locate the victim's larynx with two fingers and then slide them slightly laterally with gentle pressure to locate the carotid pulse and check it for 5 seconds.

   RATIONALE Positions the fingers over the carotid artery.

7. *ACTION* If the pulse is present but the patient is not breathing, continue rescue breathing at a rate of 12 breaths per minute (1 every 5 seconds). If there is no pulse or other signs of circulation (i.e., movement of the victim), begin chest compressions.

   RATIONALE Both respiration and cardiac pumping are essential to move oxygenated blood around the body.

8. *ACTION* Find the xiphoid process and place two fingers on the sternum above it. Place the heel of the hand closest to the victim's head next to the two fingers. Place the heel of the other hand on top of the first hand, keeping the fingers off of the chest.

   RATIONALE Positions hands for effective chest compressions and prevents damage to the liver.

9. *ACTION* With your body aligned directly over the hands, depress 1½ to 2 inches, with equal time

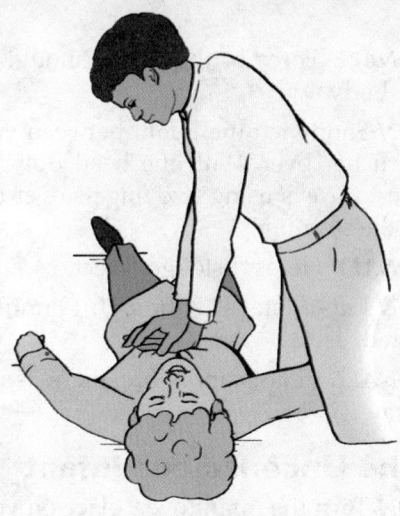

Step **8**

for compression and release. Give 15 compressions at a rate of 100 per minute (2 rescuers). For a lone rescuer, use a series of 30 compressions to 2 breaths.

   RATIONALE Pumps blood out of the heart at a rate sufficient to provide adequate oxygenation to maintain tissue life.

10. *ACTION* Stop compressions, perform head tilt–chin lift, and give two slow 2-second breaths; begin another cycle of compression.

    RATIONALE Rescue breathing opens airway and provides oxygen. Compressions circulate oxygenated blood.

11. *ACTION* Check the carotid pulse for a spontaneous heartbeat every minute (every four cycles).

    RATIONALE Spontaneous pulse indicates that chest compressions may be halted.

12. *ACTION* If the pulse is present but victim is not breathing, stop compressions but continue the breathing for the victim.

    RATIONALE Circulation of blood does little good if it does not carry oxygen.

■ Special Considerations

✓ When a second trained rescuer is present, and the patient is intubated, perform two-rescuer CPR. The compression-to-ventilation ratio is 5:1, with the second person doing the breathing. The second person is positioned opposite the first rescuer. When CPR is stopped at the end of a cycle and the first rescuer is checking the pulse for 5 seconds, the second person switches and positions hands for the chest compressions. If the first rescuer says, "No pulse; continue CPR," wait for a breath to be given by the first rescuer and then begin compressions. One breath is given for every five compressions. When you tire (after a minimum of 10 cycles), call out, "Switch on five," and count with your compressions, "one-and-two-and-three-and-four-and-switch," as you give the five compressions and then move to the patient's head; check the carotid pulse, indicate the result, and continue CPR by giving a breath.

✓ If a pulse is present, check breathing. If breathing is present, place the patient in side-lying recovery position and continue to monitor.

✓ If pulse is present but breathing is absent, continue rescue breathing at 12 per minute.

✓ If automated external defibrillator (AED) is available, use it as soon as possible if no effective heart rhythm is present.

?CRITICAL THINKING QUESTIONS

1. What do you do if the victim vomits while you are performing CPR?

2. What do you do if you come upon a motor vehicle accident victim who is still in the car, has no signs of respiration or circulation, and might have a spinal injury?

Table 28-2 | *CPR Guidelines*

MANEUVER	ADULT Lay Rescuer: >8 yr HCP: Adolescent and Older	CHILD Lay Rescuers: 1-8 yr HCP: 1 yr to Adolescent	INFANT <1 yr
Activate Emergency response number (lone rescuer)	Activate when victim found unresponsive HCP: If asphyxial arrest likely, call after 5 cycles (2 min) of CPR	Activate after performing 5 cycles of CPR For sudden, witnessed collapse, activate after verifying that victim unresponsive	
Airway	Head tilt–chin lift (HCP: Suspected trauma, use jaw thrust)		
Breaths: Initial	2 breaths at 1 sec/breath	Two effective breaths at 1 sec/breath	
HCP: Rescue breathing without chest compressions	10-12 breaths/min (approximately 1 breath q 5-6 sec)	12-20 breaths/min (approximately 1 breath q 3-5 sec)	
HCP: Rescue breaths for CPR with advanced airway	8-10 breaths/min (approximately 1 breath q 6-8 sec)		
Foreign-body airway obstruction	Abdominal thrusts		Back slaps and chest thrusts
Circulation HCP: Pulse check (<10 sec)	Carotid (HCP can use femoral in child)		Brachial or femoral
Compression landmarks	Center of chest, between nipples		Just below nipple line
Compression method (Push hard and fast) (Allow complete recoil)	2 Hands: Heel of 1 hand, other hand on top	2 Hands: Heel of 1 hand with other hand on top *or* 1 Hand: Heel of 1 hand only	1 rescuer: 2 fingers HCP, 2 rescuers: 2 thumb-encircling hands
Compression depth	1½-2 in	Approximately ⅓-½ the depth of the chest	
Compression rate	Approximately 100/min		
Compression-ventilation ratio	30:2 (1 or 2 rescuers)	30:2 (single rescuer) HCP: 15:2 (2 rescuers)	
Defibrillation AED	Use adult pads. Do not use child pads/child system. HCP: for out-of-hospital response may provide 5 cycles/2 min of CPR before shock if response >4-5 min and arrest not witnessed.	HCP: Use AED as soon as available for sudden collapse and in-hospital. All: After 5 cycles of CPR (out-of-hospital). Use child pads/child system for child 1-8 yr if available. If child pads/system not available, use adult AED and pads.	No recommendation for infants <1 yr

From American Heart Association. (2006). Highlights of the 2005 American Heart Association Guidelines for Cardiopulmonary Resuscitation and Emergency Cardiovascular Care. *Currents in Emergency Cardiovascular Care, 16*(4), 15. Copyright © American Heart Association. Reprinted with permission.
Key: *AED,* Automated external defibrillator; *CPR,* cardiopulmonary resuscitation; *HCP,* health care professional.
For the lay rescuer, an adult is any person older than 8 years, a child is between 1 and 8 years old, and an infant is younger than 1 year. For the health care provider, an adult is an adolescent or older, a child is between 1 year and adolescence, and an infant is younger than 1 year.

Patient Teaching 28-1

Deep Breathing and Coughing

Have the patient sit up on the side of the bed or in a chair leaning slightly forward so the back is not against the back of the chair. If the patient cannot sit up, raise her to a high Fowler's position. Demonstrate the following steps and then coach the patient through the steps. These exercises should be performed for at least 72 hours after surgery and during treatment and recovery from a respiratory illness.

DEEP BREATHING

- Splint an abdominal or chest incision with a small pillow.
- Inhale through the nose; hold the breath for 3 to 5 seconds and then exhale through pursed lips. Keep the shoulders level and use the diaphragm and abdominal muscles to bring air into the lungs.
- Repeat the sequence four more times, breathing slowly.
- Instruct the patient to take 5 to 10 deep breaths every 2 hours while awake.

EFFECTIVE COUGHING

- Take a deep breath through the nose, hold it for 3 to 5 seconds, and then exhale through pursed lips.
- Take another deep breath and, in short segments, forcibly exhale in a huff-cough with the mouth open. Expel one third of the expiratory volume with each huff-cough. Use a tissue to cover the mouth.
- Perform the sequence three times or until all secretions have been cleared.
- Expectorate the secretions into a tissue; dispose of the tissue in a sealable plastic bag.
- Instruct the patient to use huff-coughing technique at least once every 2 hours while awake, preferably once an hour.

breaths and then inhales deeply again. That breath is rapidly and forcibly exhaled as quickly as possible with the mouth open. This moves secretions up the bronchial tree. Repeated forceful exhalation can bring the secretions up to a point where they can be more easily coughed up (Patient Teaching 28-2).

POSTURAL DRAINAGE

Although the respiratory therapist usually is responsible for this procedure in the inpatient setting, in community and home settings the nurse must teach patients the procedure. Different positions are used to drain different segments of the lungs so that secretions can be cleared (Figure 28-4). As specific segments of the lung are drained into the bronchi, the patient is able to cough more effectively and expectorate (cough up and spit out) secretions. The lungs are auscultated before and after the procedure. Generally, the patient should assume each position for 5 to 15 minutes two to four times a day as tolerated. When preparing for postural drainage, a nebulizer (a device that dispenses liquid in a fine spray) with bronchodilator or liquefying drugs may be used as

Patient Teaching 28-2

Obtaining a Coughed Sputum Specimen

A sputum specimen is best obtained just after the patient awakens or after a nebulizer treatment because this is when there is more mucus available or when it is easier to cough up. Provide a sterile sputum cup. Teach to patient to

- Rinse the mouth with water.
- Open the sputum cup and place the lid upside down on the counter or table.
- Take several deep breaths, forcefully huff-cough to move secretions up, and expectorate produced sputum into the cup.
- Take several more deep breaths, force another huff-cough, and expectorate produced sputum into the cup.
- Repeat until about a half teaspoon of sputum is in the cup.
- Place the lid on the cup without contaminating the inside of the lid or the lip of the cup.
- Cleanse the mouth.
- Ring for the nurse, who will collect the specimen and send it to the laboratory.

inhalation therapy to thin out thick secretions and open the bronchial tree by relaxing spasm. Best results occur when the procedure is carried out in the morning and 45 to 60 minutes before a meal.

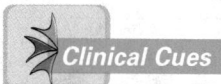

Clinical Cues

Be sure to offer mouth care after this procedure so that the appetite isn't affected by a bad taste in the mouth from coughing up secretion.

Secretions and mucus plugs may be loosened by percussion of the chest. Percussion is the rhythmic clapping with cupped hands over the thoracic area, but not over the spine or sternum. After percussion and postural drainage, the patient is assisted to cough effectively and expectorate the secretions.

Think Critically About . . . Why do you think postural drainage and percussion should not be done right before a meal or within an hour afterward?

OXYGEN ADMINISTRATION

When the patient cannot maintain a sufficient amount of oxygen in the body, supplemental oxygen is often ordered. Oxygen can be administered by cannula (tube for insertion into a cavity), mask, tent, Croupette, or catheter. Although respiratory therapists are usually

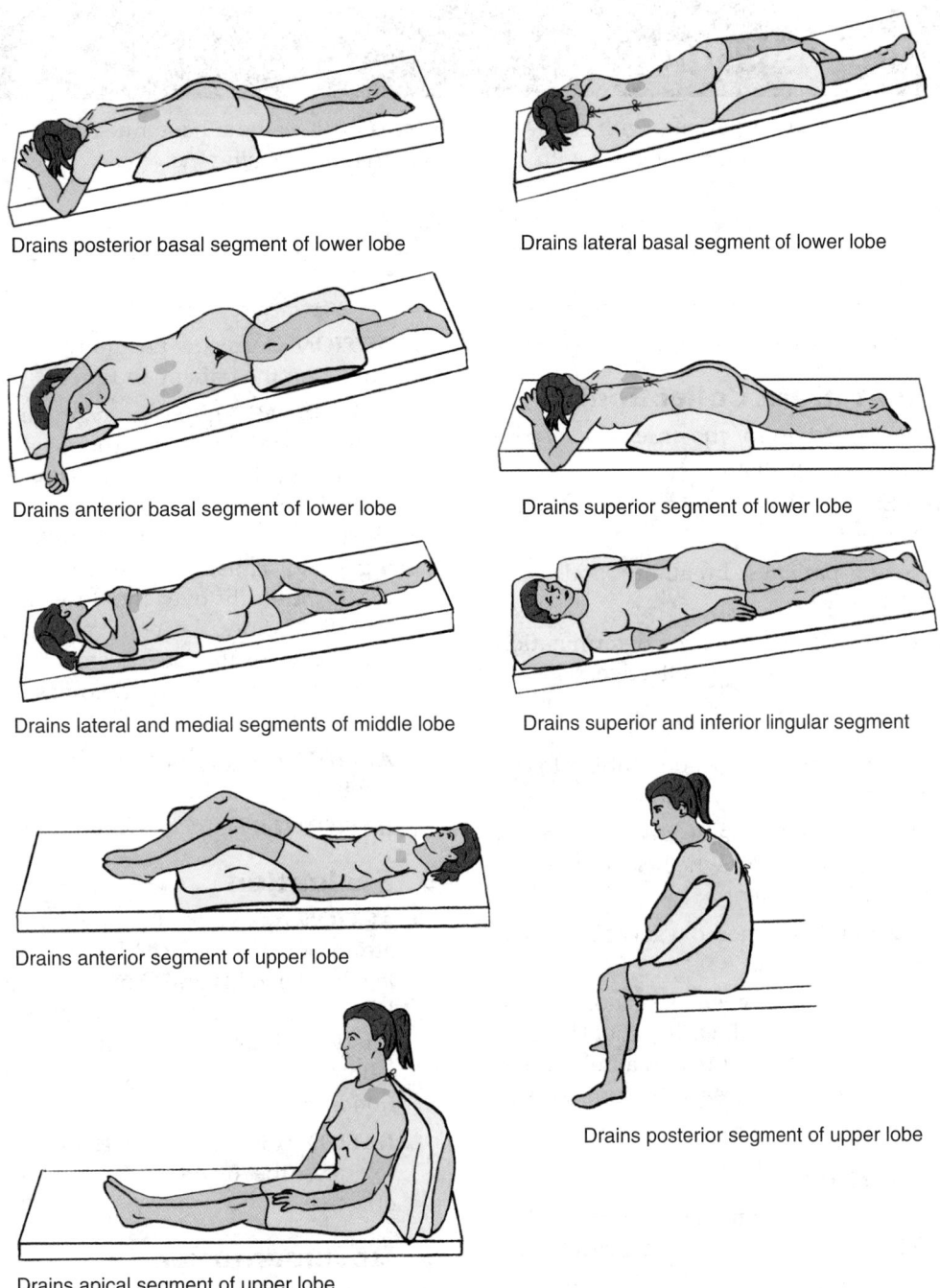

Drains posterior basal segment of lower lobe

Drains lateral basal segment of lower lobe

Drains anterior basal segment of lower lobe

Drains superior segment of lower lobe

Drains lateral and medial segments of middle lobe

Drains superior and inferior lingular segment

Drains anterior segment of upper lobe

Drains posterior segment of upper lobe

Drains apical segment of upper lobe

FIGURE 28-4 Positions for postural drainage.

responsible for setting up and supervising oxygen equipment, nurses often need to initiate therapy or supervise its use on a PRN (as-needed) basis (Skill 28-4).

Oxygen is a colorless, tasteless, and odorless gas that is present in the air. Although it is essential for life, the use of oxygen is not without its disadvantages (Safety Alert 28-1). One of the properties of the gas is that it supports combustion. High concentrations of oxygen can cause fires to burn very rapidly, and when oxygen is used medically in the treatment of patients, great care must be taken to prevent fires from occurring. Another disadvantage associated with the use of the gas is that it

is very drying to the tissues of the respiratory tract. Unless moisture is added, the dried tissues may become cracked and provide less resistance to infection.

The pieces of equipment needed for oxygen therapy are the oxygen source, the flowmeter, the humidifier (device supplying moisture) (optional), the tubing, and the appropriate appliance for the method ordered. Most hospitals have a central oxygen supply with outlets mounted in the wall near the patient's bed. The flowmeter is attached to the piped-in oxygen and regulates the amount given (Figure 28-5). The rate of flow is prescribed by the physician in terms of liters per minute

Skill 28-4 | Administering Oxygen

Oxygen therapy is ordered for patients with respiratory illnesses or those who have musculo-skeletal or neurologic problems that interfere with proper oxygenation, causing hypoxia.

■ Supplies
✓ Oxygen source
✓ Humidifier (optional)
✓ Oxygen delivery device
✓ Nasal cannula
✓ Face mask
✓ Face tent
✓ Oxygen flowmeter
✓ Connecting tubing

Review and carry out the Standard Steps in Appendix 3.

■ Assessment (Data Collection)

1. **ACTION** Check the chart for the ordered flow rate and oxygen delivery method.

   RATIONALE Ensures that patient will receive oxygen therapy as ordered.

2. **ACTION** Assess patient's breathing and lung sounds.

   RATIONALE Provides baseline for determination as to whether oxygen therapy is effective.

■ Planning

3. **ACTION** Plan amount of connecting tubing to the oxygen source needed by the patient.

   RATIONALE Length of tubing needed depends on prescribed activity level and whether O_2 needs to be continuous or intermittent.

4. **ACTION** Determine whether oxygen setup will need a humidifier.

   RATIONALE Low-flow oxygen does not need a humidifier to moisten the flow. If patient suffers from sinus problems, it is best to add a humidifier. Oxygen is drying to the mucosa. A humidifier provides moisture.

■ Implementation

5. **ACTION** Connect the flowmeter to the piped-in oxygen outlet on the wall by pressing it firmly into the outlet. Or attach the flowmeter to the oxygen cylinder.

   RATIONALE Prepares the oxygen to be dispensed in a regulated flow.

6. **ACTION** Attach the humidifier and the connecting tubing to the oxygen delivery device and turn on the oxygen, adjusting the flow to the ordered rate. Check for flow through the oxygen delivery device.

   RATIONALE Readies the delivery system for the patient. By turning the knob on the flowmeter, the metal ball inside the glass graduated gauge rises, indicating the rate of flow being delivered. The ordered rate is commonly between 2 and 5 L/min and is ordered by the physician. Feel for the flow with your fingers.

7. **ACTION** Correctly position the oxygen delivery device on the patient and secure it in place.

   RATIONALE An oxygen cannula should be positioned with the nasal prongs curved downward as they go into the nares. The tubing is looped over the ears and secured in place by raising the cinch device toward the chin. Be certain the tubing is not causing pressure on the ears. A face mask should fit over the nose and mouth. A face tent fits below the chin and rises to cover the lower part of the face. A small tent-mask fits just above the upper lip and comes to a point above the nares.

8. **ACTION** Instruct patient and visitors regarding safety during oxygen use.

   RATIONALE Helps prevent fires and injury.

■ Evaluation

9. **ACTION** Ask yourself: Is the patient able to tolerate the oxygen device? Is the oxygen flow at the level ordered? Is an "Oxygen in Use" sign posted? Does patient understand instructions regarding safety during O_2 administration? Is breathing less labored with oxygen administration? Is O_2 saturation improving?

   RATIONALE Answers determine whether patient tolerates the oxygen and whether procedure is effective.

■ Documentation

10. **ACTION** Include the reason for the oxygen therapy, the time that oxygen therapy is instituted, the type of oxygen delivery device in use, flow rate, and whether it is continuous or PRN.

    RATIONALE Verifies that oxygen is administered as ordered; data support charges for oxygen administration.

Documentation Example

11/16 0945 Spo_2 89%; O_2 ordered. Nasal cannula at 3 L/min applied.
1100 Spo_2 94%. Tolerating flow by cannula without complaint; ears not irritated by tubing.

_____

(Nurse's signature)

■ Special Considerations

✓ If patient does not tolerate oxygen delivery by one method, an order to change to another device may be needed.

✓ If oxygen is delivered PRN by cannula, instruct the patient that it is desirable to use the oxygen after meals and during activity. O_2 demands are higher when digestion or activity is occurring.

✓ Cleanse the nares regularly when oxygen is in use to prevent excessive crusting.

✓ It is important that the patient understand the reason for and potential benefits of using the oxygen before applying the delivery device; otherwise compliance with use may be low.

✓ The flow rate should be checked each time you enter the patient's room; the patient or a visitor may change it from what is prescribed.

✓ Oxygen delivery devices should be turned off when not in use; instruct the patient with PRN oxygen how to do this.

✓ Teaching safety precautions for the home care patient is especially important because there is no medical supervision when the nurse's visit is over.

? CRITICAL THINKING QUESTIONS

1. If you have a patient with a history of frequent sinusitis who is receiving oxygen by nasal cannula at 3 L/min and that patient complains about nasal stuffiness and sinus discomfort, what could you do to alleviate the problem?

2. You have a postoperative patient who is receiving oxygen by nasal cannula. The patient keeps taking off the O_2 cannula. What might you say that might convince the patient to leave the oxygen cannula in place?

⚠ Safety Alert 28-1

Oxygen Therapy Safety

- Place a "No Smoking: Oxygen in Use" sign on the patient's door and at the foot of the bed or over the head of the bed.
- Remind visitors about the hazard of smoking when oxygen is in use. Teach family to smoke only far removed from the room where oxygen is in use.
- Check all electrical devices for frayed wires and to see that they are in good working order to prevent short-circuit sparks that could cause a fire.
- Avoid the use of bedclothes and pajamas that are made of material that can generate static electricity. Cotton fabrics are best.
- Do not use oils, grease-based ointments, alcohol, ether, acetone, or other flammable materials on or near the patient when oxygen is in use in the room. If oxygen cylinders are being used, handle them with caution. Be certain they are strapped securely into stands and transport devices to prevent them from falling. Situate the cylinders away from heat and heavy traffic pathways.
- Monitor the patient for skin irritation from the oxygen delivery device.
- Assess for dry mucous membranes indicating a need for humidification to prevent tissue breakdown that can provide an avenue for infection.

---

and may range from 2 to 12 L/min. The flow rate is based on the patient's condition and on the blood gas report or pulse oximetry, which measures the amount of oxygen in the blood. Rates of 4 to 6 L/min are common (Safety Alert 28-2). The flow rate is adjusted by turning the valve to the "on" position, and continuing to turn it until the desired flow level is indicated in the gauge just above the flow adjustment valve (Figure 28-6).

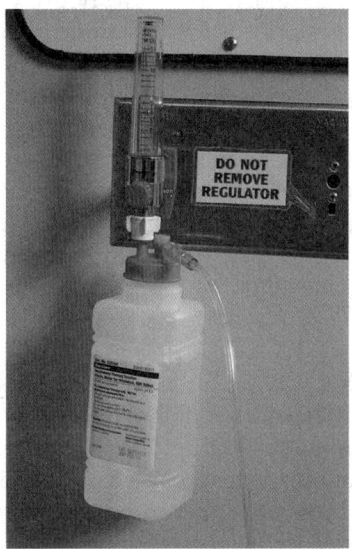

FIGURE **28-5** Wall oxygen flowmeter and humidifier setup.

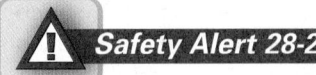

⚠ Safety Alert 28-2

Safe Oxygen Flow Rates

Patients with obstructive lung diseases should be given only 2 to 3 L/min because higher concentrations of oxygen further reduce the respiratory rate. This is because their incentive to breathe comes from oxygen levels rather than carbon dioxide levels in the blood (they have a continual high level of carbon dioxide). Check the orders carefully and verify high flow rates with the physician.

The humidifier is attached to the flowmeter and is usually situated between the flowmeter and the tubing. The oxygen bubbles through the container of water and is moisturized before entering the air passages. Check the level of fluid in the container at intervals

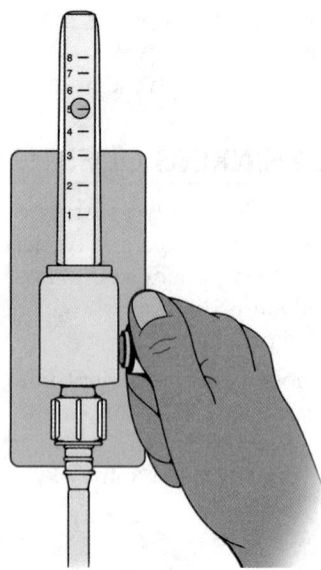

FIGURE **28-6** Adjusting the oxygen flowmeter valve control.

during the day to make sure that it is working satisfactorily. When the fluid level is low, notify the respiratory care department so that the unit can be replaced or refilled with distilled water, if this is the policy in the agency. In the home setting a portable oxygen tank is used. Portable oxygen is also used when transporting oxygen-dependent patients within the hospital.

An oxygen concentrator is frequently used in the home or long-term care setting. The machine collects and concentrates oxygen from room air, storing it for use. The machine must be plugged into an electrical outlet (Figure 28-7).

CANNULA

The nasal cannula consists of a plastic tube with short, curved prongs that extend into the nostril about ¼ to ½ inch. The cannula is held in place by looping it over the ears and cinching the tubing under the chin, and can be easily adjusted for the patient's comfort (Figure 28-8). A Velcro holder may be placed on top of the head to keep the tubing from causing pressure sores on the ears. The nares should be checked to be certain they are unobstructed and are not becoming excoriated (Assignment Considerations 28-1). A cannula is useful for patients requiring oxygen during meals.

MASKS

Various types of masks are available for the administration of oxygen in concentrations ranging from 24% to 55% at flows of 3 to 7 L/min (Figure 28-9). Oxygen concentrations above 60% are rarely used because of the danger of oxygen toxicity. Some patients may dislike this method of oxygen administration because the mask must be placed over the face and they feel that the mask will suffocate them.

Advantages and disadvantages of various oxygen devices are listed in Table 28-3. Oxygen tents are still

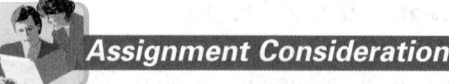

Assignment Considerations 28-1

Detecting Skin Irritation

Ask the UAPs to check the backs of the ears and the nares for tissue irritation when they assist the patient with morning care. This is especially important for the elderly, who have thin, easily damaged skin.

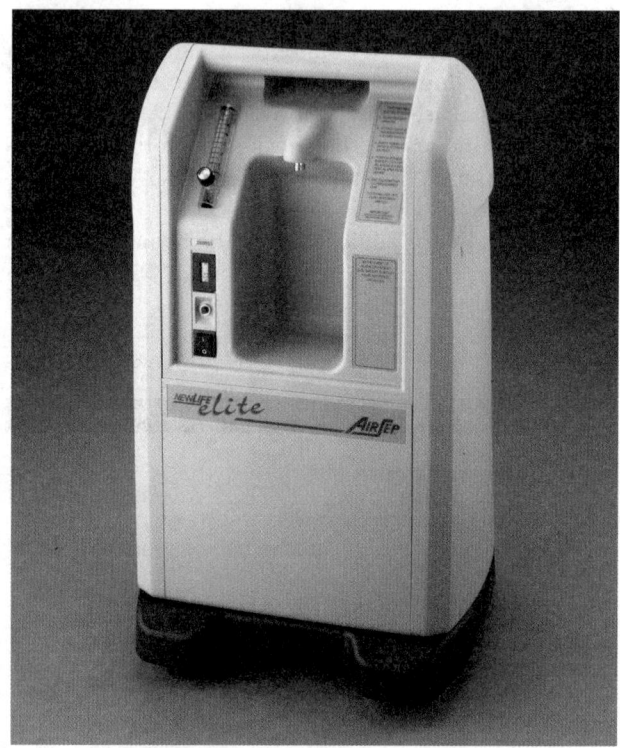

FIGURE **28-7** Oxygen concentrator.

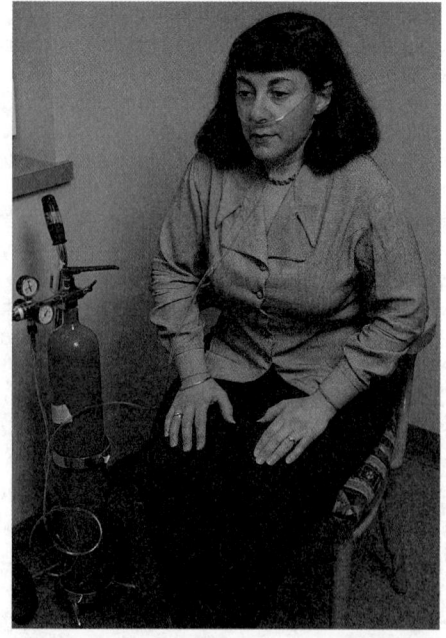

FIGURE **28-8** Oxygen cannula in use by home care patient.

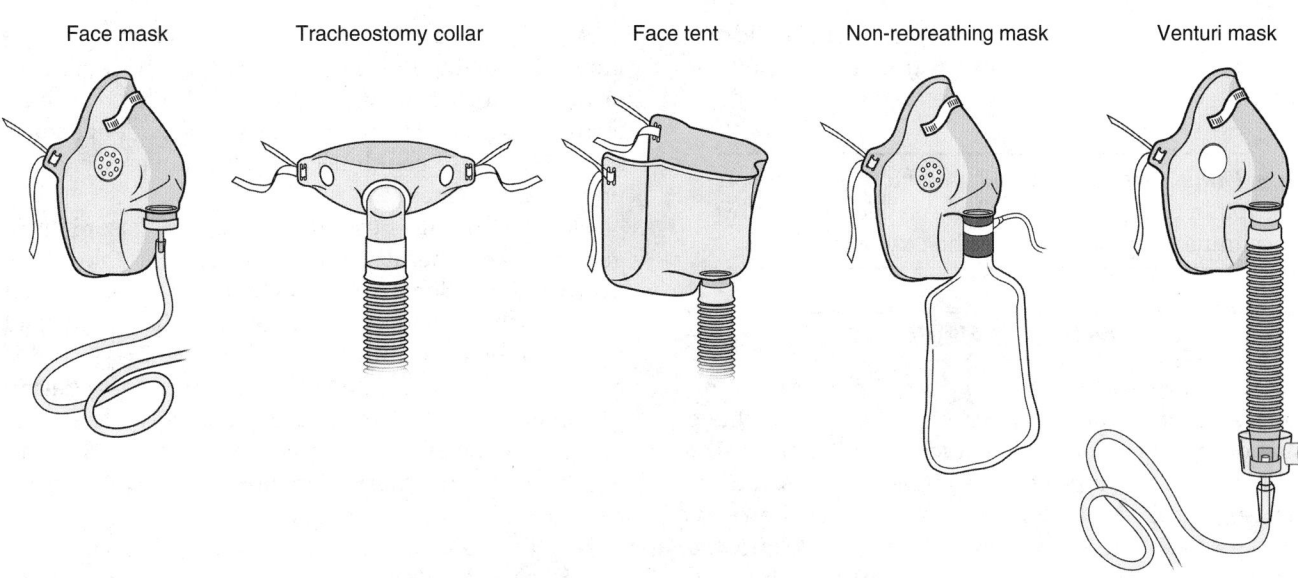

Face mask   Tracheostomy collar   Face tent   Non-rebreathing mask   Venturi mask

FIGURE **28-9** Various oxygen delivery devices.

Table 28-3 | *Advantages and Disadvantages of Common Oxygen Administration Devices*

METHOD	O₂ DELIVERY	ADVANTAGES	DISADVANTAGES
Nasal cannula (nasal prongs)	Low concentrations dependent on rate and depth of breathing FLOWS 1 L = 24% O₂ 2 L = 28% O₂ 3 L = 32% O₂ 4 L = 36% O₂ 5 L = 40% O₂ 6 L = 44% O₂	Patient can move, talk, and eat without disrupting delivery of O₂	Easily dislodged; risk of necrosis to nostrils, cheeks, and ears; irritation of nasal mucosa; cannot be used for more than 6 L/min; must be humidified if used for more than 3 L/min
Simple mask	Low to medium concentrations, 40%-60%; must use liter flow greater than 5 L/min	Higher delivery of O₂ than with a cannula	Discomfort and risk of pressure necrosis caused by tight seal between face and mask; must be removed for eating, drinking, and oral medication
Partial rebreathing mask	Higher concentrations, 60%-80%; must keep reservoir bag inflated at all times	Rebreathes ⅓ of exhaled breath that is high in oxygen	Risk of pressure necrosis; not for long-term use
Non-rebreathing mask	Highest concentrations, 80%-95%; must keep reservoir bag inflated at all times	Useful in emergency situations	Discomfort and risk of necrosis from snug fit; not for long-term use
Venturi mask	Delivers consistent Fio₂ regardless of breathing pattern; concentration and liter flow marked on apparatus; 24%-50% masks available	Useful when accuracy of delivery is essential	Discomfort and risk of skin irritation; must be removed for eating and oral medication
Tracheostomy collar	Delivers O₂ and humidification via tracheostomy; must be connected to a nebulizer; Fio₂ is set on the nebulizer 24%-100%	Adds humidity to liquefy secretions	Must drain condensation often; risk of nosocomial respiratory infection
T-bar (Briggs' adapter)	Delivers O₂ and humidification via tracheostomy; must be connected to a nebulizer; Fio₂ is set on the nebulizer 24%-100%	Adds humidity to liquefy secretions	Must drain condensation often; risk of nosocomial respiratory infection

Key: *Fio₂*, Fraction of inspired oxygen; *O₂*, oxygen.
From Monahan, F.D., & Neighbors, M. (1998). *Medical-Surgical Nursing: Foundations for Clinical Practice* (2nd ed., p. 555). Philadelphia: Saunders.

sometimes used, particularly for small children. Oxygen halos, Oxyhoods, or Croupettes are used for infants.

> **? Think Critically About . . .** How would you explain to a patient who has oxygen ordered by cannula PRN when to use the oxygen?

ARTIFICIAL AIRWAYS

Artificial airways are used for several purposes: to relieve an obstruction, to protect the airway, to facilitate suctioning, and to provide artificial ventilation.

There are two types of pharyngeal airways: the nasopharyngeal airway and the oropharyngeal airway, used to keep the tongue from falling back into the throat and frequently required for postoperative patients until they have recovered from anesthesia (Figure 28-10). These airways are used for patients who can breathe on their own.

Endotracheal tubes maintain an airway in those patients who are unconscious or unable to ventilate on their own. The tube is inserted by a physician, certified nurse anesthetist, nurse practitioner, or advanced practice nurse who is certified in the procedure; intubation is often done under emergency circumstances. The tube is generally removed after 48 to 72 hours, but it may be left in place for a week or more. If it is needed for an extended period of time, the patient should have a tracheostomy performed. An endotracheal tube may cause a mucosal ulcer after 5 to 7 days of use, depending on cuff pressures or type of cuff used.

NASOPHARYNGEAL SUCTIONING

The purpose of suctioning is to maintain a patent airway by removing accumulated secretions. When air passages are obstructed by emesis or secretions, suctioning may prove to be a lifesaving procedure. Pharyngeal suctioning involves the upper air passages of the nose, mouth, and pharynx.

Among those who may require suctioning to remove obstructing fluids are infants, gravely debilitated or unconscious patients, and those who have an ineffective cough. When at all possible, the patient should be stimulated to cough because this moves secretions up into the trachea.

Oral suctioning is usually tried before nasopharyngeal suctioning because it is a more comfortable procedure for the patient. A Yankauer suction tip is attached to the suction connecting tubing and the mouth and top of the pharynx are suctioned (Figure 28-11). If this does not remove secretions adequately, nasopharyngeal suctioning is performed. Either a portable electric machine or a wall-mounted model is used for suctioning. **The amount of suction pressure should be set between 80 and 120 mm Hg.**

Select the suction catheter based on the size of the patient's tube and the thickness of the secretions to be removed. Smaller 8- to 12-Fr. catheters are used for thin secretions; size 14- or 16-Fr. catheters are needed for an adult with tenacious (adhesive, sticky) or thick secretions. The amount of pressure for suctioning is controlled by placing the thumb over the suction port of the catheter or the open end of a Y connector between the tubing and the catheter.

When suctioning, every effort is made to prevent the introduction of pathogens into the airways. Countless microorganisms are found in the upper respiratory tract, and it is virtually impossible to maintain sterility when suctioning the nose or pharynx. Clean technique and thorough hand hygiene are essential for pharyngeal suctioning of the oral and nasal cavities, but aseptic technique is mandatory for suctioning the trachea. **It is best to use aseptic technique for all suctioning of the airway structures.**

Disposable sterile suctioning sets are widely used. A set contains a plastic catheter, a carton to hold a small amount of solution to moisten and rinse the catheter and tubing, and a sterile glove. Tap water may be used to clear secretions from the tubing in pharyngeal suctioning (Skill 28-5). **A catheter that has been used in the mouth is never used again for nasopha-**

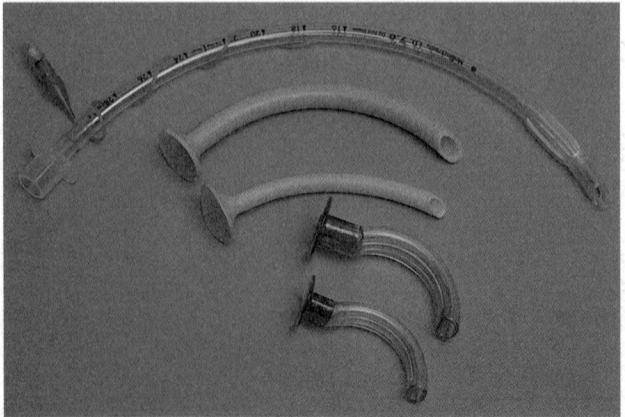

FIGURE **28-10** Types of airways *(top to bottom)*: endotracheal, nasal, and oropharyngeal.

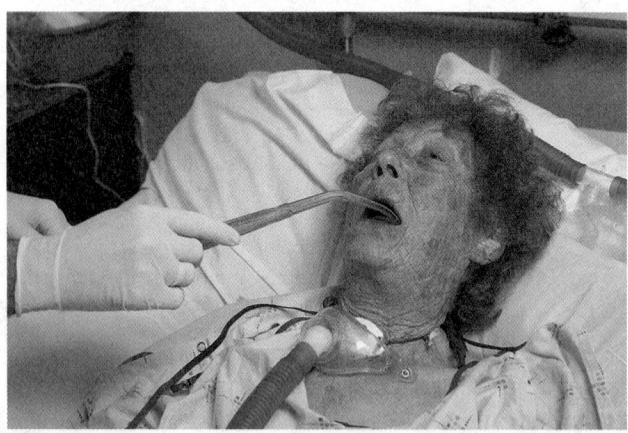

FIGURE **28-11** Yankauer suction tip is used for oral suction.

Skill 28-5 | Nasopharyngeal Suctioning

Nasopharyngeal suctioning is performed when the patient is unable to adequately clear secretions from the pharynx or when a patient cannot expectorate sputum for a diagnostic test. Suction equipment is kept at the bedside. Have patient deep breathe for several breaths before suctioning or preoxygenate.

■ Supplies

✓ Disposable sterile suction catheter
✓ Towel or sterile drape
✓ Solution container
✓ Suction connecting tubing
✓ Sterile gloves
✓ Sterile water or normal saline
✓ Suction source
✓ Water-soluble lubricant
✓ Protective eyewear

Review and carry out the Standard Steps in Appendix 3.

■ Assessment (Data Collection)

1. **ACTION** Auscultate the lungs to locate retained secretions. Assist patient to cough and expectorate if possible. If secretions cannot be cleared, continue with procedure.

   RATIONALE Determines necessity for suctioning. If secretions are cleared, suctioning is not necessary.

■ Planning

2. **ACTION** Position the patient in the semi-Fowler's position if possible.

   RATIONALE Permits an unobstructed view of the mouth and nose for correct suctioning.

3. **ACTION** Set up and check equipment to see that suction is functioning correctly. Think about placement of supplies in order to maintain sterility during the procedure.

   RATIONALE Suction must be functioning for procedure to be effective. Planning prevents contamination of sterile supplies.

■ Implementation

4. **ACTION** Open the catheter suction kit and pour the solution into the solution container; open the water-soluble lubricant. Open the catheter package; squeeze the lubricant onto the inside of the package.

   RATIONALE Prepares the equipment for sterile suctioning.

5. **ACTION** Put on sterile gloves, or one sterile glove on the dominant hand and a nonsterile glove on other hand.

   RATIONALE Reduces transfer of microorganisms.

6. **ACTION** Pick up the sterile catheter with your gloved dominant hand and attach the suction port to the connecting tubing held by your other hand (glove on nondominant hand is no longer sterile).

   RATIONALE Prepares catheter for suctioning procedure. Connecting tubing is not sterile; therefore, glove that touches it is no longer sterile.

7. **ACTION** Moisten 6 to 8 cm of the catheter with water-soluble lubricant and insert the catheter through the right naris into the nasopharynx, about 6 to 8 cm, without suction. If you meet an obstruction, remove the catheter and try the left naris. Do not force the catheter; seek assistance if you meet resistance on the left side also.

   RATIONALE Moistening the catheter makes passage through the nasal passages easier.

8. **ACTION** Intermittently close the suction port with the thumb of your nonsterile hand. Suction no more than 10 seconds at a time. Rotate the catheter while withdrawing it.

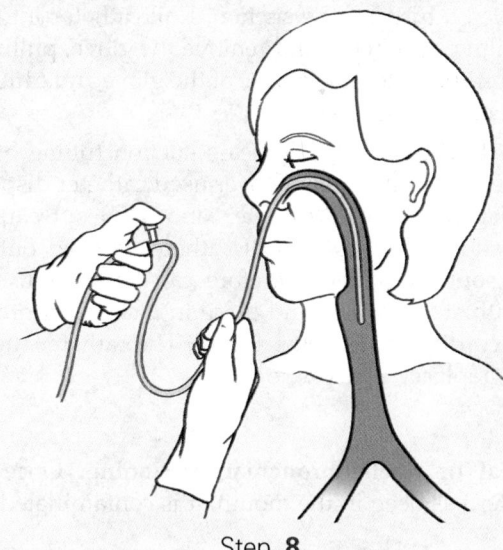

Step **8**

   RATIONALE Suctioning extracts oxygen from the patient's airway. Rotating the catheter pulls up secretions from various parts of the airway.

9. **ACTION** Rinse the catheter by placing it in a container of solution and applying suction to draw the solution through the catheter.

   RATIONALE Removes secretions from the catheter and connecting tubing.

10. **ACTION** Suction the other naris. Repeat the entire process if needed. Allow patient to rest between

Continued

suction sessions. Observe for signs of hypoxia. Talk calmly to reassure the patient and inform of each step before doing it.

RATIONALE Secretions may be copious, and several short suction sessions may be needed to clear them completely.

11. *ACTION* Ask the patient to cough.

RATIONALE Brings secretions into the back of the nose and throat, where they can be easily suctioned.

12. *ACTION* Rinse and moisten the catheter with the solution, insert it into the oral cavity toward the pharynx, and suction the pooled secretions. Suction along the outer gums and cheeks, and at the base of the tongue as needed, using 5 to 10 seconds of suction at a time for the throat area.

RATIONALE Once the catheter has been introduced into the mouth, it is **never** used to enter the nasopharynx area because it is now contaminated. Suctioning in all of these areas clears pooled secretions.

13. *ACTION* Rinse the catheter and tubing by placing the tip in the water container and applying suction briefly; turn off the suction. Roll catheter into the palm of one hand and remove the glove, pulling it over the catheter; dispose of the glove and catheter. Remove other glove.

RATIONALE Rinsing clears suction tubing of secretions. Pulling glove over used catheter disposes of contaminated catheter and gloves by using Standard Precautions. If catheter is used only in nasopharynx and therefore can be reused, rinse with sterile water and place in a closed container according to agency protocol. The catheter should be replaced every 8 hours.

■ Evaluation

14. *ACTION* Auscultate the lungs and listen to see if there is any noise indicating retained secretions.

RATIONALE Determines whether secretions have been adequately removed.

■ Documentation

15. *ACTION* Document date, time, reason for suctioning, size of catheter used, type of technique, and how patient tolerated procedure.

RATIONALE Notes reason for invasive procedure and patient's tolerance.

Documentation Example

10/20 1015 Noisy respirations 24 per minute and stopped-up nose. States cannot get secretions out. 16 Fr. catheter used to suction nasopharynx and oral cavity. Caused considerable coughing. Moderate amount of yellow secretions extracted. Respirations quiet; lungs without crackles or wheezes. Resting quietly.

_____
(Nurse's signature)

?CRITICAL THINKING QUESTIONS

1. Why do you think that moistening the suction catheter well with the lubricant makes the nasopharyngeal suctioning procedure more comfortable for the patient?

2. Why can't you substitute petroleum jelly for the water-soluble lubricant if none is on hand? What would you do if you had no water-soluble lubricant and the patient was becoming severely hypoxic?

ryngeal or tracheobronchial suctioning. Once the catheter has been in the mouth, it is contaminated.

TRACHEOBRONCHIAL SUCTIONING

Deep suctioning of the lower respiratory passages stimulates the cough reflex and removes secretions from the trachea and bronchi. This is most frequently performed when a patient has been intubated. **Sterile technique is mandatory for deep suctioning in the tracheobronchial tree and for the intubated patient.** Sterile saline or sterile water is used to wet the catheter when endotracheal (within the trachea) or bronchial suctioning is necessary. Because the patient is not receiving oxygen when you are suctioning, do not suction for longer than 10 seconds at a time.

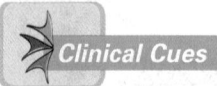
Clinical Cues

Holding your own breath while suctioning is one way to judge how long you can safely suction the patient. Another way is to count "1-1000, 2-1000," etc. to "10-1000" for determining a 10-second period.

TRACHEOSTOMY

A tracheostomy (opening into the trachea) consists of a surgical incision into the throat and insertion of a tube to aerate the lungs (Figure 28-12). It is performed on patients who have apnea (absence of breathing) or some form of respiratory obstruction. The procedure is done to prevent aspiration of secretions and blood and

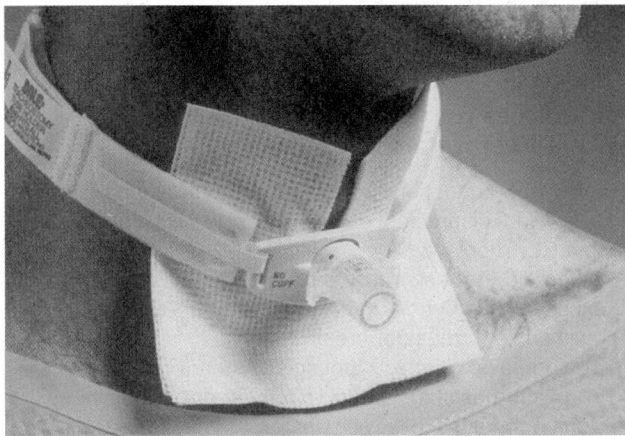

FIGURE **28-12** Patient with a tracheostomy tube and commercial tube holder.

to provide easier access to the lower airways. Intubation of the trachea with the endotracheal tube or the tracheostomy tube is performed frequently, often in order to provide mechanical ventilation. Various types of tracheostomy tubes are used depending on the purpose and the condition of the patient.

When a tracheostomy tube has a cuff, it seals the space between the tube and the tracheal wall when inflated, prevents fluid from being aspirated into the lungs, and allows only a minimal leakage of air. There may be either a foam cuff or a soft balloon cuff. Patients on a positive-pressure ventilator to treat respiratory failure must have a cuffed tracheostomy or endotracheal tube for effective use of the ventilator. When an inflated cuff is present, the pressure is checked at least every 8 hours. **Pharyngeal suctioning is carried out before deflating the cuff.** The patient is never left alone when the cuff is deflated because of the danger of aspirating fluid. When the cuff is reinflated, check for air leakage by holding a hand in front of the patient's nose and mouth and asking her to blow. If air movement is felt, the cuff seal is underinflated and it is not a minimal air leak as intended.

CHEST DRAINAGE TUBES

A chest tube is inserted by the physician as an emergency treatment or at the completion of intrathoracic surgery. It is connected to a disposable pleural drainage system (Figure 28-13). Drainage systems are used to drain air or fluid out of the pleural space and to keep it from being sucked back into the chest. When gravity drainage is inadequate to remove air and fluids from a patient with a large pleural leak, suction can be applied using either wall suction or a portable suction machine. The disposable chest drainage unit has a suction control chamber to prevent excessive negative pressure in the pleural space, as well as a water-seal chamber and a drainage chamber (Figure 28-14). If suction is used in the wa-

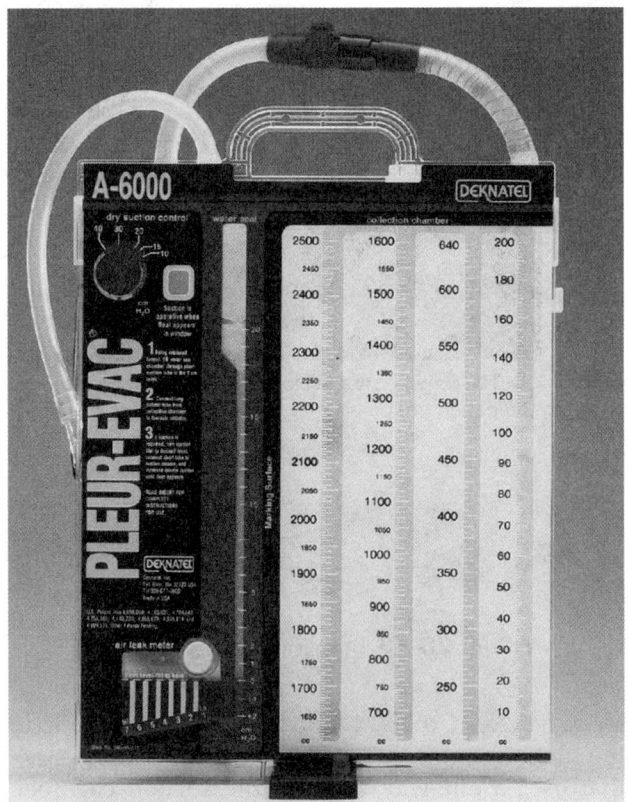

FIGURE **28-13** Disposable chest drainage unit.

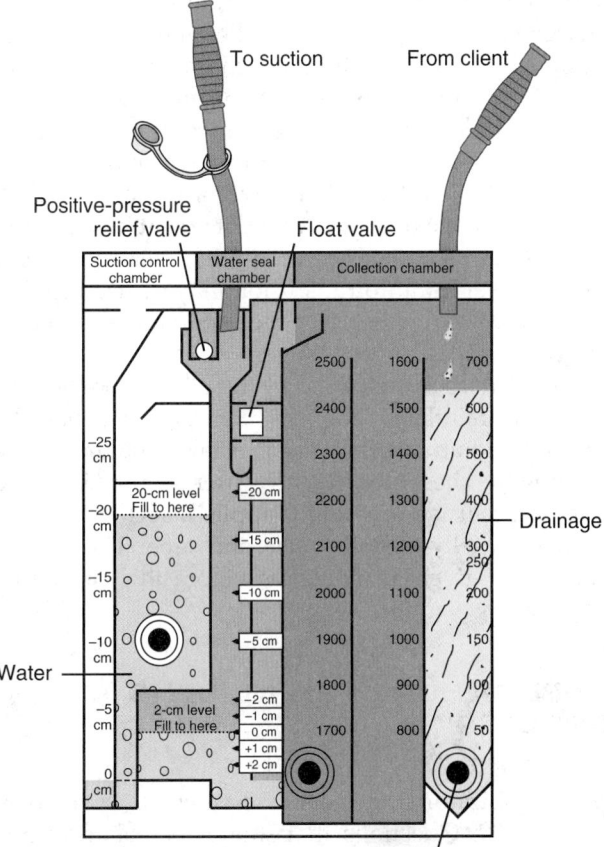

FIGURE **28-14** Suction chamber, water-seal chamber, and drainage chamber of disposable chest drainage device.

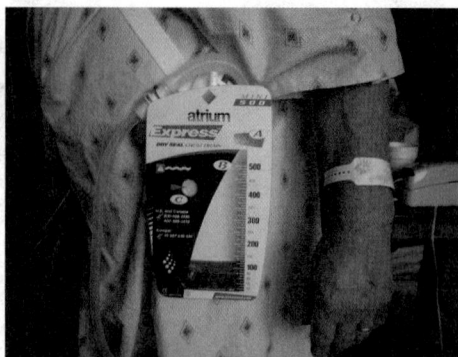

FIGURE **28-15** Small portable closed chest drainage system allowing the patient mobility.

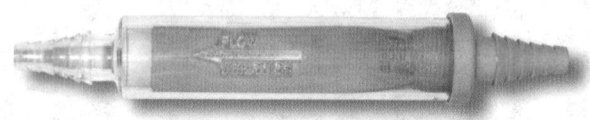

FIGURE **28-16** Heimlich chest drain valve.

ter-seal system, there should be constant bubbling in the suction chamber. There is also a waterless system that uses a one-way valve in the suction chamber. The disposable unit and the flutter valve have largely replaced the former 1-, 2-, or 3-glass bottle system for chest drainage. A number of patients are now given a mobile chest drainage unit so that they can be discharged home (Figure 28-15). The mobile devices are designed so that the drainage chamber can be emptied. A Heimlich valve may be used in place of the chest drainage unit for a small, uncomplicated pneumothorax with little or no drainage and no need for suction. The Heimlich valve, a flutter valve, allows the escape of air but prevents reentry of air into the pleural space (Figure 28-16) After surgery, a drainage set for autotransfusion may be used so that the blood drained can be processed and returned to the patient.

Chest tubes are removed by the physician when the lung has reinflated and the pleural space has decreased. A suture set is used to take out the suture holding the chest tube in place. After the tube is pulled out, an occlusive dressing is applied, such as a 4 × 4 petroleum jelly–coated gauze and tape. The patient should be given an analgesic before this procedure because it is painful.

APPLICATION of the NURSING PROCESS

Assessment (Data Collection)

Basic respiratory physical assessment is covered in Chapter 22. Questions that should be asked of any patient with a respiratory problem are listed in Focused Assessment 28-1; Focused Assessment 28-2 reviews points of assessment along with the rationales.

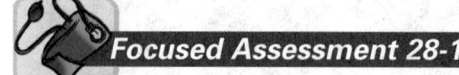

Focused Assessment 28-1

Guidelines for Interviewing the Patient with a Respiratory Problem

The following questions should be asked of any patient who has nursing diagnoses or medical diagnoses indicating a respiratory problem:

- When did the respiratory problem begin? Were you exposed to infection? What are the symptoms? Do you have any shortness of breath?
- Do you have allergies? Sinusitis? Asthma? Emphysema? Chronic bronchitis? Exposure to dust or other irritants?
- Do you smoke? How many packs per day for how many years? Have you had any exposure to industrial air pollutants? Have you been exposed to tuberculosis?
- What type of cough do you have? When does it occur? Is it productive? What color is the sputum?
- When does shortness of breath (SOB) occur? Is there any wheezing?
- What measures ease your breathing or your cough? What medications are you taking?
- How much fluid are you drinking?
- Do you have any heart problems?

The lungs should be auscultated each shift along with assessment of other respiratory status parameters. Careful documentation of findings allows other nurses to compare later data and pick up on subtle trends or deterioration. Respiratory assessment is intertwined with cardiac assessment because if the heart is not functioning properly, oxygenated blood will not be delivered to the tissues in adequate amounts. If the patient is receiving respiratory support, the equipment and settings are checked at least once a shift.

Think Critically About . . . What is the best way to develop skill in detection of all types of breath sound abnormalities?

Nursing Diagnosis

Common nursing diagnoses for patients who have respiratory problems include the following:

- Ineffective airway clearance related to muscle weakness and impaired cough; decreased level of consciousness; or thick secretions
- Impaired gas exchange related to retained respiratory secretions
- Risk for infection related to alteration in airway (tracheostomy)
- Deficient knowledge related to use of oxygen equipment, tracheostomy, ventilator, or incentive spirometer
- Risk for injury related to improper safety precautions when using oxygen

Focused Assessment 28-2

Respiratory System

ASSESSMENT	RATIONALE
Assess respirations: rate, depth, and character.	Although rate may be within normal limits, the patient may be breathing very shallowly and consequently not oxygenating well.
Auscultate lungs to assess patency of airways.	Secretions may be present that interfere with gas exchange, or areas of the lung may not be inflating.
Assess for subtle signs of hypoxemia.	Restlessness, confusion, combativeness, decreased ability to concentrate, lethargy, and headache can all indicate that the patient is not obtaining enough oxygen. Slight hypoxia may be reversed with turning, coughing, and deep breathing.
Assess mucous membranes and nail beds for signs of cyanosis.	Inside of the mouth is the best place to assess for signs of cyanosis in dark-skinned people. Hypoxia may be discovered before the patient experiences respiratory failure.
Assess character of cough, if present.	Deep rattling cough indicates retained secretions, whereas a shallow, raspy cough may indicate throat irritation.
Assess amount and character of sputum and times at which it is produced.	Sputum produced only in the morning may indicate sinus drainage rather than a problem in the lungs.
Assess patient's ability to cough effectively.	Ineffective coughing will not clear secretions or open lower airways.
Assess for factors that cause restriction of respiratory effort.	Fractured ribs, severe arthritis, and many diseases can cause restrictive respiratory disorders and, when such conditions preexist, can compound the problems of a respiratory illness.

Planning

Sample goals or expected outcomes are as follows:
- Patient demonstrates effective cough.
- Lungs are free of secretions.
- Patient demonstrates proper suctioning of the tracheostomy with aseptic technique.
- Area of left-lobe atelectasis (collapsed area of lung) is cleared with use of incentive spirometer.
- Patient demonstrates proper safety techniques when using oxygen.

More goals/expected outcomes can be found in Nursing Care Plan 28-1.

Other planning involves fitting in time for appropriate care of the respiratory patient into the daily work plan. **Each patient with a respiratory problem or the potential for one should turn, cough, and deep breathe every 2 hours.** Times for this to be done should be noted on the shift work organization sheet. Procedures such as postural drainage or tracheostomy care take time and should be planned. If a pa-

---

NURSING CARE PLAN 28-1

Care of the Patient with Impaired Gas Exchange

SCENARIO Susan Tamara, age 72, has been admitted with a bacterial pneumonia. She has been ill for a week and is quite weak because she lives alone and has not felt like preparing meals. Orders read: O_2 at 5 L/min per cannula; nebulization with albuterol q 4 hr while awake; turn, cough, and deep breathe (TC&DB), incentive spirometer q 2 hr, up in chair tid; input and output (I & O); ofloxacin (Floxin) 400 mg intravenous piggyback (IVPB) q12 hr; Robitussin 30 mL q 4 hr PRN cough; increase fluids to 2400 mL/24 hr.

PROBLEM/NURSING DIAGNOSIS *Severe chest congestion*/Impaired gas exchange r/t secretions in lungs.
Supporting Assessment Data: Subjective: Patient states, "I am short of breath and dizzy." ***Objective:*** Chest x-ray reveals bilateral lower lobe pneumonia. O_2 saturation 86%.

Goals/Expected Outcomes	Nursing Interventions	Selected Rationale	Evaluation
Oxygen saturation will reach 95% within 12 hr.	O_2 by nasal cannula at 5 L/min continuous.	Increases oxygen saturation of blood.	*Is O_2 at 95%?* O_2 sat varying from 90% to 92%. Goal partially met.
Patient will exhibit no shortness of breath by discharge.	Semi-Fowler's position except when sleeping.	Helps lungs expand more fully so that more oxygen can be absorbed.	*Is patient short of breath?* Yes, but states, "I'm less short of breath."

Continued

■

NURSING CARE PLAN 28-1

Care of the Patient with Impaired Gas Exchange—cont'd

Goals/Expected Outcomes	Nursing Interventions	Selected Rationale	Evaluation
Patient will exhibit no shortness of breath by discharge—cont'd	Assist to TC&DB q 2 hr; use incentive spirometer q 2 hr.	Clears secretions and opens alveoli; changing position prevents pooling and stagnant secretions.	Lungs with decreased sounds in bases and rales in middle lobes. Expectorating secretions.
	Albuterol nebulizer treatment q 4 hr while awake.	Albuterol assists in keeping airways open.	
	Floxin 400 mg IVPB q 12 hr.	Floxin is effective against the bacterial pneumonia.	
	Monitor oxygen saturation via oximeter q 4 hr.	Monitoring will alert nurse if oxygen saturation is dropping.	
	Up in chair tid for meals.	Sitting upright helps lungs expand completely.	Tolerating being up for meals.
	Auscultate lungs q shift.	Auscultation will tell nurse whether condition is improving or deteriorating.	
	Encourage fluids at regular intervals to provide intake of 2400 mL/24 hr.	Fluids will help thin secretions so they can be coughed up.	Consumed 1875 mL on day shift.
	Offer Robitussin for cough as needed.	Robitussin helps thin secretions.	Gave Robitussin × 2.
	Encourage to expectorate secretions in tissue and to discard tissue in plastic bag.	Secretions can spread the bacteria from the lungs. A plastic bag will contain the bacteria.	Expectorating secretions and containing tissues in bag.
	Offer mouth care q 4 hr while awake.	Infected secretions have an unpleasant taste. Mouth care improves appetite.	Mouth care provided before meals and at bedtime.
	Inspect ears for pressure areas from cannula q 4 hr.	O_2 cannula may cause pressure areas on the ears.	No signs of skin breakdown. Continue with current plan of care. Goal partially met.

❓ CRITICAL THINKING QUESTIONS

1. What is the physiologic reason that increasing fluids will help this pneumonia patient?

2. The patient is weak. Although this care plan only deals with the "respiratory" problems discussed in this chapter, what other nursing actions do you think would help the patient conserve energy and oxygen?

---

tient has copious secretions that need frequent suctioning, time must be allotted for this activity. Planning also includes seeing to it that necessary supplies for respiratory care are available at the bedside.

Implementation

The nurse has a very active role in assisting the patient to perform needed respiratory exercises, teaching respiratory care techniques, maintaining patient safety, and offering encouragement for self-care success. Your

attention to respiratory care for every patient can prevent complications and nosocomial infection and assist the patient to recovery.

First and foremost, maintain an open airway. Secretions can be removed by effective coughing, turning, and deep breathing. Splinting an incision with a small pillow and sitting on the side of the bed allow for a more effective cough (Figure 28-17; see Patient Teaching 28-1). A fluid intake of 1500 to 2000 mL/day helps thin secretions. Use suction to remove secretions and mucus when the patient is unable to cough them out.

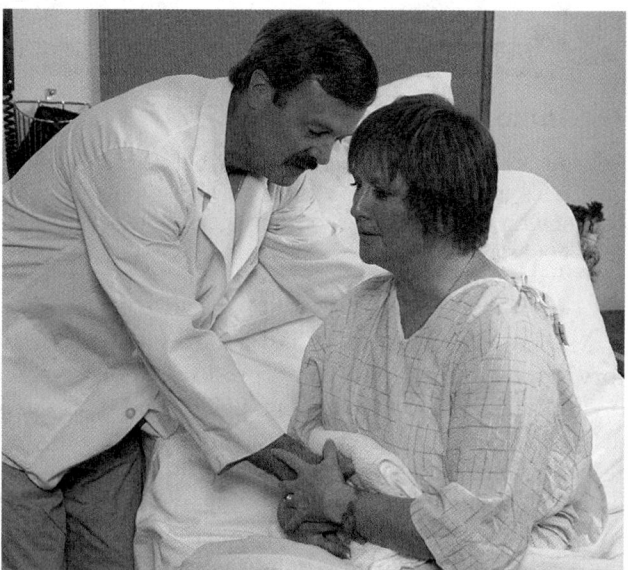

FIGURE **28-17** Teaching the patient to splint an incision while coughing.

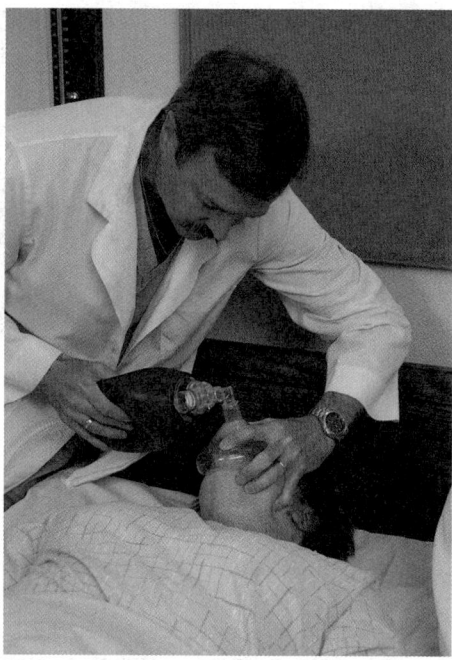

FIGURE **28-18** Use of manual resuscitator bag.

Be alert to wet, gurgling respirations in the unconscious patient and see that suctioning is done aseptically. For the unconscious or comatose patient, use an oral airway or nasal trumpet airway to keep the tongue from falling back into the throat and obstructing the passage of air. If the patient cannot breathe deeply enough to maintain adequate oxygenation, a manual resuscitator bag can be used to increase oxygenation (Figure 28-18). Use proper positioning; turn the patient frequently. Yawns and sighs are two forms of deep breaths that help expand the alveoli in the lung. A yawn is a deep, long inspiration usually due to mental or physical fatigue; a sigh is a prolonged inspiration followed by a long expiration. Encourage the use of an incentive spirometer to open alveoli and prevent or relieve atelectasis.

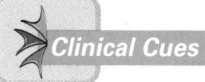 **Clinical Cues**

Remember that restlessness and irritability may be the first signs of hypoxia. In the elderly, confusion often presents as oxygen levels fall. Observe patients with respiratory problems closely for these early symptoms.

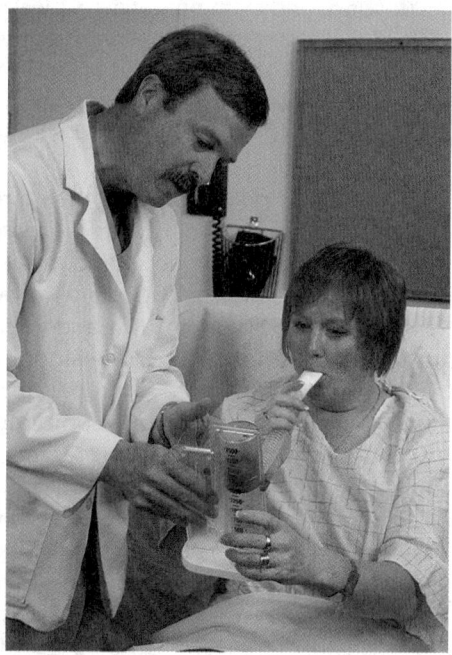

FIGURE **28-19** Teaching use of the incentive spirometer.

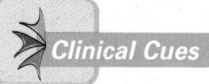 **Clinical Cues**

Making a small "pillow" with a large towel in a pillowcase and helping the patient to splint well when attempting to deep breathe or cough will help make the patient's efforts more successful. Large pillows can be unwieldy.

Patients who have undergone abdominal or chest surgery avoid using muscles in the affected areas. However, these muscles are necessary in order to take deep breaths or to cough effectively to remove accumulated secretions. Hypoxia, pneumonitis, and atelectasis are the more common conditions that pose a danger to the individual and prolong hospitalization. In atelectasis, the alveoli collapse and fail to fill with air. The condition may be acute or chronic and involve a part or all of the lung.

These common respiratory complications can be prevented by reinflating the alveoli and removing the mucous secretions. The best method to accomplish this is through a sustained maximum inspiration, or the taking of a deep breath to inflate the entire lung and

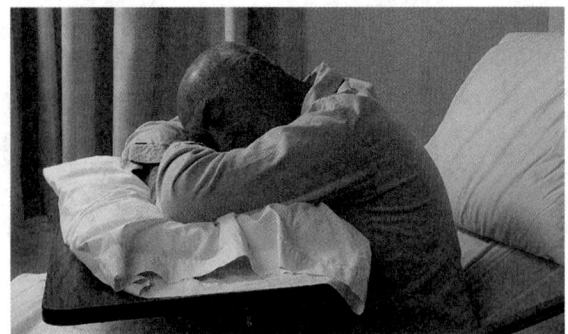

FIGURE **28-20** Position the person who is very short of breath in the orthopneic position, using pillows on the over-the-bed table.

holding the inspiration for at least 3 seconds so that the resulting pressure will keep the alveoli from immediately collapsing again. The same effect is produced by a sigh or a yawn.

Incentive spirometers encourage patients to do respiratory exercises with sustained maximum inspiration (Figure 28-19). When the patient takes a deep breath, a ball moves upward, or the amount of air is measured so the results are visible to the user. The incentive is to reach a certain volume of air and hold it for 3 seconds. Patients at risk of developing respiratory complications should be instructed to use the device and take 10 slow, deep breaths every hour when awake.

Use positioning and relaxation to optimize respiratory exchange. Additional energy and oxygen are needed when patients are anxious and have tense, rigid muscles. Nurses can help patients with dyspnea to relax, expand the chest more fully, and use less of their limited oxygen supply by good positioning. Bed patients with dyspnea are placed in proper alignment and in high Fowler's position unless contraindicated by their condition. Place the patient's forearms on pillows at the sides to relax the shoulder muscles. Patients with obstructive diseases such as emphysema breathe easier when they sit at the side of the bed or in a chair, hunch the upper body over, and rest their arms on two or three pillows placed on a table or nightstand in front of them (orthopneic position, Figure 28-20). Turning to one side helps prevent the pooling of secretions in the back of the throat of unconscious, weak, or helpless patients. Postural drainage is also used to promote the removal of secretions from the lungs.

When administering oxygen therapy, give the amount as ordered by the physician. When oxygen is in use, give oral hygiene every 3 to 4 hours because oxygen therapy is drying to the tissues, which often makes the mouth smell or taste bad. Inspect the skin around the nose and mouth for irritation from the equipment. Prevent infection by changing oxygen delivery equipment on time per agency policy. Temperature measurements should be taken tympanically, over the temporal artery, or rectally so that the patient's breathing is not impaired by an oral thermometer.

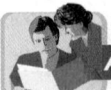

Assignment Considerations 28-2

The Intubated Patient

Remind the UAPs to be sure the call bell is within reach whenever they reposition a patient who is intubated. The patient with an endotracheal or tracheostomy tube is unable to call out for help.

Monitor the activity of the patient with a respiratory problem. Activity may produce shortness of breath, dizziness, or complaints of chest pain because activity uses up oxygen more quickly than the body at rest. Space activities and provide sufficient rest periods between activities of daily living and exercise. For the patient who is on PRN oxygen, do not discontinue the oxygen and then immediately ask the patient to get up and move to the chair or go to the bathroom. Allow time for the patient to adjust to room air before activity is increased. Observe safety measures to prevent explosion or fire (see Safety Alert 28-1).

Tracheostomy Care

When a patient has either a temporary or a permanent tracheostomy, daily care is needed. Care consists of suctioning and cleaning the skin around the stoma, changing the dressing, cleaning the inner cannula if there is one, and replacing the ties that hold the tube in place when they are soiled. Tracheostomy care is done every 8 hours or as frequently as needed to keep the secretions from becoming dried, blocking the airway.

A tracheostomy tube is a curved, hollow cannula made of plastic or metal. Some have an inner and an outer cannula so that the inner one can be removed to be cleaned while the outer one stays in place. All tracheostomy tubes come with a piece called an obturator, which is a curved guide that facilitates placement of the tube in the trachea when it is inserted; after insertion of the tube, the obturator is removed. An extra tube and obturator are often taped to the head of the bed so that they are handy should the tracheostomy tube somehow be dislodged and need to be replaced in an emergency.

Since the tracheostomy tube sits below the larynx, the patient cannot speak naturally. Provision for communication must be made with paper and pencil, magic slate, communication board, or other device. **It is vitally important for this patient to have the call bell at hand at all times.** It is frightening not to be able to call for help should it be needed (Assignment Considerations 28-2). Check on the patient frequently.

Suctioning of secretions following a tracheostomy is of prime importance in maintaining a patent airway. Patients with tracheostomies lose their ability to cough effectively. Before beginning suctioning, observe the patient's rate and quality of respiration and auscultate lung sounds. Frequency of needed suctioning varies; in the new tracheostomy patient it may be needed as

Skill 28-6 | Endotracheal and Tracheostomy Suctioning

Since it is often difficult for a patient to cough secretions out via an endotracheal or tracheostomy tube, the tube must be periodically suctioned. The tracheostomy tube must be kept free of secretions for the patient to breathe or receive oxygen. To determine when suctioning is needed, the lungs are auscultated. A face shield or goggles and mask should be used when suctioning because the patient may spray sputum when coughing.

■ Supplies
- ✓ Suction source
- ✓ Face shield
- ✓ Sterile normal saline
- ✓ Sterile catheter suction kit:
  - ✓ Solution container
  - ✓ Sterile gloves
  - ✓ Sterile suction catheter
- ✓ Resuscitation bag
- ✓ Connecting tubing

Review and carry out the Standard Steps in Appendix 3.

■ Assessment (Data Collection)

1. **ACTION** Auscultate the patient's lungs to determine if there are retained secretions present.

   RATIONALE Moist breath sounds, including gurgles and bubbling, indicate a need for suctioning.

■ Planning

2. **ACTION** Be certain all equipment is at hand and think through the procedure before opening sterile supplies.

   RATIONALE Ensures that the procedure will go smoothly.

3. **ACTION** Obtain a partner to preoxygenate the patient with the resuscitator bag if possible.

   RATIONALE The patient should be preoxygenated before suctioning so that oxygen is not seriously depleted by suctioning. The procedure is easier to perform with an assistant.

4. **ACTION** Attach the connecting tubing to suction source and turn on suction; check the pressure. Place the connecting tubing close at hand.

   RATIONALE Verify that the suction is functioning by occluding end of suction tubing with your thumb and watching pressure on gauge rise. Set pressure according to agency protocol. Wall suction unit pressure is generally set between 80 and 120 mm Hg maximum. Placing tubing nearby prepares tubing to be easily connected to the suction catheter.

■ Implementation

5. **ACTION** Perform hand hygiene; open supplies and put on sterile gloves. Set up the water container. Place sterile drape, if available across patient's chest. Pour about 100 mL sterile water into the container with the nondominant hand. With gloved dominant hand holding the catheter, attach the catheter to the connecting tubing. Be careful not to contaminate glove holding the catheter.

Hand holding the connecting tubing is no longer sterile.

RATIONALE Provides sterile field on the chest. Prepares the water for use and maintains sterility of dominant hand. Supplies catheter with suction.

6. **ACTION** Have an assistant oxygenate patient by resuscitator bag with two or three large-volume inspirations while you prepare to suction, or do this yourself. If working alone and the patient is receiving oxygen, increase the concentration to 100% for a short time, keeping hand on oxygen adjustment, or give two or three sigh breaths with the ventilator. Check agency protocol for desired way to preoxygenate the patient.

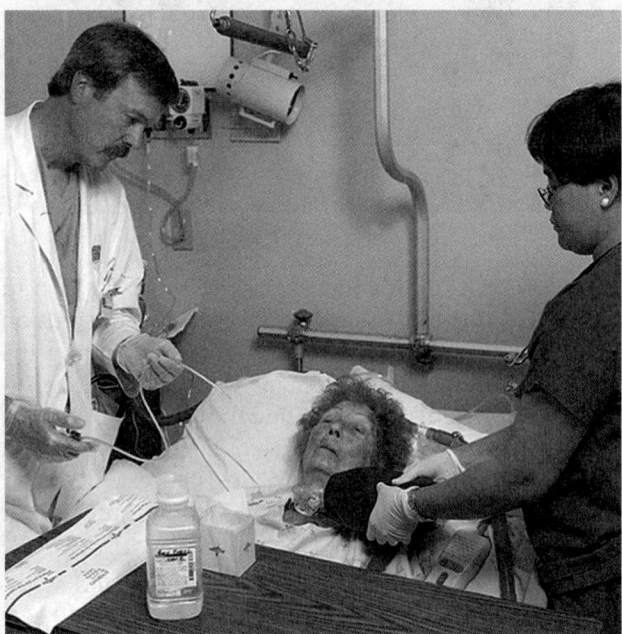

Step **6**

RATIONALE Preoxygenation prevents hypoxia during suctioning.

7. **ACTION** Moisten the catheter tip in the sterile saline solution and suction up a small bit of the solution to test the system. Disconnect the ventilator

Continued

Skill 28-6 | Endotracheal and Tracheostomy Suctioning—cont'd

tubing if ventilator is in use, and immediately introduce the catheter into the endotracheal tube or tracheostomy tube using only sterile gloved hand; do not use suction while placing the catheter. Advance catheter until resistance is met, then pull back 1 cm.

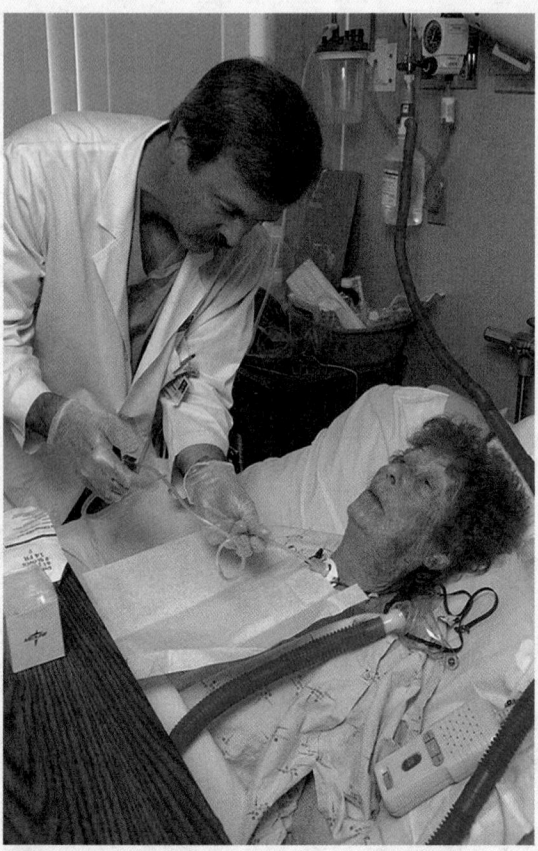

Step **7**

RATIONALE Moisture lubricates the catheter and makes it easier to introduce; testing with solution ensures suction is working properly. Holding the catheter at a 90-degree angle to the tube to enter it helps prevent contaminating the catheter by touching the patient's face or neck. Suction applied on entry draws out oxygen. Resistance will occur when the catheter reaches the carina (junction of main bronchi).

8. *ACTION* Apply suction while rotating and withdrawing the catheter. Allow no more than 10 seconds to suction and withdraw the catheter. Counting "1-1000, 2-1000," etc., while suctioning is one way to track the time.

    RATIONALE Suction draws out secretions. Rolling the catheter between your fingers rotates the catheter openings at the tip so that they will suck up secretions around the circumference of the trachea.

Suctioning for more than 10 seconds seriously depletes the patient's oxygen.

9. *ACTION* Reattach the patient's tube to the oxygen source if one has been in use, and allow a rest period before suctioning again. Keep the catheter sterile while waiting; use the nonsterile hand to reattach the oxygen source. Auscultate the lungs when finished to be certain that secretions have been adequately cleared.

    RATIONALE Suction draws out oxygen as well as secretions and may cause hypoxia. Hyperoxygenation should be done again before each suctioning.

10. *ACTION* Suction the nasopharynx if needed.

    RATIONALE Secretions may collect above the cuffed tracheostomy tube and need to be removed.

11. *ACTION* Rinse catheter and connecting tubing by suctioning up more solution. Discard the catheter by coiling it in your gloved hand and pulling the glove off over it.

    RATIONALE Connecting tubing should be cleared of secretions. A sterile catheter must be used each time tracheobronchial suctioning is performed. Sterile catheters must be kept at the bedside for immediate use. Pulling glove over the used catheter prevents spread of microorganisms.

Suctioning with a Sleeved Catheter

12. *ACTION* Open catheter package without disturbing protective sleeve covering the catheter.

    RATIONALE Sleeve maintains sterility of catheter so that it can be reused several times.

13. *ACTION* Attach catheter to endotracheal tube or tracheostomy adaptor and to suction tubing. If secretions are thick, inject sterile saline via saline port per agency protocol.

    RATIONALE Sterile saline thins secretions.

14. *ACTION* As catheter is inserted via endotracheal tube or tracheostomy, sleeve slides back; advance the catheter as far as possible.

    RATIONALE Positions catheter within trachea to carina.

15. *ACTION* Apply suction while rotating and withdrawing the catheter. Allow the sleeve to re-cover the catheter as it is withdrawn; pull it back out of the tube opening.

    RATIONALE The sleeve will prevent the catheter from becoming contaminated from environment outside the trachea. Pulling it out of the tube prevents the catheter from occluding the airway.

16. *ACTION* Remove gloves and perform hand hygiene. Turn off suction.

RATIONALE Performing hand hygiene reduces transfer of microorganisms. Suction may remain off between suctioning sessions.

■ Evaluation

17. *ACTION* Ask yourself: Did patient tolerate the procedure without drastic changes in heart rate? Are the lungs clear to auscultation? Did suctioning remove secretions? Was sterility maintained?

RATIONALE Answers provide data to determine if procedure was effective.

■ Documentation

18. *ACTION* Include number of times patient received suctioning, type of technique used, characteristics of secretions, and any problems encountered.

RATIONALE Documents procedure and any problems encountered.

Documentation Example

10/24 1430   Coughing; gurgling sounds auscultated. Suctioned × 2 with sterile technique and preoxygenation. Moderate white secretions obtained; lungs clear, tubing reattached to ventilator; no signs of dysrhythmia.

_____
(Nurse's signature)

■ Special Considerations

✓ Some patients can cough secretions out; allow patient to try before suctioning.

✓ Holding your breath while you apply suction helps judge the time the patient is without oxygen.

✓ Suction container is emptied at the end of each shift or at least every 24 hours; check agency protocol.

✓ Do not suction unnecessarily because the procedure is irritating to the tracheal tissues.

✓ In the home care situation, suction catheters can be cleaned, sterilized, and reused.

✓ The home care patient is taught to perform the suctioning procedure. The teaching plan should be consistently used by all home care nurses working with the patient.

?CRITICAL THINKING QUESTIONS

1. What is one way to hold the suction catheter to introduce it into an endotracheal tube so that it doesn't kink and hit the patient's skin or your hand and become contaminated?

2. What would you need to do before suctioning a patient if you know that this patient frequently forcibly coughs out secretions when being suctioned?

---

frequently as every 15 to 30 minutes. Older tracheostomies have less inflammation and therefore less secretion production and need to be suctioned only periodically. **Suctioning is carried out only as needed, and need is indicated by audible respirations or dyspnea** (Skill 28-6).

Use strict aseptic technique and use separate catheters and solution when both the nasopharyngeal area and the trachea are suctioned. Suctioning should be no longer than 10 seconds in length. The patient should be well oxygenated before any tracheal suctioning is attempted because the hypoxemia produced by prolonged suctioning can lead to sudden death. Sleeved or in-line catheters are available that can be reused several times for tracheobronchial or endotracheal suctioning. These catheters have an outside plastic sleeve covering that slides up to allow the catheter to be introduced into the trachea for suctioning and then is allowed to slide over the catheter as it is withdrawn. The sleeve prevents contamination of the catheter between suctioning. Continuous oxygenation is provided to the patient around the catheter, and the arterial O_2 partial pressure (Pao_2) level does not drop as low as with other suctioning.

The inner cannula of the tracheostomy tube should be cleaned as often as needed to keep it free from tenacious secretions and crusts (Skill 28-7). Aseptic technique is employed in cleaning the wound and the inner cannula to reduce the risk of infection. Work calmly and efficiently. Remember that having a tracheostomy is a very traumatic experience. **The nasopharynx is always suctioned before deflating the cuff.**

Chest Tube Care

When the patient has a chest tube, the lungs should be auscultated frequently to assess reexpansion of the involved lung. An accurate measure of the amount of drainage is done every 1, 2, 4, or 8 hours, depending on the situation; the drainage level is marked on the container along with the time noted. Observe the tube and level of drainage in the collection chamber each time you enter the patient's room (Steps 28-1). Report drainage of more than 100 mL/hr.

Nebulizer Treatments

If the patient is having difficulty bringing up mucous secretions trapped in the lung, a nebulizer treatment may be ordered. Nebulizer treatments are also used to deliver bronchodilators to the lung to relieve bronchospasm. Nurses often give these treatments in clinics and physicians' offices (Figure 28-21, p. 539).

Skill 28-7 | Providing Tracheostomy Care

Tracheostomy care is performed every 8 hours. The tracheostomy patient is taught to do this procedure before being sent home with a new tracheostomy. The soiled dressing is removed, the area around the stoma is cleaned, and if needed, the tape or ties holding the tracheostomy tube in place are changed. If there is an inner cannula, it is removed, cleaned, and replaced.

■ Supplies

✓ Normal saline
✓ Forceps
✓ Sterile gloves
✓ Hydrogen peroxide

✓ Precut tracheostomy dressing
✓ Brush or pipe cleaners
✓ Tracheostomy tape or tube fastener
✓ Scissors

✓ Sterile 4 × 4 gauze pad
✓ Cotton swabs
✓ Solution containers (2)
✓ Discard bag

Review and carry out the Standard Steps in Appendix 3.

■ Assessment (Data Collection)

1. **ACTION** Suction as needed before beginning the procedure.

   RATIONALE Clears airway. Movement of the tracheostomy tube during cleaning and care may make patient cough, loosening secretions that could block the airway.

■ Planning

2. **ACTION** Set up the equipment on a table close to the patient and plan the order in which to perform the tasks.

   RATIONALE Planning makes work more efficient.

■ Implementation

3. **ACTION** Place the patient in a low semi-Fowler's position. Perform hand hygiene, open the supplies, and put on one glove. Separate basins with gloved hand; pour solutions with ungloved hand. Use one part hydrogen peroxide to one part normal saline for the wash solution; normal saline is used to rinse.

   RATIONALE Positioning makes visualization of the tracheostomy site clear; opening supplies prepares them for use. Gloves prevent transfer of microorganisms. Some plastic cannulas are harmed by hydrogen peroxide; check manufacturer's instructions.

4. **ACTION** Put on the second glove. Undo the lock on the outer cannula, stabilizing the tube flange with the index finger and thumb, and remove the inner cannula by gently pulling it out toward you.

   RATIONALE Latch must be unlocked in order to remove the inner cannula. If tube moves, patient will cough. If difficulty is encountered, obtain assistance.

5. **ACTION** Place the reusable inner cannula in the basin of wash solution and clean the lumen thoroughly with pipe cleaners or a small brush. Cleanse the outer surface with the brush. Rinse in the basin

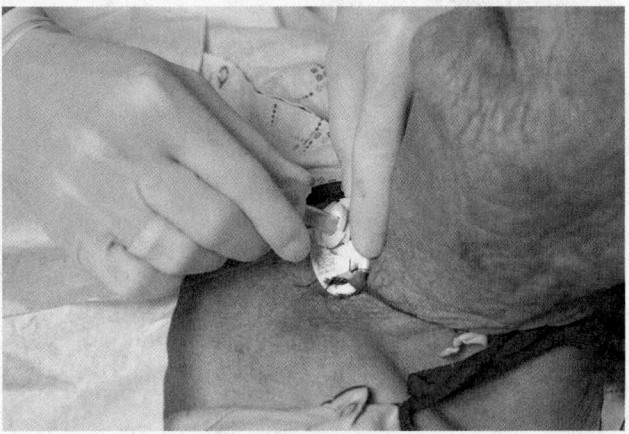

Step **4**

of normal saline or sterile water. Place on 4 × 4 gauze pad to drain. Handle silver cannulas carefully because they tend to dent easily.

RATIONALE Pushing the pipe cleaner all the way through the cannula removes secretions. Some patients will have a second inner cannula available to place into the tracheostomy tube while the one removed is cleaned. In that case, store the removed cannula after cleaning.

6. **ACTION** Reinsert the cannula after excessive moisture has been removed. Hold the face plate of the outer tube securely and, using aseptic technique, insert the inner cannula into the lumen of the outer cannula. Lock in place by turning the latch on the outer cannula one-quarter turn counterclockwise. Check to see that it is properly latched. Many hospitals use disposable inner cannulas that eliminate the need for cleaning.

   RATIONALE Excessive moisture may make the patient cough as the cannula is replaced. Cannula must be firmly locked into place so that it is not coughed out.

7. **ACTION** Remove the soiled dressing and dispose of it in the discard bag. Clean around the tube with solution required by agency protocol, using cotton swabs; rinse with saline. Move the tube as little as possible during the cleaning process.

RATIONALE Soiled tracheostomy dressings are changed as needed. The area around the tube is cleaned every 8 hours or per agency protocol. Some agencies require the use of hydrogen peroxide for cleaning; some physicians order acetic acid to be used. Moving the tube causes irritation to the trachea and is uncomfortable for the patient.

8. *ACTION* Replace soiled tracheostomy ties or tube holder. Ask an assistant to help if possible. Punch a hole in the end of the tie with the closed points of the forceps, pass the end through the flange on the side of the tracheostomy tube, and thread the tie through the hole, pulling it taut. Remove the old tie. Repeat for the other side, and tie the tapes at the side of the neck with a double square knot so that the patient need not lie on the knot. The knot should be rotated from one side of the neck to the other with each change. Commercial tracheostomy tube holders may be used in place of tracheostomy tape ties.

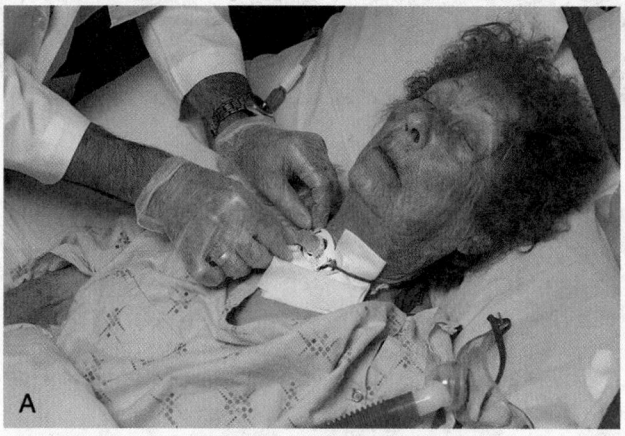

A

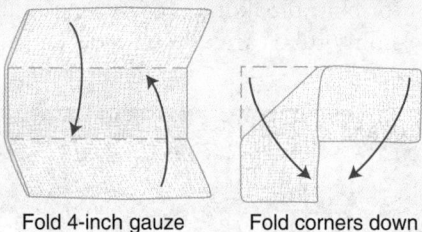

Fold 4-inch gauze square in thirds

Fold corners down to midline

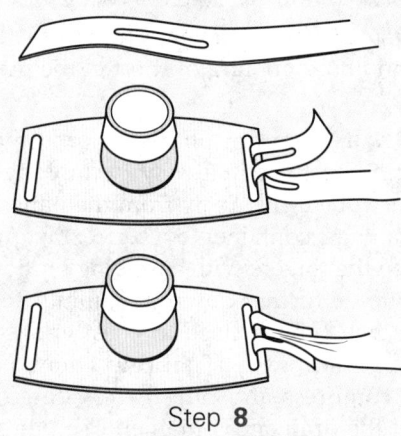

Step **8**

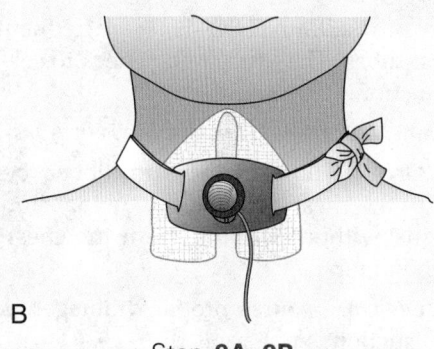

B

Step **9A, 9B**

RATIONALE Ties are replaced when soiled or at least once every 24 hours. Ties are easier to replace if done before the new dressing is applied.

9. *ACTION* Apply the precut dressing or a "V"-folded gauze. Place it under and around the outer cannula to catch secretions. Forceps may be used to manipulate the dressing into place.

RATIONALE Cutting a 4 × 4 gauze pad to use as a tracheostomy dressing should not be done because the loose gauze may fall into the tracheostomy tube and be aspirated by the patient.

■ Evaluation

10. *ACTION* Ask yourself: Did the procedure go smoothly? Was the tube moved too much, making the patient cough a lot? Are the ties smooth? Is the dressing sitting properly in place?

RATIONALE Answers to these questions determine if the procedure was done properly and efficiently.

■ Documentation

11. *ACTION* Documentation may be in narrative form or on a flowsheet. Note the care given and the condition of the tracheostomy site.

RATIONALE Notes that this nursing care was administered.

Documentation Example

10/25 1045 Tracheostomy care given with aseptic technique; reddening 1.5-cm diameter around tube, no complaints of discomfort. Inner cannula cleaned and replaced.

_____
(Nurse's signature)

Continued

Skill 28-7 | Providing Tracheostomy Care—cont'd

■ Special Considerations

✓ For patients with a permanent tracheostomy, teach all steps of tracheostomy care and suctioning. Proceed by explaining the rationale for a step and then demonstrate the step. Teach only a few steps at a time. Have patient demonstrate the procedure with coaching. Obtain a return demonstration of the entire procedure before the patient is discharged.

✓ Assess for skin breakdown each time you provide tracheostomy tube care.

?CRITICAL THINKING QUESTIONS

1. What may happen if you do not perform oral suction before deflating an inflatable tracheostomy cuff?

2. Why is it best to prepare the tracheostomy tube ties by cutting a slit in each tie before beginning tracheostomy care?

Steps 28-1 | Maintaining a Disposable Water-Seal Chest Drainage System

Disposable chest drainage systems are frequently used with chest tubes. The nurse must check to see that the unit is functioning properly.

Review and carry out the Standard Steps in Appendix 3.

1. **ACTION** The unit must be positioned below the level of the chest tube and the tubing should hang straight, without looping, from the chest tube to the container.

   RATIONALE Ensures proper drainage, especially when suction is not applied.

2. **ACTION** The water-seal chamber should be filled to the correct level; refill with sterile water as needed. Suction chamber may also require sterile solution. Check manufacturer's directions for amounts; some systems are waterless.

   RATIONALE Provides adequate water seal to act as a one-way valve and keep room air from entering the intrapleural space.

3. **ACTION** Unit should be attached to the wall suction and suction should be set to measure 20 cm on the suction control chamber gauge, or to amount ordered; there should be mild continuous bubbling in the suction chamber.

   RATIONALE Suction is not always ordered. Too much suction pressure may damage the lung. Bubbling indicates suction is working.

4. **ACTION** All connections should be taped.

   RATIONALE Prevents accidental disconnection.

5. **ACTION** There should be no kinks in the chest tube or connecting tubing.

   RATIONALE Kinks prevent proper function of the unit and allow pooling of fluid in the intrapleural space.

6. **ACTION** If there are physician orders to do so, maintain chest tube patency by milking or stripping the tube. Milk away from the patient toward the drainage container by squeezing the tubing between the fingers with a milking motion; release and squeeze further down the tubing. To strip the tube, pinch tubing close to chest and stabilize it with one hand; with a lubricated thumb and forefinger, compress and pull fingers down the tube toward the drainage container. Use petrolatum or an alcohol swab to lubricate. Let go and move farther down the tube and repeat the process, continuing the length of the chest tube.

   RATIONALE Provides gentle, intermittent suction to the chest tube. This is not needed when suction is continuous to the tube, and is not frequently ordered.

7. **ACTION** Mark and record the drainage output each shift.

   RATIONALE Measure drainage at eye level and place a mark on the drainage chamber. If drainage exceeds 100 mL/hr, report to physician.

8. **ACTION** Assist patient to deep breathe and cough and change positions at frequent intervals.

   RATIONALE Assists in reexpanding the lung.

9. **ACTION** Assess pain level and medicate as ordered when needed.

   RATIONALE Patient will deep breathe more effectively if kept comfortable. Chest tubes are uncomfortable.

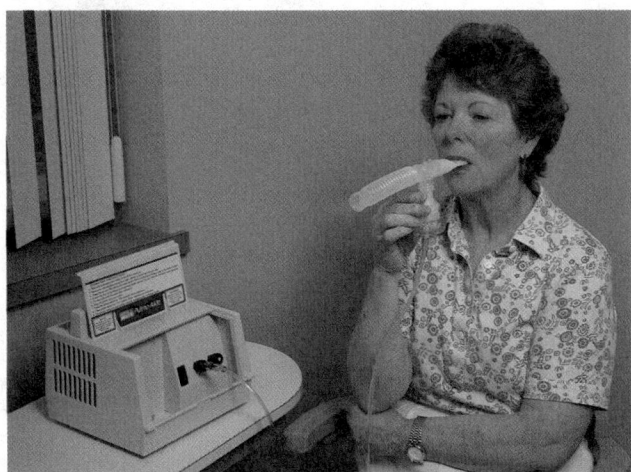

FIGURE **28-21** Patient receiving a nebulizer treatment in a physician's office.

Patient Teaching

Because many respiratory patients have chronic problems, teaching for self-care is very important to independence. The patient with a permanent tracheostomy is taught to suction properly in an aseptic manner and to care for the tube, stoma, and skin. All patients are taught to deep breathe and cough effectively.

Home care patients are taught to reduce air pollutants in the home and to avoid them elsewhere as much as possible (Home Care Considerations 28-1). Safety measures are taught to the patient and family regarding the use of oxygen. Ways to conserve energy are explained to the patient and family so that the patient can maintain independence as much as possible. Patients and family are taught suctioning techniques (Home Care Considerations 28-2).

In the home, the patient and caregiver can be taught to clean suction equipment with hydrogen peroxide, gentle soap and water, or a household bleach solution depending on the type of equipment; rinse it with sterile water; and store it in a clean container until the next use.

Evaluation

It is vitally important that the patient's respiratory status be evaluated continuously when the patient is suffering from a respiratory disorder. The lungs must be evaluated at least once a shift. The success of respiratory treatments and drugs is evaluated each day. Some sample evaluation statements are as follows:
- Effectively coughing up secretions.
- Pao_2 increased to 88 mm Hg.
- $Paco_2$ decreased to 38 mm Hg.
- Patient able to ambulate length of hall without shortness of breath.
- Lungs clear, no sign of respiratory infection.
- Patient turns off oxygen when not using it.
- Atelectasis cleared as evidenced by x-ray.

Documentation

Documentation should include the following:
- Data from the respiratory assessment
- Oxygen flow rate and method of delivery
- Amount of time PRN oxygen is used
- Time and location of blood gas sampling
- Location of oximetry probe and range of oxygen saturation
- Description of sputum expectorated
- Times patient deep breathes and coughs
- Time and result of any respiratory treatments

Suction technique is constantly evaluated, and ways to improve in delivering respiratory care should be considered. It takes considerable practice to suction efficiently.

Home Care Considerations 28-1

Preventing Respiratory Infection

- All respiratory patients are reminded to avoid places where they will be exposed to flu or respiratory infections. Crowded theaters, shopping malls, and other places where people sit close together place the person with compromised respiration at risk.
- Special care should be taken to sit a good distance away from anyone who is coughing or sneezing.

Home Care Considerations 28-2

Suctioning at Home

- In the home care situation, teach the caregiver and family members how to suction the patient using aseptic technique. Instruct in definitive signs that indicate suctioning is needed.
- Some patients can learn to suction themselves, but the procedure is uncomfortable and many cannot clear secretions adequately.
- After a suctioning session, if secretions still are not totally cleared, wait 10 minutes or so to allow patient to become fully oxygenated again before resuming suctioning.
- Note date and time on covered catheter container so that catheter will be changed on schedule after 8 hours.

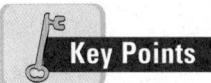

Key Points

- Respiratory insufficiency is the inability of the body to meet its oxygen needs and remove excess amounts of carbon dioxide.
- Airway obstruction is a frequent cause of hypoxia.
- One of the first signs of hypoxia is irritability or restlessness.
- Dyspnea often causes anxiety, which in turn makes the problem worse.
- Hypoxia depresses body functions and disturbs the acid–base balance of the body.
- Hypoxic patients are very susceptible to respiratory infection.

- Pulse oximetry is used for continuous, noninvasive monitoring of arterial oxygen saturation.
- The Heimlich maneuver is used to dislodge an airway obstruction when the patient suddenly cannot breathe.
- If an airway obstruction is not relieved, anoxia occurs and the heart may stop, necessitating cardiopulmonary resuscitation.
- The simplest method of clearing the air passages is to cough effectively.
- Patients must be taught to cough effectively; forced exhalation coughing helps bring up secretions.
- Postural drainage is used to drain different segments of the lung.
- Nebulizer treatments may be used to liquefy secretions and decrease bronchospasm.
- Nasopharyngeal suctioning is used to remove secretions from the nose and pharynx when the patient is too weak to expectorate them, or is unconscious.
- Nasopharyngeal suctioning should be performed aseptically; tracheobronchial suctioning is a sterile procedure.
- Oxygen may be administered by mask, cannula, tent, catheter, Croupette, or ventilator.
- High concentrations of oxygen can cause fires to burn very rapidly.
- Oxygen is ordered by the physician, and a flowmeter is used to deliver it.
- Oxygen should be humidified because it is very drying to the mucosa.
- When a patient cannot maintain respiration in a normal manner, a tracheostomy may be performed to provide an artificial airway.
- When a tracheostomy tube has an inflatable cuff, it must be deflated at least every 8 hours; inflation pressure is checked with a manometer.
- A chest drainage tube may be placed in the intrapleural space when the patient has a pneumothorax, hemothorax, or hemopneumothorax. A chest tube may drain air or fluid.
- Chest tubes are often connected to water-seal or dry drainage devices.

- The nurse must know how to care for the chest tubes and drainage system.
- Nursing diagnoses relevant to the respiratory patient are "Ineffective airway clearance," "Impaired gas exchange," "Risk for infection," "Deficient knowledge," and "Risk for injury."
- Expected outcomes are written for the specific nursing diagnoses chosen for the patient.
- Every respiratory patient should turn, cough, and deep breathe every 2 hours. These activities can prevent respiratory insufficiency and respiratory failure.
- Thorough, careful assessment is essential for respiratory patients.
- Incentive spirometry assists in regaining or maintaining open airways.
- The patient with chronic obstructive pulmonary disease (COPD), also termed *chronic airflow limitation,* should not be given oxygen at more than 3 L/min because it may depress the respiratory drive.
- Tracheostomy suctioning takes practice and is a sterile procedure.
- The patient with a permanent tracheostomy is taught how to care for the tracheostomy, including cleaning the stoma area, cleaning the inner cannula of the tube, changing the ties and dressing, and suctioning.
- All respiratory patients should avoid people with respiratory infection and avoid areas where air pollutants occur.
- Evaluation is based on assessment findings, pulse oximetry, and arterial blood gas measurements.
- The nurse, physician, and respiratory therapist work closely together when caring for a respiratory patient.

Go to your **Companion CD-ROM** for an Audio Glossary, animations, video clips, and more.

 evolve Be sure to visit the companion Evolve site at http://evolve.elsevier.com/deWit/fundamental/ for additional online resources.

NCLEX-PN® EXAMINATION-STYLE REVIEW QUESTIONS

*Choose the **best** answer(s) for each question.*

Your patient has undergone a thoracotomy with resection of the right lung. She is receiving O₂ by cannula at 5 L/min and has a chest tube in place attached to a disposable chest drainage system with suction. *(This scenario applies to questions 1 to 4.)*

1. You observe the patient for early signs of hypoxia. You know that the first signs of hypoxia include: *(Select all that apply.)*
   1. increasing restlessness or irritability.
   2. increased respiratory rate.
   3. cyanosis of the nail beds of the fingers.
   4. retraction of muscles used in breathing.

2. In providing nursing care for this patient, who is having difficulty breathing, it is important to reduce her anxiety because it:
   1. increases the pulse and blood pressure.
   2. causes tense muscles, which need more oxygen.
   3. causes needless fear and worry.
   4. delays recovery and healing of injured tissues.

3. The patient is in pain but doesn't want to take pain medication. You know that it is important to keep her comfortable because:
   1. when breathing causes pain, she won't take deep breaths to open alveoli.
   2. the surgeon ordered pain medication for her.
   3. she needs to sleep a lot in order to heal.
   4. she may become irritable and confused.

4. Regarding the disposable water-seal chest drainage unit, you know that there should be:

   1. bubbling in all the chambers of the drainage device.
   2. continuous bubbling in the suction chamber.
   3. intermittent bubbling in the suction chamber.
   4. continuous bubbling in the water-seal chamber.

5. When performing nasopharyngeal suctioning, you should: *(Select all that apply.)*

   1. raise the head of the bed 30 to 45 degrees.
   2. set suction at 100 mm Hg.
   3. deflate the cuff before deciding to do nasopharyngeal suctioning.
   4. moisten the catheter before attempting suctioning.

6. The most common cause of respiratory insufficiency is _____. *(Fill in the blank.)*

7. The most effective way to clear a patient's respiratory tract of secretions after a thoracotomy and lung resection is to:

   1. position her for postural drainage.
   2. use pharyngeal suctioning.
   3. teach her to cough effectively.
   4. use endotracheal suctioning.

8. Older people are more prone to respiratory problems because aging causes which of the following changes? *(Select all that apply.)*

   1. Thinning of the alveolar membrane
   2. Decreased elasticity of respiratory tissues
   3. Increased secretion production
   4. Decreased efficiency of the immune system

9. In normal individuals, the drive to breathe and the control of the respiratory rate are dependent on:

   1. the elasticity of the lung.
   2. the Pao_2 level in the blood.
   3. the cerebral cortex.
   4. the $Paco_2$ level in the blood.

10. One nursing measure that can prevent respiratory insufficiency is to:

    1. assist the patient to turn, cough, and deep breathe.
    2. administer low-flow oxygen continuously.
    3. allow the patient to rest as much as possible.
    4. perform postural drainage at least three times a day.

CRITICAL THINKING ACTIVITIES *Read each clinical scenario and discuss the questions with your classmates.*

Scenario A
Clara Johnson has had upper abdominal surgery. She is reluctant to deep breathe or cough.

1. How would you explain to her the importance of deep breathing and coughing after this surgery?
2. What could you do to make deep breathing and coughing less painful for her?
3. How would you teach her to use an incentive spirometer? (Be very specific with the instructions.)

Scenario B
Paul Suarez has a new tracheostomy. He is receiving oxygen by tracheostomy collar (device placed over the tracheostomy tube to deliver oxygen).

1. Describe the steps you would use to suction Mr. Suarez's tracheostomy.
2. Since Mr. Suarez cannot speak, how would you communicate with him? He is very weak and has a difficult time writing.
3. Create a plan to teach Mr. Suarez how to care for his tracheostomy at home.

evolve http://evolve.elsevier.com/deWit/fundamental/

Objectives

Upon completing this chapter, you should be able to:

Theory

1. Describe the structure and functions of the urinary system.
2. Identify abnormal appearance of a urine specimen.
3. Describe three nursing measures to assist patients to urinate normally.
4. List the purposes and principles of indwelling and intermittent catheterization.
5. Explain the rationale for using a continuous bladder irrigation system.
6. Discuss ways to manage urinary incontinence.

Clinical Practice

1. Assess a patient's urinary status.
2. Teach a patient how to obtain a "clean-catch" (midstream) specimen.
3. Perform a urine dipstick test accurately.
4. Assist patients with toileting.
5. Insert an indwelling catheter using sterile technique.
6. Perform catheter care.
7. Teach a patient how to perform Kegel exercises.

Skills & Steps

Skills

Skill 29-1	Placing and Removing a Bedpan
Skill 29-2	Applying a Condom Catheter
Skill 29-3	Catheterizing the Female Patient
Skill 29-4	Catheterizing the Male Patient
Skill 29-5	Performing Intermittent Bladder Irrigation and Instillation

Steps

Steps 29-1	Obtaining a Urine Specimen from an Indwelling Catheter
Steps 29-2	Removing an Indwelling Catheter
Steps 29-3	Continence Training

Key Terms

Be sure to check out the bonus material on the Companion CD-ROM, including selected audio pronunciations.

anuria (ă-NŪ-rē-ă, p. 544)
catheterization (kă-thě-těr-ĭ-ZĀ-shŭn, p. 554)
commode chair (kō-MŌD, p. 549)
condom catheter (KŎN-dŏm KĂ-thě-těr, p. 556)

Credé's maneuver (kră-DĀ Z mă-NŪ-věr, p. 554)
cystitis (sĭs-TĪ-tĭs, p. 545)
dysuria (dĭs-Ū-rē-ă, p. 545)
glycosuria (p. 546)
hematuria (hěm-ă-TŪ-rē-ă, p. 546)
instillation (p. 545)
ketonuria (kē-tō-NŪ-rē-ă, p. 546)
micturition (mĭk-tū-RĬSH-ŭn, p. 543)
nocturia (nŏk-TŪ-rē-ă, p. 544)
oliguria (ŏl-ĭ-GŪ-rē-ă, p. 545)
polyuria (pŏl-ē-Ū-rē-ă, p. 545)
proteinuria (prō-tēn-YŪR-ē-ă, p. 546)
pyuria (pī-Ū-rē-ă, p. 546)
residual urine (rě-ZĬ-dū-ăl Ū-rĭn, p. 544)
stricture (STRĬK-chŭr, p. 554)
suprapubic (SŪ-pră-PYŪ-bĭk, p. 555)
urinary incontinence (ĭn-KŎN-tĭ-něns, p. 544)
urinary retention (rē-TĚN-shŭn, p. 544)
urination (ūr-ĭ-NĀ-shŭn, p. 544)
urinometer (yūr-ĭ-NŎ-mě-těr, p. 545)
urostomy (yūr-Ŏ-stō-mē, p. 572)
void (VŎYD, p. 542)

NORMAL URINARY ELIMINATION

The frequency of urination varies. Infants will **void** (excrete urine) from 5 to 40 times a day. The preschool child may void every 2 hours. The adult voids from 5 to 10 times a day. On average, the adult male voids 300 to 500 mL and the adult female voids 250 mL. **There should be at least an hourly urine output of 30 mL. This reflects adequate kidney perfusion.** This amounts to 720 mL per 24 hours.

People usually have the urge to void on awakening in the morning, after each meal, at bedtime, and after drinking extra fluid. Urine production is decreased during sleep, and many people can sleep through the night without voiding. Urine is normally sterile, but provides a good medium for the growth of infectious organisms if they are introduced into the bladder.

FACTORS AFFECTING NORMAL URINATION

Urinary elimination is affected by neurologic and muscle development; alterations in spinal cord integrity; the volume of fluid intake; the amount of fluid lost by perspiration, vomiting, or diarrhea; and the amount of antidiuretic hormone (ADH) secreted by

OVERVIEW OF STRUCTURE AND FUNCTION OF THE URINARY SYSTEM

Which structures are involved in urinary elimination?

- The kidneys are bean shaped, approximately 6 cm wide, 12 cm long, and 3 cm thick, and are located at the level of L1 on the sides of the spine (Figure 29-1).

- Each kidney contains approximately 1 million nephrons, which are the working units.

- Within each nephron is a glomerulus consisting of a cluster of capillaries surrounded by Bowman's capsule, and a system of tubules.

- The ureters are hollow tubes about 25 to 30 cm long in the adult and connect each kidney to the bladder.

- The bladder is a hollow, muscular organ located in the lower pelvis.

- The urethra is a tube attached to the base of the bladder extending to the outside of the body. In the male it is about 8 inches (20 cm) long and goes through the penis, ending at its tip. This exit point is the urinary meatus (Figure 29-2). In the female, the urethra is from 1½ to 2½ inches (3 to 5 cm) in length and goes to the urinary meatus located beneath the clitoris, between the folds of the labia.

- The internal and external urinary sphincters control the flow of urine out of the body.

What are the functions of the urinary structures for elimination?

- The kidneys filter blood through the nephrons, and metabolic wastes and excess water are extracted. The kidney regulates electrolytes in the body by excreting excess amounts, and assists in acid–base balance by retaining or excreting hydrogen ions (H^+) and bicarbonate ions (HCO_3^-). The waste products are diluted with water and excreted as urine. The tubules secrete, excrete, or reabsorb electrolytes, water, and other substances.

- The kidneys manufacture 1 to 1½ L of urine on average in 24 hours. Urine output is related to the amount of fluid intake and can vary considerably.

- The ureters carry urine from the kidneys to the bladder.

- The bladder stores urine and sends a signal to the spinal cord when it becomes full to signal the need for emptying. The signal usually occurs when the bladder contains between 250 and 400 mL of urine.

- The bladder can hold 1000 to 1800 mL of urine. **Average urine output is 1000 to 1500 mL/day.**

- The urethra carries urine from the bladder to the outside of the body.

- The urinary meatus is the exit point for urination and the entrance point for a catheter.

- The internal sphincter relaxes in response to the *micturition* (urinating) reflex.

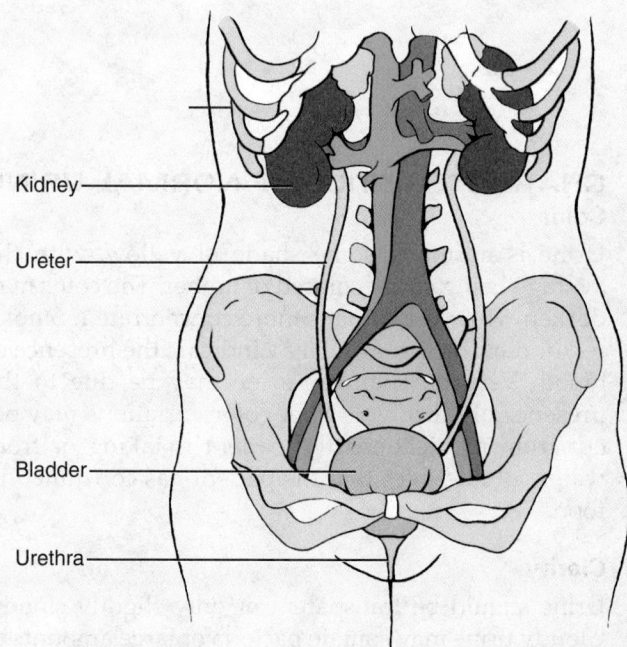

FIGURE **29-1** Structures of the urinary system.

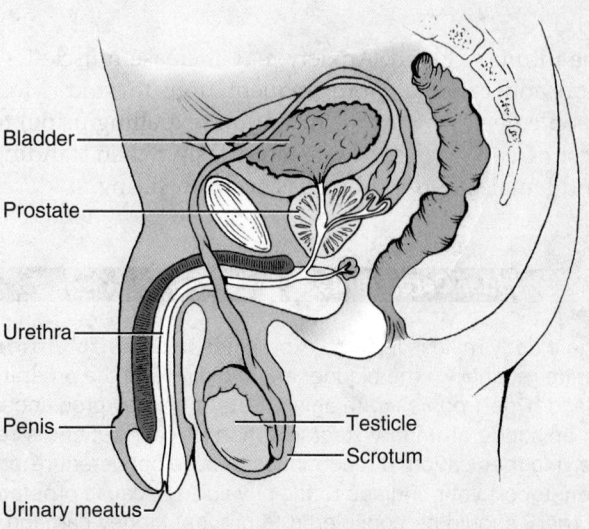

FIGURE **29-2** Tract of the male urethra.

OVERVIEW OF STRUCTURE AND FUNCTION OF THE URINARY SYSTEM—cont'd

- Voluntary contraction of the external sphincter stops the expulsion of urine. Relaxing the external sphincter starts the flow of urine for excretion.

What factors can interfere with urinary elimination?

- Total loss of the kidney's ability to manufacture urine (kidney failure) may result in anuria (absence of urine). **At least 600 mL of urine must be excreted by an adult per day to remove the waste products of the body.**

- Decreased kidney perfusion (e.g., shock or severe dehydration) can lead to kidney damage.

- Blockage of the ureters prevents the urine from traveling to the bladder. Blockage may occur due to the presence of a stone in the ureter, pressure from a tumor in the abdominal cavity, or trauma to the lower abdomen.

- Disruption of the bladder by tumor or trauma may impede the flow of urine out of the bladder or decrease its holding capacity.

- Pressure on the urethra from an enlarged prostate can make emptying the bladder difficult. Trauma to the urethra from any cause can impede the elimination of urine. Childbirth sometimes alters the position of the bladder and urethra and predisposes to incidences of urinary incontinence (inability to prevent passing urine).

- Infection in any part of the urinary system causes inflammation and may alter the flow of urine.

- Neurologic damage to the nerves that control the internal and external sphincters or the muscular wall of the bladder may cause alteration in urinary patterns.

- Prostate surgery may damage the external urinary sphincter and cause temporary or permanent urinary incontinence in the male.

What changes in the system occur with aging?

- There is a decrease in the number of functioning nephrons and a reduction in the rate of renal filtration with aging. Because of these changes, even minor body stress can cause a decrease in renal function.

- The bladder muscle tone decreases and its capacity lessens, causing nocturia (voiding during the night). Decreased muscle tone may interfere with the external urinary sphincter and predispose to incontinence. **Incontinence is not a normal part of aging.**

- Decreased bladder and muscle tone may cause incomplete bladder emptying and residual urine (urine left in the bladder after urination). Residual urine becomes stagnant and predisposes to infection.

- Lower estrogen levels in women can result in tissue atrophy in the urethra, vagina, and bladder, which predisposes to infection and incontinence.

the pituitary gland. Anxiety may increase muscle tension and cause a more frequent urge to void. Most people need privacy for urination (expelling urine) to occur freely. Males urinate more easily when standing and females find voiding easier when sitting.

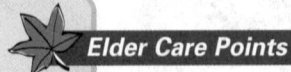

Elder Care Points

The elderly male is likely to experience **urinary retention** (urine retained in the bladder after voiding), as the prostate gland hypertrophies with aging. Retention may predispose to episodes of urinary tract infection. If your patient is receiving medication, but continues to have persistent retention, report your findings to the physician because prostate surgery should be considered to prevent kidney damage.

CHARACTERISTICS OF NORMAL URINE
Color

Urine is normally some shade of yellow, with the average being straw colored or amber. The color may darken when the urine is more concentrated. Smoky red or dark brown urine may indicate the presence of blood. Very dark amber urine may be due to the presence of bilirubin. Other color variations may occur from medications the patient is taking or from water-soluble dyes that the patient has consumed in food.

Clarity

Urine should be transparent or only slightly cloudy. Cloudy urine may contain bacteria or large amounts of protein.

Odor

Normal urine smells faintly like ammonia. If the odor is foul, infection may be present. If the odor resembles acetone, ketones are probably present. Other odors may occur depending on what foods the person has eaten or what vitamins have been taken.

Specific Gravity

Specific gravity is the thinness or thickness of the urine. It may be measured by an instrument called the urinometer, an instrument that reads the amount of light the urine absorbs, or by the use of a chemical dipstick. **The normal range is 1.010 to 1.030, but conditions such as dehydration and fluid excess may extend the range slightly in either direction.**

pH

The acidity or alkalinity of urine is measured in units called *pH*. **The pH of normal urine is slightly acid, ranging from 5.5 to 7.0.**

Think Critically About ... Your elderly patient is upset and concerned because his urine is a different color. What are some questions you could ask him to obtain more information about the color change?

ALTERATIONS IN URINARY ELIMINATION

Alterations in urinary elimination patterns are listed in Box 29-1. A common urinary tract infection is cystitis (inflammation of the bladder). Cystitis may be caused by irritation of highly concentrated urine, pathogenic bacteria, injury, or instillation (putting in a solution) of an irritating substance. A break in aseptic technique when inserting or caring for an indwelling catheter is a frequent cause of cystitis. *Escherichia coli* is often the bacterium responsible for cystitis, especially in females. **Symptoms of cystitis are frequency, urgency, dysuria, (painful urination), burning, malaise, foul-smelling urine, and a slight temperature elevation.** Health Promotion Points 29-1 and Complementary & Alternative Therapies 29-1 include useful information to help your patients prevent cystitis.

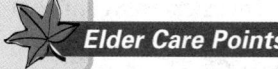

Elder Care Points

Your elderly patient may develop an infection and not manifest a fever. In fact, the temperature may be lower than normal. However, subtle changes in mental status may be the first symptom of an infection, so monitor your elderly patients closely for changes in alertness and orientation.

Box 29-1 | *Alterations in Urinary Elimination Patterns*

- **Anuria** is present when less than 100 mL of urine is excreted in 24 hours. It may be due to *urinary suppression*, in which the kidneys are not forming urine, or to the retention of urine (all urine is not expelled from the bladder during voiding).
- **Dysuria** (painful or difficult urination) occurs when there is inflammation present in the bladder or urethra and is usually due to infection or trauma.
- **Incontinence** (involuntary release of urine) occurs with a variety of pathologic conditions. When it is due to decreased muscle tone, special exercises (see Patient Teaching 29-3) may prevent it.
- **Nocturia** occurs when the person must get up to void during the night more than twice.
- **Oliguria** (decreased amount of urine output) occurs when urine output falls below 400 mL in 24 hours. It may be a sign of kidney failure, blockage of urine outflow somewhere in the system, or retention.
- **Polyuria** (excessive urination) occurs when there is no cause for large amounts of urine to be voided and there is an output of greater than 1500 mL in 24 hours. It is usually associated with either diabetes mellitus, in which there is an absence of insulin, or diabetes insipidus, in which there is a decrease in production of antidiuretic hormone.

 Health Promotion Points 29-1

How to Prevent Recurrent Cystitis

Episodes of recurrent cystitis predispose to kidney infection and consequent kidney damage. In accordance with *Healthy People 2010*, measures should be taken to prevent long-term kidney disease. Cystitis and other urinary tract infections may be avoided by

- Increasing fluid intake to 2500 to 3000 mL/day.
- Avoiding citrus fruits and juice because they cause alkaline urine; bacteria grow more readily in alkaline urine.
- Always wiping the rectal area from front to back after a bowel movement. This is especially important in female patients.
- For the female patient, avoiding wearing tight clothing and nylon pantyhose that cause continual perineal moisture; wear cotton underwear.
- Not sitting around in a wet bathing suit for extended periods.
- For the female patient, not using bubble bath or feminine hygiene sprays.
- For the female patient, emptying the bladder promptly after intercourse and drinking two glasses of water to flush out microorganisms that may have entered the bladder.
- Emptying the bladder every 2 to 3 hours to prevent stasis and potential for bacteria to multiply if present.

Vitamin C and Fruits to Prevent Bladder Infections

Acidifying the urine by taking a vitamin C supplement daily and increasing the intake of prunes, plums, cranberries, or cranberry juice to decrease the urine pH will help to combat urinary tract infections.

APPLICATION of the NURSING PROCESS

Assessment (Data Collection)

Obtain a history of the patient's usual pattern of urinary elimination. Inquire if there are ever incidences of incontinence. Ask if there is a need to urinate frequently, burning when urinating, or a sense of urgency in finding a toilet quickly. Does the patient need to get up to urinate at night frequently? Have there been changes in the appearance of the urine? At what times of the day does the patient usually void? Is the bladder usually completely emptied or is there a need to void again in less than 2 hours? How much fluid is taken in a 24-hour period? Does the patient have a urinary catheter in place? Is there a history of previous urinary problems? What is the patient's total 24-hour intake and output? Is it normal? Assess the patient's mobility to determine if it is safe to allow ambulation to the bathroom unassisted. Note when the patient last voided. **Each patient should void at least every 8 hours unless an indwelling catheter is in place.** If voided amounts are small and intake is normal, gently palpate the bladder to see if it is distended. To do this, feel with the palm of the hand for a bulge indicating a full bladder above the symphysis pubis.

Urine Specimen Collection

Voided Specimen for Urinalysis. Inspection of the urine is the next step in the assessment. Various types of specimens may be collected depending on the patient's symptoms. For a simple voided specimen for urinalysis, ask the patient to void into a clean bedpan, urinal, collection bottle, or plastic "hat" collection device placed inside the front of the toilet (Figure 29-3). Provide privacy for the patient. Explain to the female how to hold the urine bottle or cup so that it surrounds the urethra. She should stand in a slightly squatting position, or sit over the toilet and hold the collection container steady to catch the urine as she voids. Explain to both men and women that only about 1½ inches of urine is needed. It is not necessary to fill the container. If the specimen is to go to the laboratory, transfer it to the specimen container, label it properly, and send it to the laboratory within 5 to 10 minutes. **Urine that stands for 15 minutes or more changes characteristics, and the urinaly-**

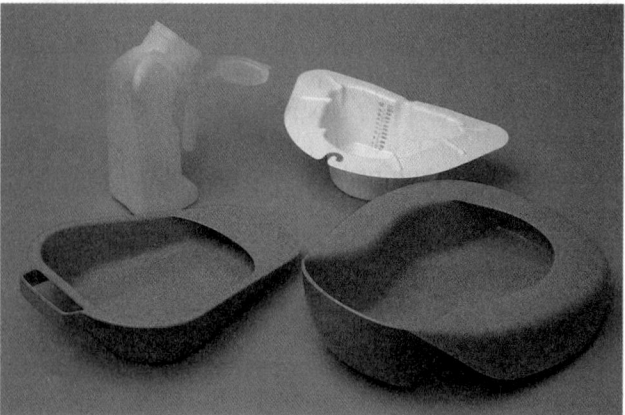

FIGURE **29-3** Urine collection devices: fracture pan *(left front)*, standard bedpan *(right front)*, urinal *(left rear)*, and in-toilet "hat" *(right rear)*.

Box 29-2 *Abnormalities Commonly Found in Urinalysis*

- Glycosuria (glucose in the urine) is present when there is too much glucose in the blood (hyperglycemia), or when the renal threshold for glucose is lowered for some reason.
- Proteinuria (protein in the urine) occurs at times of stress, when infection is present, when there has been recent strenuous exercise, or when there is a disorder of the glomeruli.
- Hematuria (blood in the urine) occurs from bleeding somewhere in the urinary system.
- Pyuria (pus in the urine) occurs when there is a bacterial infection present in the kidney or bladder. Bacteria will be present in the urine in large numbers.
- Ketonuria (ketones in the urine) occurs when the patient is in ketoacidosis. This occurs in uncontrolled diabetes mellitus.
- **Casts** occur in increased numbers in the presence of bacteria or protein, and indicate urinary **calculi** (stones) or renal disease.
- **Red blood cells** in the urine greater than 0 to 2 per high-power field of the microscope may indicate a stone, tumor, glomerular disorder, **cystitis** (bladder inflammation), or bleeding disorder.
- **White blood cells** in the urine mean there is an infectious or inflammatory process somewhere in the urinary tract.
- **Bilirubin** in the urine suggests liver disease or obstruction of the bile duct.

sis will not be accurate. Box 29-2 shows some common abnormalities found by urinalysis.

Dipstick tests, containing chemical reagents, are routinely performed in most physicians' offices and outpatient clinics. They may test for a variety of components, including glucose, ketones, protein, blood, specific gravity, pH, nitrate, bilirubin, and leukocytes. If a dipstick test is to be performed, follow the directions on the side of the bottle of test strips. **Exact timing for checking each component is essential for accuracy of the result** (Figure 29-4).

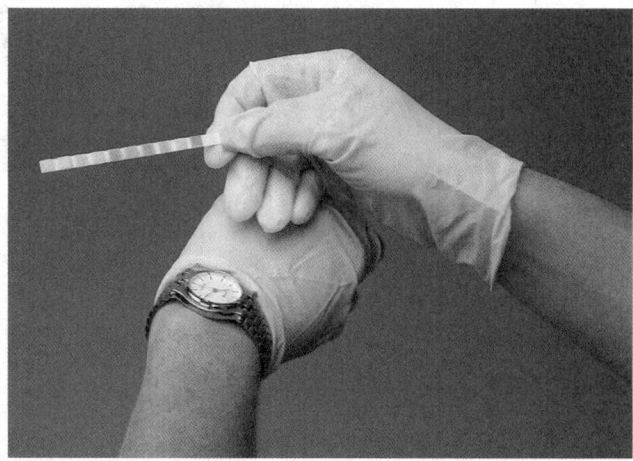

FIGURE **29-4** Timing the reading of a urine dipstick.

Midstream (Clean-Catch) Urine Specimen. This procedure is used to obtain a specimen for a culture and sensitivity test when a urinary tract infection is suspected. The purpose is to obtain a specimen that is relatively free from external contamination (Patient Teaching 29-1).

? *Think Critically About . . .* Your patient is voiding only 100 mL of urine at a time. What further assessments should you make? What questions should you ask this patient?

Specimen from an Indwelling Catheter. A specimen may be obtained from the self-sealing port of an indwelling catheter system or from the lumen of a latex catheter (Steps 29-1, Figure 29-5).

Sterile Catheterized Specimen. When a sterile specimen is ordered and the patient does not have an indwelling catheter in place, the patient is catheterized with a straight catheter (no balloon) that may be attached to a small collection bag, or the urine may be collected by placing the distal end of the catheter into a sterile specimen container.

24-Hour Urine Specimen. All urine voided during the 24-hour period is collected in the designated container and stored on ice if necessary. The laboratory analysis is done to determine the amount of a specified chemical that is excreted through the urine in a 24-hour period. If some urine is accidentally thrown out, the test is invalid and must be started over. A sign should be

Patient Teaching 29-1

How to Obtain a Midstream Urine Specimen

FOR THE FEMALE PATIENT
- Perform hand hygiene.
- Open the midstream kit and remove the lid of the specimen container, being careful not to touch the inside of the container; place the lid upside down on the sink or counter.
- Sit on the toilet. The labia need to be held apart during cleaning and until the specimen is obtained.
- Open the packets of cleaning swabs.
- With the index finger and thumb of the nondominant hand, spread the labia apart.
- Clean the right side of the area from front to back in one stroke; discard the swab.
- With a new swab, clean the left side of the area from front to back in one stroke; discard the swab.
- With another swab, clean down the center of the area from front to back in one stroke; discard the swab.
- Pick up the specimen container by the outside; void a small amount of urine into the toilet; catch the middle portion of urine by moving the container into the stream. Collect about an ounce of urine. Do not let the specimen container touch the skin or pubic hair. Set the container on the sink, being careful not to touch the inside or the rim. Finish voiding into the toilet.
- Place the lid on the container tightly; do not touch the inside of the lid.
- Rinse and dry the outside of the container.
- Perform hand hygiene.

FOR THE MALE PATIENT
- Perform hand hygiene.
- Open the midstream kit; remove the lid of the specimen container and place it on the sink or counter upside down; be careful not to touch the inside of the container or the lid.
- Open the packets of cleansing swabs.
- If you are uncircumcised, retract the foreskin. Cleanse the end of the penis: start at the urinary meatus (opening) and work outward in circles; throw the swab into the trash.
- Repeat the cleansing process with one more swab.
- Pick up the specimen container; with the foreskin still retracted, begin urinating and pass a small amount of urine.
- Move specimen container into the stream and collect about 1 ounce of urine without touching the container to the skin. Put the container down on the sink or on a paper towel.
- Finish urinating into the toilet. Replace the foreskin.
- Replace the lid on the container, being careful not to touch the inside of the container or lid.
- Rinse and dry the outside of the container.
- Perform hand hygiene.

FOR THE PATIENT AT HOME
- Label the container with name, date, time, and physician's name.
- Take the specimen to the physician's office or laboratory, or place it in a plastic bag and refrigerate until the specimen can be transported.

Steps 29-1 Obtaining a Urine Specimen from an Indwelling Catheter

If it is suspected that the patient is developing a urinary tract infection, the physician may order a urine culture and sensitivity test. The specimen is taken from the port on the catheter or connecting tubing using sterile technique.

Review and carry out the Standard Steps in Appendix 3.

1. ***ACTION*** Clamp the catheter below the aspiration port with a catheter clamp or double it over and secure it with a rubber band. Note the time. Leave it clamped for 15 to 30 minutes per agency policy.

   RATIONALE Ensures that there will be urine in the catheter for the removal of the specimen.

2. ***ACTION*** Perform hand hygiene and don gloves. Wipe the aspiration port of the drainage tubing with an alcohol or antimicrobial swab.

   RATIONALE Maintains asepsis and prevents contamination of catheter.

3. ***ACTION*** Insert a 25-gauge needle attached to a 5- to 10-mL syringe into the aspiration port at a 30- to 45-degree angle.

   RATIONALE Use of small-bore needle and angle ensures that the port will reseal following removal of the needle.

4. ***ACTION*** Aspirate 3 mL of urine by gently pulling back on the plunger of the syringe. Remove the needle from the port. Swab the aspiration port with the alcohol or antimicrobial pad.

   RATIONALE Pulling too hard on the plunger causes excessive pressure and may collapse the catheter, preventing urine from flowing into the syringe.

5. ***ACTION*** Empty the syringe into the sterile specimen container without touching the needle to the container. Dispose in sharps container. Close and label the container. **Unclamp the catheter.**

   RATIONALE Keeps the specimen sterile. Proper labeling is essential to obtain desired report. Unclamping the catheter allows free flow of urine again.

6. ***ACTION*** Ensure that specimen goes to the laboratory within 15 minutes or refrigerate the specimen.

   RATIONALE Changes can occur in urine that sits at room temperature for more than 15 minutes.

7. ***ACTION*** Remove gloves and perform hand hygiene.

   RATIONALE Reduces transfer of microorganisms.

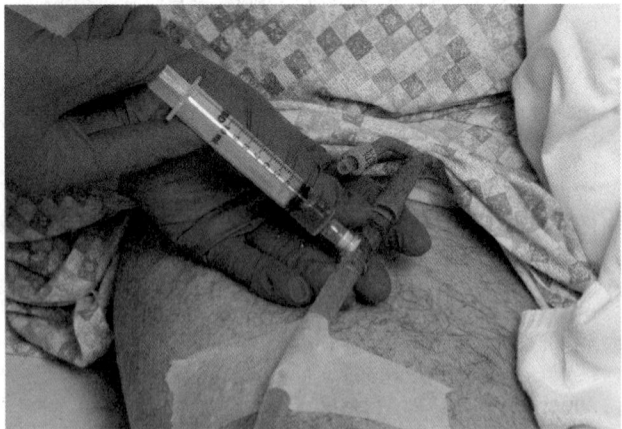

FIGURE **29-5** Aspirating urine from drainage port.

posted over the bed and over the toilet indicating that all urine is to be saved. The patient's bladder should be empty at the beginning and at the conclusion of the test. **The patient empties the bladder just before beginning the collection and the urine is discarded. At the ending time, the patient voids and the urine is added to the collection container.** Check with the laboratory before beginning the test to be certain the right container with preservative is on hand and to see whether the specimen must be kept cold during the 24-hour period (see Chapter 24).

Urinary Collection Bag. This device is used to obtain a urine specimen from an infant or toddler. It attaches to the skin by an adhesive backing and is placed so that it surrounds the genitals. When sufficient urine has collected in the bag for a specimen, the bag is carefully removed and the urine is poured into a specimen container.

Strained Specimen. If it is suspected that the patient has a urinary stone, all urine is strained when voided. Usually a fine sieve is used. If a stone is found, it should be saved and sent to the laboratory for analysis.

Nursing Diagnosis

Nursing diagnoses for patients with problems of urinary elimination are as follows:

- Urinary elimination, impaired
- Urinary retention
- Urinary incontinence (urge, stress, total, reflex, overflow, or functional)
- Body image, disturbed
- Infection, risk for
- Pain (acute or chronic)
- Injury, risk for (to kidney from urine blockage)

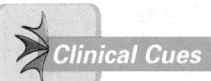

Cultural Cues 29-1

Cultural Awareness for Toileting Preferences

Rather than using toilet paper, patients from other cultures may feel more comfortable if a source of flowing water (e.g., pericare bottle or bidet) is available to clean the perineal area after toileting.

- Self-care deficit, toileting
- Risk for impaired skin integrity
- Knowledge, deficient

The specific defining characteristics are added to the diagnosis stem for the individual patient.

Planning

The data gathered during assessment will give you the information needed to plan time to assist the patient needing help with toileting. If a patient has been prone to urinary tract infections (UTIs), you can specifically plan to increase fluids, unless they are contraindicated, at set intervals and to reinforce patient teaching regarding ways to prevent further UTIs. You should plan for time to collect any needed urine specimens, and should tell the patient that one will be needed sufficiently ahead of time for the patient to be able to produce the urine. When you are planning care for your patient, remember to be culturally sensitive in helping your patient to achieve toileting needs (Cultural Cues 29-1).

For the patient prone to urinary retention, you can plan to note the amount of each voiding and to palpate the bladder for distention if output falls below normal.

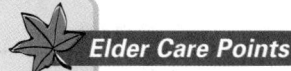

Clinical Cues

Every patient who has an abnormality of urinary elimination should be placed on intake and output (I & O) recording. You should plan ahead by placing an I & O recording sheet by the patient's bed and by placing a 24-hour I & O sheet in the chart. All urine voided is recorded as output.

If the patient is in need of assistive devices for toileting, place a bedpan and/or urinal in the bedside stand or obtain an order for the device needed. Discharge planning includes ensuring that arrangements are made before the patient goes home for devices such as grab bars by the toilet, a commode chair (chair with a container inserted to catch urine or feces), or a raised toilet seat (Figure 29-6).

Keep in mind that urinary elimination is usually an independent function and it is embarrassing to most people to have assistance. The insertion of a catheter causes a disturbance in body image even if the catheter

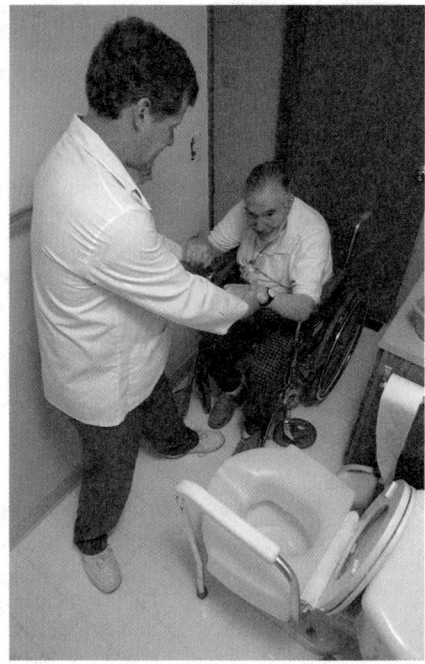

FIGURE **29-6** Grab bars and raised toilet seat in home.

is temporary. Plan to show extra sensitivity when caring for these patients. Some examples of expected outcomes can be found in Nursing Care Plan 29-1.

Implementation

Assisting patients with urinary elimination is a basic nursing function. Patients who can ambulate can be assisted to the bathroom to use the toilet. Others may use a commode chair. This is a chair with an opening in the seat and a large receptacle beneath it. It is usually placed by the bedside or a short distance away. The patient is transferred from the bed to the commode and then back again. The receptacle is emptied after each use. The commode chair is used for bowel movements as well as urination. Another assistive device is a raised toilet seat. This is usually a frame device that fits over the toilet bowl and has a toilet seat attached to it at a higher point than is usual. Patients who have difficulty with hip flexion or who have had a hip replacement need to use such a device.

Elder Care Points

The elderly may experience incontinence as a result of mobility problems or neurologic deficit. Timed toileting can be helpful in keeping these patients dry.

Patients on bed rest are provided with a bedpan for elimination. It is made of metal or plastic (see Figure 29-3). Each patient has an individual bedpan stored in the bedside stand during the hospital stay. The female uses it for both urine and bowel elimination, whereas the male uses it for bowel elimination only. The bed-

NURSING CARE PLAN 29-1

Care of the Patient with Cystitis

SCENARIO Ms. Juarez, age 33, comes to the outpatient clinic. She states that she has been experiencing burning, urgency, and lower pelvic discomfort for 3 days. She needs to urinate several times an hour. She has had a bladder infection before and is afraid that she has one again. "How do I get these infections? What should I do?" Her blood pressure and pulse are normal, but her temperature is 100.8° F (38.2° C). You ask her to obtain a midstream urine specimen and provide the instructions for this. You check her urine with a dipstick and it shows that she has leukocytes in the urine. The physician examines the patient and concludes that she does have cystitis. Norfloxacin (Noroxin) and phenazopyridine HCl (Pyridium) are prescribed.

PROBLEM/NURSING DIAGNOSIS *Burning and lower pelvic discomfort*/Pain related to burning with urination and lower pelvic discomfort.
Supporting Assessment Data: **Subjective:** Discomfort in lower pelvic area × 3 days; states, "It burns." **Objective:** Urine is cloudy and malodorous.

Goals/Expected Outcomes	Nursing Interventions	Selected Rationale	Evaluation
Pain will be lessened within 6 hr. Pain will be relieved within 72 hr.	Review the instructions for taking phenazopyridine HCl (Pyridium). Explain that it will turn the urine red or orange.	Patient might be frightened if red or orange urine is not expected.	*How did the patient respond to the treatments?* After taking the medications and fluids for 24 hr, stated in follow-up phone call that the discomfort is almost gone.
	Encourage the patient to increase fluid intake to 3000 mL a day to keep the urine dilute and lessen bladder irritation.	Increasing fluid intake keeps the bladder flushed out and decreases the bacteria population, decreasing irritation.	
	Explain that hot sitz baths with water up to the umbilicus taken for 20 minutes two or three times a day help increase blood flow to the bladder and lessen bladder irritation and pain.	Hot water increases circulation in the pelvic area.	
	Encourage the patient to take Norfloxacin (Noroxin) prescribed exactly as directed to kill the causative organism.	A steady amount of the antibiotic in the bloodstream is essential to kill the bacteria in the bladder.	Meeting expected outcomes.

PROBLEM/NURSING DIAGNOSIS *Does not know how to prevent infection*/Deficient knowledge related to factors that predispose to urinary tract infection.
Supporting Assessment Data: **Subjective:** Asks, "How do I get these infections? What should I do?" **Objective:** Unable to state how much fluid she should drink in a day. Unable to identify any factors that predispose to urinary tract infection when asked.

Goals/Expected Outcomes	Nursing Interventions	Selected Rationale	Evaluation
Patient will verbalize five ways to help prevent recurrence of urinary tract infection (UTI) at follow-up visit in 10 days.	Instruct to: • Continue to drink at least 2500 mL of fluid per day.	Understanding risk factors and measures to prevent infection is essential in following a regimen that will keep her from getting another bladder infection.	*Was the patient able to verbalize ways to prevent recurrent UTIs?* Verbalized five measures to prevent UTIs during follow-up visit. Urine is clear of bacteria.
	• Void immediately after intercourse and drink at least a full glass of water.	Voiding after intercourse flushes bacteria from the urethra.	

NURSING CARE PLAN 29-1

Care of the Patient with Cystitis—cont'd

Goals/Expected Outcomes	Nursing Interventions	Selected Rationale	Evaluation
	• Refrain from wearing clothing that is tight in the groin area.	Tight clothing creates a warm moist environment for bacteria growth.	
	• Bathe daily and thoroughly cleanse the perineal area.	Keeping the perineal area clean prevents bacteria from traveling up the urethra.	
	• Always wipe the perineum from front to back only.	Prevents feces from coming into contact with the urethra.	
	• Drink cranberry juice, eat a few prunes or plums daily.	Acidifies the urine, which is unfriendly to bacteria.	
	• Empty the bladder at least every 3 hours while awake.	Stagnant urine creates a medium for bacterial growth.	Met expected outcomes.

? CRITICAL THINKING QUESTIONS

1. Why do you think that many women develop cystitis after having intercourse?

2. What is the rationale for asking a patient to have another urine specimen checked a day after finishing a course of treatment for cystitis?

---

pan should be covered if it must be carried outside the patient's room. Paper towels or a small hand towel may be used.

The *fracture pan* (see Figure 29-3) is used when patients are unable to sit on a regular-sized bedpan. It is smaller in surface area and height than the regular bedpan. It is used for patients with musculoskeletal problems. The flat end with the wide rim is placed under the patient's buttocks. It is placed under the patient by separating the patient's legs and slipping the pan under the buttocks. A little powder on the flat rim helps when the patient is unable to raise the hips to assist. The greater depth at the front of the pan helps keep the urine from spilling on the bed. Remove the pan carefully so that urine is not spilled on the bed. Skill 29-1 presents instructions on how to place and remove a bedpan.

Skill 29-1 | Placing and Removing a Bedpan

The female patient who is very weak or who has bed rest ordered uses a bedpan to void or to have a bowel movement. The male uses a urinal to void, but uses the bedpan to evacuate the bowel. If the patient is in traction or cannot raise the hips or turn for placement of the normal bedpan, a fracture pan may be used.

■ Supplies

✓ Bedpan
✓ Toilet tissue
✓ Hand hygiene equipment
✓ Gloves
✓ Powder
✓ Underpad

Review and carry out the Standard Steps in Appendix 3.

■ Assessment (Data Collection)

1. **ACTION** Inquire if the patient needs to void.

   RATIONALE Checks for bladder distention and establishes need to void.

2. **ACTION** Determine mobility to see if the patient can use a full-size bedpan or if a fracture pan is needed.

   RATIONALE Fracture pan use prevents further injury from turning or raising the hips.

Continued

Skill 29-1 | Placing and Removing a Bedpan—cont'd

■ Planning

3. *ACTION* Gather equipment; warm the metal bedpan with warm water and dry it. Raise the bed to proper working height.

   RATIONALE Displays good time management and work organization. A warm bedpan is more comfortable for the patient. Raising the bed prevents back strain.

4. *ACTION* Provide privacy by closing the door and/or the privacy curtains.

   RATIONALE Protects the patient's right to privacy and reduces embarrassment.

■ Implementation

5. *ACTION* Perform hand hygiene and don gloves.

   RATIONALE Reduces transfer of microorganisms.

6. *ACTION* Lower the side rail if up, and raise the top linen enough to determine location of the hips and buttocks.

   RATIONALE Provides access to place for bedpan.

7. *ACTION* Ask patient to bend the knees and press down with the feet while you slip one hand under the lower back for assistance; place an absorbent pad under the hips and buttocks. Ask patient to repeat this maneuver and place bedpan under the patient with the back rim at the end of the sacrum.

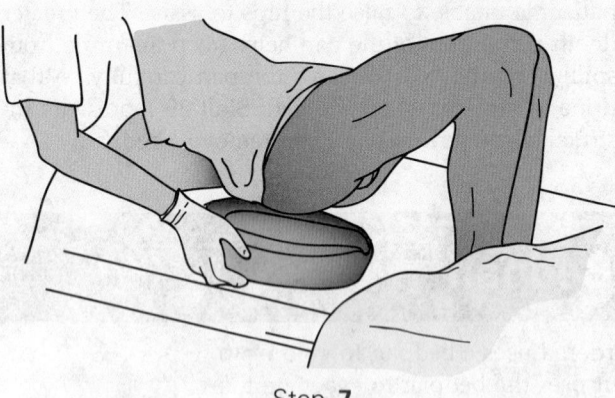

Step **7**

   RATIONALE Helps raise the patient's hips for placement of the bedpan. Placing your hand palm up under the small of the back and your elbow on the mattress helps lift the patient onto the bedpan. The buttocks will form a seal along the rim of the pan.

8. *ACTION* Raise the head of the bed to 30 degrees if not contraindicated. Place the toilet tissue and call light within reach.

   RATIONALE A sitting position makes voiding easier. Patient can signal when finished or in need of assistance.

9. *ACTION* Ask the patient to flex the knees, place the feet on the mattress, and raise the hips. Remove the bedpan. Place it on the chair or the floor.

   RATIONALE Maneuver allows for removal of the bedpan. If urine is to be measured, provide another receptacle for the used toilet tissue so it is not placed in the bedpan.

For the Helpless Patient

10. *ACTION* Turn the patient on one side; face the patient's back and lightly powder the buttocks and lower back area; place the bedpan firmly against the buttocks with the top of the bedpan at the top

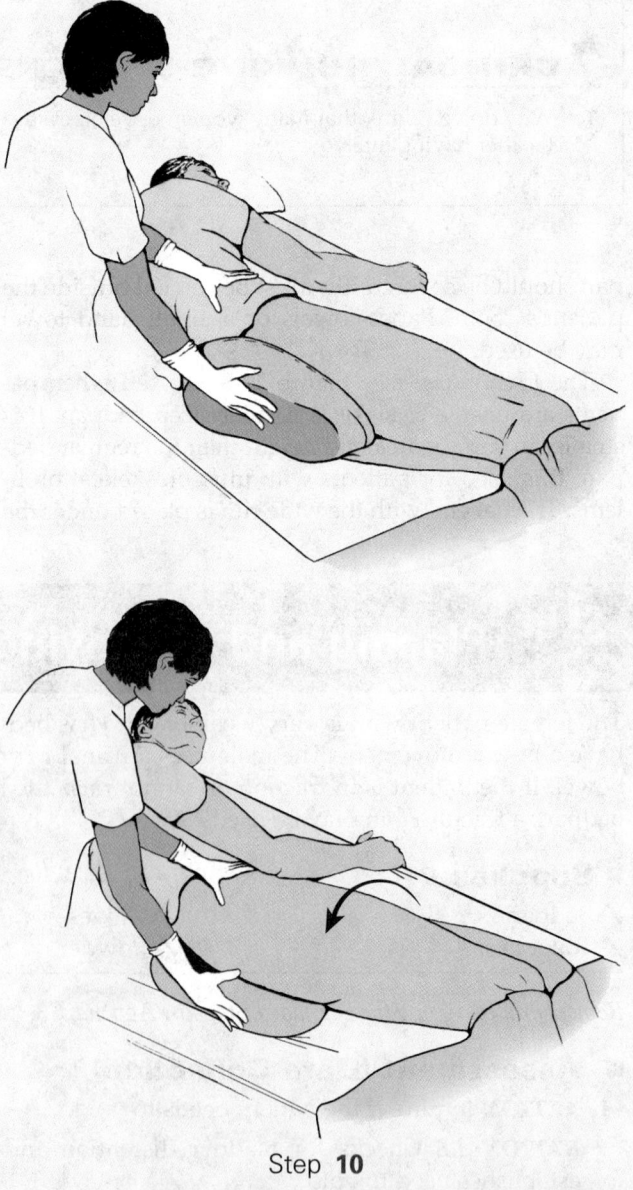

Step **10**

of the fold of the buttocks. Place one hand on the hip and hold the bedpan in place with the other hand. Roll the patient onto the bedpan and check its position for comfort.

RATIONALE Allows bedpan placement for the weak patient who cannot assist. The powder keeps the bedpan from sticking to the patient's skin and aids in removal of the pan.

11. *ACTION* Raise the head of the bed.

RATIONALE Sitting is an easier position for voiding.

12. *ACTION* When the patient is finished, lower the head of the bed and assist the patient to turn to the far side of the bed. Hold the bedpan to prevent spilling. Remove the bedpan and set it on the floor or chair.

RATIONALE Aids removal of the bedpan without spilling urine.

13. *ACTION* Wipe the perineal area dry with toilet tissue, stroking from the front of the vulva to the anus. Reposition patient for comfort.

RATIONALE Cleansing from front to back prevents contamination of the urinary meatus and vaginal area.

14. *ACTION* Measure the urine, note unusual characteristics, and record the amount on the intake and output record as needed. Discard the urine and clean and dry the bedpan and store it in its proper place.

RATIONALE Notation documents output accurately. Unclean bedpans are odorous and provide a place for growth of bacteria.

15. *ACTION* Have the patient perform hand hygiene. Remove your gloves and perform hand hygiene.

RATIONALE Reduces transfer of microorganisms.

16. *ACTION* Lower the bed and restore the unit. Place the call light within reach; raise side rails.

RATIONALE Makes the patient comfortable and institutes safety measures.

■ Evaluation

17. *ACTION* Ask patient if bladder feels empty. Was there spilling of urine? If so, what would you do

differently next time? Has the patient performed hand hygiene? Is the patient comfortable?

RATIONALE Helps determine whether procedure went smoothly and accomplished the goal.

■ Documentation

18. *ACTION* Document on the flow sheet or in the nurse's notes depending on agency policy. Note time, amount of voiding, and characteristics of the urine.

RATIONALE Verifies patient's voiding pattern.

Documentation Example

5/19 0800   Voided 240 mL clear, pale yellow urine in bedpan.

_____
(Nurse's signature)

■ Special Considerations

✓ When the patient cannot raise the hips or turn to the side, a fracture pan is used. It can be slid into place from between the patient's legs. The rim of the pan fits under the buttocks. A trapeze bar is of great assistance in helping patients position themselves on a bedpan. Using the trapeze bar does require some upper arm strength.

Elder Care Points

• The elderly patient may be especially reluctant to have the nurse cleanse the perineum; be matter of fact and protect dignity, but get the patient clean.

?CRITICAL THINKING QUESTIONS

1. What would you do to make placing and removing a bedpan for a patient who is in full leg traction as easy as possible?

2. How would you make sure the patient who cannot turn to the side is properly cleansed after a bowel movement?

For the ambulatory patient who needs urinary output recorded, place a plastic "hat" device toward the front of the toilet bowel between the bowl and the seat. The inside is graduated so that you can record the amount of output after each voiding and then empty, rinse, and replace the container so that it is ready for the next voiding.

Whatever method is used for urinary elimination, provide an opportunity for hand hygiene (Cultural

Cues 29-2). The patient is made comfortable with side rails replaced and the call bell within reach.

Assisting with Use of a Urinal

When a male is unable to use a urinal unassisted, the nurse helps. If the patient can stand by the side of the bed, this is the most desirable position. The male urinal is a plastic or metal bottle with a round neck, a handle, rectangular sides, and a flat base (see Fig-

Hand Hygiene After Eliminating

For nurses, hand hygiene is second nature, but for many people this is not an automatic behavior. For example, patients who come from the Republic of Uzbekistan may not be in the habit of using soap to wash their hands after eliminating because of the general expense of soap products in that country (D'Avanzo, 2008). In accordance with *Healthy People 2010*, improvements in personal and domestic hygiene are needed to reduce the global incidence of disease.

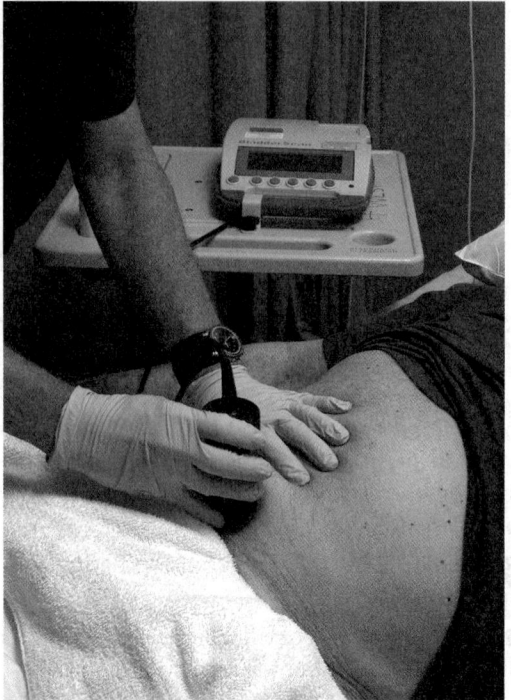

FIGURE 29-7 Using a bladder scanner to determine amount of urine in the bladder.

ure 29-3). It may or may not have a lid. The urinal can be used by the patient who is confined to bed, in any one of four positions: lying supine, lying on either the right or the left side, or in Fowler's position. Provide privacy by closing the door or the privacy curtain, don gloves, lower the side rail, and ask the patient to spread his legs. Hold the urinal by the handle and direct it at an angle between the legs so that the flat side rests on the bed. Lift the penis and place it well within the urinal. After urination, carefully remove the urinal and empty it immediately, measuring and recording the urine voided. Be sure the penis is dry. Clean the urinal and return it to the proper place.

Assisting a Patient to Urinate

Patients often have difficulty urinating after surgery and anesthesia, childbirth, or other trauma to the perineum. All efforts are made to help the patient void naturally before resorting to catheterization (insertion of a tube into the bladder). Some methods of helping patients initiate the voiding reflex are as follows:

- Run water in a nearby sink so the patient hears the sound.
- Have the patient deep breathe, relax, and visualize a peaceful place with a bubbling brook.
- Assist the male to stand by the side of the bed (with a physician's order).
- Have the female blow through a straw in a glass of water, causing bubbling, while sitting on the toilet or bedpan.
- Pour warm water over the perineum while the patient attempts to void. Measure the water volume so you can subtract it from the total volume to determine how much the patient voided.
- With a physician's order, gently but firmly use Credé's maneuver over the bladder (massage from top of bladder to bottom by starting above the pubic bone and rocking the palm of the hand steadily downward).

- Obtain an order for a sitz bath and have the patient sit in the warm water. Encourage the patient to void while in the bath. Cleanse the perineum afterward.

When a patient cannot empty the bladder naturally for a period longer than 8 hours, a bladder scan may be performed using an ultrasound machine designed for that purpose (Figure 29-7). If the bladder contains a large amount of urine, an order is obtained for catheterization. The bladder scan can also disclose the amount of residual urine in the bladder after a patient voids. This tells the physician whether the bladder is emptying sufficiently. If needed, the physician orders either a straight "in-and-out" catheterization or the insertion of an indwelling (Foley) catheter. Other reasons for catheterization include

- Preparing a patient for a surgical procedure or obstetric delivery
- Keeping the genitalia and perineum clean after obstetric or surgical procedures
- Dilating a urethral stricture (narrowed lumen)
- Splinting the urethra following surgery on the urethra
- Measuring the amount of residual urine in the bladder (this is also accomplished by a using a portable ultrasound bladder scanner)
- Monitoring hourly urine output or to obtain exact measurements of total output
- Performing irrigation or instillation and drainage of chemotherapeutic solutions into the bladder
- Assisting with the re-toning of the bladder muscle after surgery on the bladder

Single lumen

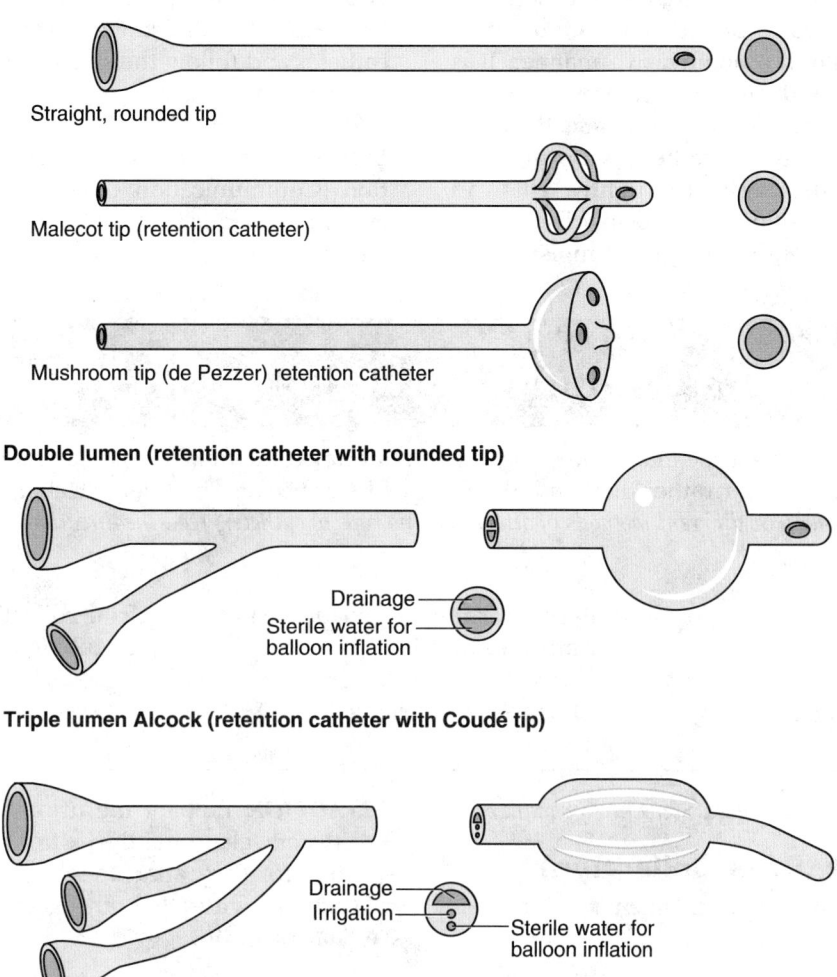

Straight, rounded tip

Malecot tip (retention catheter)

Mushroom tip (de Pezzer) retention catheter

Double lumen (retention catheter with rounded tip)

Drainage
Sterile water for
balloon inflation

Triple lumen Alcock (retention catheter with Coudé tip)

Drainage
Irrigation
Sterile water for
balloon inflation

FIGURE **29-8** Common urinary catheters.

Think Critically About . . . You have a patient who returned from surgery at 10:30 A.M. She has been awake since she returned to the unit. She had spinal anesthesia, but has recovered the feeling in her lower extremities. It is now 7 P.M. and she still has not voided since her return to the unit. What would you do to assist her to void? If she has not voided by 8 P.M., what would you do?

Types of Urinary Catheters

Catheters come in several sizes and shapes and are either rubber or plastic. Some are Teflon coated. They are sized by the French system, with the average size used for an adult female being 14 to 16 Fr. and for the male 18 to 20 Fr. (Figure 29-8). A straight catheter (e.g., the Robinson) is used to relieve retention when a patient is temporarily unable to void, or obtain a sterile specimen. The Foley is the most common indwelling catheter, the type that remains in the bladder for an extended period. It is sometimes referred to as a "re-tention" catheter because it is retained in the bladder. A Foley catheter has two lumens, one to drain urine and one for inflation of the balloon that holds the catheter in the bladder to prevent it from slipping out the urethra. The balloon usually holds 5 to 10 mL of sterile water. This catheter is used for continuous drainage, particularly postoperatively, and can also be used for suprapubic (above the pubic bone) drainage.

The Coudé catheter, a variation of the Robinson catheter, is curved and has a rounded or bulbous tip that is easier to insert into the male urethra when the prostate is enlarged.

The Alcock catheter, used for continuous bladder irrigation following prostate or bladder surgery, is a Foley-type catheter with two eyes. It has three lumens, one for urine drainage, one for inflation of the balloon, and one for the instillation of the irrigation fluid.

The de Pezzer catheter, which has a tip shaped like a mushroom, is used for suprapubic drainage. The Malecot catheter, which has a large single tube with a tip shaped like wings, is often used as a nephrostomy tube; it is placed into the pelvis of the kidney.

A condom catheter consists of a condom with a tube attached to the distal end that is attached to a drainage bag. It is used to provide continuous urine drainage for the male in a noninvasive manner. It is applied to the penis and, since it is noninvasive, it is less likely to predispose to urinary tract infection.

When applying a condom catheter, care must be taken not to apply the sheath too tightly. This can cause a decreased blood flow to the penis. The sheath must be checked frequently for signs of moisture ac-cumulation as this can lead to skin breakdown. Unless applied carefully and correctly, a condom catheter will leak. Read the directions that come with the specific catheter and follow the steps in Skill 29-2.

Performing Catheterization

Explain the procedure and elicit the patient's coopera-tion (Communication Cues 29-1). Sterile equipment and strict aseptic technique must be used to catheter-ize a patient. **Any break in aseptic technique causing**

Skill 29-2 | Applying a Condom Catheter

A condom catheter is used for the male who is incontinent but can void on his own. It is prefer-able to use a condom catheter rather than an indwelling catheter because bladder infection is less likely to occur. *There are different methods of attaching this type of catheter; read the directions on the package.*

■ Supplies
- ✓ Condom catheter
- ✓ Gloves
- ✓ Adherent elastic tape strip
- ✓ Basin, warm water, soap, wash-cloth, and towel
- ✓ Skin prep pads or solution
- ✓ Clippers for hair removal if needed
- ✓ Urine collection bag with drain-age tubing or leg bag and straps

---

Review and carry out the Standard Steps in Appendix 3.

■ Assessment (Data Collection)

1. *ACTION* Assess need for and patient's willingness to use a condom catheter.

   RATIONALE If unwilling, the patient will detach the condom catheter.

2. *ACTION* Assess condition of skin on penis.

   RATIONALE Urine incontinence places the skin at risk for breakdown.

■ Planning

3. *ACTION* Gather equipment and prepare the work-ing space by raising the bed to proper height.

   RATIONALE Promotes work efficiency and pre-vents back strain.

4. *ACTION* Close the door and/or draw the privacy curtains.

   RATIONALE Protects the patient's privacy.

5. *ACTION* Explain the procedure.

   RATIONALE Promotes cooperation and reduces anxiety.

6. *ACTION* Lower the side rail if up. Place the patient in a supine position, drape the upper torso with a bath blanket, and then fold the sheet down so it covers the legs and can be lowered to expose the genitalia.

   RATIONALE Provides comfort, conserves body heat, and prevents unnecessary exposure.

7. *ACTION* Prepare the urinary drainage collection system, clamping the exit port and positioning the bag for easy attachment to the condom catheter. Roll the wider tip of the condom sheath toward the narrower tip.

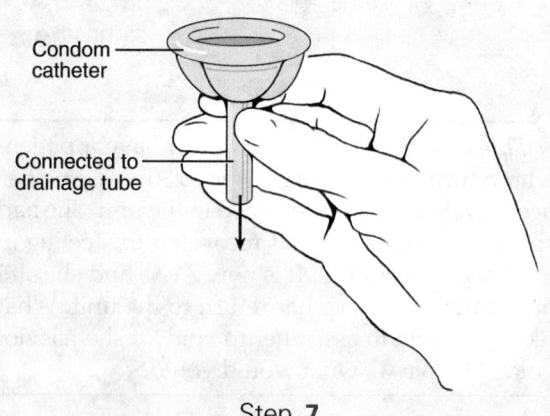

Condom catheter

Connected to drainage tube

Step **7**

RATIONALE Prepares the system for use.

■ Implementation

8. *ACTION* Perform hand hygiene and don gloves.

   RATIONALE Prevents transfer of microorganisms.

9. *ACTION* Wash and dry the penis and surrounding skin, clip the hair at the base of the penis, apply the skin prep, and allow to dry.

   RATIONALE Washing cleanses the skin before ap-plication of the condom device. The skin prep helps protect the skin against urine and provides an adherent surface on which to apply the condom catheter.

10. **ACTION** Apply the double-sided elastic tape in a spiral fashion from the base of the penis downward.

    RATIONALE Provides a surface on which the condom catheter can be attached without impeding circulation in the penis. *Some condom catheters attach with a Velcro strip over the sheath.*

11. **ACTION** Grasp the penis along the shaft with the nondominant hand. Hold the condom sheath at the tip of the penis and smoothly roll the sheath onto the penis, leaving 1 to 2 inches of space between the tip of the penis and the drainage tube of the condom sheath.

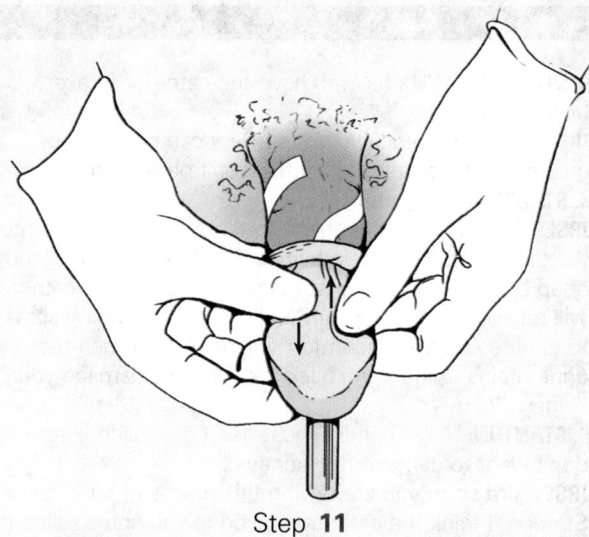

Step **11**

RATIONALE Positions the condom catheter on the penis. Allows free passage of urine into the collecting tube and drainage bag. Keeps penis away from collecting urine. Secures the condom sheath to the penis.

12. **ACTION** Gently press the sheath to the underlying adhesive strip with the palm of the hand in a grasp, being careful not to wrinkle the rubber sheath. Hold for 1 minute. Explain the rationale for holding x 1 minute to the patient.

    RATIONALE Wrinkles in the sheath may cause urine leakage. The warmth of the hand over 1 minute activates the adhesive.

13. **ACTION** Position the penis downward and connect the drainage tube to the collection bag.

    RATIONALE Allows urine to flow into the collection bag.

14. **ACTION** Return bed to low position and make patient comfortable; place call light within reach. Raise side rails.

RATIONALE Prevents accidents and provides comfort and security.

15. **ACTION** Check the penis after 30 minutes and then every 2 hours and ensure that the catheter is not twisted so that urine can drain freely.

    RATIONALE Ensures that the catheter is not too tight and impairing circulation; twisting of catheter impedes urine flow.

16. **ACTION** If a leg bag is used, empty it when it is partially filled with urine.

    RATIONALE Prevents the weight of the collected urine from dislodging the catheter from the penis.

17. **ACTION** Remove gloves and perform hand hygiene.

    RATIONALE Reduces transfer of microorganisms.

▪ Evaluation

18. **ACTION** Does the catheter fit smoothly and firmly adhere to the penis? Is there evidence of irritation to the skin or impaired circulation? Is urine draining into the bag? Is there any leakage of urine?

    RATIONALE Determines whether system is functioning effectively without problems.

▪ Documentation

19. **ACTION** Note date, condition of genital area, size and type of catheter applied, type of skin prep used, type of drainage collection attached to catheter, amount of urine obtained in bag and its color and character, and patient's tolerance of the procedure.

    RATIONALE Documents use of condom catheter.

Documentation Example

2/22 1630   Skin on genitals slightly reddened from contact with incontinent urine. Area cleansed, prepped, and condom catheter applied with Velcro strip. Patient states does not feel too tight. Attached to leg bag. Draining clear, yellow urine.

_____

(Nurse's signature)

▪ Special Considerations

✓ If the condom catheter is the newer self-adhesive type, apply catheter as in Step 11 and apply gentle pressure around the penile shaft for 10 to 15 seconds to secure the catheter.

✓ The catheter must be checked frequently because the end of the sheath is prone to twist, preventing the urine from flowing into the drainage tube. Care must be taken not to allow pulling on the drainage tubing when repositioning or ambulating the patient because this may dislodge the condom catheter.

✓ Remove and change the catheter daily or more often if it fits improperly.

✓ Wash the used catheter and collection bag with mild

Continued

Skill 29-2 | Applying a Condom Catheter—cont'd

soap and water, rinse with a 1:7 strength vinegar solution, and allow to completely dry.

✓ If the rolled-over portion at the base of the penis seems too tight, clip the roll a tiny bit to loosen it. It should not constrict the penis and interfere with blood flow.

✓ Indications that the catheter is too tight are swelling or discoloration of the penis and complaints of discomfort.

❓CRITICAL THINKING QUESTIONS

1. If an elderly male resists the idea of a condom catheter, and the only other option is to insert an indwelling catheter, what might you say to him that might make him accept the condom catheter?

2. How would you tell if the condom catheter is too tight?

Communication Cues 29-1

Talking to the Patient About Catheter Insertion

James Stanton is suffering from urinary retention. He is in the emergency room because he can't urinate and is in pain. His physician ordered a Foley catheter to be inserted. Mr. Stanton has expressed reluctance about having a catheter. The nurse explains the procedure to him.

NURSE: "Hi, Mr. Stanton; I'm Karen. How are you feeling?"

MR. STANTON: "I'm very uncomfortable."

NURSE: "Can you tell me about your discomfort?"

MR. STANTON: "I can't pee and I have an ache down low." *(Nurse gently palpates the lower abdomen above the symphysis pubis.)*

NURSE: "Mr. Stanton, your bladder is very full. The doctor has ordered a catheter so that the urine can drain. Have you ever had a catheter inserted before?"

MR. STANTON: "No; isn't that like a tube of some sort?"

NURSE: "Yes, it is a tube. Since you've been having so much trouble urinating, the doctor wants me to insert the catheter and leave it there so urine will drain. In addition, we will be trying to determine why you are having trouble passing your urine."

MR. STANTON: "Will I have to have the catheter forever? I don't want that."

NURSE: "Usually medication or surgery can correct the problem, and then the catheter won't be needed.."

MR. STANTON: "Will it hurt?"

NURSE: "It may be a little uncomfortable when it is put into the bladder. You can help by relaxing and by doing some deep breathing when I instruct you to do so. The catheter will relieve the pain you are feeling from not being able to urinate and the discomfort will go away. When the urine drains, there is no backup that could damage your kidneys."

MR. STANTON: "OK. Then let's just get it over with. I sure don't want to damage my kidneys."

NURSE: "I'm sorry you are having this problem, Mr. Stanton. I think the catheter will bring you some relief. I will drape your groin area, cleanse the penis with iodine solution, which feels cool, and then insert the catheter. It will be hooked up to a bag to collect the urine. Are you allergic to iodine?"

MR. STANTON: "No, I'm not."

NURSE: "OK, then I'll go ahead and get started."

---

contamination must be corrected before continuing with the procedure. Each catheter kit is suitable for catheterizing a male or female. The procedure for male and female catheterization is similar except for variations in the positioning, draping, and cleansing of the urinary meatus. In the male, the catheter is inserted farther (about 7 to 8 inches). **When inserting a catheter, gently insert until you see the urine flow and then insert 1 to 2 more inches.** This will ensure the balloon will not damage the urethra during inflation. Skill 29-3 and Skill 29-4 (p. 563) give the steps for catheterization of the female patient and the male patient, respectively. The Foley catheter system should be maintained as a closed system to lessen the risk of infection. The procedure for inserting a straight or Foley

catheter is similar. The difference is that with the Foley, the balloon must be inflated and there is a connecting tube to a drainage bag. Information on straight catheterization is presented in the Special Considerations at the end of Skills 29-3 and 29-4.

It is a good idea to identify the urethral meatus in the female before beginning the procedure. This may be done before gathering the equipment or just before opening the sterile catheterization kit. When the patient is in the dorsal recumbent position and draped, put on exam gloves, use adequate light, and spread the labia minora to reveal the inner anatomy. The urethral meatus is usually slightly above the vaginal opening and often looks like a dimple or fold in the mucous membrane.

Skill 29-3 Catheterizing the Female Patient

An indwelling or retention catheter is used when continuous drainage of urine is desirable because the patient cannot void or cannot stay dry because of constant incontinence. This type of catheter is also used when it is necessary to track urinary output closely hour by hour. The catheter is held in the bladder by a small inflated balloon. Catheter insertion is a sterile procedure, and the student must be supervised when performing catheterization.

■ Supplies

✓ Foley catheter kit with appropriate-size catheter (adult female: 14 to 16 Fr.)
✓ Sterile 4 × 4 gauze
✓ Bath blanket
✓ Basin with warm water
✓ Towel and washcloth
✓ Mild soap
✓ Tape or catheter holder
✓ Extra light (standing lamp or flashlight)

Review and carry out the Standard Steps in Appendix 3.

■ Assessment (Data Collection)

1. **ACTION** Check the physician's order for type and size of catheter.

   RATIONALE Catheterization is only done by medical order.

2. **ACTION** Assess patient's knowledge of catheterization and use of a catheter.

   RATIONALE Considers the patient's knowledge level before beginning needed teaching.

3. **ACTION** Assess whether patient is allergic to iodine or tape.

   RATIONALE Povidone-iodine is often used to cleanse the perineum before catheterization.

4. **ACTION** Assess female patient's ability to assume the dorsal recumbent (lithotomy) position.

   RATIONALE If the female cannot assume the dorsal recumbent position, a side-lying position may be used.

■ Planning

5. **ACTION** Check the patient's identification band, gather equipment, and prepare the working space by raising the bed to proper height and positioning the over-the-bed table for use.

   RATIONALE Ensures that the procedure is performed on the correct patient; promotes work efficiency and prevents back strain.

6. **ACTION** Close the door and/or privacy curtains.

   RATIONALE Protects the patient's right to privacy; helps prevent embarrassment.

7. **ACTION** Explain the procedure.

   RATIONALE Decreases fear of the unknown; prepares the patient for what will occur.

■ Implementation

8. **ACTION** Perform hand hygiene and don disposable gloves.

   RATIONALE Reduces transfer of microorganisms.

9. **ACTION** Assist patient to assume the dorsal recumbent position, with thighs relaxed so that hips can externally rotate, and drape with a bath blanket or sheet.

   RATIONALE Positions patient for ease of viewing the meatus and inserting the catheter into the bladder.

10. **ACTION** With the use of good lighting, inspect the perineum. Wash the area if needed. Spread the labia with your nondominant hand and locate the urinary meatus.

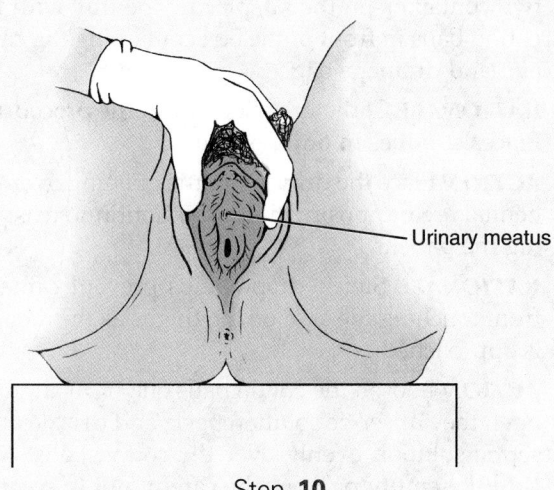

Step **10**

   RATIONALE An assistant may be needed to hold a flashlight with the beam directed at the perineum. This step ensures greater success in placing the catheter into the bladder on the first attempt.

11. **ACTION** Remove gloves and perform hand hygiene.

   RATIONALE Reduces transfer of microorganisms.

12. **ACTION** Open the plastic covering of the catheter kit by tearing along the lined perforated edge. Use the plastic cover as a discard bag and place it to the side of the field or toward the foot of the bed for waste disposal.

Continued

Skill 29-3 | Catheterizing the Female Patient—cont'd

RATIONALE Provides a receptacle for used supplies.

13. *ACTION* Remove the paper-wrapped catheter tray and place it on the bed between the patient's legs, near the perineum (8 to 12 inches away).

   RATIONALE Provides a workspace.

14. *ACTION* Fold back the corner of the bath blanket drape to expose the perineum. With clean hands, using sterile technique, open the wrapper and use it as a sterile field.

   RATIONALE Provides a sterile field within which to work.

15. *ACTION* Pick up the sterile absorbent underpad by one corner and, while holding two corners turned over your fingers, slip it under the patient's buttocks, plastic side down, while asking her to lift the buttocks. Touch only the corners and underside of the sterile underpad.

   RATIONALE Keeps solution from soiling the bedding. Keeps the center of the pad sterile.

16. *ACTION* Put on the sterile gloves and separate the two containers in the kit, placing the tray with the cotton balls in front of the box containing the catheter and drainage bag.

   RATIONALE Catheterization is a sterile procedure. Places supplies in order of use.

17. *ACTION* Place the drape with the opening over the genital area, exposing the labia. Continue reassuring the patient.

   RATIONALE Sterile drape helps prevent catheter from touching the skin on the thighs as the meatus is approached.

18. *ACTION* Loosen the cotton balls one from another, open the antiseptic solution pack, and drizzle antiseptic solution evenly over the cotton balls. Discard the empty package. Be careful not to splatter the solution.

   RATIONALE Prepares the cotton balls to be picked up individually with the forceps.

19. *ACTION* Open the package of lubricant, or remove the stopper from the syringe containing it, and squirt it into an open area of the tray.

   RATIONALE Lubricant may be squirted into the tray and the catheter tip then rotated in it to lubricate.

20. *ACTION* Place the sterile specimen bottle on the side of the tray or discard it.

   RATIONALE Bottle may be discarded if no specimen is required.

21. *ACTION* Remove the plastic sleeve on the catheter by tearing it down the perforated side while carefully controlling the catheter. Place the catheter within the sterile tray where it can be easily reached.

   RATIONALE Prepares the catheter for use. An uncontrolled catheter may strike a nonsterile surface, contaminating it. Wrapping the catheter around a gloved hand while tearing the sleeve helps prevent a break in sterile technique.

22. *ACTION* Attach the sterile water-filled syringe to the balloon port on the catheter and gently insert the water to test the patency of the balloon. Omit pretesting if the balloon is prefilled or if contraindicated by the manufacturer.

   RATIONALE Ensures balloon patency before the catheter is introduced into the bladder.

23. *ACTION* After the test, draw the water back into the syringe, leaving the syringe attached to the catheter balloon port.

   RATIONALE Makes it easier to inject the water into the balloon at the right moment.

24. *ACTION* With the forefinger and thumb of the nondominant hand, separate the labia minora, exposing the meatus. Pull slightly upward (see figure with Step 10). Leave this hand in place, holding the labia open until the catheter is inserted.

   RATIONALE Exposes the urinary meatus so that the catheter can be introduced. Using a sterile 4 × 4 gauze between the fingers and the inner labia helps prevent the fingers from slipping. *Remember:* The hand holding open the labia is now contaminated and must not be used to handle sterile objects.

25. *ACTION* Using the forceps, pick up one saturated cotton ball at a time and cleanse down one side of the labia majora and then the other, discarding each used cotton ball after one stroke. Cleanse one side of the labia minora and then the other. Cleanse last over the meatus with a slow downward stroke. *Do not allow the labia to close over the meatus after cleansing.*

   RATIONALE Removes microorganisms from the perineal area and urinary meatus. *Take care not to pass over the sterile field with used cotton balls when discarding them because this contaminates the sterile field.*

   a. *ACTION* If solution is obscuring the meatus, a dry sterile cotton ball can be used to sponge up the excess solution.

RATIONALE This allows better visualization of the meatus.

b. *ACTION* Dispose of the forceps in the discard bag.

RATIONALE Contaminated forceps must be discarded.

26. *ACTION* Pick up the catheter about 3 inches from the tip, lubricate it well, and gently insert it into the meatus while pointing the catheter slightly toward the umbilicus. Insert it about 2 to 3 inches or until you visualize urine flow. After you see the urine flow, insert the catheter an additional 1 to 2 inches. There may be slight resistance as the catheter passes the internal urethral sphincter. If urine does not flow, rotate the catheter gently and carefully insert it another inch farther. Do not use force. If resistance is encountered, ask the patient to take a deep breath, and twist and advance the catheter as the patient does so; this relaxes the sphincter. If the catheter has been inserted into the vagina by mistake, leave it there as a marker for the vaginal opening, rescrub, and begin the procedure again with a sterile kit.

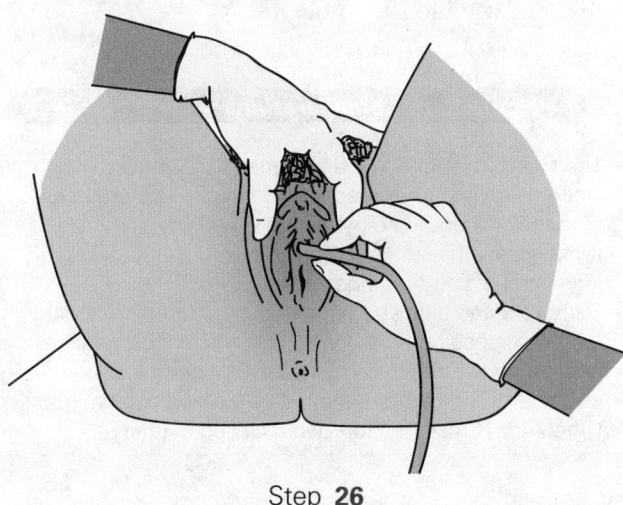

Step **26**

RATIONALE Technique eases insertion into the bladder. Leaving marker catheter in place ensures vaginal opening is not mistaken for urinary meatus.

27. *ACTION* Hold the catheter in place with the dominant hand while instilling the water into the balloon with the nondominant hand. Remove the syringe from the port after inflation and discard it. A prefilled balloon is filled by unclamping the port. Gently pull on the catheter to see if it is anchored securely, and then gently push it into the bladder about 1½ inches. *Watch the patient's face for an expression of discomfort while inflating the balloon to be certain that the balloon is not in the urethra.*

RATIONALE Inflated balloon keeps the catheter from slipping back into the urethra. If the balloon sits at the neck of the bladder after inflation, it causes pressure and a greater urge to urinate.

28. *ACTION* Cleanse the antiseptic solution from the perineum and remove the underpad.

RATIONALE Prevents the antiseptic solution from irritating the skin and makes the patient more comfortable.

29. *ACTION* Attach the drainage bag to the stationary part of the bed frame along the side of the bed close to the middle. Remove the drapes, dry the genital area, dispose of used supplies, remove gloves, and perform hand hygiene.

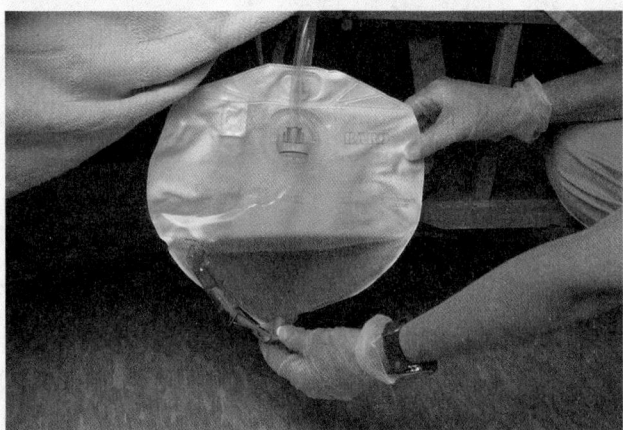

Step **29**

RATIONALE Attaching bag to bed frame keeps bag from coming into contact with the floor. Use the plastic or metal hook to attach the bag to the bed.

30. *ACTION* Attach the catheter to the thigh with tape or a catheter holder.

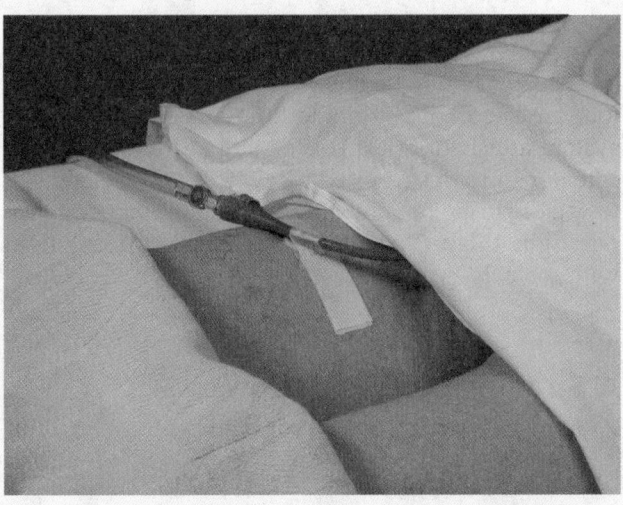

Step **30**

RATIONALE Secures the catheter so that there is no tension on the internal urethral sphincter. Tension on the catheter causes pressure on the internal urethral sphincter and may damage it.

Continued

Skill 29-3 | Catheterizing the Female Patient—cont'd

31. **ACTION** Coil the excess drainage tubing on the bed so that the last portion hangs straight to the drainage bag and secure it.

 RATIONALE The catheter will drain better if no tubing is hanging below the level of entry into the drainage bag.

32. **ACTION** Restore the unit, lower the bed, and place the call light within reach.

 RATIONALE Protects the patient; call light provides a sense of security.

■ Evaluation

33. **ACTION** Ask yourself:

 Was sterile technique maintained?

 Is urine draining, indicating proper placement in the bladder?

 Is the patient having any pain associated with the procedure?

 Is there anything you would do differently next time?

 RATIONALE Determines whether the procedure was done correctly and whether the catheter system is patent. Helps improve technique.

■ Documentation

34. **ACTION** Note date, time, size and type of catheter, amount of water instilled into balloon, type of technique used, and color and characteristics of the urine.

 RATIONALE Documents catheter insertion.

Documentation Example

2/23 1030   No. 16 Fr. Foley with 10 mL water into balloon inserted with sterile technique. Closed drainage system attached. Pt expressing slight discomfort with catheter in place. Approximately 230 mL of dark yellow, clear urine obtained in bag. Catheter taped to inner right thigh. Bed into lowest position, call light within reach.

_____

(Nurse's signature)

■ Special Considerations

✓ Some physicians may order lubricant with local anesthetic.

✓ Once the catheter has touched the patient's skin, it should not be introduced into the urinary meatus because it is contaminated. Anytime the catheter becomes contaminated, the procedure is stopped and begun again with a sterile catheter and kit.

✓ **For Straight Catheterization:** There is no balloon to inflate and no drainage bag. The distal end of the catheter is left in the tray so that urine will drain into it. If a specimen is required, prepare the specimen bottle by labeling and opening it; place the lid upside down on a clean surface. After urine has started to flow, pinch off the catheter with the nondominant hand and place the end of the catheter above the specimen container. Allow 1 to 2 oz of urine to flow into the container. Pinch off the flow, replace the catheter in the tray, and drain the remaining urine from the bladder. Pinch off, remove, and discard the catheter. Measure and record the amount of urine on the intake and output record. Place lid on container, label, and send to laboratory.

Home Care Considerations

- The working height of the bed may be awkward.
- Good planning and placement of supplies before beginning the procedure helps ease back strain.
- If necessary, have the caregiver assist by steadying the legs and holding the knees apart.
- Catheters and drainage bags may be reused. Cleanse with mild soap and rinse well. Deodorize the drainage bag with a rinse of 1 part vinegar to 7 parts water and allow to dry. The catheter should be boiled for 20 minutes. When dry, it may be stored in a closed container.

❓CRITICAL THINKING QUESTIONS

1. If you cannot tell where the urinary meatus is located by looking for it, what would you do?

2. If you have a patient who has difficulty keeping her knees apart for the catheterization procedure, what would you do?

Skill 29-4 | Catheterizing the Male Patient

An indwelling or retention catheter is used when the patient cannot void or when it is desirable to track urinary output closely. A small inflated balloon holds the catheter in the bladder. Supervision of the student is required for this sterile invasive procedure.

■ Supplies
✓ Foley catheter kit with appropriate size catheter (adult male: 18 to 20 Fr.)
✓ Basin with warm water
✓ Bath blanket
✓ Mild soap
✓ Towel and washcloth
✓ Tape or catheter holder
✓ Extra light if needed

Review and carry out the Standard Steps in Appendix 3.

■ Assessment (Data Collection)

1. **ACTION** Check the physician's order for type and size of catheter.

   RATIONALE Ensures that the right patient is catheterized.

2. **ACTION** Assess patient's knowledge of catheterization and use of a catheter. Assess whether patient is allergic to iodine or tape.

   RATIONALE Povidone-iodine is often used to cleanse around the meatus. It must not be used on allergic individuals.

■ Planning

3. **ACTION** Check the patient's identi-band, gather equipment, and prepare the working space by raising the bed to proper height and positioning the over-the-bed table for use.

   RATIONALE Ensures that the procedure is performed on the correct patient. Promotes work efficiency and prevents back strain.

4. **ACTION** Close the door and/or privacy curtains.

   RATIONALE Protects the patient's right to privacy; helps prevent embarrassment.

5. **ACTION** Explain the procedure.

   RATIONALE Decreases fear of the unknown; prepares the patient for what will occur.

■ Implementation

6. **ACTION** Perform hand hygiene.

   RATIONALE Reduces transfer of microorganisms.

7. **ACTION** With the patient supine and knees slightly apart, drape by fan-folding the bedcovers down to cover the lower legs, exposing the perineal area. Use a bath blanket to cover the trunk.

   RATIONALE Draping keeps the patient warm and reduces embarrassment. *Bunching the bath blanket a bit over the abdomen obstructs the patient's view and may decrease his embarrassment. It is not unusual for an erection to occur when the penis is handled.*

8. a. **ACTION** Open the catheter tray by tearing open the plastic cover at the perforated line. Place the kit on the bed between the legs.

   RATIONALE Supplies must be within reach.

   b. **ACTION** Use the plastic cover as a discard bag by placing it to the side of the field or toward the foot of the bed.

   RATIONALE Provides a receptacle for used supplies.

9. **ACTION** Place the absorbent pad under the penis; place the opening of the sterile drape over the penis and onto the perineum, touching only the outer corners.

   RATIONALE Provides a sterile field within which to work.

10. **ACTION** Separate the two parts of the kit and remove the plastic sleeve from the catheter by tearing it down the perforated side while controlling the catheter. Test the balloon unless it is prefilled or testing is contraindicated by the manufacturer.

    RATIONALE Prepares the catheter for use. Controlling the catheter prevents it from touching contaminated surfaces and ensures sterility. Testing is done to detect leaks in the balloon.

11. **ACTION** Lubricate around the first 3 to 4 inches (5 to 7 cm) of the catheter if the lubricant comes in a foil package. *If it is in a syringe, squirt it directly into the urethra.*

    RATIONALE Lubricant prevents undue trauma when inserting the catheter into the urethra. It is recommended practice to place the lubricant into the urethra of the male. When difficulty is encountered with insertion of the catheter, obtain an order for Xylocaine gel. Squirting this into the urethra immediately relaxes muscle spasm and allows easier entry for the catheter.

12. **ACTION** Retract the foreskin if necessary to expose the head of the penis.

    RATIONALE Foreskin interferes with adequate cleansing.

    Continued

Skill 29-4 | **Catheterizing the Male Patient**—cont'd

13. **ACTION** Using forceps and a saturated cotton ball, grasp the glans below the tip with the nondominant hand, hold the penis erect, and cleanse the glans in a circular motion moving outward from the meatus.

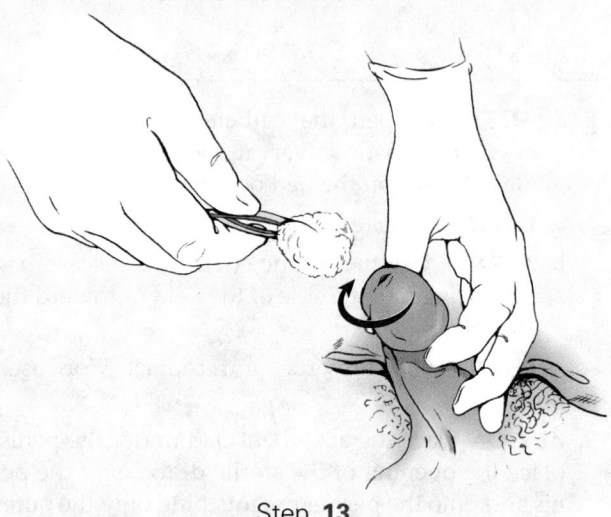

Step **13**

RATIONALE Reduces the number of microorganisms around the meatus.

14. **ACTION** Discard the used cotton ball and cleanse again with two more cotton balls. Continue to hold the shaft of the penis.

RATIONALE Be careful not to cross the sterile field when discarding the used cotton ball because this contaminates the field.

15. **ACTION** Pick up the catheter with the dominant hand 3 to 4 inches (8 to 10 cm) below the tip. With the penis perpendicular to the body, pull it slightly upward, ask the patient to bear down as if trying to urinate, and insert the catheter into the meatus until you reach the catheter bifurcation using a rotating motion. Urine should flow.

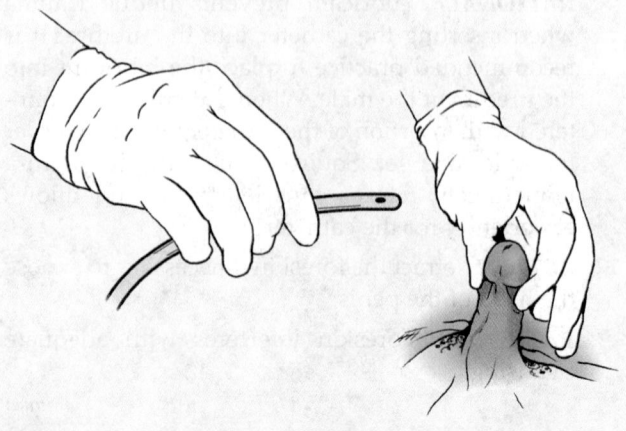

Step **15**

RATIONALE Elevating and putting slight traction on the penis straightens the urethra and makes it easier to insert the catheter into the bladder.

16. **ACTION** If resistance is met, twist the catheter and ask the patient to take a deep breath, and or to turn feet soles inward and wiggle the toes to relax the muscles. If resistance persists and the catheter will not advance without difficulty, remove it and notify the physician.

RATIONALE The internal sphincter relaxes when a deep breath is taken. Forcing the catheter to advance when continued resistance is met may cause trauma.

17. **ACTION** **After urine starts to flow, insert the catheter an additional 1 to 2 inches** and then hold the catheter in place, inject the contents of the prefilled syringe into the balloon, and detach the syringe while holding the plunger all the way down. If the catheter has a prefilled balloon clamp at the drainage end, release it.

RATIONALE Holding the catheter in place guides the balloon away from the sphincter, preventing pressure on the neck of the bladder. Filling the balloon ensures that the catheter will remain in the bladder. Holding down the plunger of the syringe that is used to fill the balloon keeps the water from flowing back into the syringe.

18. **ACTION** Pull gently on the catheter to check that the balloon is inflated. Then push it back in slightly.

RATIONALE Ensures that the catheter will not fall out. Relieves pressure on the internal sphincter.

19. **ACTION** Clean the antiseptic solution from the penis and remove the drape by tearing it toward the penis on one side.

RATIONALE Prevents irritation of the skin and makes the patient comfortable.

20. **ACTION** Reposition the foreskin if it was retracted.

RATIONALE If not repositioned, the foreskin can constrict the penis, causing circulation difficulties and swelling.

21. **ACTION** Tape the catheter to the abdomen if it is to remain in place for an extended period. Alternatively, it may be taped to the top of the thigh for short-term use.

RATIONALE Secures the catheter so there is no tension on the internal urinary sphincter. Taping the catheter to the abdomen helps prevent pressure on the penoscrotal angle.

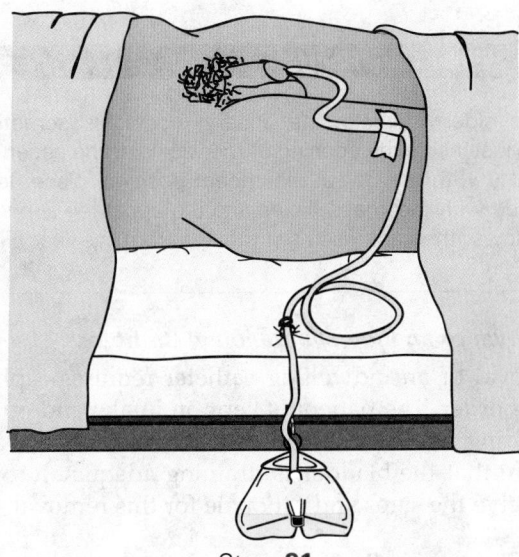

Step **21**

22. *ACTION* Attach the drainage bag to the bed frame (not the side rail). Coil the excess drainage tubing on the mattress and secure it.

RATIONALE The drainage bag must be kept below the level of the bladder for drainage to occur. Tubing should not hang below the level of entry into the bag.

23. *ACTION* Remove the drape, make the patient comfortable, lower the bed, and restore the unit, placing the call light within reach.

RATIONALE Provides for patient comfort and safety.

24. *ACTION* Dispose of used supplies in the appropriate waste container.

RATIONALE Patient's unit wastebasket should not be overfilled with used supplies.

25. *ACTION* Note the initial amount and character of urine in the bag.

RATIONALE Provides output data and a baseline for further assessments of urine character and output.

26. *ACTION* Remove gloves and perform hand hygiene.

RATIONALE Reduces transfer of microorganisms.

■ Evaluation

27. *ACTION* Was sterile technique maintained? Was urine obtained? Were any problems encountered? Would you do anything differently next time?

RATIONALE Questions help determine success of the procedure and ways to improve the technique.

■ Documentation

28. *ACTION* Note date, time, size and type of catheter inserted, amount of water in balloon, any prob-

lems encountered, and amount and character of urine obtained initially.

RATIONALE Documents procedure, catheter size, and amount of water in balloon for future reference.

Documentation Example

2/23 1630   18 Fr. Foley inserted with sterile technique; 10 mL water in balloon. Slight resistance encountered, but catheterization successful. Approximately 300 mL dark yellow, cloudy urine obtained. Bed into lowest position, call light in reach. States is comfortable.

_____

(Nurse's signature)

■ Special Considerations

✓ The ambulatory patient who needs an indwelling catheter may use a leg bag for urine drainage. This needs to be emptied when partially full so that the weight does not become burdensome.

✓ **For Straight Catheterization:** There is no balloon to inflate and no drainage bag. The distal end of the catheter is left in the tray so that the urine will flow into the tray. All urine is drained unless there is an agency policy to clamp the catheter for a time after 800 to 1000 mL has drained. If a specimen is needed, the urine flow is started, and the catheter pinched off with the nondominant hand and then held over the opened sterile specimen container. As soon as an ounce or two of urine is in the specimen container, the catheter is replaced in the tray and the urine is completely drained from the bladder. The catheter is pinched off, removed, and discarded. The urine is measured and the amount entered on the intake and output record. The specimen is labeled and sent to the laboratory.

✓ Catheterization in the home may be a clean technique rather than a sterile one. The patient's bladder should be resistant to the organisms normally found in the home. The drainage bag can be washed in mild soap and water, rinsed, and rinsed again with a solution of 1 part vinegar to 7 parts water to deodorize it. It should be allowed to dry before reuse. Catheters should be washed with mild soap, rinsed well, and allowed to dry before boiling for 20 minutes. Store them in a closed container when dry.

?CRITICAL THINKING QUESTIONS

1. What is the best thing to do if you simply cannot get the catheter into the bladder?

2. What should you do as you inflate the balloon after catheterizing the male patient?

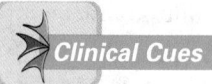

Clinical Cues

If there is difficulty in identifying the urinary meatus, the patient is asked to cough or bear down as if to pass urine. The meatus will usually pucker. If there is still doubt as to which dimple is the meatus, exploring each dimple gently with a sterile cotton swab can aid in identification.

The catheter is taped to the thigh of the female, preferably the inner thigh, and to the top of the thigh or the abdomen of the male. Allow a little slack in the catheter before taping it to the skin so that there is not constant tension on the internal sphincter by the balloon. All patients with an indwelling catheter are placed on intake and output recording.

The perineum is cleaned during the daily bath, and the external portion of the catheter is washed at that time if it is soiled. No special cleansing of the urinary meatus is recommended. Box 29-3 provides suggestions for caring for the patient with an indwelling catheter.

Box 29-3 | *Care of an Indwelling (Foley) Catheter*

- Ensure that the patient takes in adequate fluid to flush bacteria and sediment from the urinary system.
- Maintain a closed drainage system.
- Accurately measure and record the urinary output at least every 8 hours.
- Empty the urine bag via the spout at the bottom, being careful not to contaminate the spout. Wipe the spout with a clean antiseptic swab before returning it to the storage sleeve. Use a separate collection container to empty the bag for each patient.
- Observe the drainage tubing and amount of urine in the bag each time the patient is seen. Keep the drainage tubing above the level of entrance to the collection bag. Check to see that the patient is not lying on the catheter or tubing.
- Keep the drainage bag below the level of the catheter in the bladder. Clamp the tubing before raising the bag above the level of the bladder when moving the patient to avoid backflow into the bladder. (Remember to unclamp the tube after patient is repositioned.)
- Provide perineal care at least twice daily. Cleanse the genitalia and the area around the meatus and 7 to 10 inches down the catheter with soap and rinse well, or follow the agency's policy for cleansing.
- Keep the catheter firmly attached to the leg or to the abdomen of the male to prevent pulling on the catheter at the meatus, which causes irritation.
- Cleanse the insertion site of the suprapubic catheter twice a day according to agency policy.
- Expect at least 30 mL/hr urine output. Less than this is abnormal unless there is a physiologic reason. Check for kinked tubing, bladder distention, or a wet bed. If no reason is found, report the decreased flow to the physician.

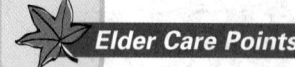

Elder Care Points

In the elderly female, the urinary meatus is sometimes found just inside the opening of the vagina. If the patient has difficulty with the dorsal recumbent position, place her on her side with the knees flexed and the upper leg supported by pillows, then approach the meatus from the rear (Figure 29-9).

Removal of an Indwelling (Foley) Catheter

Removal of an indwelling catheter requires a physician's order. The patient is kept on intake and output recording for 12 to 24 hours after catheter removal to ensure that the bladder is draining adequately. Steps 29-2 give the steps and rationale for this removal.

The Suprapubic Catheter

A suprapubic catheter may be used for urine drainage following gynecologic and bladder surgery. It is inserted through the abdominal wall by the surgeon. The suprapubic catheter is sutured to the skin at the time of insertion (Figure 29-10).

Intermittent Self-Catheterization

Intermittent self-catheterization is used for patients who regularly experience incontinence or urinary retention. In accordance with 2009 National Patient Safety Goals, patients should be taught and encouraged to participate in their own care (Patient Teaching 29-2). Often these patients have a spinal cord problem

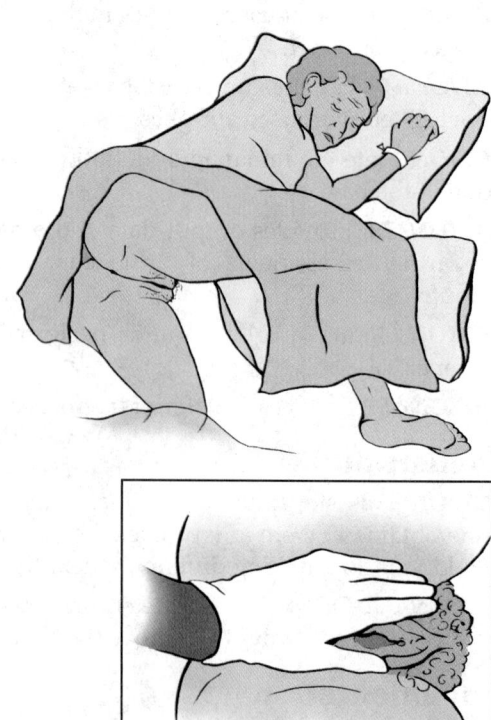

FIGURE **29-9** Side-lying position for catheterization.

Steps 29-2 | Removing an Indwelling Catheter

When the physician writes the order to discontinue the indwelling catheter, the catheter is removed. The catheter and bag should be disposed of in the dirty utility room, not left in the patient's room trashcan.

Review and carry out the Standard Steps in Appendix 3.

1. ***ACTION*** Check the order on the patient's chart.

   RATIONALE Prevents removing a catheter from the wrong patient.

2. ***ACTION*** Obtain a 5- to 10-mL syringe, depending on the size of the balloon noted in the chart and on the balloon port of the catheter, and an absorbent towel.

   RATIONALE The water in the balloon must be withdrawn prior to removing the catheter.

3. ***ACTION*** Perform hand hygiene, don gloves, and check the patient's identi-band while explaining the procedure. Warn the patient that there may be slight discomfort as the catheter is removed.

   RATIONALE Correctly identifies the right patient; reduces fear of the unknown.

4. ***ACTION*** Place the absorbent towel on the mattress under the catheter and attach the syringe to the balloon port. Withdraw the water from the balloon until resistance is met. **Never cut the catheter.**

   RATIONALE Protects the mattress; deflates the balloon. Cutting the catheter will sever the access to the balloon. If the catheter will not come out, it will have to be surgically removed.

5. ***ACTION*** While holding the absorbent towel in your nondominant hand in front of the perineum, pinch off the catheter near the meatus and pull it steadily out onto the absorbent towel until the end is retrieved. It should slip out easily. Hold the catheter at an upward angle to the drainage tubing so that any urine in it will drain into the drainage bag.

   RATIONALE Prevents soiling by spilled urine.

6. ***ACTION*** Inspect the catheter to make certain it is intact. If it is not, notify the physician immediately.

   RATIONALE Ensures that a piece of catheter is not left in the bladder.

7. ***ACTION*** Measure the output in the drainage bag. Enter the output on the input and output record. Empty the urine into the toilet and clean the measuring equipment.

   RATIONALE Adds the urine drainage to the output for the shift. Reduces transfer of microorganisms.

8. ***ACTION*** Remove gloves, perform hand hygiene, and make the patient comfortable. Instruct the patient to drink extra fluid and warn that there may be mild burning with the first few voidings.

   RATIONALE Reduces transfer of microorganisms. Extra fluid helps to flush the bladder. Irritation of the mucosa in the urethra may cause burning with voiding.

9. ***ACTION*** Document the time of removal and time by which patient should have next voided.

   RATIONALE Sets guideline by which all nurses will know when to check to see if the patient has voided.

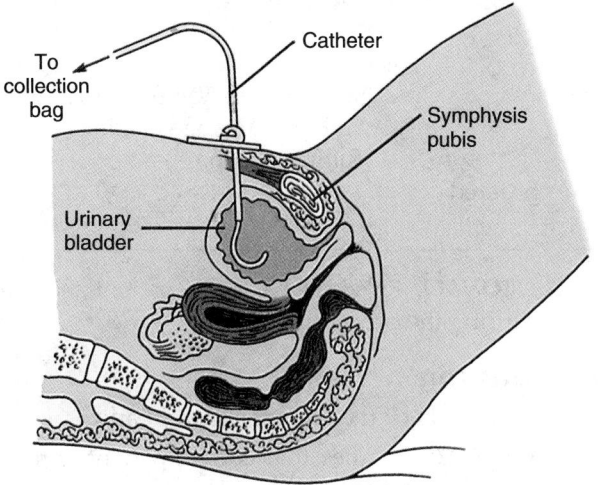

FIGURE **29-10** Suprapubic catheter.

that prevents proper function of the nerves that control the bladder and urinary sphincters. This procedure, most often performed outside of the hospital, is a "clean" rather than a "sterile" procedure and does not require the use of a sterile catheter.

Bladder Irrigation or Instillation

Irrigation or instillation is performed on patients with indwelling catheters to

- Wash out residual urine or sediment from the bladder
- Remove clots and stop oozing of blood after prostate or bladder surgery
- Soothe irritated bladder tissues and promote healing
- Ensure that the lumen of the indwelling catheter is open and draining
- Instill medication into the bladder

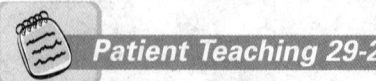

Self-Catheterization

- Catheterize as frequently as necessary to maintain a residual urine volume as indicated by your physician or nurse.
- Gather equipment, use a good light source, and if female, remove a tampon if one is in use.
- Perform hand hygiene.
- Place lubricant on a paper towel. Lubricate the catheter 2 inches for the female; inject lubricant into the meatus for the male. Place supplies within reach.
- Assume a comfortable position such as semi-reclining in bed or sitting on a chair or the toilet. Men may wish to stand.
- Cleanse the urinary meatus with a towelette or a soapy washcloth; rinse with a wet washcloth; pat dry. If female, hold the inner labia open and stroke down and back to prevent fecal contamination of the meatus.

- For the female, locate the meatus by touch. Place the index finger of your nondominant hand on the clitoris. Place the third and fourth fingers at the vaginal opening and locate the meatus between the index and third fingers. Separate the labia.
- For the male, lift the penis to about a 60- to 90-degree angle to straighten the urethra before inserting the catheter.
- With the drainage end over a basin or the toilet, insert the catheter into the meatus. For the female, direct the angle toward the umbilicus. Twist the catheter as you advance it. If resistance is met, take a deep breath while trying to advance the catheter.
- Hold the catheter in place until all urine stops draining.
- Pinch and withdraw the catheter slowly.
- Wash the catheter in warm soapy water, rinse, and dry with a clean towel. Place it in a plastic container. Catheters may be boiled in water for 20 minutes to kill bacteria.

Bladder irrigation or instillation is best done via the injection port on the drainage tubing. The tubing is clamped distal to the port and the medication or solution is introduced via a needle placed in the port. The solution is then allowed to drain. If medication is instilled, the catheter is clamped for a designated period of time before unclamping it so drainage can occur. For irrigation, continue instilling 30 to 50 mL of solution, depending on the medical order, and allow it to drain until the return is clear (Skill 29-5).

? *Think Critically About . . .* The nurse applies a clamp to a urinary catheter after instilling a medication and she forgets to remove the clamp at the designated time. In fact, she leaves the hospital at the end of her shift and never remembered to undo the clamp. What are the patient complications that could result from this error?

Skill 29-5 | Performing Intermittent Bladder Irrigation and Instillation

Bladder or catheter irrigation is performed when the system is clogged and urine will not drain through the catheter. A bladder instillation is performed to place a medicated solution in the bladder. The catheter and drainage system should not be opened for irrigation unless closed irrigation has not corrected the problem.

■ Supplies
✓ Sterile irrigation set
✓ Basin
✓ For open irrigation: Sterile tubing cap

✓ Clean and sterile gloves
✓ Absorbent pad
✓ Antiseptic swabs
✓ Sterile normal saline or ordered irrigation solution

✓ Sterile 30- to 50-mL syringe with a 19- or 23-gauge needle
✓ Tubing clamp

Review and carry out the Standard Steps in Appendix 3.

■ Assessment (Data Collection)
1. **ACTION** Check the order and the patient's care plan.

   RATIONALE Provides data about the type and amount of solution to be used.

2. **ACTION** Determine what the patient knows about bladder irrigation or instillation.

   RATIONALE Provides basis for patient teaching regarding the procedure.

■ Planning
3. **ACTION** Check the patient's identi-band.

   RATIONALE Verifies that correct patient is to receive the irrigation.

4. **ACTION** Gather the equipment and set up the workspace, raising the bed to working height.

RATIONALE Promotes work efficiency and prevents back strain.

5. *ACTION* Plan sufficient time to perform the irrigation without neglecting other patients.

   RATIONALE Demonstrates good work organization.

6. *ACTION* Explain the procedure to the patient.

   RATIONALE Decreases fear of the unknown and enlists the patient's cooperation.

7. *ACTION* Provide privacy by closing the door and/or privacy curtains.

   RATIONALE Protects patient's right to privacy.

■ Implementation

8. *ACTION* Perform hand hygiene and lower the side rail if up.

   RATIONALE Reduces transfer of microorganisms. Eliminates obstacle to reaching work area.

9. *ACTION* Have patient assume a dorsal recumbent position and fan-fold the linen to expose the catheter without exposing the patient. Use a bath blanket to cover the trunk of the body.

   RATIONALE Exposes work area and protects patient's dignity. Keeps the patient from becoming chilled.

10. *ACTION* Check the bladder for distention by palpation.

    RATIONALE Ensures that fluid will not overdistend the bladder.

11. *ACTION* Open the sterile irrigation set and place beside the patient's thigh or between the legs. Maintain sterility.

    RATIONALE Keeps supplies within reach.

12. *ACTION* Place the absorbent pad under the catheter drainage tubing connection, handling only the corners of the pad.

    RATIONALE Provides a field within which to work. Protects the bedding.

13. *ACTION* Don gloves.

    RATIONALE Reduces transfer of microorganisms.

14. *ACTION* For a bladder irrigation or instillation, clamp the drainage tubing distal to the catheter connection.

    RATIONALE Clamping directs the solution toward the bladder and prevents the solution from draining into the collection bag.

15. *ACTION* Determine the amount of urine in the drainage bag before beginning the irrigation.

    RATIONALE The amount of urine must be subtracted from the total drainage at the end of the procedure to determine if all the irrigation solution is returned.

16. *ACTION* Pour 100 to 200 mL of irrigating solution into the sterile container using aseptic technique.

    RATIONALE Amount depends on medical order.

17. *ACTION* Remove the cap from the syringe and draw up 30 to 40 mL of solution while maintaining sterility. Expel any air and attach the sterile needle.

    RATIONALE Thirty to 40 mL of solution at a time is normal for irrigation of the adult bladder. Air in the bladder causes discomfort.

18. *ACTION* With an antiseptic swab, wipe the port on the drainage tubing or the place on the lumen of the catheter for instilling solution.

    RATIONALE Reduces contamination of the system by microorganisms.

19. *ACTION* Insert the needle into the port and gently instill the solution.

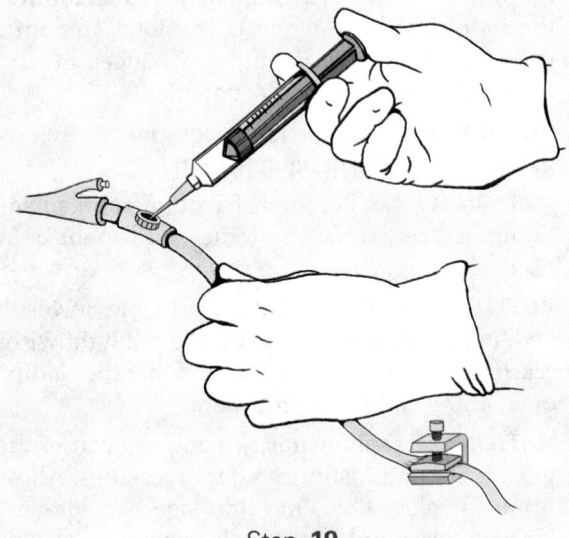

Step **19**

RATIONALE Gentle instillation prevents injury to the lining of the bladder and helps prevent bladder spasms.

20. *ACTION* Remove the needle from the port and cleanse the port with an antiseptic swab. Place the needle and syringe where it will remain sterile.

    RATIONALE Keeps the needle sterile so that the procedure can be repeated until the full amount of irrigant has been instilled.

21. a. *ACTION* For irrigation, immediately unclamp the tubing and lower the catheter so that the fluid runs into the drainage tubing.

      RATIONALE Allows return of the irrigating fluid and any debris that was clogging the catheter.

    b. *ACTION* For a bladder instillation, leave the tubing clamped for the ordered amount of time, then unclamp it and allow the fluid to run into the drainage container.

      RATIONALE Allows medicine to remain in contact with the bladder wall before draining.

Continued

22. **ACTION** Repeat the process until all of the ordered solution has been used or until the catheter is clear and the bladder is draining clear urine.

    RATIONALE Accomplishes purpose of the irrigation or instillation.

23. **ACTION** Empty the urine drainage bag and measure the output. Note the color and characteristics of the drainage. Enter the amount on the intake and output record.

    RATIONALE Irrigation solution must be deducted from the total output to determine actual urine output. Amount of irrigant is entered as input on the input and output sheet. The total amount of drainage is entered as output. Changes in urine color or clarity must be documented.

24. **ACTION** Dispose of used equipment, remove gloves, and perform hand hygiene.

    RATIONALE Reduces transfer of microorganisms. Equipment is no longer sterile and cannot be re-used.

25. **ACTION** Make the patient comfortable, lower the bed, raise side rails, and place the call light within reach. Double check to make sure that the clamp is open at the end of the treatment.

    RATIONALE Demonstrates caring and concern for the patient and institutes safety measures. Allows urine to freely flow into drainage bag; prevents blockage that could damage kidneys.

■ Evaluation

26. **ACTION** Assess for changes in discomfort. Ask yourself: Is the catheter draining properly now? Is the urine clear and without clots?

    RATIONALE Determines whether the procedure was effective.

■ Documentation

27. **ACTION** Note date, time, how irrigated, amount of solution used each time, appearance of return fluid, how patient tolerated the procedure, whether catheter is now patent.

    RATIONALE Verifies ordered procedure was carried out.

Documentation Example

2/24 0930 Foley tubing clamped and catheter irrigated × 4 per orders with 40 mL sterile saline using sterile syringe and needle. Unclamped between irrigations. Return cloudy with debris × 2, then cleared. Draining adequate urine; no bladder distention. Voiced only mild discomfort with first irrigation. Resting comfortably; bed into lowest position, call light in reach.

_____
(Nurse's signature)

Variation: Open System Irrigation

28. **ACTION** After patient and workspace are prepared (Steps 1 through 16 on pp. 568 and 569), perform hand hygiene and don sterile gloves. Be certain there is an order or valid reason for performing an open irrigation.

    RATIONALE Performing hand hygiene and gloving reduces transfer of microorganisms. Catheter drainage system should not be opened unnecessarily.

29. **ACTION** With an antiseptic swab, disinfect the junction of the catheter and drainage tubing.

    RATIONALE Reduces chance of contamination of the lumen of the catheter or drainage tubing.

30. **ACTION** Placing your fingers at least 1 inch from the junction, separate the catheter and tubing and place a sterile tube cap over the end of the drainage tubing.

    RATIONALE Keeps the end of the drainage tubing sterile.

31. **ACTION** Draw the 30- to 40-mL solution into the sterile irrigation syringe (could be a bulb syringe) and carefully fit the irrigation tip into the end of the catheter.

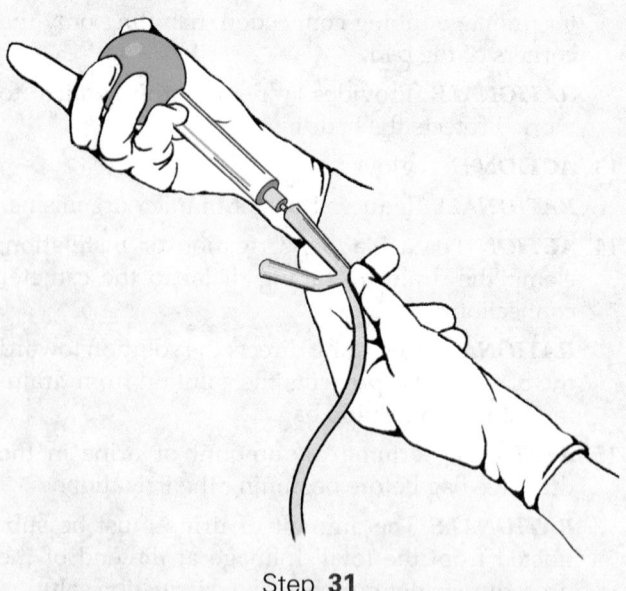

Step **31**

RATIONALE Prepares the solution for instillation.

32. *ACTION* Gently instill the solution into the catheter by squeezing the bulb of the syringe or pressing on the plunger.

RATIONALE Too much force may damage the bladder lining or cause bladder spasms.

33. *ACTION* Remove the syringe and allow the fluid to run from the catheter into the sterile drainage receptacle. Repeat until the fluid is running freely or the purpose of the irrigation is accomplished.

RATIONALE Provides avenue for drainage of fluid. A clogged catheter may take several irrigations before it is unclogged.

34. *ACTION* Carefully remove the cap on the drainage tubing and reattach it to the catheter, keeping both ends sterile. Swab the connection with an antiseptic swab.

RATIONALE Restores the closed drainage system without contaminating either the catheter or the tubing. Removes any leakage of urine.

35. *ACTION* Remove gloves, perform hand hygiene, and follow the remaining steps as for closed irrigation.

RATIONALE Reduces transfer of microorganisms.

■ Special Considerations

✓ When there is no specific solution or amount of solution ordered for the irrigation, check the agency's policy and procedure manual for the accepted protocol.

✓ Although it is always preferable to use a closed irrigation technique, using the open irrigation method in the home is less likely to lead to an infection than if done in the hospital because there are fewer resident microorganisms in the average home.

?CRITICAL THINKING QUESTIONS

1. What may happen if the irrigation solution is introduced into the bladder too rapidly?

2. Where should you clamp the Foley system when doing a closed bladder irrigation?

Continuous irrigation is performed after prostate or bladder surgery via the "three-way" indwelling (Foley) catheter system where the irrigation solution is hooked up to the irrigation port of the catheter. The solution container is positioned on an intravenous (IV) pole. Using sterile technique, solution is run through the tubing to remove air and then the tubing is connected to the irrigation port of the catheter. When using a three-way catheter consult the package instructions to determine which port should be attached to the irrigating solution and which port is designated for the drainage bag connection. (Note: The inner lumen with the largest diameter should be used for the drainage because of the potential for clots or debris that are washed from the bladder.) The third port is for inflating the "balloon" and will appear similar to a standard Foley catheter port. The order is checked for the flow rate. Generally, the irrigation solution is set to flow just fast enough to prevent clots from forming in the bladder (Figure 29-11). The return should be pink to light red. The irrigation solution container is changed at least every 24 hours.

When the drainage system must be opened for irrigation, **strict asepsis must be maintained.** Take special care not to contaminate the end of the drainage tubing or the end of the catheter.

The amount of solution to be introduced is ordered by the physician. If there is no specific amount ordered, follow agency procedure. All irrigation fluid is subtracted from the amount of output.

Assisting the Patient Who Is Incontinent

There are at least six types of incontinence: urge, stress, total, overflow, functional, and reflex (Box 29-4). The effect on the patient is much the same. The incontinent

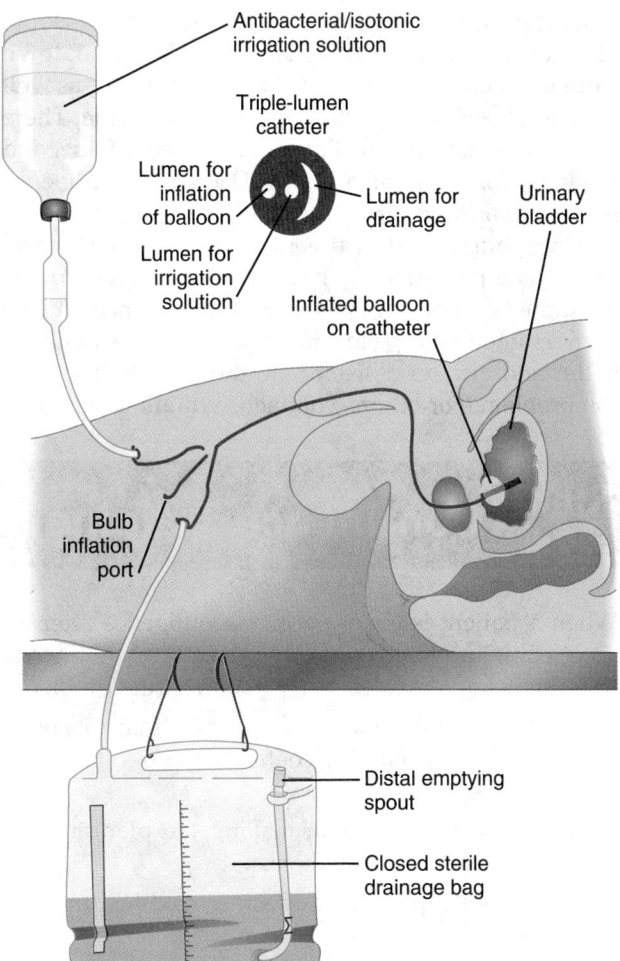

FIGURE **29-11** Continuous bladder irrigation.

Box 29-4 *Types of Incontinence*

- **Urge incontinence:** There is involuntary loss of urine in response to a strong sensation of need to empty the bladder (urinary urgency).
- **Stress incontinence:** There is urethral sphincter failure; often associated with increased intra-abdominal pressure, as occurs with sneezing, laughing, coughing, and aerobic exercise.
- **Total incontinence:** A combination of different types such as stress and urge incontinence.
- **Overflow incontinence:** There is poor contractility of the detrusor muscle of the bladder, obstruction of the urethra as in prostate enlargement in the male, or genital prolapse or abnormality in the female.
- **Functional incontinence:** Caused by cognitive inability to recognize the urge to urinate, extreme depression, or dementia. Inability to reach the bathroom due to restraints, side rails, or an out-of-reach walker can also result in this type of incontinence.
- **Reflex incontinence:** Caused by disorders of the neurologic system such as multiple sclerosis, spinal cord injury, or stroke.

patient suffers a body image disturbance over the loss of a normal function. There is risk of skin breakdown from moisture and waste products in the urine, as well as worry over being wet and smelling of urine. There is also the risk of infection because urine is a good medium for bacterial growth. Urinary incontinence may be temporary or it may be permanent.

Management and treatment of incontinence is complex; some patients may have more than one form of incontinence. For example, stress incontinence is often accompanied by urge incontinence. For some patients, better and quicker assistance to the toilet will resolve the problem. For others, continence training may help

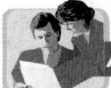

Assignment Considerations 29-1

UAPs Can Assist with Continence Training

If continence training is in progress, time must be planned to work with the patient and the nursing assistant on this task. Instruct the nursing assistant about timed interval toileting and work together as a team to clean up accidents.

(Steps 29-3) (Assignment Considerations 29-1). Regularly performing Kegel exercises may greatly reduce or stop incontinence in patients (Patient Teaching 29-3). Several surgical procedures can be used for patients who choose to correct a specific physiologic problem. For those incontinent patients for whom there is no cure, such as people with neurologic damage that prevents sphincter control, you must help the patient stay dry and clean and preserve his dignity (Legal & Ethical Considerations 29-1). Condom catheters are often used for the incontinent male. Adult briefs containing material similar to diapers are used for females. Absorbent pads similar to sanitary napkins may be used for either sex.

Urinary Diversion Care

Urinary diversion is necessary when the bladder must be removed or bypassed for some reason. When urinary diversion is performed, one or both ureters are implanted into the abdominal wall, the bowel, or a portion of bowel that forms a pouch. When the ureter exits on the abdominal wall, discharging urine through the opening, it is called a **urostomy** (opening through which urine drains). The nurse is concerned with collection of the draining urine and care of the skin around the urostomy. Unless the urostomy is con-

Steps 29-3 | Continence Training

When a patient is experiencing incontinence after an illness or injury that is possibly correctable, continence training is implemented to try to correct the problem.

1. **ACTION** Determine the cause of urinary incontinence and whether a continence program is appropriate.

   RATIONALE Assists in making the plan and increases the chance of success.

2. **ACTION** Keep a record of actual voiding times for 3 days.

   RATIONALE Provides data about the patient's usual voiding times.

3. **ACTION** Establish a 2-hour voiding schedule timed before the patient's usual voiding times.

   RATIONALE Having the patient void prior to bladder overfilling prevents incontinence.

4. **ACTION** Encourage the intake of 2000 to 3000 mL of fluid between awakening and 6 P.M.

   RATIONALE Provides sufficient urine for hydration and scheduled voidings. Stopping liquids at 6:00 P.M. decreases nighttime incontinence.

5. **ACTION** Toilet just before bedtime; do not awaken for toileting except before time when patient has been consistently incontinent during the night.

   RATIONALE Empties the bladder and prevents nighttime incontinence.

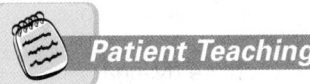

Patient Teaching 29-3

Pelvic Muscle (Kegel) Exercises to Correct Female Incontinence

- Concentrate on stopping the flow of urine when voiding by tightening the pelvic muscles. If you cannot identify the correct muscles this way, place a finger inside your vagina or rectum and try to squeeze around the finger. These are the same muscles you use to stop from expelling gas or a bowel movement. If you are contracting your abdominal muscles, you are doing the exercise incorrectly. Do not hold your breath while contracting and holding.
- To do the exercise, squeeze the muscle you identified and hold for a count of 10 seconds. Relax for a count of 10 seconds. At first you may not be able to hold the contraction for the full 10 seconds. With practice you will build up to the full 10 seconds, usually over a 2-week period.
- Do the exercise three times a day. Try to do 15 repetitions in the morning, 15 in the afternoon, and 20 at night. Or exercise for 10 minutes three times a day. Set a timer. Try to work up to 25 repetitions at one time. It will take at least 2 weeks of consistent exercise to notice a difference. Within a month of regular exercise, you should notice a decrease in instances of incontinence.

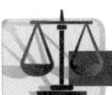

Legal & Ethical Considerations 29-1

Preserving Patients' Dignity and Rights in Toileting

The British Geriatrics Society launched a campaign in April 2007 (Hairon, 2007) that addresses rights and dignity of vulnerable patients to use the toilet in private. In addition, patients deserve to use clean facilities or equipment in a timely, safe fashion, and attention should be given to their views and preferences.

structed with an internal pouch and valve, urine drains constantly. This presents a challenge when changing the urostomy bag. Place a tampon in the opening while you clean the skin and prepare the clean urostomy bag. The urostomy with an internal pouch is emptied by the insertion of a catheter. Urine contains ammonia, which is very irritating to the skin, and a skin barrier is applied before attaching the collection appliance. Because bowel ostomies are more common than urostomies, particulars of skin care and changing the ostomy bag (appliance) are presented in Chapter 30.

Evaluation

Review the expected outcomes written during the planning phase in order to properly evaluate the effectiveness of interventions for the patient's problems.

Determining whether the patient can urinate normally without urgency, dysuria, or frequency, plus a urinalysis performed after treatment is complete or when a Foley catheter is removed, indicates whether infection has been eliminated or avoided. Noting intake and output records and comparing them from day to day indicates whether fluid intake is sufficient and output is adequate. Noting the condition of skin in the perineal area of the patient who has been incontinent provides information as to whether measures to protect the skin are sufficient. Evidence that the patient has had fewer episodes of incontinence over a period of days indicates that the continence training program is helpful. Checking the appearance of the urine for normal characteristics is another evaluation tool.

Obtain feedback for all patient teaching performed. Can the patient tell you measures to take to prevent urinary tract infection? Can the patient needing intermittent catheterization self-catheterize successfully? Does the patient, or the family member of the patient at home, know how to care for the catheter and empty the collection bag properly? Is the patient in the long-term care facility who has functional incontinence now receiving the needed assistance? Nursing Care Plan 29-1 provides some specific examples of evaluative statements for expected outcomes on the plan.

Documentation

When a patient voids normally and without problems in adequate amounts, include a short note of "voiding quantity sufficient." If a patient has been having a problem with some aspect of urinary elimination, the number of voidings per day is charted along with the urinary output and the appearance of the urine. When a patient is catheterized, a note is made regarding the appearance of the urine returned from the catheter and any problems encountered during the procedure. The size and type of catheter are charted and the amount of water instilled in the Foley balloon is noted. A description of the urine should be documented on the computer or chart flow sheet or nurse's notes at least once a day when a patient has an indwelling catheter, along with assessment data that indicate no urinary tract infection is present (unless one was present before the catheter was inserted).

For the incontinent patient, a note regarding the number of times the patient voided normally is made along with a description of the time and circumstances of any incontinent voidings. The assessment of the skin in the perineal area is charted at least once a shift.

Documentation of all patient teaching is done in the nurse's notes or on a patient education flow sheet. All diagnostic tests and specimens obtained and sent to the lab are noted on the daily activity flow sheet. Urostomy care is documented on the flow sheet as well. A note regarding the condition of the stoma and the surrounding skin should be placed in the nurse's notes.

If a bladder irrigation or instillation is performed, it is documented in the nurse's notes stating the amount of solution instilled, whether aseptic technique was maintained, the time the fluid remained in the bladder, the amount and description of the outflow, and any problems encountered. When an indwelling catheter is removed, document the time, date, and amount of urine in the drainage bag. Add a note as to the time by which the patient should void (within 8 hours). Document any problems the patient has voiding after catheter removal.

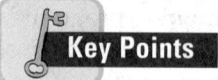 **Key Points**

- The kidneys, ureters, bladder, and urethra make up the urinary system and function to rid the body of waste and excess fluid. Fluid balance is a primary function of the kidneys.
- Infection, severe dehydration, shock, destruction of tissue, blockage, pressure, and lack of neurologic innervation can interfere with proper function of the urinary system.
- Kidney function and bladder muscle tone decrease with age. In males, the prostate gland can enlarge and may lead to urethral obstruction.
- Urination is under voluntary control. The adult voids 5 to 10 times a day, ridding the body of an average of 1000 to 1500 mL urine a day.

- The characteristics of a person's urine can help diagnose or rule out many disorders.
- Symptoms of urinary dysfunction are dysuria, urgency, anuria, polyuria, oliguria, retention, and difficulty starting the urinary stream.
- Urine specimens are obtained in different ways (e.g., clean catch, catheterization) for a variety of diagnostic tests (e.g., culture and sensitivity).
- An indwelling urinary catheter is inserted for a variety of reasons (e.g., urinary stricture, bladder irrigation). The closed urinary catheter and drainage system should be kept sterile.
- It is best to perform closed intermittent irrigation, rather than opening the drainage system, to prevent microorganisms from entering the bladder.
- There are at least six types of incontinence (e.g., functional, stress, urge).
- When the patient has a urinary diversion, the focus is on collection of the urine and care of the skin around the urostomy.
- Comparison of daily intake and output is a part of the evaluation process.

 Go to your **Companion CD-ROM** for an Audio Glossary, animations, video clips, and more.

evolve Be sure to visit the companion Evolve site at http://evolve.elsevier.com/deWit/fundamental/ for additional online resources.

NCLEX-PN® EXAMINATION-STYLE REVIEW QUESTIONS

*Choose the **best** answer(s) for each question.*

1. A patient underwent a hernia repair in the same-day surgery department. He is awake and alert, but has not been able to void since he returned from surgery 4 hours ago. He cannot be discharged until he voids. He has had 1000 mL of IV fluid. Which intervention would be the most likely to help this patient to urinate?
   1. Give more liquids by mouth.
   2. Wait a least 3 more hours.
   3. Assist him to stand by the side of the bed to void.
   4. Call the physician and obtain an order for a Foley catheter.

2. The physician prescribes phenazopyridine HCl (Pyridium) for a patient with cystitis. What is a correct teaching point for this medication?
   1. The medication helps to flush the bladder.
   2. The medication acidifies the urine.
   3. The medication turns the urine orange or red.
   4. The medication prevents resistance to organisms.

3. The nurse is obtaining a urine specimen for a patient who has an existing Foley catheter. Below are the steps for the procedure. Place these steps (1 though 6) in the correct order.
   _____ 1. Wipe the aspiration port of the drainage tubing with an alcohol pad.

   _____ 2. Aspirate 3 mL of urine by gently pulling back on the plunger.
   _____ 3. Clamp the catheter below the aspiration port.
   _____ 4. Empty the syringe into the sterile container; needle should not touch the container.
   _____ 5. Close and label the container. Unclamp the catheter.
   _____ 6. Insert a 25-gauge needle attached to a syringe into the aspiration port.

4. Which statement by the patient indicates a need for additional patient teaching about cystitis?
   1. "I should increase fluids, including orange and grapefruit juice."
   2. "I should avoid use of bubble bath and feminine hygiene sprays."
   3. "I should empty my bladder every 2 to 3 hours."
   4. "I should wipe my perineal area from front to back."

5. The nurse has just collected a midstream urine specimen from a patient. Which urine characteristic would be of the greatest concern?
   1. Urine smells slightly of ammonia.
   2. Urine is an amber color.
   3. Urine is slightly cloudy.
   4. Urine is dark brown.

6. A patient in a long-term facility has a retention catheter in place. The nurse identifies Risk for infection as a nursing diagnosis. Which urine abnormality supports the choice of this diagnosis?

   1. Glycosuria
   2. Ketonuria
   3. Presence of casts
   4. Presence of bilirubin

7. A patient is admitted with urinary retention. There is an order to insert a Foley catheter into his bladder. He attempts to void and passes 100 mL of urine. Before catheterization, the nurse should:

   1. use a condom catheter with a leg bag.
   2. wait 2 hours and have him try to void again.
   3. have him drink 2 to 3 glasses of water.
   4. perform a bladder scan to determine amount of urine retained.

8. The nurse is catheterizing a male patient, who is confused. He moves several times during the procedure despite repeated verbal instructions to remain calm, quiet, and still. Which nursing diagnosis is the priority related to the presence of the catheter for this patient?

   1. Risk for injury
   2. Risk for infection
   3. Noncompliance
   4. Deficient knowledge

9. The nurse is catheterizing a male patient. Resistance is met. The nurse should:

   1. apply more pressure with a twisting motion to insert the catheter.
   2. obtain a new sterile kit and try again with a sterile Coudé catheter.
   3. ask him to take a deep breath and slowly exhale as the catheter is inserted.
   4. discontinue the procedure and try again after the patient relaxes.

10. A fracture pan is generally used for a patient who has:

    1. bowel and bladder incontinence.
    2. musculoskeletal problems.
    3. obesity and immobility.
    4. weakness and cardiac failure.

11. Which urine characteristic suggests that the patient might be dehydrated?

    1. Urine specific gravity of 1.035
    2. Urine pH of 6.0
    3. Urine is straw colored
    4. Urine is positive for bilirubin

12. The patient complains of urinary frequency, urgency, and burning. Which nursing action should be done *first?*

    1. Obtain an order for a urinalysis.
    2. Check the patient's temperature.
    3. Encourage the patient to take fluids.
    4. Notify the RN or the MD about the problem.

13. The purpose of clamping the catheter tubing when irrigating the bladder is to:

    1. prevent urine from draining into the bag.
    2. hold the solution in the bladder.
    3. prevent the solution from going directly into the bag.
    4. prevent urine from being drawn back into the catheter.

14. Which of the following statements by the patient indicates that she understands how to perform the clean-catch method for a urine specimen?

    1. "I should clean my genital area first, pee into the cup, and then re-clean myself."
    2. "I should fill the cup completely and save it in the refrigerator."
    3. "I should keep the contents of the kit sterile at all times."
    4. "I should clean myself first, pee a little into the toilet, and then pee into the cup."

15. The patient had a resection of the prostate gland yesterday and has a three-way catheter for continuous irrigation. The draining urine is very red. This means that the nurse needs to:

    1. notify the physician immediately.
    2. increase the rate of flow of the irrigation solution.
    3. increase his fluid intake to 4000 mL per 24 hours.
    4. empty the drainage bag to prevent clotting.

16. A 24-hour urine specimen is ordered for a patient. The UAP discards some of the urine that should have been saved. Which is the most appropriate nursing action?

    1. Verbally reprimand the nursing assistant.
    2. Make a note to extend the urine collection period.
    3. Continue the urine collection and label the specimen.
    4. Notify the RN about the incident and restart the test.

17. A nurse is caring for a patient who is incontinent. What is the priority action?

    1. Assist the patient to void every 2 hours.
    2. Decrease the fluid intake, especially in the evening.
    3. Gather data to find the cause of incontinence.
    4. Encourage expression of feelings such as embarrassment.

CRITICAL THINKING ACTIVITIES *Read each clinical scenario and discuss the questions with your classmates.*

Scenario A

What assessment data would you need to determine whether the patient has a urinary tract infection?

Scenario B

How would you explain to a patient what a catheterization procedure is like?

Scenario C

What measures would you use to assist a patient to urinate?

Objectives

Upon completing this chapter, you should be able to:

Theory

1. Describe the process of normal bowel elimination.
2. Identify abnormal characteristics of stool.
3. Discuss the physiologic effects of hypoactive bowel and nursing interventions to assist patients with constipation.
4. List safety considerations related to giving a patient an enema.
5. Describe three types of intestinal diversions.
6. Discuss the stoma and peristomal assessment and skin care.
7. Discuss the psychosocial implications for a patient who has an ostomy.

Clinical Practice

1. Use nursing measures to promote regular bowel elimination in patients.
2. Collect a stool specimen.
3. Perform a focused assessment of the bowel.
4. Assist RN in identifying appropriate nursing diagnoses for a patient with bowel problems.
5. Prepare to administer an enema.
6. Assist and teach the patient who is incontinent with a bowel retraining program.
7. Provide ostomy care, including irrigation and changing the ostomy appliance.
8. Assist a patient to catheterize a continent diversion.

Skills & Steps

Skills

Skill 30-1 Administering an Enema
Skill 30-2 Changing an Ostomy Appliance

Steps

Steps 30-1 Removal of a Fecal Impaction
Steps 30-2 Catheterizing a Continent Ileostomy
Steps 30-3 Irrigating a Colostomy

Key Terms

Be sure to check out the bonus material on the Companion CD-ROM, including selected audio pronunciations.

anus (Ā-nŭs, p. 577)
appliances (p. 590)
atrophy (Ā-trō-fē, p. 577)

bile (p. 578)
bowel training program (p. 588)
chyme (KĪM, p. 577)
colostomy (kŏ-LŎS-tō-mē, p. 590)
constipation (p. 578)
defecate (DĔF-ē-kāt, p. 577)
diarrhea (dī-ā-RĒ-ā, p. 580)
effluent (ē-FLŪ-ĕnt, p. 590)
excoriation (ĕks-kŏr-ē-Ā-shŭn, p. 584)
fecal impaction (FĒ-kăl ĭm-PĂK-shŭn, p. 579)
fecal incontinence (ĭn-KŎN-tĭ-nĕns, p. 580)
feces (FĒ-sēz, p. 577)
flatus (FLĀ-tŭs, p. 579)
gastrocolic reflex (găs-trō-KŎL-ĭk RĒ-flĕks, p. 577)
hemorrhoid (HĔM-ō-rŏyd, p. 578)
ileostomy (ĭl-ē-ŏ-ŎS-tō-mē, p. 590)
melena (MĔL-ĕh-nă, p. 578)
occult (ō-KŬLT, p. 578)
ostomy (ŎS-tō-mē, pp. 576, 590)
periostomal (pĕr-ĭ-Ō-stō-mŭl, p. 592)
peristalsis (pĕr-ĭ-stăl-sis, p. 577)
rectum (RĔK-tŭm, p. 577)
sphincter (SFĪNK-tĕr, p. 577)
steatorrhea (STĒ-ā-tō-RĒ-ā, p. 578)
stoma (STŌ-mă, p. 590)
stool (p. 576)
vagal response (VĀ-găl rĕ-SPŎNS, p. 588)
Valsalva maneuver (văl-SĂL-vă mă-NŪ-vĕr, p. 577)

The term *bowel* refers to the intestine. Bowel elimination, the excretion of solid waste, is the final step in the process of digestion. The processing of nutrients through digestion was discussed in Chapter 26. In this chapter, normal functions of the intestinal tract are reviewed and conditions that affect the composition and appearance of stool (waste eliminated from the colon) are discussed. Ways to assist the patient in achieving and maintaining regular elimination of waste matter from the bowel and procedures to alleviate problems related to alterations in elimination are presented. When an alternative for waste elimination is needed due to disease of the intestine, an ostomy (opening into the intestine) may be performed. The basic nursing care for such a procedure completes this chapter.

OVERVIEW OF STRUCTURE AND FUNCTION OF THE INTESTINAL SYSTEM

Which structures of the intestinal system are involved in waste elimination?

- The small intestine—consisting of the duodenum, the jejunum, and the ileum—carries chyme (liquefied food and digestive juices) from the stomach to the large intestine.

- The small intestine attaches to the large intestine at the cecum. The ileocecal valve controls the progress of substances into the large intestine.

- The large intestine has four main portions: the ascending colon, transverse colon, descending colon, and sigmoid colon. It is larger in diameter than the small intestine but only about 1.5 m (59.5 inches) long (Figure 30-1).

- The rectum (distal portion of the large intestine where feces are stored) connects to the anus (opening of the rectum at the skin).

- The walls of the intestines have four layers: mucosa, submucosa, muscular layer, and a serous layer called serosa.

What are the functions of the intestines?

- The small intestine further processes chyme into a more liquid state. Food substances are absorbed into the bloodstream from the villi on the walls of the small intestine.

- In the large intestine, water, sodium, and chlorides are reabsorbed and waste material is propelled to the anus.

- The large intestine contains bacteria that break down waste products. Water is extracted from the waste during transit.

- Peristalsis (wavelike movement through the intestines) moves chyme and gas formed by bacterial action through the intestines. The circular, longitudinal, and oblique muscle layers of the intestine expand and contract to accommodate and move the chyme.

- The movement of liquid and gas causes the rumbling noise of bowel sounds. It takes about 18 to 72 hours for food to move from the mouth to the anus.

- Feces (intestinal waste material) is stored in the sigmoid until it moves into the rectum for expulsion through the anus.

- As the rectum fills, the pressure on the sphincter (circular muscle that closes an orifice) of the anus increases until the urge to defecate (expel feces) occurs.

- The abdominal muscles contract to help force the evacuation of the rectum.

- The internal anal sphincter, located at the top of the anal canal, is under involuntary control; the external sphincter at the end of the anal canal is controlled voluntarily.

- The gastrocolic (stomach to colon) reflex initiates peristalsis, which in turn initiates the urge to defecate; it is stimulated by eating. Reflex emptying of the rectum can be stopped by tightening the voluntary anal sphincter.

- Intra-abdominal pressure increases when a person holds the breath, closes the glottis, and tightens the abdominal muscles. This initiates voluntary defecation and is called the Valsalva maneuver.

- The vermiform appendix attaches to the cecum of the ascending colon and has no known digestive function.

What effect does aging have on the intestinal tract?

- Atrophy (decrease in size) of the villi in the small intestine may decrease the total absorptive surface. It has not been proven that decreased absorption of nutrients, other than fats and vitamin B$_{12}$, actually occurs.

- Sometimes twisting of blood vessels supplying the large intestine compromises the blood flow to the large intestine. Motility in the large intestine may decrease in some individuals, but bowel habits do not change with aging in the healthy individual.

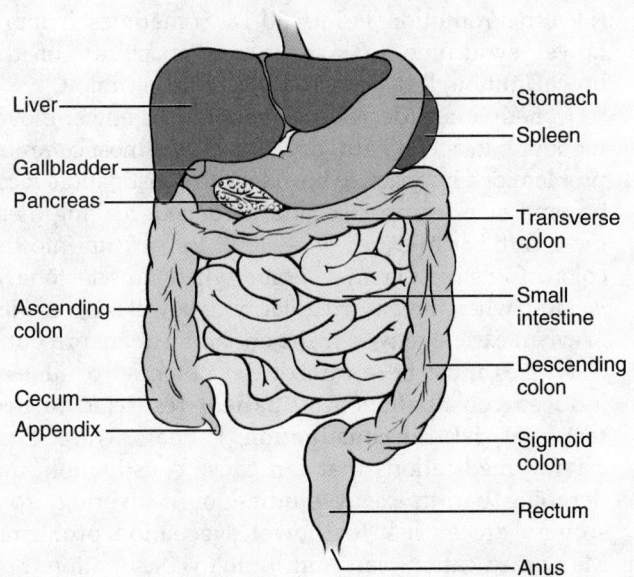

FIGURE **30-1** The intestinal system.

CHARACTERISTICS OF STOOL

Stool is another term for *feces*. Normal feces are one quarter solid material and three quarters water. The solid material consists of about 30% dead bacteria and 70% undigested roughage from carbohydrate, fat, protein, and inorganic matter. The appearance of stool is influenced by diet and metabolism.

NORMAL CHARACTERISTICS OF STOOL

Normal stool is light to dark brown, soft, and formed in children and adults. Infant stool may be a dark yellow depending on the type of feedings. The light to dark brown color is caused by bile (orange or yellow digestive fluid produced by the liver). The color of feces may be changed by certain vitamins, drugs, or diet. Stool is usually tubular in shape and has a diameter of about 2.5 cm (1 inch).

ABNORMAL CHARACTERISTICS OF STOOL

The most serious abnormality is blood in the stool. Fresh blood in the stool is easily visible as bright red on the surface of the stool. Occult (hidden) or old blood is suspected when the stool changes from a normal brown appearance to a dark black color with a sticky appearance. The observance of blood in the stool should be reported promptly and recorded on the patient's chart.

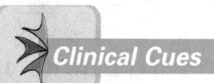
Clinical Cues

A small amount of bleeding from a hemorrhoid (an enlarged vein inside or just outside the rectum) or an irritation caused by straining to defecate may clear up without any treatment. Ask your patient to describe the color and appearance of the stool. For example, formed brown stool (normal) that has small streaks of red blood on the outer surface of the stool suggests that the blood is associated with a hemorrhoid.

Serious causes of blood in the stool include hemorrhage from ulcers in the stomach or duodenum; severe inflammation or irritation, as in ulcerative colitis or diverticulitis; cancer; and other diseases that cause hemorrhage. Collection of a stool specimen and testing for occult blood are presented in Chapter 24.

Bright red blood in the stool is a sign of a recent gastrointestinal (GI) hemorrhage or bleeding that occurred in the large intestine. The color indicates that the blood has not undergone digestion in the upper part of the bowel, nor has it been in the intestinal tract for hours. As blood moves through the stomach or small intestine, it undergoes partial digestion, which changes it to a dark, tarry substance (melena). Eating beets may make the stool appear red, but this should not be confused with blood.

Pale white or light gray stool indicates an absence of bile in the intestine. This is usually due to an obstruction in the bile or common duct leading to the intestine from the liver and gallbladder. This finding should be reported to the physician.

Other abnormal characteristics of feces are the presence of large amounts of mucus, fat, pus, or parasites, such as worms. Unusual amounts of mucus in the stool indicate an irritation or inflammation of the inner surface of the intestines. The mucus coats the stool and gives it a slimy appearance. The presence of pus indicates drainage of an ulcer that is inflamed or infected. The most common parasitic worms found in the intestines are the tapeworm, pinworm, and roundworm. Stools with an abnormally high fat content (steatorrhea) are usually foul smelling and float on water.

The first signs of colorectal cancer are changes in bowel patterns and stool characteristics; in accordance with the *Healthy People 2010* goal (3.5) to reduce colorectal cancers, patients should be encouraged to report these changes and to participate in colon cancer screening programs.

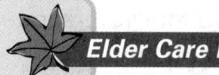
Elder Care Points

Because cancer of the colon is a common problem of the elderly, all people over age 50 should undergo sigmoidoscopy at regular intervals.

HYPOACTIVE BOWEL AND CONSTIPATION

An absence or reduction of peristaltic movement of the bowel results in a hypoactive bowel. Some injuries and diseases cause a hypoactive bowel, but often this condition is a complication of immobility. In the normal person, lack of sufficient fiber in the diet and decreased exercise may produce a sluggish or hypoactive bowel (Health Promotion Points 30-1). Sometimes irritable bowel syndrome (IBS) causes hypoactivity of the bowel, although hyperactivity is more common.

Constipation (decreased frequency of bowel movement or passage of hard, dry feces) is the most common problem of a hypoactive bowel. With constipation, feces become more compacted and hardened, making them more difficult to expel. Feces tend to back up into the colon. Constipation may occur when muscle tone is lacking, when there is irregularity of bowel movements, or when excessive worry, anxiety, and fear are present.

Nurses must be aware of the potential of illness-induced constipation. **Any patient restricted to bed rest is at risk for constipation.** Patients who are receiving medications that can cause constipation, undergoing barium x-ray studies, or recovering from surgery are at risk for bowel evacuation problems. Many medications can contribute to constipation (Box 30-1). It is extremely important that every nurse be

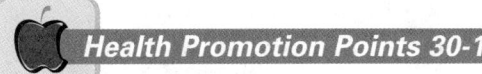

Health Promotion Points 30-1

Promoting Regular Bowel Elimination

Instruct the patient to do the following:

• Pay attention to the urge to defecate; frequently postponing defecation interferes with normal bowel evacuation and can lead to constipation.
• Eat a diet high in fiber. Foods that provide fiber are bran, whole-grain cereals, nuts, prunes, and other raw fruits and vegetables; cooked vegetables provide some fiber. Avoid excessive amounts of constipating foods such as cheese, pasta, eggs, and lean meat.
• Drink at least eight 8-oz glasses of liquid per day.
• Exercise every day; walking is very good for bowel function.
• Attempt to defecate when the gastrocolic reflex is strongest (e.g., after breakfast).
• Use aids such as a hot cup of coffee, hot water and lemon juice, or prune juice to aid defecation.
• Establish a pattern by attempting defecation at the same time each day.

Box 30-1 | *Medications that May Cause or Contribute to Constipation*

• **Narcotic analgesics,** especially codeine, morphine, and meperidine, depress central nervous system (CNS) activity and slow peristalsis.
• **General anesthetics** slow peristalsis by depressing CNS activity.
• **Diuretics** rid the body of fluid.
• **Sedatives** slow CNS activity and peristalsis.
• **Antidepressants** alter CNS activity, and have a drying effect.
• **Anticholinergics** interfere with muscle activation, causing decreased tone in and motility of the gastrointestinal tract and have drying effects.
• **Calcium channel blockers** (verapamil [Calan]) cause a blockade of calcium channels, which affects the smooth muscle of the intestine.

---

alert to patients at risk for constipation in order to prevent its occurrence (Concept Map 30-1).

Abdominal distention is caused by flatus (gas) accumulation in the intestinal tract when peristalsis is reduced or absent. Just as fecal matter will collect in the hypoactive bowel, so will flatus. Distention and gas pains occur frequently after abdominal surgery. The discomfort and pain are caused by the stretching of the intestinal wall and spasm of the muscle layers.

?*Think Critically About . . .* Your elderly female patient had abdominal surgery yesterday. You need to know when she starts passing gas and the frequency and consistency of bowel movements, but she says she would be too embarrassed to talk about this even with a nurse. What could you say to her?

Elder Care Points

• Elderly people who live alone tend to eat more processed convenience foods and do not take in sufficient fiber to prevent constipation; diet alterations should be considered.
• Many elderly patients decrease fluid intake because they have urinary urgency or stress incontinence. The underlying problem may have to be addressed to establish better fluid intake and softer stool.
• Elderly people who have been regularly taking mineral oil to aid evacuation must be told that mineral oil interferes with vitamin absorption. Bulk-forming laxatives containing psyllium are a better choice. Products such as Metamucil and FiberCon are readily available without prescription. **A large amount of fluid should be taken with these products to prevent constipation and** fecal impaction (rectum and sigmoid colon become filled with hardened fecal material). Box 30-2 lists common medications used for constipation.

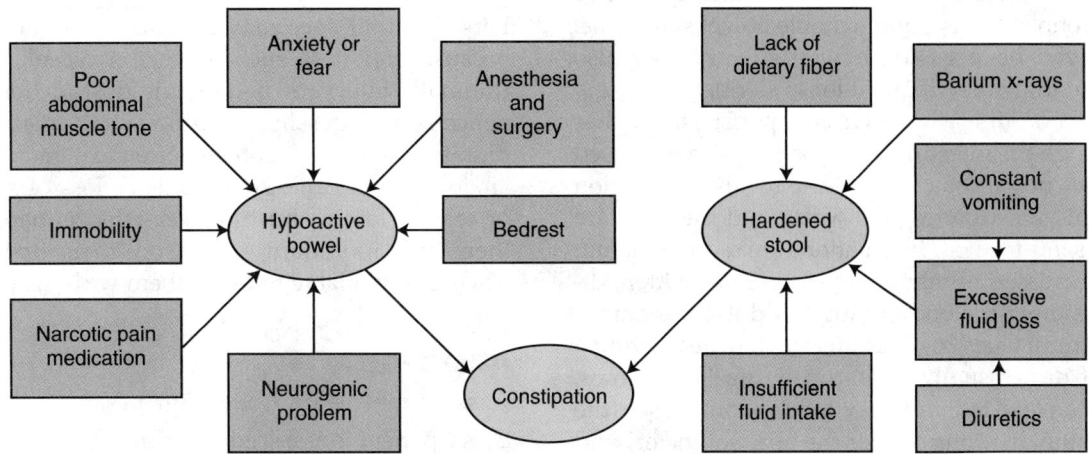

CONCEPT MAP **30-1** Factors contributing to constipation.

> **Box 30-2** *Common Medications Used for Constipation or Diarrhea*

MEDICATIONS USED FOR CONSTIPATION

Stool Softeners
- Docusate sodium (Colace)
- Docusate calcium (Surfak)
- Docusate potassium (Dialose)
- Polyethylene glycol–electrolyte solution (MiraLax)

Bulk-Forming Laxatives
- Polycarbophil (FiberCon)
- Psyllium (Metamucil)
- Methylcellulose (Citrucel)

Irritant or Stimulant Laxatives
- Bisacodyl (Dulcolax)
- Cascara sagrada
- Castor oil (Neoloid)
- Phenolphthalein (Ex-Lax, Correctol)
- Senna (Senokot)

Saline Laxatives
- Citrate of magnesia
- Magnesium hydroxide (Milk of Magnesia)
- Sodium phosphate (Phospho-Soda)

New Laxative for Chronic Constipation
- Lubiprostone (Amitiza)

MEDICATIONS USED FOR DIARRHEA (ANTIDIARRHEALS)
- Diphenoxylate hydrochloride with atropine sulfate (Lomotil)
- Loperamide hydrochloride (Imodium)
- Difenoxin hydrochloride with atropine sulfate (Motofen)
- Paregoric
- Opium tincture

HYPERACTIVE BOWEL AND DIARRHEA

An increase in motility of the gastrointestinal tract or increased peristalsis results in a hyperactive bowel. Causes of a hyperactive bowel include inflammation in the gastrointestinal tract, certain drugs, infectious agents, and diseases such as diverticulitis, ulcerative colitis, Crohn's disease, and irritable bowel syndrome. Patients who have gastric bypass surgery may also experience diarrhea (frequent loose stool).

Diarrhea occurs when increased peristalsis pushes food through the intestinal tract too fast. The increased speed does not allow enough time for the absorption of nutrients, electrolytes, and water, and the feces are liquid or semi-formed. Evacuations are more frequent, with an increased number of stools per day. Often, diarrhea is simply the body trying to rid itself of pathogens (Cultural Cues 30-1). Moderate diarrhea lasting a couple of days usually clears up by itself. At times, diarrhea can lead to temporary fecal incontinence (the lack of voluntary control over the anal sphincter) and inability to retain feces. See Box 30-2 for a list of common antidiarrheal medications.

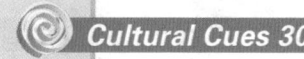
Cultural Cues 30-1

Hand Hygiene to Prevent Diarrhea

Two million children die of diarrheal disease each year. Preventing transmission of diarrheal organisms through good handwashing is essential. Scott et al. (2007) conducted a study to determine motivators for handwashing in Ghana. They found that nurturance, social acceptance, and disgust of feces, latrines, and smells were motivators. However, protection from disease was not a key motivator! Use of culturally relevant information is important when conducting patient teaching even for basic measures such as good handwashing.

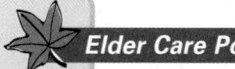
Elder Care Points

- The elderly patient becomes dehydrated more quickly than younger adults. Observe closely for signs of dehydration and fluid imbalance when diarrhea occurs. Commercial beverages such as Gatorade that contain sodium and potassium taken in small amounts (1 to 2 oz at a time) will help replace electrolytes if the patient has continuing diarrhea. If the person becomes confused as well as dehydrated, a trip to the emergency room for fluid replacement may be necessary.
- Sometimes diarrhea may be caused by spoiled food if the patient forgets how long something has been in the refrigerator or forgets to place leftovers into the refrigerator in a timely manner after a meal.

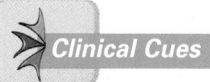
Clinical Cues

The bowel can be rested by consuming only clear liquids and avoiding solid food for a day or two. Resumption of solid foods should begin with bland, low-fiber foods, gradually adding other foods as the diet is tolerated. Cottage cheese, gelatin, applesauce, and bananas are usually tolerated well.

FECAL INCONTINENCE

Persons of all ages may become incontinent of feces because of illness such as cerebrovascular accident, traumatic injury, or neurogenic dysfunction. Incontinence is a distressing condition that causes a loss of dignity. Incontinent patients often feel embarrassed or anxious. They can also experience loss of self-respect or fear of loss of control over what is happening to them. It is important to reassure them that there are programs available to assist them with the problem.

APPLICATION of the NURSING PROCESS

Assessment (Data Collection)

Every patient is assessed regarding bowel status every day in an inpatient facility. Home care nurses assess bowel status at each visit. The patient is questioned

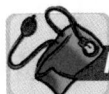

Focused Assessment 30-1

Assessment of the Bowel

Whether or not the patient has a bowel problem, the following points should be considered or questions asked:

HISTORY

- Determine the usual bowel pattern, time of defecation, and measures used to promote defecation, if any (e.g., a cup of coffee, breakfast, dose of Metamucil).
- Inquire about use of enemas, laxatives, suppositories, and stool softeners.
- Assess for changes in stool characteristics: alternating diarrhea and constipation, changes in shape of stool, changes in color of stool, stool floating in commode, foul odor.
- Determine usual eating habits and dietary intake. Is there sufficient fiber in the diet? Does the patient drink sufficient fluids?
- How much exercise does the patient get?
- Is the patient taking medications that are constipating or that may cause diarrhea?
- Does the patient have a chronic disorder that contributes to constipation or diarrhea?

- Has there been any exposure to parasites or helminths (especially travel outside the United States)?
- Does diarrhea occur after eating milk products (may indicate lactose intolerance)?
- Does diarrhea occur after eating wheat and other gluten products (may indicate sprue or gluten intolerance)?
- Does the patient have any food sensitivities? Do spicy foods cause gas discomfort or diarrhea?
- Has incontinence been brought on by a neurologic condition or cerebrovascular accident?
- Is the incontinent patient receptive to a bowel training program?

PHYSICAL ASSESSMENT

- Observe the shape of the abdomen with the patient supine.
- Auscultate for bowel sounds in all four quadrants.
- Percuss for presence of excessive air/gas in the bowel.
- Gently palpate for masses or tenderness in all four quadrants.

---

about the regularity of bowel evacuation, problems, and any abnormal characteristics in the appearance of the stool. If possible, the stool is visually examined. Focused Assessment 30-1 provides guidelines for bowel assessment. Many people think that it is abnormal not to have a bowel movement every day, but it is normal for many people to have a bowel movement only every 2 to 3 days. Look at all the factors that affect bowel function and the patient's normal pattern before determining whether there is a problem (Cultural Cues 30-2).

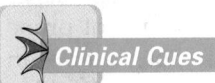

Place the patient in a supine position. Auscultate for bowel sounds in all four quadrants. Absent or few bowel sounds indicate decreased motility and potential for constipation, or may signal an abnormal bowel blockage. Active bowel sounds are associated with the increased motility that occurs after eating. Hyperactive sounds can occur with diarrhea.

Distention is revealed by an abdomen that is rounder and tighter in appearance than normal. The patient's abdomen is assessed for distention by percussion, and the nurse gently palpates the four quadrants of the abdomen to check for tenderness and masses. The patient may complain of abdominal discomfort and often describes it as gas pain. Percussion is used to detect abnormal amounts of gas. Areas of gas produce a drum-like, hollow tone. Review assessment of the abdomen in Chapter 22.

Cultural Cues 30-2

Cultural Use of Laxatives

If your patient is from the Central African Republic (D'Avanzo & Geissler, 2003), there is a culture-based practice of using laxatives to "wash out illness." Assess your patient for any excessive use of laxatives that could lead to electrolyte imbalances.

Nursing Diagnosis

When assessment data indicate an intestinal problem, the correct nursing diagnosis is chosen from the NANDA-I list. Possible choices are as follows:

- Constipation related to hypoactive bowel
- Diarrhea related to food intolerance
- Bowel incontinence related to loss of anal sphincter control
- Pain related to abdominal distention
- Self-care deficit, toileting related to traction
- Disturbed body image related to bowel incontinence
- Deficient knowledge related to factors that contribute to constipation

The full diagnosis is written using the related cause particular to each patient.

Planning

A plan is developed for the patient's care by writing expected outcomes for each nursing diagnosis chosen. Outcomes must be realistic and can be both short and

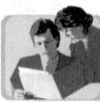

Assignment Considerations 30-1

Patient Ambulation

The task of assisting with ambulation is frequently assigned to the nursing assistant. If the patient is resistant to the idea of getting out of bed or ambulating, support the nursing assistant by giving the patient some concrete examples of the benefits (e.g., getting up and walking decreases the risk of pneumonia, deep vein thrombosis, pressure ulcers, and constipation). Remember to thank the assistant for his hard work and contributions to the patient's well-being.

Cultural Cues 30-3

Toileting Practices

Using a bedpan, a bedside commode, or even a typical American-style toilet may be unfamiliar or uncomfortable to your patient, because in many other countries, squatting is a more typical position for elimination. A careful cultural assessment will help to identify potential issues. With the help of a translator, explain the use and purpose of required and available equipment.

long term. Sample expected outcomes for the previous nursing diagnoses are as follows:

- Constipation will be relieved by walking a mile a day.
- Episodes of diarrhea will decrease within 3 days.
- Patient will improve bowel control within 2 months of starting a retraining program.
- Pain from distention will be decreased within 24 hours.
- Patient will maintain as much independence as possible in toileting by using an over-the-bed trapeze and a urinal during this shift.
- Body image will improve as incontinence lessens.
- Patient will identify foods to add to diet to increase fiber during this shift.

See Nursing Care Plan 30-1 for further examples of expected outcomes.

Another aspect of planning is to provide time in the shift work schedule for the administration of ordered treatments such as enemas. Time must be planned to carry out a bowel retraining program if that is part of the care plan for the incontinent patient. When an incontinent patient is assigned, more time must be allotted for attempts at toileting and for cleaning the patient (Assignment Considerations 30-1).

Implementation

You must assist the bed rest patient with use of the bedpan or bedside commode. **Privacy is of great importance in making the patient comfortable enough to defecate.** Patients are often embarrassed by the

Safety Alert 30-1

Side Rails Can Be Hazardous

Side rails are intended to be a safety measure; however, studies (Capezuti, 2004) demonstrate that side rails can actually increase the risk for injury for confused patients, because they attempt to crawl around or over the side rails to get out of bed. Also be aware that many incontinent patients are often reluctant to call for help even if they understand and acknowledge the use of the call button because "I didn't want to bother you again." Check on patients every 2 hours or offer toileting on a set schedule, to decrease unassisted attempts to get out of bed.

sounds and smells accompanying defecation of feces. Patients should be assisted to as much of a sitting position as their condition allows (Cultural Cues 30-3). The abdominal muscles and gravity can then assist with defecation. Gloves are always worn when helping the patient off the bedpan. Check to see that the patient is thoroughly cleaned, especially if the patient cannot lift up off of the pan in order to clean the anus and surrounding area. The bedpan should be thoroughly cleansed and dried and put away. The bedside commode should be emptied and cleaned promptly after use (Safety Alert 30-1).

When the average patient has not experienced bowel evacuation within 3 days, measures should be taken to assist elimination. Assessment data guide the measures to be implemented. The least invasive measures are used first. Encouraging and monitoring activity, adequate fluid intake, and a diet with sufficient fiber may lead to regular bowel elimination. Noninvasive measures that can be used to promote bowel elimination include the consumption of 1 to 3 tablespoons of bran mixed with applesauce, small amounts of prune juice, warmed prune juice and cola, hot water with lemon juice, or stewed or dried prunes. Be careful because some people are particularly sensitive to the effects of prunes, and diarrhea may develop.

If these actions are not successful, more invasive measures to promote bowel elimination should be implemented. These measures include the administration of medications to soften the stool, suppositories to stimulate the urge to defecate, laxatives to stimulate bowel activity, and enemas to empty the rectum. All of these measures require a physician's order for inpatients. **Measures to rid the bowel of barium are essential after a patient has had barium x-rays.** Encourage an increase in fluid intake of 3500 mL/day for the next 24 hours unless contraindicated. A laxative is often recommended.

Home care patients are encouraged to phone the nurse if they have not had a bowel movement in 3 days. Impaction may be prevented if constipation is treated early. The caregiver for the patient is given in-

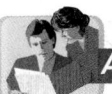

Assignment Considerations 30-2

Teamwork for Better Hygienic Care

Hygienic care is usually assigned to the nursing assistant; however, when a bedridden patient has continuous diarrhea, make an effort to help the assistant to clean the patient. The task of repeated cleaning is exhausting for the caregiver and the patient; it is much easier for two people to accomplish the job. In addition, the patient's skin needs frequent assessment and this is a nursing responsibility that cannot be delegated.

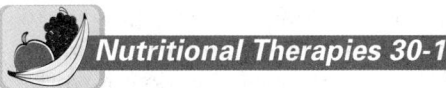

Nutritional Therapies 30-1

Yogurt and Buttermilk

Many antibiotics kill the normal bacteria that reside in the bowel, and this leads to diarrhea. Patients who experience diarrhea from antibiotics should be counseled to begin eating yogurt, drinking buttermilk, or taking acidophilus when they begin taking antibiotics. Replacing the normal bacteria with those contained in these food products reestablishes the right balance and stops the diarrhea.

NURSING CARE PLAN 30-1

Care of the Patient with Constipation

SCENARIO Martina Svoboda, age 64, fractured her left hip in a fall a month ago. Her hip is healing, but she still has difficulty walking. While in the hospital, her usual bowel pattern became disrupted. She has had difficulty with constipation ever since (*"having difficulty with bowels."*). She is presently staying at her daughter's home. The stool is hard and dry; she has a BM every third day.

PROBLEM/NURSING DIAGNOSIS *Bowel movement pattern changed since hospitalization/*Constipation related to immobility.
Supporting Assessment Data: Subjective: States . . . "is having difficulty with bowels." ***Objective:*** Bowel movement only every third day; stool hard and dry.

Goals/Expected Outcomes	Nursing Interventions	Selected Rationales	Evaluation
Constipation will be relieved by medication within 2 days.	Obtain history of bowel pattern prior to accident and hip fracture.	History provides baseline for choosing interventions.	*Is the patient making progress toward reestablishing the usual bowel pattern?*
Usual bowel pattern will be reestablished within 1 month.	Assess dietary and fluid intake.	Assists in determining if enough fluid and fiber is being consumed.	
	Teach ways to increase fiber in the diet (e.g., raw fruits and vegetables, whole-grain breads).	Knowledge promotes correct food choices.	States will have oatmeal for breakfast with fresh fruit.
	Increase fluid intake to 2500 mL/day.	Fluid keeps stool soft.	Dislikes drinking too much water: "I don't like plain water."
	Use stool softeners at bedtime for 1 week.	Stool softeners promote softer stool.	Taking stool softener each evening.
	Encourage walking and abdominal muscle setting exercises.	Muscle strengthening assists with evacuation efforts.	Attending PT 3 × per week. Starting exercise program.
	Work with family in providing regular, morning, unhurried bathroom time.	Helps to establish a daily evacuation pattern.	Progressing toward expected outcomes. Continue plan.

? CRITICAL THINKING QUESTIONS

1. Since the patient still has trouble walking, how can you promote exercise that will strengthen abdominal muscles and assist with bowel evacuation?

2. Ms. Svoboda tells you she doesn't like to drink water. She loves tea. What would you suggest in the way of increased fluid intake?

struction on how to insert a suppository or how to give a small-volume enema so that these measures might be carried out if less invasive measures do not work.

When the patient experiences incontinence, cleansing should occur as soon as possible (Assignment Considerations 30-2). Skin care must be thorough and gentle because feces are irritating to the skin and can cause excoriation (abrasion of the skin). The patient who is having diarrhea stools may need a skin protectant around the anus to prevent skin breakdown and considerable discomfort. Products such as petroleum jelly, A & D ointment, cod liver oil ointments with zinc oxide, and commercial skin barrier products are helpful to protect the skin. Gentle washing with soap and water, rinsing, and patting dry are essential to protect the skin. Baby wipes are useful during diarrhea episodes.

When diarrhea is thought to be caused by bacteria or a virus, the physician may want to let it run its course for at least 24 hours so that the body has a chance to rid itself of the offending organism. Diarrhea from other causes simply leads to fluid and electrolyte loss and should not be allowed to continue for long periods of time. Treatment involves placing the patient on a clear liquid diet to rest the bowel, replacing fluids and electrolytes, and seeking medication to stop the loose stools. **Observe for signs of dehydration when the patient has severe diarrhea: decreased skin turgor, dry mucous membranes with thick saliva, and increased thirst. Self-medication for diarrhea should not continue for more than 48 hours without consulting a physician** (Nutritional Therapies 30-1).

Evaluation

Evaluation for patients with problems of bowel function is based on whether expected outcomes and goals have been met. If outcomes and goals are not being met, the plan needs to be reconsidered and revised. Examples of evaluation statements might be as follows:

- Patient is walking 1 mile a day.
- Patient has increased fluid intake to 3500 mL, is eating bran at breakfast, and is producing stool every other day.
- Bowel movement occurs every morning despite continued use of pain medication.
- Patient has been continent of stool for 6 days.
- Patient is feeling better about self since bowel regimen has produced continent stool for 3 days in a row.
- Patient identified foods high in fat and milk products as causing diarrhea.

Nursing Care Plan 30-1 provides other examples of evaluation.

Documentation

Any changes in bowel habits should be documented: stool characteristics, episodes of constipation or diarrhea, and measures taken to remedy the problem. The teaching plan is documented along with times of

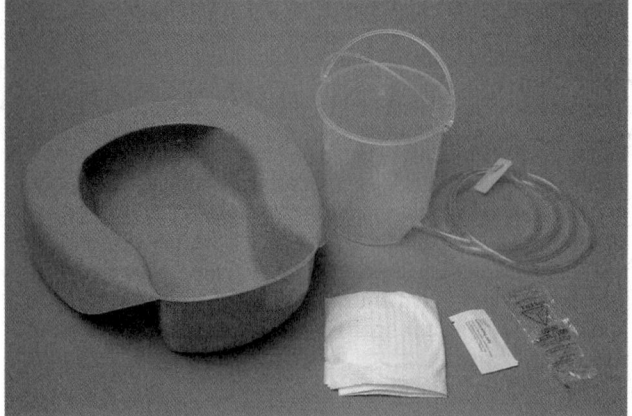

FIGURE **30-2** Enema equipment.

each teaching session and material covered. Evaluation of teaching is also noted. All measures to promote bowel elimination must be documented. The number and approximate amount of diarrhea stools are charted on the appropriate flow sheets (intake and output and daily activity sheets).

RECTAL SUPPOSITORIES

Rectal suppositories used to promote bowel movements are glycerin and bisacodyl suppositories. Suppositories that promote bowel evacuation do so by (1) stimulating the inner surface of the rectum and increasing the urge to defecate, (2) forming gas that expands the rectum, or (3) melting into a lubricating material to coat the stool for easier passage through the anal sphincter. See Chapter 34 for the procedure to insert a rectal suppository.

?
Think Critically About . . . What time of day would be best for administering a rectal suppository to stimulate defecation?

ENEMAS

An enema is the introduction of fluid into the rectum and colon by means of a tube. Enemas are given to stimulate peristalsis and the urge to defecate or to wash out the waste products or feces. Cleansing enemas are given when the bowel is to be examined by x-ray, colonoscopy, or sigmoidoscopy or when the bowel is distended by flatus. The volume of a cleansing enema depends on the age of the patient: infant or toddler, 50 to 150 mL (normal saline only); ages 3 to 5, 200 to 300 mL; school age, 300 to 500 mL; adult, 500 to 1000 mL. Figure 30-2 shows the equipment used for a cleansing enema. An enema kit will contain either a bag or a bucket for the solution. The commercially disposable enema, such as the Fleet enema, is convenient and easy to use when only a small amount of

Table 30-1 *Types of Enemas and Their Actions*

TYPES OF ENEMAS	EXAMPLES	ACTIONS
Retention enema	Mineral oil	Softens stool as oil is absorbed
Cleansing enema	Soapsuds (5 mL castile soap in 1000 mL of water) Tap water Saline (500-1000 mL normal saline)	Stimulates peristalsis through distention and irritation of colon and rectum
Distention reduction enema	Carminative (30 g magnesium sulfate, 60 g glycerin, and 90 mL warm water)	Relieves discomfort from flatus causing distention
Medicated enema	Kayexalate (removes potassium) Neomycin (reduces bacteria)	Solution with drugs to reduce bacteria or remove potassium
Disposable enema (small volume)	Sodium phosphate (Fleet)	Stimulates peristalsis by acting as irritant

fluid is needed to stimulate a bowel movement. Enemas can be given at any time, but it is best to try to give them before the morning bath and bed linen change.

TYPES OF ENEMAS

The type of enema to be given is prescribed by the physician and will vary depending on the patient's age and condition, the purpose of the enema, and the preference of the physician (Table 30-1). The type of solution is specified, and you are expected to know how to prepare it unless a commercial enema has been ordered. The commercially packaged enema may require more lubricant on the nozzle; other supplies needed are the same as for any type of enema. When other types of enemas are ordered, consult the hospital's procedure manual for the ingredients and the proportions to use.

Retention Enema

Often an oil-retention enema is ordered for a patient who is constipated. The oil must be retained in the rectum to soften and coat the hardened feces. Between 120 and 180 mL of warm oil is instilled rectally in the same manner as the cleansing enema, except that **the oil should be retained at least 20 minutes.** Prepackaged enemas are usually used for this purpose, but mineral oil or olive oil can be used.

AMOUNT AND TEMPERATURE OF SOLUTION

Disposable enema units contain about 240 mL of solution (Figure 30-3). They may be given at room temperature, but work best when slightly warmed (Safety Alert 30-2). No special preparation is needed; they are ready for use when taken from the package. With the patient in the left Sims' position, the prelubricated nozzle is inserted into the rectum, and the solution is instilled by squeezing the flexible plastic bottle. Rolling the bottle up from the bottom aids in instilling the entire contents.

The amount of solution used for a cleansing enema for adults is between 500 and 1000 mL; smaller amounts are used for children (Safety Alert 30-3). Hold the container approximately 12 to 18 inches above the patient's anus and allow the warm solution to run in

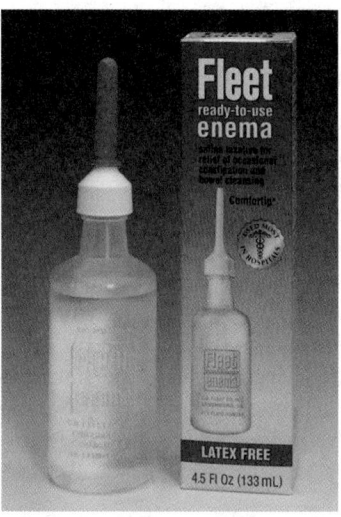

FIGURE **30-3** Disposable enema.

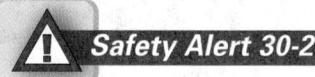

Not Too Hot, Not Too Cold

The temperature of the enema solution should be about 105° F (40.5° C). If a bath thermometer is not available, test the temperature of the fluid by pouring a small amount over the inner wrist. It should be warm to the touch but not hot. Solution that is too cool usually cannot be retained; hot solutions may damage the tissues of the rectum.

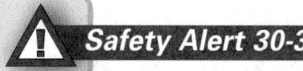

"Enemas Until Clear"

When an order to "give enemas until clear" is written, it means that the return fluid must not have any fecal matter in it; however, **no more than three large-volume enemas are given without checking with the physician.** Repeated enemas may deplete electrolytes and can be dangerous.

slowly; a greater height creates too much pressure because the fluid runs in too rapidly and causes painful distention of the rectum and colon. This stimulates the urge to defecate immediately, so that the patient cannot retain the fluid.

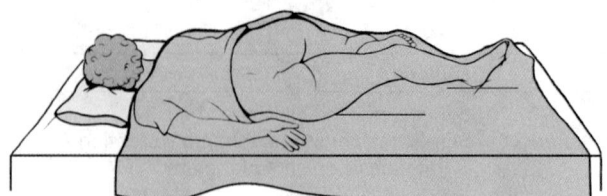

FIGURE **30-4** Position for giving an enema.

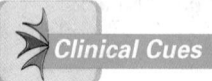

If your elderly patient has trouble holding an enema, take a baby bottle nipple, cut off the tip and insert the enema tube through the nipple. Gently support the outer rim of the nipple with your gloved hand; this helps to provide a temporary "plug" that helps the patient to retain the enema.

RECOMMENDED POSITION

The position of choice when giving an enema is the left Sims' position with the hips slightly elevated (Figure 30-4). This allows the fluid, aided by the force of gravity, to flow downward along the natural curve of the rectum and descending colon. If the patient is unable to turn to the side, the supine position can be used (Skill 30-1).

RECTAL TUBE

When a patient is uncomfortable because of flatus in the lower bowel, a rectal tube can be inserted in the anus. The tube is similar to the enema tubing. This allows the gas to be expelled without the patient's straining to open the anal sphincter. Oral medications to reduce gas have mostly eliminated the use of this tube.

FECAL IMPACTION

Fecal impaction means that the rectum and sigmoid colon become filled with hardened fecal material. The most obvious sign of fecal impaction is the absence of (or only a small amount of) bowel movement for more than 3 days in a patient who usually has a bowel movement more frequently. Impaction occurs in patients who are very ill, are on bed rest, or are not fully aware of their surroundings due to a state of confusion. The very young and very old are more prone to fecal impaction.

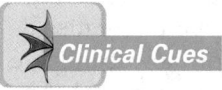

Passage of small amounts of liquid or semisoft stool onto the bed linens is a sign of fecal impaction. Bacterial action on the hardened surface of the fecal material causes liquefaction.

Skill 30-1 | Administering an Enema

An enema is given to evacuate the bowel. Tap water, soapsuds, or saline solution of 500 to 1000 mL is given to the adult with an enema bucket or bag. A disposable enema, consisting of 120 mL of hypertonic solution, may be ordered. An oil-retention enema may be required to soften stool so that evacuation can occur more easily.

■ **Supplies**
- ✓ Enema container and tubing with clamp, or disposable enema
- ✓ Bedpan or bedside commode
- ✓ Underpad or Chux
- ✓ Lubricant
- ✓ Gloves
- ✓ Enema solution and additives as ordered
- ✓ Bath blanket
- ✓ Paper towel and toilet tissue

Review and carry out the Standard Steps in Appendix 3.

■ **Assessment (Data Collection)**

1. ***ACTION*** Check the physician's order. Determine what patient knows about the enema procedure. Check to see that a bedpan or bedside commode is on hand.

   RATIONALE Ensures that an enema order has been written. Determines how much explanation is needed. Bedpan or bedside commode is desirable.

■ **Planning**

2. ***ACTION*** Plan time to give a large-volume enema without interruption.

RATIONALE A large-volume enema procedure may take as long as 30 minutes if the order is "enemas until clear."

■ **Implementation**

3. ***ACTION*** If possible, place the patient in the left Sims' position and drape with the bath blanket. Place the underpad under the buttocks.

   RATIONALE Solution travels up the colon more easily when the patient is lying on the left side. Underpad will protect the linens from moisture or soiling.

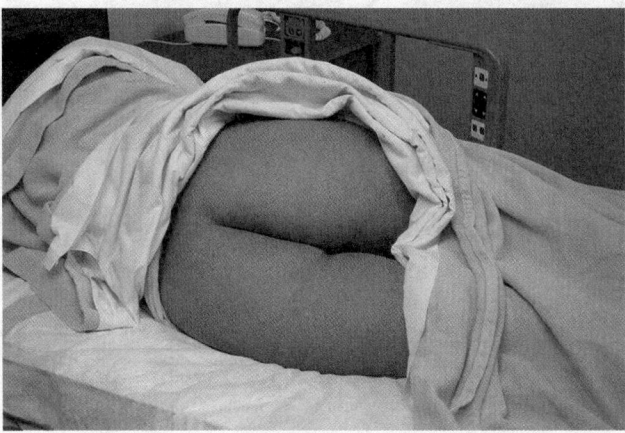

Step **3**

For Large-Solution Enema

4. *ACTION* Put on gloves. Fill the enema bag with the correct solution; temperature of the water should be between 100° and 105° F (37.8° and 40.5° C). Expel air from the tubing by opening the clamp and allowing the solution to run through. Use the bedpan or sink to collect the solution; reclamp the tube.

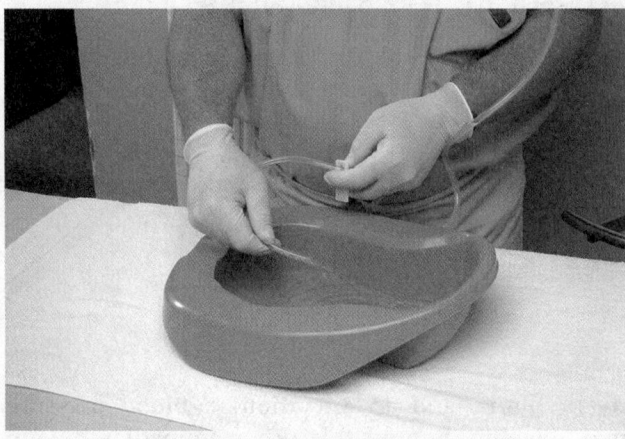

Step **4**

RATIONALE Gloves prevent transfer of microorganisms. The physician orders the type of solution. Water that is too hot may burn the patient; water too cool may cause cramping. Expelling air from tube prevents air from being introduced into the colon, which could cause the patient discomfort.

5. *ACTION* Position the bedside commode or put the bedpan close at hand. Generously lubricate the end of the enema tube and, while the patient takes a deep breath, gently insert it about 4 inches in the adult anus. Direct the tube toward the umbilicus. Ask the patient to take a deep breath through the mouth to relax the anal sphincter. Twisting the tube gently helps it pass through the sphincter.

RATIONALE Bedpan or bedside commode will be needed as soon as all the fluid has been instilled. Generous lubricant is needed if the patient has

hemorrhoids. It is possible to perforate the wall of the rectum with the tube if force is used; gentle pressure and slow advancement are best.

6. *ACTION* With the container about 12 to 18 inches above the anus, open the clamp on the tube, steady the tube in place, and allow the solution to flow slowly into the bowel over 5 to 10 minutes. Lowering slightly and again raising the container to this height will regulate the speed of the flow. Slight pressure on the tubing with the clamp can also slow the flow. When the patient expresses discomfort, stop the flow by kinking the tubing or clamping it, and instruct the patient to take deep breaths by mouth until the cramping and urge to expel the fluid pass. Continue until the patient can retain no more or the container is empty. Clamp the tubing and withdraw it, asking the patient to squeeze the sphincter shut; place the soiled tube on a paper towel.

RATIONALE Too forceful a flow may damage the bowel. Instilling the fluid slowly prevents cramping and usually obtains the best result with the least discomfort. Some patients can hold only a few hundred milliliters of solution at a time; others can tolerate the entire volume.

For Disposable or Oil-Retention Enema

7. *ACTION* Add extra lubricant to the tip if the amount of prelubrication seems insufficient. Insert the tip into the anal opening as directed previously. Gently squeeze the bottle, and roll it up from the bottom as the contents enter the bowel. Squeeze as much of the fluid into the patient as possible. Remove the tip slowly and hold the buttocks together.

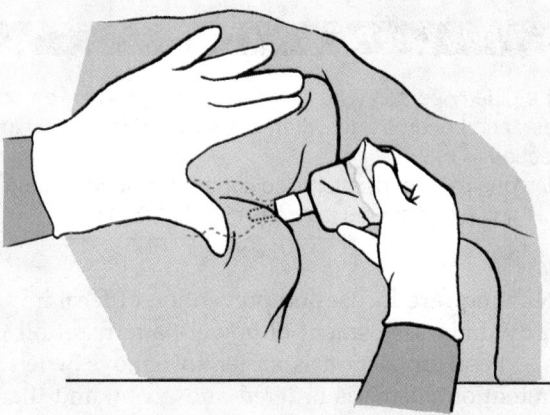

Step **7**

RATIONALE The lubricant on the tip sometimes dries out. Disposable enemas contain approximately 120 to 240 mL of solution. Slow instillation achieves the best result. An oil-retention enema is given in the same manner, but the patient should retain it for 20 minutes to 2 hours so that it will soften the stool.

Continued

Skill 30-1 | Administering an Enema—cont'd

For Both Types of Enema

8. **ACTION** Assist the patient onto the bedpan or bedside commode. If the patient uses the toilet, request to see the result before flushing. If a bedpan is used, raise the head of the bed to a sitting position. Place call bell and toilet paper within reach.

   RATIONALE This provides a container for collection of enema return and the opportunity to observe characteristics of stool expelled.

9. **ACTION** When the bowel contents have been expelled, assist the patient in cleaning the anal area; observe the results of the enema, noting the color, amount, and consistency of the stool. Remove and clean the bedpan or bedside commode.

   RATIONALE Results of the enema are judged by the stool expelled.

10. **ACTION** Restore the patient unit, lower the bed, and place the call bell within reach.

    RATIONALE Shows consideration for the patient and provides safety.

■ Evaluation

11. **ACTION** Ask yourself: Was the patient able to hold sufficient enema fluid to flush the bowel? Did all the fluid seem to return? Was there a normal amount of stool expelled? Does the patient feel relief from fullness and flatus?

RATIONALE Answers determine whether enema was successful.

■ Documentation

12. **ACTION** Note date, time, type of enema and amount of fluid instilled; describe the result and how the patient tolerated the procedure.

    RATIONALE Documents the invasive procedure and its results.

Documentation Example

10/12 0930   1000 mL tap water enema given 500 mL at a time. No c/o severe cramping. Produced large amount of brown formed stool and returned fluid. States feels much better. Bed down, call bell in reach. Resting.

_____
(Nurse's signature)

? CRITICAL THINKING QUESTIONS

1. Why do you think that a patient who is taking a diuretic and is now in the hospital may become constipated and need an enema?

2. When an enema is ordered, how would you organize your work for the day if you are working the day shift?

 **Elder Care Points**

- The elderly person who is ill, has fever, is mostly on bed rest, and becomes dehydrated is very prone to fecal impaction.
- Narcotic pain medication also contributes to impaction in this group of patients, as does diuretic therapy.

Nursing care focuses on prevention of fecal impaction by daily assessment of bowel patterns of all patients. Fecal impaction is easier to remove when an oil-retention enema is ordered and given, and then a cleansing enema is given 2 to 3 hours later. Sometimes the physician will order the impaction to be digitally broken up after the oil has had time to soften the stool (Steps 30-1).

Removal of a fecal impaction digitally must be done gently and the patient watched for signs of vagal response (activation of the vagal nerve) from stimulation of the sphincter and rectal wall (Figure 30-5). **The vagal response may cause a slow pulse and cardiac dysrhythmia, and an alteration in blood pressure may develop. Should this occur, immediately stop the procedure, place the patient in a supine position, monitor vital signs, and notify the physician.** A dose of atropine may be ordered to counteract the vagal response.

BOWEL TRAINING FOR INCONTINENCE

The treatment for incontinence is training for bowel control. This is a long process, but it helps the patient regain self-esteem. A special effort should be made to help the very elderly patient overcome incontinence.

A bowel training program is based on the principles for establishing regular bowel elimination: adequate diet, sufficient fluids, adequate exercise, and sufficient rest (Box 30-3). A regular time for evacuation should be established. A reasonable goal is to achieve defecation within 1 hour of the established time. Factors that will help establish the time include prior

Steps 30-1 | Removal of a Fecal Impaction

When a patient has impacted stool that cannot be flushed out with an oil-retention enema followed by cleansing enemas, manual removal of the impaction is required. The patient should be given analgesia before carrying out this procedure because it is painful.

Review and carry out the Standard Steps in Appendix 3.

1. **ACTION** Assess when the last bowel movement occurred, check risk factors that contribute to constipation, assess the abdomen, and determine if small amounts of liquid stool have been passed.

    RATIONALE Assessment data help in determination as to whether fecal impaction has occurred.

2. **ACTION** Have patient assume a left lateral or Sims' position. Put on gloves and arrange the bedpan and toilet tissue on a chair by the bed within reach. Lubricate the index finger.

    RATIONALE Lubrication prevents injury to the anal and rectal mucosa as the finger is introduced. Generous lubricant makes it easier for the finger to slide up and around the hardened stool. An oil-retention enema 20 minutes to 3 hours prior to impaction removal is helpful.

3. **ACTION** Insert the index finger into the anus and along the wall of the rectum in a slightly curving motion. As the finger comes in contact with feces in the rectum, note the consistency; then move the finger into the lower portion of the fecal mass, again noting the consistency.

    RATIONALE This provides data about the amount and consistency of the stool in the rectum.

4. **ACTION** With the examining index finger, dislodge or break off a small amount of fecal material and gently remove it, placing it in the bedpan. Lubricate the finger as needed. Continue removing as much fecal material as you can reach with your finger or until the patient's discomfort, or adverse effects such as palpitations or dizziness, warrant discontinuing the procedure. After the patient has rested, re-glove and remove the remaining fecal material. Cleanse the rectal area. Remove gloves and dispose of them properly.

    RATIONALE The stool is broken up so that it can be removed with less discomfort to the patient and without damage to the rectal mucosa.

5. **ACTION** Make the patient comfortable, lower the bed, raise side rails, and restore the unit.

    RATIONALE Shows consideration for the patient; provides safety.

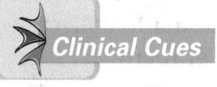

FIGURE **30-5** Removing a fecal impaction.

bowel habits of the patient or the nurse's observation of when incontinent movements tend to occur. Many bowel retraining programs are timed around a triggering meal when gastrocolic reflexes are the strongest.

Clinical Cues

After breakfast seems to be the most common time for a bowel movement to be triggered.

After a regular time for evacuation has been established, all efforts must be made to provide the patient with an environment that is conducive to evacuation. Privacy and adequate time are only two parts of the environment that are considered. The patient must also feel safe in the environment and know that if a problem occurs, the nurse is available to provide assistance. In anticipation of a successful evacuation, provide the patient with toilet tissue and remember to plan for hand hygiene after the evacuation (Safety Alert 30-4; see also Safety Alert 17-1).

Some patients with a neurogenic dysfunction may require digital stimulation to relax the anal sphincter. Using a gloved and lubricated finger, insert the finger 1 to 2 cm into the rectum and gently rotate the finger for 30 to 60 seconds.

Suppositories, stool softeners, and bulk laxatives may be used to assist in establishing a normal, regular bowel pattern. The type of suppository used will depend on the physician's order. As a rule, suppositories are inserted about 1 hour before the triggering meal or the established evacuation time. In some bowel retraining programs, a suppository is used every day for the first week, then every other day for the second and third weeks, and thereafter only as needed to maintain a regular movement every 2 to 3 days.

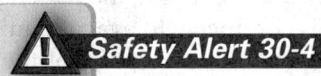

Box 30-3 | *Interventions for Bowel Training*

- Assess for fecal impaction, which may be causing incontinent diarrhea. Remove impaction if present.
- Ensure that the patient's diet is high in bulk and fiber. Attention should be given to teeth or properly fitting dentures if oral condition is a reason for low fiber intake.
- Increase fluids to 2500 mL/day unless contraindicated due to congestive heart failure, renal insufficiency, potential for increased intracranial pressure, or other disorder.
- Perform a thorough assessment for 1 week to determine intake and output patterns, usual time of incontinent stool, and previous bowel pattern before incontinence began, including frequency of bowel movement, time of day, and surrounding events (e.g., while drinking coffee; use of commode, toilet, or bedpan).
- Encourage regular toileting after meals. Toileting should be performed just before the time at which incontinent defecation has been occurring.
- Use positive reinforcement for continent defecation. Refrain from use of negative reinforcement (shaming, scolding, etc.) at any time.
- Provide privacy for toileting; position the patient comfortably on the commode, toilet, or bedpan with feet supported.
- If diarrhea is present, assess and remedy the cause with diet or medications as ordered.
- Begin an exercise program for the patient to strengthen abdominal muscles.
- If other measures do not work, obtain an order for a suppository or an enema every 2 to 3 days to stimulate peristalsis and produce controlled defecation.

⚠ Safety Alert 30-4

Attention to Hand Hygiene

To comply with The Joint Commission 2009 National Patient Safety Goals, nurses should practice and encourage hand hygiene according to the Centers for Disease Control and Prevention guidelines, which include use of alcohol-based cleaning agents and/or soap and water. Wash before and after gloving and avoid artificial nails. Additional information can be obtained from the Hand Hygiene Guidelines Fact Sheet at www.cdc.gov/od/oc/media/pressrel/fs021025.htm.

When stool softeners and bulk laxatives are used as part of a bowel training program, remember that a fluid intake of at least 2500 mL per day is required. In most cases, stronger types of laxatives and enemas are not considered part of a bowel training program.

BOWEL OSTOMY

Disease or trauma can damage the intestinal system and require surgical intervention, which alters the process of elimination. A diversion of intestinal con-

tents from the normal path is called an ostomy. An ostomy results in the formation of an external stoma (opening into the intestine), or an internal tissue pouch with a valve nipple opening. The internal pouch forming the continent ostomy is usually constructed from a segment of bowel (Figure 30-6). This type of ostomy is emptied with a catheter (Steps 30-2). Patients with stoma ostomies use various appliances (devices to gather and contain output) and special procedures to aid in effective, controlled elimination through the stoma.

Human elimination is a subject that many adults view with embarrassment or distaste. Physical conditions that create the need for an ostomy carry a heavy psychosocial burden for the patient as well as many new demands in handling elimination. Soiling, wetness, and the presence of odor from feces are all socially unacceptable in adult society, and the possibility of such things is often of grave concern to the new ostomy patient. There is also concern about ability to care for oneself and to return to work and recreation activities performed before surgery. You must keep your body language neutral and not display any sign of distaste when caring for the ostomy patient. An attitude of acceptance is very important.

Conditions that can require ostomy include cancer, abdominal trauma, congenital malformation of the bowel, and severe chronic Crohn's disease or ulcerative colitis. Patients facing an ostomy frequently experience fear, concern, and denial followed by information seeking. Fear may focus on the loss of a normal body function and change in body image, the possibility of rejection by others, the loss of physical or sexual attractiveness, or the prospect of death from the underlying disease.

The patient may be helped by a visit from a member of the United Ostomy Association, which is a support network of persons with ostomies. The patient needs a support system in place before discharge from the hospital. The local office of the American Cancer Society is a good source of information about ostomy support groups or visitors in the area, as is the United Ostomy Association, which can be reached at (800) 826-0826 or on the Internet at www.uoaa.org.

OSTOMY CARE

An ileostomy is an opening surgically created at the ileum to divert intestinal contents. This is done because lower portions of the bowel have been surgically removed. Effluent (fecal matter) from an ileostomy is liquid. A colostomy is an opening into the colon. The stoma is the entrance to the opening. An appliance is the apparatus that attaches to the skin plus a pouch (bag) worn over the stoma to collect effluent (Figure 30-7). Colostomy effluent is more formed. Patient care involves providing skin care around the stoma, applying the appliance, or if there is a continent ileostomy, draining it with a catheter.

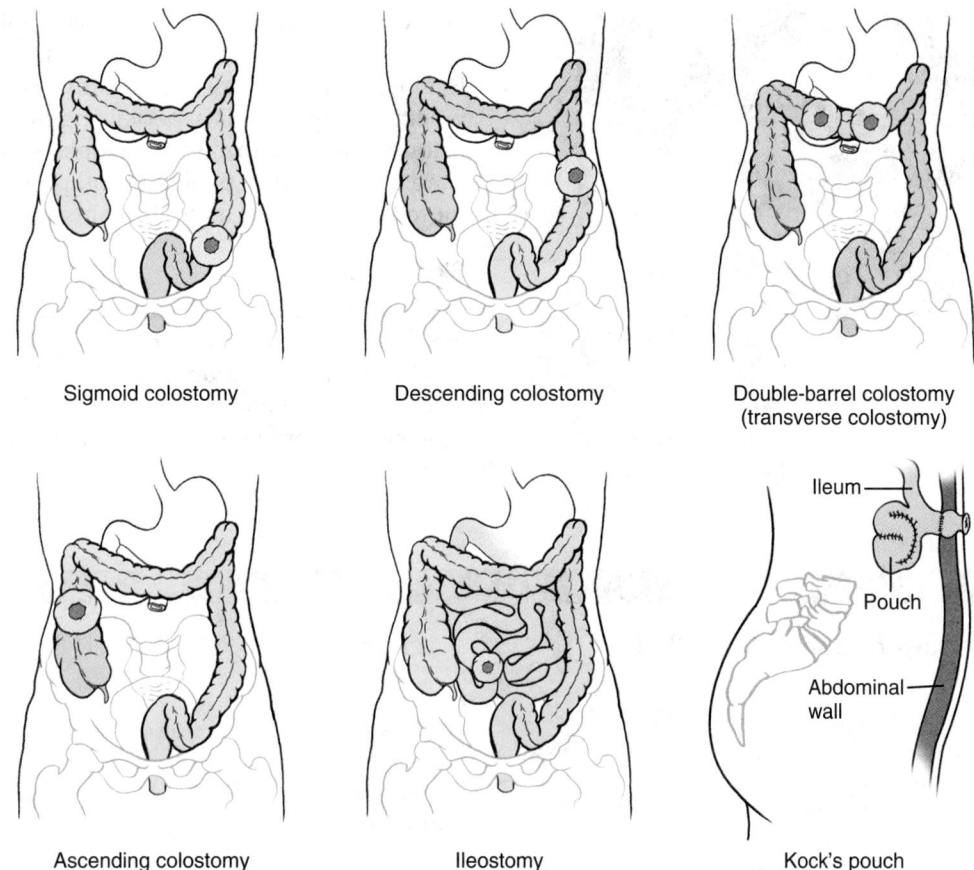

Sigmoid colostomy   Descending colostomy   Double-barrel colostomy (transverse colostomy)

Ascending colostomy   Ileostomy   Kock's pouch

Ileum

Pouch

Abdominal wall

FIGURE **30-6** Types of bowel ostomies and intestinal diversions.

Steps 30-2 | Catheterizing a Continent Ileostomy

A continent bowel diversion such as Koch's pouch, has a nipple valve attached to the abdomen through which the waste contents of the internal reservoir can be drained of stool. Initial catheterization of a fresh continent ileostomy should be done only by a trained enterostomal therapist (ET) nurse or the physician. Thereafter, another nurse may assist the patient as needed.

Review and carry out the Standard Steps in Appendix 3.

1. ***ACTION*** Assist patient to comfortable position on toilet, commode, or chair.

   RATIONALE Patient will be able to relax abdominal muscles if comfortably positioned.

2. ***ACTION*** Perform hand hygiene, put on gloves, and remove and discard any covering over nipple valve.

   RATIONALE Reduces transfer of microorganisms; prepares nipple valve for catheterization.

3. ***ACTION*** Lubricate the catheter with water-soluble lubricant.

   RATIONALE Allows easier entry of catheter into pouch.

4. ***ACTION*** Place distal end of catheter into waste drainage container or toilet. Slowly insert the cath-

eter through the nipple valve and into the internal reservoir until stool begins to drain.

   RATIONALE Places catheter into reservoir, allowing waste drainage. When the catheter meets the resistance of the internal valve, ask the patient to take a deep breath and apply gentle pressure to open the valve.

5. ***ACTION*** Allow about 5 minutes for the catheter to drain the stool in the reservoir fully.

   RATIONALE Empties the reservoir.

6. ***ACTION*** Ask the patient to cough three or four times to expel any remaining waste. Remove the catheter and rinse in warm water, then wash in mild soap and rinse again. Lay catheter on a towel to dry.

   RATIONALE Prepares the catheter for the next use.

7. ***ACTION*** Clean the nipple valve and surrounding area with water or towelette as necessary and cover with 4 × 4 gauze if needed.

   RATIONALE Cleanses the area and prevents dripping.

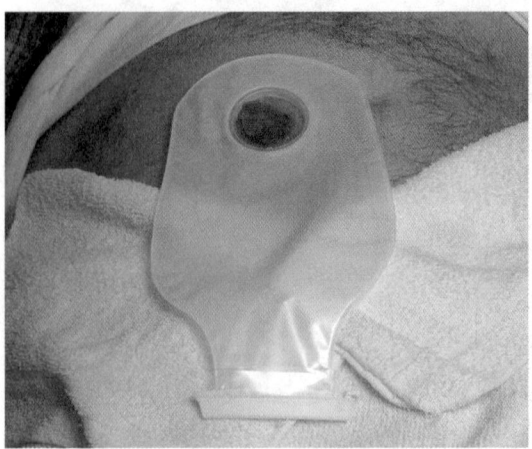

FIGURE **30-7** Ostomy collection device in place.

Diet can adversely affect the ostomy patient and is an important part of teaching (Patient Teaching 30-1). Evaluation of care for the ostomy patient hinges on whether the patient is experiencing problems with the ostomy, the skin around the stoma, or the appliance. Care of the ostomy patient is complex and is covered more thoroughly in a medical-surgical nursing text.

Skin Care

Periostomal (around the stoma) care includes assessment of the health of the stoma and skin surrounding it. The stoma should appear pink or red, which indicates adequate blood supply. It should look like healthy mucous membrane, such as the membrane inside the mouth.

 Patient Teaching 30-1

Dietary Guidelines for the Ostomy Patient

ILEOSTOMY
- Eat a diet high in protein, calories, and vitamins.
- Avoid foods that irritate the intestine or require excessive intestinal activity, such as milk products, spicy or fried high-residue foods, raw vegetables and fruits, and whole-grain cereals.
- Avoid carbonated, caffeinated, and alcoholic beverages because they increase intestinal activity.
- Avoid extremely hot or cold foods and fluids because they cause gas.
- Eat small, frequent meals.
- Drink 8 to 10 cups of fluid per day.

COLOSTOMY
- Control the consistency of the stool with diet.

To Control Diarrhea, Increase Intake of:
- Ripe bananas
- Rice
- Creamy peanut butter
- Cheese
- Potatoes (no skin)
- Applesauce
- Tapioca

To Soften Consistency of Stool, Increase Intake of:
- Beans
- Caffeinated beverages
- Leafy vegetables
- Apple juice
- Prune juice or prunes
- Fresh fruits (except bananas)
- Raw vegetables
- Spicy or highly seasoned foods
- Green beans
- Broccoli
- Fluids

These Foods May Increase Stool or Urine Odor:
- Beans
- Fish
- Eggs
- Asparagus
- Coffee
- Onions
- Cabbage
- Turnips
- Cucumbers
- Broccoli
- Beer

These Foods May Decrease Stool Odor:
- Parsley
- Beet greens
- Buttermilk
- Yogurt

These Foods Increase Flatus:
- Beer
- Carbonated beverages
- Dried beans and peas
- Strong-flavored cheeses
- Onions
- Broccoli, cabbage, brussels sprouts
- Radishes
- Cucumbers
- Eggs
- Turnips
- Corn
- Spicy foods

Avoid These Foods Because They May Cause Obstruction:
- Popcorn
- Chinese vegetables
- Raw fruits
- Pineapple
- Whole-kernel corn
- Celery
- Tomatoes
- Nuts
- Coconut
- Fruits with seeds
- Tough meats, shrimp, lobster

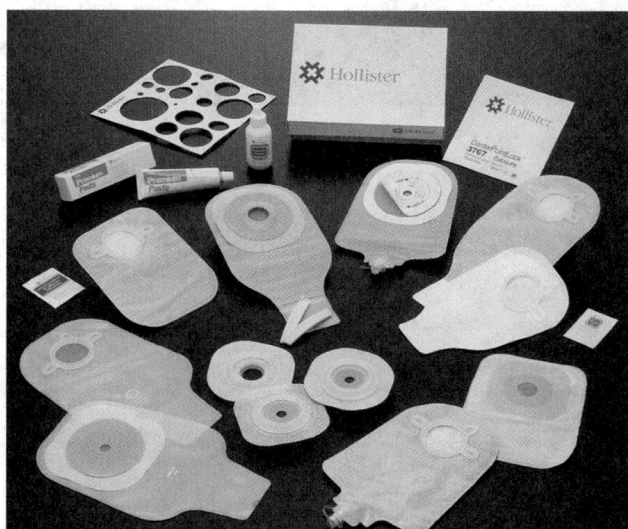

FIGURE **30-8** Ostomy application and supplies.

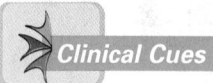

A pale or dusky stoma indicates compromised blood supply and should be reported to the physician.

Assess the skin around the stoma for signs of irritation or breakdown. With an ileostomy, enzymes in the effluent can quickly cause excoriation. When changing the faceplate (every 3 to 5 days), the stoma and skin are washed with mild soap and water and patted dry. A skin barrier paste is applied, with care to prevent any of it from getting on the stoma. Skin barriers are commercially available along with other ostomy supplies (Figure 30-8). A karaya ring may be attached to the

skin to hold the faceplate in place; it is often part of the faceplate. Karaya is a plant material that becomes gelatinous (soft and sticky) when wet; it helps prevent excoriation.

Applying an Ostomy Appliance

There are many different sizes and types of ostomy appliances. All appliances have a faceplate, or disk, that attaches to the abdomen, and a pouch for collecting effluent. The appliance is positioned with the stoma protruding through the opening in the center of the faceplate. **It is essential that the appliance be the correct size for the patient's stoma.** The stoma must be measured so that the right-size appliance can be chosen. The pouch attaches over the stoma and is fastened onto the faceplate. Some patients wear a belt that also supports the pouch so that it is not pulled loose from the faceplate as effluent fills the pouch. A clamp at the bottom of the pouch allows effluent to be drained. Pouches are simply emptied and rinsed as needed and are detached and replaced only every few days. It is best to empty stool from the pouch when it becomes one third to one half full so that the weight of the effluent does not pull the appliance loose (Skill 30-2).

Irrigating a Colostomy

To irrigate a colostomy, a solution is instilled into the colon via the stoma; it is similar to giving an enema (Steps 30-3).

Think Critically About . . . What concerns do you have about caring for an ostomy patient for the first time?

Skill 30-2 | Changing an Ostomy Appliance

You will initially change the ostomy appliance, but should take each opportunity to teach the patient this skill. An ostomy pouch is changed when adherence to the skin is no longer adequate or every 2 days if the skin condition is compromised. The type of pouch applied depends on the type of ostomy.

■ **Supplies**

✓ Washcloth or premoistened towelettes
✓ Plastic disposal bag

✓ Clear plastic stoma measuring template
✓ Clean pouch and faceplate
✓ Gloves
✓ Skin barrier paste

✓ Pouch closure device
✓ Scissors
✓ Tissues or portion of tampon
✓ Tape or belt

Review and carry out Standard Steps in Appendix 3.

■ **Assessment (Data Collection)**

1. *ACTION* Assess for type of ostomy and location. Assess stoma for color and appearance. Assess size of stoma using stoma measuring device. Assess skin condition around stoma.

RATIONALE Stoma measuring device provides data regarding stoma size for choice of correct appliance. If the stoma is more than 6 months old, a precut appliance of the correct size may be used. Red or dark pink color indicates adequate blood supply. Stoma should not be receding or protruding. Skin breakdown may be caused by stool ac-

Continued

tion on skin, improperly fitting pouch, perspiration, irritation to skin from appliance, allergic reaction, or bacterial or fungal infection.

■ Planning

2. *ACTION* Gather appropriate supplies needed to apply the new pouch/appliance.

   RATIONALE Ensures that all needed items are on hand before beginning.

■ Implementation

3. *ACTION* Measure the stoma with the stoma measuring device. Prepare the skin barrier or pouch with faceplate by cutting an opening in the center approximately ⅛ inch (for urostomy) to ¼ inch (for colostomy) larger than the stoma. Smoothing the cut edges with your finger will help prevent irritation or leakage around the stoma.

   RATIONALE Drawing the pattern on the paper side of the plate and cutting out on top of the line will ensure more accurate sizing. The edges of the pouch can injure or irritate the stoma if the opening is too small. Too small an opening may restrict blood flow or prevent correct adherence of the appliance to the skin.

4. *ACTION* Put on gloves. Empty old pouch.

   RATIONALE Prevents transfer of microorganisms. Prevents the weight of the pouch contents from loosening the pouch and spilling.

5. *ACTION* Remove old pouch by stabilizing the skin with one hand and pulling the backing from the skin with the other hand; discard the old pouch in the plastic bag. Save the tail closure clip.

   RATIONALE Readies the area for new pouch application.

6. *ACTION* Clean the stoma and skin gently with warm water and soft cloth. Dry the skin well by patting. Place tissue or piece of tampon at stoma opening to prevent leakage.

   RATIONALE Cleaning and drying prepares skin for attachment of new appliance. Tissue or tampon will absorb any leakage.

7. *ACTION* Change gloves. Remove paper from skin barrier on back of appliance. Apply skin barrier paste to periostomal area. Wet fingers, and spread paste around the stoma, but not on it.

   RATIONALE Reduces transfer of microorganisms. Prepares an adhesive surface on the skin for attachment of pouch appliance.

8. *ACTION* Center and carefully apply the pouch appliance while having patient push out the abdomen.

RATIONALE This prevents skin wrinkles from occurring while pouch is pressed into place.

9. *ACTION* Gently press down the skin barrier ring around the stoma while abdomen is pushed out by patient. Check that seal is wrinkle free.

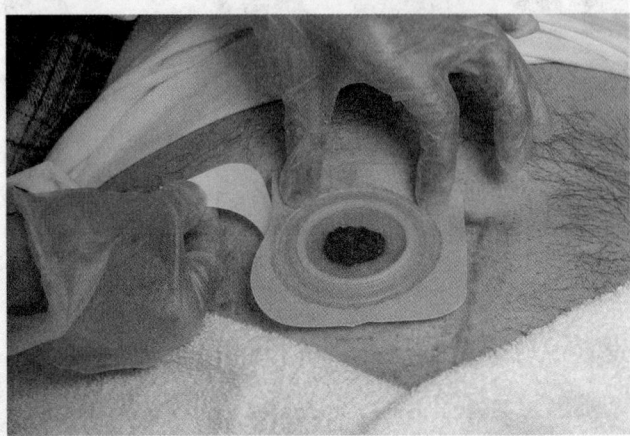

Step **9**

RATIONALE Adheres appliance to skin without causing wrinkles. Good adherence prevents leakage.

10. *ACTION* Reinforce ring with tape as needed.

   RATIONALE Balances weight of pouch and prevents edges from loosening during showering.

11. *ACTION* Instruct patient to lie quietly or sit still for 5 minutes to allow body heat to seal pouch well.

   RATIONALE Body heat activates the skin barrier and causes it to adhere to the skin.

12. *ACTION* Place deodorant inside pouch if patient desires.

   RATIONALE Various types of ostomy deodorants are available commercially.

13. *ACTION* Attach and secure pouch tail closure so that bow of clip fits curve of abdomen. Allow a 1-inch fold-over of pouch before closing the clip.

   RATIONALE Closes pouch; when bow fits curve of abdomen, clip is less noticeable through clothing.

14. *ACTION* Attach belt to faceplate of pouch if belt is to be worn.

   RATIONALE If stoma is flush to the skin, a belt may be needed to prevent leakage from the pouch.

15. *ACTION* Remove gloves and perform hand hygiene.

   RATIONALE Reduces transfer of microorganisms.

16. *ACTION* Assist patient to replace gown or clothing and position for comfort. Restore the area.

RATIONALE Makes patient comfortable and provides safety.

■ Evaluation

17. **ACTION** Ask yourself: Is the appliance applied without wrinkles? Is it attached securely? Is the bottom of the pouch closed securely? Was the old pouch disposed of properly? Is there any leakage from the pouch?

RATIONALE Determines whether appliance/pouch was applied correctly.

■ Documentation

18. **ACTION** Note date, time, condition of stoma and periostomal area. Indicate type of skin barrier used, size of opening cut for new appliance, treatment of skin, and new pouch applied.

RATIONALE Documents nursing action and provides data for next pouch change to health care team.

Documentation Example

10/14 0920 Colostomy stoma red and moist; periostomal skin intact; cleaned with warm water and dried. Stomahesive applied around stoma; 2⅛" opening cut in faceplate; new pouch applied without wrinkles. States has had no leakage problems.

_____
(Nurse's signature)

■ Special Considerations

✓ Patient is draped during procedure to prevent chilling.
✓ Old pouch must be disposed of as hazardous waste. Plastic discard bag should be closed securely before discarding.
✓ Some pouches can be washed and reused. Rinse with tepid water, wash with warm soap and water, rinse with vinegar solution (1 part water, 7 parts vinegar), and allow to dry.

?CRITICAL THINKING QUESTIONS

1. How would you handle a patient with a new colostomy who doesn't even want to look at the stoma, much less change the appliance?

2. What are possible consequences of using an ostomy appliance that is too small?

Steps 30-3 | Irrigating a Colostomy

When the colostomy patient has difficulty evacuating the bowel during times of illness or immobility, an irrigation is used to promote evacuation.

Review and carry out the Standard Steps in Appendix 3.

1. **ACTION** Assist patient as needed to assume comfortable position on the toilet or commode chair. Place patient on bed rest in side-lying position.

RATIONALE If patient is confined to bed, assisting into a side-lying position will permit irrigation with evacuation into a bedpan or bedside commode.

2. **ACTION** Put on gloves and remove the old pouch and place it in plastic disposable bag.

RATIONALE Pouch may be cleansed and reused or discarded. Supporting the skin around the appliance during removal will prevent pulling.

3. **ACTION** Cleanse skin and stoma with tepid water and pat dry. Observe the condition of skin and stoma.

RATIONALE Determines whether any problems with stoma and skin exist.

4. **ACTION** Apply irrigating sleeve and secure with belt. Direct the sleeve between the thighs or over side of the bed and into the toilet, bedside commode, or bedpan.

RATIONALE The sleeve is the correct length if it reaches water level in the toilet; cut off any excess.

5. **ACTION** Hang irrigation container filled with approximately 1 quart of warm water so that the base of the container is level with the patient's shoulder or 18 inches above bed.

RATIONALE Cold water causes cramping, and hot water can burn the intestinal mucosa. More than 1000 mL of water overdistends the bowel. Hanging the container too high results in too much force of the water and causes cramping. If the container is too low, there will not be sufficient flow to irrigate adequately.

6. **ACTION** Allow enough water to flow through irrigation tubing to remove air. Close the clamp.

RATIONALE Air entering the colon can cause gas pains.

7. **ACTION** Lubricate the cone tip and gently insert it through hole in top of irrigation sleeve into stoma; use gentle pressure to hold the cone in place.

RATIONALE Lubrication makes insertion easier. Cone should fit snugly to hold water in bowel; do not force. Cone prevents backflow.

8. **ACTION** Open control clamp and allow the solution to flow into patient (takes about 5 to 10 min-

Continued

Steps 30-3   **Irrigating a Colostomy**—cont'd

utes). If there is no flow, rotate the cone. Initially 500 mL may be used. If water won't flow, the cone may be against the bowel and require repositioning. If repositioning does not result in better flow, there may be kinks in tubing or hard stool blocking the stoma.

RATIONALE A slow flow gently distends the bowel without causing cramping.

9. **ACTION** If cramping occurs, slow or stop the flow of fluid.

RATIONALE When cramps occur, fluid must be stopped until they subside. Have patient take deep breaths through the mouth to relax the abdominal muscles.

10. **ACTION** When all irrigation fluid has been instilled, close the flow control clamp and remove the irrigation cone from the stoma. Close the top of the irrigation sleeve. Make certain end of irrigation sleeve is in toilet or appropriate container.

RATIONALE Return of stool takes 10 to 20 minutes. Proper positioning of sleeve prevents spillage of feces.

11. **ACTION** After initial evacuation is complete, close end of irrigation sleeve with the clip. Patient may get up and walk around, shower, shave, etc.

RATIONALE Further evacuation occurs in about 30 minutes. Exercise stimulates evacuation.

12. **ACTION** Have patient resume position on toilet and open sleeve into the bowl or container until drainage is complete.

RATIONALE Directs feces and fluid into toilet.

13. **ACTION** Remove the irrigation sleeve and rinse it well and hang up to dry if it is reusable. Cleanse the skin as needed and apply skin barrier and clean pouch as appropriate (see Skill 30-2).

RATIONALE Many irrigation sleeves are reusable. Pouch prevents accidental leakage of feces.

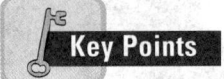

Key Points

- The small and large intestines are involved in waste production and elimination (see Figure 30-1).
- The appearance of stool is affected by diet and metabolism; normal stool is light to dark brown, soft, and tubular in shape, with a diameter of about 1 inch.
- Occult blood is suspected when stool appears dark black with a sticky consistency.
- Black, sticky stool indicates bleeding in the upper intestinal tract; bright red blood indicates bleeding in the large intestine.
- Pale white or light gray stool indicates an absence of bile in the intestine.
- Constipation is the most common problem of a hypoactive bowel; feces become compacted and hardened. Any patient restricted to bed rest is at risk for constipation.
- The elderly may develop constipation from a lack of fiber or from decreasing fluid intake.
- If a laxative is needed, a bulk-forming type is best.
- Diarrhea occurs when increased peristalsis pushes food through the intestinal tract too fast; infants or elderly patients with diarrhea can become dehydrated very quickly.
- Fecal incontinence may affect persons of all ages due to illness, injury, or neurogenic dysfunction.
- Bowel status should be assessed for every patient every day (see Focused Assessment 30-1).
- Measures to assist elimination are needed if a patient has not had a bowel movement for more than 3 days.

- For regular bowel movements, encourage exercise, dietary fiber, and at least 2500 mL of fluid per day.
- Patients undergoing barium x-rays need to flush the bowel after the test to prevent impaction.
- Diarrhea caused by a virus or bacteria is usually not treated with medication for 24 to 48 hours. The patient is given clear fluids and allowed to rest.
- If diarrhea does not clear within 48 hours after starting medication, the doctor should be consulted.
- Rectal suppositories are used to stimulate a bowel movement.
- Enemas are given to cleanse the bowel, deliver medication, relieve distention, or soften stool.
- Use a left Sims' position for enema administration; enema fluid should not be warmer than 105° F (40.5° C).
- Fecal impaction is first treated by oil-retention enema followed several hours later by a cleansing enema; if this does not relieve it, digital removal must occur.
- No more than three large-volume enemas are given without checking with the physician about additional enemas.
- A bowel training program takes 2 to 3 months or longer.
- A bowel ostomy is performed when fecal diversion is necessary (see Figure 30-6); an ostomy can cause a serious disruption to body image.
- An ileostomy produces very liquid effluent, whereas a colostomy produces more formed stool.

- A pale or dusky stoma indicates compromised blood supply and should be reported to the physician.
- An ostomy appliance must be cut to the correct size or it will not fit correctly over the stoma.
- Ostomy pouches should be emptied when one third to one half full to prevent excessive pulling on the faceplate of the appliance.

 Go to your **Companion CD-ROM** for an Audio Glossary, animations, video clips, and more.

evolve Be sure to visit the companion Evolve site at http://evolve.elsevier.com/deWit/fundamental/ for additional online resources.

NCLEX-PN® EXAMINATION-STYLE REVIEW QUESTIONS

*Choose the **best** answer(s) for each question.*

1. Based on an understanding of normal physiology, the nurse knows that functions of the large intestine are to: *(Select all that apply.)*
   1. absorb sodium and chlorides.
   2. aid in the digestion of foods.
   3. reabsorb water.
   4. transport waste products.
   5. produce and carry chyme.

2. The nurse is doing preprocedural teaching with a patient who is scheduled to have a barium enema. Which of the following statements by the patient indicates a need for additional teaching?
   1. "I will have to increase my fluid intake after the procedure."
   2. "The barium increases my risk for diarrhea."
   3. "I may receive a laxative after the procedure."
   4. "My stool may be chalk-colored for several days."

3. A nurse is preparing to give a patient an enema. The patient should be placed in the left Sims' position because:
   1. it is the most comfortable position.
   2. bringing the knee to the abdomen straightens the colon.
   3. fluid will flow along the natural curve of the rectum.
   4. the prone position is too uncomfortable.

4. If the solution for an enema is too cool,
   1. the solution runs in too slowly.
   2. cramping and discomfort may occur.
   3. bubbling and flatus occur in the bowel.
   4. bowel constriction prevents evacuation.

5. Which abnormal stool characteristics is the cause for the greatest immediate concern?
   1. Dark black, sticky stool
   2. Pale white or light gray stool
   3. Mucus-coated; slimy appearance
   4. Foul-smelling and floating

6. Which statement by the patient indicates an understanding of the information that was taught for self-care related to diarrhea?
   1. "I should consume clear liquids for 2 days and then try applesauce."
   2. "I should increase my consumption of fruits and vegetables."
   3. "I should eat small, frequent meals that include high-quality proteins."
   4. "I should try over-the-counter antidiarrheals for at least 3 days."

7. The nurse is attempting to manually remove a fecal impaction. What is the most serious complication that can occur during the procedure?
   1. Vagal response causes severe pain in the rectal area.
   2. Vagal response causes semiliquid stool and cramping.
   3. Vagal response predisposes to future episodes of reimpaction.
   4. Vagal response causes slow pulse and cardiac dysrhythmias.

8. The nursing student is reviewing the procedure for how to administer a cleansing enema solution. Which statement by the student indicates a correct understanding of the procedure?
   1. "The amount of solution for an adult, is between 1000 and 1500 mL."
   2. "The enema tube should be inserted about 6 to 10 inches into the anus."
   3. "The temperature of the solution should be between 110° and 120° F."
   4. "If the physician orders 'enemas until clear,' three is the maximum."

9. The nurse is changing the stoma appliance for a patient who has an existing colostomy. Below are the steps for the procedure. Place these steps (1 though 7) in the correct order.
   _____ 1. Center and carefully apply the pouch appliance.
   _____ 2. Remove old pouch by stabilizing the skin with one hand.
   _____ 3. Instruct patient to lie quietly or sit still for 5 minutes.
   _____ 4. Apply skin barrier paste to periostomal area.
   _____ 5. Clean the stoma and skin gently with warm water and soft cloth.
   _____ 6. Gently press down the skin barrier ring around the stoma.
   _____ 7. Attach and secure pouch tail closure.

10. An elderly patient living in an extended care facility has a nursing diagnosis of Bowel incontinence related to confusion. Which intervention would be the best for this patient?

1. Use positive reinforcement for incontinence episodes.
2. Obtain a physician's order for a low-fiber diet.
3. Have the patient drink 1000 mL of fluid unless contraindicated.
4. Assist the patient to the toilet, especially after meals.

CRITICAL THINKING ACTIVITIES *Read each clinical scenario and discuss the questions with your classmates.*

Scenario A
Lana Jakubowsky had a stroke and has been incontinent of feces. Her condition is improving and she is regaining muscle tone in her left arm and leg.

1. How would you go about devising a bowel training program for her?
2. How long do you think it might take for her to be continent of stool again?

Scenario B
Von Troung, age 78, has had the flu and diarrhea for 3 days. He is confused, and the skin around his anus is very inflamed.

1. How would you determine whether Mr. Troung is experiencing an electrolyte imbalance?
2. What would you do about skin care for Mr. Troung?
3. What measures should be taken to treat Mr. Troung's diarrhea?

Scenario C
Carol Tweed is to have a hip replacement. She also has a colostomy.

1. Create a care plan for her nursing diagnosis of Risk for constipation related to intestinal diversion, narcotic analgesics, and NPO status.
2. What extra precautions would need to be taken in the early postoperative period for this patient?

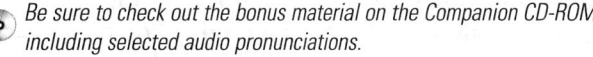

http://evolve.elsevier.com/deWit/fundamental/

Objectives

Upon completing this chapter, you should be able to:

Theory

1. Discuss the application of The Joint Commission pain standards in planning patient care.
2. Explain why pain is considered the "fifth vital sign."
3. Explain the physiology of pain using the gate control theory.
4. Describe the use of a variety of nursing interventions for pain control, including biofeedback, distraction, guided imagery, massage, and relaxation.
5. Describe the need for normal sleep.
6. Discuss how the need for sleep changes over the life span.
7. Delineate factors that can interfere with sleep.
8. Define the sleep disorders insomnia, sleep apnea, and narcolepsy.

Clinical Practice

1. Assist the patient in accurately describing sensations of pain and discomfort.
2. Accurately and appropriately record the patient's report of pain using clear, descriptive terms.
3. Evaluate the effects of various techniques used for pain control.
4. Assist the patient using a transcutaneous electrical nerve stimulation (TENS) unit.
5. Evaluate the effects of pain medication, and accurately report and record observations.
6. Assist with the care of patients receiving patient-controlled analgesia (PCA) or epidural analgesia.
7. Assess a patient regarding sleep difficulties.
8. Develop a plan designed to assist the patient in getting adequate sleep.

Skills & Steps

Skills

Skill 31-1   Operating a Transcutaneous Electrical Nerve Stimulator Unit
Skill 31-2   Setting Up (or Monitoring) a PCA Pump

Steps

Steps 31-1   Monitoring an Epidural Catheter and Changing the Dressing

Key Terms

Be sure to check out the bonus material on the Companion CD-ROM, including selected audio pronunciations.

analgesic (ăn-ăl-JĒ-zĭk, p. 610)
biofeedback (p. 608)
bolus (p. 610)
continuous positive airway pressure (CPAP) (p. 616)
distraction (p. 608)
endorphins (ĕn-DŌR-fĭnz) (p. 601)
epidural analgesia (ĕ-pĭ-DŪ-rŭl, p. 613)
gate control theory (p. 600)
guided imagery (Ĭ-măj-rē, p. 608)
hypnosis (p. 608)
insomnia (p. 616)
massage (p. 608)
meditation (p. 608)
narcolepsy (p. 616)
non–rapid eye movement (NREM) sleep (p. 613)
nonsteroidal anti-inflammatory drugs (NSAIDs)
   (nŏn-stē-RŌY-dăl ĂN-tĭ-ĭn-FLĂ-mă-tō-rē, p. 609)
pain (p. 599)
patient-controlled analgesia (PCA) (ă-năl-JĒ-sē-ă, p. 610)
rapid eye movement (REM) sleep (p. 613)
relaxation (p. 607)
sleep apnea (p. 616)
transcutaneous electrical nerve stimulation (TENS)
   (trăns-kū-TĀ-nē-ŭs, p. 605)

PAIN AND DISCOMFORT

Pain (feeling of discomfort strong enough to be intrusive and to affect or interfere with normal activity) is experienced by the majority of patients sometime during their health care experience. Surgical patients experience postoperative pain, and the condition requiring surgery may also cause pain. Many medical conditions, ranging from a headache to a myocardial infarction (heart attack), can cause pain. Fever causes generalized discomfort. Cancer, infection, fractures, cuts and abrasions, indeed the majority of illnesses and conditions are accompanied by varying degrees and types of pain.

There is no accurate objective measurement of pain. An electrocardiogram can indicate whether or not a patient's heart is beating correctly, and an electroencephalogram can verify abnormal brain activity, but there are no such tests for pain. It can only be assumed that patients will experience pain based on their diagnosed condition. Pain has historically been regarded as a symptom of a condition to be diagnosed and treated, thus eliminating the pain. For example, based on past experience, it was understood that patients with appendicitis experience severe pain. Following surgery, it was expected that they would experience significant incisional pain for the first day or two, following which the amount of pain would steadily decrease with each passing day until it ceased altogether. Using this model, continued severe pain was judged either as an indication of complications, or, in the absence of such complications, as drug-seeking behavior in a patient who has become addicted to the pain medication. Now, however, experts in the field regard pain as a condition rather than a symptom, and ideas about pain and its management are changing.

In the past, pain control measures were based on the health care providers' understanding of how much pain the patient should have, based on the diagnosis. The physician ordered what was believed to be an appropriate amount of pain medication, and it was dispensed in response to the patient's request and the nurse's assessment of the actual degree of need. For example, the physician might order hydromorphone (Dilaudid) 2 to 4 mg every 4 to 6 hours subcutaneously for pain as needed, and the nurse would then determine how frequent and how large a dose within these limits would keep the patient comfortable.

The approach to pain control has changed. The establishment of pain assessment and treatment standards and the expansion of pain management options are two factors that have contributed to these changes. In 1999, The Joint Commission established standards related to pain that focus on the patient. The standards relative to direct patient care state the following:

- Patients have the right to appropriate assessment and management of pain.
- Pain is assessed in all patients.
- Patients are educated about pain and managing pain as part of treatment, as appropriate.
- The discharge process provides for continuing pain care based on the patient's assessed needs at the time of discharge.

Pain assessment is now performed along with each assessment of vital signs, and pain is now considered the "fifth vital sign." Documentation of the findings must be completed. Hospitalized patients are now frequently using patient-controlled analgesia (PCA) machines. These allow patients to administer medication within safe boundaries based on their perception of pain. Medication is administered intravenously, with the patient controlling when administration occurs, within boundaries prescribed by the physician. There is also an increased use of nonpharmacologic methods of pain relief, such as biofeedback, distraction, guided imagery, massage, and relaxation techniques, each of which is discussed in this chapter. Other complementary treatments, such as chiropractic, acupuncture, and acupressure, are also being used (see Chapter 32).

The fentanyl patch is a newer method for controlling chronic pain. It is replaced every 72 hours and can be managed at home by the patient. For postsurgical patients, a new form of pump allows the patient to administer pain medication directly to the incision site, rather than systemically.

THEORIES OF PAIN

Pain is defined as a feeling of discomfort, distress, or suffering caused by the stimulation of nerve endings. Acute pain is often a warning of potential or actual tissue damage, and allows the sufferer to withdraw from the source or to seek help in relieving symptoms.

Pain is transmitted to the brain through the nervous system. This is done through afferent (sensory) neurons leading to the spinal nerves, and then to the brain. Once the signal is interpreted, the brain sends out a message to the body to respond (Figure 31-1).

Gate Control Theory

The gate control theory was first described by Melzack and Wall in 1965. Pain transmission is viewed as being controlled by a gate mechanism in the central nervous system (Figure 31-2). Stated in the simplest terms, opening the gate allows the transmission of pain sensation and closing the gate blocks this transmission. Several ideas that impact nursing practice are part of the gate control theory, including

- The gate may be opened by activity in the small-diameter nerve fibers from such things as tissue damage. Activity in the large-diameter nerve fibers, such as that provided by massage or vibration, seems to close the gate.
- Brainstem impulses caused by a high sensory input seem to close the gate, whereas a lack of this input allows the gate to open. This may be why people who are bored or lonely can experience a greater intensity in their pain than when they are occupied or distracted by such things as visitors or a particularly interesting program or activity.
- The cerebral cortex and thalamus play a role by opening the gate with impulses originating from an increase in anxiety, or by closing it with impulses originating from a decrease in anxiety. For example, fear that the pain will get worse and

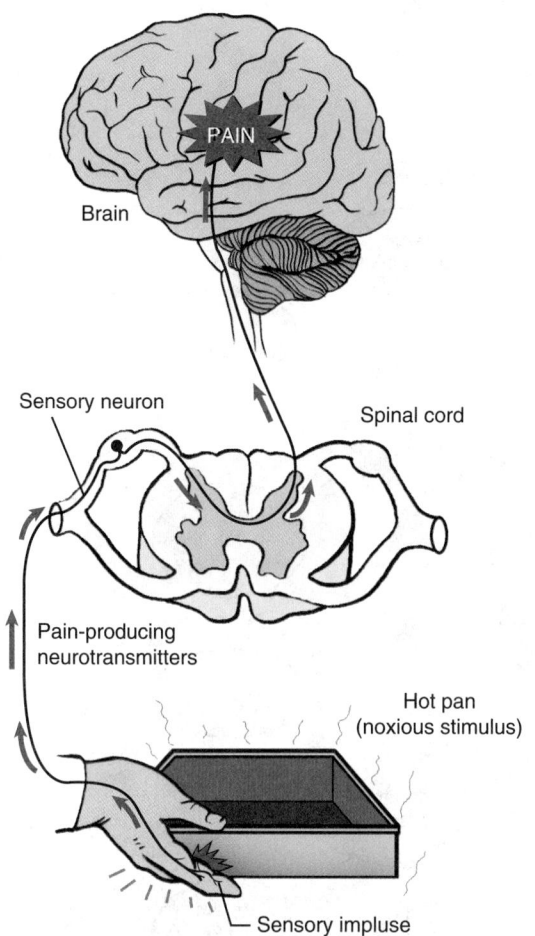

FIGURE **31-1** Pain transmission.

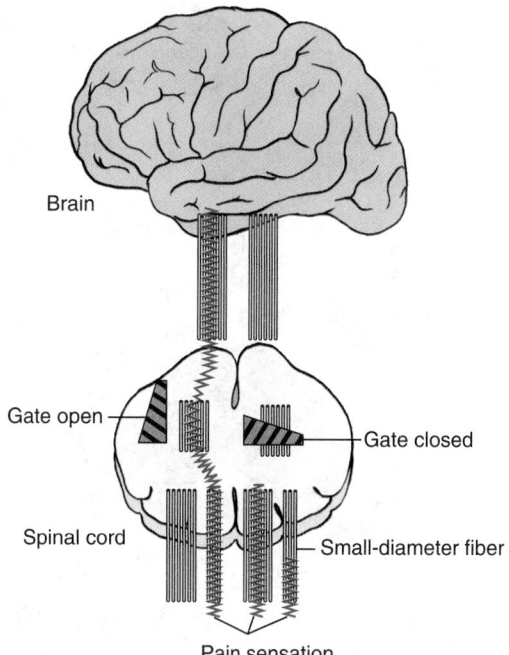

FIGURE **31-2** The gate control theory of pain.

not be controlled can increase the intensity; knowing that pain can be and is being controlled can reduce the intensity.

Endorphins

Endorphins are endogenous, naturally occurring, opiate-like peptides that reduce or block the perception of pain. The word "endorphin" comes from "morphine" and "endogenous" (from within). Like morphine, endorphins attach to nerve endings in opioid receptors and block pain transmission. Both physiologic and psychological stressors can release endorphins, resulting in a reduction in pain and an increase in the sense of well-being.

TYPES OF PAIN

The type and intensity of pain the patient is experiencing will assist in selecting methods that will best relieve the patient's discomfort. The patient's verbal description of pain, nonverbal signs of pain, and physiologic indicators of pain may vary according to the type of pain the patient is experiencing. **Treatment decisions should be based on assessment that considers all of these factors.** Concept Map 31-1 depicts the various types of pain.

Acute Pain

Acute pain is usually associated with an injury, medical condition, or surgical procedure. It is of short duration, lasting from a few hours to a few days. Injuries causing acute pain may include burns, bone fractures, and muscle strains. Medical conditions causing acute pain may include pneumonia, sickle cell crisis, angina, herpes zoster, inflammations, infections, and blockages. Acute pain may be described as aching, throbbing, or searing. The patient may be agitated or restless, and may protect the painful area by *splinting*, or supporting the area. Pain may also be accompanied by an increase in heart rate, blood pressure, and respiratory rate. **Acute pain may worsen in the presence of anxiety or fear.** The cause is usually easily determined, and the pain well controlled with analgesics (pain medications), surgery, or other techniques. Once the cause is removed, acute pain will be relieved.

Chronic Pain

Chronic pain may continue for months or possibly years. Chronic pain is associated with ongoing conditions, such as arthritis and back problems. There are many medical problems that can cause chronic pain. The limitations imposed by chronic pain can cause long-lasting psychosocial effects for the patient, due to necessary changes in lifestyle. Chronic pain may be described as dull, constant, shooting, tingling, or burning. The increased heart rate, blood pressure, and respiratory rate seen with acute pain are often absent with chronic pain. A combination of pharmacologic and nonpharmacologic treatments is recommended to

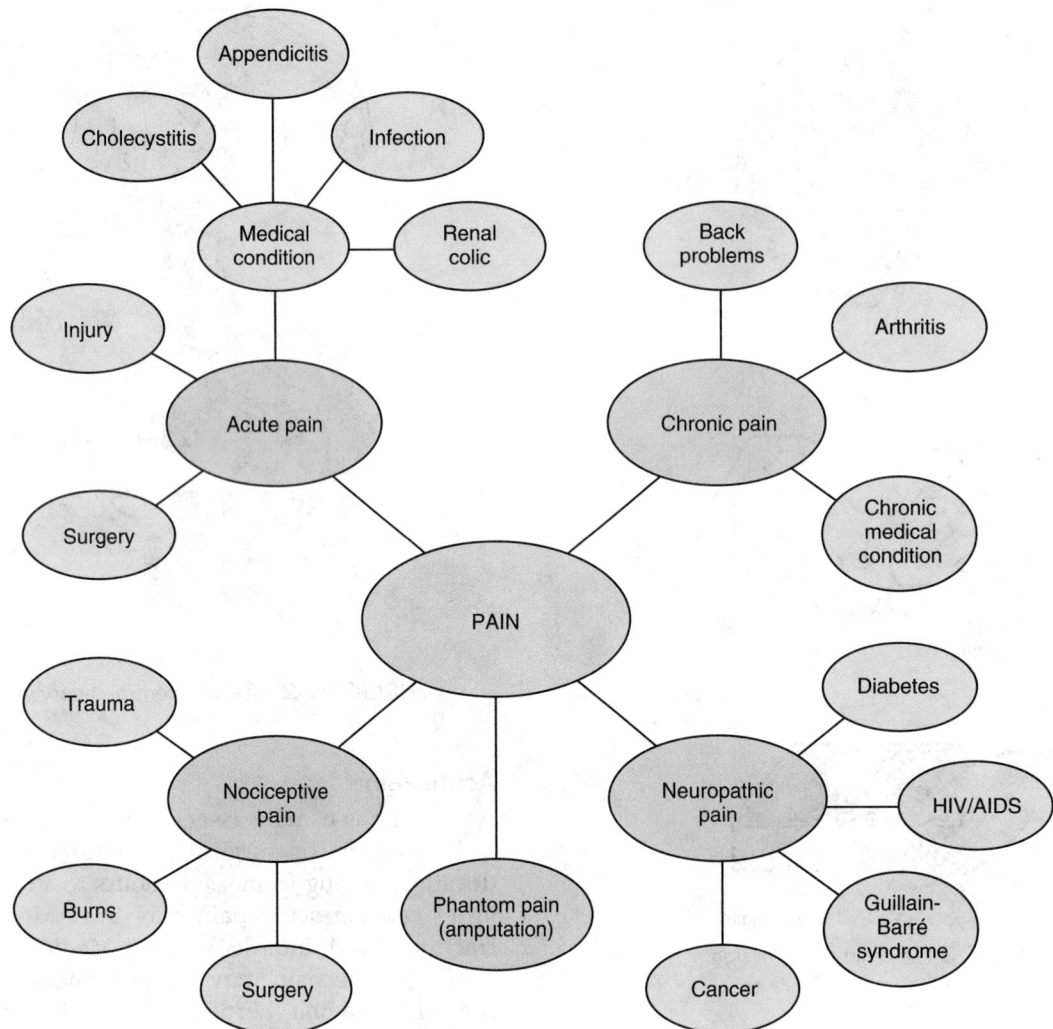

CONCEPT MAP **31-1** The various types and causes of pain.

alleviate chronic pain. This would include combining medication with treatments such as guided imagery, application of heat and cold, and massage (see Concept Map 31-1).

Nociceptive Pain

Nociceptive pain involves injury to tissue in which receptors called *nociceptors* are located. Nociceptors may be found in skin, joints, or organ viscera. Injuries triggering nociceptive pain may be caused by trauma, burns, or surgery. There are four phases of pain associated with nociceptive pain. *Transduction* is the first phase and begins when tissue damage causes the release of substances that stimulate the nociceptors and start the sensation of pain. *Transmission* is the second phase and involves movement of the pain sensation to the spinal cord. *Perception*, the third phase, occurs when pain impulses reach the brain and the pain is recognized. The fourth phase, *modulation*, occurs when neurons in the brain send signals back down the spinal cord by release of neurotrans-

mitters. Treatment of nociceptive pain may be directed toward one or all of the four phases. Nonsteroidal anti-inflammatory drugs (NSAIDs) work by blocking the production of the substances that trigger the nociceptors in the transduction phase. Drugs that interfere with the transmission phase include opioids. Nonpharmacologic treatments such as distraction and guided imagery may be effective during the perception phase. Drugs that block neurotransmitter uptake work in the modulation stage.

Neuropathic Pain

Neuropathic pain is usually associated with a dysfunction of the nervous system, specifically an abnormality in the processing of sensations. Pain receptors in the body become sensitive to stimuli and send pain signals more easily. Nerve endings grow additional branches that send stronger pain signals to the brain. As the branches grow, they influence touch and warmth receptors and these receptors begin to send pain signals. In some cases, the pain signal that normally moves from the periphery toward the brain reverses and is sent in the opposite direction. These changes in the nervous system are often associated with medical conditions rather than tissue damage. Diabetes, Guillain-Barré syndrome, cancer, HIV, and nutritional deficiencies are examples of medical conditions that are associated with neuropathic pain. Analgesics and opioids usually do not relieve neuropathic pain. Neuropathic pain is sometimes managed with common analgesics such as those in the NSAID family, but also increasingly with adjuvant medications such as tricyclic antidepressants, anticonvulsants, and corticosteroids.

Phantom Pain

Phantom pain occurs after the loss of a body part from amputation. The patient may "feel" pain in the amputated part for years after the amputation has occurred. If this is not controlled with conventional methods, pain may be controlled by the use of continuous electrical stimulation from electrodes surgically implanted in the thalamus.

Think Critically About . . . What conditions might involve chronic pain and what might cause acute pain?

APPLICATION of the NURSING PROCESS

Assessment (Data Collection)

According to pain specialists, **"pain is whatever the experiencing person says it is, existing whenever he says it does"** (McCaffery and Pasero, 1989). In other words, only the patient knows what hurts and how much, and interventions must be based on the patient's own assessment of the degree of pain and the need for pain relief.

Perception of Pain

One of the most difficult aspects of pain management is the assessment of pain and the evaluation of the effectiveness of interventions. Cultural background influences how people may show pain (Cultural Cues 31-1). Some cultures teach that outward expressions of pain are to be avoided. Men in some cultures may believe that denying the presence of pain shows bravery and strength. Care must be taken to ensure that adequate pain management is provided. The elderly may not express pain because they mistakenly believe it is a logical consequence of aging, because they don't want to be a bother, or because they have been culturally trained not to complain about pain.

Observable indicators of pain include moaning, crying, irritability, inability to sleep, grimacing or frowning, restlessness, and a rigid posture in bed. Remember that these things can also indicate sorrow,

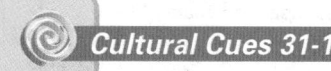
Cultural Cues 31-1

Perception of Pain

People from other cultures may have differing ideas about pain, both how to react to pain and what to do about it. It is important to understand these differences, and equally important not to assume someone believes a certain way because they belong to a particular cultural group.

Table 31-1 *Descriptive Terms for Pain*

TYPE OF DESCRIPTION	SPECIFIC TERMS
Degree of pain	Absent, minimal, mild, moderate, fairly severe, very or extremely severe, exquisite, excruciating
Quality of pain	Crushing, throbbing, pulsating, twisting, pulling, burning, searing, stabbing, tearing, biting, blinding, nauseating, debilitating
Area of pain	Name of affected body area or part (e.g., right foot, right lower abdomen)
	Localized, radiating, generalized
Frequency of pain	Constant, intermittent, occasional

worry, fear, and fatigue. In addition, some stoic patients may show none of these outward expressions of pain. Other detectable signs of pain can be an elevation in blood pressure, heart rate, and respirations or the presence of nausea or diaphoresis. Fully assess the patient's pain, and encourage the patient to express the perception of the pain being experienced. **Some patients may perceive pain to be less than or greater than what you may have seen before for the same condition.**

Alert adult patients may be able to use specific words to describe their pain. However, even for adults, it can be difficult to describe and tell how much pain is present. Table 31-1 gives some terms that can be used to describe pain. Be aware of any communication blocks that may prevent the patient from adequately describing the pain. For example, patients who speak a foreign language may require a translator to adequately describe their pain.

Pain Scales

A variety of pain scales are available to assist patients in communicating their pain level. A number scale is often used to assist the patient to rate the level of pain, with 0 being pain free and 10 being the worst pain imaginable (Figure 31-3). When requesting pain medication and when assessing the degree of relief following the dose, the patient can refer to the number scale. For example, David Randel, who had an appendectomy this morning, may describe his incisional pain as being 8 on a scale of 0 to 10, or very bad, but not the

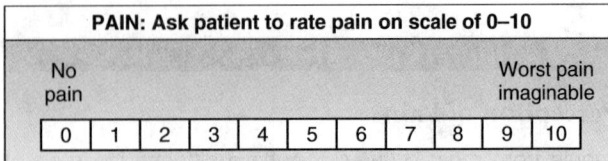

FIGURE **31-3** Pain number rating scale.

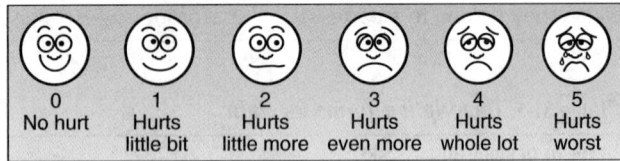

FIGURE **31-4** Wong-Baker FACES Pain Rating Scale for children.

worst possible pain. One hour after receiving his medication, he may describe his pain as being a 3, not gone but greatly reduced, allowing him to move about and rest in reasonable comfort.

Children, as well as some adults, may find a number scale difficult to use. A picture scale showing faces in varying degrees of pain can also help assess pain (Figure 31-4). The FLACC (Face, Legs, Activity, Cry, and Consolability) scale is used for preverbal or noncommunicative children (Assignment Considerations 31-1). For infants, one of several scales is used: the NIPS (Neonatal Infant Pain Scale), CRIES (Crying, Requires oxygen to maintain saturation, Increased vital signs, Expression, and Sleeplessness), and PIPP (Premature Infant Pain Profile).

For the confused patient, nonverbal cues that pain is being experienced may include restlessness, rocking, pacing, rigidity, guarding, wincing, crying, grimacing with movement, new inability to sleep, hypersensitivity to touch, withdrawal from usual contact with others, moaning, and grunting. Family or close friends may be able to provide input on how the individual has expressed pain in the past.

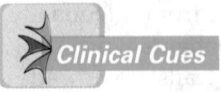

Management of acute pain, such as postsurgical pain, may be more difficult for patients who have been on opioid medications to control chronic pain. Because they already have an underlying degree of constant pain being controlled by routine medication, they often require higher and/or more frequent doses of analgesia than other patients. This is not a sign of addiction, but rather a legitimate need for a greater degree of analgesia being needed to achieve relief of the additional acute pain.

The scale selected to assist in determining the presence and intensity of pain must be indicated on the patient care plan so that it is used consistently by staff.

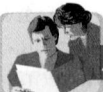

Assignment Considerations 31-1

Reporting Signs of Pain

Remind assistive personnel to report nonverbal signs of pain in patients such as wincing when being turned, rigid posture, grimacing with movement, or crying with repositioning.

| Box 31-1 | *Nursing Diagnoses for the Patient with Pain* |

- Readiness for enhanced comfort
- Acute pain
- Chronic pain
- Fatigue
- Self-care deficit
- Deficient knowledge
- Sleep deprivation
- Anxiety
- Fear

Think Critically About . . . How would you assess pain in a nonverbal patient? How would you assess pain relief?

Nursing Diagnosis

Accurate nursing diagnosis for the patient with pain is based on the patient assessment. Because pain is an individual experience, the reported pain may vary from patient to patient, even though they share a similar medical diagnosis. Box 31-1 gives examples of possible nursing diagnoses for the patient with pain.

Planning

The plan of care must include pain assessment and management. This should include realistic goals with specific time frames for achieving results. A possible goal might be "patient will report pain at a level of less than 3 on a 0-to-10 scale within 2 days." Goals should be realistic; a patient with a chronic condition may not be pain free, even with the use of analgesics.

Implementation

Pain is an individual experience. **Medications or treatments that prove effective for one patient may not relieve symptoms as well for another patient.** Different methods may need to be tried alone or in combination before the patient has effective pain relief (Nursing Care Plan 31-1).

Nonmedicinal Methods of Pain Control

Just as an individual may get better relief from one medication than another, there will be a variation in the effectiveness of nonmedicinal pain control methods. Appropriate use of nonmedicinal methods of pain control in some cases can greatly reduce the amount of

NURSING CARE PLAN 31-1

Care of the Patient in Pain

SCENARIO Sara Reynolds, a 45-year-old patient with a history of rheumatoid arthritis, has been admitted to the unit following a right total hip replacement performed this morning. Orders include morphine sulfate via patient-controlled analgesia (PCA) pump, which has just been started. Ms. Reynolds has complained of pain at 8 on a 0-to-10 scale. Her blood pressure and pulse are slightly elevated, but her temperature and respirations are normal. She has been restless and grimaces frequently. You implement the following portion of her plan of care.

PROBLEM/NURSING DIAGNOSIS *Hip replacement*/Pain related to surgical procedure.
Supporting Assessment Data: Subjective: Patient reports pain at 8 on a 0-to-10 scale. **Objective:** Hip replacement today. BP and pulse slightly elevated; grimacing and restless.

Goals/Expected Outcomes	Nursing Interventions	Selected Rationale	Evaluation
Patient will report pain at 0 to 4 on a 0-to-10 scale within 2 hr.	Teach to use the PCA pump.	Knowledge of how to use the pump allows the patient to use it correctly.	*Is pain at 0 to 4?* Yes. Using pump correctly.
	Encourage relaxation techniques; provide diversionary activities such as television and reading.	Relaxation and diversion are known to lessen pain by focusing the mind elsewhere.	Taught relaxation exercise. Does not wish to watch TV at present.
	Encourage use of the PCA before ambulation, or exercise.	Medicating before activity reduces pain from the activity.	Medicated before PT visit.
	Splint abdomen with pillow when coughing or using spirometer.	Splinting reduces pain associated with movement of the abdomen.	Taught splinting technique.
	Observe frequently for pain relief and side effects of medication.	If pain is inadequately relieved, other measures to relieve it can be employed. Knowing if side effects are occurring allows measures to be taken to alleviate or prevent them.	No side effects noted other than drowsiness. Pain at 3. Progressing toward expected outcomes.

❓ CRITICAL THINKING QUESTIONS

1. What factors might influence a child's report of pain?

2. What factors might lead to undertreatment of pain in the elderly population?

---

medication needed. However, this does not mean that the patient should be denied medication to control the pain. As patients gain control and as changes in their condition reduce overall pain, they will voluntarily reduce the use of medications.

Transcutaneous Electrical Nerve Stimulation. Transcutaneous electrical nerve stimulation (TENS) uses a small electrical stimulator attached to electrodes to block pain. This therapy is available in high-frequency stimulation and low-frequency stimulation. Acute pain may be treated with conventional high-frequency TENS therapy, whereas low-frequency TENS therapy is more effective in the treatment of chronic pain. The electrodes are placed on the skin around the area of pain. Low-level current running between the electrodes acts to block the pain sensation. The patient can control the intensity and interval of the current with the dials on the stimulator (Figure 31-5). A health care professional trained in its use should initiate the

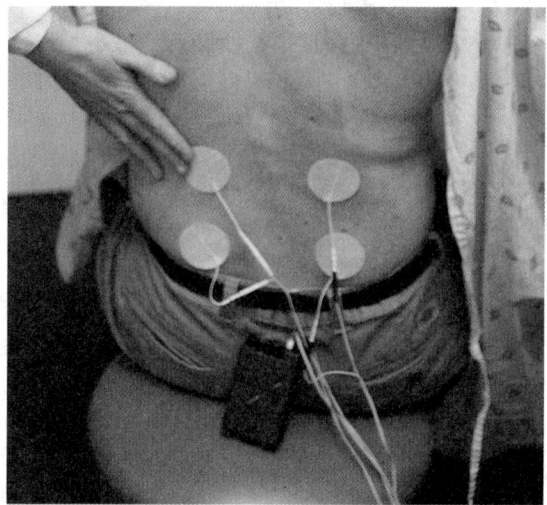

FIGURE **31-5** TENS unit blocks pain signal transmission.

application of the TENS unit. This may be a physical therapist, but may also be a nurse or physician.

The use of TENS requires a physician's order. TENS for the relief of postoperative pain is generally most effective when the patient has received instructions on the use of the device before surgery. Postoperative pain and analgesic medications make teaching more difficult than it would have been before surgery for most patients. TENS may also be ordered following traumatic injuries. The occasional patient will not tolerate TENS stimulation well. If this is the case, discontinue treatment and notify the physician (Skill 31-1).

Percutaneous Electrical Nerve Stimulation. A treatment showing promise for relief of lower back pain, such as that due to sciatica, and for relief of some severe headaches is percutaneous electrical nerve stimulation (PENS). An electric current is sent through thin needle probes positioned in the soft tissues and muscles of the back. A series of intermittent treatments using the electric current are given.

Binders. Binders are cloths wrapped around a limb or body part. They are effective in relieving pain associated with strains, sprains, and surgical incisions. They support the surface and internal tissues during

---

Skill 31-1 | Operating a Transcutaneous Electrical Nerve Stimulator Unit

Transcutaneous electrical nerve stimulation, or TENS, uses low-level electric current via electrodes to block pain sensation. Patients need to be properly instructed in the use of the TENS unit.

■ Supplies

✓ TENS unit
✓ Electrodes

✓ Conductive jelly (if electrodes are not precoated)

✓ Tape (if electrodes are not self-adhesive)

Review and carry out the Standard Steps in Appendix 3.

■ Assessment

1. **ACTION** Check the physician's orders. Check to see where electrodes are to be placed.

   RATIONALE Ensures proper placement of electrodes and appropriate TENS settings.

■ Planning

2. **ACTION** Assemble equipment.

   RATIONALE Avoids interruptions and provides for good time management.

3. **ACTION** Identify the patient.

   RATIONALE Ensures correct patient receives the TENS.

4. **ACTION** Explain the procedure to the patient.

   RATIONALE Decreases patient anxiety and increases cooperation.

■ Implementation

5. **ACTION** Make sure the TENS unit is turned off; check to see that the electrodes are properly connected to the unit.

   RATIONALE Avoids premature stimulation of the site.

6. **ACTION** Spread the conductive jelly on the electrode pads, if electrodes are not precoated.

   RATIONALE Provides for correct electrical conduction.

7. **ACTION** Place the electrode pads against the patient's skin in the designated places. Use tape if necessary to secure.

   RATIONALE Ensures good conduction; provides stimulation in prescribed places.

8. **ACTION** Position the patient comfortably.

   RATIONALE Comfort enhances effectiveness of the TENS treatment.

9. **ACTION** Explain to the patient that a tingling sensation will be felt.

   RATIONALE Explanations decrease patient anxiety.

10. **ACTION** Turn the TENS unit on.

    RATIONALE This begins the treatment.

11. **ACTION** Increase the amplitude of the TENS unit according to the response of the patient. Check frequently to see how the patient is tolerating the procedure.

    RATIONALE Patients should not receive TENS stimulation to the point of discomfort.

12. **ACTION** Turn off the TENS unit and remove the electrodes at the end of the ordered treatment time.

    RATIONALE Follows the prescribed treatment.

13. **ACTION** Assist the patient in cleaning the jelly off the skin and rearrange clothing.

    RATIONALE Provides for comfort and good hygiene.

■ Evaluation

14. ACTION Assess how the patient tolerated the procedure. Assess level of discomfort.

RATIONALE Evaluates effectiveness of procedure.

■ Documentation

15. ACTION Document the date, time, amplitude and length of time of the procedure, how the patient tolerated the procedure, and current level of pain.

RATIONALE Documents use of TENS unit and response to treatment.

Documentation Example

6/2 1000   TENS unit applied to right shoulder at amplitude of 5 for 20 minutes, tolerated well. Patient states pain at a level of 1 on 0-10 scale following the procedure.

_____

(Nurse's signature)

?CRITICAL THINKING QUESTIONS

1. In what patient population might TENS therapy be contraindicated?
2. What safety precautions should be considered for the patient receiving TENS therapy?

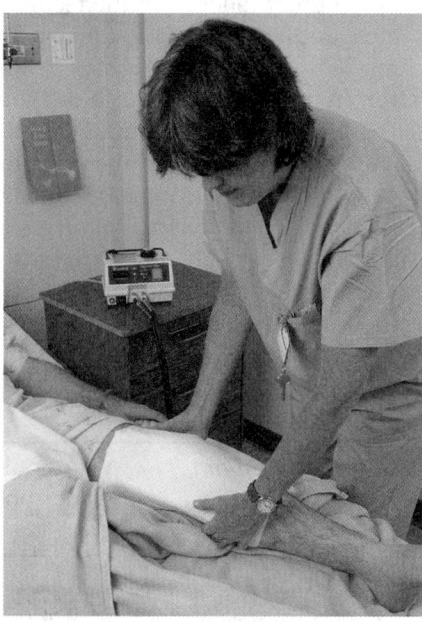

FIGURE **31-6** An Aquathermia K-Pad is used to help relieve pain in the knee.

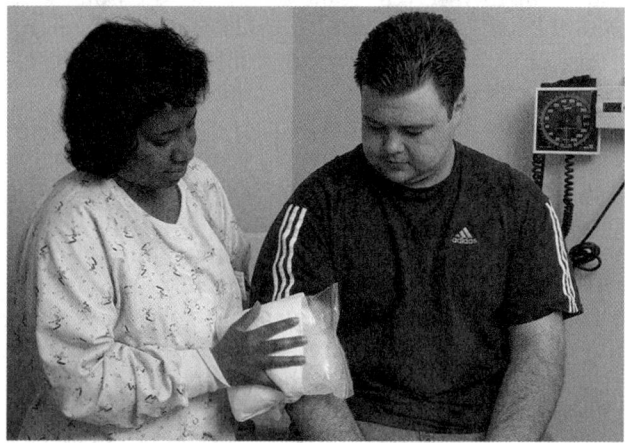

FIGURE **31-7** A cold pack reduces pain as well as swelling.

movement, coughing, and other activities. For example, an abdominal binder may be ordered to give additional support and provide comfort after abdominal surgery (see Chapter 38, Figure 38-11).

Application of Heat and Cold. The application of heat or cold, or the alternate application of first one and then the other, can often soothe or relieve pain from muscular strain or overwork. It is also effective in reducing pain associated with healing tissues.

Sources of warmth include warm water compresses, warm blankets, Aquathermia K-Pads, tub and whirlpool baths, and chemical self-heating packs (Figure 31-6). The use of heat-producing equipment may require a physician's order. When applying heat, check the temperature carefully to avoid burning the patient. Remember that very young and very old patients have skin that is more sensitive to heat damage. In addition, patients with altered levels of consciousness, impaired movement and feeling, or poor circulation may not be aware when something is too hot. These patients can suffer severe

burns in a short period. All patients should be closely monitored if heat applications are being used.

Cold is particularly helpful in reducing swelling and can also be effective in calming muscle spasms and reducing the pain in joints and muscles from a variety of causes (Figure 31-7). Gentle ice massage of painful muscles can be done using ice that has been frozen in a paper cup. The edge of the cup is torn away to expose the ice, the remaining cup is used as a handle, and the area is massaged with the ice surface. A bag of frozen peas can be used as an ice pack. Cold is most frequently applied in the form of cold or iced compresses. Some patients will have a poor tolerance for cold treatment, so be alert to the patient's response when using cold applications. Occasionally, patients will have an increase rather than a decrease in pain when ice is applied. To prevent skin damage, ice should be in contact with the skin for only a few minutes at a time, under direct supervision. Ice packs should be applied with a towel or other barrier between the pack and the skin, and not left in place for more than 15 to 20 minutes.

Relaxation. Relaxation or tension release is helpful in reducing pain and in allowing the patient to obtain greater relief from pain medications. It is a physical technique that involves conscious relaxation of muscle groups. Before beginning, the patient should be made comfortable in a quiet environment. Many people find that a darkened environment helps them relax. The patient is instructed to first tighten and then release the muscles. Initially, the patient is encouraged to pay close attention to the difference in the feeling of tension versus relaxation. Frequently, relaxation is done progressively. Have the patient begin by tensing and relaxing (or just relaxing) the toes and feet and then the ankles, calves, knees, thighs, lower abdomen (or stomach), upper abdomen (or chest), shoulders, arms, hands and fingers, neck, face, and head. These directions are given slowly, one body area at a time, with a short space of quiet between each directed relaxation. After a session or two, most patients can do this technique for themselves. Some people with chronic tension-related pain go to sleep this way every night. There are a variety of relaxation tapes available to assist patients who find this technique helpful.

Biofeedback. Biofeedback is a specialized relaxation technique using a machine that measures the degree of muscular tension with skin electrodes. The machine has colored lights that change (usually red to yellow to green) and a tone that changes in pitch from higher to lower as the patient relaxes muscular tension. The patient learns to use relaxation techniques or imagery to decrease tension. The degree of relaxation is measured by the biofeedback machine, causing the lights and the frequency tones to change, giving the patient immediate feedback on the degree of relaxation being achieved.

Distraction. Distraction assists the patient to focus on something other than the pain. Patients frequently do this inadvertently, such as when they joke with visitors and for the moment forget their pain. Unfortunately, nurses sometimes take this as proof that the patient is not in pain at all and see the patient's request for medication as drug-seeking behavior. In fact, the patient still hurts but is just focusing elsewhere.

Television, radio, playing a game, conversing with a friend or volunteer, reading, playing cards, using a computer, or even thinking about something else may all act as distractions. However, remember that the distraction does not make the pain go away; it merely diverts the attention elsewhere for a time. After the distraction is over, such as at the end of the television program or a visit, the patient may be more aware than ever of the pain. Distraction may be particularly helpful while waiting for an administered dose of medication to take effect. By the time the distraction ends, the pain has begun to be relieved by the analgesic.

? *Think Critically About . . .* What methods could you use to distract a patient in the hospital? In a long-term care facility? Being cared for at home?

Guided Imagery and Meditation. These methods differ from relaxation in that they are mental rather than physical techniques. In guided imagery (verbally guiding the patient to imagine something) as it is used for pain control, patients are assisted to form mental images of a pleasant environment where they are comfortable and happy, such as a favorite vacation place. Patients undergoing painful procedures, such as bone marrow aspiration, can learn to use imagery to "leave" the procedure and mentally go somewhere else while it is occurring. Some people have great difficulty seeing things in their minds and will need verbal direction to hear or feel pleasant sensations, such as the rustle of leaves or the feel of a breeze as it brushes across their cheeks. Many people who do not visualize well can still get great relief from the technique when it calls on their auditory and kinesthetic abilities (Patient Teaching 31-1).

Meditation (focusing on an image or thought) can provide the same relief from a painful situation, but it relies on the use of a focus point rather than the mental creation of an alternate environment. During meditation, individuals focus on a visual point, a sound, or a repeated phrase, or just the pattern of their own breathing. This focuses attention away from the pain or a painful situation and, for many people, induces profound physical relaxation and reduction in blood pressure and respiratory rate.

? *Think Critically About . . .* What could you suggest to a patient to use as a visual point for meditation?

Music. Music can be used alone as a source of distraction from pain, and is frequently used effectively in conjunction with other methods. Meditation and relaxation techniques can be done to restful music, and massage can be greatly enhanced by the presence of soft, soothing sound. Also effective is the use of nature sounds, such as tapes of the ocean, a flowing stream, or the sounds of the wind and birds in the trees. Listening with headphones allows patients to enjoy their own preferences in music without disturbing others.

Hypnosis. Hypnosis is also called therapeutic suggestion. It involves inducing a trance-like state using focusing and relaxation techniques and giving the patient suggestions that may be helpful after the return to an alert state of consciousness. Hypnosis should be done by someone trained in the technique. Hypnosis is only possible and effective when the individual is able to cooperate with the technique; it is pointless to urge it on someone who truly does not want to be hypnotized.

Massage. Massage has long been used to induce relaxation and bring relief from muscle and structural pain. A nightly back rub can bring much comfort to the bedridden patient. Long firm strokes, softer circular

Pain Control Through Guided Imagery

1. PREPARATION
- Assist the patient to a comfortable position.
- Lower the lights to a comfortable level, but not completely dark.
- Eliminate any distractions, such as television or radio.
- Close the door. Post a note asking not to be disturbed.

2. READ THE IMAGERY SCRIPT
- Read slowly, in a soft but easily heard voice. Pause frequently to allow the patient to form mental images. The script may be changed to incorporate a place or sensations specific to the patient.
- **Imagery Script:**
  - Relax, and gently close your eyes.
  - Take a deep, slow breath in through your nose. *(Pause)* Now slowly exhale through your mouth. Let your tension leave your body as you exhale. *(Pause)* Continue this with each breath. *(Pause)*
  - Imagine you are walking along a forest path. *(Pause)* Smell the fresh air. *(Pause)* Feel the breeze against your face. *(Pause)* Hear the crunch of leaves under your feet.
  - The path leads to your favorite place. It may be a beach, the mountains, or a favorite room in your home. *(Pause)* This is a special place, one where you feel relaxed and secure. *(Pause)*
  - Listen to the sounds around you. *(Pause)* Smell the air. *(Pause)* Take in the comforting sensations of your special place. *(Pause)*
  - Relax even more as you enjoy your surroundings. A feeling of peace and security wraps around you. *(Pause)* Tension leaves as you take in the sensations of this place. *(Pause)*
  - It is now time to leave this place. Get ready to leave, and head back to the forest path. *(Pause)*
  - You feel relaxed and at peace as you return to this room. *(Pause)* You know that you can return to your special place any time. *(Pause)*
  - When you are ready, open your eyes.

3. AFTER THE IMAGERY EXPERIENCE
- Allow the patient to share with you if desired. Accept that some patients will not want to share.

strokes, and gentle pounding stimulate circulation, relax muscles, and increase the patient's sense of well-being. This gift of direct comfort from nurse to patient, perhaps more than any other, demonstrates the caring relationship so important to good nursing care. The use of lotion warmed between the hands and then applied to the patient's back refreshes the skin and relieves dryness and itching (Figure 31-8).

Conditions such as a healing surgical wound or inflammation of the tissues or vessels may preclude direct massage to the area of pain. In such cases, firm massage to another area of the body may allow the patient to focus away from the area of pain. Also, massage distal or proximal to the point of pain may relieve

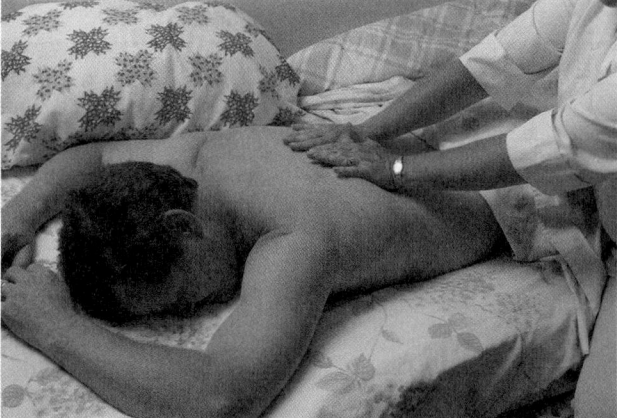

FIGURE **31-8** Massage is used to relax muscles and relieve pain.

pain while avoiding direct stimulation to an injured site.

Chiropractic, acupuncture, and acupressure therapies are also used for pain management. These are discussed in Chapter 32.

Medical Methods of Pain Control

Analgesic Medications. When pain medications are ordered for patients experiencing pain, you are responsible for monitoring the patient's pain level and administering the medication as ordered. The patient must also be monitored for effectiveness of the medication after administration. The time frame for reassessment will vary depending on the route of administration.

There are four basic categories of medications for the relief of pain. They are (1) nonopioid pain medications, a category that includes nonsteroidal anti-inflammatory drugs (NSAIDs); (2) cyclooxygenase-2 (COX-2) inhibitors; (3) narcotics or opioids; and (4) adjuvant analgesics. This fourth group includes drugs not primarily regarded as analgesics but that have been proven to be effective in the relief of certain types of pain; or that work with standard analgesics to produce better pain control. COX-2 inhibitors are a type of drug that selectively blocks the COX-2 enzyme, thought to play a role in the cause of arthritis pain. They do not block the COX-1 enzyme, which protects the gastrointestinal system. Therefore, these drugs are not supposed to cause the GI side effects such as gastritis and ulcers that NSAIDs may cause. Table 31-2 gives examples of the drugs in these four categories.

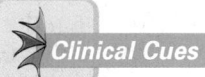
Clinical Cues

One of the most common side effects of analgesia is constipation. Patients on pain-relieving drugs should be encouraged to increase their fluid intake if not otherwise contraindicated, and they should be assessed daily regarding bowel function.

Table 31-2	*Categories of Analgesic Medications*	
TYPE OF DRUG	**PRIMARY MODE OF ACTION**	**EXAMPLES**
Non-narcotic analgesics, including NSAIDs	Block pain at the peripheral nervous system level	Over-the-counter: aspirin, acetaminophen, ibuprofen (nonprescription dose) Prescription: ibuprofen (prescription dose), naproxen, indomethacin
COX-2 inhibitors	Block the COX-2 enzyme, which plays a role in arthritis pain	Anti-inflammatories: celecoxib (Celebrex) currently only FDA approved COX-2 inhibitor
Narcotics or opioids	Block pain at the central nervous system level	Narcotic agonists: morphine, oxycodone, hydrocodone, hydromorphone, codeine, levorphanol, oxymorphone, meperidine (used less frequently in recent times due to significant side effects)
Adjuvant analgesics	Various methods of action	Anticonvulsants: phenytoin, carbamazepine Antidepressants: amitriptyline, imipramine Stimulants: caffeine, dextroamphetamine

Key: *COX-2*, Cyclooxygenase-2; *FDA*, U.S. Food and Drug Administration; *NSAIDs*, nonsteroidal anti-inflammatory drugs.

Analgesic (pain-relieving) medications, whether prescription or nonprescription, are ordered by the physician for the patient. Check the name of the drug, dosage, route, and frequency. If the medication is ordered "as needed" (PRN), the order must include the circumstances under which the drug may be given, such as "PRN for back pain." Analgesics may be given by a number of routes, including oral, intramuscular (IM) injection, intravenous (IV) injection or infusion, PCA, and epidural infusion.

Oral Medications. Oral medications have been traditionally used for mild to moderate pain. Recent advances, however, have made available products such as time-released oral morphine, which may be used effectively for severe pain. This dosage form is particularly helpful for patients with chronic severe pain, such as occurs in patients with cancer. The use of this type of medication has allowed many individuals with severe chronic pain to return to work and a near-normal life for long periods of time despite serious illness.

Topical Medications. Various topical creams, such as capsaicin creams, may provide relief for muscle or joint pain. Medication patches, such as fentanyl (Duragesic) patches, allow the analgesic medicine to be absorbed slowly through the skin. Lidoderm patches are often helpful for neuropathic pain. Fentanyl is approved for relief of severe chronic pain only.

Injected Medications. Intramuscular or subcutaneous injection of pain medication is usually used for severe pain and only for a relatively short time. Medication given by this method has the advantage of lasting several hours, but administration is painful for the patient, and prolonged use can be detrimental to the tissues. Many individuals, particularly children, are fearful of injections. Small children and elderly adults also have relatively few sites with adequate muscle tissue; therefore, they can only safely receive medication by this route for a short time. Intramuscular injection requires careful technique to avoid nerve injury.

Intravenous Medications. Intravenous pain medication may be given as a bolus (concentrated dose given rapidly); as a slow push (over a few minutes); as an intermittent infusion; or by continuous infusion. These techniques are discussed in Chapter 36.

Recent studies have shown that continuous infusion of opioids is less effective at pain control and may more easily result in overmedication. Administration via PCA (discussed in the next section) has become the preferred route for most patients, although continuous infusion may still be the route of choice for control of severe chronic pain, such as that experienced by some terminally ill cancer patients.

Intramuscular injections are used less today than in the past. The dose given is larger than that given IV, and the length of time the medication is effective is extended as a result of the slow absorption from the muscular tissue. They are more commonly used for immediate relief of severe pain when an IV line is not in place, although some physicians and patients still prefer the IM route (Assignment Considerations 31-2).

Patient-Controlled Analgesia. Currently, the most common method used for injectable opioids in acute care is patient-controlled analgesia (PCA) (analgesia doses

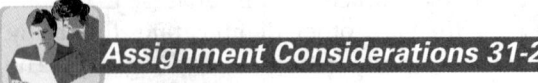

Assignment Considerations 31-2

Monitoring Patients on Narcotic Analgesics

Because many analgesics are constipating, ask assistive personnel to carefully monitor patients who are receiving a narcotic analgesic by any route. Bowel movements need to be tracked and when there is a deviation from the patient's normal pattern, it should be reported to the nurse right away.

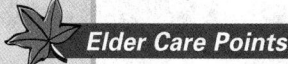

Elder Care Points

Due to the normal changes of aging, the older adult may respond differently to analgesics than a younger adult. The older adult should be monitored closely for side effects, such as excessive sedation and constipation.

controlled by the patient). This method uses one of a variety of programmable pumps (Figure 31-9). The medication comes in special cartridges or syringes, prediluted to an appropriate strength. The pump is programmed to administer the prescribed dose each time the patient pushes a button, within limitations set by the physician. The doctor's order will specify the size of the dose and the minimum time between doses. The pumps are programmed by the RN or pharmacist. The physician may also order an initial dose or even a continuous infusion dose to be programmed along with the intermittent dose. Within the limits set by the physician's order, the patient can then choose how often to receive the medication. Studies show that this level of control greatly reduces patient anxiety about

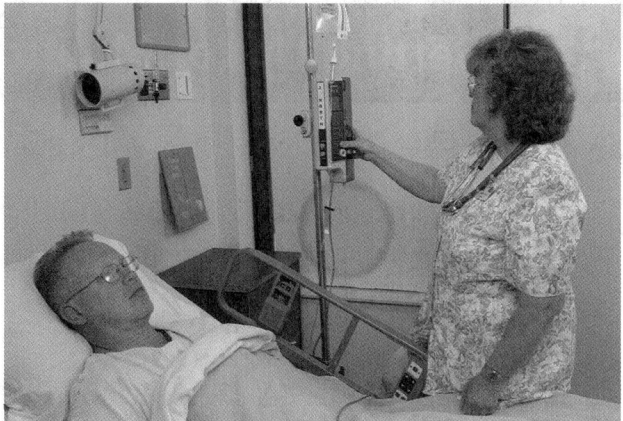

FIGURE **31-9** Portable PCA pump in use by a patient.

pain by putting the patient in more control, and that most patients actually use less rather than more medication. Before caring for a patient with a PCA pump, it is important to understand how it is programmed, how the medication is inserted, and how the machine is locked to prevent anyone from tampering with the medication or the programming (Skill 31-2).

Skill 31-2 | Setting Up (or Monitoring) a PCA Pump

Although the primary responsibility for a patient-controlled analgesia (PCA) pump usually lies with the RN, a LPN/LVN may be required to assist or monitor. Close attention needs to be paid both to the intravenous (IV) site and for side effects of medications.

■ Supplies
✓ PCA pump
✓ IV solution
✓ Medication vial
✓ IV administration set
✓ PCA tubing
✓ IV start kit and catheter (if needed)

Review and carry out Standard Steps in Appendix 3.

■ Assessment
1. *ACTION* Check the physician's orders.

   RATIONALE Ensures correct medication dosage and administration.

2. *ACTION* Assess the patient's knowledge of PCA usage.

   RATIONALE Patients need adequate teaching to use PCA correctly.

■ Planning
3. *ACTION* Assemble the equipment.

   RATIONALE Avoids interruption of the procedure, provides good time management.

4. *ACTION* Identify the patient.

   RATIONALE Ensures correct patient receives the PCA.

5. *ACTION* Explain the procedure to the patient.

   RATIONALE Decreases patient anxiety and increases cooperation.

■ Implementation
6. *ACTION* Start an IV if one does not already exist.

   RATIONALE Intravenous access is necessary for standard PCA administration.

7. *ACTION* Prepare the PCA medication vial following instructions on the vial.

   RATIONALE Proper assembly ensures accurate medication administration.

8. *ACTION* Attach PCA tubing to the medication vial.

   RATIONALE Allows for medication administration.

9. *ACTION* Flush air out of the tubing.

   RATIONALE Decreases possibility of air embolism, provides for accurate dosage administration.

Continued

10. **ACTION** Close the slide clamp on the PCA set.

    RATIONALE Prevents leakage of medication.

11. **ACTION** Connect the primed IV administration set to the "Y" adapter of the PCA set.

    RATIONALE Allows for administration of medication through existing intravenous site.

12. **ACTION** Insert the medication vial into the pump according to the pump directions.

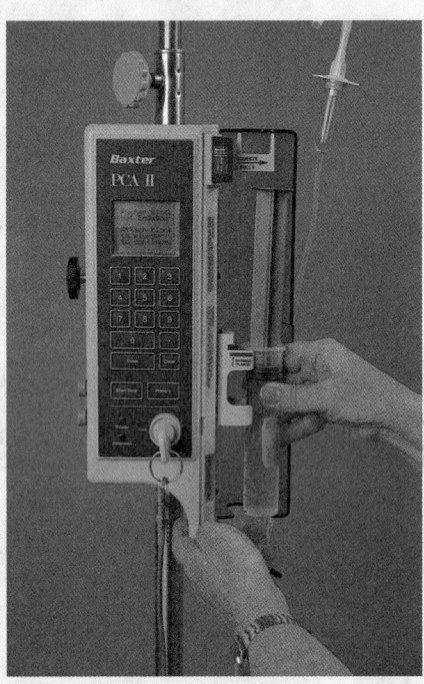

Step **12**

    RATIONALE Allows for administration of medication via the pump.

13. **ACTION** Plug the PCA pump into a power source.

    RATIONALE Provides a continuous power source; prevents unnecessary drain on the internal battery.

14. **ACTION** Set the PCA pump according to physician's orders.

    RATIONALE This ensures proper drug administration.

15. **ACTION** Open all slide clamps.

    RATIONALE Allows for PCA administration.

16. **ACTION** Review use of the PCA with the patient.

    RATIONALE Reinforces previous teaching. Ensures proper use of equipment for pain control.

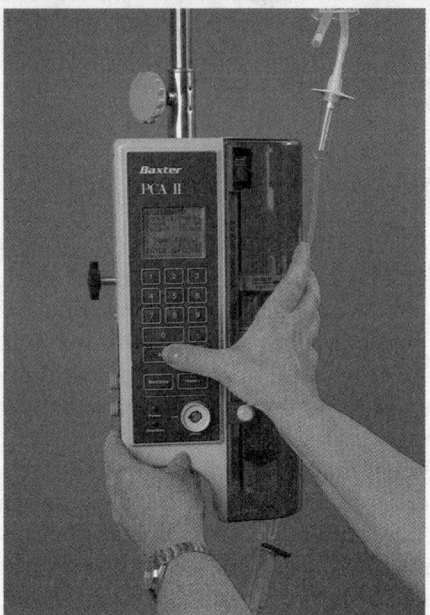

Step **14**

■ Evaluation

17. **ACTION** Assess the patient frequently for ability to use the PCA, effectiveness of medication, and side effects. Assess the IV site for redness, drainage, swelling, or tenderness.

    RATIONALE Ensures patient comfort, decreases complications.

■ Documentation

18. **ACTION** Document on the patient's chart the date and time PCA started, medication, pump settings, observations of the IV site, effectiveness of medication, and patient teaching.

    RATIONALE Documents use of PCA pump and patient response.

Documentation Example

6/2 0800 Morphine sulfate via PCA started, 1 mg every 10 minutes, not to exceed 4 doses per hour. No redness, swelling, drainage, tenderness at IV site. Instructions on PCA use given to patient; able to self-administer a dose. States pain at 3 on a 0-10 scale.

_____

(Nurse's signature)

?CRITICAL THINKING QUESTIONS

1. How do your beliefs about addiction to pain medication affect the care you provide?

2. What would you teach a patient who expresses a concern about opioid addiction?

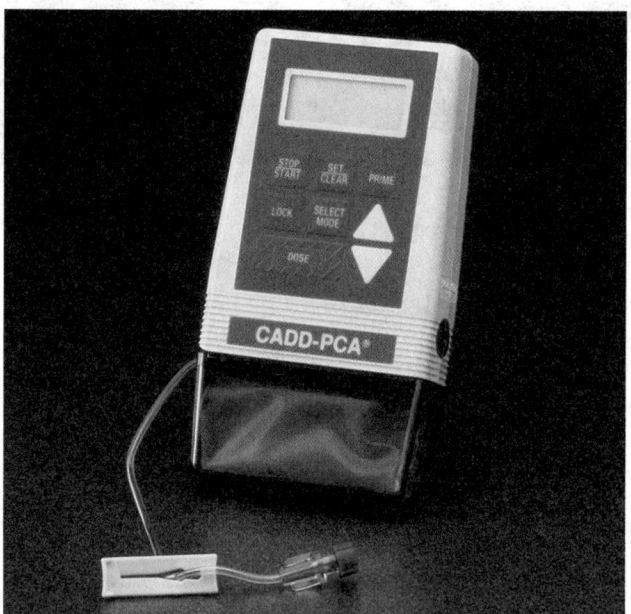

FIGURE **31-10** CADD portable PCA pump.

PCAs are commonly attached to an IV line, but the medication may also be injected into the subcutaneous tissue on the abdomen. This second method is often seen when the pumps are used to administer medication to nonhospitalized patients using small, portable pumps. These pumps may also be used for nonhospitalized patients with IV lines or ports (Figure 31-10).

? *Think Critically About* . . . What type of teaching would you do for a patient using a PCA pump for the first time?

Epidural Analgesia. The epidural route has been used for anesthesia for a number of years. Epidural analgesia, however, is one of the newest forms of pain control. An anesthesiologist or nurse anesthetist places a fine catheter in the epidural space near the base of the spine, then connects the catheter to a small battery-operated programmable pump. The pump administers an opioid analgesic into the epidural space (outside the dural space), either as a bolus followed by a continuous infusion or as repeated bolus doses, as ordered by the physician. **This method is effective in controlling pain while allowing the patient to remain alert.** Its uses include pain relief for obstetric patients in labor, postoperative patients, and patients with cancer. Possible side effects from the opiate component of the infusion include respiratory depression, pruritus, nausea and vomiting, constipation, urinary retention, low pulse rate, and hypotension. Because of the infrequent but possible occurrence of potentially dangerous side effects, particularly respiratory depression, patients receiving epidural analgesia are monitored closely. This often includes being placed on an apnea monitor and/or a pulse oximeter for the first 12 hours. The primary

responsibility for caring for the epidural catheter lies with the RN. The LPN/LVN will monitor the patient for response to the medication (Steps 31-1).

? *Think Critically About* . . . How does monitoring a patient with an epidural catheter for pain differ from monitoring a patient with a PCA?

Evaluation

Frequent evaluation of pain control measures is important. As the patient's condition changes, so may the need for pain control. A patient's perception of pain may increase with anxiety, which can be caused in part by ineffective pain control measures. As the patient's condition improves, various interventions, such as medication, may need to be tapered or discontinued.

SLEEP

Proper rest and sleep are important, and may be interrupted for patients due to pain, fear, or stress, or as a side effect of medications and necessary treatments. An important nursing action is to assist the patient in obtaining enough sleep to aid in healing and maintaining health.

FUNCTIONS OF SLEEP

Although much of the actual function of sleep is not known, it is clear that adequate rest and sleep are important factors in general health and recovery from illness. These activities also play a major role in pain control. Being rested increases pain tolerance and allows an improved response to analgesia.

People who do not get adequate rest often suffer from daytime drowsiness and fatigue. Irritability, depression, and a decrease in concentration and memory are also common. There is an increase in the frequency of both accidents and illness.

STAGES OF SLEEP

Normal sleep follows a course through two states, non–rapid eye movement (NREM) sleep and rapid eye movement (REM) sleep. REM sleep is time in which you dream, and is a period of a high level of activity. Heart rate, blood pressure, and respirations are similar to that when awake. NREM sleep is believed to be the time when the body receives the most rest. During this stage, heart rate, blood pressure, and respirations decline. During the course of the night, a person will go through these two states in 90-minute cycles, repeating the cycles five or six times a night.

NREM sleep is divided into four stages. The first is a transition stage. As a person falls into a light sleep, the muscles relax. This stage usually lasts a few minutes, followed by stage 2. In stage 2 the person falls into a deeper sleep. Brain wave activity becomes

Steps 31-1 | Monitoring an Epidural Catheter and Changing the Dressing

A patient may be given an epidural catheter for control of some types of pain. Although an RN or physician will start the administration, other members of the health care team need to closely monitor the patient, both for problems with the catheter and for side effects of medications. The analgesia may be infused by an infusion pump or be given by bolus injection.

Review and carry out the Standard Steps in Appendix 3.

1. **ACTION** Assess the patient for adequate pain control without signs of oversedation, including decreased level of consciousness or depressed respirations. Be certain that naloxone (Narcan) is immediately available to use in case of an adverse reaction to the analgesia. Monitor vital signs.

   RATIONALE Ensures that pain control is effective and that patient is not experiencing severe central nervous system depression.

2. **ACTION** Assess mobility and motor and sensory function before allowing patient out of bed.

   RATIONALE Prevents injury from falling that may occur from sedation, weakness, or postural hypotension.

3. **ACTION** Know the facility's policy and procedure for epidural dressing changes. Always change the dressing when soiled, wet, or loose. Gauze and tape dressings should be changed every 48 to 72 hours, and transparent semipermeable dressings at least weekly.

   RATIONALE A clean, dry, adherent dressing reduces the chances of infection.

4. **ACTION** Perform thorough hand hygiene before beginning assessment of the site.

   RATIONALE Prevents the spread of microorganisms; infection at the site could travel into the central nervous system.

5. **ACTION** Position the patient comfortably so that the epidural site is exposed.

   RATIONALE Allows for access to the epidural site, provides for patient comfort.

6. **ACTION** Put on gloves; remove the old dressing and discard, being careful not to dislodge the catheter.

RATIONALE Provides for access to the epidural site. Movement of the catheter could result in the need for reinsertion.

7. **ACTION** Observe for signs of infection such as redness, swelling, warmth, tenderness, or drainage.

   RATIONALE Allows for prompt intervention.

8. **ACTION** Perform hand hygiene. Open sterile dressings and prepare sterile field. Don sterile gloves.

   RATIONALE Sterile technique reduces possibility of introduction of microorganisms into skin or epidural space.

9. **ACTION** Using aseptic technique, cleanse the site with alcohol × 3, using a circular motion, starting in the center and working out.

   RATIONALE Alcohol removes dirt and body oils.

10. **ACTION** Repeat the cleansing with povidone-iodine (Betadine) × 3. Allow the solution to air dry.

    RATIONALE Allows for the destruction of microorganisms on the skin surface.

11. **ACTION** Apply the sterile dressing using proper aseptic technique.

    RATIONALE Prevents contamination of epidural site, and prevents infection.

12. **ACTION** Adhere the epidural catheter securely to the skin.

    RATIONALE Securing the catheter prevents it from becoming dislodged or migrating into the subarachnoid space.

13. **ACTION** Remove soiled supplies and dressings and restore the unit. Perform hand hygiene.

    RATIONALE Preserve clean, sanitary patient environment.

14. **ACTION** Document assessment of the site and the procedure.

    RATIONALE Verifies dressing change and condition of epidural catheter site.

15. **ACTION** If an infusion pump is in use, check it for proper function and for correct settings for analgesia infusion.

    RATIONALE Ensures that ordered dosage of analgesia is infused.

larger, and there are bursts of electrical activity. This stage lasts 10 to 20 minutes.

As stage 3 begins, the person enters a period called delta sleep or slow-wave sleep, named for the high-voltage slow brain waves that occur. Respirations and heart rate slow in this stage, and the body becomes immobile. This stage lasts 15 to 30 minutes, resembling a coma, after which the person enters stage 4. This is the deepest stage of sleep. During this stage, it is difficult to arouse the sleeping person. This stage lasts approximately 15 to 30 minutes.

This is followed by a period of REM sleep. Brain waves become active, almost the same as when awake. This is the stage in which dreams occur, and it lasts approximately 20 minutes. About 25% of the night is spent in REM sleep, and the duration will increase with each sleep cycle during the night.

NORMAL SLEEP REQUIREMENTS

The amount of sleep an individual needs varies from person to person, and the amount of sleep needed also changes as a person passes through the life cycle.

Newborns require at least 16 hours of sleep per day, but this is distributed throughout the 24 hours rather than a having a true sleep cycle. They also spend about 80% of the time in REM sleep. It is speculated that the neural activity occurring during REM sleep is necessary for brain maturation. By 2 to 3 months of age, they begin to develop a true sleep cycle and REM sleep falls to about 50%. By age 1, the child is sleeping 12 to 14 hours per day, and continues to need this amount of sleep until reaching the age of preschool, when the amount needed drops to 11 to 13 hours.

School-age children require 10 to 11 hours of sleep per night. REM sleep decreases and deep sleep increases, allowing for necessary repair of damaged cells and the growth of new cells. Insufficient sleep can hamper both normal growth and daytime learning activities.

Growth hormone is secreted during deep sleep in both children and adolescents. Adolescents, however, have very different sleep patterns from younger children and adults. Although they need to get 9 to 10 hours of sleep a night, their internal clock does not trigger feelings of sleepiness until late at night due to a natural shift in circadian rhythms that occurs at this period in development. Because school hours demand that they waken by 6:30 or 7 A.M., many teens are chronically sleep deprived, affecting temperament, academic performance, and ability to stay awake at critical times, such as when driving a car.

Most adults require approximately 8 hours sleep a night, but many get less. Deep sleep time decreases, and REM sleep occurs for about 20% of the night. Mild to severe sleep disorders plague many adults, including varying degrees of insomnia, and waking multiple times during the night. Sleep difficulties increase during middle age, and can be particularly difficult for menopausal women.

It is a common misconception that the elderly need less sleep. However, such things as nocturia, joint pain, and other physical conditions may interrupt the sleep cycle with increasing frequency. The elderly also tend to have what is called advanced sleep onset—they go to bed earlier and get up earlier than during their younger years. They may also nap during the day. This again represents a shift in the circadian rhythm.

FACTORS AFFECTING SLEEP

Many things can cause disruption of the normal sleep cycle. People who work evening and night shifts often have difficulty in sleep during the day. Workers who change shifts during the month will have even more difficulty in adjusting in order to get enough rest. Students often spend nights studying and find that getting enough sleep can be a problem. Travelers may suffer from jet lag as they go through different time zones. Exposure to sunlight for several hours seems to help reset one's internal clock. People who snore, or have partners who snore, may find that they are awakened frequently. People who snore also have an increased incidence of sleep apnea, which is linked to an increased frequency of cardiac ailments.

Lifestyle can affect the ability to sleep. Caffeine, nicotine, and alcohol consumption can interrupt normal sleep patterns. Caffeine and nicotine can delay sleep, and alcohol may cause nocturnal awakenings.

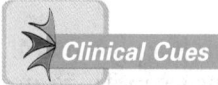
Clinical Cues

If a patient reports sleeping difficulties, ask if he often drinks something with caffeine in it after 3 P.M. Many drinks contain caffeine, including a number of carbonated beverages, and it is important to check ingredient labels.

Regular exercise can help a person sleep, but exercise too close to bedtime may be overstimulating and keep a person awake. Taking a nap during the day may also disrupt nighttime sleep, and should be particularly avoided if the individual suffers from insomnia.

Stress and illness may also affect sleep. Nighttime worry may keep a person awake or cause awakening in the middle of the night. Illness or discomfort may prevent a person from resting well. An old mattress may contribute to sleeplessness because it is lumpy or no longer properly supportive.

Environmental factors, such as a room that is too hot or too cold, noisy, or with ambient light can also affect sleep. Patients in the hospital have an increase in interruptions of regular sleep due to hospital routines that can cause noise or require turning on lights, or the need to be awakened for such things as medications.

SLEEP DISORDERS

Disorders of sleep can interfere with a person's quality of life and affect health. Accidents may occur due to a lack of sleep. **People with sleep disorders should be treated by a health care practitioner if lifestyle changes or relaxation techniques fail to increase the quality of sleep.** Referral to a sleep disorder clinic for testing may prove helpful.

Insomnia

Insomnia is difficulty in getting to sleep or staying asleep at night. This may be short term, lasting only a few nights, or chronic, lasting a month or longer.

Transient insomnia may be caused by stress, excitement, or a change in sleeping arrangements, such as occurs when traveling. The sleep pattern will usually normalize as the life situation settles back to routine.

Chronic insomnia may be the result of an underlying medical, behavioral, or psychiatric problem. Depression can often cause insomnia. Persons suffering from chronic insomnia may require treatment from a health care provider specializing in sleep disorders.

Sleep Apnea

Sleep apnea is a condition in which the person will stop breathing for brief periods during sleep. There are three types of sleep apnea: obstructive, central, and mixed-complex. They can be further classified as mild, moderate, and severe.

Obstructive apnea is the most common type. It is caused by a relaxation of the soft tissues, which allows partial to total obstruction of the airway. The condition may be further complicated by tissue or bony structure abnormalities. A person with obstructive apnea will have visible respiratory effort, but may not be able to move air past the obstruction, causing him to arouse sufficiently to draw breath before falling back into sleep. These individuals often do not remember waking, although it will occur multiple times through the night, even multiple times per hour.

Central apnea occurs due to a failure of the brain to communicate with the respiratory muscles. This results in cessation of breathing with no observable respiratory effort. As the oxygen saturation decreases, the individual resumes breathing. This is much less common than obstructive apnea. Mixed-complex sleep apnea is, as the name implies, a combination of obstructive and central sleep apnea.

Obstructive apnea may be treated with a continuous positive airway pressure (CPAP) device. This uses a small compressor to maintain airflow via a mask or nasal prongs while the patient sleeps. A dental appliance may be prescribed to reposition the tongue or jaw at night. Central apnea does not respond to CPAP, but other treatments are available. Apnea is a problem that should be treated by a specialist.

Snoring

Snoring, or breathing during sleep accompanied by harsh sounds, is caused by vibration and/or obstruction of the air passages at the back of the mouth and nose. This may result from poor muscle tone, excessive tissue, or deformities such as a deviated septum. Obstructed airways due to colds or allergies can also cause snoring. Snoring may be simple, but can also be a symptom of sleep apnea. Heavy snorers may disrupt their own sleep, as well as the sleep of others.

The mild snorer should exercise to develop good muscle tone, and lose weight if needed. Sleeping on the side instead of on the back may help. Remember that snoring can be a symptom of airway obstruction and should be taken seriously. Referral to a physician or sleep disorder specialist may be necessary.

Narcolepsy

Narcolepsy is sudden-onset, recurrent, uncontrollable, brief episodes of sleep during normal hours of wakefulness in a well-rested person. These sudden sleep periods may occur at any time and last from a few seconds to more than 30 minutes. For example, patients may fall asleep while reading a book, watching TV, attending a meeting, engaging in conversation, or driving. Symptoms usually begin by the age of 25 and may start as excessive daytime sleepiness. There is currently no cure, but drug and behavioral therapies have proven helpful. Regular exercise and exposure to bright light are recommended. Stimulant medication is often used to prevent daytime sleepiness. The diagnosis of narcolepsy is by clinical evaluation, sleep logs or diaries, and the results of sleep laboratory tests. Most narcolepsy is not inherited.

APPLICATION of the NURSING PROCESS

Assessment (Data Collection)

Adequate assessment of the patient having difficulty sleeping is necessary to provide effective interventions. A thorough history of any problems the patient has had related to sleep in the past should be completed. Any current illness or injury should be discussed in relation to comfort and disruption of sleep.

Encourage patients with sleep difficulties to keep a sleep diary. Information to be recorded includes the time they went to bed, when they woke up, and any time they awoke during the night; usual diet; and all medications taken, including sleep aids. They should also include information about where they sleep and anything that disturbs sleep, such as neighborhood noise, a snoring partner, wakeful children, or pets who demand attention in the night.

Nursing Diagnosis

Assessment of the patient allows identification of various nursing diagnoses for the patient with sleep problems. These may be related to the patient's health as well as sleep disturbances. Box 31-2 lists possible nursing diagnoses for the patient with sleep disturbances. Sleep pattern disturbances may be related to many things, including environmental factors such as noise, health issues, and the necessity of shift work.

Planning

When setting up goals related to sleep disturbances, attention should be paid to the amount of sleep the individual patient needs. A possible goal might be that the patient will sleep undisturbed for 6 hours each night, or awake in the morning feeling rested.

Implementation

Assisting the patient to adjust lifestyle and bedtime habits can allow the patient to obtain a sufficient amount of sleep. Avoiding caffeinated beverages for 6 hours before bedtime will eliminate stimulants that may be interfering with sleep. Eliminating alcohol or nicotine for at least 2 hours before bedtime can also help the patient get to sleep and stay asleep. Encourage the patient to exercise regularly, but not immediately before bedtime. Patients should try to establish a routine time for going to bed and getting up, and avoid taking naps during the day. Going to bed hungry or overly full can interfere with sleep. Reading in bed should be avoided.

Sleep experts agree that the bedroom should be a refuge, with the bed used for sleep and for sexual relations. Reading, watching television, and discussing the day's problems in bed are all disruptive to the sleep cycle. Many advise that when sleep does not come within 30 minutes, the individual should get up, go into another room, and read or engage in some restful activity until the feeling of sleepiness returns. It is also important that the room be at a comfortable temperature, and the mattress comfortable and properly supportive.

Patients in a health care facility are especially prone to environmental disruptions. The use of earplugs or a "white noise" machine may help block out noise. **Many patients will sleep better if they have a favorite pillow or blanket from home.** Take care to avoid

---

| Box 31-2 | *Nursing Diagnoses for the Patient with Sleep Difficulties* |

- Readiness for enhanced sleep
- Sleep deprivation
- Fatigue
- Readiness for enhanced comfort
- Acute pain
- Chronic pain
- Anxiety
- Ineffective breathing pattern
- Impaired spontaneous ventilation

---

waking patients unless absolutely necessary. Procedures such as vital signs and dressing changes should be scheduled together to avoid waking a patient repeatedly. If possible, close the patient's room door, and avoid talking in the hallway during the night hours.

Think Critically About . . . What would be the difference between interruptions in sleep for the patient in a health care facility and the patient at home? How can you decrease sleep interruptions for a patient in the hospital?

Medication such as sedatives and hypnotics are sometimes prescribed to promote sleep. These should be used only for short-term relief. Over-the-counter sleep medications often contain antihistamines that induce drowsiness. If using medications, the patient should take the dose early enough to allow time for absorption before bedtime. Patients should be instructed about potential side effects of any medications.

Evaluation

An ongoing evaluation of the effectiveness of interventions is important to adequately assist the patient in achieving sufficient rest. The amount of time the patient slept, number and types of interruptions, and patient assessment of quality of sleep should be recorded.

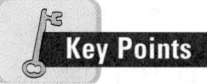 **Key Points**

- Pain is a subjective experience; there is no objective way to measure pain.
- The major types of pain are acute, chronic, nociceptive, neuropathic, and phantom.
- Pain is what the patient says it is.
- Observable indicators of pain include moaning, crying, irritability, inability to sleep, grimacing or frowning, restlessness, and a rigid posture in bed.
- Pain assessment should include the use of a pain scale.
- Pain is the "fifth vital sign" and is assessed whenever vital signs are measured.
- Pain management can include analgesic medications, TENS, binders, heat and cold application, relaxation,

- biofeedback, distraction, guided imagery and meditation, music, hypnosis, and massage.
- Although the actual function of sleep is unknown, adequate rest is necessary for good general health and recovery from illness.
- The two states of sleep are non–rapid eye movement (NREM) sleep, which is divided into four stages, and rapid eye movement (REM) sleep, when we dream.
- The amount of sleep needed varies throughout the life span.
- Factors affecting sleep include shift work; jet lag; caffeine, nicotine, and alcohol consumption; exercise; environmental factors; stress; and illness.
- Sleep disorders include insomnia, sleep apnea, and narcolepsy.

- Keeping a sleep diary or journal can help in assessing the patient experiencing sleep difficulties.
- Medications should be used only for short-term relief of sleeping problems.

 Go to your **Companion CD-ROM** for an Audio Glossary, animations, video clips, and more.

evolve Be sure to visit the companion Evolve site at http://evolve.elsevier.com/deWit/fundamental/ for additional online resources.

NCLEX-PN® EXAMINATION-STYLE REVIEW QUESTIONS

*Choose the **best** answer(s) for each question.*

1. There are several nonpharmacologic interventions for pain. The one that uses a machine to measure learned responses is _____.
(Fill in the blank.)

2. Endorphins modulate pain by:
   1. acting on small-diameter nerve fibers.
   2. acting on large-diameter nerve fibers.
   3. inhibiting impulses originating in the thalamus.
   4. attaching to nerve endings in opioid receptors.

3. Your patient, a 27-year-old computer programmer, is suffering pain in her right ankle due to a fracture received in a skiing accident. This type of pain would be considered:
   1. acute.
   2. chronic.
   3. phantom.
   4. controlled.

4. Intramuscular injections of pain medication may be contraindicated in patients:
   1. who have large, well-developed muscles.
   2. who require long-term pain management.
   3. who have no fear of needles.
   4. who have poor cognitive abilities.

5. When monitoring the patient for responses to opioid medication administered via an epidural catheter, the nurse knows that complications may include: *(Select all that apply.)*
   1. urinary retention.
   2. hypertension.
   3. pruritus.
   4. photosensitivity.

6. Epidural analgesia is used:
   1. during active labor.
   2. routinely in hospital environments for patients in pain.
   3. to induce general anesthesia.
   4. very rarely and only as a last resort to manage pain.

7. A 55-year-old patient is receiving analgesia postoperatively via a PCA pump. He expresses concern about accidentally overdosing himself. Appropriate information to give the patient includes: *(Select the two best responses.)*
   1. "Even though I am not giving you the medication, I do assess your tolerance of the ordered dose at regular intervals."
   2. "The doctor doesn't order enough medication that you would be able to overdose."
   3. "I can ask the doctor to adjust your medication if you are worried."
   4. "The PCA has a lockout mechanism that prevents you from giving yourself too much medication."

8. Patients for whom warm packs carry an increased risk of skin damage include: *(Select all that apply.)*
   1. a middle-aged patient.
   2. an elderly patient.
   3. a male patient.
   4. a female patient.
   5. an infant.

9. Factors that can adversely affect sleep include: *(Select all that apply.)*
   1. consistent nighttime routines.
   2. alcohol consumption near bedtime.
   3. rotating shift work.
   4. quiet environments.
   5. a television in the bedroom.
   6. reading in bed.
   7. discussions of the day's problems in bed.

10. Patients should be advised that medications to promote sleep should be: *(Select all that apply.)*
    1. used as needed.
    2. used for short periods only.
    3. used on a routine basis.
    4. never used.
    5. used according to instructions.

CRITICAL THINKING ACTIVITIES *Read each clinical scenario and discuss the questions with your classmates.*

Scenario A
Patients in a hospital or long-term care facility may wake up in the middle of the night and find it difficult to go back to sleep. What interventions might the nurse provide to assist the patient to return to sleep?

Scenario B
What helps you go to sleep? Compare your notes with those of other students. What techniques identified could be used to assist a patient?

Scenario C
When assessing a patient with postoperative pain, what questions would you ask to understand your patient's level of distress? How would this differ for a patient with chronic pain from arthritis?

Scenario D
What type of assessments would be necessary for a patient receiving opioid analgesics?

Scenario E
What actions might be the most helpful to assist a child to sleep in the hospital?

Scenario F
What would you do if a patient is not able to maintain comfort despite receiving analgesic medication as ordered by the physician?

Objectives

Upon completing this chapter, you should be able to:

Theory

1. Discuss the use of complementary and alternative medicine (CAM) in integrative medicine.
2. Identify therapies that are considered part of CAM.
3. Discuss five commonly used complementary and alternative therapies.
4. Name four mind–body therapies.
5. Direct patients to information needed to make a decision on whether to use an herbal remedy.
6. Describe the desired outcome of spinal manipulation during chiropractic treatment.

Clinical Practice

1. Assess the use of complementary and alternative therapies by assigned patients.
2. Direct patients to information about complementary and alternative therapies.
3. Assist patients to use relaxation and imagery.

Key Terms

Be sure to check out the bonus material on the Companion CD-ROM, including selected audio pronunciations.

acupuncture (ĂK-ū-pŭnk-chŭr, p. 621)
alternative therapies (p. 620)
aromatherapy (ă-RŌ-mă thĕr-ă-pē, p. 625)
chiropractic (kī-rō-PRĂK-tĭk, p. 626)
complementary therapies (p. 620)
herbal (ĔR-băl, p. 623)
imagery (Ĭ-măj-rē, p. 622)
phytotherapy (FĪ-tō-thĕr-ă-pē, p. 623)
Qi Gong (kē gŏng, p. 621)
Reiki (RĪ-kē, p. 626)
yoga (p. 620)

This chapter will give you a broad overview of complementary and alternative therapies. Becoming well versed in the therapies discussed here requires many hours of exploration and reading. Learning to provide these services to others involves hundreds of hours of training, and some practitioners, such as chiropractors, must complete a formal training program and pass licensure examinations.

Complementary and alternative medicine (CAM) comprises those therapies that are not presently considered to be part of conventional medical practice. The term complementary therapies is used when these practices are utilized *in conjunction with* conventional medical treatment. An example would be the use of relaxation therapy along with pain medication to increase a patient's comfort. They become alternative therapies when they are used *in place of* mainstream medicine. An example would be eating a special diet to treat cancer rather than undergoing the surgery, radiation, or chemotherapy that has been recommended by one's physician.

In recent decades, there has been a significant increase in the use of complementary and alternative therapies. There are a variety of reasons for this. For some, it is related to an overall effort to live a healthier lifestyle, which includes alterations in diet and the adoption of specific practices such as yoga (ancient Hindu art for harmonizing the body, mind, and spirit) or daily meditation. Other concerns that lead individuals to investigate or begin alternative practices include a desire to decrease or eliminate the use of standard pharmaceuticals, or the failure of conventional medicine to address their health issues, such as chronic pain. Many people cite the impersonal approach and the focus on cure rather than prevention found in standard Western medicine as the primary reason they sought an alternative or integrative practitioner.

Cost is not a major factor in the decision. Many of the alternatives can be expensive and frequently are not covered by insurance. For a variety of reasons, many people make the decision to invest some or all of the money they have for health maintenance into alternative rather than conventional care.

A growing number of conventional medical providers practice integrative medicine. This means they are providing complementary and alternative care along with conventional medicine and providing a holistic approach with more personalized care and easy access to alternative therapies.

The National Center for Complementary and Alternative Medicine (NCCAM) has been established to provide evidence-based research regarding the efficacy of the various complementary and alternative therapies, and to provide information for the public. The NCCAM website is nccam.nih.gov. NCCAM classifies complementary and alternative therapies into five major categories:

- *Alternative medical systems,* which are complete systems of theory and practice that often developed apart from and earlier than conventional Western medicine.
- *Mind–body interventions,* composed of a variety of techniques designed to enhance the mind's capacity to affect bodily functions and symptoms.
- *Biologic-based therapies* using substances found in nature, such as herbs, foods, and vitamins.
- *Manipulative and body-based methods* such as chiropractic, osteopathic manipulation, and massage.
- *Energy therapies* involving the use of bodily energy fields. These are one of two types:
  - Biofield therapies that are intended to affect energy fields that are believed to surround and penetrate the human body.
  - Bioelectromagnetic-based therapies that use pulsed, magnetic, alternating current, or direct current fields.

Examples of these therapies are discussed later in this chapter.

ALTERNATIVE MEDICAL SYSTEMS

Homeopathy, naturopathy, traditional Chinese medicine, and Ayurveda (traditional medicine from India) are examples of alternative medical systems. Each of these is briefly described below.

HOMEOPATHIC MEDICINE

Homeopathy teaches that symptoms are signs of the body's effort to get rid of disease and that disease can be cured by giving small doses of substances that produce symptoms of the disease or disorder in a healthy person. This process stimulates the person's natural defenses, alleviating the problem. Homeopathy is based on three principles: (1) like cures like; (2) the greater the dilution of the remedy, the greater its potency; and (3) illness is specific to the individual. Homeopathic remedies are derived from plants, animals, or minerals.

NATUROPATHIC MEDICINE

Naturopathic medicine is a philosophy directed at the prevention of disease. Its basis is the use of natural means to promote health. Lifestyle management, natural foods, massage, and substances such as botanicals, light, and fresh air are used along with regular exercise to maintain the body at a high level of wellness through use of the body's inherent healing ability.

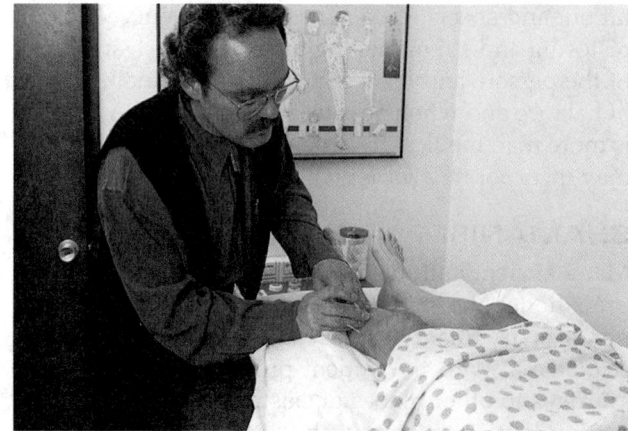

FIGURE **32-1** Patient undergoing acupuncture for relief of pain.

TRADITIONAL CHINESE MEDICINE

Traditional Chinese medicine is a comprehensive system based on the opposition of polarities (yin and yang); the elements of wood, fire, earth, metal, and water; and the flow of energy or Q*i* in the body. It focuses on looking for underlying causes of imbalances and patterns of disharmony in the body. Chinese medicine uses over 50,000 medicinal plants, acupuncture, and massage. Tai Chi, a form of stretching exercise that promotes relaxation and increased circulation, and Qi Gong, another type of exercise and stimulation therapy emphasizing breathing, coordination, and relaxation, are also recommended.

Acupuncture

Acupuncture is a branch of traditional Chinese medicine. Very fine needles are used to stimulate certain points on the body along lines called meridians to increase or disperse the flow of energy (Figure 32-1). Studies by the National Institutes of Health have found that acupuncture can be an effective method to treat pain. Acupuncture is also used to increase immunity. It is very important that only sterile needles be used for acupuncture because of the danger of infection and transmission of HIV or hepatitis.

Qi Gong

Qi Gong is a form of Chinese exercise-stimulation therapy that seeks to improve health by redirecting mental focus, controlling breathing, improving coordination, and promoting relaxation. Activation of the natural electric currents that flow along meridians in the body helps to rebalance the body's own healing capability. Qi Gong has been effective for many people for the management of chronic disease.

AYURVEDA

Ayurveda is the traditional Indian system of medicine dating from before the first century A.D. It uses combinations of herbs, minerals, purgatives, massage, meditation, and special diets. The focus of Ayurveda is on restoring and strengthening the body, mind, and spirit of the person, and its healing focus is on maintenance of balance and wholeness to prevent illness. Ayurveda is more than medical treatment—it is a way of life, and may incorporate a variety of other practices.

SHAMANISM

Many ancient cultures practice shamanism. A trained practitioner, the **shaman,** uses techniques to achieve a nonordinary reality, or a "shamanic" state of consciousness. With the patient present, the practitioner journeys to other planes of existence to retrieve information that is necessary for the healing process. The patient and the shamanic practitioner work together to make use of the information obtained. The shaman may perform various ceremonies, including the burning of particular plants and herbs, to bring about the rebalancing of the individual with nature.

FOLK MEDICINE

Folk medicine practices are seen in many cultures. In Mexico, it is called *curanderismo.* In this practice, illness is seen as an imbalance. This may be between hot and cold in the body, between the patient and the environment, between parts of the body, or between the patient and the spiritual realm. Folk medicine combines many healing practices and is prevalent throughout Latin America. Biologic compounds, foods, and herbs are used to treat the physical components of the illness. The *curandero* also treats the supernatural components. *Susto* (fear) is thought to cause the soul to separate from the body, resulting in illness. *Mal de ojo* (evil eye) generally is thought to affect children and causes fever, irritability, headache, and weeping. *Empacho* is a gastrointestinal disorder thought to be caused by a blockage in the stomach or intestine. Practitioners are believed to have a *don* or God-given talent for specific healing and usually specialize in treating those areas of illness related to their *don.*

AMERICAN INDIAN MEDICINE

In American Indian medicine, healing herbs and ceremonies combined with a spiritual emphasis are used to treat ailing patients. The therapies are based on the belief that spirit, mind, and emotions all interact with the environment. A patient's disease or disorder is believed to be caused by a disharmony in the patient's connection to nature, Mother Earth, and the spirit world. The focus of treatment is bringing the patient back into harmony.

There are a variety of forms of therapy that include the sweat lodge ceremony, the sacred pipe, and sacred sage, sweet grass, cedar, and other herbs burned and wafted over the patient with the use of a feather. Herbs may also be used in tea or in a bath, or burned with the smoke inhaled. Shaking of rattles helps break up blocks of dead or jammed energy, and drums align the heartbeat of Mother Earth with the patient's spirit. All thera-

pies are performed by highly trained medicine people. Specific treatments, ceremonies, and beliefs vary throughout the many tribal cultures that are contained within the designation of Native American. Mainstream medical therapies may be used by the patient as well.

MIND–BODY INTERVENTIONS

Mind–body therapies use a variety of techniques aimed at enhancing the mind's ability to affect the body. Relaxation therapy and therapies that use creative outlets, such as imagery, music, art, or dance, as well as meditation and prayer, are considered to be mind–body interventions.

RELAXATION THERAPY

Relaxation techniques are used to ease stress and are helpful for a variety of chronic illnesses, including headache, irritable bowel syndrome, hypertension, dysrhythmias, inflammatory bowel disease, and musculoskeletal pain. Relaxation induces a light state of altered consciousness through refocusing, conscious breathing, and body awareness. Chapter 31 describes some specific relaxation techniques.

IMAGERY

Imagery uses a visual stimulus to produce a particular physiologic change that can decrease stress or promote healing. It is useful in decreasing pain, and can be particularly helpful to patients undergoing painful procedures such as bone marrow aspiration. Imagery may produce a physiologic effect on all of the major systems of the body. Chapter 31 contains an imagery scenario.

MEDITATION

Meditation involves focusing attention on a single repetitive stimulus, thereby decreasing all other stimuli. It alters consciousness and can bring a beneficial mind–body response. Meditation induces a restful state and lowers heart and respiratory rates, and may reduce anxiety. It has been helpful for people with asthma, hypertension, diabetes, and other disorders. Meditation can improve productivity and mood and reduce irritability.

BIOFEEDBACK

Biofeedback is a technique that trains the patient to lessen symptoms by learning to control particular internal physiologic processes that normally occur involuntarily, such as heart rate or blood pressure. It has also been successful in managing pain and controlling panic attacks. The internal activity can be measured with electrodes and shown either visually on a screen or as a sound, giving the patient and the practitioner feedback about the internal workings of the body. The person, with practice, can use this information to gain control over the "involuntary" activity. Biofeedback is used effectively for many conditions, but is particularly successful in treating tension or migraine headaches and chronic pain.

HYPNOTHERAPY

Hypnotherapy is used to alter behavior, retrieve memories, and induce anesthesia. A hypnotic state is created in which suggestions are implanted that remain during the posthypnotic period. Many physiologic responses have been observed with patients under hypnosis. Hypnotherapy has had moderate success in helping people to quit smoking and to lose weight. On occasion, people who were not good candidates for general anesthesia have been hypnotized into a deep trance state and were thereby able to undergo a necessary surgical procedure. Not all people are able to be hypnotized.

MUSIC, ART, AND DANCE THERAPY

An artistic medium is used to help the individual neutralize conflict or work through a problem. Art therapy has proven helpful when the person has difficulty expressing feelings verbally. Music therapy is beneficial for the expression of feelings, reduction of stress and anxiety, and enhancement of relaxation, or as a distraction to aid in pain management. Dance therapy promotes recognition of feelings and awareness of the body. Its goal is to integrate body and mind and promote self-esteem.

YOGA

Yoga, a word derived from the Sanskrit meaning "union," is a spiritual practice that combines exercise, controlled breathing, posture, and mental focus to bring about positive effects on the body and mind (Figure 32-2). It began as part of the ancient medicine system of India, Ayurveda. Yoga has been effective for regulating blood pressure and heart rate, increasing circulation, aiding digestion, healing chronic back pain, and helping with other disorders. Yoga may also be practiced for exercise and stress reduction without a spiritual connotation.

HUMOR

Humor has proven to be very helpful as a complementary treatment. It can speed the course of healing and decrease pain. Watching movies or comedy sketches or reading humorous literature is distracting, and laughter seems to have a positive effect on the body (Cultural Cues 32-1). Humor generally will raise spirits and help to bring about a more positive outlook.

PRAYER

The offering of prayers to a higher power helps reduce stress, promotes healing, and may arrest disease. Prayer or spiritual healing may be practiced individually or in groups as intercessory prayer. Prayer chains, in which different people pray for a set time for an individual's recovery over a period of hours or days,

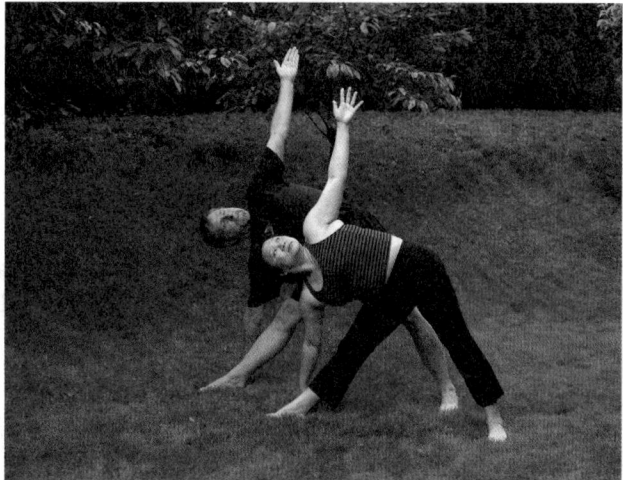

FIGURE **32-2** Yoga is a complementary therapy that focuses on posture, muscles, breathing, and focused consciousness.

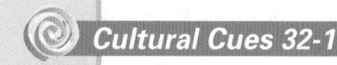

Cultural Cues 32-1

Humor

Nurses should be circumspect about using humor of their own, as some humor may be considered disrespectful. It is important to understand how humor is viewed within the patient's culture before initiating its use.

are considered beneficial by many people. Research has shown that prayer can be effective in healing. Chapter 14 presents further information on the spiritual aspects of healing.

BIOLOGIC-BASED THERAPIES

Biologic-based therapies use natural substances, such as foods and herbs. Dietary supplements and vitamins also fall into this category. Many of these therapies are as yet medically unproven. Various clinical trials and research projects are under way at the National Institutes of Health to verify the effectiveness of various herbs and supplements. Vitamins, supplements, and herb therapies are used by many patients.

HERBAL THERAPY

Herbal therapy, or phytotherapy (plant therapy), is used by more than 70% of the world's population as a major form of treatment for disorders of the mind and body. Herbal medicines contain plant material as their active ingredients and are used to treat a wide variety of health conditions. There are far too many herbs to discuss each one here. There are handbooks and texts about herbs, and much information can be found on the Internet. There are many safe and effective herbs, but others can be dangerous. Herbs may interact with various prescription drugs. **Contraindications to taking an herb should be checked before use is started.**

Table 32-1 lists some herbs determined to be safe, mostly by research through the German E Commission. Table 32-2 lists the herbs known to be unsafe. Herbal preparations are not regulated by the U.S. Food and Drug Administration (FDA), but are regarded as food supplements and subject to those regulations. Only a few have been scientifically researched in the United States as to efficacy and safety.

Increasing concerns about both the cost of prescription drugs and their toxic side effects are causing many patients to turn to herbal remedies to treat their maladies. Echinacea is used to combat cold symptoms, and ginkgo biloba is taken to improve memory. Some older men take saw palmetto to shrink the hypertrophy of the prostate gland that comes with age. St. John's wort is used to combat mild to moderate depression. Many

Table 32-1 *Safe or Effective Herbs as Determined by Non–U.S. Regulatory Authorities*

COMMON NAME	EFFECTS	EXAMPLES OF USES
Aloe	Antiinflammatory Acceleration of wound healing Alkalinization of digestive juices	Minor burns Wound healing Gastrointestinal (GI) disorders
Astralagus	Stimulant of immune system	Cancer
Bilberry	Improvement of microcirculation in eyes Mild antiinflammatory	Myopia Retinal problems GI disorders
Cat's claw	Stimulant of immune system Antioxidant Antiinflammatory Lowering of blood pressure	Cancer GI disorders Hypertension Infections
Chamomile	Antiinflammatory Antispasmodic Antiinfective	Inflammatory disease of GI and upper respiratory tracts Inflammation of skin and mucous membranes GI spasms
Dong quai	Antispasmodic Vasodilation Balancing effects of estrogen Mild sedative effect	Menstrual cramps Premenstrual syndrome Menstrual irregularities Hot flashes Vaginal dryness
Echinacea	Stimulant of immune system Antiinflammatory Antibacterial	Upper respiratory tract infection Allergic rhinitis Wound healing
Feverfew	Antiinflammatory Inhibition of serotonin and prostaglandins Vasodilator	Migraine headaches Arthritis
Garlic	Lowering of lipids Inhibition of platelet aggregation Antibacterial	Elevated cholesterol levels Hypertension Diabetes Infections
Ginger	Antiemetic	Nausea and vomiting Motion sickness
Ginkgo biloba	Memory improvement Increasing blood flow Antioxidant Increased metabolism efficiency	Alzheimer's disease Dementia Eye disease Heart disease Poor circulation Varicose veins Anxiety Age-related diseases
Ginseng	Increased physical endurance "Balancing" of body Resistance to stress	Fatigue Headaches Decreased libido Hot flashes
Goldenseal	Antiinflammatory Antibacterial Laxative	Respiratory and GI infections Gallbladder inflammation Cirrhosis of liver
Hawthorn	Increased O_2 utilization by heart Lowering of cholesterol Peripheral vasodilator	Angina Coronary artery disease

Adapted from Lewis, S.L., Heitkemper, M.M., Dirksen, S.R., et al. (2007). *Medical-Surgical Nursing: Assessment and Management of Clinical Problems* (7th ed.). St. Louis: Mosby.

Table 32-1 *Safe or Effective Herbs as Determined by Non–U.S. Regulatory Authorities—cont'd*

COMMON NAME	EFFECTS	EXAMPLES OF USES
Milk thistle	Stimulation of production of new liver cells Protection of liver from damage	Liver disease
St. John's Wort (hypericum)	Inhibition of monoamine oxidase (MAO) and serotonin reuptake Antiviral Antibacterial *Warning:* Avoid foods containing tyramine, such as aged cheese, red wine.	Mild to moderate depression Viral infections Wound healing
Saw palmetto	Prevention of conversion of testosterone to dihydrotesterone (needed for prostate cell multiplication) Balancing of sex hormones	Benign prostatic hyperplasia Urinary problems
Valerian	Minor tranquilizer Central nervous system (CNS) depression	Sleep disorders Restlessness

Table 32-2 *Unsafe Herbs*

COMMON NAME	USE/EFFECT	COMMENTS
Borage	Diuretic Antidiarrheal	Contains toxic pyrrolizidine alkaloids
Calamus	Fever Digestive aid	Contains varying amounts of carcinogenic *cis*-isoasarone; Indian type most toxic; North American type nontoxic
Chaparral	Anticancer	No proven efficacy; may induce severe liver toxicity
Coltsfoot	Antitussive Demulcent	Contains carcinogenic pyrrolizidine alkaloids
Comfrey	Wound healing	Contains large number of toxic pyrrolizidine alkaloids; may induce veno-occlusive disease
Ephedra (Ma Huang)	CNS stimulant Anorectic Bronchodilator Cardiac stimulation	Unsafe for people with hypertension, diabetes, or thyroid disease; avoid consumption with caffeine
Germander	Anorectic	Causes hepatotoxicity because of diterpenoid derivatives
Life root	Menstrual flow stimulant	Hepatotoxic; contains toxic pyrrolizidine alkaloids
Pokeroot	Antirheumatic Anticancer	May be fatal in children
Sassafras	Stimulant Antispasmodic Antirheumatic	Volatile oil contains carcinogenic safrole

From Lewis, S.L., Heitkemper, M.M., Dirksen, S.R., et al. (2007). *Medical-Surgical Nursing: Assessment and Management of Clinical Problems* (7th ed.). St. Louis: Mosby.

women rely on black cohosh rather than hormone replacement therapy to treat the hot flashes and mood swings of menopause. Ephedra, or Ma Huang, once a common ingredient in weight-loss preparations, is a cardiac stimulant and can cause a variety of adverse side effects, including death. Sale of weight-loss products that contain ephedra have been banned by the FDA, and patients should be counseled to stay away from this herb. Information on various herbs and supplements can be found on the Internet. One database is at www.herbmed.org. Information on supplements is available from the Food & Nutrition Information Center at www.nal.usda.gov/fnic/resource_lists.shtml.

AROMATHERAPY

Aromatherapy uses oils from plants that are either absorbed through the skin during massage or inhaled. The aromatic properties of certain herbs are thought to act on the brain to evoke pleasant feelings related to past experiences and emotions.

Think Critically About . . . What type of complementary therapy might be effective for the teenager who is experiencing a lot of pain after an automobile accident?

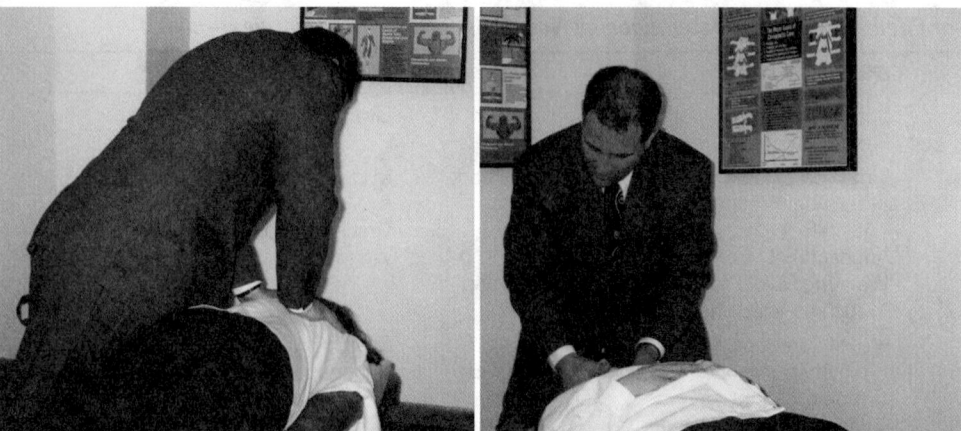

FIGURE **32-3** Chiropractic adjustment for relief of back pain.

MANIPULATIVE AND BODY-BASED THERAPIES

These therapies involve some form of manipulation, movement, or touch performed on parts of the body. Chiropractic manipulation, massage, reflexology, and acupressure are body-based therapies. Reflexology uses pressure points on the feet and sometimes the palms and ears to relieve symptoms. **Acupressure** is similar to acupuncture, except it uses pressure points rather than needles.

CHIROPRACTIC

Chiropractic uses manipulation of the spine for symptomatic relief and improved functioning by bringing the spinal components back into correct alignment, thereby decreasing or eliminating pain (Figure 32-3). Exercise, ice, heat, electrical stimulation, and massage may be used in conjunction with spinal manipulation. The treatment does not usually include the use of drugs. Chiropractic is becoming more mainstream as health care providers refer patients to a doctor of chiropractic medicine. Health insurance will often pay for this therapy.

MASSAGE THERAPY

Massage therapy uses soft tissue manipulation to improve health. Stroking, kneading, friction, and vibration are the techniques used to relieve muscle pain and promote comfort. There are several varieties of massage, with each using specialized ways of manipulating the soft tissue.

ENERGY THERAPIES

The use of energy fields is the core of energy therapies. Biofield therapies are supposed to affect energy fields that surround and penetrate the human body. Such energy fields have not yet been scientifically proven to exist. Examples include Qi Gong, Reiki, and therapeutic touch. Bioelectromagnetic-based therapies are based on the use of electromagnetic fields. A therapy may use pulsed fields, magnetic fields, or alternating or direct current. The use of magnets on a body part to relieve pain is an example of a bioelectromagnetic therapy. The research showing the effectiveness of the therapy is largely historical or anecdotal, but there are some studies validating the notion that magnets reduce pain for some people.

REIKI

Reiki stems from the Japanese word meaning "universal life force energy." A practitioner acts as a conduit for healing energy that is directed into the person's energy field or body. The practitioner channels energy to the person and the person's body does the healing. Energy flows through receptors in the crown, forehead, throat, heart, stomach, abdomen, and groin.

THERAPEUTIC TOUCH

Therapeutic touch is a technique used to alter body energy fields to restore natural healing powers. The hands of the practitioner are passed over the client to ascertain where tensions or excessive energies exist. Touch may be used to redirect energies and reestablish energy balance. Although energy therapies seem to help some individuals, there is a lack of controlled scientific studies validating that the techniques work.

? *Think Critically About* . . . Which complementary or alternative therapies do you think might help an elderly gentleman who is experiencing considerable stress and a consequent rise in his blood pressure?

THE NURSE'S ROLE IN COMPLEMENTARY AND ALTERNATIVE THERAPIES

The nurse should be knowledgeable about the various types of complementary and alternative therapies so that basic information can be given to patients if they ask. It is vital for health care providers to know if patients are taking over-the-counter herbal or homeopathic substances, because these may interact with prescription medications. For example, ginkgo biloba prolongs bleeding time, and this can cause an interaction for a patient who is receiving warfarin (Coumadin). Mixing fluoxetine (Prozac) with St. John's wort can cause toxicity.

Patients may request a referral to a CAM practitioner. Referrals to a specific practitioner are not part of the role of the nurse. You can and should explain the necessity for determining the educational background, qualifications, and certification of any practitioner before seeking services. Whenever a patient is using any of these therapies, the health care provider should be informed.

Patients should be questioned about the use of a CAM therapy in a nonjudgmental manner. It is not the nurse's place to encourage or discourage the patient's use of alternative or complementary therapy. This is a decision that must be made by the individual patient. The nurse should only guide the patient on where to find information about the therapy and how to choose a practitioner. The patient should find out about how many treatments will be required, the cost of treatment, and the possible benefits.

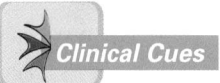
Clinical Cues

Patients often do not discuss their use of CAM with their physicians. Some feel that, because what they are doing or taking is natural, it does not interfere with prescribed medicine. Others are afraid their physician will disapprove and insist they cease the alternative practice or that they use prescription medications instead of other supplements and herbs. It is important that the nurse assist patients in understanding why it is necessary that the doctor know what supplements and alternative treatments they are utilizing.

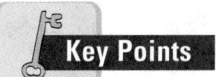
Key Points

- Complementary therapies are used along with conventional medical treatments.
- Alternative therapies are those used instead of conventional medical treatment.
- The National Center for Complementary and Alternative Medicine (NCCAM) is researching the efficacy of various therapies.
- There are five categories of complementary and alternative therapies: (1) alternative medical systems, (2) mind–body interventions, (3) biologic-based therapies, (4) manipulative and body-based methods, and (5) energy therapies.
- Homeopathic medicine, naturopathic medicine, traditional Chinese medicine, and Ayurveda are examples of alternative medical systems.
- Herbs and other supplements may interact with prescription medications.
- Many herbs may be safely taken (Table 32-1).
- Some herbs are known to be unsafe (Table 32-2).
- The nurse should be prepared to direct patients to information about complementary and alternative therapies.
- The nurse should encourage the patient to check qualifications and certification of an alternative or complementary therapy practitioner.

 Go to your **Companion CD-ROM** for an Audio Glossary, animations, video clips, and more.

evolve   Be sure to visit the companion Evolve site at http://evolve.elsevier.com/deWit/fundamental/ for additional online resources.

NCLEX-PN® EXAMINATION-STYLE REVIEW QUESTIONS

*Choose the **best** answer(s) for each question.*

1. Your patient asks you what phytotherapy means. You respond that it refers to:
   1. plant, animal, or mineral substances given in small amounts used to diminish symptoms.
   2. plant-based prescription drugs used to treat allergies.
   3. homemade remedies handed down from generation to generation.
   4. herbs compounded into medicines.

2. Biofeedback is considered a type of _____ therapy. *(Fill in the blank.)*

3. It is important to know if a patient is using herbal therapies because:
   1. certain herbs can interact adversely with prescription drugs.
   2. herbs block the action of most prescription drugs.
   3. herbs often cause odd side effects that may mimic disease.
   4. no one should take herbs while ill.

4. Chiropractic therapy: *(Select all that apply.)*
   1. is rarely covered by insurance.
   2. is usually used in combination with pain-relieving medications.
   3. uses spinal manipulation to relieve pain and restore function.
   4. may be combined with exercise, ice, heat, and electrical stimulation massage.

5. The practice of using complementary and alternative therapies along with mainstream medicine is called:
   1. duo-medicine.
   2. integrative medicine.
   3. homeopathic medicine.
   4. osteopathic medicine.

6. A logical choice of a complementary therapy for a person who has difficulty expressing her feelings might be:

1. acupuncture.
2. Reiki therapy.
3. relaxation therapy.
4. art therapy.

7. An herb once commonly used in weight-loss preparations and now banned by the FDA is:

1. valerian.
2. ginseng.
3. ginger.
4. ephedra.

CRITICAL THINKING ACTIVITIES *Read each clinical scenario and discuss the questions with your classmates.*

Scenario A
What would you say to a patient who has been suffering with back pain who wants to try a Reiki practitioner?

Scenario B
A woman who wants to stop taking hormone replacement therapy for menopausal symptoms is seeking alternative therapies. What alternative therapies are available about which you could suggest she explore information?

Scenario C
Your patient is a young adult who is experiencing chronic pain and who doesn't like to take pain medication. What complementary therapies might you suggest be explored?

33 Pharmacology and Preparation for Drug Administration

evolve http://evolve.elsevier.com/deWit/fundamental/

Objectives

Upon completing this chapter, you should be able to:

Theory

1. Describe how drugs are classified.
2. Explain the legal implications for administration of drugs by nurses.
3. Trace the general actions of drugs in the body.
4. Discuss areas of concern regarding medication administration to children or the elderly.
5. Describe issues of medication administration in home care.
6. List three reasons why patients may be noncompliant with drug treatment.
7. Discuss measures used to prevent medication errors.

Clinical Practice

1. Locate information about a drug, including action, use, usual dosage, side effects, interactions, recommended routes of administration, and nursing implications.
2. Identify information the patient must be taught to safely use a drug.
3. Demonstrate a method for accurately calculating a drug dosage.
4. Demonstrate safe practices in administration of medications.
5. Demonstrate the correct procedure for documenting medication administration.

Key Terms

Be sure to check out the bonus material on the Companion CD-ROM, including selected audio pronunciations.

adverse effects (p. 633)
agonists (ĂG-ŏ-nĭsts, p. 634)
anaphylaxis (ă-nă-fă-LĂK-sĭs, p. 634)
antagonists (ăn-TĂG-ŏ-nĭsts, p. 634)
contraindications (kŏn-tră-ĭn-dĭ-KĂ-shŭns, p. 642)
degrade (dĭ-GRĀD, p. 633)
drug interactions (p. 630)
generic name (jĕ-NĔR-ĭk, p. 630)
half-life (p. 633)
Institute for Safe Medication Practices (p. 630)
medication administration record (MAR) (p. 642)
medication reconciliation (p. 642)
noncompliance (nŏn-kŏm-PLĪ-ăns, p. 640)
nursing implications (p. 629)
peak action (p. 633)

pharmacodynamics (făr-mă-kō-dĭ-NĂM-ĭks, p. 633)
pharmacokinetics (făr-mă-kō-kĭ-NĔT-ĭks, p. 632)
PRN (p. 639)
side effects (p. 633)
stat (p. 639)
synergistic effect (sĭn-ĕr-JĬS-tĭk, p. 634)
therapeutic range (thĕr-ă-PŪ-tĭk, p. 634)
toxic effects (p. 634)
trade name (p. 630)
unit dose (p. 639)

PHARMACOLOGY

The variety of drugs used in the treatment of diseases has increased tremendously in the past decade. New drugs continue to appear as medical researchers discover more chemicals that produce highly sophisticated effects on specific tissues and cells. Although some drugs, such as opium and castor oil, have been in use since 1600 B.C., the majority of drugs currently used are of more recent origin. For example, insulin was discovered by Banting in 1922, sulfanilamide was introduced in 1937, and the first patient was treated with penicillin in 1942.

Along with physicians and pharmacists, **nurses are held legally responsible for the safe and therapeutic effects of the drugs.** Medication errors account for a great number of occurrence reports.

In this chapter, the practical information needed to administer drugs competently and safely is presented. The chapter is not intended to supply all the information needed about how drugs work or to provide comprehensive practice for drug calculations; consult additional medication references and math workbooks. **To prepare for medication administration, you need to (1) be able to locate the information about each drug, (2) consistently calculate drug dosages accurately, (3) devise a method for using the Five Rights and five "rules" of medication administration consistently, and (4) recognize the** nursing implications (points you need to remember about the drug or teach to the patient) **for each drug administered.**

For pharmaceutical medical treatment to be effective, the patient must be compliant with the medication regimen. We assume that compliance increases when patients are knowledgeable about the medication. It is your responsibility to teach the patient about drugs and to acquire the information that you and the patient need to know about each medication.

The vast increase of pharmaceutical agents used for medical treatment, and the multiple drugs that many patients take, mean that nurses must be knowledgeable about possible drug interactions (one drug modifies the action of another). For the patient to receive the full benefit of the drug, nurses must also be aware of foods that interfere with the desired uptake or action of the medication.

Issues of cost containment demand that nurses be aware of how drugs affect diagnostic testing. If a drug causes a false-positive result, then unnecessary and expensive treatment may be erroneously ordered. Likewise, a drug that causes a false-negative result may lead a physician to overlook a disease condition until great damage has been done to the patient.

USES FOR DRUGS

Drugs or medications are substances used in the treatment, palliation, diagnosis, cure, and prevention of disease. Physicians, dentists, osteopaths, and veterinarians prescribe medications; physicians' assistants, nurse practitioners, and advanced practice nurses (APNs) prescribe medications in collaboration with physicians and under written protocols or standing orders. Drugs may be dispensed and administered by pharmacists as well as those prescribing them. In accordance with *Healthy People 2010*, pharmacists and prescribers should provide counseling for patients about the risks and uses of medications. Nurses must support this effort by reinforcing the teaching and encouraging patients to ask questions.

Although drugs may have three names—a chemical name, a generic name (name not protected by trademark), and a trade name (name protected by a trademark)—usually knowing the generic and trade names is sufficient for the nurse. The chemical name provides a description of the chemical composition of the drug. Some drugs have many different trade names because they are manufactured by several different companies. For example, the generic-named drug ibuprofen may be marketed under the trade names of Advil, Motrin, and others.

Drugs come in a variety of forms and types of preparations. The form of a drug determines its route of administration. The composition of a particular form is designed to enhance its absorption and metabolism in the body. Many drugs come in several forms, such as tablets, capsules, ointments, solutions, suspensions, and suppositories (Safety Alert 33-1).

CLASSIFICATION OF DRUGS

Learn to categorize medications with similar characteristics by their class. Classifications may be defined by the effect of the drug on a body system (example: anticon-

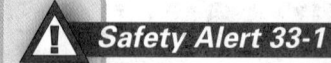

Safety Alert 33-1

Appropriate Form of the Drug

You must be certain to administer the appropriate form of each drug. For example, if the physician orders two 325-mg tablets of acetaminophen for a patient, you cannot substitute the liquid form without a change in the physician's order. Also, be vigilant in reading the labels of drugs. For example, the Institute for Safe Medication Practices (ISMP), which is an organization devoted to safe medication practices and the prevention of errors, has reported that numerous mistakes have been made when nurses did not notice the warning on the label for methylprednisolone *acetate* (Depo-Medrol), which is **NOT** for IV use, compared to methylprednisolone *sodium succinate* (Solu-Medrol), which can be used for IV administration.

vulsants), the symptoms the drug relieves (example: antihypertensives), or the drug's desired effect (example: analgesics). Similar types of problems are treated by the same class of drug, although the class may be broken into subgroups depending on how the drug works in the body to produce the desired overall effect. A drug may also have a variety of properties and effects and therefore may belong to more than one class. A common example is aspirin, which has antipyretic, antiinflammatory, analgesic, and anticlotting effects.

Another way is to learn the drugs by groups categorized by their generic drug name endings. Drugs with the same name ending often have similar characteristics and are for the same type of problem (Table 33-1).

It is extremely important to learn the general characteristics of each drug classification and the **nursing implications, which are your guide to safe and effective medication administration.** The role of the nurse in drug therapy is to administer an individual dose of a medication at a specified time. You must be aware of state statutes regulating the type and forms of drugs you may administer because this varies somewhat from state to state.

LEGAL CONTROL OF DRUGS

The public health, safety, and welfare of citizens are concerns of state and federal governments. The Pure Food and Drug Act of 1906 was the first federal statute regulating drug use. It sought to combat misuse of narcotics and to prevent the manufacture of adulterated or misbranded foods, drugs, and liquors. The federal Food, Drug, and Cosmetic Act of 1938 updated earlier laws, especially those dealing with labeling. Federal laws have since been passed that extend and refine controls on drug distribution, sales, testing, naming, and labeling. The Comprehensive Drug Abuse Prevention and Control Act of 1970 further regulates dispensing and handling of all controlled substances (Table 33-2). This act defines a drug-dependent person

Table 33-1 *Major Drug Categories by Generic Name Endings*

GENERIC NAME ENDING	TYPE OF DRUG	COMMON ACTION
"Prils" (e.g., lisinopril)	ACE inhibitors	Antihypertensive that relaxes arterial vessels
"Sartans" (e.g., losartan)	Angiotensin receptor blockers	Antihypertensive that blocks action of vasoconstriction effects of angiotensin II
"Olols, alols, and ilols" (e.g., atenolol, labetalol, carvedilol)	Beta blockers	Antihypertensives/antianginals that block beta adrenergic receptors in vascular smooth muscle
"Statins" (e.g., atorvastatin)	Antilipemics	Inhibit HMG-COA reductase enzyme reducing cholesterol synthesis
"Dipines" (e.g., amlopidipine)	Peripheral vessel calcium channel blockers	Antihypertensives/antianginals that produce relaxation of coronary smooth muscle and vascular smooth muscle; dilate coronary arteries
"Afils" (e.g., sildenafil)	Erectile agents	Peripheral vasodilator that promotes a penile erection
"Floxacins" (e.g., ciprofloxacin)	Broad-spectrum antiinfectives	Inhibits bacteria by interfering with DNA
"Prazoles" (e.g., esomeprazole)	Proton pump inhibitors	Suppress gastric secretions preventing gastric reflux and gastric and duodenal ulcers
"Tidines" (e.g., famotidine)	Block histamine-2 receptors	Inhibits histamine at H_2 receptor sites decreasing gastric secretions
"Azoles" (e.g., fluconazole)	Antifungals	Cause direct damage to fungal membrane
"Cyclovirs" (e.g., acyclovir)	Antiherpetic	Interferes with DNA synthesis causing decreased viral replication

Adapted from a presentation by Barb Bancroft at the California Vocational Nurse Educators Conference in Sacramento, CA on April 25, 2008,

Table 33-2 *Schedule of Controlled Drugs*

CLASSIFICATION	CRITERIA AND EXAMPLES OF CONTROLLED DRUGS
Schedule I	Drugs with no accepted medical use, a high potential for abuse, and lacking accepted safety measures. Group includes some opioids, psychedelics, cannabis derivatives, methaqualone, and phencyclidine. *Examples: heroin, lysergic acid diethylamide (LSD), phenolsulfonphthalein (PSP), and peyote*
Schedule II	Drugs with a medical use, a high potential for abuse, with severe psychological or physical dependence. Group includes many opioids, psychostimulants, barbiturates, and cannabinoids. *Examples: secobarbital (Seconal), amobarbital (Tuinal), amphetamine, meperidine, morphine, and methadone*
Schedule III	Drugs that are medically useful but with less potential for abuse that lead to moderate or low physical and high psychological dependence. Group includes lesser opioids, stimulants, some barbiturates, miscellaneous depressants, and anabolic steroids. *Examples: paregoric, butabarbital, and acetaminophen with codeine*
Schedule IV	Drugs that are medically useful, but with less potential for abuse than the Schedule III drugs, their abuse causing limited physical or psychological dependence. Group includes some lesser opioids, stimulants that suppress appetite, some barbiturates, benzodiazepines, and miscellaneous depressants. *Examples: tranquilizers such as chlordiazepoxide (Librium), diazepam (Valium), fenfluramine, temazepam, and chloral hydrate*
Schedule V	Drugs with medical use, low potential for abuse, and producing less physical dependence than the Schedule IV drugs. Group includes a few opioids. *Examples: mixtures with small amounts of narcotics (e.g., cough syrup containing codeine)*

in terms of physical and psychological dependence. It classifies drugs according to their medical usefulness as well as their potential for abuse. Because many controlled substances are used daily in health care agencies, you must know how to comply with regulations and agency policies to prevent misuse of these drugs.

In the hospital, the responsibility for the security of controlled drugs is shared by the pharmacists and the nurses. Stock supplies of controlled drugs are stored in the pharmacy safe and dispensed as needed to the nursing units.

In a majority of hospitals, Schedule II and III drugs are dispensed in limited amounts to the nursing units, where they are stored in a locked narcotics drawer, compartment, or automated dispensing unit. **The licensed nurse is responsible for the security of these medications and must account for each dose that is used.** Although the method of accounting varies among hospitals, a record is kept on which the nurse notes each dose that is given, to whom, and when. Other information may be included, such as the patient's room and hospital number or the name of the physician. A proof-of-use record would be used to account for each dose dispensed to the nursing unit. Information is recorded when the dose is administered to the patient. When the contents of the locked narcotics drawer are counted at the change of shifts, there should be a record of each dose given, a dose of the drug remaining for each unrecorded line, and the total remaining. To ensure the accuracy of this inventory, it is common practice for two nurses from consecutive shifts to count the drugs together. The completed proof-of-use records are eventually returned to the pharmacy and must be kept for a specified period of time. Automated dispensing units track doses removed by each nurse by computer.

? *Think Critically About* . . . What would you do if you noticed that there are frequent discrepancies in the proof-of-use record whenever Nurse A is working?

Drug Standards

Standards for drug quality, purity, packaging, safety, labeling, and dose form were set by the Pure Food and Drug Act of 1906. The standards are published in the *United States Pharmacopeia* (USP) and the *National Formulary*. The *British Pharmacopoeia* (BP) sets similar standards for drugs in Canada. For a drug to pass U.S. Food and Drug Administration (FDA) approval and be marketed, it must meet standards in five areas: purity, potency, bioavailability, efficacy, and safety (Table 33-3).

Health care institutions establish individual policies to prevent health problems resulting from drug administration. An example would be the automatic discontinuation of an antibiotic order after a certain number of days of therapy. The order may be renewed, but the physician should review the status of the patient and effectiveness of the antibiotic prior to doing so; physicians are alerted to the need for renewal.

BASIC CONCEPTS OF PHARMACOLOGY
Drug Action and Pharmacokinetics

Drugs are potent chemicals that affect the body by acting on body cells. Any drug can be either beneficial or harmful, depending on the cellular reaction. Essentially, cell functions are either stimulated or depressed, and these reactions can be achieved in various ways. Digoxin, for example, stimulates heart muscle fibers to contract more powerfully, and its effect on the heart's electrical properties causes changes in rate and rhythm. Barbiturates depress the function of cell groups in the central nervous system, causing drowsiness. Antineoplastic drugs, such as vincristine, have the ability to block cell division. Although the exact effect on cellular function is not known for all drugs, such information is continually expanding.

The study of how drugs enter the body and reach their site of action, and how they are metabolized and excreted, is called pharmacokinetics. Knowledge of pharmacokinetics is used by nurses in timing drug administration. Nurses judge the patient's risk for alterations in drug action considering physiologic condition and other drugs the patient is taking.

Absorption. To reach the cellular level, solid drugs in the form of capsules, pills, or powders must be dissolved within the body before the medication is absorbed into the bloodstream and distributed to the tissues. Drugs already in solution, such as oral liquids

Table 33-3 *Drug Standards that Must Be Met by Manufacturers*

STANDARD	DESCRIPTION
Purity	Types and concentrations of substances other than the drug that can be in the tablet, capsule, suspension, etc.
Potency	Amount of active drug in the preparation contributing to its strength
Bioavailability	Drug's ability to dissolve, be absorbed, and be transported in the body to its desired site of action
Efficacy	Laboratory studies indicative of proof that the drug is effective for its intended use
Safety	Sufficient studies completed to indicate potential side effects, adverse effects, and toxic reactions; safety is determined from the data

Table 33-4 *Differences in Absorption by Route*

ROUTE	RATE OF ABSORPTION
Skin (transdermal)	Slow absorption
Mucous membranes	Quick absorption
Respiratory tract	Quick absorption
Oral	Slow absorption (liquids are faster than pills, tablets, or capsules)
Intramuscular	Depends on form of the drug: aqueous is quicker than oil, which slows absorption
Subcutaneous	Slow absorption
Intravenous	Most rapid absorption

or injections, are generally absorbed more rapidly. Absorption may be affected by the patient's physical status. Differences in absorption by route are shown in Table 33-4.

The rate of absorption is determined by many factors. Body weight, age, sex, disease conditions, genetic factors, immune mechanisms, and physiologic and emotional factors modify reactions to a given drug. Even such a factor as hot or cold weather affects the absorption rate. Infants display a lower tolerance for drugs than children; this relates to the immaturity of organs needed to detoxify and excrete the drugs.

Distribution. Distribution to tissues and the cellular site of action depends on the chemical and physical properties of the drug and the physical status of the patient.

Other Factors Affecting Drug Action. A direct relationship exists between the amount of drug administered and the amount of body tissue in which it is distributed. An increase in the percentage of body fat tends to cause a slower distribution of the drug. **The less a patient weighs, the more concentrated the drug will be in the tissues, and consequently the more powerful the effect.**

The rapidity with which concentration at a target site occurs depends on the blood supply to the site. Local vasodilation or vasoconstriction affects the rate of blood flow. Biologic membranes affect the distribution of drugs. The blood–brain barrier is permeable only to fat-soluble drugs, and only these drugs can reach the brain and cerebrospinal fluid. **Most drugs cross the placental barrier and affect the fetus.**

The protein-binding capacity of a drug affects distribution. Most drugs bind to the protein albumin to some extent. Only the unbound portion of the drug in the bloodstream is then distributed to the target tissue. **If a patient is taking two drugs that are protein bound, one or the other drug may have a higher concentration in the unbound state than it would if it had been given alone.** This is because the drug with the lower unbound concentration has a greater ability to bind to available protein, leaving less protein to bind to the other drug.

At the site of action, the drug is soon metabolized into an inactive form that can be more easily excreted (Cultural Cues 33-1). This occurs when enzymes detoxify, degrade (break down), and remove the active drug chemicals. Most drugs are metabolized in the liver, but the lungs, blood, intestines, and kidneys contribute to metabolism. **When there is a decrease in liver function from disease or aging, a drug may be eliminated more slowly than usual, resulting in an accumulation of the drug that could lead to toxic levels.**

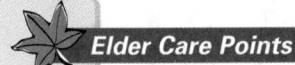
Elder Care Points

- The elderly often have a decreased level of albumin. This causes a greater potential for unbound drug in the system and a risk for increased drug activity and toxicity.
- Changes in the neurologic system, metabolic rate, and liver function of the elderly patient indicate a need for smaller doses of a drug than for the middle-aged patient.

Drugs are mainly excreted by the kidneys, but some excretion occurs via the bowel, liver, lungs, and exocrine glands. Alcohol and gaseous and volatile compounds such as anesthetics are excreted through the lungs. Deep breathing and coughing help the postsurgery patient rid the body of anesthetic more rapidly. Drugs metabolized in the liver may be excreted into the intestine in the bile. The chemicals may be reabsorbed through the intestines. Therefore, an increase in peristalsis accelerates drug excretion and factors that slow peristalsis may prolong the drug's effect. Some drugs are excreted by the kidney unchanged, but most drugs are metabolized and then excreted by the kidney. If kidney function declines, drug excretion drops, placing the patient at risk for drug toxicity. **Adequate fluid intake (50 mL/kg/day) is essential for the patient to eliminate drugs properly.**

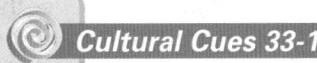
Cultural Cues 33-1

Ethnopharmacology

Ethnopharmacologic research shows that different ethnic groups may metabolize drugs differently. For example, Asian patients may require lower doses of antipsychotic medications. For African American patients, angiotensin-converting enzyme (ACE) inhibitors, such as captopril (Capoten), are less effective than for white patients (Munoz et al., 2005).

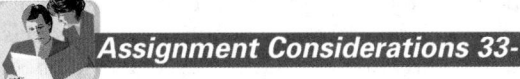
Assignment Considerations 33-1

Alert UAPs About Possible Medication Side Effects

When your patient is taking a medication that may cause secondary effects such as dizziness, inform the UAP so that she will be alert when assisting with ambulation or hygiene.

Drug Response and Pharmacodynamics

The study of a drug's effect on cellular physiology and biochemistry and its mechanism of action is known as pharmacodynamics. Response to a drug can cause a primary or secondary physiologic effect, or both. The primary effect is the desired effect; the secondary effect may be desirable or undesirable, causing side effects (unintended actions) or adverse effects (very undesirable effects with more serious consequences) (Assignment Considerations 33-1). Antihistamines such as diphenhydramine hydrochloride (Benadryl) compete with histamine at receptor sites, producing a primary antihistamine effect. A secondary effect is the inhibition of central acetylcholine, which produces a sedative effect. The secondary effect is undesirable when driving a car, but might be desirable at bedtime.

Onset, peak, and duration of action differ for each drug. Peak action occurs when the highest blood or plasma concentration of the drug is achieved. **The length of time the drug exerts a pharmacologic effect is the duration of action.** The onset of drug action begins when the drug reaches a minimum effective concentration level. Each drug has a serum half-life, or the time it takes for excretion to lower the drug concentration by half. The next dose of a drug is scheduled at the time the previous dose should reach its half-life, thus sustaining a therapeutic level of the drug.

When giving sequential doses of a drug, it is important that the doses be timed so that the concentration level of the drug in the blood never drops below the minimum effective concentration level. However, if doses of a drug are given too close together, the peak may be exceeded, causing a toxic concentration of the drug in the body.

Drugs work by attaching to receptor sites on cells or preventing other substances from attaching to those sites. The action of many drugs is dependent on their ability to attach to specific receptor sites. The better the drug fits the receptor site, the better the drug's intended action. Most cell receptors are protein in structure. Drugs that produce a response are agonists and drugs that block a response are antagonists.

Most drugs do not bind only to specific or selective sites. For this reason they produce multiple side effects as a result of binding at other sites as well as the intended ones. For example, a drug that binds to and therefore blocks cholinergic receptors will produce anticholinergic responses. The drug may be intended to dry up secretions by blocking gland secretion before surgery, but may also cause urinary retention due to effects on the bladder. An anticholinergic drug will also affect the heart, lungs, and eyes. For this reason, **if you know how a drug works, you can usually figure out what its side effects will be.** Those side effects depend on which receptor sites the drug is stimulating or blocking. Some drugs work nonselectively and affect multiple types of receptor sites. Epinephrine is such a drug; it acts on alpha$_1$, beta$_1$, and beta$_2$ receptors. Other drugs produce a response by stimulating or inhibiting enzymes or hormones and do not act on receptor sites at all.

There are four types of drug action:
1. *Stimulation* or *depression* (direct action on a receptor site), such as when the rate of cell activity is stimulated or secretion from a gland is increased, or cell activity is depressed and the function of a specific organ is reduced.
2. *Replacement,* such as injected insulin for people who do not produce their own.
3. *Inhibition* or *killing* of organisms, such as the action of an antibiotic when it blocks synthesis of the bacterial cell wall.
4. *Irritation,* such as that produced by a laxative on the colon wall, resulting in peristalsis and defecation.

The less specific the action of the drug, the more side effects the drug may have. Most drugs have some side effects. The drowsiness produced by an antihistamine is a side effect because the intended effect is to suppress allergic reaction. Sometimes side effects include *adverse effects.* An example of an adverse reaction is nausea produced by an antibiotic when its desired action is to kill pathogenic organisms. Another type of adverse effect is an allergic reaction. Developing a rash or hives after taking penicillin is an example of an allergic reaction. When an allergic adverse reaction occurs, the patient is cautioned never to take the drug again because an allergic response will become more severe the next time a drug is encountered and could cause anaphylaxis (severe allergic reaction), which could lead to death. **The possibility of adverse drug effects, side effects, allergic reactions, and undesirable interactions with other drugs and foods, increases with the number of drugs administered.**

The therapeutic range is the range of levels of the drug in the blood that will produce the desired effect

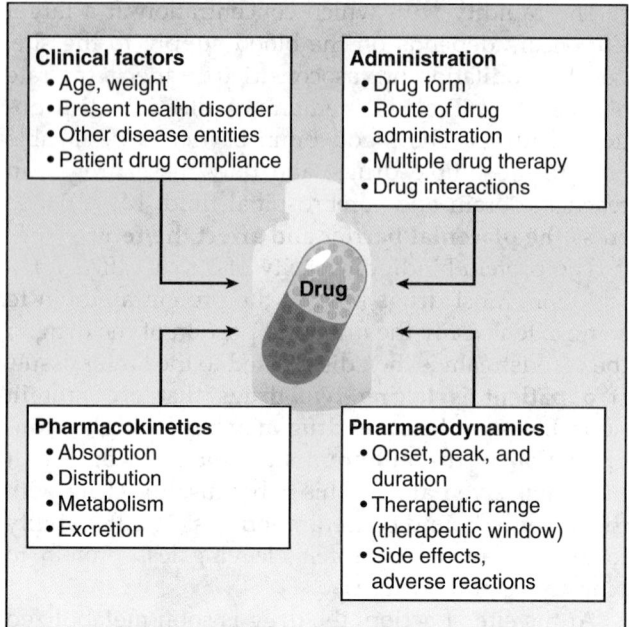

FIGURE 33-1 Factors affecting drug therapy.

without causing toxic effects. Toxic effects (harmful effects) occur when the blood level of a drug rises above the therapeutic range and causes unintended damage to normal cells. For drugs that have a narrow therapeutic range, blood levels are monitored to prevent toxicity. For example the therapeutic range of phenytoin (Dilantin), an anticonvulsant, is 10 to 20 mcg/mL of blood serum. Toxic effects occur if the blood level rises above 30 mcg/mL. Figure 33-1 reviews the factors that affect drug therapy.

A drug interaction may result in an increase or a decrease in the action of the other drug, or may alter the way in which the drug is absorbed, metabolized, or eliminated from the body. A synergistic effect (combined interaction) may occur when the action of the two drugs combined is increased or greater than the effect of the drugs given separately. Alcohol has a synergistic effect when combined with any drug that depresses the central nervous system (CNS) because it is also a CNS depressant.

Drug and Food Incompatibilities

Medications that have been taken orally can be affected by food in the digestive tract. The presence of food in the stomach can affect the drug in many ways: It can speed up, reduce, or even prevent the absorption of the drug into the bloodstream. Food delays the emptying of the stomach and so may delay the onset of the therapeutic effects of the drug. The acidic gastric juices may affect the rate of breakdown of tablets and may prevent the drug from reaching the intestinal wall, where it can be absorbed.

In addition, some drugs are incompatible with others. When such drugs are given at the same time, their effects are changed. Some drug actions are accentuated by other drugs, others have an additive effect,

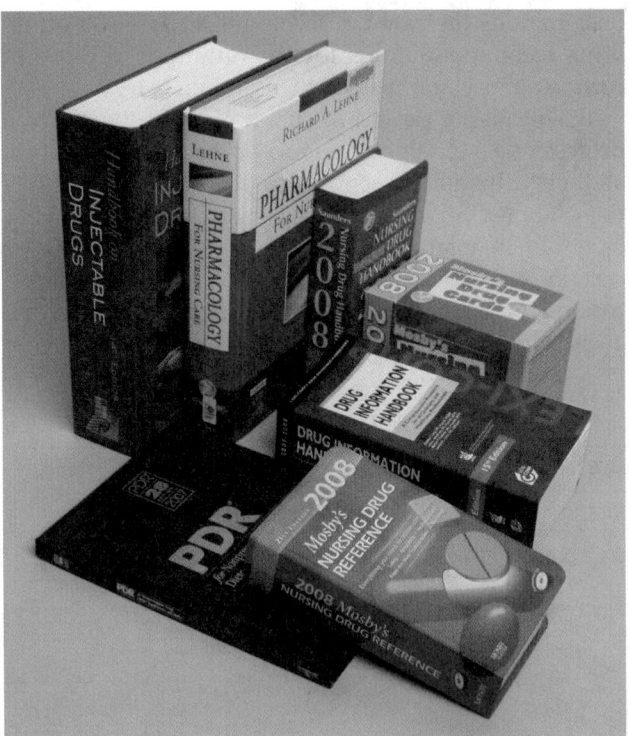

FIGURE **33-2** Drug reference books and resources.

and still other drugs may be inactivated by the other medication. The nurse is responsible for knowing the factors affecting the use of each medication given. For updated information on food and drug incompatibilities, consult drug handbooks, pharmacology books, professional journals, or the drug package insert, or check with the pharmacist (Figure 33-2). Many prescription drugs include precautions on how the drug

is to be taken in relation to food and liquids as part of the label for the patient's information.

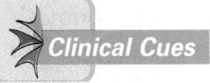

A patient may be using over-the-counter (OTC) medications, herbal remedies, or illicit substances. He may not report these, because he thinks that "they are not real drugs from a doctor"; these substances can cause drug–drug interactions. So question your patients specifically about OTC drugs, herbals, and illicit substances when taking a drug history.

MEDICATION ADMINISTRATION AND SAFETY

When a prescription or order is created for a drug to be dispensed or administered to a patient, the drug name, the amount of the drug per dose, the number of doses (tablets, capsules, etc.), the route by which to administer the drug, and the frequency or number of times a day the drug is to be taken is written by the physician or qualified person. **You must analyze the order and determine if the drug, dose, and timing of the drug are appropriate for the patient.** For this reason, you must be aware of the usual dosages for an adult or for a child for each drug. Sometimes the route ordered is not appropriate; this might happen when a patient is experiencing nausea and vomiting, but has a medication order for an oral route. If the drug comes in a rectal suppository form or an injectable form, you can consult with the physician and have the order changed. Table 33-5 presents the various routes of administration.

Table 33-5 *Routes for Drug Administration*	
ORAL ROUTES	
Oral (PO)	Medication is given by mouth and swallowed with fluid.
Sublingual	Drug is placed under the tongue, where it readily dissolves. Should not be swallowed.
Buccal	Solid medication is placed in the mouth against the mucous membrane of the cheek until it dissolves. Should not be chewed or swallowed.
PARENTERAL ROUTES	
Intradermal	Medication is injected into the dermis just under the epidermis.
Subcutaneous	Medication is injected into the tissues just below the dermis of the skin.
Intramuscular (IM)	Medication is injected into a muscle.
Intravenous (IV)	Medication is injected into a vein.
Epidural	Medication is injected into the epidural space of spinal column.*
Intrathecal	Medication is injected into the intrathecal space of spinal column.*
SKIN	
Topical	Medication is applied to the skin, eye, or ear for local effect.
Transdermal	Medication is applied in a small area for slow systemic absorption.
MUCOUS MEMBRANES	
Vaginal	Medication is inserted into vagina for local treatment.
Rectal	Medication is inserted into rectum for local or systemic effect.
Inhalation	Medication is inhaled into the nose or lungs for local and systemic effect.

*Medication administration via these routes is beyond the scope of LPN/LVN practice, but you may see this type order.

The nurse is also responsible for monitoring laboratory results related to drug administration. For example, if a patient is taking furosemide (Lasix), it would be appropriate to check the potassium level prior to administering the drug. In addition, the Institute for Safe Medication Practices (ISMP) suggests that lab values must be reported directly to licensed personnel.

Medication errors occur far more often than they should. According to the 2009 National Patient Safety Goals (2B), health care facilities should "standardize a list of abbreviations, acronyms, symbols, and dose designations that are not to be used." Table 33-6 presents recommendations for discontinuing the use of certain abbreviations in dosage orders.

It will take a period of time before all health care professionals eliminate the use of these abbreviations, so they will still be seen in drug orders. When one of these abbreviations appears, consider the order very carefully in relation to the patient's condition to be certain you understand its meaning. Developing a routine for safely giving medications and sticking to it each time you do the procedure can help you avoid

Table 33-6 *The Joint Commission's Dangerous Abbreviations or Dose Designations—Not Recommended*

OFFICIAL "DO NOT USE LIST"		
DO NOT USE	**POTENTIAL PROBLEM**	**USE INSTEAD**
U (unit)	Mistaken for "0"(zero), the number "4" (four) or "cc"	Write "unit"
IU (international units)	Mistaken for "IV" (intravenous) or the number "10" (ten)	Write "International Unit"
Q.D., QD, q.d., qd (daily) Q.O.D., QOD, q.o.d., qod (every other day)	Mistaken for each other Period after Q mistaken for "I" and "O" mistaken for "I"	Write "daily" Write "every other day"
Trailing zero (X.0 mg)	Decimal point is missed	Write X mg
Lack of leading zero (.X mg)		Write 0.X mg
MS	Can mean morphine sulfate or magnesium sulfate	Write "morphine sulfate" Write "magnesium sulfate"
MSO_4 and $MgSO_4$	Confused for one another	

IN ADDITION TO THE "MINIMUM REQUIRED LIST"		
ABBREVIATION	**POTENTIAL PROBLEM**	**PREFERRED TERM**
µg (for microgram)	Mistaken for mg (milligrams) resulting in one thousand-fold dosing overdose.	Write "mcg"
H.S. (for half-strength or Latin abbreviation for bedtime)	Mistaken for either half-strength or hour of sleep (at bedtime) q.H.S. mistaken for every hour. All can result in a dosing error.	Write out "half-strength" or "at bedtime"
T.I.W. (for three times a week)	Mistaken for three times a day or twice weekly resulting in an overdose.	Write "3 times weekly" or "three times weekly"
S.C. or S. Q. (for subcutaneous)	Mistaken as SL for sublingual, or "5 every"	Write "Sub-Q", "subQ", or "subcutaneously"
D/C (for discharge)	Interpreted as discontinue whatever medications follow (typically discharge meds).	Write "discharge"
c.c. (for cubic centimeter)	Mistaken for U (units) when poorly written.	Write "mL" for milliliters
A.S., A.D., A. U. (Latin abbreviation for left, right, or both ears).	Mistaken for each other (e.g., AS or OS, AD or OD, AU for OU, etc.).	Write: "left ear," "right ear" or "both ears;"
O.S. O. D., O. U. (Latin abbreviation for left, right, or both eyes)		"left eye," "right eye", or "both eyes"

ADDITIONAL ABBREVIATIONS, ACRONYMS, AND SYMBOLS (FOR POSSIBLE FUTURE INCLUSION IN THE OFFICIAL "DO NOT USE" LIST)		
DO NOT USE	**POTENTIAL PROBLEM**	**USE INSTEAD**
> (greater than)	Misinterpreted as the number "7"(seven) or the letter "L"	Write "greater than"
< (less than)	Confused for one another	Write "less than"
Abbreviations for drug names	Misinterpreted due to similar abbreviations for multiple drugs	Write drug names in full
Apothecary units	Unfamiliar to many practitioners Confused with metric units	Use metric units
@	Mistaken for the number "2" (two)	Write "at"

making a medication error. Should an error be made, it must be reported immediately to your clinical instructor and/or charge nurse. A medication error can be a life-threatening event for a patient, and patient safety must come first (Safety Alert 33-2). In addition, the ISMP publishes a newsletter that provides educational information for health care providers related to safe medication administration (*www.ismp.org/Nursing Articles/list.htm*). There is also a phone number to report medication errors to the ISMP (1-800-FAIL-SAF[E]). Reporting errors is an opportunity to improve individual practice and health system policies. Reviewing Box 33-1 and Concept Map 33-1 will help you keep in mind all the information you need to safely administer medications.

⚠ Safety Alert 33-2

Look-Alike, Sound-Alike Drugs

Look-alike drugs and packaging and sound-alike names increase the likelihood of mistakenly giving the wrong medication. In accordance with the 2009 National Patient Safety Goals, institutions should make an effort to minimize their stock of these types of drugs. If you identify this type of problem on your unit, call it to the attention of the unit manager.

CONSIDERATIONS FOR INFANTS AND CHILDREN

Differences in size, age, weight, surface area, and organ maturity all affect the ability to absorb, metabolize, and excrete drugs. Drug dosages are lower for infants and children than for adults and must be very carefully calculated and administered. **Doses are based on age, size, and weight of the child and are not given in a standardized amount.** Each dose is calculated very carefully.

Check with the child's parents for the most effective, least traumatic way to give the child a medication. Sometimes it is best to let the parent administer the oral medication while you supervise. You should explain in short sentences with simple language at the child's level of understanding what the drug is for and how it is to be given. Be supportive, and approach the child with confidence and an attitude of expecting cooperation.

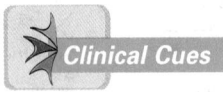
Clinical Cues

When giving medication to young children, do not say the medication is like "candy"; simply say that it will help him or her get well. After the medication has been given, praise the child and offer a simple reward such as a sticker.

Box 33-1 Safety Guidelines to Prevent Medication Errors

When preparing to administer medications:
- Plan ahead and do not rush when preparing medications for administration.
- Prepare medications for administration in as distraction-free an environment as possible.
- Follow the five "rights" every time you prepare and give medications.
- Clarify with the prescriber any illegible writing in a drug order.
- Do not administer a drug if it is not clearly and correctly labeled with name and amount of the drug contained.
- Check any questionable order or unfamiliar drug or dosage with the pharmacist.
- If an ordered drug dosage seems odd, question it and check the order with the pharmacist or physician.
- If a dosage calculation has to be made, have the calculation repeated by another nurse and compare the result.
- Review the patient's MAR for any possible drug interactions.
- Determine if the patient is receiving more than one drug with the same action. If so, question the order.
- Ask another nurse to double-check the order and dose you are going to give of any high-risk drug such as IV potassium, heparin, IV cardiac drugs, and insulins.
- Keep the drug in its original container. Discard leftover portions of unused medication from single-dose packages.
- Question the pharmacist whenever multiple tablets or vials are needed to prepare a single dose of medication.

- Become aware of drugs with similar names and carefully check the original order and why the patient is receiving the drug before administering it.
- Question an excessive dosage increase in a patient's medication.
- Be familiar with every drug you administer. Look it up if you can't remember the information you need to safely administer it.
- Check each medication with the order thoroughly three times before giving it to the patient.

At the time of medication administration to the patient:
- Always have the patient state his or her full name and verify the name and number on the patient's armband with the information on the MAR. Ask about allergies each time you administer medications to the patient.
- Check each drug at the bedside with the patient's MAR before administering the medication.
- Sign that a medication has been given only after the patient has received it.
- Do not leave a medication dose at the patient's bedside.

Working with the patient for error prevention:
- Teach the patient about the drugs he or she is taking and the importance of proper identification of the patient before a drug is taken.
- Familiarize the patient with the color and shape of each medication.
- Obtain a complete drug history from the patient.

If a medication error does occur, always report it.

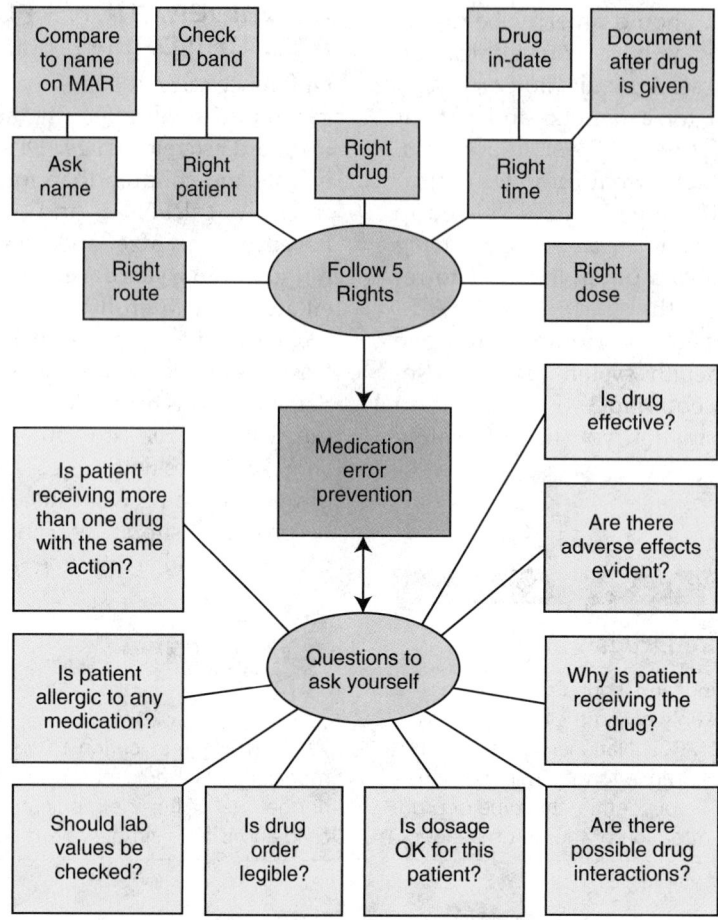

CONCEPT MAP **33-1** Steps to medication error prevention.

CONSIDERATIONS FOR THE ELDERLY

The following points should be considered before administering medications to an elderly person:

- Elderly patients may have chronic medical conditions and may be taking multiple medications; check drug interactions carefully.
- Metabolism of drugs is slowed in the elderly, and normal doses may build to toxic levels when liver or kidney function is decreased. Elderly patients experience twice as many adverse reactions as younger people; observe the patient closely for signs of adverse reaction.
- Older patients who are on long-term anti-inflammatory therapy for arthritis should be monitored for gastrointestinal bleeding and anemia.
- Elderly patients may need a pill organizer to help them remember which drugs to take and to remind them whether they have taken a dose of medication.
- Elderly patients are likely to have greater blood pressure fluctuations with position changes and are more susceptible to falls when taking drugs that can cause orthostatic hypotension.
- Elderly patients may become quickly dehydrated and experience electrolyte imbalances when taking diuretics; these drugs also may increase uric acid levels, making the patient susceptible to gout.

- Elderly patients who have decreased kidney function are particularly susceptible to digoxin toxicity and should be carefully watched for early signs of this condition, which include appetite loss, confusion, fatigue, and depression.
- Patients with limited financial resources may not be able to afford the purchase of needed medication; a tactful inquiry is sometimes necessary.
- Some elderly patients have very limited vision and can misread the label on medication containers; encourage the patient to have another person verify or color-code medications.
- With age, swallowing muscles weaken, and the patient is more susceptible to choking; position the patient upright and, if the person is not on fluid restrictions, have him take a sip of water and then the oral medication with more water.
- If the patient has had a stroke causing weakness on one side, be certain that the medication is placed on the strongest side of the mouth (always assess swallowing ability before giving anything by mouth to a patient who has had a stroke or neurologic problem causing weakness).
- Many older patients have difficulty opening "childproof" caps on medication bottles; they can request that medication be placed in bottles with caps that are easy to remove and replace.

• Approximately one third of elderly patients are noncompliant with their medication regimens because of confusion, forgetfulness, poor vision, and other socioeconomic reasons. In such cases, help is needed to promote understanding of the drug regimen and to provide a reliable method of adhering to a medication schedule.

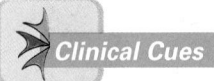
Clinical Cues

When assessing your patient's ability to swallow, put him in a high Fowler's position. Ask him to swallow as you observe movements in his throat and his ability to follow instructions. Gently place your thumb and finger over the larynx and ask him to swallow again as you feel the swallow movement. Next, try giving him 1 teaspoon of water and observe as he swallows.

CONSIDERATIONS FOR HOME CARE

For home care patients, be certain that the patient or caregiver can open the medication bottles or dispenser. A pill organizer may need to be set up for the patient to ensure that medications are taken on schedule. Written instructions about what to report to the physician should be left with the patient. If possible, observe the caregiver or patient as he or she prepares medication to validate the process of administration that is being used. Verify that the patient can obtain the needed medications; if not, notify the physician. Caution patients about keeping medications out of the reach of children. Check medicine cabinets for medications that are out of date and see that they are discarded.

If a caregiver is to administer the medications, thorough teaching must be performed. Obtain feedback that indicates the caregiver understands what each medication is for, when it is to be given, side effects to monitor, and adverse effects to report to the physician.

Think Critically About . . . You are providing home care for an elderly patient who is taking multiple medications prescribed by several different specialists. You notice that some of the medications could have drug–drug interactions. Why might this occur? What would you do about this situation?

TYPES OF ORDERS

There are four common types of medication orders based on the frequency of drug administration.

• A standing order is carried out until it is canceled by the physician or until the prescribed number of doses has been given. "Ceftin 250 mg po bid × 10 days" is an example of a standing order.
• A PRN (as-needed) order is an order written for when the patient requires it. The nurse and patient determine the patient's need. The physician sets time limits for the interval between doses. An example of a PRN order is "Morphine 4 mg IM q 4 hr PRN pain."
• A one-time (single) order is written for a drug to be given just the one time. Such orders are common preoperatively or before a diagnostic procedure. An example is "Valium 10 mg IM on call to G.I. lab."
• A stat (immediate) order is for a single dose of a medication to be given right away without delay. A stat order is used in emergencies when the patient's condition has suddenly changed. An example is "Benadryl 50 mg IM stat" to help counteract an allergic reaction.

There are many abbreviations and symbols used in medication orders that you must know. Although it is recommended that use of some of these abbreviations and symbols be discontinued, you should learn all of them because they are still in use in some areas. The most common ones are given in Table 33-7.

DISTRIBUTION OF DRUGS

Health care facilities providing nursing care have a particular way of stocking and dispensing drugs. A medication room; a rolling, locked drug cart; a computerized drug cabinet; and individual storage units in the patient's room are some of the methods used.

Stock supply drugs are in large, multidose containers, and each patient dose must be individually prepared. This is a time-consuming, costly method of dispensing drugs. An individual patient supply of drugs is usually kept in a bin or drawer labeled with the patient's name. The pharmacist oversees placement in the drawer or bin of only the amount of a drug the patient will use for 12 to 72 hours. The patient is given only the drugs from the individual supply bin or drawer.

Unit dose refers to drugs packaged in single, individual doses (Safety Alert 33-3). Each unit dose contains the medication the patient is to receive at one particular time. Each dose is wrapped individually. In the unit-dose systems, the pharmacy will deliver a 24-hour supply of drugs for each patient. The patients' medications are then stored in a drawer or a cart. The medications are refilled by the pharmacy each day. The cart or storage area may also contain a locked compartment with a select supply of common PRN and stock drugs for special needs. The system, when used properly, reduces medication errors and is time efficient.

A computer-controlled dispensing system such as the Pyxis system is especially useful for the delivery and control of narcotics and other scheduled drugs. Each nurse is assigned a security code allowing access to the system. The patient's identification number must be entered and then the desired drug, dosage, and route are entered. The system gives the drug to the nurse, records it, and charges it to the patient. Sometimes a bar code system is used in conjunction with the dispensing system.

Table 33-7 *Abbreviations and Symbols Used in Medication Orders*

ABBREVIATION	MEANING	ABBREVIATION	MEANING
ac	before meals	**ERROR-PRONE ABBREVIATIONS***	
ad lib	freely	cc	cubic centimeter
B.I.D. or bid	twice a day	DC	discontinue
g or gm	gram	3	dram
gtt	drops	gr	grain
H	hour	h.s.	at bedtime
I.D.	intradermal	♏	minim
I.M.	intramuscular	OD	right eye
I.V.	intravenous	OS	left eye
I.V.P.B.	intravenous piggyback	OU	both eyes
kg	kilogram	qd, q1d	each day
K.V.O.	keep vein open	qh	every hour
L	liter	qod	every other day
mcg	microgram	SC, SQ, subq	subcut or subcutaneous
mEq	milliequivalent	ss	sliding scale (insulin)
mL	milliliter	SSRI	sliding scale regular insulin
MDI	metered-dose inhaler	SSI	sliding scale insulin
NGT	nasogastric tube	U or u	unit
oz	ounce		
PCA	patient-controlled analgesia		
pc	after meals		
PR	per rectum		
PRN or prn	as needed		
q	every		
Q.I.D. or qid	four times a day		
Rx	take		
STAT or stat	immediately		
S.L.	sublingual		
SR	sustained release		
T.I.D. or tid	three times a day		
tsp	teaspoon		
T or tbsp	tablespoon		

*Although the apothecary system and some other abbreviations are being discontinued because of medication safety concerns, these symbols and abbreviations are included because they are still sometimes encountered. For additional information and other error-prone abbreviations see www.ismp.org/tools/errorproneabbreviations.pdf.

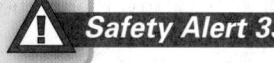

Unit-Dose System

Use the unit-dose system to avoid errors. If you find that the dosage that you are preparing exceeds three unit-dose packets, question if the ordered dose is too high, or if you have made an error in interpreting the order or making the dosage calculations.

PROBLEMS OF NONCOMPLIANCE

There are many reasons why patients do not take the drugs that are prescribed for them on the schedule that is indicated by the prescription (noncompliance). One reason is that the patient does not comprehend the action of the drug or why it is being taken. There is no understanding that a steady blood level is needed for it to work effectively. Understanding is needed to convince the patient to continue taking the drug when symptoms are gone.

Another reason for stopping a drug is that the patient cannot tolerate a side effect of the drug. In the male, urinary retention and sexual dysfunction are common reasons for noncompliance. Often a dosage adjustment or change in the drug prescribed will alleviate these problems. Otherwise if the drug is vital to the patient's health, another medication may be used to ease the undesirable side effect in question.

Inability to purchase a medication is another reason for noncompliance. Medication is expensive, and many people do not have the extra money required to purchase their prescriptions. Patients often stop taking blood pressure medication because they cannot afford to buy more and, after taking the first round of the prescription, are feeling fine. Thorough patient teaching is needed so the patient understands that the medication is essential. Once the patient understands what can happen without medication, medication purchase may receive higher priority in the budget.

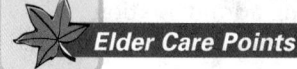

Particularly for the elderly patient, an inability to remember when a dose of medication is due is another problem. Some new pill organizers have an alarm built into them. Setting the alarm as a reminder that a dose of medication is due can be very helpful for some people.

NURSING CARE PLAN 33-1

Care of the Patient Who Is Noncompliant

SCENARIO Richard Paloni was diagnosed with hypertension and started on enalapril (Vasotec) 5 mg PO daily. When he came into the clinic for a follow-up visit, his blood pressure was 166/96. It is determined that Mr. Paloni does not understand his disease or the need for continuous medication. He had not been taking the medication since his prescription had run out. When asked why he had quit taking his medication, he stated he thought the medicine had cured his blood pressure problem since he feels fine.

PROBLEM/NURSING DIAGNOSIS *Does not understand disease or need for medication*/Deficient knowledge related to effects and control of hypertension.
Supporting Assessment Data: Subjective: States, "thought the medicine had cured my blood pressure problem since I feel fine." Has not been taking medication since his prescription ran out. *Objective:* BP 166/96.

Goals/Expected Outcomes	Nursing Interventions	Selected Rationale	Evaluation
Patient will verbalize possible outcomes of uncontrolled hypertension during next visit.	Assess patient's knowledge of how hypertension affects the body.	Establishes knowledge base about his disease process.	*What does the patient know about his hypertension?* States, "My doctor told me I had high blood pressure."
	Instruct regarding effects of hypertension on the body (i.e., possible kidney damage). Advise of potential complications of uncontrolled hypertension (i.e., increased risk for stroke).	Promotes understanding of damage uncontrolled hypertension can do.	*What information was given to patient?* Pamphlet regarding high blood pressure control and complications reviewed with patient. Agrees to read material and ask questions tomorrow.
Patient will verbalize action of antihypertensive medication and importance of taking it as scheduled by next visit.	Discuss how enalapril (Vasotec) works in the body to lower the blood pressure.	Knowledge of how a drug works and an understanding of what it is expected to do promote compliance.	*What was the patient able to recall about medication teaching?* Knows to take enalapril (Vasotec) every day. States, "Medication helps to block sodium." Outcomes partially met. Continue with plan.

PROBLEM/NURSING DIAGNOSIS *Not taking medication*/Noncompliance related to lack of understanding about his disease and medication.
Supporting Assessment Data: Subjective: "I didn't see the need to refill the prescription." Quit taking medication after prescription ran out. *Objective:* BP 166/96.

Goals/Expected Outcomes	Nursing Interventions	Selected Rationale	Evaluation
Patient will take antihypertensive as it is prescribed on a continuing basis.	Explain that when blood pressure is down to normal when taking the medication, it is because the medication is working in the body.	Understanding of how medication works promotes compliance.	*Is the patient taking his medication as ordered?* Reports, "I'm taking my medicine every day."
	Explain that the medication must be taken every day for it to remain in the bloodstream, where it can work to lower the blood pressure.	Taking the drug on a set daily schedule keeps a steady amount in the bloodstream that will maintain the blood pressure at a lower level.	Discussed maintaining blood level of the drug by taking it regularly. Reports, "I'm feeling better, and proud of myself for remembering to take care of myself."

Continued

NURSING CARE PLAN 33-1

Care of the Patient Who Is Noncompliant—cont'd

Goals/Expected Outcomes	Nursing Interventions	Selected Rationale	Evaluation
Patient will take antihypertensive as it is prescribed on a continuing basis.	Explore whether patient can afford to buy the medication. Establish how patient will routinely take the medication.	Must be able to obtain the drug in order to take it to lower the blood pressure.	States, "I understand the need for regular doses of the medication." States, "Insurance will cover most of the cost," and "I will take it each morning when I brush my teeth." Progressing toward expected outcome. Continue with plan.

? CRITICAL THINKING QUESTIONS

1. What specifically would you teach Mr. Paloni about the possible consequences of uncontrolled hypertension?

2. What type of antihypertensive is enalapril (Vasotec)? How does it work? How would you explain this to Mr. Paloni?

Some people do not like to have to depend on a chemical to get well or to maintain health. When alternative ways of alleviating their health problems can be found, they should be used. Otherwise good patient teaching is a tool available to increase compliance (Nursing Care Plan 33-1).

APPLICATION of the NURSING PROCESS

Assessment (Data Collection)

Assessment of the patient's condition and medication history is essential before administering a medication. In accordance with 2009 National Patient Safety Goals, all health care staff should be participating in medication reconciliation. Medication reconciliation is a process of identifying all the patient's medications and communicating this information to the patient and staff. This is particularly relevant when the patient is transferred to different providers, facilities, or units or discharged home. The process includes the following:

1. Listing all current medications
2. Listing all medications to be prescribed (i.e., preoperative medications)
3. Comparing lists for interactions
4. Using information to make clinical decisions
5. Communicating information to all caregivers

When you know about the patient's medical problems, you can correlate the reason for the prescribed drug. When assessing for allergies, check all locations where allergies are listed on charts in your facility; *also question the patient.* You must know whether there are any contraindications (reasons not to administer) for giving the drug ordered by the route ordered. **If giving a medication that affects vital signs,** know the current readings prior to administration in order to determine if it will be safe to give the drug. If the drug

has a narrow therapeutic range, it is important to assess the serum blood level of the drug. Check lab results for a serum drug level and determine whether it is within safe and therapeutic limits.

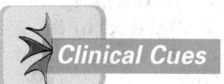
Clinical Cues

Get in the habit of asking about allergies to medication **every time** you give a drug, even if you have already asked the patient about allergies earlier in the day. Later in your career, this habit will be in place when you are caring for multiple patients at a very fast pace.

Assess information about each drug, noting how the drug works, its purpose, usual dosages, routes of administration, side effects, and the nursing implications for administration and monitoring the patient. Look at the other drugs listed on the medication administration record (MAR) (sheet listing medications prescribed and times to be given) and determine if there are any possible drug interactions with the drug you are about to give. Assess for any food interactions and counsel the patient appropriately.

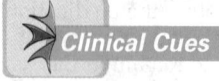
Clinical Cues

Make friends with the pharmacist and have that number at your fingertips. The pharmacy can help you with all types of information, including drug interactions and compatibilities.

Other factors to assess include whether the patient can swallow an oral medication, or has sufficient muscle tissue to absorb an intramuscular injection, and what site will be best to use for such an injection. Assess for side or adverse effects from previous doses of the drug. Determine the patient's attitude about drugs because this may provide data about whether the patient is likely to be compliant with the medication regimen.

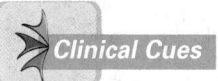

When you are at the bedside doing your third and final medication check, ask the patient if he is noticing any ill effects that he associates with taking his medications. For example, "Sir, this is your antibiotic medication. Does this medication seem to be causing any problems for you?" [Such as diarrhea or nausea?] This is one method for assessing the patient's subjective response to the medication. Of course, you are also responsible for evaluating relevant laboratory values and observing for effects that the patient may not cognitively associate with the medication.

When working in a home care or clinic situation, assess for any patient limitations that might make self-administration difficult, such as poor eyesight, weakness or paralysis, or confusion and forgetfulness. If such limitations exist, assess for ways that the patient might receive the medications in a safe manner. Assess the patient's knowledge about the drug therapy to determine areas of needed instruction.

Nursing Diagnosis

Possible nursing diagnoses for patients receiving drug therapy include the following:
- Deficient knowledge related to use and adverse effects of prescribed drugs
- Noncompliance with medication regimen

Planning

Examples of expected outcomes are as follows:
- Patient verbalizes reason he is taking the drug.
- Before discharge, patient lists signs of adverse effects to report to physician.
- Patient will take medications as prescribed.

Safely and accurately administering drugs requires preplanning. **Unfamiliar drugs should be verified in reference handbooks before the scheduled time to give them.** A medication administration schedule should be incorporated into the daily work organization plan. Specific planning is required to properly evaluate whether signs and symptoms of adverse effects are present in the patient. Time is planned for teaching the patient the information needed to safely take each drug prescribed.

Before administering a drug, check the **Five Rights** of medication administration (Safety Alert 33-4). Be sure you have the following:
- **The right drug**
- **The right dose**
- **The right route**
- **The right time**
- **The right patient**

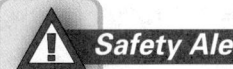

Patient Identifiers

In accordance with the 2009 National Patient Safety Goals, at least two patient identifiers must be used to ensure that the medication is administered to the correct patient. Say to the patient, "State your name for me, please." (Do not call the patient by name; some patients who do not hear well will say "yes"; confused patients may answer to any name.) Look at the patient's identification armband or number. Some facilities may also require validation of the birth date.

During the 1990s, five more rules for safe administration of drugs were added to the Five Rights. They are as follows:
- **Teach the patient about the drugs.**
- **Take a complete drug history.**
- **Assess the patient for drug allergies.**
- **Be aware of potential drug interactions with other drugs or foods.**
- **Document each drug you administer after giving it.**

Plan ahead whether you will need to take juice or milk and crackers to the patient in order for a particular drug to be taken. If a patient needs a drug crushed and mixed in applesauce or something else, take the supplies to the bedside with you. This saves a trip back to the workroom. If your patient will need to be helped to sit upright or has difficulty taking medications, plan to take extra time for that patient's medication administration.

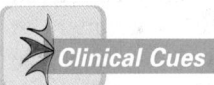

Plan to give routinely scheduled medications to those needing extra help last. Always give the most important medication first, for example, give digoxin first and a multivitamin last.

Before preparing medications for your assigned patients, verify which patients are NPO (nothing by mouth) for surgery or tests and which have an order to "hold breakfast." Check with the charge nurse about giving these patients their medications when tests are completed. Dialysis patients also may need to have medications held, especially blood pressure medications, but this may vary by physician preference.

Check and replenish supplies such as medication cups, straws, water cups, and so forth on the medication cart before heading to patient rooms with the cart.

Implementation

When giving medications, the nurse is guided by many principles. Facility policies vary, but you will safely and accurately give medications if you follow these principles:

- Medications are given by the person who prepared them. If not given, the drug should not be returned to the drug cabinet or cart unless it is still in the unopened, labeled unit-dose package.
- Medications are not to be left at the bedside because they may be forgotten, lost, or taken by another patient. Exceptions may be made for drugs such as antacids, nitroglycerin, or birth control pills when so ordered in writing by the physician. Monitor their use and document the doses taken.
- Narcotics and other controlled drugs are kept in locked cabinets. You are legally responsible for the security of these cabinets and must account for each dose used.
- Check medication orders before giving drugs. Routinely compare medication records or medication cards with those drugs listed on the MAR to see that there are no errors or omissions. If there is a question about the accuracy, refer to the original order on the physician's order sheet.
- Avoid distractions or interruptions when preparing or administering medications. Concentrate on the task to be done.
- Know about the drugs being given. Research information on unfamiliar drugs concerning their action, dosage, and any precautions to be followed.
- **Observe the Five Rights and five rules when administering drugs.**
- Observe the principles of aseptic technique. Perform hand hygiene before beginning to dispense medications and after patient contact. Avoid touching the inside of medication containers or cups. Dispose of pills dropped on the floor. Do not handle or touch medications; pour the pills or tablets into the bottle cover and then transfer them into the medication cup (Figure 33-3).
- Obtain a complete medication history from the patient and look for possible drug interactions among the medications the patient is taking.
- Is the medication order consistent with the patient's diagnosis and plan of treatment? If the answer is no, or if there is doubt, check it out with the charge nurse or physician.
- Is the medication similar in action to another medication the patient has been receiving? Is he still getting the other drug? If so, question both orders.
- Check the chart and MAR for listed patient allergies and ask the patient about allergies whenever you are administering medication; look for an allergy identification band.
- Teach the patient about the drug: what it looks like, its intended action, possible side effects, and how to take it. Explain why it should be taken with food or on an empty stomach and why it is

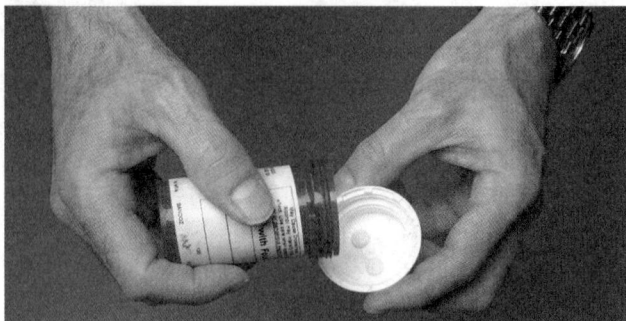

FIGURE **33-3** Pour pills from the patient's own supply into the vial cover.

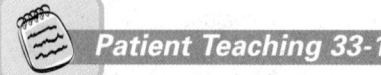

Patient Teaching 33-1

Drug Information

The following points should be taught to the patient about each prescribed drug:

- Why the drug is prescribed and what it is supposed to do
- How long it will be before results of the drug will be evident
- Signs and symptoms of adverse effects to be observed for, and which ones to report to the physician immediately
- How to deal with common side effects
- The dosage and schedule for taking the drug
- The reason for taking the drug as scheduled
- The amount of fluid that the patient should drink while taking the drug
- Whether the drug should be taken with food
- What to do if a dose is accidentally forgotten
- Foods that should be avoided while taking the drug
- Any special instructions pertinent to the drug, such as weighing daily, eating high-potassium foods, or avoiding salt
- The need to consult with the physician before taking any over-the-counter medications
- Over-the-counter drugs that might interfere with the drug's action
- The importance of any needed periodic laboratory tests

important to take it on schedule (Patient Teaching 33-1).

- Check all MAR entries with the original order for accuracy at least once every 24 hours.
- If the patient questions the dose or the medication you are about to give, *stop* and verify the order.
- Check pertinent laboratory values and assess for side effects of the drug before giving the next dose of a medication.
- Avoid contamination of your own skin or inhalation to minimize chance of allergy or development of drug sensitivity.
- Document after the drug is given. Note the route, time, and site (if pertinent). Information about assessment for side effects from previous doses of the drug should be documented also. Include any patient teaching that was done about the medication, dosage schedule, or precautions.

Evolving technologies will contribute to safe and accurate medication administration. For example, eMedPass is a new user-friendly system that incorporates a touch screen of patient photos and medication icons. A nurse fingerprint identification process allows easy access while ensuring patient privacy. The nurse scans the medication bar code prior to administration and the system automatically documents this on an electronic MAR and reorders medications as needed.

> **?** *Think Critically About* ... Another nurse asks you to obtain a drug for her patient from the medication cart while you are getting medications for your patients. Discuss some of the problems that could occur.

Calculating the Drug Dosage to Be Given

Several methods can be used to accurately calculate the dosage to be given for a particular drug order. An example is given here as a refresher, because this information is usually covered in a nursing mathematics or pharmacology course.

Examples of Conversion Problems. Sometimes it is still necessary to convert from one system of measurement to another, for example, from the metric to the apothecary system. The apothecary system is not exact for measurements. **Current recommendations for safety in medication administration state not to use the apothecary system, but change in physician habits for prescribing medication comes slowly.** There is variation of measurement conversion to the metric system. For example, one grain varies from 60 to 65 mg. The conversion should not vary by more than 10%. The equivalents must be memorized first (Box 33-2).

To set up a conversion problem, let us assume that grains need to be converted to milligrams. The order requests that 5 grains of medication be given *(dose desired)*. On hand are tablets that contain 300 mg of medication *(dose on hand)*. The following formula is used:

(Formula: Dose desired/dose on hand)
Dose desired = grains

First convert milligrams to grains. The conversion problem is

$$60 \text{ mg} = 1 \text{ grain}$$

Then calculate the total dose desired in milligrams. Dose on hand is 300 mg/tablet.

$$300 \text{ mg} = ? \text{ grains}$$

Cross-multiply:

$$\frac{1 \text{ grain}}{60 \text{ mg}} \bowtie \frac{5 \text{ grains}}{x \text{ mg}}$$
$$x = 300 \text{ mg} = 1 \text{ tablet}$$

Give one tablet because one tablet is equivalent to 5 grains.

Box 33-2 *Approximate Measurement Equivalents*

VOLUME EQUIVALENTS
Metric to Apothecary System*
1 mL = 15 or 16 minims (♏)
30 mL = 1 fluid ounce (℥)
500 mL = 1 pint (pt)
1000 mL = 1 quart (qt)
Metric to Household
1 mL = 15 gtt (gtt)
5 mL = 1 teaspoon (tsp)
15 mL = 1 tablespoon (Tbsp, T)
30 mL = 1 ounce (oz)
240 mL = 1 pint (pt)
960 mL = 1 quart (qt)
3840 mL = gallon (gal)

WEIGHT EQUIVALENTS

Metric	Apothecary
1 mg =	1/60 grain
60-65 mg =	1 grain
1000 mg = 1 g =	15 grains
30 g =	1 ounce
500 g =	1.1 pound (lb)
1000 g = 1 kg =	2.2 lb

MISCELLANEOUS EQUIVALENTS
1 gtt = 1 ♏*
3 teaspoons = 1 tablespoon (household)

*Although the apothecary system is being phased out, measurement equivalents are listed because they are still sometimes encountered.

This method can also be used to convert within a measurement system, such as when grams need to be converted to milligrams. The order reads:

$$1.5 \text{ g of sulfisoxazole orally stat}$$

The order calls for 1.5 g of medication (amount desired). First convert the 1.5 g to milligrams. The conversion problem is:

$$1.5 \text{ g} = x \text{ mg (amount desired)}$$

Cross multiply:

$$\frac{1000 \text{ mg}}{x \text{ mg}} \bowtie \frac{1 \text{ g}}{1.5 \text{ g}}$$
$$x = 1500 \text{ mg (amount desired)}$$

On hand are 500-mg tablets. The dosage problem then would be:

$$1500 \text{ mg} = x \text{ tablets}$$

Cross-multiply:

$$\frac{1500 \text{ mg}}{500 \text{ mg}} \bowtie \frac{x}{1 \text{ tablet}}$$
$$500x = 1500$$

Divide both sides by 500:

$$\frac{500x}{500} = \frac{1500}{500}$$
$$x = 3 \text{ tablets}$$

One tablet contains 500 mg (amount on hand); 3 tablets = 1500 mg, or 1.5 g.

Drug Problem Formula. You have an order for glipizide (Glucotrol), 2.5 mg to be given orally (D = dose desired). On hand you have Glucotrol, 5 mg per tablet (H = amount on hand). Set up the problem putting the unknown factor on top. (D and H need to be measured in like units, so do conversion problem first.)

$$D/H = x$$

Now cross-multiply, ignoring the units until the end.

$$\frac{2.5 \text{ mg}}{5 \text{ mg}} \diagtimes \frac{x \text{ tablets}}{1 \text{ tablet}}$$
$$5x = 2.5$$

Divide both sides by 5:

$$\frac{x}{5} = \frac{2.5}{5}$$
$$x = 0.5 \text{ tablet}$$

(Because the x was in front of tablets, then x = 0.5 tablets.) Give ½ tablet.

For liquid medications, follow the same formula.

The order specifies guaifenesin, 75 mg PO tid. On hand is guaifenesin syrup, 100 mg per 5 mL. The problem is set up as follows:

$$D/H \times \text{Volume}$$

Cross-multiply:

$$\frac{75 \text{ mg}}{100 \text{ mg}} \diagtimes \frac{x}{5 \text{ mL}}$$
$$100x = 375$$

Divide both sides by 100:

$$\frac{x}{100} = \frac{375}{100}$$
$$x = 3.75$$

Give 3.75 mL of guaifenesin syrup.

For an injection, use the same formula.

The order reads meperidine, 35 mg IM q 4 hr PRN pain. On hand is meperidine, 50 mg per mL. Cross-multiply:

$$\frac{35 \text{ mg}}{50 \text{ mg}} \diagtimes \frac{x}{1 \text{ mL}}$$
$$50x = 35$$

Divide both side by 50:

$$\frac{x}{50} = \frac{35}{50}$$
$$x = 0.7 \text{ mL}$$

Give 0.7 mL.

Practicing the Five Rights

1. Give the Right Drug. Check MARs against the physician's original orders on the chart periodically to make certain that the order was transcribed correctly.

This task is usually done by the registered nurse during the night shift. Each time a drug dose is administered, the order is checked against the drug label for the correct name of drug. *Check the expiration date of the drug at this time.* If the spelling is different on the MAR or medication card than on the drug label, the original order is checked. If there is a discrepancy, the physician should be consulted. The patient is told the name of the drug and shown the medication before taking it.

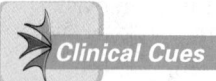
Clinical Cues

Always double-check if the patient tells you the pill looks different or makes any other comment that causes doubt that this medication is correct. Sometimes, a medication order is written on the wrong chart or you might have made in error when preparing the medication.

Many nurses are now using a palm-held device (PHD) to quickly access drug information or do dosage calculations. Drug information software is available that can be installed and updated on these little computers.

2. Give the Right Dose. Carefully compare the dose you are about to give with the dose indicated, as ordered on the MAR or medication card. The oral doses are supplied in standard amounts per pill or capsule. When the dose ordered is in milligrams rather than in capsules, tablets, or milliliters, a mathematical calculation is needed to ensure accuracy (Safety Alert 33-5). Many medication errors occur because the dosage given to the patient is not the dosage ordered.

3. Give the Right Drug by the Right Route. If a drug is ordered intramuscularly, it must be given that way or the physician should be consulted and asked to change the order. The fact that the patient does not feel the need for pain medication by injection anymore does not mean that the nurse can give it in oral form. The order must be changed for the drug to be legally given orally.

⚠ Safety Alert 33-5

Watch That Decimal Point!

A very common dosage error is a mistaken decimal point or a floating zero. For example, the physician writes "030 mL of medication." One nurse says use 3/100 mL, one nurse says use 3/10 mL, one nurse says use 3 mL, and one nurse says use 30 mL. Who is correct? Where is the error? Another physician writes "5.0 mg of medication." One nurse says use 5 mg and another nurse says use 50 mg. Who is correct? Where is the error?

In some cases, a drug is ordered to be given orally, but the patient cannot swallow the capsule or tablet. Look for how the drug is supplied to determine the safety of crushing. For example, sublingual, buccal, enteric-coated, and extended-release products and products with carcinogenic potential should not be crushed. The list of such drugs is extensive, covering several pages, and cannot be included here. When in doubt, check with the pharmacist. Certainly when a liquid form of the drug is available, a more exact dosage is achieved than with a crushed pill; a liquid dose is also more time-efficient for the nurse. When a liquid form is available, ask the physician to change the order.

4. Give the Right Drug at the Right Time. The times at which patients are to receive medications should be written down on the work organization sheet. This is particularly important when a medication is slated to be given at a time other than the most common medication times during the shift.

Day-shift medications are most commonly given at 9 A.M. and 1 A.M.; medications ordered for 7:30, 8, 9:30, or 11 A.M., or any other nontraditional time, should be highlighted on the work sheet so that they are not forgotten. The agency protocol may state that a drug may be given within 30 minutes of the time ordered simply because it is not possible to give all the drugs ordered for a particular time to all patients exactly at the appointed time. In some acute care agencies, this flexibility means that the drug may be given from 30 minutes before the ordered time to 30 minutes after that time. Other agencies require that the drug be given within a 30-minute window from 15 minutes before the ordered time to 15 minutes after the time.

Nurses must remember that drug scheduling is for the purpose of maintaining a consistent level of the drug in the blood. For that reason, drugs should be given as close to the ordered time as possible. Antiarrhythmic heart medications in particular should be given very close to the appointed time. **Document at the right time.** Too often, nurses are in the habit of signing off on medications when they are taken from the medication cart drawer or bin. Frequently, the patient is not available to take the drug when the nurse reaches the room and, if things become hectic on the unit, the dose is forgotten. The patient may be off the floor, in the shower, severely nauseated, or in the middle of a respiratory treatment. Never document that a dose was given until it is in the patient. When a dose is *not* administered, it should also be noted on the MAR.

5. Give the Right Drug to the Right Patient. Even though you are working with the patient continually throughout the shift and are very familiar with the person, **you must identify the patient correctly by checking the armband information.** It is safest to check the identification band for both name and identification number, verifying that these match the imprint on the MAR sheet.

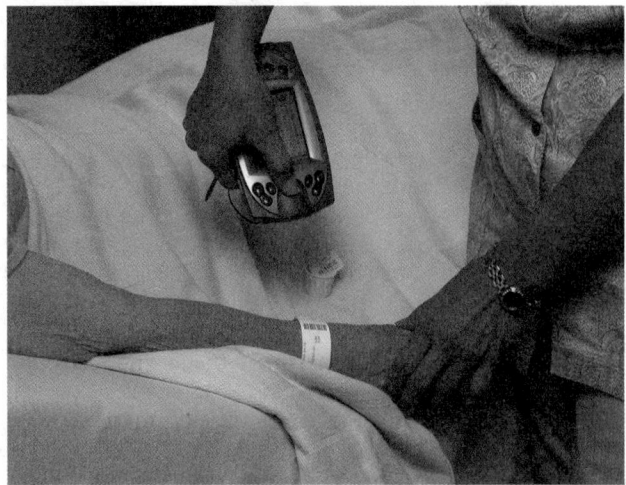

FIGURE **33-4** The nurse checks the bar code on the patient's bracelet and on the medication packet.

A new method designed to prevent medication errors is using a bar code system. The FDA has formally recommended that the bar code method be adopted by all hospitals. The patient is issued a bracelet with an individual bar code on it. The same bar code is placed on the patient's MAR and on each unit-dose medication dispensed by the pharmacy. The nurse scans the patient's bracelet when administering medications. The scanner verifies that the same code is on the patient's bracelet and on the medication packet (Figure 33-4). The nurse may also scan the bar code on her own identification tag and the system then documents that this particular nurse gave the medication.

To prevent medication errors, it is best to check each medication three times. Each of the Five Rights should be checked all three times. The third check should be done at the bedside before opening the unit-dose package. Because unit-dose systems have become the standard, nurses do not seem to check medications as carefully as they did when they used a stock drug supply. One method for instituting three checks using the Five Rights for each medication is listed in Box 33-3.

Oral medications should be given with the patient in as upright a position as possible and with sufficient fluid to carry the pills to the stomach. If the patient must remain recumbent, the side-lying position should be used to prevent aspiration.

Injection sites should be chosen carefully using anatomic landmarks and considering the size and physical condition of the patient. Sterility of medication and injection equipment must be maintained. **To maintain Standard Precautions, gloves must be worn for administration of all injections.** Intravenous medications must be given diluted in the recommended amount of fluid and administered no faster than the time recommended. Otherwise, toxicity or tissue damage may occur.

Box 33-3 *Performing the Five Rights*

For safety, check the Five Rights *three* times: Take out the patient's medication drawer or bin and place it alongside the medication administration record (MAR) sheet containing the drug orders. Verify that the patient name on the drawer corresponds to the name on the MAR sheet. Count the number of medications to be administered at this particular time. For example, there are three drugs scheduled to be administered at 0900.

1. **The right drug:** Locate the first drug on the MAR list that is to be given at 0900. Remove it from the drawer and carefully compare the drug name on the label with the drug name on the MAR sheet. Ask yourself why the patient is receiving this medication. If the answer is not apparent, stop and check.
2. **The right dose:** Check the dosage on the MAR sheet and compare it with the dosage you have in your hand. Verify correct dosage by calculation if needed. Determine if the dosage is within normal recommendations. Check the expiration date. If outdated, discard the medication and obtain another dose. Place the correct dosage unopened in a medication cup or on a medication tray.
3. **The right route:** Check the route ordered with the type of medication you have prepared.
4. **The right time:** Verify that the time the drug is scheduled is this date and this hour (0900). Remember that some drugs are ordered on an every-other-day or every-third-day schedule. *Perform the second check of the medications.* Put the drawer or bin away and then for each drug, meticulously check the drug, dose, time, and route against the MAR again.
5. **The right patient:** Check the patient's identity by comparing the name and hospital number on the patient's identification band with the imprint on the MAR sheet or medication card. Ask the patient to state his or her name. Verify that the patient has no allergy to the medication before administration. Assess for adverse effects the patient might be experiencing from previous doses of each medication. *Perform the third check* by checking the drug, dose, time, and route one more time before opening the medication package and administering the dose. For medications such as antibiotics, it is wise to verify that the patient is not allergic to the medication for each dose administered. Once given, the dose cannot be retrieved. If you cannot take the MAR sheet into the room (e.g., patient is in contact isolation), make or obtain a label to ensure proper patient identification.

Clinical Cues

The prudent nurse will ask another nurse to check the prepared doses of certain drugs before administering them. All insulin is double-checked in this manner; anticoagulants, injectable digoxin, and any other drugs that have a potentially toxic or lethal effect on the patient are double-checked. Many agencies have a list of drugs that require a check by two different nurses before the drug is given.

Evaluation

Evaluation of drug therapy is related to whether the desired therapeutic effect is occurring. For example, when antibiotics are being given, the temperature, the white blood cell count, and perhaps other laboratory values are assessed along with an evaluation of the patient's general condition (e.g., how the patient feels). For other drugs, determine if the condition being treated is improving. Evaluation is also necessary regarding the occurrence of side effects of medications. Each patient is assessed for the signs and symptoms of side effects for every drug being administered.

Evaluate whether the expected outcomes listed on the nursing care plan or critical pathway are being met. If they are not, the plan of care must be revised.

Documentation

Record the drug given, dose, time, route, and your initials when documenting on an MAR. When documenting a PRN medication in the chart, write the date, time, reason the medication was given, dose and route, and location if it was given by injection, and sign with first initial, last name, and designation (student vocational nurse; SVN, SPN). When the medication has had sufficient time to take effect, the patient's response to it should be documented. The PRN medication is also recorded on the MAR, noting the date, time, vital signs if required, and your initials.

Any time the patient has an adverse reaction or suffers from a side effect of a drug, a notation should be made in the chart. Any type of allergic reaction should be noted in all locations in which allergies are recorded in the patient record. Any patient concerns about the drug therapy should also be mentioned when documenting care. The patient is taught to carry allergy information in a billfold or to wear an allergy bracelet.

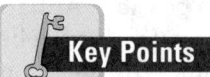

Key Points

- Nurses are legally responsible for the safe and therapeutic effects of drugs they administer.
- Drug therapy is used for treatment of, palliation of, cure of, prevention of, or diagnosis of disease.
- The form of a drug determines its route of administration.
- The general characteristics of each class of drugs should be learned along with the nursing implications for the class.
- Controlled drugs are kept in locked compartments, and each dose must be accounted for at all times.
- The Food and Drug Administration sets the standards for drug quality, purity, packaging, safety, dose form, and labeling.
- Drugs are absorbed at different rates depending on their form and physical factors within the body.
- Distribution of a drug is affected by the chemical and physical properties of the drug and the physical status of the patient.

- If an individual has a greater percentage of body fat, drug distribution is slower; the less a patient weighs, the more concentrated the drug is and the more powerful its effect.
- If a drug is highly protein bound, very little of it is distributed to the target tissue.
- The elderly often have decreased albumin, causing an increase in unbound drug circulation; this causes increased drug activity and possible toxicity.
- Most drugs are metabolized in the liver and excreted by the kidneys.
- Most drugs produce a primary and a secondary effect. The primary effect is the intended effect; the secondary effect may be desirable or undesirable. Secondary effects are often the side effects of the drug.
- Drug doses must be given on schedule to maintain a therapeutic level of the drug in the blood serum of the patient.
- Drugs that produce a response are named agonists; drugs that block a response are called antagonists.
- There are four types of drug action: stimulation or depression, replacement, inhibition or killing, and irritation.
- The therapeutic range of a drug is that which produces the desired effect without causing toxic effects.

- Drugs tend to interact, altering the way a drug is absorbed, metabolized, or eliminated from the body.
- Alcohol has a synergistic effect when combined with drugs that depress the central nervous system.
- Foods can affect the absorption or action of drugs.
- The five rights must be followed when administering drugs.
- When giving medication to children, the dose is based on age, weight, and size.
- Noncompliance can be related lack of information, financial problems, health beliefs, unpleasant side effects, or cognitive issues.
- Evaluation of drug therapy requires data about the response of the patient to the drug. Side effects are also evaluated.
- Every dose of every drug administered must be documented.

 Go to your **Companion CD-ROM** for an Audio Glossary, animations, video clips, and more.

evolve   Be sure to visit the companion Evolve site at http://evolve.elsevier.com/deWit/fundamental/ for additional online resources.

NCLEX-PN® EXAMINATION-STYLE REVIEW QUESTIONS

*Choose the **best** answer(s) for each question.*

1. The patient is to receive sequential doses of a drug. Based on your knowledge of pharmacologic action, the drug must be administered as close to the time scheduled as possible to:
   1. maintain a minimum concentration of the drug in the patient's bloodstream.
   2. follow hospital policy and procedure and the physician's orders.
   3. help the patient understand the importance of taking drugs at regular intervals.
   4. determine if side effects or adverse effects of the drug are going to occur.

2. The physician orders a medication blood level after making an adjustment in a patient's prescribed dose of antiseizure medication. The purpose of monitoring this level would be because:
   1. there are synergistic effects with other drugs.
   2. the patient is suspected of noncompliance.
   3. the drug has a narrow therapeutic range.
   4. there is danger of anaphylaxis and other adverse effects.

3. When an elderly patient is taking an anti-inflammatory drug for arthritis on a continuing basis, the nurse would:
   1. ask questions about whether constipation is occurring.
   2. caution the patient to stay out of the sun because the skin is more sensitive.

   3. ask about any recent changes in appetite.
   4. monitor the patient for gastrointestinal bleeding.

4. The physician has just written several medication orders for several different patients. Which order has the highest priority?
   1. Hydrocodone/acetaminophen (Lortab) 5 mg PO q 4-6 hr PRN pain
   2. Lorazepam (Ativan) 2 mg IV bolus stat
   3. Gentamicin (Garamycin) 200 mg IV q 8 hr
   4. Cefazolin (Ancef) 250 mg IVP on call to OR

5. The surgeon orders 500 mg PO tablets q 8 hr. The pharmacy delivers the medication in tablet form, but the patient tells the nurse that he cannot swallow the tablets and that his family doctor always gives him liquid medications. What is the most appropriate nursing action?
   1. Gently encourage the patient to take the medication that the surgeon has ordered.
   2. Call the pharmacy and ask them to send the liquid form of the medication.
   3. Call the patient's family doctor to verify what the patient usually takes.
   4. Call the surgeon, explain the situation, and ask for the order to be changed.

6. A nurse has completed teaching a patient about several medications that he must use at home. These include Coumadin, vitamin C supplement, and a blood pressure medication. Which statement by the patient indicates an understanding of the medication teaching?

   1. "If I need a follow-up blood test, the office nurse will call me."
   2. "I'll take the medication because my doctor told me to."
   3. "My wife knows what to do if I miss a dose."
   4. "I know which foods to avoid while I am taking the medication."

7. The nurse must give a medication to a child. The medication is ordered in mg/kg. The child weighs 44 lb. Convert the child's weight to kilograms. _____

8. The pharmacy delivers a 6-oz bottle of take-home medication for a patient. The patient needs to take 25 mL of the medication every morning. The patient wants to know how many days the bottle will last. _____days

CRITICAL THINKING ACTIVITIES *Read each clinical scenario and discuss the questions with your classmates.*

Scenario A
George Hamarabi, age 72, is receiving Ceftin 250 mg bid for his pneumonia.

1. What would you need to teach Mr. Hamarabi about this antibiotic?
2. He has been on the medication for 4 days. How would you evaluate whether the medication treatment is effective?

Scenario B
Florence Simoneski, age 78, is receiving Ecotrin, an enteric-coated aspirin, for her arthritis. She is hospitalized with dehydration and is very weak. She cannot swallow the Ecotrin tablets. What would you do?

Scenario C
Jacob Giovanni, age 5, has come to the clinic with his mother to get the immunizations he will need to enter kindergarten. He is calm at the moment, but appears scared. You must give him four injections. How would you handle the situation and interact with Jacob?

Scenario D
Calculate the necessary drug dosages.

1. Potassium chloride, 10 mEq is ordered; 40 mEq/10 mL is the preparation available. How many milliliters will you give?
2. The order reads 400 mg IM. The vial reads 1 g/2 mL. How many milliliters will you give?

evolve http://evolve.elsevier.com/deWit/fundamental/

Objectives

Upon completing this chapter, you should be able to:

Theory

1. Describe the legal and professional responsibilities of the LPN/LVN related to medication administration.
2. List the different classifications of drugs based on their specific actions.
3. Identify the parts of a valid medication order.
4. Compare and contrast various medication record systems such as the medication administration record (MAR), medication cards, and computerized systems.
5. Discuss medication dispensing and delivery systems.
6. Discuss the advantages and disadvantages of the unit-dose system and the prescription system.
7. Consider special needs when administering oral and topical medications to an elderly patient.
8. Identify four principles to be followed when giving a medication through a feeding tube.
9. Discuss your responsibilities in the event of a medication error.

Clinical Practice

1. Demonstrate the accounting of doses of controlled drugs that must be withdrawn from the locked narcotics cabinet or dispensed from an automatic dispensing unit.
2. Give oral and topical medications using the Five Rights and five rules.
3. Prepare and apply topical medications such as eye ointments, eardrops, nasal medications, transdermal patches, and topical ointments.
4. Teach a patient to use a metered-dose inhaler.
5. Instill a vaginal and a rectal suppository safely and effectively.
6. Write a care plan for a patient who is receiving medication to include patient specific data, an identified nursing diagnosis, and interventions that you used.
7. Document medication administration and your patient's response to the therapy.

Skills & Steps

Skills

Steps

Key Terms

 Be sure to check out the bonus material on the Companion CD-ROM, including selected audio pronunciations.

buccal (BŬK-ăl, p. 663)
douche (doosh, p. 671)
meniscus (mĕ-NĬS-kŭs, p. 663)
metered-dose inhalers (MDIs) (p. 670)
ophthalmic (ŏf-THĂL-mĭk, p. 663)
otic (Ō-tĭk, p. 667)
PO (p. 654)
PRN (p. 656)
spansule (p. 661)
stat (p. 656)
sublingual (sŭb-LĬNG-wăl, p. 663)
topical (TŎP-ĭ-kăl, p. 656)
transdermal (trăns-DĔR-măl, p. 673)

NURSING RESPONSIBILITIES IN MEDICATION ADMINISTRATION

Accuracy during all steps of medication administration is extremely important. Medications are chemicals that alter actions performed by cells of the body. If the wrong medication is given to a patient, it could have serious consequences. All procedures related to medication administration should be followed exactly to promote safety and avoid making a medication error. However, should an error be made, report it promptly in accordance with agency policy and take appropriate action to promote patient safety and well-being.

To administer medications, you must be able to interpret the medication order correctly and then give the correct medication to the patient. The procedures for administering medications accurately using the various routes can be mastered with practice. Attentiveness to each step of the task is essential when administering medications. Nurses are legally responsible for being knowledgeable about each medication they administer to patients: the correct dose, the route by which it should be given, desired effects, side effects, interactions with other medications, and any contraindications. **Medication orders that are unclear, incomplete, or ambiguous should be questioned to avoid errors.** Assessment of the patient after medication has been administered provides data for evaluating the effectiveness of the drug and guiding health teaching. On discharge from the health care facility, patients need to know how often to take each drug, if the medication should be taken before or after meals, if certain foods or fluids should be avoided, the expected effect, what to do about side effects if they occur, and what to do if they forget to take a dose at the prescribed time. In accordance with 2009 National Patient Safety Goals, involving and educating patients and families in care and treatment is a safety measure.

? *Think Critically About* . . . You are a new nurse. The physician has written a medication order, but it is very difficult to read. You call for clarification, but the physician abruptly states, "It's my standard order" and hangs up. What would you do in this situation?

The Five Rights of medication administration provide a framework for safe delivery of drugs to patients (see Chapter 33). Box 34-1 presents pertinent National Patient Safety Goals of The Joint Commission as they relate to medication administration. Practice in the clinical setting helps establish a consistent, efficient routine for giving drugs. Concept Map 34-1 depicts the nurse's responsibilities when administering medications.

Box 34-1 *Safe Medication Administration Guidelines*

- Ask yourself why this drug is prescribed for this patient. Know the drug, the patient, and all the patient's medical conditions.
- Always record a verbal order clearly in its entirety and "read back" for verification that you heard the order correctly.
- Become familiar with the "high-alert drug list" from your facility's pharmacy. Be extra careful when administering a drug that is on this list. Be attuned to look-alike and sound-alike drug names.
- Become familiar with the list of abbreviations that are no longer to be used and ask for verification from the prescriber as to what is intended by the abbreviation if it appears in an order.
- If the patient is a child or an older adult, review any special precautions to be considered.
- If you need to administer more than three tablets or capsules, check with the pharmacist to verify the amount is correct per the order.
- Before crushing a drug, check to see whether it can be safely administered after crushing.
- Do not unwrap a unit-dose drug before you are at the patient's bedside and ready to administer the medication.
- Check two patient identifiers each and every time before administering drugs to a patient.
- Always report every medication error so that medication safety can be improved.
- Be alert for look-alike or sound-alike medication and advocate that these be kept to a minimum.
- Label all medications if removed from original container (e.g., syringe or medication cup).
- Be especially alert to prevent complications for patients on anticoagulant medications.

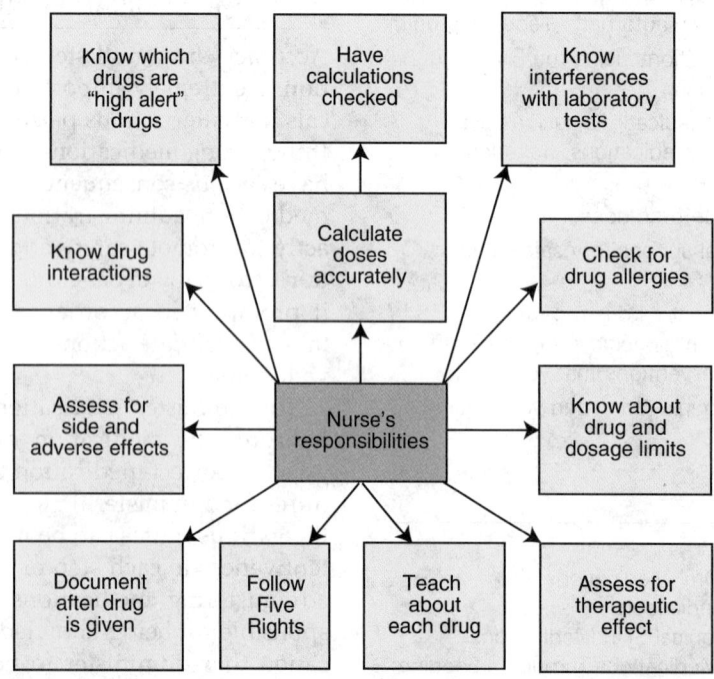

CONCEPT MAP **34-1** Nurse's responsibilities in medication administration.

CLASSIFICATION OF DRUGS

As mentioned in Chapter 33, drugs are classified in various ways. It is an advantage to learn drugs by the class to which they belong. To learn the possible side effects of each medication, begin by learning drugs by classification and then learn the most common side effects of the classification to which the drug belongs. Drugs are classified in various ways; one of the most useful is based on the effect of the drug on the body (Table 34-1). In this system, drugs that reduce pain and discomfort are classified as analgesics; those that control severe pain are potent analgesics or opioid narcotics, which may produce a stuporous state as a result of their effect on the central nervous system. For a complete list of drug classifications, consult a drug handbook or pharmacology textbook. The classification index in the *Physicians' Desk Reference* also serves as a convenient reference.

Although there may be subdivisions within a class of drugs, the major side effects within that class will be the same. By learning the side effects of one major drug in the class, you will know what the major side effects of other similarly acting drugs in the class will be. This prevents the necessity of memorizing a multitude of separate facts about drug side effects. Different classifications and some examples of medications within each group are shown in Table 34-1.

Table 34-1 *Selected Groups of Drugs Classified by Action*

CLASSIFICATION	ACTION	EXAMPLES
CIRCULATORY SYSTEM AND HEART		
Anticoagulants	Inhibit clotting of blood	Sodium warfarin, heparin
Antianginals	Increase blood flow to the heart	Nitroglycerin, isosorbide dinitrate, diltiazem
Antidysrhythmics	Regulate the heart rate	Lidocaine, atropine, amiodarone
Antihypertensives	Control high blood pressure	Atenolol, enalapril maleate, captopril, clonidine
Antilipidemics	Lower abnormal blood lipid levels	Lovastatin, atorvastatin
Antiplatelets	Inhibits platelet aggregation	Clopidogrel bisulfate
Cardiotonics	Strengthen the contraction of the heart	Digoxin, digitalis
Diuretics	Reduce edema and increase urinary output	Furosemide, chlorothiazide, bumetanide
Hemostatics	Promote clotting of blood	Vitamin K_5, absorbable gelatin sponge (Gelfoam)
EMOTIONAL AND MENTAL STATES		
Hypnotics, sedatives	Relieve anxiety, reduce activity, and promote sleep	Chloral hydrate, secobarbital, flurazepam, zolpidem tartrate
Stimulants	Increase mental alertness and function	Caffeine, methylphenidate, dextroamphetamine, modafinil
Tricyclic antidepressants	Relieve depression	Amitriptyline, doxepin
Selective serotonin reuptake inhibitors	Relieve depression	Paroxetine, fluoxetine, citalopram, sertraline
Anxiolytics	Relieve anxiety	Lorazepam, buspirone, diazepam
Antipsychotics	Relieve psychotic symptoms	Aripiprazole, haloperidol, olanzapine, ziprasidone
MUSCULAR SYSTEM AND INTEGUMENT		
Antihistamines	Reduce congestion and allergic reactions	Diphenhydramine, chlorpheniramine
Muscle relaxants	Control muscle spasms and tension	Baclofen, carisoprodol
NEUROLOGIC SYSTEM		
Analgesics	Relieve pain	
Narcotics (opioids)	Relieve moderate to severe pain	Morphine, codeine, meperidine, hydromorphone, fentanyl, oxycodone,
Non-narcotics (nonopioids)	Relieve mild pain	Aspirin, acetaminophen
Nonsteroidal anti-inflammatory drugs	Reduce inflammation and pain	Ibuprofen, naproxen, sulindac
Alzheimer's disease drug	Slows progression of disease	Donepezil, rivastigmine
Antiepileptics	Control epileptic seizures and tremors	Phenytoin, paramethadione, phenobarbital
RESPIRATORY SYSTEM		
Antitussives	Relieve cough	Codeine, dextromethorphan, guaifenesin
Bronchodilators and expectorants	Relieve obstruction of air passages	Terbutaline, albuterol, metaproterenol

Continued

Table 34-1 *Selected Groups of Drugs Classified by Action—cont'd*

CLASSIFICATION	ACTION	EXAMPLES
ENDOCRINE SYSTEM		
Adrenal hormones	All hormones act to regulate body growth, function, and metabolism	Corticotropin, aldosterone, epinephrine, cortisone
Female hormones		Estrogen, estrone, progestin, ethinyl estradiol
Male hormone		Testosterone
Pancreatic hormone	Reduces blood sugar	Regular insulin, isophane insulin, Humalog, Humulin (NPH), lente insulin
Hypoglycemics	Reduce blood sugar	Glyburide, metformin, chlorpropamide
GASTROINSTESTINAL SYSTEM		
Antacids	Neutralize stomach acids	Aluminum hydroxide, magaldrate, aluminum carbonate
Antisecretories	Decrease gastric acid secretion	Ranitidine, omeprazole, pantoprazole, lansoprazole
Anticholinergics	Reduce spasms and secretions of stomach	Propantheline
Antidiarrheals	Reduce bowel irritability and movements	Diphenoxylate, kaolin and pectin, loperamide, octreotide
Antiemetics	Relieve nausea and control vomiting	Promethazine, metoclopramide, dolasetron mesylate, ondansetron
Cathartics, laxatives	Promote bowel movements	Bisacodyl, magnesium hydroxide, senna
Stool softeners	Add water or bulk to stool and aid defecation	Docusate calcium, docusate sodium
INFECTIONS		
Antibiotics	Inhibit the growth of or kill microorganisms	Erythromycin, cephalosporin, penicillin, vancomycin, ciprofloxacin, clarithromycin

MEDICATION ORDERS

The physician prescribes the type of treatment in a series of instructions written on the physician's order sheet of the hospital chart. The written prescription for a drug is called the *medication order* or the *drug order*. Physicians' orders are part of the patient record.

Medication orders must meet certain standards specified by state law and by regulations established by inspecting agencies. **A complete drug order must include the full name of the patient, the name of the drug, the dosage to be given, the route of administration, how often it is to be given, the date and time written, and the signature of the prescriber.** Some orders also specify the total number of doses that are to be given. Examples of medication orders are given in Table 34-2. Oral and topical medications come in many different forms (Table 34-3).

DOSAGE OF MEDICATIONS

In Canada, the metric system is the only system of weight and measurement; although it is the primary system of measuring medication dosage in the United States, the apothecary system is still occasionally used. The apothecary system was brought to America from England during colonial times. You must be familiar with this system because it has not been fully phased out as yet. Although use of the metric system is the standard, you still need to be able to convert values from one system to the other. It is helpful to keep a table of conversion values in the area where medications are prepared to ensure accurate calculations (Table 34-4).

Table 34-2 *Examples of Drug Orders*

ORDER	MEANING
Digoxin 0.25 mg PO daily	Digoxin (a drug that strengthens the heart) in a dose of 0.25 mg to be given orally every day
Methylprednisolone 4 mg PO qid	Methylprednisolone (a type of cortisone) in a dose of 4 mg to be given orally four times a day
Maalox 30 mL PO q2h when awake	Maalox (an antacid) in a dose of 30 mL to be given orally every 2 hours during waking hours

Each dose of medication should be taken from a labeled package or container clearly stating the name and dosage of the drug. There is widespread use of medications supplied as unit doses, with each dose packaged separately with its own label.

Checking any conversions and calculations for a divided dose with another colleague is recommended at all times as a medication safety measure. Consult pediatric textbooks for additional information about how to confirm dosages and to prepare divided doses of medications for infants and children.

ROUTES OF MEDICATION ADMINISTRATION

The selected route of administration depends on several factors: the condition of the patient, the nature of the drug (taste, stability, and so on), and the rate of absorption via one route versus another. The oral route (PO, or *per os*, which means "by mouth") is used for many solid and liquid medications because it is the

Table 34-3 *Oral and Topical Medications*

FORM OF DRUG	CHARACTERISTICS	PRESCRIPTION ABBREVIATION	USE
ORAL MEDICATIONS			
Tablet	Powder compressed into a tablet with a binding substance	Tab	Given by mouth
Capsule	Powder placed in a capsule	Cap	Given by mouth
Spansule	Time-release pellets placed in a capsule shell	Span	Given by mouth (do not open)
Enteric coated	Tablet with a coating that does not dissolve until it is in the intestine	EC	Given by mouth (do not crush)
Elixir	Sweetened flavoring substance with an active medicinal ingredient	Elix	Given by mouth or feeding tube
Lozenge	Medicated tablet or disk		Given by mouth to be sucked on until it totally dissolves
Sublingual	Tablet formulated to quickly dissolve under the tongue	Subling	Given by mouth by placing under the tongue (not to be swallowed)
Buccal	Tablet formulated to dissolve when placed in the inner cheek of the mouth	Bucc	Given by mouth by placing in the inner cheek pocket (not to be swallowed)
Syrup	A thick sugar solution combined with a medicinal ingredient	Syr	Given by mouth or by feeding tube; often used for children's medication preparations and cough medicines
Suspension	Medication particles suspended rather than dissolved in a liquid substance	Susp	Given by mouth or by feeding tube. Antibiotics are often prepared this way for children
TOPICAL MEDICATIONS			
Lotion	A liquid suspension		Applied to the skin
Ointment	A semisolid, thick preparation containing a medicinal agent	Oint	Applied to the skin or mucous membrane
Cream	A semisolid, thin preparation containing a medicinal agent		Applied to the skin or mucous membrane
Tincture	Medication dissolved in alcohol	Tinct, tr	Applied to the skin
Drops	Liquid medication provided in a dropper bottle or a bottle with a detachable dropper	gt, gtt	Usually formulated for the nose, eye, or ear, although infant vitamins and other medications are made as drops
Patch	An adhesive substance with medication bonded to it that is slowly absorbed into the skin		Applied to the skin for up to 7 days for transdermal absorption
Inhalant	A liquid placed in a pressurized container or a squeeze bottle so that it will form an aerosol when activated		Inhaled through the mouth or the nose
Suppository	Solid medication mixed with a viscous substance that dissolves at body temperature	Supp	Placed in the vagina, rectum, or urethra depending on the type of suppository

Table 34-4 *Selected Metric Doses and the Apothecary Equivalents*

METRIC	WEIGHT MEASURES: APOTHECARY EQUIVALENT (APPROXIMATE)	METRIC	LIQUID MEASURES: APOTHECARY EQUIVALENT (APPROXIMATE)	HOUSEHOLD MEASURES EQUIVALENT (APPROXIMATE)
5 g	75 grains	960 mL	32 fluid oz	1 quart
1 g	15 grains	480 mL	16 fluid oz	1 pint
0.6 g	10 grains	240 mL	8 fluid oz	1 cup
0.1 g	1½ grains	120 mL	4 fluid oz	½ cup
60 mg	1 grain	60 mL	2 fluid oz	
30 mg	½ grain	30 mL	1 fluid oz	2 tablespoons
15 mg	¼ grain	15 mL		1 tablespoon
10 mg	⅙ grain	5 mL		1 teaspoon
8 mg	⅛ grain			
1 mg	1/60 grain			
0.6 mg	1/100 grain			
0.4 mg	1/150 grain			
0.3 mg	1/200 grain			

simplest, most convenient, and least expensive (see Table 34-3). Those patients who have difficulty swallowing pills must have them crushed and given mixed in some food or juice. Some pills cannot be crushed because this changes their effect on the body. In this case, ask the physician to order the medication in liquid form.

Topical medications are instilled in the form of eyedrops or eardrops, or applied as ointments, pastes, or lotions to the skin or mucous membrane. The rectal route is often used to give medications to children or for patients who are vomiting. (Skills detailing the procedures for giving solutions as enemas can be reviewed in Chapter 30.) A number of medications affecting the respiratory system are given as inhalants. Parenteral routes are used for injecting medications into the body tissues, commonly via subcutaneous, intramuscular, intravenous, percutaneous, and intradermal routes. These are described in detail in Chapters 35 and 36.

REGULARLY SCHEDULED MEDICATION ORDERS

To maintain the desired level of medication in the bloodstream, the drug may be given several times a day. The physician's order will specify how often the medication is to be given, such as three times a day (tid), every 4 hours (q4h), and so forth.

Each health care agency has policies that designate the time of day corresponding to the frequency ordered by the physician. It is imperative that the agency policy be followed. For example, on some nursing units the schedule of times might be as follows:

Order	Schedule
daily	0900
bid	0900 and 1700
tid	0900, 1300, and 1700
qid	0900, 1300, 1700, and 2100
q4h	0100, 0500, 0900, 1300 (and so on)

❓ *Think Critically About* . . . Can you correctly interpret the following medication orders? "Cefprozil 500 mg PO q12h × 10 days." "Ferrous sulfate 300-mg tabs PO bid." "Digoxin 0.125 mg PO daily."

PRN MEDICATION ORDERS

Medications taken "as needed" (PRN or prn) are given in response to a patient's request or when the need is indicated. Examples of these medications usually include analgesics (to control pain), tranquilizers or sedatives (for restlessness), and laxatives (for constipation). Some PRN medication orders specify when or how often the medication can be given (e.g., at bedtime PRN, meaning "at bedtime as needed" and q 4 hr PRN, meaning "as often as every 4 hours as needed"). Table 34-5 shows two examples of PRN orders.

Table 34-5 *Examples of PRN Orders*

ORDER	MEANING
Oxycodone HCl, 5 mg PO q6h PRN pain	Oxycodone (an analgesic) 5 mg given by mouth every 6 hours as needed for pain
Milk of magnesia, 30 mL PO at bedtime PRN	Milk of magnesia (a laxative) 30 mL by mouth given at bedtime as needed for constipation

STAT AND SINGLE-DOSE MEDICATION ORDERS

Numerous occasions arise when a stat medication or a single dose of a drug must be given. The stat (give immediately) or single-time order may consist of more than one drug, or it may involve spacing the drops or tablets over a short period of time, such as when giving radiopaque tablets in preparation for a gallbladder series or eyedrops to dilate the pupils for refraction. Preoperative medications are prime examples of drugs given one time. **Stat orders indicate that the order has top priority and the medication must be administered without delay.** In emergencies, many orders are on a stat basis. The following are examples of stat and single-dose orders:

- Nembutal 100 mg PO at 2200
- Ancef 500 mg on call to OR
- Potassium chloride 20 mEq in 200 mL 5% dextrose in water IVPB (intravenous piggyback) over 2 hours stat

RENEWAL ORDERS

Drugs are potent and are capable of causing adverse reactions as well as the desired effects. Many drugs can result in drug addiction or drug dependency. Therefore, many hospitals have medication policies limiting the time for which certain types of medication orders are valid. Opiate analgesics generally have a 48- or 72-hour limit, sedatives and antibiotics may have a 5- or 7-day limit, and a 30-day limit may be imposed by some agencies on all medications. At the end of the specified period, the order is no longer considered valid, and no additional doses of the drug may be given. If you think the medication will need to be continued, phone the physician and obtain a new order rather than just holding the drug. The physician must give or write a renewal order to continue the medication.

STOP OR DISCONTINUE ORDERS

Medications are given to the patient until the specified number of doses has been administered or until the order has expired or has been canceled. Usually a change in medication is ordered by the physician, who writes a stop or discontinue order for one drug and then prescribes a new one. Examples of stop orders are "stop gentamicin" or "discontinue probenecid." **All**

medication orders are automatically canceled whenever a patient undergoes surgery or general anesthesia. New orders must be rewritten after surgery, even for routine medications.

MEDICATION RECORDS

After the physician writes a medication order on the patient's chart, it is transcribed onto the medication administration record (MAR). Medication orders are usually transcribed onto the patient's MAR, on the computer-generated care plan, and/or on medication cards (Figure 34-1). Sometimes medications are listed on the patient's Kardex card also.

MEDICATION ADMINISTRATION RECORD (MAR)

One of the forms commonly used to record a patient's medications is the MAR, on which nurses record the doses of drugs administered each day. A copy of the MAR is placed on the patient's chart. For added convenience, the forms may be in binders or in a special Kardex kept in the medication area and referred to when giving regularly scheduled and PRN medications.

MEDICATION CARDS

Medication cards are rarely used now, but may be encountered in small long-term care facilities or rehabilitation centers. For each patient, one card is made for each medication ordered. The card is used when the dose is prepared, at the bedside to help identify what is being given, and to chart after the medication is given. Information on the card includes patient's name; room number; physician's name; name of drug; dose, route, and time of administration; the date the order was written; and the initials of the person making the card.

MEDICATION ADMINISTRATION AND TECHNOLOGY

There is a rapid increase in the use of technology, such as computerized physician order entry (CPOE) systems, bar code scanners, and personal digital assistants (PDAs), to improve medication administration safety. In the CPOE system, the prescriber directly enters the medication order in the computer; this de-

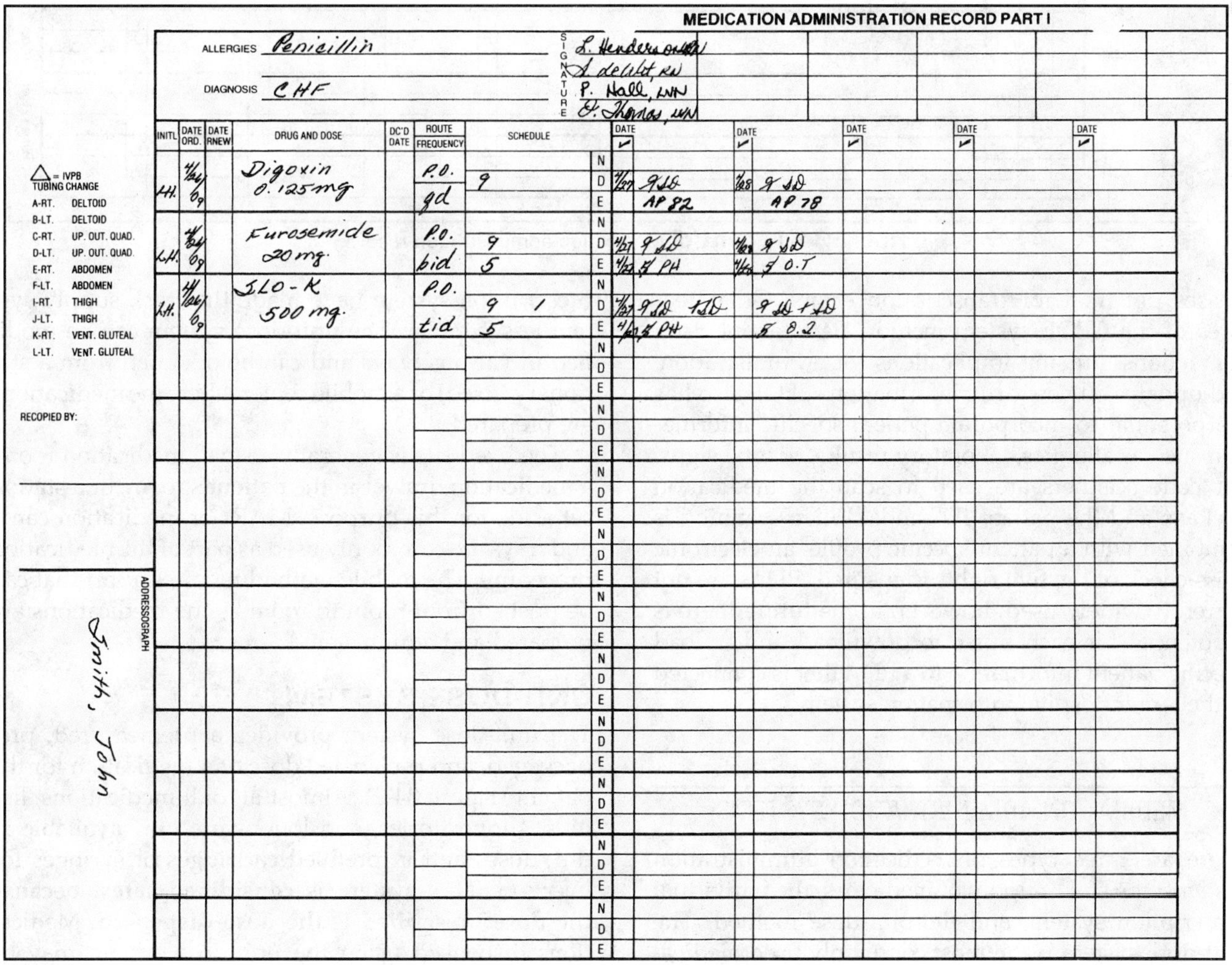
MEDICATION ADMINISTRATION RECORD PART I

ALLERGIES Penicillin
DIAGNOSIS CHF
SIGNATURE: L. Henderson RN; A. deWitt, RN; P. Hall, LVN; D. Thomas, LVN

△ = IVPB TUBING CHANGE
A-RT. DELTOID
B-LT. DELTOID
C-RT. UP. OUT. QUAD.
D-LT. UP. OUT. QUAD.
E-RT. ABDOMEN
F-LT. ABDOMEN
I-RT. THIGH
J-LT. THIGH
K-RT. VENT. GLUTEAL
L-LT. VENT. GLUTEAL
RECOPIED BY:
ADDRESSOGRAPH: Smith, John

INITL	DATE ORD.	DATE RNEW	DRUG AND DOSE	DC'D DATE	ROUTE FREQUENCY	SCHEDULE		DATE	DATE	DATE	DATE	DATE
LH.	4/26	09	Digoxin 0.125 mg		P.O. qd	9	N					
							D	4/27 9 LD	4/28 9 LD			
							E	AP 82	AP 78			
LH.	4/26	09	Furosemide 20 mg.		P.O. bid	9 5	N					
							D	4/27 9 LD	4/28 9 LD			
							E	4/27 5 PH	4/28 5 O.T			
LH.	4/26	09	SLO-K 500 mg.		P.O. tid	9 1 5	N					
							D	4/27 9 LD 1 LD	9 LD 1 LD			
							E	4/27 5 PH	5 O.T.			

FIGURE **34-1** Medication administration record.

Continued

FIGURE **34-1, cont'd** Medication administration record.

creases potential for transcription errors. Other features of the CPOE system include alerts about drug interactions, nursing implications for administration, and updates on new drug information. CPOE also has the potential to incorporate patient-specific information such as allergies, laboratory results, or vital signs. Bar code scanners are used to scan the medication package and the patient ID bands. When scanning is combined with a patient-specific profile, an electronic cross-check of the five rights is ensured. PDAs are not currently widely used; however, in the future there is a potential for each nurse to download and upload specific patient information to a PDA that is connected to the larger hospital information system.

MEDICATION ADMINISTRATION SYSTEMS

There are three types of medication administration systems: the stock supply of medicines, the individual prescription system, and the unit-dose method. The unit-dose system is the most commonly used medication administration system in health care agencies. The advantages of the unit-dose system and the individual prescription system have made the stock supply system less popular. The unit-dose system can be modified in various ways and can be operated from a stationary (fixed) or a mobile center where the medications are prepared.

The fixed site is generally a small medication room, a medication drawer in the patient's room, or a station set aside for this purpose. MARs or medication cards and trays are commonly used as part of the medication procedure. The mobile method requires a cart that can be pushed from room to room as the medications are prepared and administered.

UNIT-DOSE SYSTEM

The unit-dose system provides a premeasured, prepackaged, and prelabeled dose of a medication for the patient (Figure 34-2). Almost all oral medications, liquids, suppositories, and lotions are now available in unit doses and in prefilled cartridges or syringes for injection. **This system is considered safest because the dose prescribed is the dose dispensed.** Medications dispensed using the unit-dose system may be administered from a mobile cart or from the fixed medication preparation center. The medication is

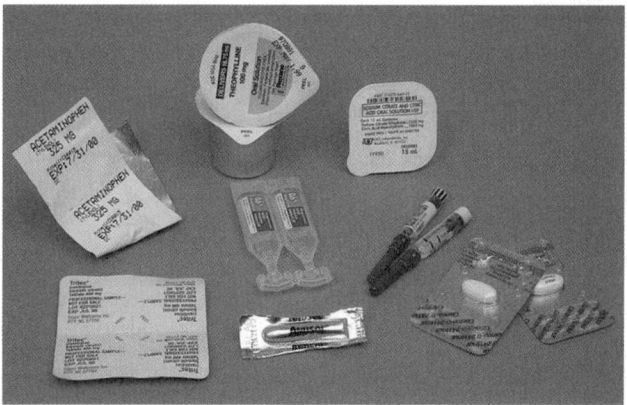

FIGURE **34-2** Unit-dose medications.

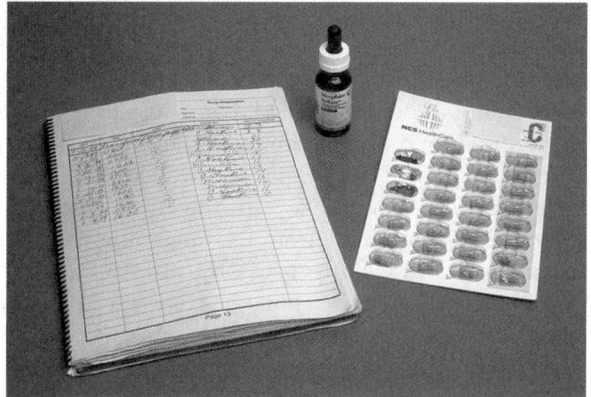

FIGURE **34-3** Tracking doses of controlled drugs.

opened at the bedside. It is customary to keep medication records in a binder or Kardex file on top of the cart from which medications are administered.

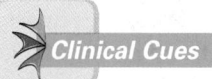

The unit-dose packaging can help you avoid drug dosage errors. For example, if the order calls for 1 gram and the drug comes in a unit-dose package of 0.25-mg tablets, you would need 4000 tablets! Whenever you are preparing medications, **if three or more unit-dose packages are required to achieve the dose, recheck the order and your calculations.** Call the prescriber, as appropriate, for clarification.

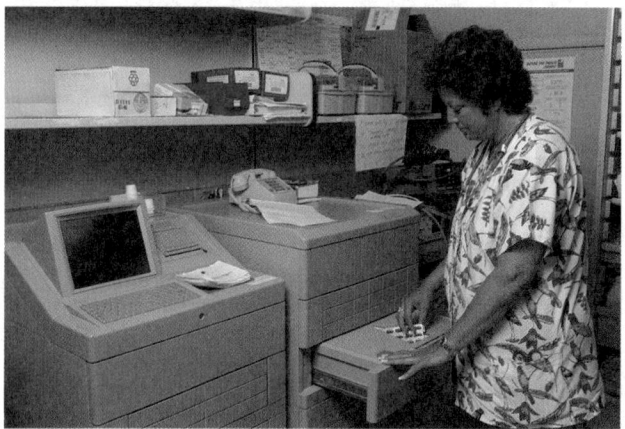

FIGURE **34-4** Nurse obtaining medication from automated dispensing unit.

The unit-dose system provides a number of benefits. The pharmacy supplies the exact dose of medication ordered, and each dose is administered at the bedside, enhancing patient safety and reducing medication errors. The system also saves time for the nurse. Another benefit is that the patient is charged only for medications that are used. Finally, this system allows keeping a minimum amount of drugs on the nursing units.

PRESCRIPTION SYSTEM

The prescription system is similar to the unit-dose system except that a sufficient number of doses for several days are supplied. This system is used in pharmacies in the community and in outpatient clinics. As the name implies, a prescription is written for each drug ordered and is filled by the pharmacist, who then provides individual containers holding doses for several days.

The prescription system can be used in connection with a fixed or a mobile preparation site. Its advantages include the fact that only a limited amount of drugs needs to be kept on the nursing units. In the long-term care facility, a week's or month's supply of each medication is often provided in a bubble pack. Each day's dose is pushed out of a bubble on the pack as needed. Home care patients use prescription system–prepared drugs from the local pharmacy or by-mail pharmacies.

PREPARATION OF ORAL CONTROLLED SUBSTANCES FROM A DISPENSER

A controlled dispensing system is used for distributing opiate analgesics and hypnotics (Figure 34-3). **Legally controlled substances must be under lock and key at all times.** Automated controlled-substance dispensing machines are often used in the clinical setting to monitor and control narcotic use (Figure 34-4). A significant advantage of this type of system is that a code number is used to enter the system. This eliminates the problem of having to find the nurse who has the keys to the locked cabinet and increases efficiency. Each nurse has a password by which to gain entry to the system.

When not in a dispensing machine, the drugs are supplied in a controlled dispenser or a commercially prepared package. Most medications are supplied in small pull-strip boxes with a roll of numbered doses of a particular medication. These often have 25 tablets or capsules per box. The first pill to be dispensed is numbered "25," so that there is an accurate count of the remaining pills in the box. Tablets or capsules may be prepared in plastic sectioned containers, usually with 25 compartments clearly marked on top of the container as number 25, 24, 23, and so forth. The top surface of the container is movable, so that when the small opening in the cover is centered over one of the compartments, the container can be inverted over the medicine cup and the tablet or capsule falls into the cup without being handled. Each dose given must be accounted for and the number remaining verified at the time each shift counts the controlled substances before handing over the keys to the compartment to the next shift. One nurse from the oncoming shift and one nurse from the shift going off duty do the count together. Any discrepancy must be resolved before the nurses on the ending shift leave the unit.

As soon as the medicine has been dispensed, verify the label on the dispenser with the patient's medication record. Replace the dispenser. Record the medication on the proof-of-use form and administer the drug to the patient. At the end of the shift, the remaining controlled drugs are counted, or a computerized count is obtained from the dispensing machine.

? *Think Critically About . . .* If a patient decides not to take a dose of a controlled medication that is in an unopened unit-dose package, how do you think the situation would be handled?

TOPICAL DRUGS

Topical drugs are applied externally to the skin and the mucous membranes; they may also have a systemic effect. Drug solutions instilled in the eye, ear, and nose are topical and act locally on these tissues. Other common forms of topical drugs include ointments, creams, pastes, liniments, and lotions that are used to treat local conditions. Drops and ointments for the eye must be sterile and nonirritating to the tissues. Solutions to be instilled in the eye, ear, or nose are generally prepared in dropper bottles.

Ointments are medicines manufactured in an oily base, such as petrolatum or lanolin, which keeps the drug in prolonged contact with the skin surface to obtain a soothing and anti-inflammatory effect. To protect against local infections, many contain antibiotics. *Pastes* are stiffer in consistency than ointments and do not melt at body temperature. Aluminum paste and zinc oxide are examples of pastes that are used to absorb secretions and protect the skin. *Lotions* and *liniments* are topical drugs in liquid form, such as calamine lotion, which are used to cool, soothe, and reduce inflammation or itching of the skin. Lotions are patted on gently, whereas liniments are rubbed into the skin. Liniments provide temporary relief of pain or soothing warmth by their action, which dilates the superficial blood vessels.

Suppositories are small cylinder-shaped, semisolid substances that are inserted into body orifices, such as the rectum, vagina, urethra, or ostomy stoma. Suppositories contain medication that is absorbed through mucous membranes.

Medications can also be dissolved in solutions and applied topically in the form of *irrigations*. Vaginal irrigations are the most common type of medicinal irrigation. Irrigations are presented in Chapter 38.

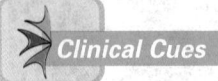
Clinical Cues

When you apply a topical skin medication such as nitroglycerin ointment, always wear gloves; otherwise you may accidentally absorb some of the medication through your skin.

APPLICATION of the NURSING PROCESS

Assessment (Data Collection)

First check the order for each medication, noting the patient's name, drug name, dosage, route, time, and the date the order was written to be certain it is still valid. Check the patient record for allergies. Determine why the patient is receiving the drug. If previous doses have been given, assess for therapeutic effect (the drug is working as intended). Assess for interactions among the drugs the patient is receiving. Check lab values and determine if there is any contraindication to taking the drug.

Assess what the patient knows about each medication and define learning needs. Assess for side effects to the drug if previous doses have been given. Decide whether the route in which the drug is ordered will be effective for the patient. For example, if the patient is nauseated, an oral dose may not be retained. Assess for drugs that must be given with food or on an empty stomach so that timing of the dose will be appropriate. When topical medications are to be applied, assess for adverse effects such as inflammation, swelling, redness, or discharge.

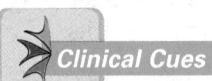
Clinical Cues

Always determine what the blood pressure is before administering an antihypertensive drug. The apical heart rate is assessed before giving a digitalis preparation.

Nursing Diagnosis

Look at the classification of each medication and determine how nursing diagnoses are related to each prescribed medication. A hospitalized patient has acute problems, but other chronic problems may also be present for which the patient is receiving medication. These chronic problems need to be addressed with nursing diagnoses on the care plan. For example, a patient who had a colon resection may also be diabetic and hypertensive. Patient care is often very complex. By looking at the medications patients are receiving that are unrelated to the primary condition for which they are hospitalized, chronic conditions can be uncovered and addressed. For example, if the patient is in the hospital for a hip replacement and the major nursing diagnosis on the care plan is Impaired physical mobility related to hip replacement, but the medication administration record includes digoxin (Lanoxin) as a scheduled medication, then the patient may also have the nursing diagnosis of *Decreased cardiac output*. Digoxin is given to increase contractility of the heart. A few examples of nursing diagnoses for which medications are part of the treatment plan include the following:

- Pain (analgesics)
- Ineffective tissue perfusion related to increased blood pressure (antihypertensives)
- Ineffective tissue perfusion related to cardiac arrhythmia (antiarrhythmics)
- Impaired tissue integrity related to wound infection (antibiotics)
- Imbalanced nutrition: less than body requirements related to nausea (antiemetics)
- Deficient knowledge related to action or side effects of prescribed medications

Elder Care Points

A thorough medication history should be obtained from the elderly patient, who may be receiving prescriptions from more than one physician and filling them by mail as well as at the local pharmacy. Encourage patients to use one pharmacy if possible.

Planning

Plan and incorporate times for medication administration into the daily shift work schedule. A grid on the daily worksheet for assigned patients and the times of their medications is very useful. Plan to take juice or crackers to the room when a patient's medication is scheduled between meals and needs to be taken with food. If a patient has difficulty swallowing, plan time to sit the patient upright and coach in the swallowing process. Plan to assess for side effects of the medication before giving the next scheduled dose. The overall goals of medication administration are as follows:

- All medications ordered will be safely administered to each patient on time.
- Serious side effects of medication will be identified quickly.
- The medication will be effective.
- No allergic reaction to the medication will occur.
- The patient will understand why the drug is prescribed, adhere to the medication schedule, and report serious side effects.

Expected outcomes for the previous nursing diagnoses might be:

- Pain will be relieved for 3 hours after administration of analgesic.
- Blood pressure is controlled within normal limits by antihypertensive medication within 1 week.

- Heart rate is regular and without signs of atrial fibrillation while taking antiarrhythmic medication.
- Wound culture will be negative at the end of antibiotic therapy.
- Patient will eat a meal without nausea with antiemetic 30 minutes prior to the meal.
- Patient will verbalize the reason for the medication and the side effects that might occur before discharge.

Elder Care Points

Elderly patients sometimes hold oral medication in the buccal (inner cheek) area rather than swallowing it; check the mouth to be certain that the medication has been swallowed if in doubt.

Implementation

When preparing any medication, remember to check the label three times and to follow the five rights of medication administration. Always check for patient allergy to the medication before giving it, and document *after* administering the drug. Patient teaching is an integral part of medication administration (Communication Cues 34-1 and Nursing Care Plan 34-1).

Elder Care Points

For elders with visual acuity deficits, make a chart using large dark letters on a white background. Include the name, dose, time, and purpose of the drug. If the patient cannot read, tape a sample pill to the chart.

Oral Medication

Oral drugs may be supplied as a tablet, capsule, spansule (time-released pellets put into a capsule), lozenge, or as a liquid in the form of a syrup, elixir, or suspension (Cultural Cues 34-1). When giving a drug in tablet or capsule form, be sure to offer sufficient water with which to swallow the medication. Some people want to take all their pills at once; others will want to take them one at a time.

Cultural Cues 34-1

Color, Size, and Milligrams of Pills

Some of your patients may believe that the size or color of a pill, or the dose, is related to efficacy. For example, your patient may voice a preference for a red pill, or your Cambodian patient may believe that a large pill contains a large dose. A comparative Western belief would be that your American patient believes that a large number of milligrams is related to therapeutic effect.

NURSING CARE PLAN 34-1

Care of the Patient Discharged with a New Medication

SCENARIO Phillip Hertog suffered a myocardial infarction and is being discharged home tomorrow. He has nitroglycerin ordered and has never used this medication and doesn't "understand the directions."

PROBLEM/NURSING DIAGNOSIS *Never used medication, doesn't understand*/Deficient knowledge related to prescription for nitroglycerin sublingual tablets.
Supporting Assessment Data: *Subjective:* States has never used nitroglycerin and does not "understand the directions." *Objective:* Has an anxious expression and is picking at the bedcovers.

Goals/Expected Outcomes	Nursing Interventions	Selected Rationale	Evaluation
Patient will verbalize correct way to take nitroglycerin by discharge.	Explain: • When chest pain occurs, he should lie down.	A supine position decreases the work of the heart.	*What was the patient able to recall about taking nitroglycerin?*
	• Place a sublingual tablet under the tongue.	"Sublingual" means under the tongue.	States, "Place a tablet under the tongue."
	• If pain has not eased within 5 minutes, place another sublingual tablet under the tongue.	A larger dose of nitroglycerin may be needed.	
Patient will state how many tablets he can use when he has chest pain.	• Repeat × 2 at 5-minute intervals if the pain has not eased.		*Does the patient know how many tablets to use for chest pain?*
	• Instruct not to swallow the pill.	Stomach acid may inactivate the medication and it will not be absorbed as rapidly.	States, "Maximum of 3 tablets should be taken."
Patient will state what to do if the medication does not relieve the pain.	• Call 911 if the pain continues after the three tablets have been used.	Chest pain may indicate a myocardial infarction is occurring.	*Does the patient know what to do if the medication does not relieve pain?*
	• Tablets are to be kept in an airtight, lightproof container.	Light makes tablets deteriorate and become ineffective	Knows to contact EMS if pain continues unrelieved.
	• Tablets should be carried with him at all times and should be by the bed at night.	Tablets must be at hand when chest pain occurs.	
	• Answer any questions.		
	• Leave printed instructions with him.	Printed instructions reinforce verbal instructions and are at home for later referral.	
	• Obtain verbal feedback from him regarding the instructions before discharge.	Verbal feedback, when correct, indicates understanding of procedure to follow.	Correctly verbalized all points covered. Meeting expected outcomes.

? CRITICAL THINKING QUESTIONS

1. What would you say to Mr. Hertog if he complains that the nitroglycerin tablets give him a terrible headache?

2. What instructions would you give Mr. Hertog about the side effects of nitroglycerin?

Communication Cues 34-1

Patient Education to Increase Compliance

Rita Sanchez is being discharged after hospitalization for a bacterial pneumonia. Her physician has prescribed clarithromycin (Biaxin) tablets for her to take at home to finish clearing the infection. You go to instruct her about this medication and find that she has taken it before and did not like the side effects.

MS. SANCHEZ: "Biaxin makes my mouth taste terrible and I lost my appetite the last time I took it."

NURSE: "Why was it prescribed for you the last time?"

MS. SANCHEZ: "I had bronchitis."

NURSE: "I'm sorry it caused such an unpleasant side effect. Did it cause stomach pain or diarrhea?"

MS. SANCHEZ: "No, I didn't have those problems with it."

NURSE: "It is important that you take the medication. Your doctor has prescribed it because it is the best one to treat the infection."

MS. SANCHEZ: "But I'm not going to get my strength back if I can't eat."

NURSE: "I understand your concern. You might try brushing your teeth several times a day and using a mild mouthwash every 2 hours while you are awake to get rid of the taste in your mouth."

MS. SANCHEZ: "Do you really think that will help?"

NURSE: "There is a good chance that it will help. Chewing gum between meals may also decrease the bad taste. We need for you to eat your meals. If your appetite seems really off, trying eating six small meals a day until the medication is gone."

MS. SANCHEZ: "Are you sure there isn't another medication that I can take instead of this one?"

NURSE: "Well, your sputum culture showed that this medication was the most effective at treating the bacteria responsible for the infection. I will speak with the physician and tell him your concerns and see if there is anything else you might take."

MS. SANCHEZ: "Why, thank you very much."

Remember: Any water that is used must be entered on the intake sheet if the patient is on intake and output recording (Skill 34-1). It is important to assess for side effects of the drug before giving another dose of the medication.

When preparing liquid medications, pour the dose into a graduated medicine cup. The exact level of the dose is read at the lowest point of the meniscus (curved upper surface) of the liquid in the cup when held at eye level (Figure 34-5). Always pour the liquid out the side of the bottle away from the label so that any residual liquid will not run down the label and distort the words on it.

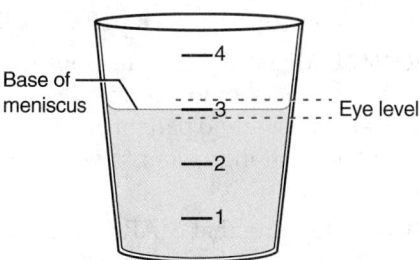

FIGURE **34-5** Reading the dose prepared at the meniscus of the liquid.

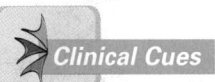

Elder Care Points

If elderly patients have difficulty swallowing a pill, instruct them to take a sip of water and swallow it; then place the pill toward the back of the tongue. Have them take a large sip of water, place the tongue on the roof of the mouth, and with the chin tilted slightly downward, swallow; follow with more water. If difficulty with swallowing persists, crush the pill unless contraindicated or ask the physician for a liquid form of the drug.

Clinical Cues

For infants, measure oral liquid medication with an oral syringe (Safety Alert 34-1). Mother or nurse cuddles the infant in an upright position on the lap. Insert the tip of the oral syringe on the side of mouth and give slowly. An alternative method for infants who can bottle feed is to use a Medibottle, which allows the attachment of a medication syringe to a nipple.

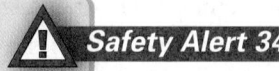

Safety Alert 34-1

Oral Syringes for Safety

Small amounts (less than 30 mL) of oral medications can be measured with a syringe. To increase safety, use an **oral syringe** to prevent accidental IM, IV, or Subcut administration of oral medications.

Sublingual medications are placed under the tongue. They should never be swallowed. The drug dissolves in the sublingual pocket and is quickly absorbed by the vessels in the oral mucosa. Buccal medications are placed in the pocket between the teeth and the cheek. Swallowing these medications alters their absorption and may make them totally ineffective.

Eye and Ear Medications

Ophthalmic (eye) medications may be in the form of drops, ointment, or an eye disk. An error with an eye medication can cause significant damage, and it is imperative to check each medication very carefully be-

Skill 34-1 | Administering Oral Medications

The unit-dose system of medication administration is the most commonly used system in health care facilities today. Each medication is usually packaged in a single-dose package. These packages are either commercially prepared or prepared in the facility pharmacy. Most nursing units have at least one unit-dose cart containing drawers in which each patient's medications are stored. However, some hospitals have started installing an individual patient medication drawer in the patient's room. Ideally, the cart is taken to each room and the medications are distributed to the patients. Medications may also be in a central location, such as the medication room. In this situation, the nurse must carry the MAR to the bedside to properly identify the patient when giving medications. Patients are identified by at least two identifiers. The keys to successful implementation of any system are following the principles of medication administration and the consistent use of the MAR when checking and giving medications.

■ Supplies
✓ Unit-dose cart stocked with medications
✓ Medication cups
✓ Disposable gloves
✓ Straws
✓ Drinking cups
✓ Tongue blades
✓ Water or juice

Review and carry out the Standard Steps in Appendix 3.

■ Assessment (Data Collection)

1. **ACTION** Verify that the medication record has been compared with the physician's orders within the past 24 hours. Check each patient's allergies.

   RATIONALE Mistakes are sometimes made when transcribing orders onto the MAR. Checking on allergies ensures that no patient is given a medication containing an ingredient to which the patient is allergic.

2. **ACTION** Determine that MARs are present at the cart for all patients to receive medications.

   RATIONALE Sometimes the unit secretary has a MAR for order changes.

3. **ACTION** Assess for side effects of previously given doses of the drug(s). Question the patient or assess the area where a topical medication was applied and is to be given.

   RATIONALE Prevents potential adverse effect of the drug.

■ Planning

4. **ACTION** Assess supplies on cart and restock as necessary.

   RATIONALE Drinking cups, disposable gloves, and medication cups for liquid medication are needed.

5. **ACTION** Determine which patients are NPO (including those who are scheduled to have dialysis) and which are off the floor for procedures or surgery.

   RATIONALE Patients who are NPO must not receive oral medications, although sometimes a medication will be ordered preoperatively to be taken with one sip of water. (Some medications, such as antihypertensives, are held before dialysis.) Knowing which patients are off the unit helps plan medication administration time.

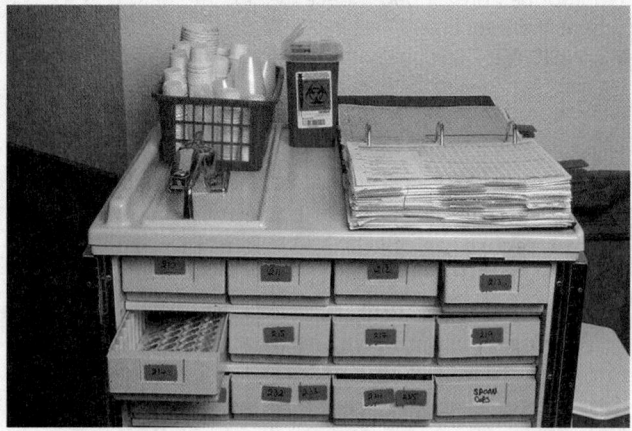

Step **4**

6. **ACTION** Calculate any doses that are not individual unit doses.

   RATIONALE Ensures that the correct amount of drug will be administered as ordered.

■ Implementation

7. **ACTION** Perform hand hygiene.

   RATIONALE Medications must be administered using aseptic technique.

8. **ACTION** Take the medication cart to the patient's room.

   RATIONALE Unit-dose medications are administered to one patient at a time, with the cart at the door of the room.

9. **ACTION** Verify that the patient is present to receive medications.

   RATIONALE The patient may be in the shower, undergoing a respiratory treatment, or severely nauseated, which could prevent or delay the taking of oral medications.

10. **ACTION** Remove the patient drawer containing the medications, and place it on the work space on

top of the cart. Position the MAR sheet beside the drawer. Perform the first check of each medication due at this hour by removing the medication from the drawer and checking the package label with the MAR order. Note the following:

a. Drug name

b. Dosage

c. Date and time to be given

d. Expiration date of the drug and the order

Place the package beside the information on the MAR and proceed to the next medication ordered for this time. Review signs and symptoms of adverse effects for which you must assess; look up any medication with which you are unfamiliar.

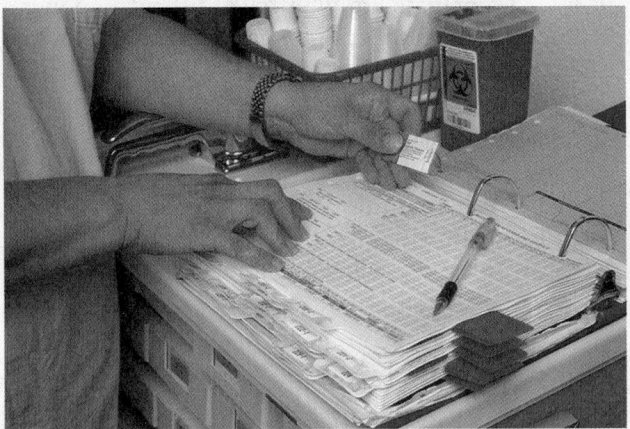
Step **10**

RATIONALE This completes the first check in following four of the Five Rights of medication administration. Legally you must know the action, normal dosage, adverse effects, interactions, and nursing implications for every drug you give.

11. ***ACTION*** Return the drawer to its place in the cart, and then carefully check each medication a second time with the MAR, checking the following:

a. Drug name

b. Dosage

c. Route ordered

d. Date and time to be given

Place each package into the medicine cup, unopened, as the second check is finished.

RATIONALE This completes the second check of medication using the Five Rights. Counting the number of medications on the MAR to be given at the designated time (e.g., 0900) and then counting the medications you have out can prevent overlooking a dose. All MAR sheets must be checked; some patients have orders continued on a second and even a third sheet. Unit-dose packages are not to be opened until after the third medicine check, when you are with the patient.

12. ***ACTION*** Pour the liquid medication dose into a medication cup unless it is in a dose-measured cup already; carefully check the dosage amount. Do not pour over the MAR sheet because a spill may occur. To pour a liquid medication from a multi-dose bottle, read the dosage from the bottom of the meniscus, the lowest point. When liquid medications are supplied in a premeasured cup, remove the lid carefully at the bedside so as not to spill the contents. If a multidose bottle is supplied, measure the dose accurately.

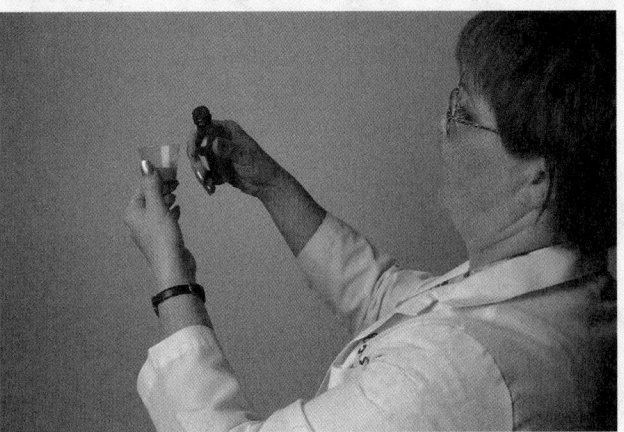
Step **12**

RATIONALE A spill on the MAR sheet will require that the sheet be recopied.

13. ***ACTION*** Take the medications and the MAR sheet in to the patient. Identify the patient by comparing the information on the armband with the information imprinted on the MAR, and by asking the patient to state his or her name; explain the procedure, thereby completing the Five Rights check.

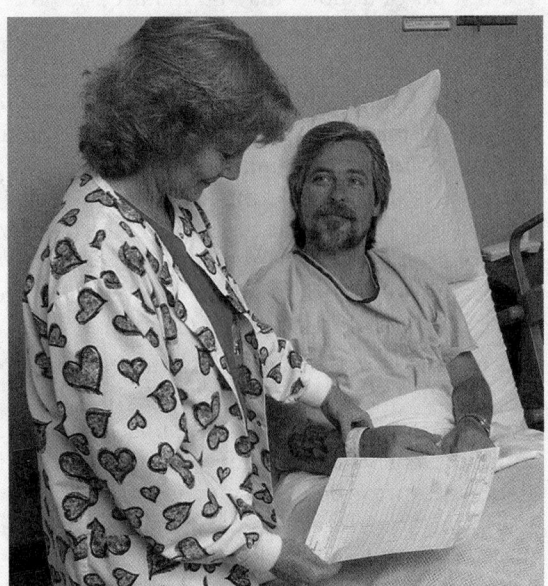
Step **13**

Continued

Skill 34-1 | Administering Oral Medications—cont'd

RATIONALE Comparison of the patient's full name and hospital number is the most fail-safe method of identification. Asking the patient to state her name provides the second required identification check. The patient should be told why you need to check the identification band.

14. *ACTION* Check each medication for the third time as you prepare to open it to give to the patient. Tell the patient what the medication is (i.e., "your heart medication"). Check the following:

   a. Drug name
   b. Dosage
   c. Route ordered
   d. Date and time

   If the patient does not recognize the medication or indicates that no "heart medication" has ever been taken, stop and recheck the original order. If there is no question, open the medication and place it in the medicine cup.

   RATIONALE When the drug is kept in its wrapper until it has been checked the third time and verified with the patient, it can be returned to the drawer if the patient refuses it or if it is not the correct medication. The third check of the medicine provides an added safety check for following the five rights of medication administration. Many medication errors are made because the date and time were not also checked along with the drug name and dosage. Even though drugs are dispensed in unit-dose packages, more than one package or part of a tablet may be required for the ordered dose.

15. *ACTION* Pour water for the patient to use to take the pills; perform any assessment necessary before the patient takes the medication (e.g., take an apical pulse rate before administering digitalis preparations, assess the blood pressure before giving an antihypertensive medication; record the data). Assess for adverse effects from previous doses of the medications you are about to give. Assess to see if any PRN medications are needed at this time.

   RATIONALE Liquid is necessary for the swallowing of pills. The heart rate and rhythm must be known before digitalis is administered; certain antihypertensive medications are withheld if the blood pressure is below a specified level. You must assess for adverse effects of a drug before giving another dose. Giving PRN medications while in the room saves time.

16. *ACTION* Give the medications to the patient with water or other acceptable liquid. Adhere to fluid-

restriction requirements for patients whose intake of fluid is restricted.

   RATIONALE Some medications cannot be taken with particular foods. Patients whose intake of fluid is restricted must space their fluid intake over 24 hours and are not allowed unlimited fluid for taking medications.

17. *ACTION* Observe the patient take the medications, and for those patients who have difficulty swallowing, put on a glove and check the inside of the mouth to see that the pills were actually swallowed. For patients who have difficulty in swallowing, placing the pill as far back on the tongue as possible before taking a sip of water helps.

   RATIONALE Sometimes pills fall onto the bed or floor when the patient places the medicine cup or hand to the mouth with the pills. A pill may remain in the mouth for the patient who has difficulty swallowing. Medication may not work correctly unless it reaches the stomach.

18. *ACTION* Initial the doses given and sign your name on the MAR according to agency policy. If the medicine is not given, circle the time of the dose and follow agency policy regarding further charting.

   RATIONALE Documentation of an administered dose is done **after** the patient has taken the medication. The MAR may need to be flagged so that a dose not given may be given at a later time when the patient returns to the floor or is no longer restricted to taking nothing by mouth.

19. *ACTION* Proceed to prepare and administer medications to the next patient.

   RATIONALE Each patient should receive medications within 30 minutes of the time scheduled.

20. *ACTION* Return the unit-dose cart and supplies to the central area.

   RATIONALE Returning the cart makes it available for the delivery of medications by the pharmacy or for use by another nurse.

■ Evaluation

21. *ACTION* For each medication given, ask yourself whether the patient had any signs or symptoms of adverse effects. Evaluate whether the medication appears to be effective in treating the condition for which it is prescribed. Recheck each MAR for the time you are giving medications to ensure that every medication scheduled for that time has been signed off.

   RATIONALE Ensures that further doses of a medication are not given without consulting the physician if the patient is experiencing adverse effects. If a medication is not effective, its use needs to be questioned. Rechecking ensures that no dose has been overlooked.

■ Special Considerations

✓ If medications are prepared for administration in the medication room, complete the two checks for each drug ordered before going to the patient's room; perform the third check at the bedside.

✓ Patients should be sitting up as high as possible to swallow medications. Instruct not to hyperextend the neck when swallowing, but to slightly tuck in the chin instead. Offer a straw if the patient has difficulty drinking from a cup.

✓ When a patient is on intake and output (I & O) recording, the amount of water used to take medications must be noted on the I & O sheet.

✓ Consider each MAR and think about possible drug interactions among the drugs ordered for the patient.

✓ If a patient is quite weak, check the swallowing reflex by offering a sip of water first, before giving medications to swallow.

✓ Tell the patient not to swallow a sublingual or buccal medication and explain why it must be left under the tongue or in the cheek pocket.

✓ If the patient is weak or has poor hand-eye coordination, place a large clean towel or sheet across the patient's chest to catch "dropped" pills.

?CRITICAL THINKING QUESTIONS

1. What would you check to verify that the patient is not allergic to a medication?

2. What will you do if the patient looks at the pill you are administering and says, "I don't recognize this pill. Is it really ordered for me?"

---

fore instilling it. The word *ophthalmic* must be clearly visible on the medication container and the medication must be in date. Skill 34-2 shows the steps for instilling eyedrops and eye ointment. Eye medications must be kept sterile. Careful hand hygiene is necessary before beginning the procedure.

Otic (ear) medication is mostly used in children to decrease the pain of otitis media, but may also be used to treat external otitis and to soften cerumen (earwax) so that it can be removed more easily. Otic medication administration is presented in Steps 34-1, p. 670. For the child younger than 3 years, pull the ear lobe downward to straighten the canal; in the adult, pull the top of the pinna out and upward (Figure 34-6).

Nasal Medications

Nasal medications come in soft plastic atomizer or dropper bottles. An atomizer bottle contains decongestant, antihistamine, antibiotic, or steroid, depending on the patient's need. To use an atomizer bottle, have the patient clear the nose as much as possible. While holding one nostril shut, insert the top of the atomizer into the other nostril. The patient squeezes the bottle while breathing in. The process is repeated on the other side (Safety Alert 34-2). One or two squirts per nostril is the usual dosage. The top of the bottle should be wiped clean before the cap is replaced.

When nose drops are prescribed, the patient should lie down face up, with the head off the bed and the neck hyperextended. The drops are pulled into the dropper by depressing the rubber top of the dropper while the stem is in the liquid and letting go. The tip of the dropper is held just above the nostril and the correct number of drops is gently expelled into the nostril by lightly squeezing the rubber top (Figure 34-7). The

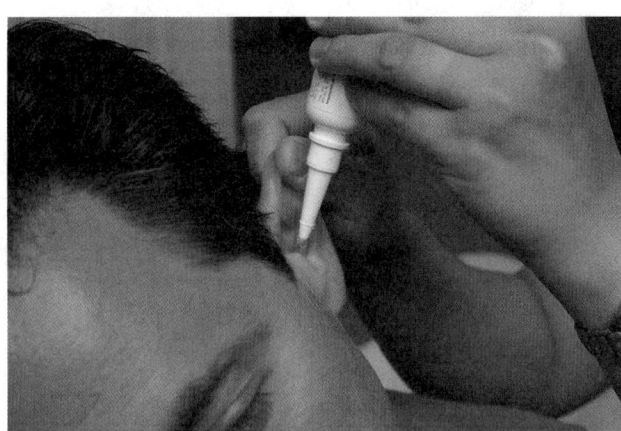

FIGURE **34-6** Straightening the ear canal for otic drops.

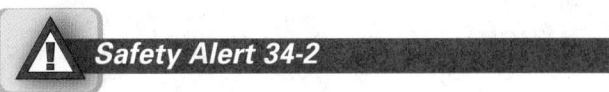

Safety Alert 34-2

One or Both Nostrils?

Nasal medications that are intended for local effect on the nasal mucosa, such as saline nose drops or drops for seasonal allergies, are administered in both nostrils. Nasal medications that are intended for systemic effects, such as sumatriptan (Imitrex), should be given in one nostril only.

patient should remain in the head-back position for a few minutes.

Inhalation Medications

Inhalation therapy is used for patients with respiratory conditions, which can originate in any area from the nasal passageways to the deep lung tissues. Drugs

Skill 34-2 | Instilling Eye Medication

Eye medications are used to control glaucoma, treat eye infections, decrease inflammation, provide moisture to the eye, and cleanse the eye. Each medication is ordered for an individual patient and should never be used for more than one patient. Cotton balls or tissues may be used to catch the excess solution. Hand hygiene must be performed before instilling eyedrops, and disposable gloves are worn.

■ Supplies

✓ Ophthalmic solution or ointment (as ordered)

✓ Disposable gloves
✓ Medical administration record (MAR)

✓ Tissues

Review and carry out the Standard Steps in Appendix 3.

■ Assessment (Data Collection)

1. *ACTION* Determine that the ordered eye medications are on hand and that the patient is ready for them to be instilled.

   RATIONALE Assists in smooth procedure performance.

2. *ACTION* Check the eye medication with the MAR, following the principles in the five rights of medication administration, twice before performing hand hygiene and once after identifying the patient. Double check if the instillation is for the right eye, left eye, or both eyes.

   RATIONALE Prevents medication errors.

3. *ACTION* Assess the eye(s) for inflammation, swelling, discharge, and change in vision.

   RATIONALE May be an adverse effect of medication.

■ Planning

4. *ACTION* Consider the order in which the eye medications are to be instilled if there is more than one.

   RATIONALE Some types of medications must be instilled before other types.

5. *ACTION* Plan sufficient time to instill the medications as ordered. You may need to remove a dressing, clean the eye, and instill drops over a set time period.

   RATIONALE Instilling eye medication often takes longer than giving an oral medication.

■ Intervention

6. *ACTION* Check the patient's ID band, comparing it with the MAR. Ask the patient to state her name. Perform hand hygiene and don gloves.

   RATIONALE Ensures that the medication is given to the right patient. Prevents transfer of microorganisms.

Eyedrop Application

7. *ACTION* Remove the cap from the bottle of medication; place it upside down on the table.

   RATIONALE Prepares the dropper bottle for use and protects sterility of the cap.

8. *ACTION* Place the patient in a sitting or reclining position. Ask the patient to look at the ceiling and tilt the head slightly to the side of the affected eye. With a tissue beneath the fingers, retract the lower lid over the bony orbit by pulling it downward to expose the conjunctival sac. If the patient is sitting in a chair, stand beside the chair.

   RATIONALE Allows easier visualization of the eye and easy retraction of the eyelid. Looking upward inhibits the desire to blink.

9. *ACTION* Stabilize the container above the eye over the conjunctival sac and drop the designated number of drops directly into the conjunctival sac without touching the surface of the eye. Do not place drops on the cornea. Block the entrance to the lacrimal gland by placing a finger over it.

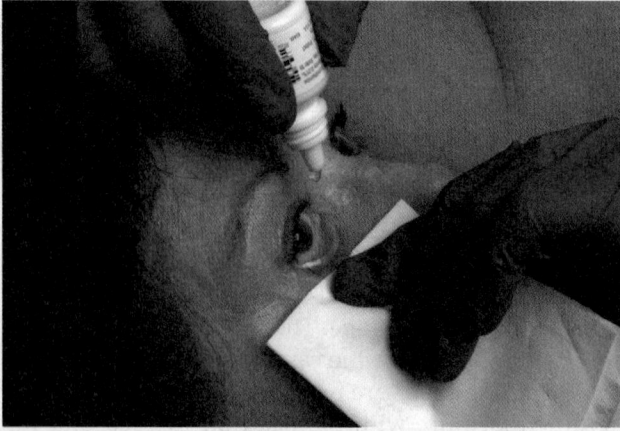

Step **9**

RATIONALE Only the amount of drops ordered is to be instilled. Drops on the cornea cause discomfort and/or damage. Some medications have adverse effects if they enter the systemic circulation through the lacrimal gland.

10. **ACTION** Replace the cap on the bottle without contaminating the dropper tip or the rim of the top. If the dropper tip becomes contaminated, replace the medication with a new bottle.

    RATIONALE If the dropper tip becomes contaminated, the medication will be contaminated.

Eye Ointment Application

11. **ACTION** For eye ointment, remove the cap from the tube and set it down on a table upside down. Expose the conjunctival sac, and apply a thin ribbon of ointment along the entire length of the visible conjunctival sac. To end the ribbon, simply twist the tube with a lateral movement of the wrist without touching the eye or the lid. Recap the tube and return it to storage.

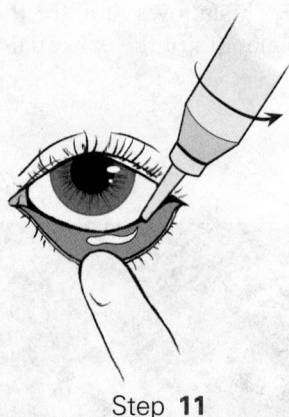

Step **11**

    RATIONALE The ointment tube tip will be contaminated if it touches the eye. Drops and ointment placed in the conjunctival sac will spread over the entire eye.

12. **ACTION** Ask the patient to close the eyelid gently and to move the eyes side to side and up and down with the eyelids closed to distribute the medication.

    RATIONALE Closing the eyelid tightly causes the medication to be pushed out. Rolling the eyeball around distributes the ointment over the entire eyeball.

13. **ACTION** With a tissue or a cotton ball, gently remove the excess medication from the outside of the lid and discard it into a designated container.

    RATIONALE Removes excess medication from the face.

For Eyedrops and Ointment

14. **ACTION** Remove gloves and perform hand hygiene. Return the medications to their storage location.

    RATIONALE Reduces transfer of microorganisms. Prepares medications for next use.

■ Evaluation

15. **ACTION** Assess for desired effect of the eye medication and for adverse effects.

    RATIONALE The signs to assess will depend on the type of medication. If adverse effects occur, the medication may need to be changed.

16. **ACTION** Evaluate own technique and consider any changes to be made for next instillation.

    RATIONALE Provides feedback on technical skill.

■ Documentation

17. **ACTION** Document the doses given on the MAR.

    RATIONALE Verifies that medication was given.

■ Special Considerations

✓ If a dressing was removed, reapply a dressing using aseptic technique.

✓ If the eye has crusting or debris is present, clean the lids and lashes with sterile normal saline and sterile cotton balls before instilling the medication. Wipe from the inner canthus at the nose to the outer canthus near the temple. Use a clean cotton ball for each wiping stroke.

✓ Eye medications should be at room temperature for administration; eye ointment will flow more easily at room temperature.

✓ If eyedrops are to be sent home with the patient for continued instillation, be certain that the patient can identify the different bottles correctly, if there is more than one medication.

✓ Assess the area for inflammation, swelling, pain, and discharge; determine if a change in vision has occurred.

?CRITICAL THINKING QUESTIONS

1. How can you mark multiple eyedrop bottles that the patient will be using at home, so that there is no mistake about when to use them and in what order?

2. Why do you think you should not drop eyedrops on the cornea?

Steps 34-1 | Instilling Otic Medication

Ear medications are used to treat infection or inflammation of the canal, to decrease the pain of otitis media, and to dissolve cerumen (earwax). A cotton ball is placed in the ear after the drops have been instilled to prevent medication from dripping out and soiling clothes.

Review and carry out the Standard Steps in Appendix 3.

1. ***ACTION*** Position the patient supine and in the lateral position so that the affected ear is uppermost.

   RATIONALE Drops will flow into the ear by gravity.

2. ***ACTION*** Draw medication into the medicine dropper by depressing the bulb and letting it go.

   RATIONALE Prepares the medication for instillation into the ear.

3. ***ACTION*** Straighten the ear canal by drawing the pinna upward and toward the back of the head. For children younger than 3 years, draw the earlobe slightly down and back. Insert the tip of the medicine dropper into the external ear canal; instill the medication and withdraw the dropper (see Figure 34-6).

   RATIONALE Places medication in the intended location.

4. ***ACTION*** Place cotton in the external meatus to prevent the medication from escaping. Have patient remain in the lateral position for 5 to 10 minutes.

   RATIONALE This allows time for the medicine to penetrate the length of the ear canal.

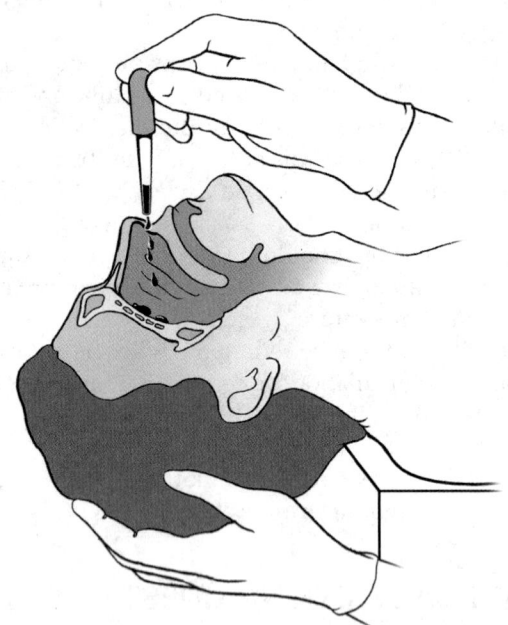

FIGURE **34-7** Instilling nose drops (Proetz's position).

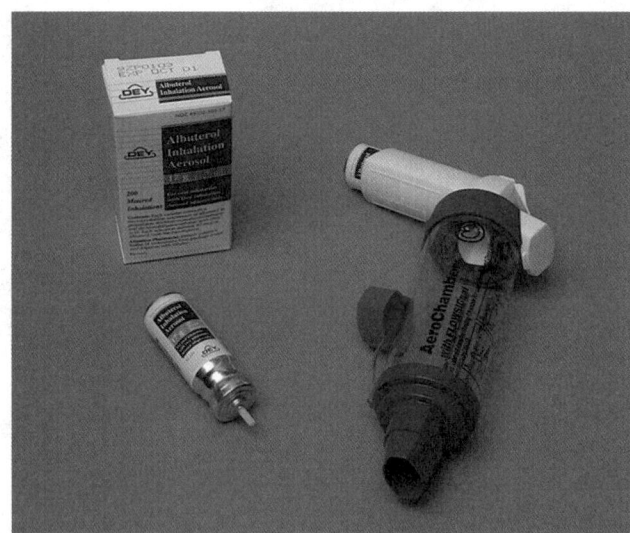

FIGURE **34-8** Metered-dose inhaler, medication canister, and spacer.

used for inhalation therapy are always water soluble to ensure quick absorption into the respiratory system without creating tissue inflammation. Various mechanical devices are designed for aerosol treatment, such as atomizers, sprays, and hand-held metered-dose inhalers (Figure 34-8).

Metered-dose inhalers (MDIs) and nasal sprays come in containers labeled with directions for use. The MDI is held in front of the mouth, the cylinder for the inhalant is depressed, and a spray of medication is released. A variety of drugs are available in MDI form: antispasmodics, bronchodilators, mucolytic agents, proteolytic enzymes, and anti-inflammatories. Using a spacer with the device enhances delivery of the medication deeper into the bronchioles. Patients must be taught how to properly use an MDI (Figure 34-9 and Patient Teaching 34-1).

Short-acting insulin (Exubera) is now available in a new inhaled form. For type 2 diabetes, it may be used alone or in conjunction with dietary modifications, oral antidiabetic drugs, or injected insulin. For type 1 diabe-

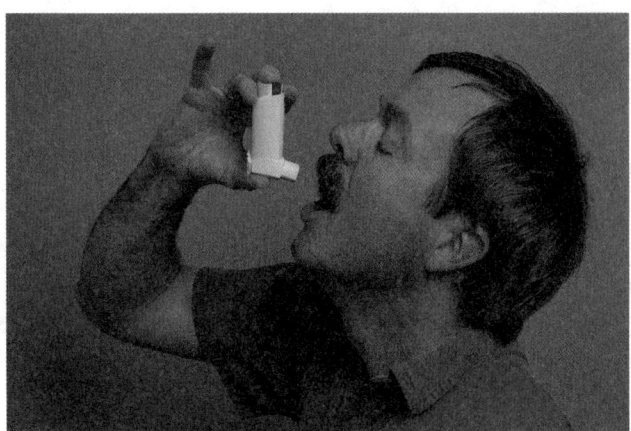

FIGURE **34-9** Using a metered-dose inhaler.

tes, this inhaled form maybe used along with injected intermediate or long-acting insulin. Exubera is contraindicated for patients with pulmonary disease or those who smoke. The medication is administered 10 minutes before a meal. Teach your patient that the medication is available in 1-mg and 3-mg blister packages; however, she should not substitute three 1-mg blisters for one 3-mg blister. This will result in an overdose. For additional information, consult www.exubera.com.

Five groups of drugs are commonly dispensed in inhalers for treatment of the lungs (Table 34-6). The patient should not take more than one drug from any one of the groups.

Vaginal Medications

A vaginal irrigation is also called a douche. Topical solution is introduced into the vaginal cavity for the following purposes:

- To cleanse the vagina in preparation for surgery
- To supply antiseptics to reduce bacterial growth
- To remove odors or foul discharge
- To apply heat or cold to soothe inflamed tissues or reduce oozing of blood

The normal secretions of the vaginal tissues are naturally acidic, which helps protect against vaginal infection. Vaginal irrigations are considered a clean procedure, except when given postoperatively or after childbirth, then principles of surgical asepsis are followed. Medicated solutions used for vaginal irrigations are 2% sodium bicarbonate solution, diluted hydrogen peroxide, povidone-iodine solution, a weak solution of acetic acid (1 tablespoon vinegar to 1000 mL of fluid), or a medication that is diluted in water. The amount of solution ranges from 1500 to 2000 mL, given slowly over a period of 10 to 15 minutes at a temperature of 100° to 105° F (37.7° to 40.5° C) unless the purpose is to

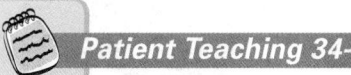

Patient Teaching 34-1

How to Use a Metered-Dose Inhaler (MDI)

When a patient is taking both a corticosteroid and a bronchodilator, teach her to take the bronchodilator first to open the airways so that the corticosteroid will be absorbed. Instruct the patient to use the following steps:

- Always sit or stand to use the MDI.
- Attach the medication canister by holding the long end of the mouthpiece and inserting the stemmed top of the canister into it.
- Shake the canister several times to mix the medication with the propellant, and remove the mouthpiece cap.
- Breathe out through the mouth, emptying the lungs.
- With the bottom of the canister pointing up, place the mouthpiece 1 to 2 inches (2.5 to 5 cm) in front of the mouth. If using a spacer attachment or an Azmacort or Advair inhaler, place the mouthpiece in the mouth and close the lips around it.
- Breathe in slowly through the mouth. While starting to inhale, press the canister down to release the medication. Keep inhaling slowly until a full breath is taken. Hold the breath for 10 seconds and try not to cough. This allows the medication to penetrate the lung mucosa.
- If a second puff is ordered, wait at least 1 minute by the clock before repeating the procedure. This allows the first dose to be fully absorbed before the second is given.
- If you can't inhale slowly or are unable to depress the canister while inhaling, a spacer or extender can be added to the mouthpiece. The spacer encloses the dose and then delivers it to the lungs when inhalation occurs.
- When using a spacer, place the lips around the mouthpiece, completely exhale through the nose, depress the canister to release the medication into the spacer, and then inhale slowly and hold the breath for 10 seconds. Exhale through the nose and take two or three short breaths to obtain the remaining medication in the spacer.

Table 34-6 | *Inhalant Drugs for Respiratory Problems*

DRUG	EXAMPLE
Beta-agonist drugs (stimulants) that open the small airways	Metaproterenol (Alupent), albuterol (Proventil, Ventolin), and terbutaline (Brethaire)
Anticholinergics used to decrease bronchospasm and open the large airways	Atropine, ipratropium (Atrovent)
Corticosteroids used to decrease inflammation	Beclomethasone (Beclovent, Vanceril), triamcinolone (Azmacort), and flunisolide (AeroBid)
Leukotriene modifiers for maintenance therapy of chronic asthma	Montelukast (Singulair)
Antiallergics used to decrease mucosal response to allergens	Cromolyn sodium (Intal)

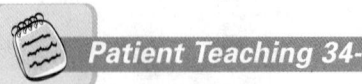
Patient Teaching 34-2

How to Perform Vaginal Irrigations and Instill Vaginal Medications

A vaginal douche works best when done in a dorsal recumbent position in the tub, but can be done when sitting on a commode. Medications are most easily inserted when the person is in the dorsal recumbent position. The bladder should be emptied before beginning a vaginal irrigation or instilling a medication. Medication is best instilled at bedtime to enhance retention of the medication for a prolonged time.
Instruct the patient to do the following:

FOR IRRIGATION WITH A VAGINAL DOUCHE
- Wash the hands.
- Prepare the douche solution per the directions with the medication.
- Fill the douche bag, run a small amount of fluid through the tubing to clear the air in the tube, and close the clamp.
- Hang the douche container no more than 18 inches above the level of the hips. Otherwise the pressure of the fluid will be too great. A coat hanger placed on a bathroom hook or towel rack may work for hanging the bag.
- Gently insert the irrigating nozzle, directing it downward or backward to the back of the vagina.
- Holding the labia closed around the nozzle, unclamp the clamp, allowing the solution to flow slowly into the vagina. When the pressure becomes slightly uncomfortable, ease your grip, allowing the solution to flow out of the vagina. Hold the labia closed again until the vagina fills; repeat the process until all the irrigating solution has been used. *With the labia closed, the solution will distend the folds of the vagina, reaching all areas.*
- The nozzle may be rotated during the irrigation.
- Close the clamp and remove the nozzle. Dry the perineum.
- Rinse the equipment and wash the nozzle with soap and warm water and rinse it well. Hang the bag upside down to drain and dry.

FOR INSERTION OF A VAGINAL SUPPOSITORY
- Wait at least an hour after a vaginal irrigation before inserting medication so that residual irrigation fluid does not wash the medication away.

- Wash hands thoroughly.
- Remove the wrapper from the suppository. Lubricate the rounded end of the suppository with a small amount of water-soluble lubricant such as K-Y jelly for easier insertion.
- Lie down, bend the legs, and spread the knees, or bend a leg and prop a foot on a chair seat or the commode.
- Gently open the labial folds with the nondominant hand.
- Insert the rounded end of the suppository into the vagina with the dominant hand and direct it toward the posterior wall, placing it the full finger's length into the vaginal vault so it will not be easily expelled. Use a vaginal applicator according to package directions if one was supplied with the medication.
- Withdraw the finger or applicator and wash hands and applicator thoroughly.
- Use a panty liner or sanitary pad to collect drainage from the medication to avoid staining of clothing.

FOR INSTILLATION OF VAGINAL CREAM OR FOAM
- Wash hands thoroughly.
- Fill the cream or foam applicator according to the directions on the package insert.
- Lie down, bend the knees, and spread the legs.
- Gently separate the labial folds with the nondominant hand.
- With the dominant hand, gently insert the applicator about 2 to 4 inches and press the plunger to deposit the medication into the vagina.
- Remove the applicator and wipe excess cream from the labia.
- Remain recumbent for at least 10 minutes to allow medication to disperse.
- Clean the applicator and wash hands thoroughly.
- Use a panty liner or sanitary napkin to catch medication drainage to avoid staining of clothing.
- Report any persistent burning or irritation to the physician because this may indicate an adverse reaction.

---

apply heat; then it should be 110° F (43° C). The patient should receive instruction in the correct way to perform the irrigation (Patient Teaching 34-2).

Other topical medications applied to the vagina are suppositories, ointments, and creams prescribed to treat infections and inflammation (Cultural Cues 34-2). Applicators are used for inserting the smaller vaginal suppositories at the distal end of the vagina. An applicator is also required for vaginal ointments. The applicator fits the top of the tube and enough medication is squeezed into the barrel to fill it, after which the applicator is inserted into the vagina, where the plunger deposits the ointment (Figure 34-10). After use, the applicator is washed with soap and water and stored for the patient's future

Cultural Cues 34-2

Touching the Genital Area

Muslim patients may prefer to have a nurse of the same gender if there is a need to touch the genital area during medication administration (D'Avanzo & Geissler, 2003).

---

use, or it is discarded. The patient may be instructed on how to insert the medication herself. After medication has been inserted, a small pad or panty shield may be worn to keep from soiling clothing or bedding.

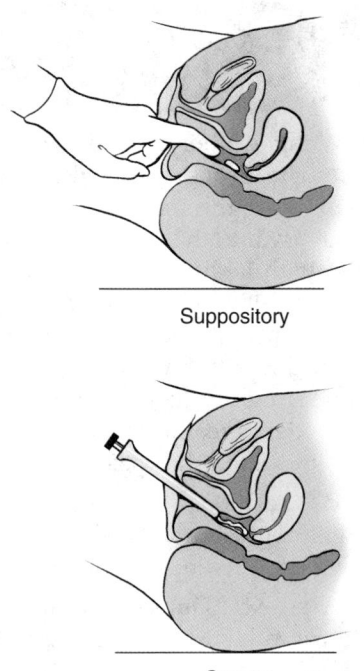

Suppository

Cream

FIGURE **34-10** Inserting vaginal medications.

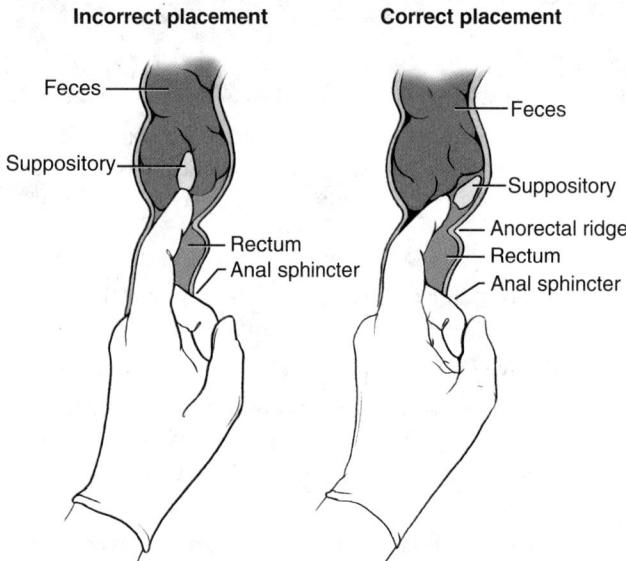

FIGURE **34-11** Inserting a rectal suppository.

Rectal Medications

Rectal medications are dispensed in the form of suppositories (Figure 34-11). There are suppositories to prevent vomiting, soothe hemorrhoids, prevent bladder spasms, promote bowel evacuation, and reduce fever. See Steps 34-2 for the procedure to insert a rectal suppository.

Topical Skin Medications

Many types of topical medications can be applied to the skin. These types include lotions, ointments, creams, and patches. The steps for medication administration must be followed when applying any topical medication. Ointments, oils, lotions, and creams are combinations of skin emollients and a medication and are applied by rubbing into the skin. Skill 34-3 provides the steps for applying a topical skin preparation.

Transdermal (through the skin) medications are supplied in a sustained-release patch that is applied to clean, dry, hairless skin and left in place, or as a paste that is spread on a small area of skin. The drug is slowly absorbed through the skin and is absorbed into the bloodstream. Several types of drugs are now available in skin patch form: nitroglycerin to dilate coronary arteries, scopolamine to relieve motion sickness, estrogen to combat symptoms of menopause, nicotine to assist smoking cessation, and fentanyl, an opioid analgesic, for severe chronic pain. Skin patches should be applied to areas where there is adequate circulation, such as the chest, shoulders, or upper arm. Scopolamine patches are placed behind the ear. Each new patch should be applied to a different area so as not to irritate the skin. Hair should be removed

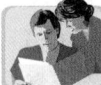

Assignment Considerations 34-1

Coordinating Hygienic Care and Topical Medication Administration

When your patient must receive a topical medication such as ointment or a transdermal patch, try to coordinate with the UAP so that showering or bathing does not interfere with the medication absorption. Remove the old patch, assess the area, and then have the UAP assist the patient with showering or bathing before applying the new medication. If the new medication has been applied before hygiene, instruct the CNA to cover the area with a plastic protector.

before applying a patch. The effect of the medication from a skin patch will begin in about 30 minutes and may remain in the system for 30 minutes after the patch is removed. The patch should be dated and initialed so it is evident when it was applied (Assignment Considerations 34-1).

Nitroglycerin also is dispensed as a paste. It is applied to the skin, but not rubbed in. A ribbon of the ointment in the amount prescribed is applied to the measuring applicator, and the paper is folded to distribute the paste or a wooden applicator is used to spread the paste over a 2¼ × 3½-inch (5.6 × 8.8-cm) area of the paper. The paper is placed paste side down on a clean, nonhairy area of skin and taped into place. When one applicator is removed, the skin is cleansed and the next applicator is applied in a different, clean area.

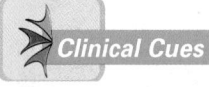

Clinical Cues

Wear gloves when preparing and applying topical medications to avoid receiving any medication.

Steps 34-2 | Inserting a Rectal Suppository

A rectal suppository may be inserted to stimulate a bowel movement, to deliver a medication when the patient cannot take it another way, or to treat hemorrhoids.

Review and carry out the Standard Steps in Appendix 3.

1. **ACTION** After checking the order, obtain the suppository, gloves, and water-soluble lubricant.

   RATIONALE Needed supplies are readily at hand.

2. **ACTION** Perform hand hygiene, identify the patient, provide privacy, explain the procedure, raise the bed to working height, and lower the near side rail if up.

   RATIONALE Ensures correct patient receives suppository. Teaches patient purpose of suppository. Allows easy access to the patient.

3. **ACTION** Place the patient in the left Sims' position and fold the top bedding obliquely back over the hips to expose the buttocks. Lower the pajama pants or fold the gown out of the way; turn on light so that anus will be easily visualized.

   RATIONALE Provides for easier insertion of suppository into rectum.

4. **ACTION** Put on gloves and open lubricant, squeezing it onto a paper towel. Remove foil wrapper from suppository and dip the point into the lubricant, being careful not to get it on your gloved fingers.

   RATIONALE Prepares suppository for insertion.

5. **ACTION** With the other hand, draw the top gluteal fold upward to expose the anus. Ask patient to take a deep breath through the mouth as you place the suppository into the anus (directed toward the umbilicus) with a slight twisting motion. Gently push the suppository along the wall of the anus up into the rectum with your index finger as far as you can reach. Withdraw your finger and hold both buttocks tightly together for a few seconds while the patient breathes deeply and the urge to expel the suppository has passed.

   RATIONALE Positions suppository above sphincter so it will not be immediately expelled. Urge to expel it will pass in a minute or so.

6. **ACTION** Wipe excess lubricant from anus. Instruct patient to try to hold the suppository in place for at least 20 minutes.

   RATIONALE Suppository will melt and deposit medication or stimulate the bowel within this time frame.

7. **ACTION** Remove the gloves and wrap them in the soiled paper towel; discard in proper waste container. Perform hand hygiene.

   RATIONALE Reduces transfer of microorganisms.

8. **ACTION** Document administration of the suppository and the outcome of its use.

   RATIONALE Provides data on success or failure of treatment.

Skill 34-3 | Administering Topical Skin Medications

Many types of topical medications can be applied to the skin. Lotions, ointments, creams, and patches are all used on the skin. The steps for medication administration must be followed when applying any topical medication.

■ Supplies

✓ Medication
✓ Disposable gloves

✓ Medication administration record (MAR)

✓ Tongue blade
✓ Waste container

Review and carry out the Standard Steps in Appendix 3.

■ Assessment (Data Collection)

1. **ACTION** Determine that ordered medication is on hand and that patient is available for the application and has already bathed.

   RATIONALE Saves time; prevents medication from being washed off.

2. **ACTION** Assess for any side or adverse effects of the medication.

   RATIONALE Further doses should not be applied if there is an adverse reaction.

■ Planning

3. **ACTION** Gather any dressing materials that may be needed.

   RATIONALE Promotes work efficiency.

4. **ACTION** Plan sufficient time to perform the application without interruption.

RATIONALE Time required for application depends on whether dressings are involved and the area to be treated.

■ Implementation

5. *ACTION* Check the medication against the MAR twice following the five rights of medication administration.

   RATIONALE Ensures giving the right drug in the right dose and applying it on the right location.

6. *ACTION* Identify the patient by checking the identification band with the MAR. Ask the patient to state her name.

   RATIONALE Ensures that the right patient receives the medication.

7. *ACTION* Perform hand hygiene and don gloves.

   RATIONALE Reduces transfer of microorganisms. Gloves also protect the nurse from absorbing medication through the hands.

To Apply Lotion

8. *ACTION* Place the medication bottle and supply of gauze dressings or cotton balls on a convenient working surface. Shake the bottle well; perform the third drug check with the MAR; remove the cap and place it upside down on the working surface.

   RATIONALE Prepares supplies for application. Third check of the drug helps prevent medication error.

9. *ACTION* Pick up a gauze dressing or cotton ball. With the bottle in your nondominant hand with the label facing upward, carefully pour the lotion onto the applicator. Catch excess solution in a basin, paper wrapper, or waste container.

   RATIONALE Keeping the label facing upward prevents soiling if some of the medicine drips down the side of the bottle while pouring. Applying the lotion to the gauze or cotton ball prevents spills.

10. *ACTION* Apply the lotion to the affected area by patting it on lightly. Do not rub. Repeat steps 9 and 10 until the area is covered, using a new applicator each time. Observe the skin for change in color, swelling, rash, and so on.

    RATIONALE Rubbing makes pruritus (itching) worse. Friction irritates lesions. Skin assessment must be documented.

11. *ACTION* Discard the gauze or cotton balls in the designated container; remove gloves and replace the cap on the lotion.

    RATIONALE Disposes of potentially infectious waste; preserves the medication.

For Application of Cream or Ointment

12. *ACTION* Apply the medication with a gloved finger or tongue blade to dry skin. Apply thin film in the direction of hair growth.

    RATIONALE A glove protects the nurse from absorbing the medication. A tongue blade will spread an even layer of ointment.

13. *ACTION* Apply a dressing if ordered.

    RATIONALE A dressing helps keep the cream or ointment on the skin.

For Antianginal Ointment

14. *ACTION* Measure out the correct amount of ointment on a paper measuring guide.

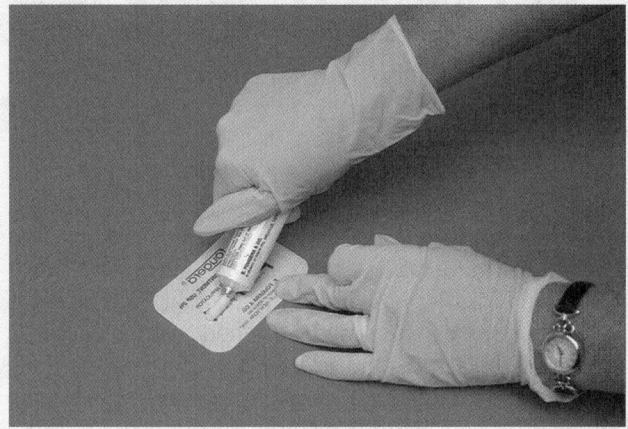

Step **14**

    RATIONALE The measurement must be exactly what is ordered.

15. *ACTION* Wash off any remaining ointment from a previous application.

    RATIONALE Remaining ointment would increase the dosage the patient is receiving.

16. *ACTION* Gently apply the paper to the patient's skin, distributing the ointment over about a 2-inch area, but not rubbing it into the skin. Rotate the site with each application; use the chest and upper arms so as to apply over as hairless an area as possible. Tape the paper in place around the edges, or place a piece of plastic wrap over the paper and tape it into place.

    RATIONALE Medication will slowly disperse into the skin and bloodstream. Hair may prevent contact of the ointment with the skin, decreasing absorption. Taping and/or covering the paper with plastic wrap protects the patient's clothing.

17. *ACTION* Remove gloves and perform hand hygiene; return medication to storage area.

    RATIONALE Reduces transfer of microorganisms; prepares medication for next use.

Continued

Skill 34-3 | Administering Topical Skin Medications—cont'd

■ Evaluation

18. **ACTION** Evaluate the skin for tolerance of the medication; assess for adverse effects. Assess for systemic therapeutic effect of antianginal ointment.

   RATIONALE Medication should not be continued if it is totally ineffective or if adverse effects occur.

■ Documentation

19. **ACTION** Document the medication dose on the MAR. Document the condition of the skin in the patient's chart.

   RATIONALE Verifies that the medication dose was given. Provides data for evaluation of effectiveness of medication.

Example

4/26 1045   Old nitroglycerin ointment removed from right anterior chest. Skin cleansed. No redness, or irritation noted. Patient advised that sites should be rotated and condition of the skin should be noted at each medication application change.

_____
(Nurse's signature)

?CRITICAL THINKING QUESTIONS

1. Why is it important to check the previous skin site where the medication patch was applied?

2. If the chest is covered with hair, where else can you apply the paste? Why should the previous area of application be wiped clean before applying the paste to a new spot?

Administering Medications via Feeding Tube

Many oral medications can be given through a feeding tube. Liquid medications are best, but if a tablet is crushable or a capsule can be opened and the contents mixed with liquid, or the liquid within the capsule can be aspirated with a needle and syringe, then the medication can be administered through the feeding tube. **Medications that should not be crushed and administered through the tube are sublingual or** **buccal, enteric-coated, or sustained-release preparations or products with a carcinogenic potential** (e.g., antineoplastics). For a small-bore tube, medications must be well dissolved in the liquid before administration. Do not mix the medication with a tube feeding because many things can interrupt or prevent delivery of the entire dose of medication. Skill 34-4 provides the steps for administering medications through a feeding tube.

Skill 34-4 | Administering Medications Through a Feeding Tube

When the patient cannot take anything by mouth, but has a feeding tube in place, oral medications can be administered through the tube. Liquid medications are best, but many medications may be crushed and mixed with water for administration. The medication dose must be followed by more water to irrigate the tube so that clogging does not occur. Each medication is mixed with water individually; medications are not combined so as to prevent clumping.

■ Supplies

✓ Medicine cup
✓ Pill crusher
✓ Warm water

✓ Syringe and needle
✓ Large irrigation syringe
✓ Disposable gloves

✓ Medication administration record (MAR)
✓ Medication(s)

Review and carry out the Standard Steps in Appendix 3.

■ Assessment (Data Collection)

1. **ACTION** Follow beginning procedures for the administration of oral medications by checking the order and assessing for allergies and adverse effects. Check the medications with the MAR, performing two checks before preparing each medication and one check after preparing each one.

   RATIONALE Follows the principles of the Five Rights of medication administration.

2. **ACTION** Assess for patency and position of the feeding tube.

   RATIONALE Follow correct procedure for verifying placement and patency of the feeding tube (see Chapter 27).

■ Planning

3. *ACTION* Verify that needed supplies are on hand. Fill a container with warm water.

   RATIONALE Procedure will not have to be stopped to gather supplies. Water is used to dissolve the medications.

4. *ACTION* Perform hand hygiene

   RATIONALE Medicines are prepared with aseptic technique.

5. *ACTION* Crush each medication to be given that comes in a tablet, if it can safely be crushed and administered. If medication is a liquid in a gel capsule, the liquid may be aspirated with a syringe and needle. For capsules containing powder, open the capsule and pour the powder into a medicine cup.

   RATIONALE Prepares medication for mixing with water.

■ Implementation

6. *ACTION* Mix each medication with 30 mL of warm water. Gelatin capsules may be dissolved by dropping the capsule into warm water and allowing to sit for 15 minutes.

   RATIONALE Prepares medications for administration because they must be liquid to traverse the tube.

7. *ACTION* Correctly identify the patient by checking the identification band with the name and hospital number on the MAR. Ask the patient to state his or her name if conscious and able.

   RATIONALE Prevents giving a medication to the wrong patient.

8. *ACTION* Place the patient in a high Fowler's position, unless contraindicated.

   RATIONALE Gravity helps medication progress down the tube into the stomach or small intestine. At least a 30-degree elevation of the head is essential.

9. *ACTION* Put on gloves and attach the irrigation syringe to the tube while keeping the tube pinched off.

   RATIONALE Readies the syringe to receive the water and medication. Prevents air from entering the tube.

10. *ACTION* Add 15 to 30 mL of water to the syringe and add the dissolved medication just as the water is about to finish entering the tube. If necessary, apply gentle pressure with the syringe plunger or bulb to instill the liquid.

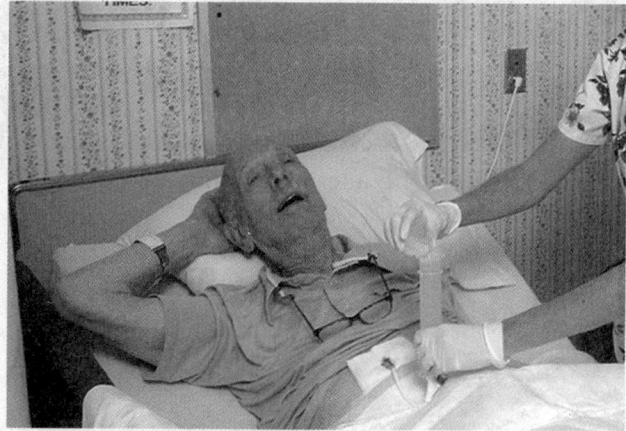

Step **10**

RATIONALE Water flushes tube feeding from the tube and decreases viscosity of fluid within the tube. Adding the medication before the syringe is empty prevents air from entering the tube. Pressure may be needed to initiate the flow.

11. *ACTION* Follow the first medication with at least 5 mL of water before administering the next one. Add next medication each time before the syringe is empty.

    RATIONALE Ensures that the various medications don't interact in the tube and clog it. Prevents air from entering the tube.

12. *ACTION* Follow the last medication with 30 to 60 mL of water. Pinch off the tube as the syringe empties.

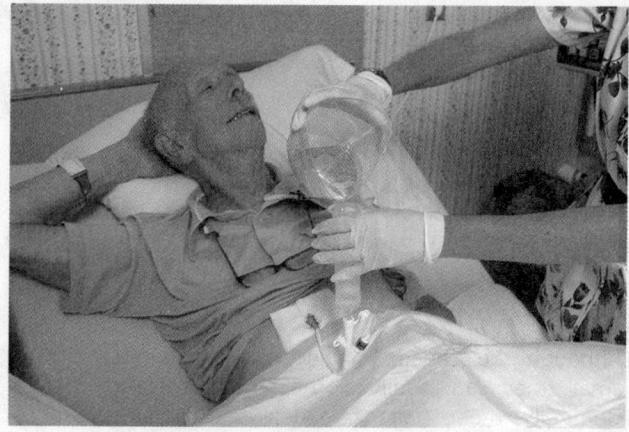

Step **12**

RATIONALE Water flushes the tube of all medication and ensures patency of tube. Pinching off the tube prevents air from entering tube.

13. *ACTION* Clamp or plug the tube for 30 minutes before reconnecting a decompression tube to suction. For a feeding tube, clamp it only if the medications cannot be mixed with food. Otherwise the tube may be reconnected to the tube feeding. If

Continued

Skill 34-4 | Administering Medications Through a Feeding Tube—cont'd

tube feedings are intermittent, the tube is simply left clamped.

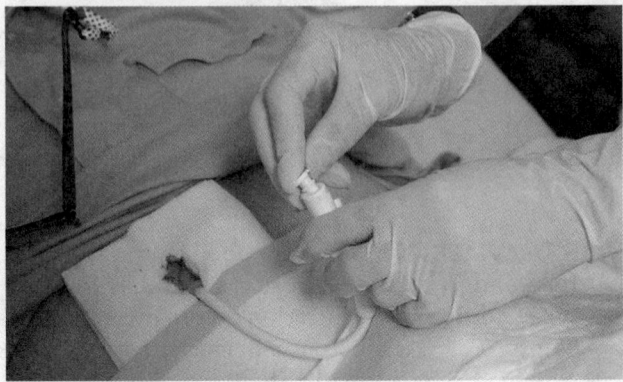

Step **13**

RATIONALE Prevents suctioning out the medication before it is absorbed. Prevents drug and food interactions. Reinitiates the tube feeding.

14. *ACTION* Leave the head of the bed elevated for at least 30 minutes, preferably for 60 minutes.

RATIONALE Prevents reflux of the medications back up the tube.

15. *ACTION* Clean up equipment, remove gloves, and perform hand hygiene.

RATIONALE Restores the unit. Reduces transfer of microorganisms.

■ Evaluation

16. *ACTION* Evaluate patency of the tube by visualizing free flow of liquid into it.

RATIONALE If liquid does not flow smoothly, tube may be becoming clogged and further irrigation may be needed.

17. *ACTION* Assess for adverse effects of the medication(s).

RATIONALE Assessment is performed before administering the next dose.

18. *ACTION* Evaluate for abdominal distention or nausea.

RATIONALE Medications may be irritating the stomach; if so, consult the physician.

■ Documentation

19. *ACTION* Document the doses given on the MAR.

RATIONALE Verifies that medications were given.

20. *ACTION* Enter the amount of fluid given on the intake portion of the I & O sheet.

RATIONALE Tracks patient's intake accurately.

21. *ACTION* Document any problems encountered in the patient's chart.

RATIONALE Records assessments and problems encountered.

?CRITICAL THINKING QUESTIONS

1. Your patient has an enteral tube in place and is to receive an enteric-coated medication. What should you do?

2. What would you do if the enteral tube becomes clogged and you can't get it to clear with the water irrigation?

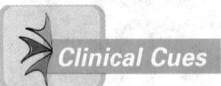

Although the "beads" inside a spansule appear very small, they can readily clog a small-bore feeding tube. Generally, these beads are designed for sustained release and should not be crushed or diluted. If your patient needs a sustained-release medication via feeding tube, consult with the pharmacist before administering the medication.

Evaluation

Only by gathering evaluation data can it be determined whether the medication is effective. Evaluation for signs of adverse effects is essential before administration of the next dose. Sometimes signs and symptoms will not appear until after the pre-scription has been finished. Evaluation statements might be as follows:

- Experienced nausea within 30 minutes of taking antibiotic.
- Refused antihistamine; itching has subsided.
- White blood cell count is 7000/mm³, temperature 99° F (37.2° C); antibiotic effective.
- Red rash on chest possibly from antibiotic; physician notified.
- Verbalizes that she will take antihypertensive even if she feels well.

Evaluation statements indicating that the expected outcomes stated earlier in the chapter have been met include:

- Pain is relieved for 3½ hours by analgesic.
- Blood pressure is within normal range (e.g., 130/74) while the patient is taking antihypertensive medication.

- Heart rate is regular and within normal limits (e.g., 70 to 85/min) while patient is taking antiarrhythmic medication.
- Wound culture is negative after 5 days of antibiotic therapy.
- No nausea when antiemetic is taken 30 minutes before eating a meal.
- Patient verbalizes that medication "controls my blood pressure."

Think Critically About . . . What would you do if your patient has been receiving an antibiotic for 6 days, but all your evaluation data indicate that the patient's condition has not improved?

Elder Care Points

Elderly patients who see more than one doctor sometimes have the same drug prescription with two different trade-name drugs. They then end up taking twice as much of the drug as they should be taking and suffer adverse effects or toxicity. Always ask to check all of the patient's prescription bottles; this contributes to the recommended process of medication reconciliation.

Documentation

Documentation of medication administration is largely done on the MAR. PRN medications, one-time doses, and preoperative medications may also be charted in the nurse's notes (follow agency policy). Data to be documented include the following:

- Medication name, dosage, route, and time administered
- Blood pressure and pulse before administration of antihypertensives and beta-blocker drugs
- Reason for a PRN medication's administration
- Assessment data regarding side effects of the medication
- Patient teaching regarding the medication (Home Care Considerations 34-1)
- Evaluation data indicative of the effectiveness of medication

MEDICATION ERRORS

In the United States, an estimated 1.5 million patients are harmed each year by medication errors (Metules & Bauer, 2007) in spite of all the safeguards. When a medication error is discovered, it is reported immediately. An incident or occurrence form is filled out for the medication error, and the agency policy for reporting drug errors is followed. After notifying the physician, orders are carried out to safeguard the patient. **All medication errors must be reported.**

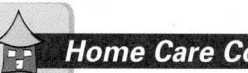

Home Care Considerations 34-1

Medication Administration for the Home Care Patient

- A 7-day medication planner container is helpful for the patient who is unreliable in taking medications or for one who has difficulty managing to remove the tops from medication vials (Figure 34-12). The patient can easily see if a medication has been taken. A friend or neighbor can be enlisted to help set up the medications once a week if the patient lives alone.
- All medication must be kept out of the reach of children. Even if children are not living in the home, this is a concern if any children visit.
- Expiration dates should be checked for all prescription and nonprescription medications in the home. Discard outdated medications.
- Assess use of over-the-counter medications when performing a medication history.
- Advise patients that if they are ordering prescriptions by mail, they need to inform the local pharmacist where they sometimes have prescriptions filled. The local pharmacy should have a complete list of everything the patient is taking so that drug interactions or overdosage can be prevented.
- If possible assess the patient's (or caregiver's) preparation of the medication to observe the methods and techniques being used.

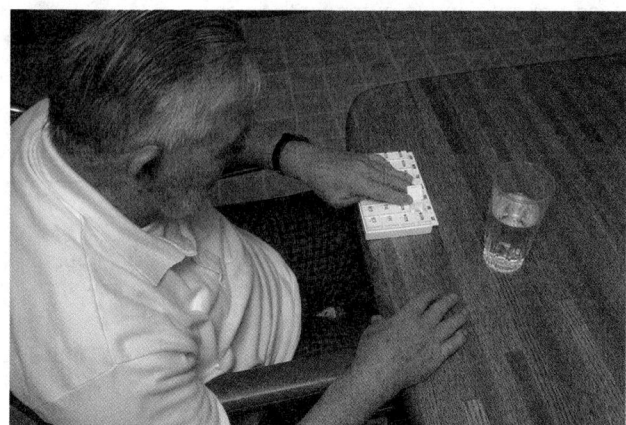

FIGURE **34-12** A 7-day medication planner helps the patient remember to take his medication.

The goal is to prevent harm to the patient from the error and to prevent similar errors from happening again. The nurse who discovers the error is the one to report it and fill out the report. Therefore, the nurse who made the error may not be the same nurse who reports it and fills out the occurrence form. In accordance with National Patient Safety Goals, health facilities and all health care workers should be supporting efforts to track and monitor adverse events to improve health care delivery systems.

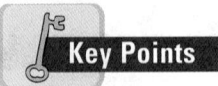
Key Points

- Because of the powerful effect medication has on the body, all medications must be administered very carefully following the five rights: the right drug in the right dose at the right time to the right patient by the right route.
- Medications should be administered only if the order is legally complete.
- You must only give the dosage of the medication ordered and it must be given by the route ordered.
- Most medications are given at routine scheduled times one, two, three, or four times a day.
- PRN medications are given at ordered intervals as the patient needs them; you may not give a lesser amount than that ordered.
- Stat orders are to be carried out immediately.
- Most narcotic orders are only good for 3 days and then must be renewed.
- All medication orders are stopped when a patient goes to surgery or undergoes general anesthesia for a procedure.
- Doses of medication administered are recorded on the MAR after the patient takes the medication.
- Medication orders are transcribed onto the MAR, the Kardex, the computer-generated nursing care plan, and/or medication cards.
- The unit-dose system is the most commonly used medication administration system in health care agencies.
- The prescription system is used in pharmacies in the community and in outpatient clinics.

- Controlled substances are kept in double-locked cabinets or drawers and are carefully counted and recorded when administered.
- Each medication should be checked three times before administering it.
- Topical medications come in the form of lotions, ointments, creams, suppositories, drops, patches, and aerosols.
- Sublingual medications are placed under the tongue; buccal medications are placed in the inner cheek pocket. These medications should not be swallowed.
- Ophthalmic medications are administered using surgical asepsis.
- Transdermal medications are administered in a sustained-release patch. The old patch should be removed before a new one is applied.
- A feeding tube is irrigated with a small amount of water between each medication and after the last medication is given. A decompression tube is clamped for 30 to 60 minutes before suction is turned back on after medications have been given.
- Medication errors should be reported promptly and actions taken to remedy the situation.

 Go to your **Companion CD-ROM** for an Audio Glossary, animations, video clips, and more.

evolve   Be sure to visit the companion Evolve site at http://evolve.elsevier.com/deWit/fundamental/ for additional online resources.

NCLEX-PN® EXAMINATION-STYLE REVIEW QUESTIONS

*Choose the **best** answer(s) for each question.*

1. The patient has returned from surgery several hours ago and is asking for pain medication. The nurse should give pain medication according to:
   1. admission orders.
   2. routine orders.
   3. postoperative orders.
   4. standing orders.

2. A nurse is caring for a patient who needs to have his morning dose of eyedrops to the right eye. Below are the steps for the procedure of instilling eyedrops. Place these steps (1 though 7) in the correct order.

   _____ 1. Document the doses given on the MAR.
   _____ 2. Stabilize the container above the eye over the conjunctival sac.
   _____ 3. Check the patient's ID band, comparing it with the MAR.
   _____ 4. Block the entrance to the lacrimal gland by placing a finger over it.
   _____ 5. Drop the designated number of drops directly into the conjunctival sac without touching the surface of the eye.

   _____ 6. Ask the patient to look at the ceiling and tilt the head slightly to the side of the affected eye.
   _____ 7. Place the patient in a sitting or reclining position.

3. The final check of a medication dose should be done:
   1. before leaving the medication cart or area.
   2. before opening the dose at the patient's bedside.
   3. after removing the medication from the drawer or supply.
   4. after administering the dose to the patient.

4. The nurse is performing the final check of the medication before administering it to the patient. Which information should be checked?
   1. Patient's name, birth date, room number, physician's name, and drug dosage
   2. Patient's name, ID number, drug name, dosage, route, time, and drug allergies
   3. Patient's name, drug classification, dosage and date, and allergies
   4. Patient's name, birth date, ID number, and admitting diagnosis

5. A nursing student is preparing to give instructions to a patient on how to use a metered-dose inhaler. Which statement by the student nurse indicates that she knows what to tell the patient?

1. "I tell the patient to wait 10 minutes between puffs."
2. "I teach him to close one nostril before depressing the canister."
3. "I have him take in a deep breath and hold it before placing the mouthpiece."
4. "I instruct him to inhale the medication and hold it for at least 10 seconds."

6. When giving ear medication to a child younger than 3 years, the technique is to:

1. draw the earlobe slightly down and back.
2. pull the top of the pinna upward and back.
3. rotate the pinna until the eardrum is visualized.
4. apply gentle pressure to the face to ease the tissue forward.

7. After preparation of a liquid medication, the patient refuses it. What is the most appropriate nursing action?

1. Record the medication as "not taken" and discard it.
2. Record the dose as taken because it must be charged.
3. Insist the patient take the medication.
4. Return the medication to the container.

8. A nurse is preparing to give morning medication and he identifies a discrepancy between what the night shift nurse said in the shift report and what is written on the medication administration record (MAR). Which action would be the most appropriate?

1. Give the medication according to the MAR.
2. Call the night shift nurse at home.
3. Consult with the pharmacist and the charge nurse.
4. Compare the MAR with the physician's order sheet.

9. An ambulatory surgery patient is to be discharged home and needs six doses of analgesic tablets for discomfort. What is the most appropriate nursing action?

1. Dispense six tablets from the controlled-substance dispenser.
2. Obtain a written prescription for the medication.
3. Call the hospital pharmacist to fill the order.
4. Ask the patient to call the physician's office for the prescription.

10. A patient reports that he is taking an aspirin every day "to prevent heart attack" as well as Ecotrin (enteric-coated aspirin). Which nursing action is the priority?

1. Tell him to stop taking either the aspirin or the Ecotrin.
2. Tell him to call his physician or his pharmacist for clarification.
3. Collect additional data about his health history.
4. Give him a pamphlet about Ecotrin and explain drug–drug interactions.

CRITICAL THINKING ACTIVITIES *Read each clinical scenario and discuss the questions with your classmates.*

Scenario A
You are in the medication room preparing medications for your patients when a nurse who is standing next to you is called to take a patient to another nursing unit. She shows you the medications she has prepared for one of her patients and asks you to please administer them so they will not be given late.

1. What do you say? How can this situation be handled so that the patient receives needed medications on time?

Scenario B
Dan Hartford is receiving ampicillin for a respiratory infection. When you go in to give him the next dose, you notice that his face seems to have a red rash on it. When you question him, he states he has been itching a little across his chest and on his legs.

1. What specifically would you do?

Scenario C
Connie Simonelli is to receive 15 mL of Mylanta II, a liquid antacid medication.

1. How would you measure the correct amount of liquid medication?

Scenario D
You go into a room to give Florence Tolstoy her medication. When you ask to check her armband, you find that she does not have one on.

1. What do you do? How can you properly identify the patient?

Administering Intradermal, Subcutaneous, and Intramuscular Injections

evolve http://evolve.elsevier.com/deWit/fundamental/

Being asked to give an injection (forcing fluid into a part) to another person makes many student nurses very apprehensive. Giving an injection means the possibility of causing pain. Focusing on the beneficial effect that the medication brings to the patient will help ease your apprehension. Developing dexterity in giving injections in the nursing skill laboratory before approaching a patient with a needle and syringe greatly decreases nervousness. Considerable practice time is required to learn how to manipulate syringes, handle vials (small bottles), accurately measure doses, and skillfully insert needles in the appropriate sites. In this chapter, you are introduced to different types of needles and syringes, the methods for withdrawing sterile solutions from vials and ampules (all-glass containers containing medication), and the sites for injections. Step-by-step procedures are outlined for the intramuscular (IM) (into the muscle), subcutaneous (beneath the skin layers), and intradermal (ID) (into the dermis) routes of administration. Intravenous administration techniques are discussed in Chapter 36.

PRINCIPLES OF PARENTERAL INJECTIONS

Parenteral (not via the gastrointestinal tract) routes require the use of a syringe and needle, or intravenous catheter, to introduce medications into the body tissues or fluids. Medications that are given parenterally must be sterile, nonallergenic to the patient, and readily absorbable. Injections are given for the following purposes:

- When the patient cannot take medication by mouth
- To hasten the action of the drug
- When digestive juices would counteract the effects of the drug if given by the oral route

Once drugs are injected into the body, they cannot be retrieved. It is therefore essential to observe these precautions:

- Ensure that the dose is accurate.
- Select the correct site to prevent damage to the tissue.
- Use sterile equipment and aseptic technique to prevent infection/sepsis.

The parenteral routes involve injecting medications into various layers of the skin or into veins. The skin is the body's protective covering, acting as a barrier between the person and the environment. The outer layer, or epithelium, is continually sloughing off dying cells. Below the epidermis is the dermis, or true skin, which contains hair follicles, sweat glands, sebaceous glands, blood vessels, and nerve endings (Figure 35-1). Combined, these layers of the skin are 1 to 2 mm in thickness. Directly below the dermis is the subcutaneous or hypodermal layer of connective tissue (also known as superficial fascia), which contains varying amounts of fat cells. In some parts of the body, the subcutaneous layer may be more than 3 cm thick. It anchors the skin to the underlying organs. While not often considered a part of the integument, the subcutaneous layer has considerable interconnectivity with the dermis. The skin has an extensive lymphatic and capillary system; the latter plays a major role in the absorption of medications. The more vascular the tissue, the quicker the medication is absorbed.

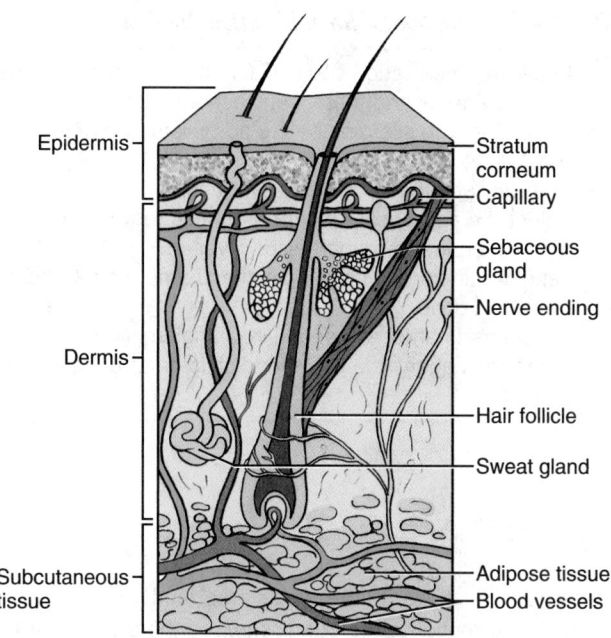

FIGURE **35-1** Structure of the skin.

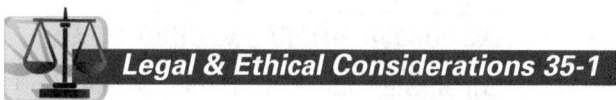

Legal & Ethical Considerations 35-1

Use of Placebos or Misrepresentation of Dosing

A **placebo** (substance that has no actual pharmacologic effect) may be ordered for your patient; however, use of placebos is highly controversial. If a patient believes that a treatment is efficacious, this belief can facilitate positive outcomes; however if the patient is not fully informed, this is a violation of his rights. "Nurses are ethically obligated to refuse to carry out a physician's orders to give a placebo if the patient hasn't been informed." (Grace, 2006, p. 60).

Another situation that you may encounter is the practice of intentional misrepresenting the dose given to the patient. For example, the patient is aware that he is allowed to have up to 3 mg of morphine for pain. The nurse draws up 1 mg, adds normal saline to the syringe to make the dose appear larger and then tells the patient that there is 3 mg of morphine in the syringe. The nurse may believe that the patient is addicted to the medication, or may fear that the patient will have ill effects from the higher dose. Regardless of the nurse's motivation, lying to the patient about the dosage is an unethical practice.

Accuracy and care must be used in preparing and administering any parenteral medication because errors can harm the patient (Legal & Ethical Considerations 35-1). The wrong site or route may cause damage to a major nerve or blood vessel. Contamination of the equipment or the medication may cause infection or abscess formation. Box 35-1 presents the principles that must be observed for safe and effective administration of parenteral medications.

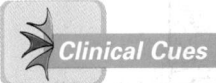

Clinical Cues

Repeated injections in the same area lead to scarring or fibrosis (formation of fibrous tissue), so the sites must be rotated.

ROUTES FOR PARENTERAL MEDICATION

The intradermal, subcutaneous, intramuscular, and intravascular routes are used for parenteral medication administration (Figure 35-2). The intravenous route is covered in Chapter 36.

INTRADERMAL ROUTE

The intradermal (ID) route, which deposits small amounts of drug solution into the dermal layer, is used extensively for skin testing, such as tuberculin testing, generally on the inner surface of the forearm. The tuberculin syringe (syringe with graduated measurements to 1 mL) is used to measure these small dosages. A fine 25-, 27-, or 29-gauge (scale of measurement) needle is used at a 5- to 15-degree angle of insertion. This creates a pool of medication under the thin layer of skin that forms a bleb (bump; visible elevation of the epidermis).

SUBCUTANEOUS ROUTE

The subcutaneous route is used for injecting medication into the tissues below the dermal layer of the skin, usually in the upper portion of the upper outer arm, the anterior surface of the thigh, or the abdomen where there are no major vessels or nerves. Small amounts of solution (0.05 to 1.0 mL in volume; see agency policy) are injected subcutaneously with either a tuberculin or 3-mL syringe. A 27-gauge, ⅜- to ½-inch, or a 25-gauge, ⅝-inch needle is used. The needle is inserted at a 45- or 90-degree angle depending on needle length and the size of the individual.

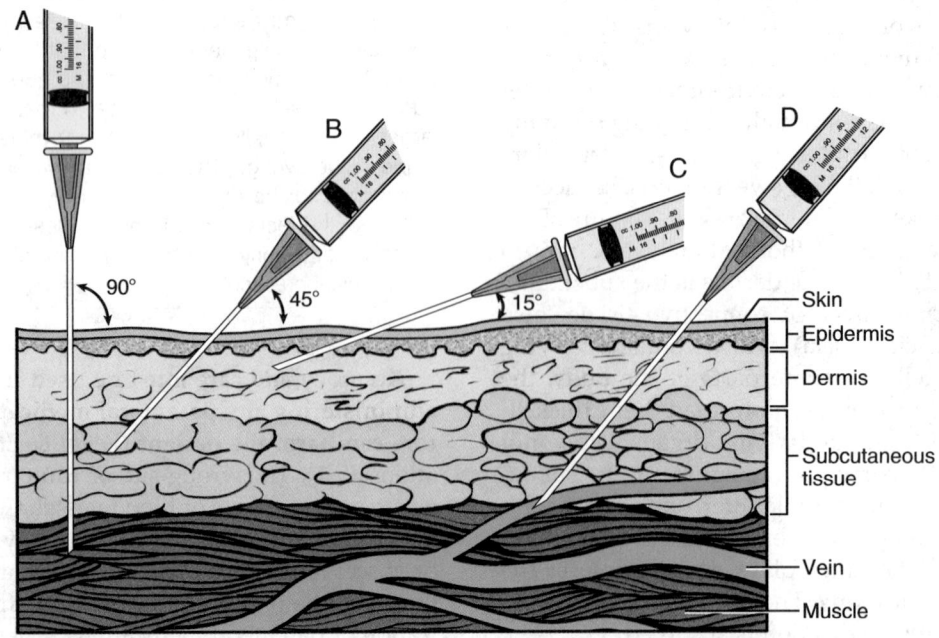

FIGURE **35-2** Injection routes. **A,** Intramuscular. **B,** Subcutaneous. **C,** Intradermal. **D,** Intravenous.

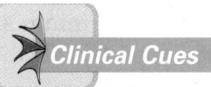
Clinical Cues

An obese person will require a longer needle than one who is normal weight; a very thin person requires a shorter needle. Evidenced-based practice (Diggle, 2007) suggests that health professionals often use needles that are too short in the mistaken belief that is it kinder to the patient; however, "problems can arise if drugs designed to be absorbed from muscle are only delivered into subcutaneous tissue" (Zaybak et al., 2007, p. 552).

Absorption time is slower than with an intramuscular injection owing to the lack of blood vessels in this area as compared with muscle. These sites are used for medications that are to be absorbed slowly for sustained action.

INTRAMUSCULAR ROUTE

Using the intramuscular (IM) route means medication is injected in the muscular layer (Cultural Cues 35-1). The most frequently used IM sites are the deltoid, ventrogluteal, vastus lateralis, and rectus femoris of the thigh. The angle of injection is 90 degrees, and depending on the size of the patient, a needle from 1 to 3 inches in length is used. For most IM injections, the nurse would aspirate for blood (pull back on the syringe plunger to create suction) before injecting the medication, to avoid injecting directly into a blood vessel. The absorption time for IM medications chiefly depends on the form of the drug; aqueous solutions are absorbed more rapidly than those in an oil suspension.

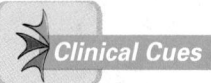
Clinical Cues

Up to 3 mL can be safely injected in the ventrogluteal, vastus lateralis, and rectus femoris sites in any patient; larger amounts may be given in one injection in a large adult muscle in some instances (see agency policy).

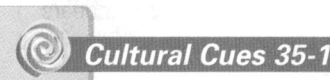
Cultural Cues 35-1

Belief in Needles

Your patient may believe that a medication is more effective if it is given as a "shot" rather than a pill or capsule.

INJECTION EQUIPMENT

TYPES OF SYRINGES

Syringes are composed of a barrel that has a tip to which the needle is attached and a plunger that fits inside the barrel (Figure 35-3). The needle, the tip, the inside of the barrel, and the sides of the plunger must be kept sterile.

Syringes are made of plastic or glass. The plastic ones are disposable, whereas glass syringes can be re-sterilized and reused. Disposable syringes are used almost exclusively in North America because they are convenient, safe, and economical (Figure 35-4). Nursing units are supplied with various sizes of syringes.

The 3-mL syringe is popular because it is large enough for subcutaneous and most IM injections given by the nurse. The U-100 syringe is used with U-100–strength insulin (Figure 35-5). The insulin needle is part of the syringe and not removable. The insulin syringe is calibrated in units, and sometimes has a milliliter scale on it as well. A minipen is available for self-administration of insulin (Patient Teaching 35-1). Tuberculin (TB) syringes are 1 mL in size and are calibrated to measure as small as 0.01-mL drug doses (Figure 35-6). They also have measurement markings for minims.

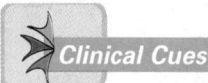
Clinical Cues

Small-gauge syringes such as the tuberculin syringe and the insulin syringe are easily confused and misread. Carefully examine the medication order and the scale on the syringe to ensure that you are interpreting the order correctly and using the right syringe and the right scale.

A number of injectable medications are supplied in unit-dose cartridge form. These require a special holder for the cartridge and needle in order to administer the injection. Typical unit-dose cartridges and holders include the Carpuject and Tubex systems.

MEASUREMENT SCALES

Each syringe is calibrated and the measurements are marked on the barrel so that the amount of medication can be measured accurately. The syringe chosen for the

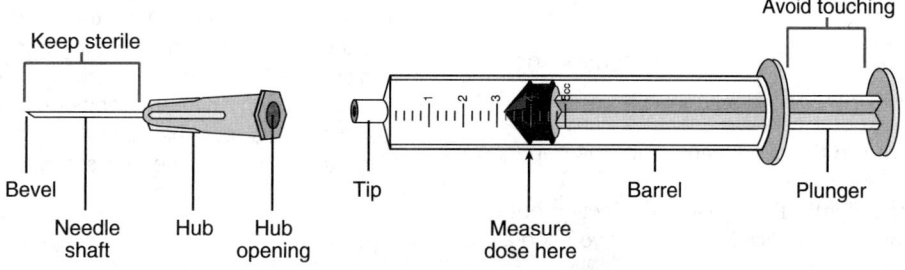

FIGURE **35-3** Parts of a syringe.

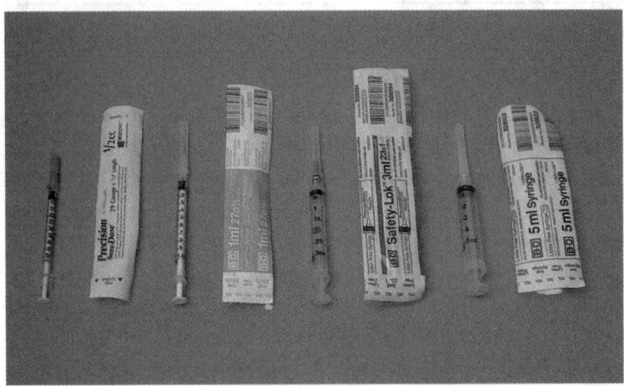

FIGURE **35-4** Disposable syringes.

injection must have a measurement scale that is appropriate for the required dose of medication. **Most 3-mL syringes have two scales: one scale measures tenths of a milliliter (0.1 mL) and the other is a minim scale** (Figure 35-7). Although the 0.1-mL scale is accurate for tenths of a milliliter, it is not appropriate or accurate to measure doses in hundredths, such as 0.25 mL. A TB syringe easily measures this amount. Because there are 16 minims per milliliter, the minim scale can be used to measure 0.25- and 0.75-mL doses

when the 3-mL syringe is used (0.25 mL = 4 minims and 0.75 mL = 12 minims). However, it is preferable to use a TB syringe for such small doses.

NEEDLE GAUGE AND LENGTH

A needle is a metal tube through which liquid medication flows. It consists of a hub fitting onto the end of a syringe, a hollow shaft (also called a **cannula**), and a bevel (slanted part of the needle tip) ending in a sharp point. The inner part of the cannula is the lumen (opening or interior diameter). Most needles are disposable and are discarded after use. Steel needles may be cleaned, sterilized, and reused.

Needles are available in standard sizes measured in gauge from 13 to 30, although each agency does not buy all sizes; Figure 35-8 shows the most commonly used sizes. **The larger the number of the gauge, the smaller the needle.** Because an intradermal injection goes under the epidermis (the outer layer of skin), a 25-, 27-, or 29-gauge needle works best. The 25-gauge needle is strong enough to puncture the skin and reach below the dermis for subcutaneous injections. Heavier-duty 20-, 21-, 22-, and 23-gauge needles are needed to penetrate the large muscle layers when IM injections are given in those sites.

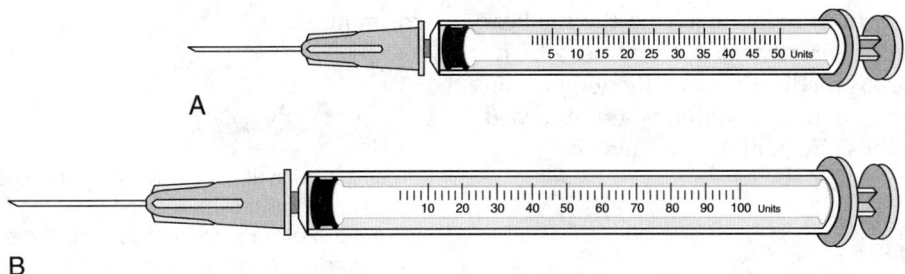

FIGURE **35-5** Insulin syringes. **A,** A 50-unit syringe. **B,** A 100-unit syringe.

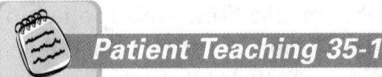

Patient Teaching 35-1

How to Use the Minipen (Humulin or Humalog)

The minipen is a convenient, safe way to administer insulin. It is lightweight, can be carried in a pocket or purse, and needs no refrigeration after the first use. The minipen is dispensed with 300 units of the most commonly prescribed insulin. To use a minipen:
- Be sure the needle is firmly attached to the pen. Use a new needle every time you use the pen for an injection.

PRIMING THE PEN
- Pull out the dose knob and turn it clockwise until a "0" appears in the dose window.
- Now turn the dose knob clockwise until a "2" appears.
- Remove the cover from the needle and point the pen upward.
- Tap the plastic barrel lightly, then push the injection button down all the way until a click is heard and you see a drop of insulin at the needle tip.

- Turn the dose knob clockwise until the arrow appears in the dose window. Pull out the dose knob. A "0" will appear in the window.
- Dial the correct number of units for your dose of insulin.
- If you dial up too large a dose, turn the dose knob backward until the correct dose appears in the dose window.

INJECTION, DISPOSAL, AND STORAGE
- Choose the injection site and insert the needle straight into the skin; press the injection button. Count to 5 slowly before you remove the needle. A click will be heard when the injection is complete.
- Replace the outer needle shield. Unscrew the capped needle and appropriately dispose of it as instructed. (Used needles are a biohazard.)
- Place the cap on the pen for storage.

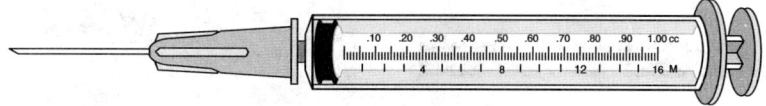

FIGURE **35-6** Tuberculin syringe.

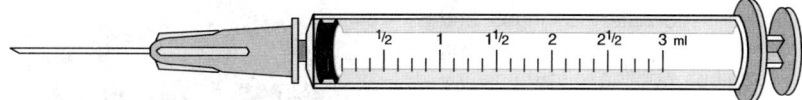

FIGURE **35-7** Measurement scale on a 3-mL syringe.

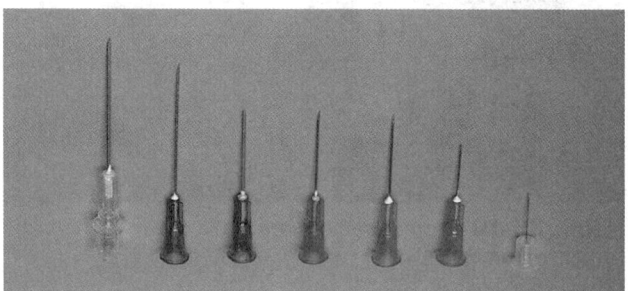

FIGURE **35-8** Various needle sizes.

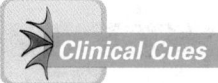

Filter needles should be used for preparing medication from an ampule because small particles of glass may fall into the medication when the ampule neck is removed. The filter in the needle traps such particles.

The length of the needle is measured from its beveled tip to the junction of the shaft and the hub. Most often 1-inch or 1½-inch needles are used for adult parenteral injections. Adult IM injections frequently use 22- and 23-gauge needles, although 20- and 21-gauge needles are preferred for viscous (sticky or gummy) solutions or medications in oil suspensions.

PREVENTING NEEDLE STICKS

A needle stick occurs any time a needle accidentally pricks the skin. The danger of the spread of human immunodeficiency virus (HIV), hepatitis B virus, and hepatitis C virus has created much concern about needle safety. Safety syringes are available that have a sheath that covers the needle as it is withdrawn from the skin, totally eliminating the possibility of a needle stick injury (Figure 35-9). There are a variety of safety syringes on the market. The Occupational Safety and Health Administration (OSHA) requires that they be used in most situations in all states. Sometimes a regular syringe and needle are used to draw up potentially irritating medications; the needle is then changed to a safety needle before injection to eliminate the possibility of depositing medication in surface tissue.

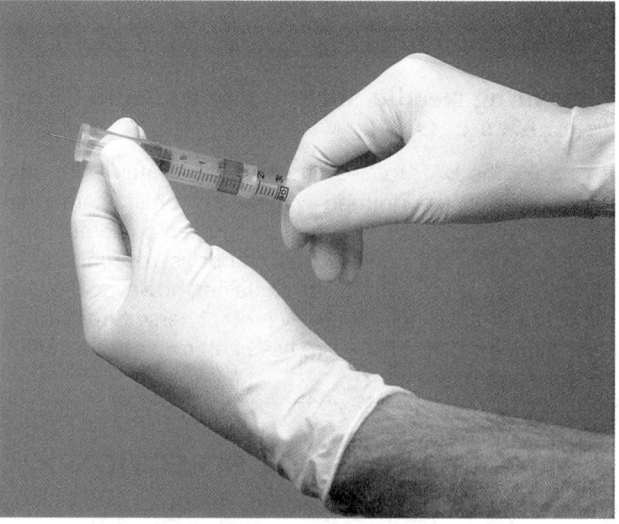

FIGURE **35-9** Needle with protective sheath.

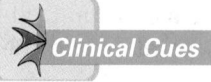

If you are in a situation in which you had to use a syringe without a safety needle and it seems more prudent to recap the needle than to transport it uncapped to another location for disposal in a sharps container, use a one-hand scoop technique. The needle cap is placed on a flat, firm surface, preferably with the closed end of the needle cover against an object. With one hand holding the syringe barrel, slide the needle into the needle cap. The cap is secured by pushing it against a vertical surface (e.g., the drawer front on the bedside table, the wall, or a door), never the other hand.

If a needle stick occurs, report to the charge nurse immediately, complete an incident/occurrence report, and follow agency policy for the incident (Safety Alert 35-1). The area of the puncture is washed thoroughly with soap and water, and agency protocol is instituted for treatment and follow-up. **You should attempt to develop a conscious awareness of where contaminated needles might be left or carried in the immediate environment by other health care workers to prevent needle stick injuries** (Assignment Considerations 35-1).

Safety Alert 35-1

Reducing Needle Stick Injuries

In *Healthy People 2010,* objective 20-10 is to "reduce occupational needle stick injuries among health care workers." To help prevent needle sticks when nonsafety syringes and needles are used, *needles are not recapped.* All syringes and needles are dropped into a sharps container immediately after use (Figure 35-10).

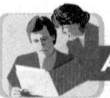

Assignment Considerations 35-1

Preventing Needle Sticks Among Health Care Team Members

If you ask the UAP to clean up or remove equipment after the physician has performed a procedure, remind her to look for sharps first, rather than to pick up used equipment in a bundle. Each person who uses sharps is responsible for placing them in the appropriate container; however, the UAP should be directed to proactively protect herself from an accidental needle stick if a sharp has been overlooked and left on the equipment tray.

SYRINGE AND NEEDLE SELECTION

In preparing to give an injection, the first step is to select the appropriate size and type of needle and syringe for the medication to be given and for the patient's age and size. Today the needle and syringe are usually supplied in a preassembled safety unit, although some agencies stock them separately and the desired types can be selected.

Guidelines for types of needles and syringes have been established for the various methods of injecting parenteral medications. For giving IM injections, the 3-mL syringe and a 22-gauge, 1½-inch needle are generally used. A tuberculin or 3-mL syringe and a 27-gauge, ⅜- to ½-inch, or a 25-gauge, ⅝-inch needle are used to give a subcutaneous injection. These sizes are modified as necessary to accommodate different medications, doses, and patient needs.

? *Think Critically About . . .* What size syringe and needle would you use to give 2 mL of medroxyprogesterone (Depo-Provera), an oil-based suspension, intramuscularly to a 135-lb female?

PREPARING THE SYRINGE FOR USE

When preparing syringes for use (Steps 35-1), you should be sure to observe these principles:

- Use aseptic technique in handling the syringe and needle. Protect the surfaces that must remain sterile: the needle, tip, inner barrel, and plunger.

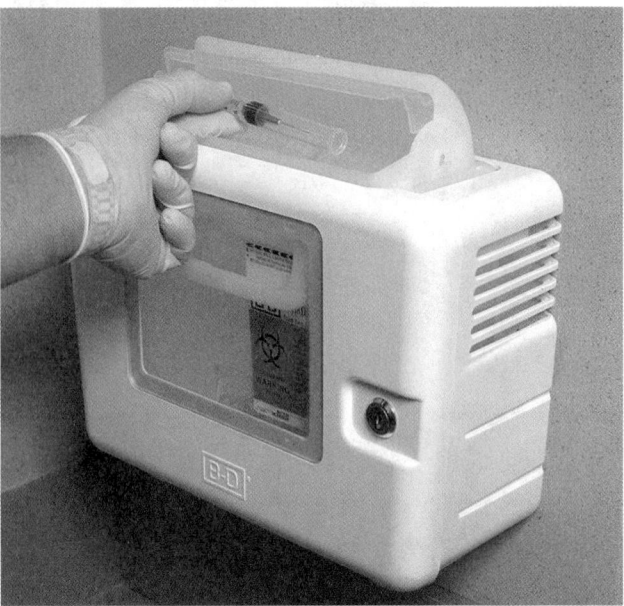

FIGURE **35-10** Drop a used syringe into a sharps biohazard container immediately.

Safety Alert 35-2

Label Syringes and Other Containers

In accordance with the 2009 National Patient Safety Goals, when medication is removed from the original container and placed in a syringe or medication cup, it should be clearly labeled. Use a piece of tape or obtain a label stamped with the patient's name and ID number, write the name of the drug and the dosage on it, and attach it to the syringe or medication cup to ensure right drug, right dose, and right patient.

- Discard the syringe or needle if it becomes contaminated during drug preparation for administration.
- Label the syringe with the patient's name, name of medication, and dose (Safety Alert 35-2).

PARENTERAL SOLUTIONS

Medications for injection are dispensed in various kinds of units: glass ampules containing a single dose, single-dose vials, mix-o-vials, and multiple-dose vials (Figure 35-11). The mix-o-vial contains powder in the base and solution in the top, which are mixed together for use. The unit-dose cartridge consists of a vial with an attached needle for use with the Carpuject or Tubex holder (Figure 35-12). Parenteral medications must be kept sterile.

Steps 35-1 Preparing a Syringe for Use

Disposable syringes are packaged in a paper wrapper or are encased in plastic to protect their sterility. The Tubex cartridge must be attached to the plunger, and the Carpuject cartridge is inserted and fastened into a syringe mechanism.

■ To Remove Protective Wrapping

1. **ACTION** Perform hand hygiene and select the desired size and type of syringe.

   RATIONALE Maintains asepsis; ensures that appropriate syringe will be used.

2. **ACTION** For a paper-wrapped syringe, peel open the wrapper while maintaining asepsis.

   RATIONALE The inside of the syringe and the needle must be kept sterile.

3. **ACTION** For a rigid plastic casing, twist the plastic cap counterclockwise and remove it; slide the cover down off of the barrel of the syringe. When ready, remove the protective cover from the needle by pulling it straight off.

   RATIONALE The barrel of the syringe and the protected needle slip out of the top of the plastic sheath.

■ For the Tubex Holder and Cartridge

1. **ACTION** Obtain the unit-dose cartridge and the cartridge holder.

   RATIONALE Both parts are needed to assemble the syringe.

2. **ACTION** Turn the ribbed collar to the "open" position until it stops.

   RATIONALE Prepares the unit to receive the cartridge.

3. **ACTION** Hold the injector with the open end up and fully insert the cartridge–needle unit. Firmly tighten the ribbed collar in the direction of the "close" arrow.

   RATIONALE Secures the cartridge in the injector.

4. **ACTION** Check that medication in the cartridge is the dose ordered and remove any excess air.

   RATIONALE Prepares the cartridge for the injection.

■ For the Carpuject System

1. **ACTION** Pull out the plunger on the holder mechanism. Insert the cartridge into the holder from the side, sliding the needle through the bottom opening.

   RATIONALE Positions the cartridge in the holder mechanism.

2. **ACTION** Twist the cartridge to lock it at the needle end.

   RATIONALE Stabilizes the cartridge in the holder mechanism.

3. **ACTION** Place the end of the plunger against the screw end of the cartridge and turn the plunger clockwise until fastened.

   RATIONALE Fastens the plunger to the cartridge so that aspiration is possible.

4. **ACTION** Remove unwanted excess medication or air from the unit.

   RATIONALE The order may not call for a full dose of the medication; excess air may be present in the cartridge.

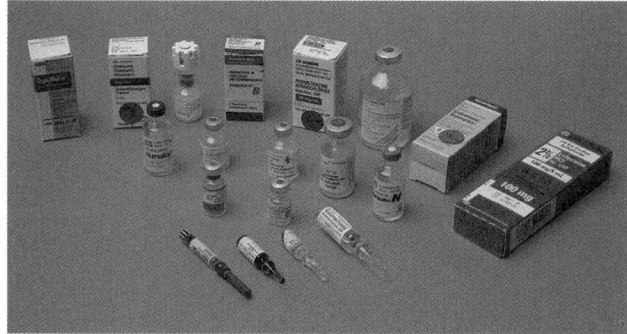

FIGURE **35-11** Containers of parenteral medication.

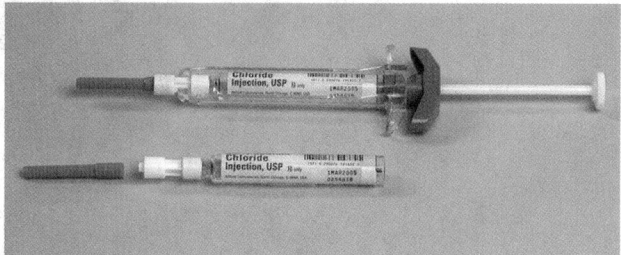

FIGURE **35-12** Carpuject cartridge and holder.

USING A MEDICATION AMPULE

Ampules are made entirely of glass or polyurethane and contain a single standard dose of the medication. Most ampules are prescored on the neck so that the glass will break more evenly with slight pressure at that portion. If the ampule is not prescored, a small file is used to etch a breaking line.

Before opening an ampule, the medication must be removed from the neck or stem of the ampule, or some will be wasted when the ampule is opened. To move the medication, tap or flick the stem several times with a finger to free the trapped solution (Figure 35-13).

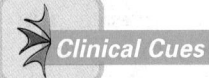

Clinical Cues

Before breaking open the ampule, you should wrap the neck with the rubber ampule guard, an unopened alcohol swab, or a gauze pad to avoid accidental cuts. The thumbs are pressed outward against the neck so the ampule will break outward away from you.

The open ampule is handled very carefully when withdrawing the medication with the filter needle (Figure 35-14). The open ampule may be stabilized on a flat surface for withdrawal of the drug when a

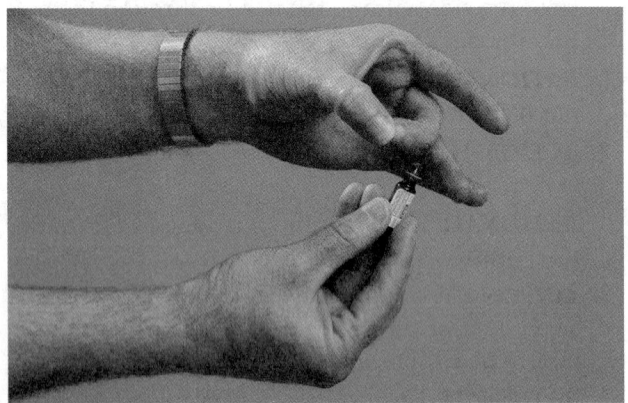

FIGURE **35-13** Moving fluid from the neck of the ampule.

long needle is used. If a short needle is used, the ampule may be inverted to withdraw the correct dose. The needle must be beneath the surface of the solution in order to withdraw it. Medication in an ampule is packaged in a specific amount per milliliter (Steps 35-2).

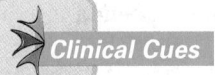

Clinical Cues

Usually an amount more than the total indicated amount is contained in the ampule in the event of spillage. **Carefully verify that the exact amount ordered is in the syringe before giving the injection.**

USING A MEDICATION VIAL

A vial is a small bottle with a rubber stopper attached by a metal band. A vial may contain one or more doses of medication. Single-dose vials are small, usually 1 or 2 mL in size; multiple-dose vials are 5, 10, 20, or 30 mL in size or larger. The desired amount of medication is removed by inserting the needle of the syringe through the rubber stopper into the liquid with the vial inverted and drawing up the solution (Figure 35-15).

When the needle is inserted into the vial, care must be taken to avoid coring the stopper. The sharp edges of the needle can create a small core (circular cut-out piece) that can be pushed into the bottle. A core can plug the needle or become a source of contamination (Steps 35-3).

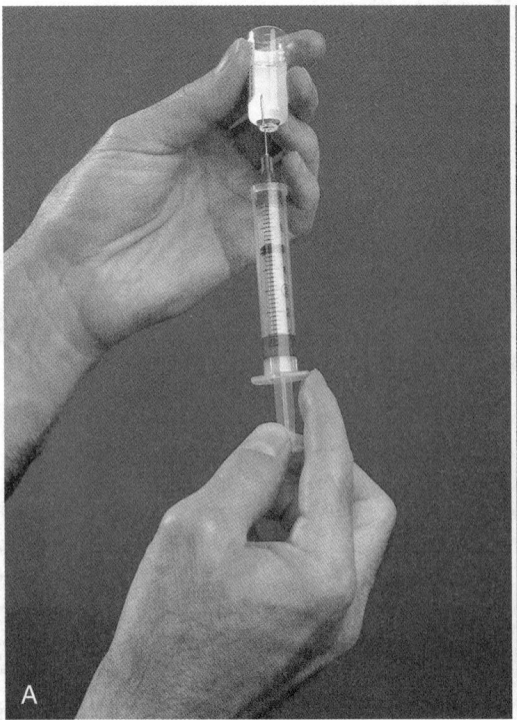

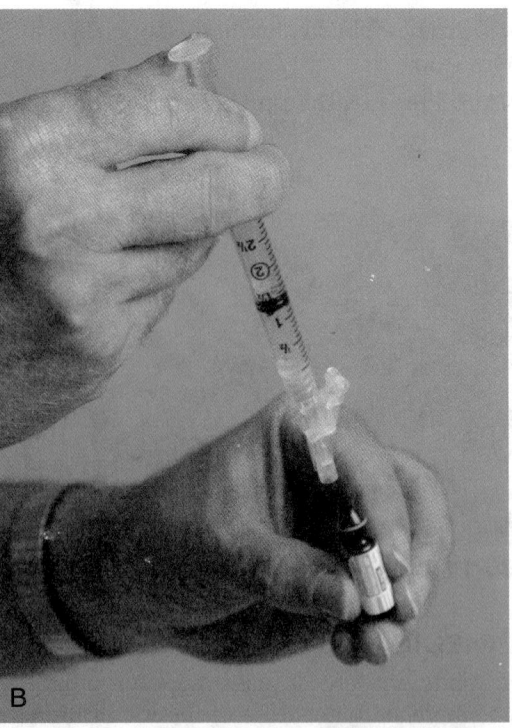

FIGURE **35-14** Withdrawing fluid from an ampule. **A,** Ampule inverted. **B,** Ampule upright and stabilized.

Steps 35-2 | Withdrawing Medication from an Ampule

A variety of medications are packaged in ampules. The ampule neck must be broken and removed to extract the medication. A filter needle must be used to withdraw the medication.

1. *ACTION* After checking the medication order and performing any calculation necessary for the correct dose, perform hand hygiene.

   RATIONALE Checking the order and careful calculation of dosage prevents medication error; performing hand hygiene reduces transfer of microorganisms.

2. *ACTION* Dislodge any fluid from the stem of the ampule by tapping the stem or by holding the ampule upside down and then quickly inverting it.

   RATIONALE These techniques move the fluid from the stem into the ampule.

3. *ACTION* Break the neck of the ampule by using an ampule breaker or wrap the neck with gauze or an alcohol swab, place both your thumbs together at the neck, and apply outward pressure to snap the top off away from you.

   RATIONALE Allows access to withdraw the medication. Breaking the neck outward prevents glass splinters from flying into the eyes or skin.

4. *ACTION* Remove the needle from the syringe and replace it with a sterile filter needle. Keep the regular needle sterile for later replacement on the syringe.

   RATIONALE Prepares the syringe and needle for drawing up medication from the ampule. The filter needle will trap any glass particles and keep them out of the syringe. The filter needle is replaced by the regular needle after the medication is drawn up.

5. *ACTION* Place the needle into the solution without touching the neck of the ampule. Keeping the bevel of the needle below the surface of the solution, pull back on the syringe plunger with your dominant hand to the correct amount line on the measuring scale.

   a. *ACTION* Place the ampule on a flat surface, insert the needle into the ampule close to the bottom of the medication, and withdraw the desired dose of medication.

   RATIONALE Prevents spilling solution from the ampule while it is inverted. This method requires a steady hand so as not to tip the ampule while drawing up the medication.

   b. *ACTION* Alternatively, hold the ampule between your thumb and middle or index finger of the nondominant hand and, with the needle inserted into the solution, invert the ampule while you grasp the syringe with your thumb and index finger of the dominant hand; rest the barrel of the syringe on the pad of the palm of the nondominant hand (Figure 33-14).

   RATIONALE This hold stabilizes the ampule while the syringe is used to draw up the medication. Keeping the bevel in the solution prevents drawing up air. This method is useful when a short needle will not reach the bottom of the ampule. Surface tension keeps the solution from leaking out of the ampule while it is inverted.

6. *ACTION* Expel air bubbles from the syringe by drawing more air into the syringe to make a larger bubble; then, holding the syringe with the needle upright, tap with your finger to move the air bubble toward the needle, and push the plunger to expel the air. Stop when one drop of liquid appears in the bevel of the needle. Ascertain that the dosage is correct.

   RATIONALE Air in the syringe interferes with preparation of the exact dosage ordered.

7. *ACTION* Change back to the sterile needle that was removed from the syringe.

   RATIONALE Prevents glass particles caught in filter needle from entering the patient.

8. *ACTION* Label the syringe with the patient's name, the name of the drug, and the dosage.

   RATIONALE When a medication is removed from the original container or vial, labeling the new container (syringe, medication cup, etc.) prevents accidentally giving the wrong drug to the wrong patient.

Clinical Cues

To avoid coring, it is recommended that the needle be inserted at a slight angle with a forward thrust while simultaneously exerting a slight lateral pressure until the needle has pierced the rubber stopper.

RECONSTITUTION OF A DRUG

Drugs that are unstable in solution are prepared in a powdered or solid form. The solute (solid material) in the vial is mixed with a diluent (specified fluid to dissolve the solute) before the drug is drawn up into a syringe. Sterile water and sterile normal saline are typical diluents. The label or the drug insert pack-

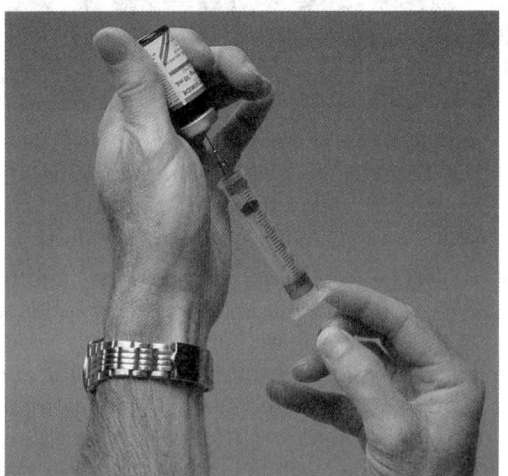

FIGURE **35-15** Drawing medication from a vial.

aged with the vial provides instructions about the type of diluent to use and the proper amount to mix with the drug. **The solute must be thoroughly mixed with the diluent before use.** The label on the vial will indicate the amount of medication per volume, such as 250 mg/mL. Follow directions with the vial for storage of the medication after reconstitution.

COMPATIBILITY OF MEDICATIONS

The number of medications that are given by injection has multiplied over the years, and not all drugs are compatible with others when mixed together. A reaction occurs when a drug combines with an incompatible drug. These reactions range from color change, precipitation, and clouding to invisible chemical changes rendering the drug inactive.

Steps 35-3 | Withdrawing Medication from a Vial

Medication may be supplied in a single-dose or a multiple-dose vial. When withdrawing from a multiple-dose vial, be careful not to allow any other medication to enter the vial when mixing drugs.

1. **ACTION** After checking the medication with the order for the correct drug and dose, select an appropriate-size syringe and needle; perform hand hygiene.

   RATIONALE Ensures that you are preparing the correct dose of the drug ordered; maintains asepsis.

2. **ACTION** Remove the plastic tab covering the vial rubber stopper and rub the stopper with an antiseptic swab. Discard the swab.

   RATIONALE This removes any residue that may have condensed on the stopper during manufacture.

3. **ACTION** Pull the plunger of the syringe back to the exact mark on the barrel of the syringe for the prescribed amount of the medication.

   RATIONALE Air equal to the amount of medication to be drawn up is drawn into the syringe.

4. **ACTION** Hold the vial between your thumb and third finger, with your index finger as a counterforce on the bottom of the vial. Insert the needle into the vial at a slight angle with lateral pressure.

   RATIONALE Inserting the needle into the vial at an angle with lateral pressure prevents coring of the stopper.

5. **ACTION** Keep the needle tip above the solution surface and push the plunger into the barrel to inject the air.

   RATIONALE The air is injected into the vial to prevent a vacuum in the vial, which may inhibit withdrawal of solution, especially in multiple-dose vials.

6. **ACTION** Invert the vial and, while holding it at eye level, pull the needle back so the tip is below the solution surface. Pull the plunger down until slightly more than the required amount of medication is in the syringe. Tap any air bubbles to the top near the needle and readjust the plunger, expelling air and excess medication, so that the exact amount of the dose is in the syringe (Figure 35-15).

   RATIONALE Keeping the bevel of the needle below the solution surface prevents air bubbles in the syringe. Expelling the air allows correct visualization of the dose in the syringe.

7. **ACTION** Verify the dose and remove the needle from the vial.

   RATIONALE The medication and dosage must be checked the third time with the MAR. Rechecking the calculation helps prevent medication errors.

8. **ACTION** Label the syringe with the patient's name, the name of the drug, and the dose.

   RATIONALE When a medication is removed from the original container or vial, labeling the new container (syringe, medication cup, etc.) prevents accidentally giving the wrong drug to the wrong patient.

9. **ACTION** For multiple-dose vials, label with the date, time, and your initials after opening the vial; use agency protocol. Refrigerate the remainder of the vial if necessary.

   RATIONALE Open medication has a specific time that it will remain usable; the amount of time varies from one medication to another. Many medications need to be refrigerated after reconstitution or opening.

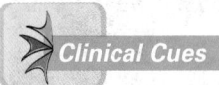 **Clinical Cues**

Before combining two or more drugs in a syringe to save the patient the discomfort of multiple injections, you should check with the pharmacist or consult a list of drugs that cites which ones can be safely combined with others.

When medications are compatible, as with insulin, you inject an amount of air equal to the desired dose of each drug into their respective vials. This reduces the vacuum inside the multidose vial and makes it easier to withdraw the medication. Air is placed in the longer-acting insulin vial first (Figure 35-16). After injecting the air into the second vial, the desired dose is withdrawn. The needle is again inserted into the first vial, into which air has already been injected, and the exact desired dose of this drug is withdrawn. If too much is drawn up, the contents of the syringe must be discarded and the medications redrawn because there is no way to separate one drug from the other when already mixed in the syringe in order to discard the excess. When mixing medications in the same syringe, care must be taken not to inject any of the medication already drawn up from the first vial into the second multidose vial (Steps 35-4).

APPLICATION of the NURSING PROCESS

Although administering an injection is part of the implementation phase of the nursing process, the other steps are also followed.

Assessment (Data Collection)

Check the physician's order for the medication. Note the patient's name, generic/trade medication name, dosage, route, and time. Careful checking prevents medication errors. The identity of the patient who is to receive the injection is carefully assessed to prevent medication errors and harm to the patient. Check the chart for indication of drug allergies and question the patient about allergies each time a parenteral medication is given. **An allergy to an injectable medication that goes into the tissue or bloodstream can have very serious consequences.**

Therapeutic effects of previous doses need to be assessed. This may include review of the patient's symptomatic response as well as checking laboratory data, such as white blood cell (WBC) count. If no improvement is seen within 2 to 3 days, the physician should be notified.

Determine the desired action of the medication, potential side effects, precautions, and recommended nursing interventions. **It is imperative to know what the medication is supposed to do (therapeutic action) and what adverse/side effects may occur in order to properly assess for their presence.** Assess the patient for signs of side effects to previous doses of the medication. If harmful side effects have occurred, the medication must be discontinued and the physician consulted.

Check the expiration date on the label of the medication container before drawing it up. Out-of-date medication should not be administered because it may have changed chemically.

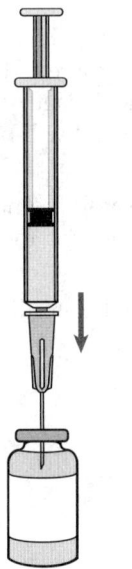
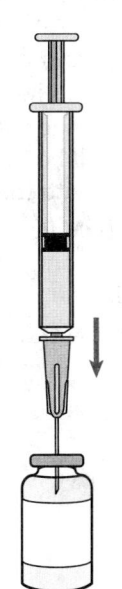
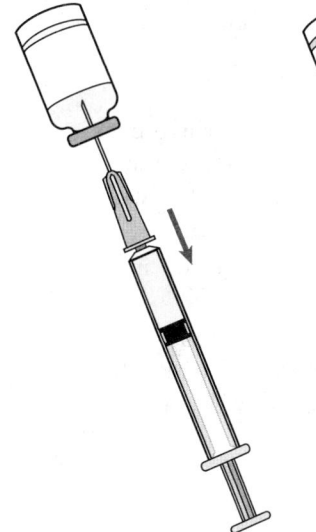
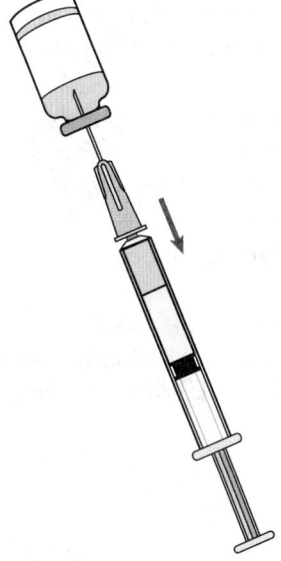

Step A:
Inject air into longer-acting (cloudy) insulin

Step B:
Inject air into short-acting (clear) insulin

Step C:
Withdraw prescribed amount of short-acting (clear) insulin

Step D:
Withdraw prescribed amount of longer-acting (cloudy) insulin

FIGURE **35-16** Mixing doses of insulin from multidose vials.

Steps 35-4 | Combining Insulins

Often short-acting insulin is ordered to be mixed with longer acting insulin. These steps are used to mix the two insulins. An insulin syringe is used to draw up the insulins.

1. *ACTION* Check expiration dates on both bottles of insulin.

   RATIONALE Outdated insulin is not reliable and should not be used.

2. *ACTION* Check for change in color, clumping, or granular appearance of insulin and discard if such has occurred.

   RATIONALE Insulin has been contaminated or exposed to heat and is no longer good.

3. *ACTION* To mix insulin suspension, swirl the vial gently or rotate between palms or roll between palm and thigh.

   RATIONALE Mixes the insulin evenly without causing air bubbles, which would interfere with accurate dosage.

4. *ACTION* Roll the vial of the long-acting cloudy insulin to distribute the insulin evenly in the suspension.

   RATIONALE Dosage will be inaccurate unless the insulin is evenly mixed.

5. *ACTION* Swab the tops of both vials of insulin with alcohol swabs.

   RATIONALE Cleans the top of the stopper, removing debris and microorganisms.

6. *ACTION* Use an insulin syringe calibrated for the concentration of insulin to be administered.

   RATIONALE Matching the syringe and the concentration in the vial ensures exact correct dosage can be drawn up.

7. *ACTION* Pull the plunger of the syringe back to the amount needed from the first bottle, the long-acting cloudy insulin, drawing in air to this measurement.

   RATIONALE Prepares air to be injected into the vial.

8. *ACTION* Insert the needle into the first vial with the long-acting cloudy insulin and inject the air into the vial. Withdraw the needle.

RATIONALE Air injected into the vial reduces the vacuum and makes it easier to withdraw the medication (see Figure 35-16).

9. *ACTION* Pull the plunger of the syringe back to the amount of insulin needed from the second vial, the short-acting clear insulin, drawing in air to this measurement.

   RATIONALE Prepares air to be injected into the vial.

10. *ACTION* Insert the needle into the second vial with the short-acting clear insulin and inject the air into the vial with the needle above the surface of the medication.

    RATIONALE Air injected into the vial prevents a vacuum, which will pull regular insulin into the long-acting insulin vial; makes it easier to withdraw the medication.

11. *ACTION* Invert the vial and, keeping the bevel of the needle beneath the surface of the insulin, withdraw the exact amount of short-acting insulin needed from this vial; tap out any air bubbles. Remove the needle.

    RATIONALE The bevel must be below the surface of the liquid in order to draw up the medication. Air bubbles interfere with measuring the exact correct dosage.

12. *ACTION* Keeping the plunger at the exact place, insert the needle into the first bottle with the long-acting cloudy insulin and withdraw exactly the amount ordered. Do not let any of the medication in the syringe enter the vial.

    RATIONALE Mixes the two insulins within the syringe in the exact amounts ordered. If fluid from the syringe enters the vial, the dosage of both insulins will be incorrect and the vial will be contaminated with the short-acting insulin.

13. *ACTION* Recap the needle if you are not with the patient and proceed to the patient to administer the insulin.

    RATIONALE Protects the needle sterility and protects others from needle sticks.

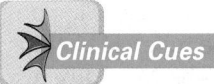

Clinical Cues

All multidose vials of medication should be dated when opened. If you see an opened multidose vial that has not been dated, it should be discarded.

Determine the reason the patient is receiving this medication. If the reason is not evident, the medication order may have been written on the wrong chart.

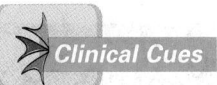

Clinical Cues

Apply your knowledge of pathophysiology and pharmacology; question a medication order that does not match your patient's condition, medical diagnosis, or symptoms.

Determine previous injection sites by consulting the medication administration record (MAR) and the patient. It is best to rotate injection sites to promote the best absorption of the medication and to decrease tissue irritation. Assess the patient's size and anatomy, and locate the appropriate landmarks at the chosen injection site. Determine if blood circulation is adequate. The needle size and length are determined by the type of injection to be given and the size of muscle tissue and the amount of fat at the injection site on the patient. Adequate circulation is essential for drug absorption.

Nursing Diagnosis

Injections are given for various reasons. The nursing diagnosis that would cover the administration of a particular medication would depend on the purpose of the drug. A few possible nursing diagnoses are as follows:

- Acute pain related to inflammation or surgery (analgesic)
- Risk for infection related to surgical procedure (antibiotic)
- Imbalanced nutrition, less than body requirements, related to inability to utilize glucose properly (insulin)
- Risk for infection related to potential for exposure to tuberculosis (purified protein derivative [PPD] test)
- Activity intolerance related to postoperative discomfort (pain medication)
- Deficient fluid volume related to vomiting (antiemetic)

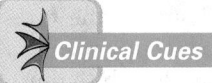

Clinical Cues

In planning for medication administration, it is important to check that patients' medications are on the unit before the time they are to be administered. Perform any calculations needed to reconstitute a drug ahead of administration time.

Planning

Sample goals/expected outcomes for the previous nursing diagnoses might be as follows:

- Pain will be relieved for 3 hours by medication.
- No signs of infection will be present at discharge.
- Blood glucose level will be maintained within normal limits.
- Patient will return for PPD test; result will be read on time.
- Patient will demonstrate willingness to ambulate, cough, and deep breathe within 30 minutes after an injection of pain medication.
- Nausea and vomiting will be controlled by antiemetic medication.

Implementation

Giving injections involves carefully checking and preparing the medication as well as skillfully administering the injection. It is necessary to choose the correct needle size and syringe for the type of injection to be given. Maintaining asepsis while drawing up and giving injections is very important. **Always follow the Five Rights when administering a medication (right drug, right route, right dose, right time, and right patient).**

Once disposable needles and syringes have been used, they must be discarded in such a way that they cannot pose a danger to others (Home Care Considerations 35-1).

Intradermal Injections

Intradermal injections are most frequently used for tuberculosis or allergy testing. **For the intradermal route, the amount of solution to be injected is very small.** Extreme care must be taken to measure the dose accurately because the solutions are capable of producing severe reactions. A tuberculin syringe and a short needle, ¼ to ½ inch in length, are used. The ventral aspect of the forearm is the customary injection site, but when this site is not available for use, the dorsal and lateral sides of the upper arm can also be used because they are readily observable. The needle is inserted at an angle of about 5 to 15 degrees between the upper layers of the skin. The injected solution will raise the epidermis to form a bleb. It is

---

🏠 **Home Care Considerations 35-1**

Disposing of Sharps in the Home Care Setting

In the home care setting, the patient may be giving himself heparin or insulin injections. Teach him to place bleach solution in a large plastic milk bottle and secure it with a screw-on cap. This container is a home substitute for a sharps biohazard container. Help him to contact the local waste management service for appropriate disposal.

then slowly absorbed from the site because the blood vessels are located in the deeper structures of the skin.

Tuberculin is a biologic product used for skin testing for exposure to tuberculosis. The test is based on the fact that a person infected with *Mycobacterium tuberculosis* develops sensitivity to certain products of this organism, which are contained in the culture extracts called tuberculins. Purified protein derivative (PPD) is the most commonly used tuberculin.

Tuberculin testing is the first step in a series to confirm that a patient is infected with the tubercle bacillus and may have clinical tuberculosis. The Mantoux test (PPD stabilized solution) is the preferred method (Skill 35-1). Box 35-2 provides guidelines for reading the results of a Mantoux test. A positive tuberculin test result denotes that exposure has occurred, but it does not signify the presence of active disease. Follow-up of a positive tuberculin test result involves a chest x-ray and possibly other tests.

Skill 35-1 Administering an Intradermal Injection

Intradermal injections are used for various skin tests, such as the Mantoux test for tuberculosis (TB). The object is to inject an antigen to determine if the patient has an inflammatory reaction, indicating that previous exposure to the antigen has caused antibodies to be manufactured by the body.

■ Supplies
✓ Tuberculin syringe with ¼- to ½-inch needle

✓ Medication to be injected
✓ Gloves

✓ Medication administration record (MAR) or order
✓ Alcohol swabs

Review and follow the Standard Steps in Appendix 3.

■ Assessment (Data Collection)

1. *ACTION* Assess if patient understands the procedure for the intradermal injection and its purpose. Assess for previous reaction to agent to be injected.

   RATIONALE Determines if teaching is needed. Alerts to possible contraindication to injection.

■ Planning

2. *ACTION* Determine when 48 to 72 hours after the injection will occur, or the proper time for reading the result will occur, and if someone will be available to read the result.

   RATIONALE Injection may need to be delayed if a weekend, or the patient's personal schedule, will interfere with proper reading of the result.

■ Implementation

3. *ACTION* Check the medication label against the MAR.

   RATIONALE Verification of the name of the medication, dose to be given, route, date, and time is necessary.

4. *ACTION* Perform hand hygiene and draw up the medication. Perform the second check per the five rights at this time.

   RATIONALE Prepares medication for injection. Helps prevent a medication error.

5. *ACTION* Clean the preparation area and take the injection and the MAR, or an identifying card, to the patient. Perform the third check of the medication with the MAR.

   RATIONALE The area should be left clean. Third check helps prevent a medication error.

6. *ACTION* Properly identify the patient. Select a relatively hairless site, usually on the inside of the forearm in a relatively hairless location. (Agency policy may specify right or left.) Have patient extend the elbow and support the forearm on a flat surface. Cleanse the site well with an antiseptic swab using firm, gentle circular motions or use soap and water. Clean an area approximately 2 inches in diameter. Allow the skin to dry.

   RATIONALE The inside of the forearm is used for intradermal injections. If the skin is still wet with alcohol when the injection is given, more stinging is experienced.

7. *ACTION* Hold the syringe vertically and verify that the exact dose is present in the syringe.

   RATIONALE The exact dose must be given.

8. *ACTION* Don gloves; stand or sit in front of the patient and turn the patient's forearm palm upward, facing you. With the index finger and thumb, pull the skin taut at the selected site on the forearm. Insert the needle, with the bevel up, at a 5- to 15-degree angle for approximately ⅛ inch (3 mm). You should be able to see the outline of the point of the needle. If you are in the dermis, you will feel resistance to the needle; if you can move the needle freely, you are in the subcutaneous tissue and must start over.

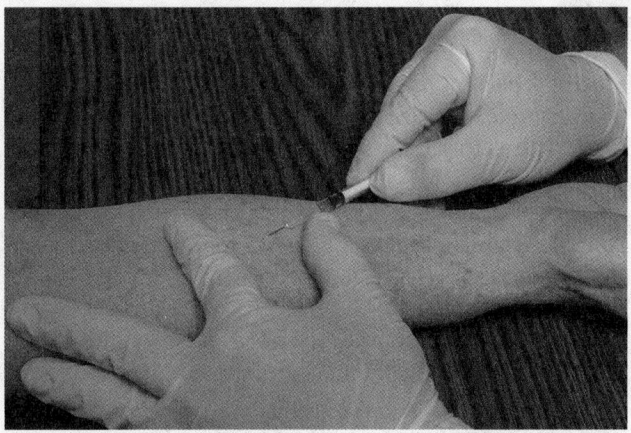

Step **8**

RATIONALE Positioning the needle bevel up minimizes resistance of the skin when the needle is inserted, decreasing discomfort. The needle must be placed sufficiently into the dermis at a 5- to 15-degree angle for the medication to form a bleb and not leak out immediately.

9. **ACTION** Lift up the needle point slightly and inject the solution slowly; a bleb or bump of 6 to 10 mm in diameter should form.

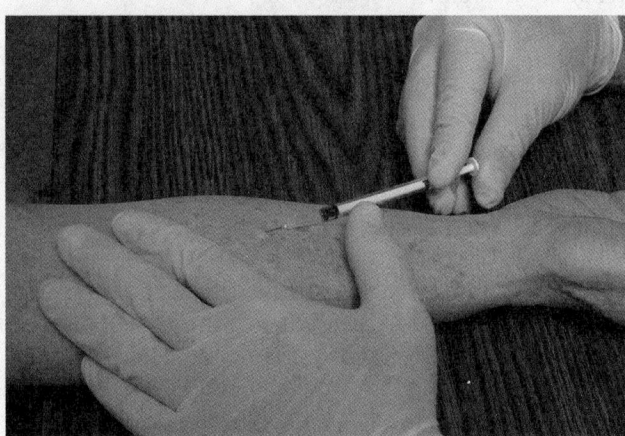

Step **9**

RATIONALE If a bleb is not formed, the medication has been deposited into the subcutaneous tissue and the test will not be valid.

10. **ACTION** Carefully withdraw the needle and wipe the skin very gently with the antiseptic swab **AFTER** you remove the needle: *do not apply pressure. Do not recap needle.*

RATIONALE Have your fingers clear of the injection site as you remove the needle to prevent accidental needle sticks. Applying pressure will force the medication back out the needle track and will nullify the injection.

11. **ACTION** Dispose of the syringe and needle by dropping them into the sharps container; remove and dispose of gloves; perform hand hygiene.

RATIONALE Prevents needle sticks to self or others. Prevents transfer of microorganisms.

12. **ACTION** Circle the injection site with a skin pencil.

RATIONALE Facilitates locating site at time of reading the reaction.

■ Evaluation

13. **ACTION** Verify that the bleb remains.

RATIONALE Procedure will have to be repeated if bleb is not visible or is less than 6 mm. If a repeat injection is necessary, select a site at least 2 inches from the original site and document as appropriate.

14. **ACTION** Read the result of the skin test at the proper interval.

RATIONALE Different antigens used for testing require different intervals before reading the result.

■ Documentation

15. **ACTION** Document the dose on the MAR and record the exact site of the injection.

RATIONALE Documenting the exact site shows where to read the result in 48 to 72 hours.

16. **ACTION** When result is read, document the findings in the patient record.

RATIONALE Records result of test on the patient record for future reference.

Documentation Example

12/2 1600   Mantoux test with 0.1 mL PPD on left inner forearm; instructed to return in 48–72 hours for reading.

_____

(Nurse's signature)

❓CRITICAL THINKING QUESTIONS

1. What would you do if a large portion of the solution for a Mantoux test leaked out of the bleb after you removed the needle from the skin?

2. How would you handle the situation if the patient states he has had a positive reaction in the past to a TB test?

Box 35-2 *Reading the Mantoux Test Result*

Locate the injection site indicated on the patient record and marked with a skin pencil. The injection site is inspected under a good light, noting any erythema. The margin of the induration is palpated. With a millimeter ruler, the transverse diameter of the indurated area is measured across the point at which the needle entered. The reading is recorded in millimeters of induration (quality of being hard). The result is read between 48 and 72 hours after injection.

POSITIVE REACTION
Tuberculosis exposure is indicated when the induration measures 5 to 15 mm. The induration, not erythema, is the key to the positive reaction.

NEGATIVE REACTION
The induration measures less than 5 mm.

Subcutaneous Injections

Medications administered by the subcutaneous route are absorbed more slowly by the body than via the intramuscular route (Skill 35-2). This route is used to give medications to patients for a variety of reasons. Insulin and heparin are given by this route, as are some preoperative medications and narcotics to relieve pain (Safety Alert 35-3). Sites that can be used for subcutaneous injections are shown in Figure 35-17. For most patients the preferred sites are the lateral surfaces of the upper arm or the anterior and lateral aspects of the thigh. Heparin is given in the abdominal subcutaneous sites (Box 35-3; Nursing Care Plan 35-1, pp. 701-702); the best site for insulin is also the abdomen because it provides the most reliable, steady absorption. In accordance with National Patient Safety Goals, you should encourage your patients to be actively involved with

---

Skill 35-2 | Administering a Subcutaneous Injection

Certain drugs must be injected subcutaneously rather than intramuscularly in order to be absorbed properly and at the desired speed. Heparin, insulin, allergy extract, and certain types of immunizations, as well as some other medications, are given subcutaneously.

■ Supplies
✓ Medication
✓ Gloves
✓ Medication administration record (MAR)
✓ Alcohol swabs
✓ Syringe and needle (preferably ⅜ to ⅝ inch in length)

Review and carry out the Standard Steps in Appendix 3.

■ Assessment (Data Collection)

1. **ACTION** Check the medication order and determine that the medication is available on the unit. Check for presence of drug allergies.

   RATIONALE Ensures that time is not lost acquiring the medication. Indicates if patient might be allergic to the medication.

2. **ACTION** Determine that the patient is in the room and ready to receive the injection.

   RATIONALE Prevents having to wait to give the injection once it is drawn up. Some drugs deteriorate in plastic syringes.

■ Planning

3. **ACTION** Plan the site at which to place the injection. Choose an appropriate syringe and needle.

   RATIONALE Consider the size and weight of the patient and the condition of the various sites in which a subcutaneous injection may be given.

■ Implementation

4. **ACTION** Perform hand hygiene and prepare the medication, checking it three times following the five rights.

   RATIONALE Checking the medication three times using the five rights helps prevent medication errors.

5. **ACTION** Identify the patient by checking the armband with the MAR and having the patient state his name. Alternatively, use a bar code device to check the bar code on the name band and on the MAR.

   RATIONALE Prevents medication errors and injury to patients.

6. **ACTION** Don the gloves, select the site for the injection, and expose the area for good visibility. Open the alcohol swab package and cleanse the selected site gently by using a circular motion until

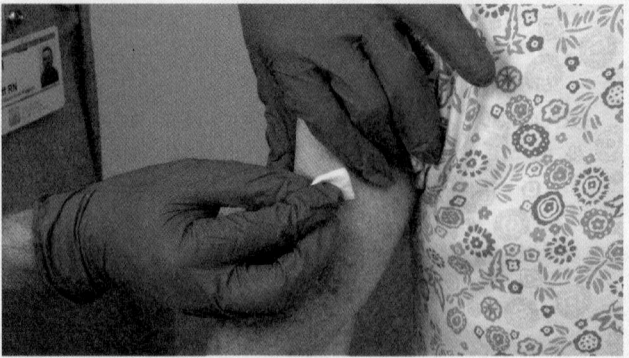

Step **6**

an area approximately 2 inches in diameter is cleansed. Place the swab between the index and middle fingers of your nondominant hand. Allow the skin to dry.

RATIONALE Cleanses the area; positions the swab for use after the injection. Vigorous rubbing increases blood flow and would increase rapidity of absorption.

7. *ACTION* Pick up the prepared syringe in one hand and remove the needle guard by pulling it straight off the needle with the other hand to avoid contaminating the needle, dulling it, or suffering a needle stick.

   RATIONALE Asepsis must be maintained.

8. *ACTION* Support the skin at the site by gently bunching up the tissue between your thumb and index finger.

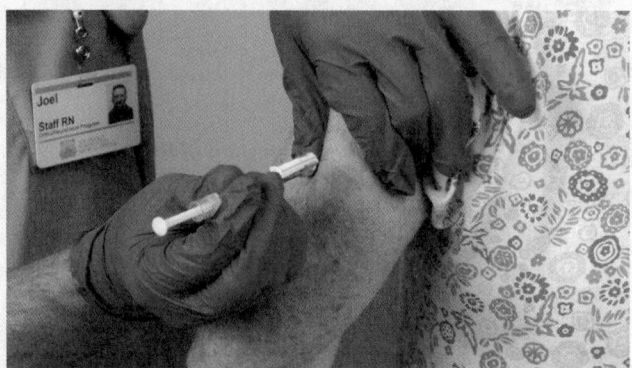

Step **8**

RATIONALE Picking up the tissue helps you assess the thickness of the subcutaneous layer into which you will inject the drug and prevents medication from being injected into the muscle.

9. *ACTION* Hold the barrel of the syringe in your hand between the thumb and index finger, bracing with the remaining three fingers. Insert the needle into the skin at a 45- or 90-degree angle depending on the length of the needle, with a firm, quick forward thrust; release the pinched-up skin.

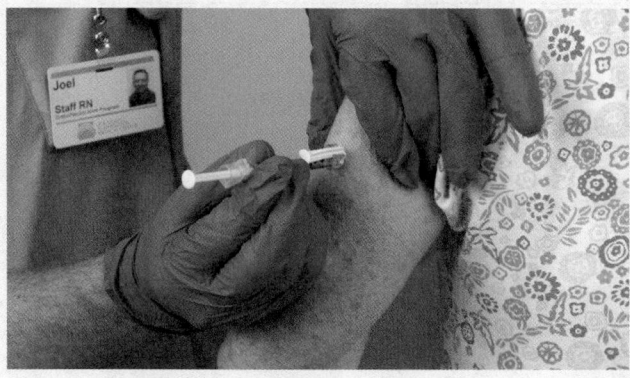

Step **9**

RATIONALE Stabilizes the tissue so that the needle will pierce cleanly. A shorter needle uses a 90-degree angle; a longer needle uses a 45-degree angle to stay in subcutaneous tissue.

10. *ACTION* Press the plunger with a smooth, slow motion until all of the medication is injected.

    RATIONALE Places medication in the tissue. Aspiration for a subcutaneous injection is not necessary because vessels in subcutaneous tissue are so small that it is unlikely that the needle would enter a vessel.

11. *ACTION* Wait 5 to 30 seconds (more time for heparin) and remove the needle by pulling it out on the angle of insertion while stabilizing the skin with the other hand. Activate the safety guard on the needle.

    RATIONALE Waiting a bit helps prevent solution from coming up needle track. Pulling the needle out quickly while stabilizing the skin causes the least discomfort for the patient. Enclosing the needle in a guard prevents needle sticks.

12. *ACTION* Rub the injection site with an alcohol swab using a gentle circular motion (except for heparin and insulin) to help disperse the medication in the subcutaneous tissue so that it will be absorbed. Do not rub an allergy extract injection site.

    RATIONALE The action of a subcutaneous injection is expected within 30 minutes.

13. *ACTION* Dispose of the needle and syringe in the sharps container. Remove gloves; perform hand hygiene.

    RATIONALE Prevents needle sticks to self or others. Reduces transfer of microorganisms.

■ Evaluation

14. *ACTION* **Check with the patient in 30 to 60 minutes to evaluate the therapeutic effect of the medication if it was an analgesic.**

    RATIONALE Analgesics should be working within 30 minutes. Allergy injection sites are checked at 30 minutes for local reaction. Immunizations cannot be visually evaluated for therapeutic effect; however, patients should be observed for untoward effects.

■ Documentation

15. *ACTION* Document the injection on the MAR or patient clinic record, noting the location in which the injection was given.

    RATIONALE Verifies that the injection was given as ordered.

Continued

■

Skill 35-2 | Administering a Subcutaneous Injection—cont'd

Documentation Example

12/8 1345 Allergy injection 0.5 mL of trees and grasses mixture, 50,000 μ/mL, in left upper outer arm subcutaneously.

_____
(Nurse's signature)

■ Special Considerations

✓ The needle angle used depends on the length of the needle and the amount of subcutaneous tissue at the site. If 2 inches (5 cm) of tissue can be grasped, insert the needle at a 90-degree angle; if only 1 inch of tissue can be grasped, use a 45-degree angle for the injection.

✓ Allergy injection sites should be rotated from one side of the body to the other.

✓ Heparin injections are given in the abdomen on both sides of and below the umbilicus outside of a 2-inch radius around the umbilicus from the lower costal margins to the iliac crests. Never aspirate before injecting the heparin.

✓ A record should be kept of where each insulin injection is given. Insulin is absorbed more quickly and uniformly when injected into the abdominal sites.

?CRITICAL THINKING QUESTIONS

1. Can you explain why you should not aspirate when giving a subcutaneous heparin injection?

2. Why should you count for 15 to 30 seconds after injecting the heparin and before removing the needle?

Safety Alert 35-3

Double-Check Insulin and Heparin Doses with Another Nurse

When you are giving insulin, heparin, injectable heart medications, or parenteral chemotherapy drugs to a patient, always have another nurse double-check for correct medication and for correct dose. Show the other nurse the medication vial and ask him or her to read the amount in the syringe. This practice should continue even after you have graduated and have many years of experience.

Box 35-3 | *Subcutaneous Administration of Heparin*

When heparin is administered subcutaneously, it requires additional precautions during administration. Because of its anticoagulant properties, it can stimulate bleeding into the tissues. Always have another nurse double-check your syringe for correct amount and the vial for correct strength and dose.

- Sites on the abdomen from below the costal margins to the iliac crests are used because this area is not involved in muscular activity, whereas the arms and legs are.
- Sites should be rotated within the abdominal area, alternating from one side to another; refrain from giving a subsequent injection too close to a previous one.
- **Do not aspirate when giving heparin** because this tends to increase bruising and needle movement could cause tissue damage.
- Do not massage the site after the drug has been injected because this may cause bruising of the tissue, bleeding, and severe **ecchymosis** (purplish area under the skin caused by bleeding).

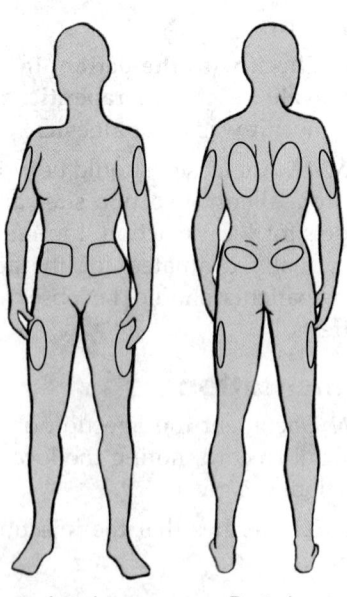

Anterior   Posterior

FIGURE **35-17** Subcutaneous injection sites.

NURSING CARE PLAN 35-1

Care of the Patient Receiving Heparin Injections

SCENARIO Lena Thomas, age 56, was admitted with a deep vein thrombosis (DVT) of the right leg. She has been receiving intravenous heparin but is to be discharged today. She was started on warfarin sodium (Coumadin) by mouth yesterday. Because it takes 3 days for the warfarin levels to be effective for maintenance of anticoagulation, she will be receiving heparin injections twice a day for 2 days. The home health nurse will give the injections.

PROBLEM/NURSING DIAGNOSIS *Has a blood clot in right leg/*Risk for injury related to potential for thrombus formation.
Supporting Assessment Data: Subjective: Injured leg. Developed swelling, redness, and pain in right leg. *Objective:* Swelling decreasing, redness diminished, pain lessened.

Goals/Expected Outcomes	Nursing Interventions	Selected Rationale	Evaluation
Patient will not display signs of emboli during recovery period.	Apply antithrombotic elastic stockings to both legs.	Elastic stockings apply pressure to tissue and vessels to encourage venous return and prevent pooling of blood in leg.	*Did the patient have any signs of emboli?* No signs of emboli (i.e., no change of mental status, denies shortness of breath [SOB] or chest pain).
	Discourage rubbing of the legs.	Rubbing an area where a thrombus is located may dislodge it and it then would become an embolus.	Agrees not to rub legs.
	Administer 5000 units sodium heparin subcutaneously in abdomen q 12 hr.	Heparin prevents DVT formation. Heparin is absorbed best from the abdominal sites.	5000 units of heparin administered Subcut in Rt. abdomen at 0900; no adverse effects.
	If bruising occurs, ice the area for 3 to 5 minutes before the next injection; do not aspirate before injecting the heparin; stabilize needle well so as not to cause bleeding in the tissues from needle movement. Count for 15 to 30 seconds after injecting the heparin and before removing the needle to allow the heparin to disperse so it will not come back up the needle track.	Cold causes vessel constriction and helps prevent bleeding that causes bruising. Aspiration may cause bruising because tissue may be pulled against needle tip. Stabilizing the needle prevents damage to tissue by needle that could cause bruising. Allowing the medication to disperse prevents it from coming back up the needle track.	No signs of bruising.
Swelling and pain will be gone within 2 weeks.	Keep leg elevated when sitting.	Elevation prevents pooling of blood and edema.	*Did the swelling and pain resolve?* Leg elevated on pillow; encouraged to change position q 2 hr. Swelling and pain decreased.
	Do not stand for long periods of time.	Standing allows blood to pool in legs.	Is aware of need to rest and elevate legs.

Continued

■

NURSING CARE PLAN 35-1

Care of the Patient Receiving Heparin Injections—cont'd

Goals/Expected Outcomes	Nursing Interventions	Selected Rationale	Evaluation
Verbalizes symptoms of thrombosis to report to physician.	Assess for signs of pulmonary crackles or shortness of breath indicating possible pulmonary emboli; assess for neurologic changes that might indicate a brain embolus; instruct to call 911 if she experiences chest pain with shortness of breath because this might indicate a coronary embolus.	Pulmonary emboli cause shortness of breath and anxiety; neurologic changes may indicate a brain embolus and stroke. A coronary embolus may cause a myocardial infarction requiring emergency treatment.	*Was the patient able to verbalize symptoms to watch for?* Patient and family verbalize signs of emboli correctly (i.e., SOB, anxiety, chest pain, or change in mental status).
	Teach family how to recognize signs of emboli.	If family has knowledge of signs and symptoms of emboli, they can obtain emergency services quickly.	Family participated in teaching session; able to state how to call 911 services. Outcomes met.

? CRITICAL THINKING QUESTIONS

1. Explain how you would evaluate the effectiveness of the heparin.

2. Explain the process of preparing and administering a heparin injection.

Home Care Considerations 35-2

Monitoring Injections Given in the Home Care Setting

- When family members or patients in the home care setting are giving injections, periodically assess if the injection is being given with correct technique by observing the injection preparation and administration.
- Be certain that used syringes and needles are being disposed of safely.
- From time to time, thoroughly review the principles of asepsis for the home care patient receiving injections.

---

medication administration. For example, teach your diabetic patients to rotate sites for insulin administration. (Home Care Considerations 35-2).

? *Think Critically About . . .* Although the abdomen is the best site for insulin, why might the nurse elect to administer the insulin in the patient's upper arm while the patient is in the hospital?

Intramuscular Injections

Intramuscular injections are used if the patient cannot take medicine orally, the medication is not prepared in an oral form, or a faster action is desired. Intramuscular injections can provide onset of action within 15 minutes because muscle tissue is highly

vascular, and drug absorption is faster than by the subcutaneous route. Drugs introduced into a large skeletal muscle mass cause less tissue irritation than drugs administered intradermally or subcutaneously.

Selection of the injection site is a critical decision. **Improper site selection can result in damaged nerves, abscesses, necrosis, and sloughing of skin, as well as pain.** Therefore, the individual's stage of development, body build, and physical condition as well as the viscosity and amount of the drug to be administered must be considered in giving an IM injection. If more than 3 mL of medication must be given at one time to an adult, such as rabies vaccine, doses should be divided in half and given in two different large muscle sites.

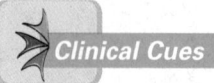
Clinical Cues

Usually intramuscular injection sites are disinfected with alcohol; however, washing visibly dirty skin with soap and water may be adequate (Practice Guide, 2007). Consult agency policies and guidelines.

The mid-deltoid muscle is a common location for IM injection; however, the actual area involved is limited because of its proximity to major vessels, nerves, and bones. The area for the mid-deltoid injection is triangular, with the base of the triangle beginning about two finger breadths below the acromion process and extending down to just above the axilla fold (Figure 35-18). The

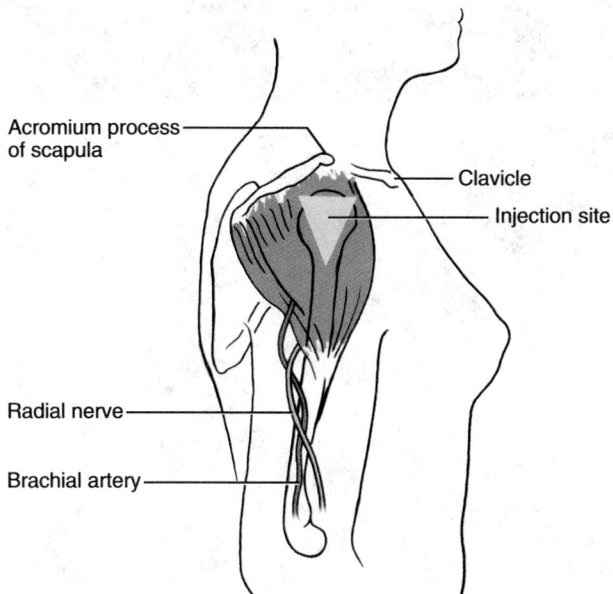

FIGURE **35-18** Locating the site for a mid-deltoid IM injection.

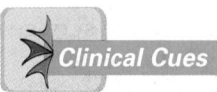

One milliliter of medication can be safely injected into the mid-deltoid site. Check agency policy before injecting a larger amount.

correct site for injection can be located by placing four fingers across the deltoid muscle with the little finger on the acromion process; the site is three finger breadths below the acromion process. This site is convenient because it is usually easily accessible; it is not used in infants or children with underdeveloped muscles.

In the past the dorsogluteal (gluteal: pertaining to the buttocks) site was used; however, it is no longer recommended because of the high potential for injury to the sciatic nerve and the blood vessels.

The ventrogluteal area is an injection site involving the gluteus medius and minimus muscles (Skill 35-3). The muscle layer is thick, and this site has a very small fatty layer. The site can be used both for adults and children and is especially helpful if patients are only able to lie on their back or turn to one side or the other. To locate the injection site, the palm is placed over the greater trochanter, the index finger is put on the anterior iliac

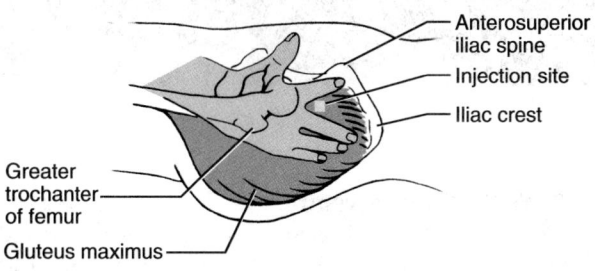

FIGURE **35-19** Locating the site for a ventrogluteal IM injection.

Skill 35-3 | Administering an Intramuscular Injection

Many drugs are given only by intramuscular (IM) injection. The site must be carefully selected to prevent injury to the patient. Intramuscular injection sites are shown in Figures 35-18 through 35-21.

■ Supplies
✓ Syringe and needle 1 to 3 inches in length
✓ Medication
✓ Gloves
✓ Medication administration record (MAR)
✓ Alcohol swabs or soap and water for cleansing
✓ Adhesive bandage (optional)

Review and carry out the Standard Steps in Appendix 3.

■ Assessment (Data Collection)
1. *ACTION* Determine that the patient is in the room and ready for the injection. Assess for allergy to the drug.

   RATIONALE Prevents having to wait on the patient after the injection is drawn up. Alerts nurse to potential contraindication to the injection.

■ Planning
2. *ACTION* Plan the site at which the injection is to be given.

   RATIONALE The deltoid, ventrogluteal, vastus lateralis, or rectus femoris sites may be used.

■ Implementation
3. *ACTION* Verify the medication label with the MAR, checking the medication three times using the five rights. Alternatively, check the bar code on the patient's bracelet and the code on the MAR.

   RATIONALE Adhering to the five rights of medication administration and checking each medication three times for drug, dose, route, date, and time prevents medication errors.

4. *ACTION* Perform hand hygiene and don gloves. Select and expose the injection site so that the view is unobstructed. For the ventrogluteal site, the patient may be supine or turned to the side.

Continued

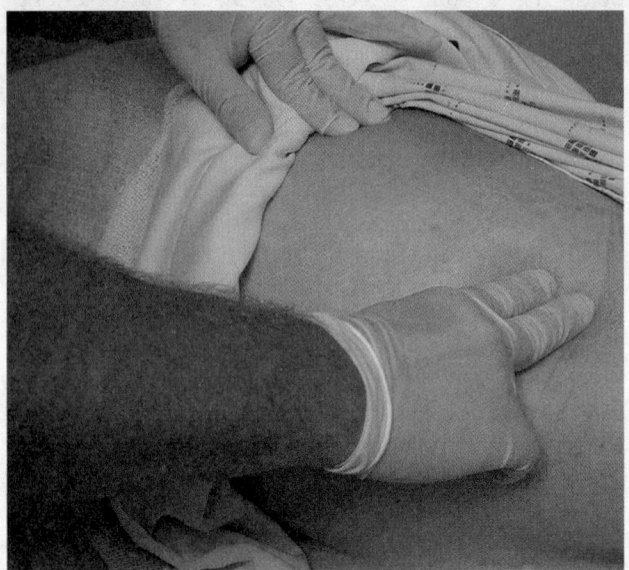

Step **4**

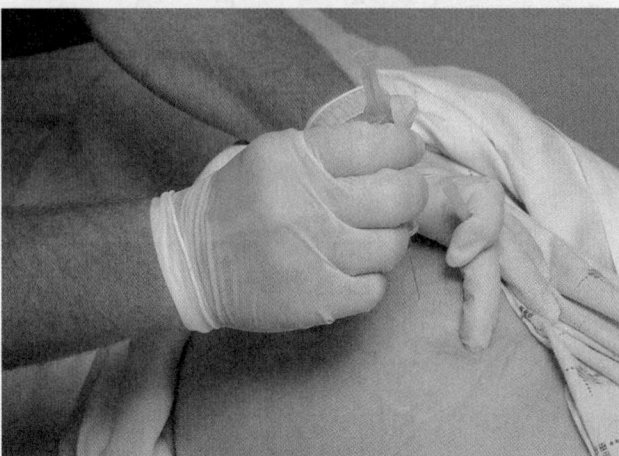

Step **7**

RATIONALE **The ventrogluteal site is the safest site. The IM site chosen must be within defined landmarks; a good view is necessary to inject at the correct location.**

5. *ACTION* Remove an alcohol swab from the package and cleanse a space 2 inches in diameter using a firm circular motion. Place the swab between the fingers of the nondominant hand for later use or place it just lateral to the site. Allow the area to dry.

   RATIONALE Prevents transfer of microorganisms. Cleanses the site. Makes swab available after the injection. Wet alcohol on the skin may cause stinging on injection.

6. *ACTION* Pick up the syringe and verify that the correct dose is in it. If an air bubble is to be used as a lock, add 0.2 mL of air. Invert the syringe so that it is perpendicular to the floor and the bubble rises to a position behind the fluid in the syringe. (Consult agency policy about using an air lock.)

   RATIONALE An air bubble is thought to seal the needle track, keeping the medication from leaking back out.

7. *ACTION* Spread the skin at the site with the nondominant hand, pressing firmly around the site to compress the subcutaneous and muscle tissues.

   RATIONALE Taut skin reduces resistance to the needle when it enters the tissues and causes less pain.

8. *ACTION* Grasp the barrel of the syringe *firmly* between your thumb and index finger, like a dart, and plunge the needle firmly into the muscle at a

90-degree angle with a quick, firm forward thrust until the desired depth is reached.

RATIONALE Holding the skin taut and the syringe steady while introducing the needle to the desired depth in one stroke causes the least discomfort to the patient.

9. *ACTION* Steady the barrel of the syringe with the nondominant hand and pull the plunger back with the dominant hand to aspirate for blood. If blood returns in the syringe, withdraw the needle and dispose of the syringe and medication. Prepare a new injection.

   RATIONALE A medication prepared for IM injection can be harmful if it is injected intravenously. Blood should not be reinjected into tissue.

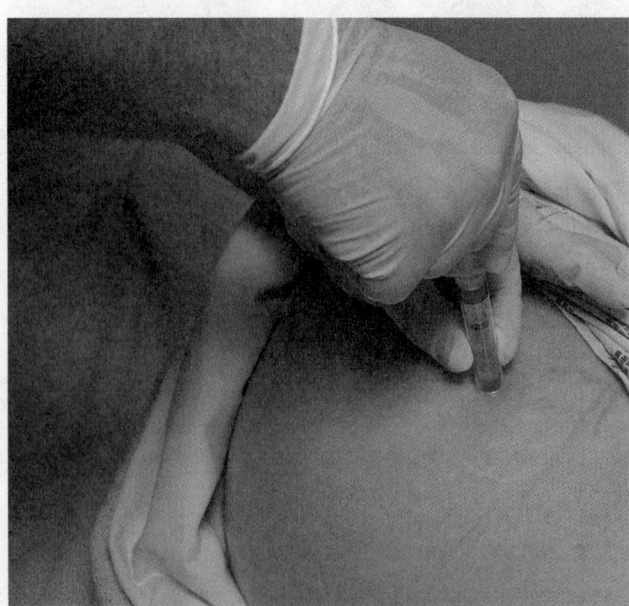

Step **9**

10. *ACTION* Inject the medication by pushing the plunger into the barrel with a slow, continuous motion. Be careful not to displace the needle from its original position as you inject.

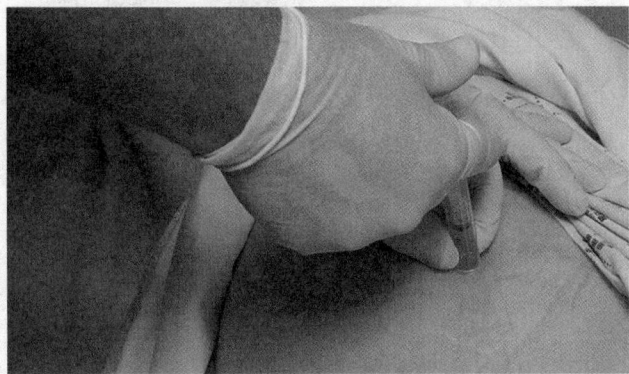

Step **10**

RATIONALE Injecting slowly is less painful because tissue has time to absorb the medication. A medication prepared for IM absorption may cause local tissue reaction if left in the fatty subcutaneous or intradermal tissue.

11. *ACTION* Quickly remove the needle, drawing it straight up with a quick motion. Activate the needle guard. Apply pressure with the alcohol swab at the needle site.

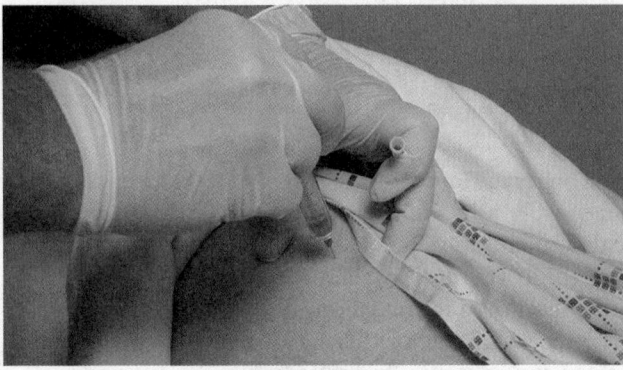

Step **11**

RATIONALE Removing the needle with a quick motion is less painful than removing it slowly. Enclosing the needle in a guard prevents needle sticks. Pressure also helps prevent the medication from leaking back up the needle track.

12. *ACTION* Massage the injection site with a gentle but firm circular motion. Apply an adhesive bandage if there is superficial bleeding.

RATIONALE Massage increases circulation and helps to disperse the medication so that it is absorbed more quickly. Blood should be contained; apply an adhesive bandage if needed.

13. *ACTION* Dispose of syringe, remove gloves, and perform hand hygiene.

RATIONALE Prevents needle sticks and decreases transfer of microorganisms.

■ Evaluation

14. *ACTION* Determine how the patient tolerated the injection. Depending on the medication injected, check for therapeutic effect of the injection at a proper interval.

RATIONALE If adverse effects of the medication occur, document them and inform the physician promptly. If the medication appears to be ineffective, discuss with the physician.

■ Documentation

15. *ACTION* Document the dose and the site on the MAR. If the medication is PRN, document in the nurse's notes.

RATIONALE The reason for the injection and the patient's response to it are documented for all PRN medications.

Documentation Examples

12/8 1020   Morphine 8 mg IM RVG (right ventrogluteal) for complaints of pain of 7 on a scale of 1 to 10 at incision.

_____
(Nurse's signature)

12/8 1100   States pain has lessened considerably; now a 4 on a scale of 1 to 10.

_____
(Nurse's signature)

■ Special Considerations

✓ The vastus lateralis site should be used for IM injections in infants less than 12 months of age.
✓ Careful consideration of the size of muscle mass in the elderly patient is necessary to choose a safe injection site. Many elderly have muscle wasting (atrophy). A shorter needle may be necessary. The vastus lateralis and ventrogluteal sites are the preferred sites in the elderly.
✓ Apply pressure to the injection site in the elderly for longer than for a younger person to prevent bleeding and hematoma formation. Clotting time is often decreased in the elderly.
✓ When the patient is receiving a series of injections, check the former sites for induration at the time of choosing a site for the next injection.
✓ If a medication causes excessive discomfort when injected, place ice over the site for 3 to 5 minutes before injecting.

?CRITICAL THINKING QUESTIONS

1. You are working with an experienced nurse who encourages you to use the dorsogluteal site to give an IM injection. What would you say to the nurse?
2. What should you do if you get a blood return on aspiration when administering an IM injection?

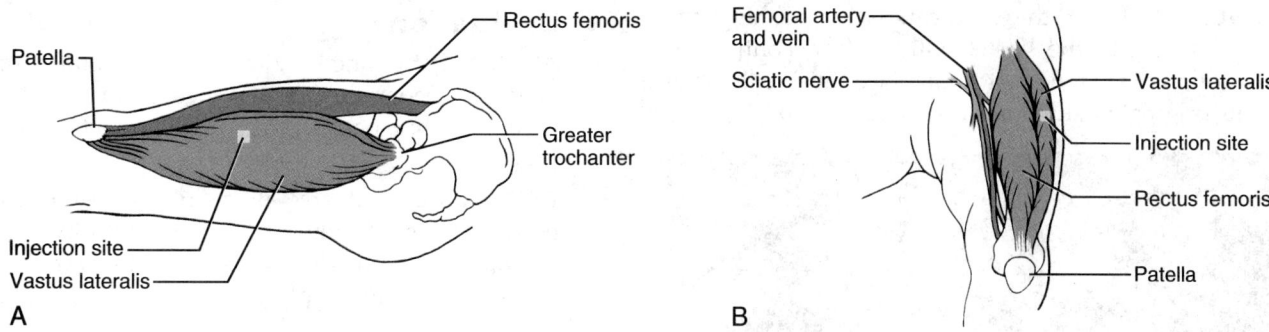

FIGURE **35-20** Locating the vastus lateralis IM injection site. **A,** Side view. **B,** Front view.

spine, and the middle finger is spread as far as possible toward the posterior iliac crest (Figure 35-19). **The center of the "V" bounded by the index and middle fingers is the precise injection site to be used.** Flexing of the knee and hip helps the person to relax the muscles.

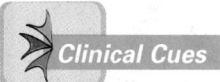

Clinical Cues

The ventrogluteal area is considered the safest IM injection site in adults to avoid damage to nerves or blood vessels. However, if you suspect that the patient might move during the procedure (i.e., confused, agitated, or unable to follow instructions), do not leave your hand in the "V" position while you are giving the injection because you want to protect yourself against an accidental needle stick. Mark the insertion site by placing an alcohol pad next to it.

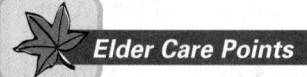

Elder Care Points

Elderly persons may have decreased muscle mass; an IM site must be chosen carefully. The body of the muscle may have to be palpated and then grasped to ensure correct needle placement within it. A shorter needle than average may need to be used.

The vastus lateralis muscle is also a preferred IM injection site for adults, children, and infants. The area extends from the anterior lateral aspect of the thigh to the midlateral thigh, a hand's width below the proximal end of the greater trochanter and a hand's width above the upper knee (Figure 35-20). The middle third of the muscle is the best site for injection. This muscle can be used when the patient is recumbent with the knee slightly flexed or in Sims' position or is sitting upright.

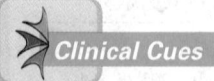

Clinical Cues

The vastus lateralis is the site of choice for infants younger than 12 months for IM injections. For children older than 13 months of age, the vastus lateralis, ventrogluteal can be used; also deltoid is appropriate unless the muscle mass is poorly developed.

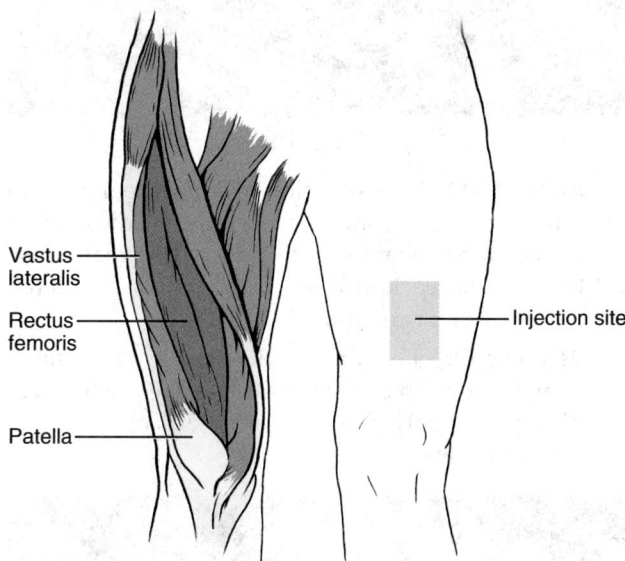

FIGURE **35-21** Locating the rectus femoris IM injection site.

The rectus femoris muscle can also be used as an IM site in the adult and when other sites are contraindicated in children. It is located on the anterior aspect of the thigh (Figure 35-21) and is used by people who give their own IM injections because it is easy to reach. The disadvantage of this site is that the injection may cause considerable discomfort.

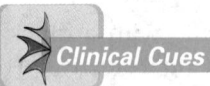

Clinical Cues

Intramuscular injections are less painful when the muscle is relaxed. Because the gluteal muscles are tense when the hip is extended or the leg is externally rotated, ask the patient to lie in prone position with the toes turned inward or to lie in Sims' position.

Air Lock Technique. An air lock can be used when giving an IM injection to clear the needle of medication and to seal the track so that the medication does not flow back up into the subcutaneous tissues. To use an air lock, after drawing up the exact amount of medication ordered, draw up a further 0.2 mL of air. When preparing to give the injection, be certain that the needle is at a 90-degree angle and the air is behind the medication so that it will be injected last. The use of an air lock is controversial; check the agency's policy on this part of the procedure.

Intramuscular Injections in Children. The site used for giving IM injections to newborns and infants is the vastus lateralis. **It is preferable to find another way to give medication to children because IM injections are painful and traumatic for the child.** Unfortunately, some pediatric immunizations must be given IM. Ways to decrease injection discomfort are listed in Box 35-4.

The needle size and the angle of the injection depend on the size of the infant or child. For infants a ⅝-inch needle is used, whereas for older children a ⅝- or 1-inch needle may be used. The angle is varied depending on the size of the child and the anatomy; the needle point must reach the desired area in the muscle. An adult may take a 90-degree angle; a child or smaller person may need a 45-degree angle for the injection. **When giving a deltoid injection to a child, the injection should be given in the thickest part of the muscle; the needle should point at a slight angle toward the shoulder.** Intramuscular immunizations for children over 13 months of age can be given in the deltoid site, unless the muscle appears poorly developed.

When giving injections to children, you must assess and understand their level of biophysical and psychosocial development. Knowledge of the various stages of child growth and development enables you to give an appropriate explanation to the child and to provide emotional support before, during, and after the injection. When it is necessary to restrain a child to give the injection safely, you should have someone hold the child. Your manner can help to reassure the child. If the child is old enough to understand, be honest and say, "It will just hurt for a minute." After the injection, talk in a soothing way and cuddle the child to reestablish trust.

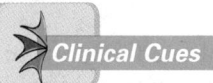
Clinical Cues

Playacting is a helpful way of explaining procedures to children in the preschool-age group. You can demonstrate the entire procedure on a doll, indicating the reasons for the injection and the way the doll responds to it, so that the child has an idea of what will happen and how to behave. Give the child an opportunity to look at or handle empty vials or syringes. Explain that the medicine will help them to get well and that then they will be able to play.

School-age children want to know how and why things work. Give a clear and simple explanation of why the injection is needed and how it is done. Compliment the child for being good about the discomfort; children thrive on praise and rewards (Communication Cues 35-1).

Teenagers may avoid expressing their real feelings of anxiety and fear as they are coping with the many changes that are hurling them toward adulthood.

Box 35-4 *Ways to Decrease Injection Discomfort*

- For a child, EMLA cream (available by prescription) can be applied to the site where the injection will be administered to numb the area. The cream is applied 1 hour before injection time.
- Apply an ice pack for 3 to 5 minutes to numb the skin.
- Use the smallest gauge needle that is appropriate.
- Select a site without signs of inflammation, lesions, or bony prominences and without large underlying vessels or nerves.
- Ask the patient to assume a prone position with the feet turned inward, or the Sims' position, to relax the muscles.
- Press down with your thumb over the injection site for 10 seconds to numb it.
- When using alcohol for cleaning the area, allow it to dry before inserting the needle to decrease stinging sensation.
- Ask the patient to deep breathe and try to relax.
- Use the Z-track method for all irritating medications.
- Instruct the patient to look away while the injection is given.
- Insert the needle smoothly and remove it quickly while applying pressure to the skin.
- Inject the medication slowly and steadily.
- Gently but firmly massage the site after withdrawing the needle (except for heparin, iron, and allergy injections).
- Encourage active use of the muscle or further massage after the injection.

Communication Cues 35-1

Communicating with Your Pediatric Patient

Jin Tang is a 5-year-old who has been brought to the clinic by his mother to have immunizations prior to entering school. He is crying as you enter the room.

JIN: "I don't want a shot! I don't want a shot!"

NURSE: "Jin, hi. My name is Sally and I am a nurse. Sit on your mom's lap and let's talk for a minute."

JIN: "Are you going to give me a shot?"

NURSE: "Right now we are just talking. Can you count numbers?"

JIN: "Yes. I can count really fast. I learned that in preschool."

NURSE: "Can you show me?"

JIN: "1, 2, 3, 4, 5, ..."

NURSE: "Wow, that was great." If you could count really fast while I give you your medicine, that would help me."

JIN: "I don't want a shot. It hurts."

NURSE: "It does hurt, just a little, but it will be quick if you'll help me. Nurse Janie will help us too. She is going to give you a big hug and you count really fast and then when we are done, your mom will come and give you a bigger hug."

Many adolescents are extremely modest, so take care to avoid unnecessary exposure of their bodies.

The Z-Track Technique. The Z-track technique (causing a needle track, or pathway, in the shape of a "Z") can be used any time an IM injection is given (Figure

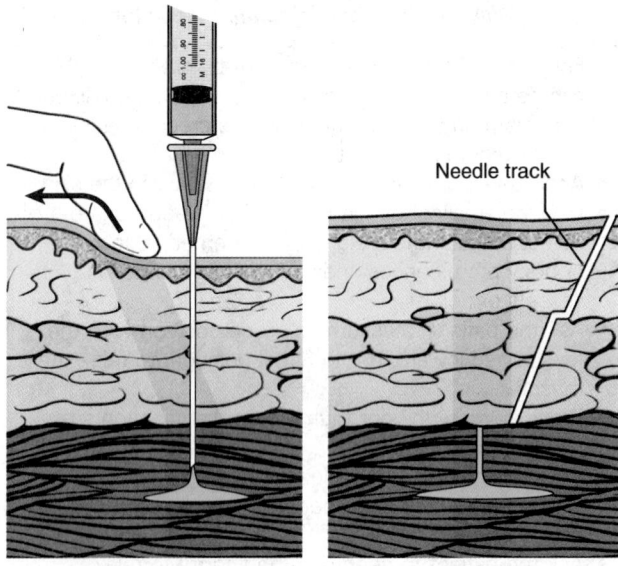

FIGURE **35-22** Z-track technique for IM injection of irritating medications.

35-22). It must be used whenever a deep IM injection of iron dextran (DexFerrum) and other irritating solutions such as hydroxyzine hydrochloride (Vistaril) and several antipsychotic agents are given (check the drug insert that comes with the medication). This method reduces the pain caused by irritating drugs that leak or escape along the track into subcutaneous tissue when the needle is withdrawn (Safety Alert 35-4). When this occurs, the tissues are stained and bruised, and it takes several weeks or longer for the tenderness to subside (Steps 35-5).

Anaphylactic Shock

When an allergen is taken in by a sensitized person, the reaction can range from mild to severe—to so severe, in fact, that death can occur within minutes. Many medications may cause this *anaphylactic* reaction, but parenteral medications are most likely to cause it because they are absorbed quickly. Symptoms of anaphylactic shock (circulatory failure from an allergic reaction) include urticaria (a reaction characterized by reddened, slightly elevated patches known as

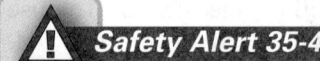

Dispose of the Cap; Do Not Contribute to Pressure Sores

As a student nurse you will be nervous as you give your first several injections. You will feel flush with success and relief after you give the medication and withdraw the needle! Before you walk away to celebrate, double check that you have not left the cap, a piece of the syringe or other debris on the bed linens. This foreign material can accidentally work its way underneath the patient and create skin irritation and breakdown.

Watch for Allergic Reactions

Critical nursing responsibilities when administering a parenteral drug are to check for allergy to the drug prior to administration and to observe the patient for 30 minutes after the drug has been given for the first time.

wheals), bronchiolar constriction that manifests as wheezing or difficulty breathing, edema, and finally, circulatory collapse. Circulatory collapse may occur as the initial symptom. Watch for signs of anaphylactic shock and, if necessary, administer immediate, lifesaving treatment. In accordance with 2009 National Patient Safety Goals (Goal 16), nurses should be vigilant for changes in patient condition and respond appropriately (Safety Alert 35-5).

Other types of allergic reactions may occur for up to 2 weeks after the medication was administered. Allergic reactions are more common the second or successive times the medication is received.

Evaluation

Administration of an injection is evaluated in terms of whether it was given properly and whether it achieved its purpose (Table 35-1). Assess for any adverse reaction to the medication and check the injection site for signs of inflammation.

Table 35-1 | *Evaluating the Effectiveness of Injections*

The main way to determine the effectiveness of injections is to assess for signs that the desired effect is taking place. This means checking to see if the signs and symptoms of the problem for which the medication is being given are subsiding, and looking at laboratory test results. Here are some specific examples:

TYPE OF DRUG	EVALUATION CRITERIA
Antibiotic	Temperature is returning to normal. Signs of infection are subsiding: decreased redness, swelling, pain, or tenderness. WBCs are returning to normal.
Antiemetic	Nausea subsides within 30-60 min; vomiting is controlled for 3 hr.
Narcotic medication	Pain subsides within 30-60 min and stays under control for 3-4 hr.
Heparin	No signs of new clots are found (negative Homans' sign). APTT lab values are within therapeutic limits.
Allergy extracts	Allergy symptoms subside: decreased sneezing, stuffy head, and runny nose.
Iron dextran (Imferon)	Red blood cell count, hemoglobin, and hematocrit rise toward normal levels.
Preoperative sedatives	Patient becomes drowsy and more relaxed.

Key: *APTT*, Activated partial thromboplastin time; *WBCs*, white blood cells.

Steps 35-5   Giving a Z-Track Injection

The Z-track technique is used when it is necessary to prevent any possibility of medication leaking up the injection track into the subcutaneous tissue. Iron dextran (Imferon) and hydroxyzine pamoate (Vistaril) must always be given by Z-track injection because they can cause excessive irritation of subcutaneous tissue.

Review and carry out the Standard Steps in Appendix 3.

1. **ACTION** Check the medication and dosage with the order; obtain the appropriate syringe with at least a 1½-inch needle and a second needle. Perform hand hygiene.

   RATIONALE Following the five rights and checking the drug and dose helps prevent a medication error. A 3-inch or longer needle is needed for the injection of iron dextran preparations. Asepsis must be maintained.

2. **ACTION** Draw up the correct amount of the medication. Add 0.5 mL of air if an air lock is desired. (The use of an air lock is controversial; check the agency's policy on this part of the procedure.)

   RATIONALE Air flushes all medication from the needle. An air lock also helps to prevent the medication from coming back up the needle track after the needle is removed.

3. **ACTION** Change the needle.

   RATIONALE The needle used to draw up the medication is not used to inject it because the medication on and in the needle might irritate the overlying tissue on its path to the muscle.

4. **ACTION** Follow the five rights, perform hand hygiene, and don gloves. Assess the patient for drug allergy. Choose a large muscle injection site.

   RATIONALE Following the five rights ensures that the right drug in the right dose will be given to the right patient at the right time by the right route. Gloves reduce the transfer of microorganisms. Checking for allergies first prevents accidentally inducing a potentially dangerous allergic reaction. Injection site selection provides a muscle large enough to absorb the medication.

5. **ACTION** With the nondominant hand, press the side of the hand down and retract the skin and tissue laterally. Cleanse the site. Insert the needle at a 90-degree angle. Maintain this hand position, with traction on the skin, until after the medication is injected.

   RATIONALE Retracting the skin and tissue provides a slanted needle track when the needle enters the tissue; layers of tissue will block the needle track after the needle is removed and tissue returns to its normal position.

6. **ACTION** Steady the syringe and aspirate for blood using your dominant hand (one-handed aspiration technique).

   RATIONALE The syringe must be steady when aspiration is done or it may not be in the same spot when the medication is injected.

7. **ACTION** If blood is aspirated, withdraw the needle and dispose of the syringe and needle. Draw up medication with a new syringe.

   RATIONALE Blood indicates needle is placed in a blood vessel, where it is contraindicated to inject the medication.

8. **ACTION** If no blood is aspirated, slowly inject the medication. Wait for 10 seconds before withdrawing the needle.

   RATIONALE Injecting medication slowly allows the tissue to absorb the medication and prevents untoward bruising. Waiting 10 seconds allows time for the medication to disperse into the tissue, helping prevent it from traveling back up the needle track.

9. **ACTION** Withdraw the needle with a slow movement while releasing the tissue. Gently wipe the injection site with the alcohol swab. **Do not massage the site.** Use alternate sites for subsequent injections.

   RATIONALE Letting go of the tissue while withdrawing the needle disrupts the needle track, preventing the medication from traveling to the skin surface. Massage might force the medication out into the subcutaneous tissue.

10. **ACTION** Document the injection was given, including the site used and the technique.

    RATIONALE Verifies that the patient received the medication and notes site in case of local reaction.

Documentation

Injection documentation should include the medication, the dosage, the route, and the site at which the injection was given. The testing substance is noted for intradermal injections. Routine injections are recorded on the MAR only. The PRN (as needed) and stat doses may also be recorded in the nurse's notes, along with the reason the medication was given and the result and duration of effect of the injection; check agency policy.

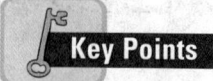
Key Points

- Parenteral routes are used when medication cannot be taken by mouth or quick drug action is desired.
- Once injected, medication cannot be retrieved; extreme care regarding dosage and route is essential.
- Correct sites for injections are extremely important because injecting outside of an accepted site may cause nerve, blood vessel, or tissue damage.
- Injections must be prepared and given using aseptic technique in order to prevent infection.
- The routes for parenteral medication include intradermal, subcutaneous, and intramuscular.
- The intradermal route deposits medication into the dermal layer of the skin. A tuberculin syringe is used for intradermal injections.
- Subcutaneous injections are placed beneath the dermis and above muscle; 0.05 to 1 mL of solution may be injected subcutaneously.
- The angle of injection for a subcutaneous medication depends on the size of the patient and the length of the needle used.
- Sites for intramuscular injections include the ventrogluteal, deltoid, vastus lateralis, and rectus femoris. The angle of injection is 90 degrees; the needle length is varied depending on the site chosen and the size of the patient.
- Three milliliters of solution may be safely injected into the ventrogluteal, vastus lateralis, and rectus femoris intramuscular sites in an adult.
- A 2- to 3-mL syringe is usually used for an IM injection with a 1- to 1½-inch needle that is 23 to 20 gauge.
- Medications for injection come packaged in ampules, vials, or individual unit-dose cartridges.
- Tuberculin and 2- and 3-mL syringes have two measurement scales: milliliters and minims.
- The minim scale is rarely used, but can be used for very small dosages.
- A filter needle is used to draw medication from an ampule; the needle is changed before administering the injection.
- The larger the number of the needle gauge, the smaller the needle and the finer the cannula.
- The selection of a gauge depends on the viscosity of the fluid to be injected.
- A needle stick from a used needle may transmit HIV or hepatitis B or C virus. Needles are generally not recapped after use, but are immediately carefully dropped into a sharps biohazard container. Use a safety syringe and needle whenever they are available.

- Air is injected in an equal amount to solution to be withdrawn to prevent creating a vacuum in a vial.
- For two medications to be mixed, they must be compatible. Check drug inserts, drug handbooks, or the pharmacist regarding the route and compatibility of drugs being administered concurrently.
- Assessment before administering an injection includes (1) checking for allergies to the medication; (2) verifying the drug, dose, route, time, expiration date, and patient identification; (3) determining why the patient is receiving the drug; and (4) checking for possible drug interactions with other prescribed and over-the-counter drugs. Use the Five Rights of medication administration.
- When a repeat injection of a drug is given, assess for side effects of the drug, previous site condition, and evidence of therapeutic effect before administration of the dose.
- Intradermal injections are mainly used for allergy testing and the administration of a PPD test for tuberculosis exposure screening.
- Rotation of sites for medications given in a series, such as heparin and insulin, prevents fibrosis of the tissue.
- Always aspirate for blood before injecting an intramuscular medication.
- The vastus lateralis site is the preferred site for IM injection in infants under the age of 12 months.
- The ventrogluteal IM injection site is the safest site to use in the adult.
- A Z-track technique is used with particularly irritating medications to decrease pain and bruising by sealing the drug in the muscle tissue.
- Injected medications are capable of causing anaphylactic shock. Symptoms of an anaphylactic reaction are urticaria, bronchiolar constriction, edema, and finally, circulatory collapse. Cardiopulmonary resuscitation and the administration of emergency drugs may be necessary.
- Each injection is documented on the MAR; PRN medications and their effect may also be documented in the nurse's notes.

 Go to your **Companion CD-ROM** for an Audio Glossary, animations, video clips, and more.

evolve Be sure to visit the companion Evolve site at http://evolve.elsevier.com/deWit/fundamental/ for additional online resources.

NCLEX-PN® EXAMINATION-STYLE REVIEW QUESTIONS

*Choose the **best** answer(s) for each question.*

1. The reasons for using the parenteral route to administer medications include:

    1. parenteral medication lasts longer than an oral medication.
    2. it is the least expensive method.
    3. it is easier to measure an accurate dose.
    4. the parenteral route allows more rapid absorption than the oral route.

2. During an intramuscular injection, the medication is absorbed quickly. This is because:

    1. the muscle tissue is more vascular.
    2. the needle is entering the dermis.
    3. there is more connective tissue.
    4. fat cells readily absorb the medication.

3. A patient needs an intradermal injection for a Mantoux test, but he currently has bilateral forearm casts in place. Which of the following would be the best alternative site?

    1. Abdomen
    2. Lateral upper arm
    3. Medial upper thigh
    4. Antecubital space

4. Which nursing diagnosis would be the priority if a patient had a severe anaphylactic reaction to a parenteral medication?

    1. Allergy response, Latex
    2. Anxiety, Death
    3. Impaired gas exchange
    4. Increased cardiac output

5. The physician orders 15 units of Humulin N (long-acting) and 5 units of regular insulin (rapid acting). Put the following steps in the correct order to properly mix two insulins in one syringe.

    _____ 1. Inject 15 units of air into the vial containing long-acting cloudy insulin.
    _____ 2. Withdraw 15 units of the long-acting cloudy insulin.
    _____ 3. Withdraw 5 units of the rapid-acting clear insulin.
    _____ 4. Inject 5 units of air into the vial containing rapid-acting clear insulin.

6. When giving a Z-track injection, the nurse would retract the surface tissue with one hand before inserting the needle. The nurse would release the tissue to return to its normal position:

    1. as the solution is slowly injected.
    2. as the needle is removed from the tissue.
    3. after the tissue is pierced with the needle.
    4. after the anatomic landmarks are palpated.

7. Which of the following is the safest place to give an IM injection for an adult patient?

    1. Gluteus maximus
    2. Ventrogluteal
    3. Deltoid
    4. Gluteus minimus

8. When the nurse is preparing a parenteral injection, medical asepsis is permissible for handling the:

    1. shaft of the plunger.
    2. needle shaft and tip.
    3. barrel of the syringe.
    4. solution in the vial.

9. The site of choice for a DTaP injection in an 8-month-old is the:

    1. upper outer quadrant of the gluteus.
    2. vastus lateralis of the thigh.
    3. inner surface of the forearm.
    4. outer surface of the upper arm.

10. The nurse has just given the patient an injection. Massaging the area is the appropriate nursing action for which medication?

    1. Heparin
    2. Insulin
    3. Morphine
    4. Iron dextran

CRITICAL THINKING ACTIVITIES *Read each clinical scenario and discuss the questions with your classmates.*

Scenario A
Choose the appropriate injection equipment to carry out the following orders:
1. 0.1 mL PPD for tuberculosis for an adult
2. 3 mL of a viscous solution for an IM injection to a 150-lb (68-kg) adult

Scenario B
Indicate which site you would most likely choose for each of the above injections.

Scenario C
Discuss special considerations when giving IM injection to elderly patients.

Scenario D
You give your patient an ordered IM injection of prochlorperazine (Compazine, an antiemetic). Within 10 minutes, the patient complains of feeling very peculiar and short of breath. What would you do?

Scenario E
Convert the following mL amounts to minims.
1. 0.125 mL = _____ minims
2. 0.25 mL = _____ minims
3. 0.50 mL = _____ minims

Objectives

Upon completing this chapter, you should be able to:

Theory

1. List four purposes for administering intravenous (IV) therapy.
2. Identify circumstances when it would be appropriate to use an infusion pump to deliver fluids or medications.
3. Describe the possible complications that can arise from the use of the IV route and the corrective actions you should take for each one.
4. State at least seven guidelines related to IV therapy of fluids or medications.
5. Discuss special considerations for elderly patients who need IV therapy.
6. Discuss the signs and symptoms of a blood transfusion reaction and the steps you should take should one occur.

Clinical Practice

1. Write a care plan for a patient who needs IV fluid therapy and include patient specific data, an identified nursing diagnosis and interventions.
2. Calculate the rate of flow of IV fluid from various IV orders.
3. Initiate IV therapy by performing venipuncture with an IV cannula (catheter over the stylet) using aseptic technique, and starting the ordered infusion.
4. Add a new bag of fluid to replace one from which the solution has infused.
5. Prepare to give medications using each of the following methods:
   a. Adding the drug to the primary IV solution.
   b. Using a second IV line as a piggyback.
   c. Using a controlled-volume device.
   d. Using an intermittent IV or a PRN (as-needed) lock.
   e. Giving the medication as a bolus.
6. Discontinue an IV infusion.
7. Safely monitor a patient receiving a blood transfusion; document your actions and the patient's response to therapy.
8. Collect data on a patient who receiving total parental nutrition; document your findings and the patient's response to therapy.

Skills & Steps

Skills

Skill 36-1 Starting the Primary Intravenous Infusion
Skill 36-2 Adding a New Solution to the Intravenous Infusion
Skill 36-3 Administering Intravenous Piggyback Medication
Skill 36-4 Administering Medication via Saline or PRN Lock
Skill 36-5 Administration of Medication with a Controlled-Volume Set
Skill 36-6 Administration of Blood Products

Steps

Steps 36-1 Adding Medication to an Intravenous Solution
Steps 36-2 Administering an IV Bolus Medication (IV Push)
Steps 36-3 Discontinuing an Intravenous Infusion or PRN Lock

Key Terms

 Be sure to check out the bonus material on the Companion CD-ROM, including selected audio pronunciations.

autologous (ăw-TŎL-ŏ-gŭs, p. 740)
bore (p. 724)
burette (bŭ-RĔT, p. 717)
catheter embolus (KĂ-thĕ-tĕr ĔM-bō-lŭs, p. 721)
epidural (p. 721)
hypertonic (hī-pĕr-TŎN-ĭk, p. 714)
hypotonic (hī-pō-TŎN-ĭk, p. 714)
infiltrated (ĬN-fĭl-trā-tĭd, p. 718)
infusion (p. 713)
infusion pump (p. 717)
insulin pump (p. 719)
intrathecal (p. 721)
intravenous (IV) (p. 713)
isotonic (ī-sō-TŎN-ĭk, p. 714)
macrodrops (p. 716)
microdrops (p. 716)
total parenteral nutrition (TPN) (p. 718)
transfusion (trăns-FŪ-shŭn, p. 716)
vascular access devices (VĂS-kū-lăr, p. 720)
viscous (VĬS-kŭs, p. 716)

INTRAVENOUS THERAPY

Basic information about intravenous equipment, the types of solutions that are used, principles related to the ordered route, and the guidelines to monitor the rate of flow is essential for all nurses.

The intravenous (IV) (via the veins) route is the main method of supplying the patient with fluids and medications when the patient is unable to take them orally or rectally. Giving a drug or solution by the IV route has the advantage of making it instantly available for circulation to all tissues. The disadvantage is that the material cannot be retrieved if an error has been made. Because the solution is injected directly through a vein into the circulation, all material must be sterile to avoid introducing bacteria. Patients who require fluids by the IV method are placed on intake and output (I & O) recording to monitor for fluid overload. IV infusion (slow introduction of fluid into a vein) amounts are recorded under parenteral fluid.

IVs are given to supply the body with needed substances or drugs that cannot be supplied as rapidly or efficiently by other means (Cultural Cues 36-1). Examples of substances delivered by the IV route include:

- Fluids and electrolytes that the patient is unable to take in orally in sufficient amounts
- Medications that are more effective when given by this route or cannot be given any other way

 Cultural Cues 36-1

Beliefs About IV Therapy

A Cambodian patient might request an IV infusion of vitamin C or B complex. This request would be based on the belief that this treatment helps to "gain energy" (D'Avanzo & Geissler, 2003).

- Blood, plasma, or other blood components
- Nutritional formulas containing glucose, amino acids, and lipids

The average adult needs 1500 to 2000 mL of fluids in a 24-hour period to replace fluids eliminated by the body. Patients whose fluid intake has decreased or those who experience an excessive loss of body fluids will require fluid replacement (Nursing Care Plan 36-1). Fluids are lost by elimination; by hemorrhage; by severe or prolonged vomiting or diarrhea; by moderate to excessive drainage from wounds, especially from burn wounds; and by profuse perspiration. Accurate recording of the patient's intake and output is needed to determine the amount of fluids necessary for daily replacement. The physician will consider laboratory tests related to electrolytes when ordering replacements of sodium, potassium, and chloride, which are the more commonly administered electrolytes.

NURSING CARE PLAN 36-1

Care of the Patient with Deficient Fluid Volume and Hyponatremia

SCENARIO Jane Weston, age 78, is admitted to your unit from the local long-term care facility. She has had the "flu" with nausea and vomiting, has not been eating, and became dehydrated. There is a question as to whether she has suffered a small stroke (cerebrovascular accident, or CVA) or is just dehydrated and has consequent electrolyte imbalance. She is receiving D_5 ½NS IV solution and is being encouraged to eat and drink. (Dehydration may increase the viscosity of the blood, which can lead to clotting in susceptible individuals.)

PROBLEM/NURSING DIAGNOSIS *Vomiting, not eating, dehydrated*/Deficient fluid volume related to nausea, vomiting, and lack of oral intake.
Supporting Assessment Data: *Subjective:* "I've been so nauseated. I don't want to eat." ***Objective:*** Tongue dry and furrowed; 4-lb weight loss; poor skin turgor, scanty urine output.

Goals/Expected Outcomes	Nursing Interventions	Selected Rationale	Evaluation
Patient will be normally hydrated within 2 days as evidenced by weight gain, normal condition of mucous membranes, and normal urine output.	Give IV solution at 125 mL/hr as ordered.	IV solution will rehydrate patient.	*How is the patient responding to therapy?* IV fluids infusing at 125 mL/hr. No redness, swelling or pain at the site. Membranes moist.
	Check laboratory values of electrolytes.	Provides data as to whether imbalances are improving.	Laboratory results not on chart yet.
	Assess lungs for signs of crackles indicating fluid overload.	Crackles in lungs may indicate fluid overload from IV infusions.	No crackles.

Continued

NURSING CARE PLAN 36-1

Care of the Patient with Deficient Fluid Volume and Hyponatremia—cont'd

Goals/Expected Outcomes	Nursing Interventions	Selected Rationale	Evaluation
Patient will be normally hydrated within 2 days as evidenced by weight gain, normal condition of mucous membranes, and normal urine output—cont'd	Perform neurologic assessment q 4 hr.	Neurologic assessment would show deterioration of neurologic function if a stroke is in progress.	Oriented to person and place, but unsure about the date. Able to follow simple commands. Speech clear and appropriate.
	Encourage oral fluids, including sodas containing sodium.	Fluids with sodium help return sodium level to normal and help rehydrate patient.	Taking 7-10 small sips of soda every 30-60 min.
	Give small amounts of fluids every 30-60 min. Assist to drink fluids. Encourage oral intake as nausea subsides.	Encourages gradual return to oral intake; helps with rehydration.	Currently denies nausea. Will take fluid with coaching, but is not independently drinking.
	Determine what the patient would like to eat.	Preferred foods may appeal to flagging appetite.	Continues to refuse offers of food.
	Initiate intake and output recording.	Comparison of input vs. output, provides information to assess fluid balance.	Intake this shift 1230 mL.
	Watch urine output closely. Report less than 30 mL/hr output to physician.	Decreasing urine flow may indicate or contribute to kidney failure.	Output: 600 mL of clear, dark yellow urine.
	Turn at least q 2 hr. Assess pressure areas each time patient is turned.	Dehydration makes skin more vulnerable to pressure areas and pressure ulcers. Turning relieves pressure over bony prominences.	Skin intact. Coached and assisted to turn q 2 hr. Progressing toward expected outcomes. Continue plan.

? CRITICAL THINKING QUESTIONS

1. What are some issues that you must consider when elderly patients need IV therapy?

2. Ms. Weston complains about the IV. What assessments should you perform?

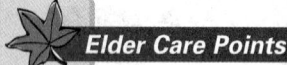
Elder Care Points

Monitor electrolyte levels closely because fluid therapy can rapidly change the fluid and electrolyte balance.

TYPES OF INTRAVENOUS SOLUTION

The physician orders the type of solution to be given, the amount to be infused, and the rate of infusion (as either the number of hours for the solution to infuse or the volume per hour). Many types of solutions are available, and still others can be prepared to meet the specific needs of the individual patient. The solutions most frequently used are those containing glucose, saline, electrolytes, vitamins, and amino acids. In addition to these, blood and blood products are given intravenously. Table 36-1 lists common IV solutions and examples of clinical uses.

Intravenous solutions are isotonic, hypotonic, or hypertonic. Isotonic solutions have the same concentration, or osmolality, as blood and are used to expand the fluid volume of the body. Hypotonic solutions contain less solute than extravascular fluid and may cause fluid to shift out of the vascular compartment. Hypertonic solutions have a greater tonicity than blood. They are used to replace electrolytes and, when given as concentrated dextrose solutions, produce a shift in fluid from the intracellular compartment to the extracellular compartment. Concentrated solutions of glucose, mannitol, or sucrose are given to reduce cerebral edema in patients with head injury because the osmotic pressure draws water out of the cells.

Table 36-1 *Common Intravenous Therapy Solutions, Tonicity, and Examples of Clinical Use*

SOLUTION	TONICITY	EXAMPLES OF CLINICAL USE
0.9% Saline	Isotonic	Trauma, diabetic ketoacidosis, with blood transfusions, hyponatremia
0.45% Saline	Hypotonic	To supply normal daily salt and water requirements
5% Dextrose in water	Isotonic	Vehicle for some IV piggyback medications, hyperkalemia
10% Dextrose in water	Hypertonic	If TPN is abruptly discontinued
5% Dextrose in 0.9% saline	Hypertonic	Early treatment of burns
5% Dextrose in 0.45% saline	Hypertonic	Postoperative; common maintenance fluid
5% Dextrose in 0.225% saline	Isotonic	Postoperative; common maintenance fluid
Ringer's lactate	Isotonic	Trauma, dehydration from severe diarrhea or vomiting
5% Dextrose in Ringer's lactate	Hypertonic	Burns, dehydration from severe diarrhea or vomiting

Key: *TPN*, Total parenteral nutrition.

? *Think Critically About . . .* You are caring for a postoperative patient who had a routine and uncomplicated surgery. Which type of IV solution (isotonic, hypotonic, or hypertonic) is the physician mostly likely to order for this patient? Why?

Solutions that are given intravenously must be sterile and free of contaminating particles. They are supplied in plastic bags in 250-, 500-, and 1000-mL amounts. Smaller bags of sterile water, dextrose in water, and normal saline are used to dissolve or dilute various drugs for parenteral use. Glass and plastic bottles are still used for a few solutions and some IV drugs. Check the expiration date and inspect the container for clarity of solution; only clear solution should be infused.

The typical IV bag (Figure 36-1) is marked with calibrations along the sides to determine the amount of fluid when the bag is hanging. A plastic cover on the tubing port is pulled off to allow the tubing spike to be inserted. A plastic or foil tab also covers the port used to add medication to the bag. The bag has a tab with a hole in it that will fit on the hanger of an IV pole.

The IV bottle is also marked with calibrations on the side. The flat metal or plastic cover on the top of the bottle is pulled off to expose a rubber stopper or diaphragm held in place by a metal rim. The diaphragm is removed, revealing a rubber stopper with an outlet

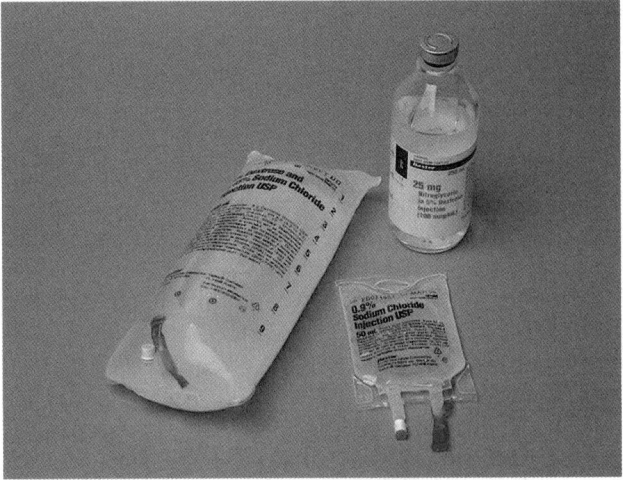

FIGURE **36-1** Intravenous solution containers.

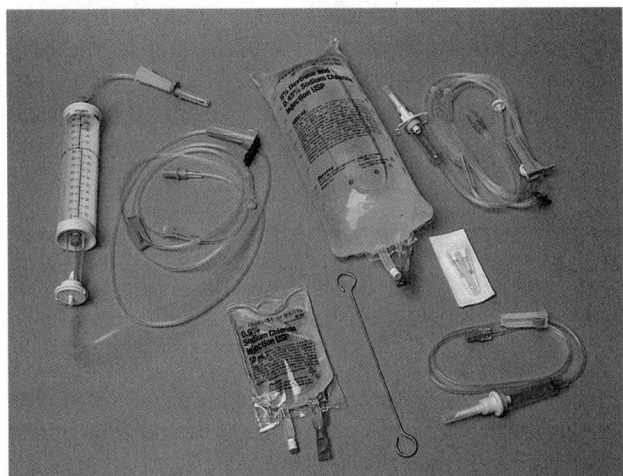

FIGURE **36-2** Intravenous fluid and medication administration sets.

vent into which the IV tubing is inserted, and an inlet for adding medications with a syringe and needle. Some IV bottles contain a tube that acts automatically as an air vent; for others, a vented tubing set must be used to let air in.

EQUIPMENT FOR INTRAVENOUS ADMINISTRATION

ADMINISTRATION SETS

There are many different types of administration sets available for IV use, some of which must be used with a particular brand of IV solution or type of bag (Figure 36-2). Administration sets can be classified as (1) primary intravenous sets, (2) secondary or piggyback intravenous sets, (3) parallel or "Y" intravenous sets, and (4) controlled-volume intravenous sets. Tubing is generally changed every 24-72 hours for infection control purposes (check the agency's policy for frequency of tubing change) and therefore should be properly labeled with the date and time. *(Refer to Steps 36-4: Changing IV Tube on the **Companion CD-ROM**.)*

Solutions can also be given intermittently through an intermittent intravenous device. Filters are recommended for the infusion of many solutions; check your agency's policy on filter use.

Primary Intravenous Set

The primary IV infusion setup consists of a bag of solution, a regular tubing set, a needleless connector, and an IV stand. A filter may be added. Tubing is either vented or nonvented. The IV tubing set consists of the spike end, which is inserted into the bag, the drip chamber, the tubing, a flow regulator or clamp, and a needle adapter. The spike and the needle adapter at the ends of the tubing are covered with plastic protectors to keep them sterile. The primary line usually has one or two injection ports on it. The primary IV infusion setup is used for any type of IV therapy except the administration of blood products, which requires a special set with a filter in the drip chamber. There are several different brands of IV administration tubing sets on the market, and you will need to check the directions for the type used in your agency.

> **?**
> *Think Critically About . . .* How would the diameter and length of IV equipment such as tubing and catheters affect the flow of fluid?

The primary IV tubing set is selected according to the size of the drop to be delivered into the drip chamber. There are three major sizes:
1. Regular drops (10 to 20 gtt/mL of fluid as specified by the manufacturer)—used for administering IV therapy to most adult patients.
2. Macrodrops (10 gtt/mL)—used for viscous (sticky or gummy) fluids, such as blood; may be used for regular fluids.
3. Microdrops (60 gtt/mL)—used when small amounts of fluid are required or when extreme care must be used to measure the exact amount; most often used for giving IV fluids to infants and children; recommended for the elderly with fragile veins.

Secondary or Piggyback Intravenous Set

Medications to be given intravenously are often added to an existing IV line by using the piggyback method. Primary administration sets have one or two inlet ports for adding medications or a second IV. When this is used, the primary infusion is interrupted to infuse medications such as antibiotics and antineoplastic drugs at regularly scheduled times. Because these drugs are diluted in amounts of 50 to 150 mL of solution, they must be given by infusion, not by bolus. **The advantage of the piggyback system is that when the solution in the smaller bag has been in-**

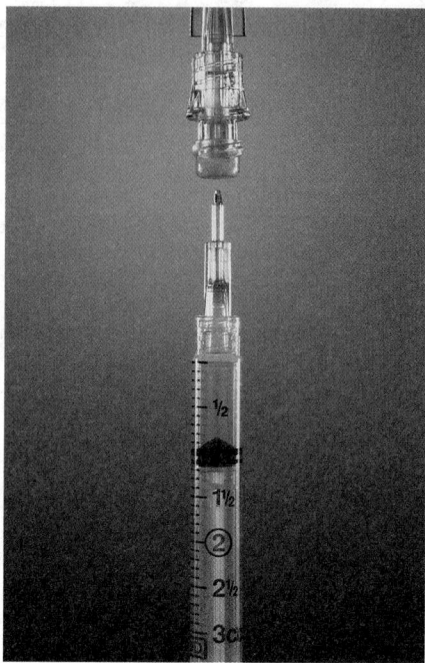

FIGURE 36-3 Needleless equipment.

fused, the primary IV begins to flow again without further adjustments.**

In accordance with *Healthy People 2010*, a primary occupational health goal is the prevention of needle sticks, which may transmit the human immunodeficiency virus (HIV), hepatitis B, or hepatitis C. Use of needleless devices for attaching secondary tubing or syringes for the infusion of medication is highly recommended to prevent injury and exposure to these diseases (Figure 36-3).

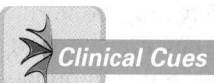
Clinical Cues

The secondary bag, containing the medication, is hung higher than the level of fluid in the primary IV so that gravity forces it to empty first. Do not clamp or alter the flow of the primary bag. If the secondary bag is positioned correctly, the primary infusion will begin to flow when the secondary bag is completed.

Parallel or "Y" Intravenous Set

A "Y"-type administration set is used to infuse certain blood products (Figure 36-4). The blood product is placed on one side, and a bag of normal saline is placed on the other side. The saline is started first, and then the blood administration is begun. The saline is stopped while the blood is running. When the transfusion (introduction of blood components into the blood stream) is complete, the tubing is flushed with the normal saline solution.

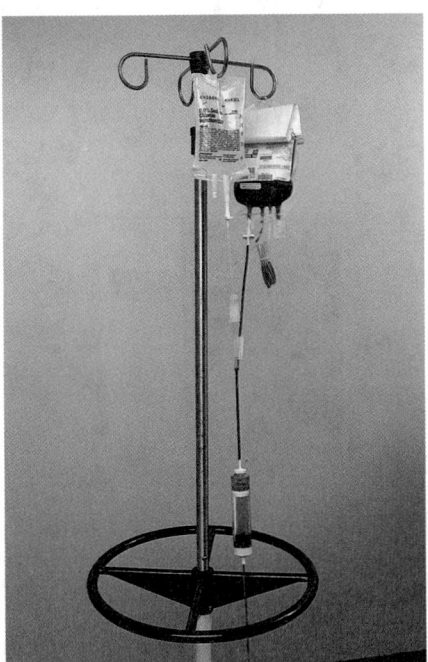

FIGURE **36-4** "Y"-type blood administration setup.

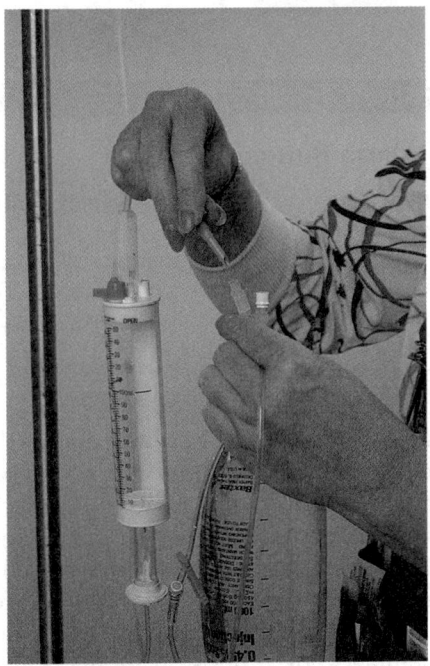

FIGURE **36-5** Controlled-volume set.

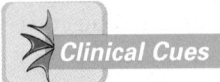

Saline is the only solution used in conjunction with infusion of a blood product. Other types of fluid may cause the cells to lyse or clump.

Controlled-Volume Intravenous Set

Another way of interrupting a primary infusion is to give a dose of diluted medication through a controlled-volume administration set. In most instances, an infu-

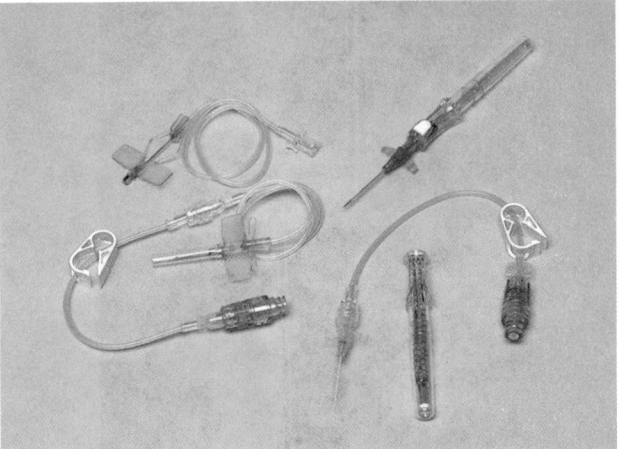

FIGURE **36-6** Intermittent intravenous device (i.e., PRN lock).

sion pump (machine that delivers IV fluids at a rate that is set by the nurse) is used to administer small volumes of fluid or medication. However, the controlled-volume system is sometimes used as a safety backup between the IV bag and the entry to the infusion pump to prevent free flow of fluid when the tubing is removed from the pump. The set contains a burette (tubelike chamber that will hold 150 mL of fluid) into which the medication is injected along with a specified volume of fluid from the primary bag, which is then clamped off. When an IV infusion pump is not used, the medication from the burette goes into the drip chamber, and the flow is regulated by a clamp on the IV tubing. The burette set is attached to the primary IV line beneath the bag of fluid (Figure 36-5). This set can also be used when a small amount of fluid is to be infused over a long period. It is often used for administration of fluids to infants, children, and the elderly.

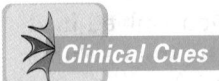

Using a controlled-volume set ensures that a fluid overload cannot occur because only a specified amount of fluid is available to be infused at any one time (e.g., 50 to 100 mL).

Intermittent Intravenous Device (Saline or PRN Lock)

Some patients do not require large amounts of fluid by the IV route but may need to receive IV medications at intervals or have an IV access in case emergency medications are needed quickly. An intermittent access device is preferred for patients who receive antibiotics, heparin, corticosteroids, antimetabolites, and some other drugs. An intermittent IV device is established by applying a Luer-Lok cap or an extension set, which is a very short piece of tubing, to the IV cannula. The peripheral device is called a saline lock, PRN lock, or INT (intermittent) lock (Figure 36-6). One advan-

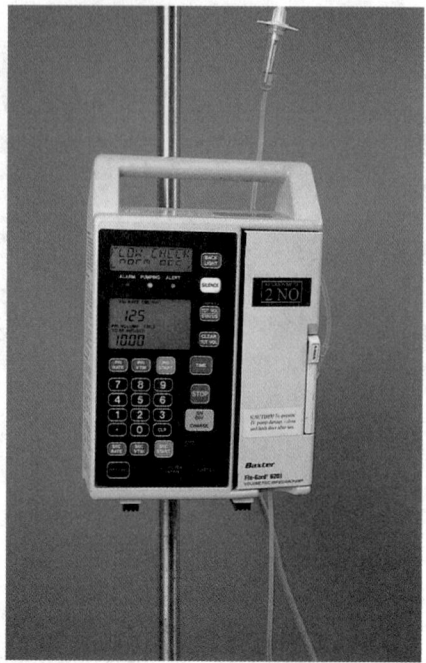

FIGURE **36-7** Intravenous infusion pump.

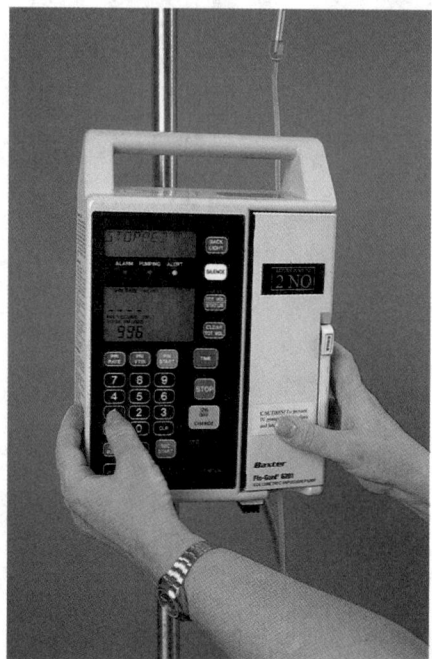

FIGURE **36-8** Setting the rate and volume on the infusion pump.

tage of this method is the freedom of movement for the patient.

Because no solution is continuously infusing through the lock, saline or a dilute heparin flush is periodically used to maintain patency by keeping a clot from forming at the tip of the catheter. Often an IV line is converted to an intermittent device when the patient no longer needs fluids but is still receiving IV medications. This is done by removing the IV tubing and attaching a catheter cap or extension set.

Filters

Filters trap small particles such as undissolved medication or salts that have precipitated from solution. They prevent such particles from entering the vein. A 0.22-micron filter is used for most solutions. For solutions containing lipids or albumin, a 1.2-micron filter is used. A special filter is needed for blood components.

INFUSION PUMPS AND CONTROLLERS

Use of infusion pumps is an added safety measure, and they are used in many facilities to regulate the flow of routine IV fluids on general medical-surgical units. Use of pumps is mandatory when patients are receiving total parenteral nutrition (TPN) (technique of providing needed nutrition intravenously) or for medications that require critical accuracy, such as heparin, insulin, cardiovascular medications, chemotherapy drugs, or medications that are used to induce labor (Figure 36-7).

Programmed infusion pumps are more accurate and provide better control over the amount of solution being infused. These pumps deliver IV fluids automatically at a rate that is calculated and programmed

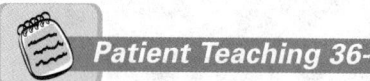

Patient Teaching 36-1

Silence Alarm Button

The patient or family may observe the nursing staff using the silence alarm button and they may push the button in an attempt "to help the nurse." Teach them to call for assistance (if it appears that no one is hearing and responding to the alarms). Reassure them that you will quickly respond to the alarms.

by the nurse (Figure 36-8). They have alarms that warn when the IV container is empty, when air is present in the tubing, or when the line is infiltrated (solution is deposited in tissue outside the vein) or occluded, depending on which model of the pump is used (Patient Teaching 36-1). Use of a pump does not replace or substitute for good nursing observation.

Disadvantages of pumps include (1) they exert pressure on the vein, (2) they are expensive, and (3) certain types of pumps require special administration sets. It is advocated that health care facilities purchase only infusion pumps that have administration sets with set-based anti–free-flow mechanisms that prevent gravity free flow by closing off the tubing when the administration set is removed from the pump. Other pumps must have a free-flow safety device attached to the tubing before it enters the pump. There are pumps that will handle multiple infusion lines that can be programmed separately for each line. Box 36-1 includes some tips for using an IV pump.

Rate controller devices operate by gravity flow. Controllers can reduce the risk of infusing fluid too

Box 36-1 | *IV Pumps: Tips for Use and Troubleshooting*

- IV pumps vary greatly by manufacturer; obtain assistance as needed to learn the specific features.
- Check the medication, calculate the correct dosage, and determine the pump setting prior to entering the patient's room (see Box 36-2, p. 724).
- For adult usage, most pumps will deliver mL/hr. Set the pump for the correct rate in mL/hr.
- Pumps usually allow you to set a total volume; the machine will alarm when it reaches that volume. (Use this feature to call you back at the end of the infusion, or sooner as needed according to your clinical judgment.)
- Before you leave the room, check to ensure the following: patient is comfortable and there is no swelling at the insertion site, appropriate clamps are open, intermittent dripping (not continuous) is observed in the drip chamber.
- Pumps can malfunction; assessment of site and equipment every 1 to 2 hours is a typical hospital policy.
- *If the IV pump is continually alarming:* Check the IV site for infiltration, clotting, etc. Check tubing for kinks. Check clamps and flow regulators. Check IV bag to see if there is fluid for infusion. Make sure the pump is plugged into an electrical source. Recheck settings on the pump. Change the position of the patient's extremity. (IV might be positional.) Try turning the pump off and resetting it. Try another pump.

quickly; however, their effectiveness can by altered by patient and mechanical factors. Rate controllers are not used for blood or viscous solutions because they are not as accurate as pumps.

> *Think Critically About . . .* Your patient needs an IV infusion and you are unable to find an IV pump. You have called central supply and several other units and were told that there were no pumps available at this time. It is the facility policy that an IV pump should always be used. What will you do?

Portable infusion pumps, such as the CADD-PCA, are often used for home care patients. This pump can be attached to a subcutaneous catheter for infusion of pain medication. Portable pumps also are available for the infusion of TPN.

Patient-controlled analgesia (PCA) pumps are commonly used in most hospitals and are also used in the home setting. This type of pump is used for pain control, and it has a remote-control button by which the patient can administer a controlled bolus of pain medication from time to time. The pump is programmed to allow only a certain limited amount of medication to be delivered during a particular period. Analgesia may be delivered continuously subcutaneously for the home care patient by the use of a CADD pump.

There are other small, self-contained pump devices that are used to deliver doses of medication, such as the insulin pump. The insulin pump is a small portable device that can be programmed to deliver a continuous infusion of regular insulin that mimics normal physiology. Use of this device requires intensive patient education and teaching; the patient must be highly motivated and capable of changing the insertion site every 2 to 3 days, refilling the pump with insulin, reprogramming the device, checking blood sugar four to six times per day, and monitoring for signs of infection.

VENOUS ACCESS DEVICES
Intravenous Needles and Catheters

New safety venous access devices decrease the risk of accidental needle sticks for the nurse. These devices have either a stylet that retracts into a closed sleeve or a plastic sleeve that advances over the stylet as it is removed from the skin. There are three basic types of IV needles and catheters used for peripheral IV fluid administration. The winged-tip or butterfly needle is meant for short-term therapy, such as to give single-dose IV medication or to obtain blood samples. After insertion, the wings are taped to the skin. These needles are supplied in odd-numbered gauges (17, 19, 23, and 25). The butterfly needle is also frequently used for pediatric infusions or for the elderly because it comes in a smaller gauge than most catheters. Because these needles are rigid, they may cause more discomfort than do other types of catheters, and mobility may be restricted to prevent dislodgement of the needle.

Over-the-needle catheters consist of a needle with a catheter sheath over it. After the device is placed into the vein and the cannula (catheter sheath) is threaded, the needle is removed, leaving the flexible catheter in the vein. Catheters of this type are thought to cause less irritation, thereby decreasing the incidence of infection and phlebitis. The size of the catheter or needle depends on the type of solution given and the size of a suitable vein. For clear aqueous solutions, a 20- to 22-gauge needle is used, but for more viscous fluids, blood products, or when the patient rapidly needs large amounts of fluid a larger (18- or 19-gauge) needle or catheter is needed. For example, a trauma patient who might need blood should have a large-bore catheter. When using the scalp veins of infants, finer-gauge needles must be used. These catheters are used when therapy will be for 7 or fewer days.

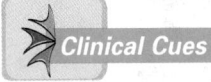
Clinical Cues

Peripheral catheters are typically replaced every 72 hours. Facility policy may dictate that catheters that are inserted in the emergency room or in the field by paramedics be replaced sooner.

A through-the-needle catheter is not recommended for short-term peripheral use. This type is used for midline catheter insertion for long-term peripheral use. Because the needle is larger in diameter than the catheter, there may be leakage when the needle is removed.

Although an arm board may be used to support and immobilize the arm during IV therapy, this is not desirable because the patient's elbow or wrist movement may be severely restricted, causing discomfort. When an arm board is the only alternative, tape or gauze secures both ends of the arm board to the arm without restricting the patient's circulation.

?
• *Think Critically About* . . . What special care do you think is needed when the patient's IV site is secured with an arm board?

Central Venous Catheters and Peripherally Inserted Central Catheters

When a peripheral vein is difficult to locate in the adult or the veins are not suitable for IV therapy, a catheter is inserted into the large subclavian vein and positioned in the superior vena cava or the right atrium. This type of catheter can be left in place for 6 to 8 weeks. The nurse assists the physician during the subclavian catheter insertion by providing the sterile catheter tray, draping the patient, opening sterile packages, and preparing the IV administration set for use. If the patient needs a central line for more than 6 to 8 weeks, a long-term catheter such as a tunneled Broviac, Hickman, or Groshong is inserted. This procedure is done in the operating room.

Peripherally inserted central catheters (PICCs), or midline catheters (MLs), are often used in children or in adults who need peripheral IV therapy that requires placement where there is high blood flow. They are also a first choice in home care IV therapy of 6 to 8 weeks. These catheters are long and are inserted in the larger basilic or cephalic vein of the upper arm. The ML ideally sits just inside the subclavian vein; the PICC may be advanced as far as the superior vena cava (Figure 36-9). Other vascular access devices (devices such as a needle, or catheter that allow direct access to the circulatory system) in the form of central venous catheters or implanted infusion ports are used for patients who need long-term drug therapy, fluid therapy, or chemotherapy. These catheters are inserted by the physician or a specially trained nurse.

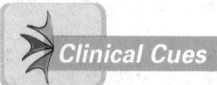
Clinical Cues

Remember not to take the blood pressure on the arm that has a PICC or ML catheter in place.

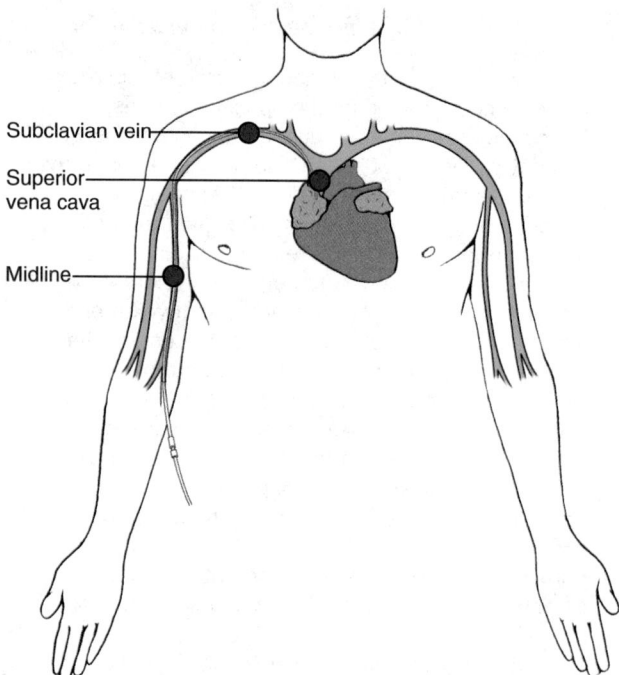

FIGURE **36-9** Placement of a PICC line.

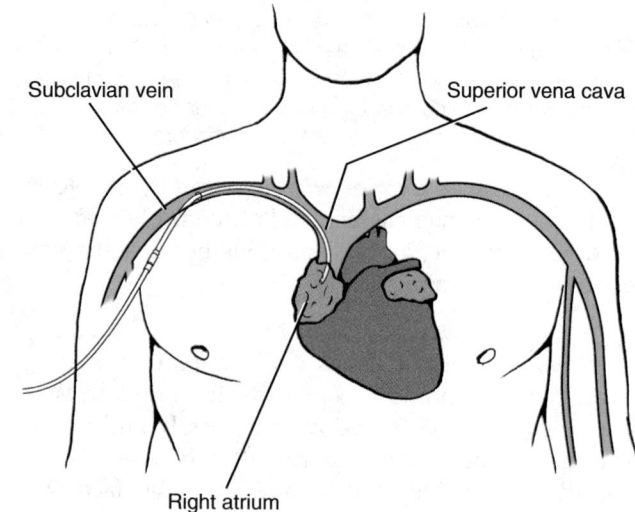

FIGURE **36-10** Placement of a subclavian central line.

Short-term central venous catheters are inserted into a large vein, usually the subclavian or jugular, by the physician. Long-term central venous catheters that are threaded to the tip of the right atrium of the heart are placed by surgical tunneling through subcutaneous tissue and then through the subclavian vein into the superior vena cava (Figure 36-10). The surgeon first enters the vein and then makes the subcutaneous tunnel or pocket. Central venous catheters range from 15 to 30 cm in length. There are several types available. Some have single lumens; others have two, three, or more lumens.

These catheters are periodically flushed, much the same as for a PRN lock, to keep the lumens patent. Agency policy will dictate specific amounts, frequency, and type of flush solution (i.e., saline or heparin) and

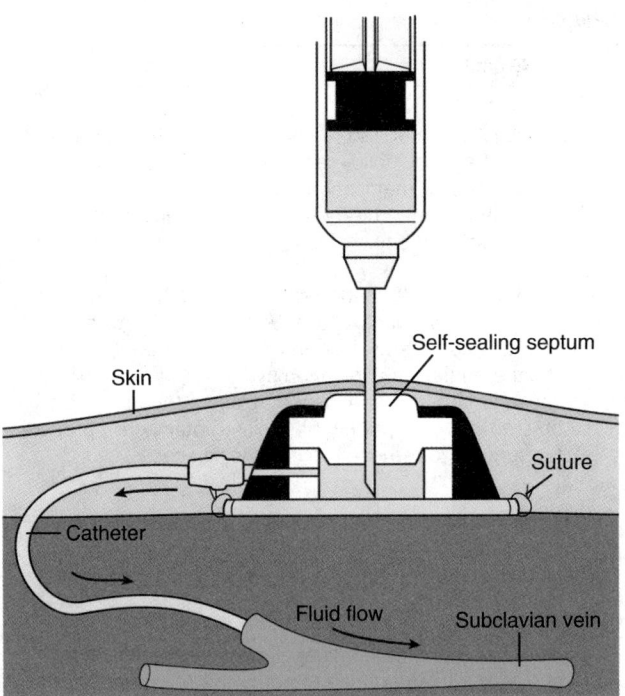

FIGURE **36-11** Implanted infusion port and Huber needle.

size of syringe (i.e., 10-mL syringe) and guidelines for when to obtain an order for special declotting solutions. Agency policy will also indicate if central line management is an RN-only responsibility. **Correct placement of subclavian catheters must be verified by radiographic studies before any fluid is infused through them.**

Infusion Port

An infusion port with a single- or dual-lumen catheter can be implanted (Figure 36-11). Most ports are placed subcutaneously on the chest beneath the right clavicle, and the catheter is threaded through a large vein and into the superior vena cava. Sometimes these ports are implanted in other areas for intraspinal or intraperitoneal infusion. Specially designed Huber noncoring needles are used to infuse solutions and medications through the port. **No other type of needle should be used because other needles cause damage to the port.**

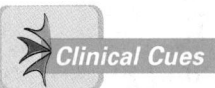

The physician may order medication to be given by the epidural (epidural space of the spinal column) or intrathecal (intrathecal space of the spinal column) route. This route of administration is beyond the current scope for LPN/LVNs; however, you should be aware that medication vials can be labeled specifically for IV, epidural, or intrathecal administration. It is not safe to interchange routes for these specifically labeled medications. **Read the labels and immediately alert the charge nurse if you find these medications are being stored together.**

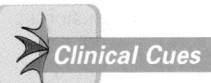

COMPLICATIONS OF INTRAVENOUS THERAPY

Complications of IV therapy are potentially very serious, such as infiltration, phlebitis, systemic infection, and catheter embolus (piece of the catheter obstructing blood flow). Ask the patient about discomfort as you visually inspect and palpate the site. Assess the flow of fluid whenever you are at the patient's bedside.

One of the most effective ways to prevent complications is to teach the patient to immediately report any changes or discomfort at the IV site. The 2009 National Patient Safety Goals advocate the active participation of the patient and the family to increase safety.

INFILTRATION

Infiltration is the most common problem. This occurs when fluid or medication leaks out of the vein into the tissue. There will often be edema around the site, and the tissue will feel cool. The skin may have a pale appearance. Flow can be slow and sluggish when infiltration has occurred; however, this is not a definitive sign, particularly in the early phase of infiltration when the fluid can be progressively leaking into the surrounding tissue. If infiltration has occurred, the infusion is discontinued and another site is initiated to continue therapy. Fluid that is in the tissue will usually reabsorb within 24 hours. Follow agency policy for treatment.

PHLEBITIS

Phlebitis is caused by irritation of the vein by the needle, catheter, medications, or additives in the IV solution. The typical signs of phlebitis are erythema, warmth, swelling, and tenderness. The IV must be discontinued and another site found for reinitiating therapy. Application of warm compresses to the inflamed site will decrease discomfort.

BLOODSTREAM INFECTION

Bloodstream infection *(septicemia)* occurs when infectious pathogens are introduced into the bloodstream. This may occur from breaks in sterile technique during cannula insertion or any time the system is opened to change the bag or tubing. Signs and symptoms are fever, chills, pain, headache, nausea, vomiting, and extreme fatigue. Blood cultures are ordered and aggressive antibiotic therapy is started. The IV site is immediately discontinued.

OTHER COMPLICATIONS

There are several additional serious complications of IV therapy. Catheter embolus can occur when a piece of the catheter breaks off and travels in the vein until

Table 36-2 *Complications of Intravenous Therapy and Nursing Interventions*

COMPLICATION	MANIFESTATIONS	NURSING CARE
LOCAL		
Infiltration	Arm swollen, tender, cool to touch; may or may not have blood return	Remove IV catheter and restart IV in the other extremity. (Consult agency policy regarding care for certain IV solutions or medications.)
Phlebitis	Vein hard with skin red, swollen, tender, warm; blood return present; IV infusion may or may not be sluggish	Remove IV catheter, notify the physician, and apply warm packs to the IV site.
Thrombophlebitis	Site red, tender, warm; IV infusion sluggish	Never irrigate the IV catheter; remove the IV catheter, notify the physician, restart IV in opposite extremity.
IV site infection	Site hot, red, painful but not hard or swollen; IV infusion sluggish	Remove IV catheter, restart in opposite extremity and change entire administration system.
Catheter embolus	Decrease in BP; pain along vein; weak, rapid pulse; cyanosis of nail beds; loss of consciousness	Remove IV catheter and inspect, place a tourniquet high on limb of IV site, notify physician, obtain x-ray, prepare for surgery to remove the catheter pieces.
SYSTEMIC		
Infection	Fever, chills, general malaise	Change the infusion system, notify the physician, and obtain cultures as ordered.
Speed shock	Flushed face, severe headache, chest pain, irregular pulse, decreased BP, loss of consciousness, cardiac arrest	Stop the infusion, notify the physician, and monitor vital signs frequently.
Circulatory overload	Increased BP, distended neck veins, rapid breathing, dyspnea, moist cough, crackles	Elevate head of the bed, keep warm, assess for edema, slow the infusion rate, and notify the physician.
Air embolus	Sudden drop in BP, increase in pulse	Place on left side and lower head of the bed, inspect IV infusion system for disconnection or leak, and notify the physician.
Allergic reaction	Catheter: red streak along vein, pain at IV site Medication: site red, itching, rash	Remove IV catheter, restart IV using different type of IV catheter, notify the physician; discontinue the medication.

Key: *BP,* Blood pressure.
From Leahy, J.M., & Kizilay, P.E. (1998). *Foundations of Nursing Practice: A Nursing Process Approach* (p. 822). Philadelphia: Saunders.

it lodges. *Air embolus* can occur when changing bags, or when opening the line of a subclavian catheter. *Speed shock* occurs when fluids or medications given by bolus are administered too rapidly. Table 36-2 lists all the complications with their signs and symptoms and the necessary nursing interventions.

IV sites must be checked at least once an hour. In accordance with The Joint Commission's 2009 National Patient Safety Goals, health care professionals are tasked "to improve recognition and response to changes in the patient's condition." Your documentation should reflect an absence of complications. If you identify a problem, document your observations and document your follow-up actions that address the problem.

> **?**
> *Think Critically About . . .* Your charting demonstrates that you observed and documented signs of infiltration or phlebitis related to your patient's IV site. You corrected the problem but forgot to chart your actions. Several years later the patient retains a lawyer and attempts to sue the hospital for a variety of issues. What are the implications of your missing documentation.

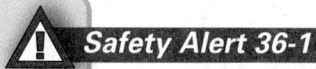
Safety Alert 36-1

Making IV Connections

When working with IV tubing connections, make sure that you trace the tube to the patient's body to ensure that you are making the correct connection. There have been incidents in which IV tubing was inadvertently attached to the inflation cuff of a tracheostomy tube. In other cases, enteral feeding tubing was mistakenly attached to central line ports and the automatic blood pressure tubing was attached to an IV. These incidents resulted in patients' deaths (Eakle et al., 2005).

APPLICATION of the NURSING PROCESS

All nurses monitor IV therapy and add IV solutions without medication to existing IV setups (Safety Alert 36-1). Depending on the state nurse practice act and the training program, many practical nurses hang IV piggyback medications, add medications to IV solutions, calculate IV infusion rates, and initiate IV therapy by inserting a catheter. Often an extra course is required for certification to perform IV therapy and to start IVs. Because of the diverse training needs of LPNs/LVNs, all basic IV skills are presented here.

Assessment (Data Collection)

A primary nursing responsibility is to check the patient's chart and verify the IV orders. Each nurse is responsible for determining that the correct IV solution is hanging. The patient who has IV fluids infusing must have the site assessed periodically, preferably hourly during the shift, to ensure that the site is patent and that the solution is infusing correctly. The flow rate must be assessed to determine that the fluid is running at the prescribed rate. Assessment is performed for the various complications of IV therapy (see Box 36-3 on p. 725).

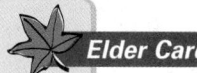

Elder Care Points

The elderly must be frequently assessed to determine that fluid overload is not occurring. Auscultate the lungs at least once each shift for sounds of crackles that can indicate fluid overload. Rapid pulse, shortness of breath, and distended neck veins are other possible signs of fluid overload.

When giving IV medications, the order must be carefully checked. Review the drug's action, possible side effects, correct dosage, and nursing implications before preparing the drug. Assess for drug allergies before preparing the IV piggyback medication. Check for possible drug–solution incompatibilities. If incompatibilities exist, the IV line must be flushed with sterile saline before the other drug or solution is started and flushed again when the infusion or injection is finished. Assess for potential drug interactions when more than one drug is being administered. **Always assess the patient for adverse or side effects of previously administered doses of IV or piggyback medications before administering the next dose.** Assess the existing IV site and catheter size before beginning an infusion of a blood product. The site must be free of any signs of infection or inflammation.

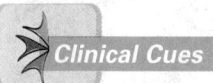

Clinical Cues

Blood products are not infused into the same IV line as medications or other fluids. Obtain baseline vital signs before starting the infusion of blood products. This allows assessment of the patient's condition and response to the product infused during and after therapy.

Nursing Diagnosis

Common nursing diagnoses for patients who are undergoing various types of IV therapy might include the following:

- Deficient fluid volume related to inability to take fluids by mouth (fluid replacement)
- Risk for infection related to invasive procedure (IV drug therapy)

Assignment Considerations 36-1

Protecting IV Sites During Showering and Bathing

When caring for a patient with a peripheral IV, plan additional time for bathing, turning, and assisting with daily activities. Advise the UAPs about which patients have IVs. There are commercial plastic sheaths that can be used to cover an IV site on an extremity, or a clean plastic bag can be taped to protect the site.

- Imbalanced nutrition less than body requirements, related to inability to take oral foods or fluids (TPN)
- Ineffective tissue perfusion (cardiopulmonary) related to loss of red blood cells/fluid volume (blood product transfusion)

Planning

Allow time for the care of the patient's IV site, hanging of solutions, and needed assessments in the daily work schedule (Assignment Considerations 36-1).

Sample goals/expected outcomes for the previous nursing diagnoses are as follows:

- No signs of dehydration are displayed.
- The patient will display no signs of postoperative infection.
- The patient's nutritional status will improve as evidenced by a weight gain of 0.5 lb per week and protein levels will be within normal limits.
- The patient's hemoglobin level will be 11.5 g/dL before discharge.

Calculation of Flow Rates

Another aspect of planning is calculating the rate of flow at which an IV solution or medication is to infuse. To calculate the flow rate, you must know how many drops are contained in each milliliter as it passes through the drip chamber of the tubing, because the size of the drops varies for different types of administration sets. The standard set produces 10 to 20 gtt/mL, the pediatric or microdrip chamber produces 60 gtt/mL, and the macrodrip of the transfusion-type sets gives 10 gtt/mL. For the purpose of demonstrating rate calculations, 10 gtt will be used for the macrodrip, 15 gtt for the regular drip, and 60 gtt for the microdrip chamber.

> **?**
> *Think Critically About* . . . Why is the microdrip set safer for pediatric patients? Can you identify other types of patients or health conditions for which a microdrip set would be a good choice?

If there are questions about how to calculate the IV drop rate, check with the instructor. Charts are avail-

---

Box 36-2   *Calculating the IV Flow Rate*

- Formula for flow rate calculation:

$$\frac{\text{Amount of solution (in mL)} \times \text{No. drops/mL}}{\text{Time (in min)}} = \text{Drops/min}$$

- When the order reads "1000 mL of D$_5$W over 10 hours," use a regular drip set (15 gtt/mL):

$$\frac{1000\ \text{mL} \times 15\ \text{gtt/mL}}{10\ \text{hr} \times 60\ \text{min}} = \frac{15,000}{600} = 25\ \text{gtt/min}$$

- When the order reads "D$_5$ ½NS at 125 mL/hr," use:

$$\frac{125\ \text{mL} \times 15\text{gtt/mL}}{60\ \text{min}} = \frac{1875}{60} = 31.25\ \text{or}\ 31\ \text{gtt/min}$$

- Formula for using a standard adult pump (mL/hr):

$$\frac{\text{Amount of solution (in mL)} \times 60\ \text{min/hr}}{\text{Time (in min)}} = \text{mL/hr}$$

- When the order reads "250 mg of medication in 100 mL, deliver over 30 minutes," use:

$$\frac{100\ \text{mL of solution} \times 60\ \text{min/hr}}{30\ \text{min}} = 200\ \text{mL/hr}$$

---

able that have precalculated rates for the various drip chambers and for the period of time that the infusion is ordered to run in standard amounts, such as 1000 mL. If these charts are not available, it is necessary to solve the problem mathematically. The basic formula for calculating the rate of flow is given in Box 36-2.

When IV therapy is administered, the fluid enters the circulation immediately. The adult adapts best to fluids at a steady rate of 20 to 60 regular gtt/minute—in other words, 80 to 250 mL/hour. Larger amounts of fluids increase the work of the heart, and the fluid overload could lead to congestive heart failure.

Factors that influence the rate of flow of an IV solution are the size of the catheter, the height of the solution container, and the viscosity of the fluid. Fluids flow less rapidly through a catheter with a small bore (internal diameter) than through a catheter with a larger bore. The higher the container is held, the faster is the flow of fluid. Packed red blood cells (RBCs) are more viscous and require a larger catheter.

The physician generally orders 1000 mL of IV fluids to infuse over an 8-, 10-, or 12-hour period. **This amount should infuse at an even rate so that equal amounts are given each hour.** When the number of hours is stated, you should prepare a time tape to be placed on the bag that shows the amount to be infused each hour and the level of the solution remaining in the bag at 0900, 1000, 1100 and so forth (Figure 36-12). To correctly determine the amount of fluid left in the bag, hold the bag on both sides and gently stretch the plastic. At eye level, read the volume of the meniscus for the remaining solution (Figure 36-13). Time tapes are not always placed on the bag when an IV pump is used.

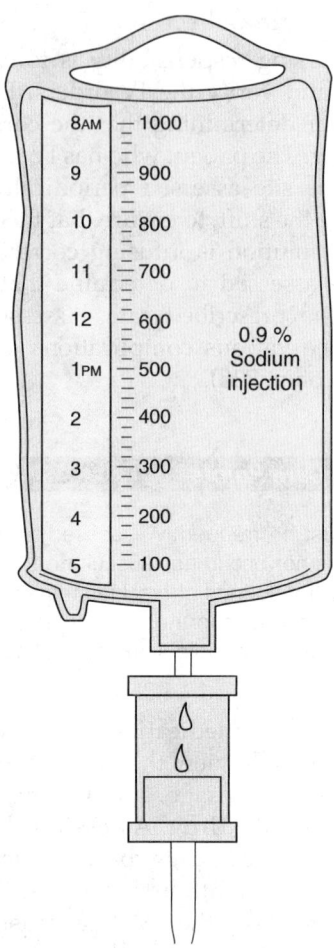

FIGURE **36-12** Time tape label for an intravenous fluid container.

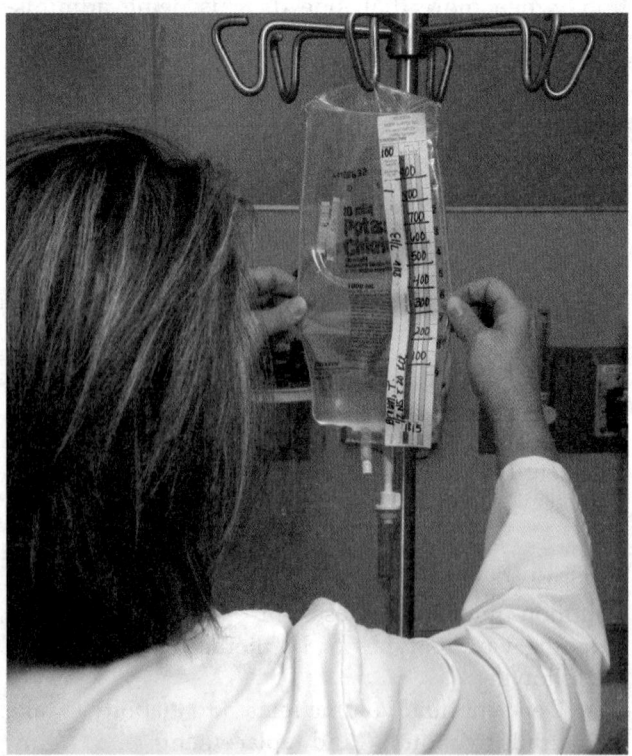

FIGURE **36-13** Gently stretch IV bag to get an accurate reading of fluid remaining.

Table 36-3 *Troubleshooting: IV Flow*

CHECK	RATIONALE
Height of infusion container	Patient may have changed position. The container should be at least 36 inches above the heart.
System vent	Air vent may be absent or occluded, which will prevent the flow.
Position of tubing	Tubing may be kinked, obstructing flow. Tubing may be hanging below the bed, interfering with the gravity flow.
Position of the extremity where the site is located	Flexion of the extremity may have compressed the vein, slowing the flow.
Any possible obstruction to flow	A protective device on the limb may be too tight. Tape may be compressing the circumference of the extremity.
When filter was changed	Filter may be occluded.
Position of the catheter within the vein	Catheter may be lying against the vein wall, obstructing flow. Slightly turning the catheter to reposition the tip may cure the problem.
If other measures have not opened the line, attempt to aspirate blood from the catheter.	A small clot may be obstructing the catheter. Aspiration may withdraw the clot.
Never force flush an IV catheter	Forcefully flushing a catheter sends the clot into the bloodstream. This creates an embolus that could lodge anywhere in the body, including the brain, heart or lungs.

Box 36-3 *Intravenous Therapy Guidelines*

- **Keep IV fluid sterile.** Make sure that everything coming into contact with the solution is sterile, including the inside surface of the catheter hub, and all connecting points between the bag and drip chamber and between the tubing and the needleless connector.
- **Protect the catheter site from contamination to avoid possible infection.** An airtight, transparent dressing is used over the catheter site; the Infusion Nurses Society now recommends that catheters be secured with a manufactured catheter stabilization device, rather than by taping.
- **Keep tubing free of air.** Clear tubing of air before connecting to the catheter. Do not allow the current bag to run dry before changing to the next one.
- **Hang fluids at the correct height.** Fluids flow through the tubing by the force of gravity. If there is negative pressure in the IV line, blood will flow back into the tubing. Keep the bag of fluid sufficiently above the level of the catheter site to maintain flow, but avoid having it too high because this significantly increases the effect of gravity.
- **Carefully regulate the rate of flow.** If the IV is behind schedule, do not open up the clamp and run in a large amount of fluid at one time to catch up. Rather, recalculate either (1) the span of time for the infusion or (2) the rate of drops per minute for the fluid to run at the ordered rate.
- **Track intake and output when a patient is receiving IV fluids or blood.** Keep accurate intake and output records and compare intake with output over 24 hours.
- **Hang the solution to run in first the higher.** When a second bag is attached piggyback to a primary IV line, lower the primary bag without clamping the tubing so it will begin to flow when the piggyback has run in. Attach the piggyback tubing to a port beneath the roller clamp on the primary tubing.
- **Assess the site frequently for signs of complications.** Infiltration, swelling at the IV site, irritation of the vein, formation of a clot stopping the flow, or systemic reaction should be identified quickly. Signs of infiltration are pain or discomfort at the site caused by dislodgement of the catheter or puncture out of the vein. Vital signs should be taken several times a day to detect early signs of infection or adverse reaction.
- **Observe closely for transfusion reactions.** Reactions to blood transfusion usually occur shortly after the start of the transfusion (within 5 to 15 minutes). Reactions are most common when packed red cells or whole blood is given. Signs of reaction include hives, itching, facial flushing, chills, back pain, apprehension, and fever. If any of these signs occur, stop the transfusion, start normal saline, and contact the physician for further orders.

Keep the IV on time by regulating the drip rate. If IV fluids are infusing behind schedule, recalculate or reschedule the time in consultation with the charge nurse or the physician. Check to see that the IV is infusing on time every 30 to 60 minutes, particularly if the fluid is not being administered by an infusion pump. If the infusion will not flow at the ordered rate, a variety of factors may be responsible. Table 36-3 indicates steps for attempting to get sluggish IV flow corrected.

Implementation

The implementation phase of the nursing process includes all the tasks involved in caring for the patient undergoing one of the various types of IV therapy. With practice, the new nurse will become adept at connecting IV tubing, changing old tubing for new, calculating flow rates, adjusting the roller clamp to the correct drop rate, starting the IV, and detecting complications. Nursing guidelines for intravenous therapy are presented in Box 36-3.

The patient who has a peripheral IV will be a bit more limited in performing usual tasks. Help may be needed to open containers on the dietary tray, and if the IV is in the dominant hand, assistance may be required for many of the tasks of daily living.

Initiating Intravenous Therapy

Considerable preparation is necessary before venipuncture is performed: gather the equipment, obtain or prepare the IV infusion (with or without medication), select the most appropriate vein, and prepare the site (Skill 36-1). The sites most frequently used for peripheral IVs are the veins of the forearm and hand. The foot veins are used only when no other site is available. The veins that are so prominent in the antecubital space are not used extensively for IV infusions because movement causes irritation or damage to the vein, and keeping the arm extended may cause muscle or nerve damage. Scalp or umbilical veins are frequently used in infants because the veins of the arms are too small or may be too difficult to locate or enter with the catheter.

It is necessary to be able to feel or see the vein before initiating venipuncture. If there is difficulty detecting the vein, a device called the venoscope can be used to illuminate the tissue and outline the vein. Agency policy will provide guidelines for IV catheter insertion.

Skill 36-1 | Starting the Primary Intravenous Infusion

Before an IV catheter is inserted, the solution to be infused is set up so that it will be immediately ready to be infused when the IV access is initiated. Be especially careful to maintain aseptic technique when handling IV fluids and tubing, as an IV site provides access for bacteria to enter the bloodstream.

■ Supplies

- ✓ IV solution with prepared time tape
- ✓ IV administration set
- ✓ IV cannula
- ✓ Scissors
- ✓ IV infusion pump (according to agency policy)
- ✓ IV stand or pole
- ✓ IV start kit (usually includes: chlorhexidine swabs, alcohol swabs, label, tape, transparent dressing, tourniquet)
- ✓ Gloves
- ✓ Commercial device to secure site
- ✓ Towel or underpad
- ✓ Arm board (optional)
- ✓ Medication administration record (MAR)

Review and carry out the Standard Steps in Appendix 3.

■ Assessment (Data Collection)

1. **ACTION** Inspect the patient's hands and forearms, and select the site for venipuncture. Choose the most distal site possible.

   RATIONALE If repeated infusions are required, it is best to start the IV in the most distal vein, and progress proximally with each successive site.

■ Planning

2. **ACTION** Verify that the patient is ready for the procedure and gather all equipment. Explain what you will do.

   RATIONALE Prepares the patient and prevents time loss.

■ Implementation
Preparing the IV Infusion

3. **ACTION** Obtain the correct IV solution; check the solution with the order.

   RATIONALE Following the five rights of medication administration applies to IV fluids and to additives.

4. **ACTION** Remove the covering from the IV bag, and check the solution for clarity, leaks, and particulate matter. Note the expiration date.

   RATIONALE If the sterility or safety of the solution is in question, it must not be infused. The solution must not be out of date.

5. **ACTION** Open the administration set, and position the roller clamp where it will be easy to reach and regulate while watching the drops in the drip chamber. Close the roller clamp, and remove the pull tab over the IV bag spike port. Be careful to keep it sterile while removing the cap on the tubing spike. Insert the spike, being careful not to touch the spike to anything but the inside of the spike port.

   RATIONALE If the roller clamp is not closed, the fluid will run quickly through the tubing and out when the bag is inverted. If a break in aseptic technique occurs, the tubing or solution must be discarded.

6. **ACTION** Squeeze the drip chamber while raising the bag and then place the container on a hook or IV stand. Allow the drip chamber to fill partially.

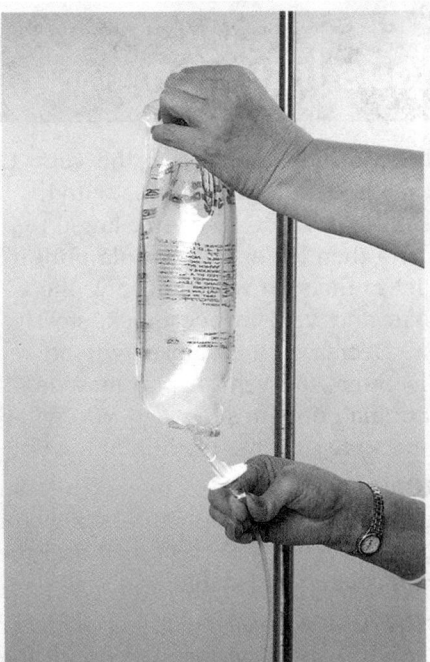

Step **6**

RATIONALE Filling the drip chamber in this manner reduces the amount of air bubbles that enter the IV tubing.

7. *ACTION* Remove the air from the tubing by slowly opening the roller clamp after loosening the protector cap over the needle adapter to allow the air to escape; allow a small amount of fluid to escape from the tubing, verifying that all air is removed. Close the roller clamp and retighten the cap.

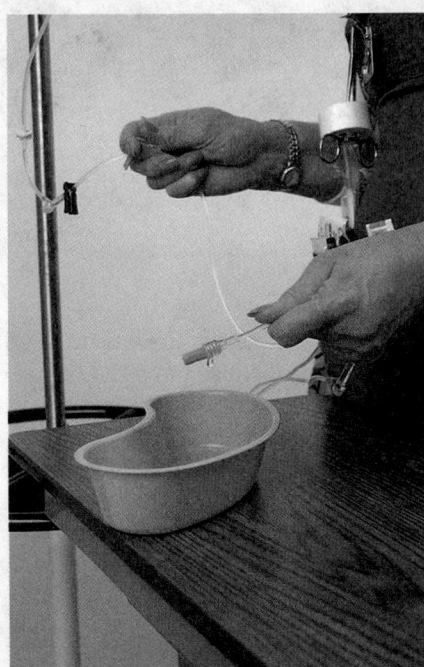

Step **7**

RATIONALE Any air left in the tubing might infuse into the patient and cause an air embolus. Although several milliliters of air must accumulate before se-

rious damage could occur, patients are very conscious of the possibility of a problem with air in the tubing, and for psychological reasons, as much air as possible should be removed from the tubing.

8. *ACTION* Place a time tape label on the IV container, and mark it in gradations of the amount of fluid to be infused every 1 to 2 hours.

   RATIONALE When time markings are indicated at different fluid levels, it is easy to see at a glance if the IV is flowing correctly according to the rate ordered.

9. *ACTION* Verify the IV solution and additives, if any, with the MAR. Take the IV solution and the MAR to the patient's bedside.

   RATIONALE Following the Five Rights prevents medication errors. The MAR is necessary to identify the patient and to perform the third medication check.

10. *ACTION* Verify the patient's identification. Prepare commercial securement device or three or four pieces of tape, and place them conveniently.

    RATIONALE Proper patient identification prevents medication errors. Tape is needed to secure the IV tubing to the patient.

Placing the IV Catheter and Starting the Infusion

11. *ACTION* Remove excess hair from the site if necessary by clipping (do not shave) the area around the chosen site and where the adhesive will be applied.

    RATIONALE Hair harbors microorganisms and can contribute to infection; the patient experiences discomfort when adhesive is removed if it is placed over hair.

12. *ACTION* Turn on the examination light, allow the extremity to hang down off the bed for a short time, or wrap it in a warm moist pack for 15 minutes to distend the vein. Prepare the IV start equipment and perform hand hygiene.

    RATIONALE Good light is necessary to visualize the vein adequately. The vein must be distended to introduce the cannula.

13. *ACTION* Apply the tourniquet and check the site suitability. The tourniquet should be positioned on the mid-forearm if the dorsum of the hand is to be used. If the forearm area is to be used, the tourniquet is placed on the upper arm or at least 4 to 6 inches above the site. Do not place the tourniquet so tightly as to restrict arterial flow. Release the tourniquet.

    RATIONALE Identifies best site. The venous flow must be restricted in the vein for it to distend enough to introduce the cannula. Releasing tourniquet promotes comfort while preparing equipment.

Continued

Skill 36-1 | Starting the Primary Intravenous Infusion—cont'd

14. **ACTION** Put down a protective pad under the extremity, and cleanse the site according to agency policy. Usually, this is done with chlorhexidine. (Povidone-iodine and alcohol may also be used.) Start at the center, and work in a circular motion outward for 2 inches. Allow the area to dry. Do not wave your hands or blow on the area to dry it.

RATIONALE A protective pad will prevent bedding and other surfaces from becoming soiled with the cleansing solution or contaminated with blood. Microorganisms, if left on the skin, may cause infection. (After cleaning area with povidone-iodine, allow area to dry completely and wipe area with an alcohol swab if you have trouble visualizing vein.) Waving over the area or blowing on it deposits microorganisms on the newly cleansed skin.

15. **ACTION** Don gloves, reapply the tourniquet; ask the patient to open and close the fist a couple of times, and then hold it closed. Stabilize the skin below the IV site by placing your thumb about 2 inches directly below the insertion site. A local anesthetic at the insertion site is sometimes allowed by agency policy.

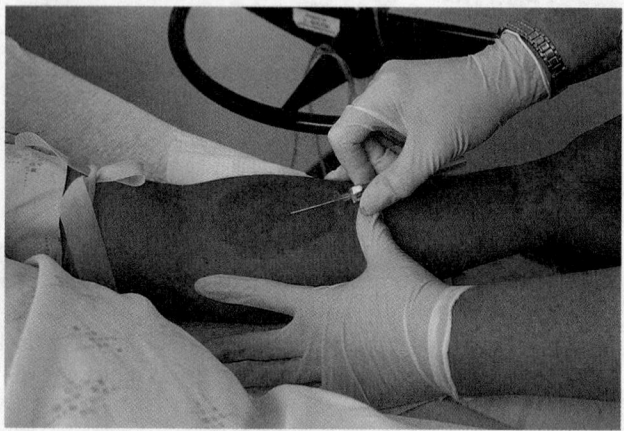

Step **15**

RATIONALE Gloves are required when contact with blood is possible. Using a tourniquet and opening and closing of the fist distend the vein. For the cannula to enter the vein smoothly, the skin must be taut. This also causes the least discomfort for the patient. The use of a local anesthetic is controversial. Either a physician's order or an agency protocol is necessary before using an anesthetic.

16. **ACTION** Insert the IV cannula into the vein by either the indirect or the direct method. Using the *indirect* method, first insert the cannula into the subcutaneous space directly parallel to the side of the vein, then move the tip toward the vein, and gently ease the cannula into the vein. Using the *direct* method, hold the cannula with the bevel upright and at a 15- to 25-degree angle to pierce the skin, and then lower the cannula until it is nearly parallel to the skin when piercing the vein. Enter the skin and vein in one quick, steady, forward thrust. Decreased resistance will be felt as the needle enters the vein. A pop may be felt. When the cannula punctures the vein, you will see blood (flashback) return into the hub of the unit.

RATIONALE The indirect method of cannula insertion has less chance of pushing completely through the vein. The direct method is best when the vein is large and stable.

17. **ACTION** After you see the flashback, insert the cannula an additional ⅛ inch and then slide the catheter off the stylet into the vein for its full length while keeping the stylet steady. Remove the tourniquet and ask the patient to open the fist. If you go through the vein wall, remove the tourniquet, withdraw the whole unit, and apply pressure.

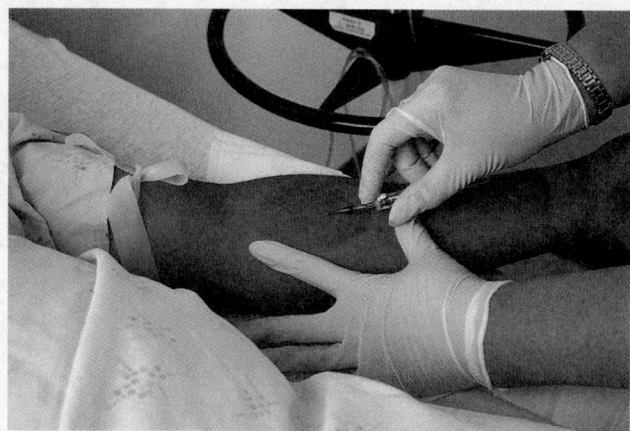

Step **17**

RATIONALE Advancing the cannula when it is not in the vein will cause pain and tissue damage. The stylet should not be advanced after the catheter is positioned through the vein wall; only the catheter should be advanced into the vein. Otherwise, the stylet may go through the vein. The tourniquet will impede the flow of IV solution. Pressure may be applied to the vein with one hand to prevent bleeding while the tubing is attached. If the IV stylet or the catheter goes through the vein, this site cannot be used because fluid will leak out of the vein.

18. **ACTION** Remove the protective cap over the needle adapter on the IV tubing, attach the tubing to the catheter hub, and open the clamp to begin the

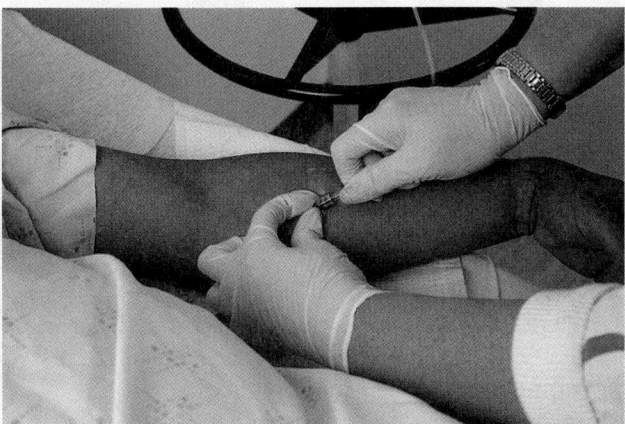

Step **18**

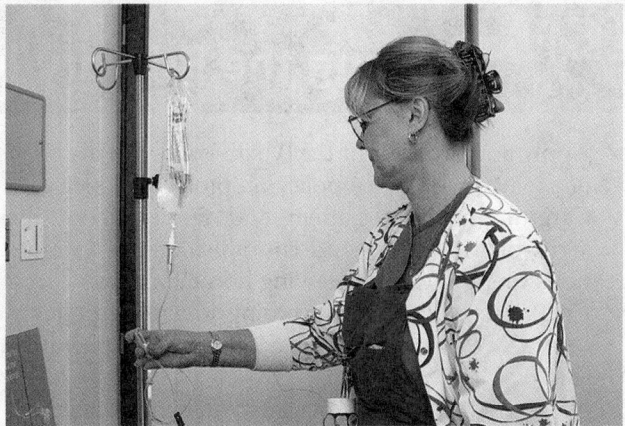

Step **20**

infusion slowly. Observe the site for swelling or leaking, indicating that the site is not patent.

RATIONALE Starting the solution flowing slowly establishes the patency of the IV before much fluid is infused. If the IV is not patent, little fluid will infiltrate the tissue. The solution is stopped and the catheter is removed if the site is not patent.

19. *ACTION* If the site is patent, secure the catheter with a manufactured catheter stabilization device. (This is a new recommendation from the Infusion Nurses Society; use of nonsterile tape around the insertion site is not considered an acceptable method.) Apply a transparent dressing. Loop the IV tubing on the extremity, and secure it again with tape. Supply an arm board as needed to immobilize or support the IV area. Label the dressing with the date and your initials.

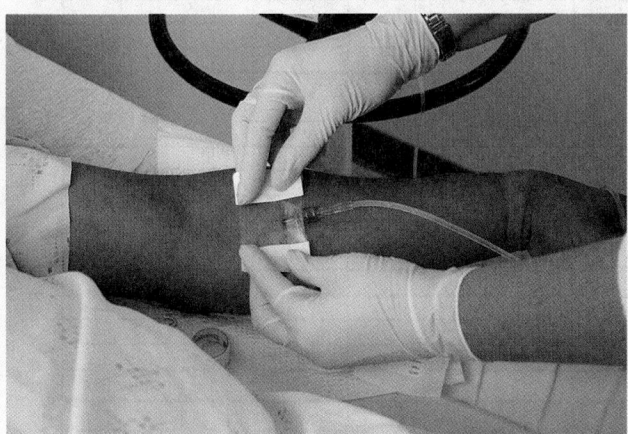

Step **19**

RATIONALE A transparent dressing protects the site from microorganisms while allowing visualization of the site. Taping the IV tubing prevents direct pull on the catheter, which could possibly dislodge when the patient moves around.

20. *ACTION* Regulate the solution flow according to the order by adjusting the roller clamp and count-

ing the drops per minute (or set the infusion pump to infuse at the correct rate).

RATIONALE The position of the arm, movement, and securing the catheter to stabilize it in the vein can alter the rate of flow.

■ Evaluation

21. *ACTION* Verify that the solution is running at the correct rate into the vein without pain and that the IV catheter is held securely in place.

RATIONALE Ensures that the IV is patent and secure.

22. *ACTION* Clean up used supplies and make patient comfortable. Remove gloves and perform hand hygiene.

RATIONALE Prevents spread of microorganisms and facilitates patient well-being.

■ Documentation

23. *ACTION* Documentation should include the location of the site, the type of catheter inserted, and the solution started. In some agencies, this information is charted on an IV flow sheet.

RATIONALE Documents when catheter was inserted so that it can be changed at the appropriate time.

Documentation Example

11/28 0630   #18 Angiocath × 1 inch inserted in L interior forearm with aseptic technique. IV 1000 mL of D_5W infusing at 125 mL/hour. Transparent dressing applied.

_____
(Nurse's signature)

■ Special Considerations

✓ Verify patient allergies before cleansing the skin at the insertion site or touching patient with a latex glove.

✓ If unsuccessful with venipuncture after two tries, ask another nurse to attempt the venipuncture.

Continued

Skill 36-1 | Starting the Primary Intravenous Infusion—cont'd

✓ Apply an arm board if the IV site is close to the bend of a joint. (See agency policy on protective devices.)

✓ Carefully instruct patient and family about the signs of infiltration and complications of intravenous therapy when receiving home therapy.

✓ An IV site is changed according to agency policy—every 72 hours is recommended for a peripheral IV site.

✓ Never perform venipuncture in an extremity where there is a hemodialysis access shunt or on the side of a mastectomy or paralysis.

✓ If the solution is running too slowly, check the site for infiltration. Adjusting the securing device or dressing over the catheter may help. Slightly rotating the catheter may move the tip away from the vein wall.

? CRITICAL THINKING QUESTIONS

1. Why would you never reinsert the same IV cannula in a slightly different spot when you have missed getting into the vein the first time?

2. What measures would you take if you could not see or feel a vein in the area chosen for IV cannula insertion?

STATUS CODES:
A = Patient w/o redness, pain or other problems.
B = DC'd w/ cannula intact.
C = Converted to Saline Lock.
D = Not patient, restart.
E = Other - See Nursing documentation.
* Paramedic

INTRAVENOUS ADMINISTRATION PROFILE

DIRECTIONS: Document each site start and end date.

Doe, John E.

Addressograph

Rev: 08/97
H8720-74

Int	Dt	Solution/Amt/Additive	Rate	Time/mt	Dt		Dt	Dt	Dt	Dt	Dt
JR	9/14/09	#1 D5 ½ NS 1000 mL			N						
			125/hr.	14 05	D						
					E						
RS	9/15/09	#2 D5 ½ NS 1000 mL c̄ 20 mEq KCl	125/hr.	22 20	N						
					D						
					E						
					N						
					D						
					E						
					N						
					D						
					E						

Start Dt / Tm / Int	Site# &Loc	Type/Sz	End Dt / Tm / Int		Site Status	Site Status	Site Status	Site Status	Site Status
9/14/09 1405 JR	#1 @ hand	20 ga 1¼"		N					
				D	Patent				
				E	Patent				
9/15/09				N					
				D					
				E					
				N					
				D					
				E					
				N					
				D					
				E					

Int	SIGNATURE	Int	SIGNATURE	Int	SIGNATURE	Int	SIGNATURE	Int	SIGNATURE	Int	SIGNATURE
JR	J. Reena, LVN										
RS	R. Schultz, RN										

FIGURE **36-14** Parenteral infusion record.

Students must have supervision when performing a venipuncture. Gloves must be worn and strict asepsis must be maintained when performing venipuncture to prevent infection. Whenever an IV site is initiated or changed, or an intravenous solution is hung, it is documented on the parenteral infusion record (Figure 36-14).

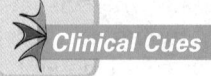
Clinical Cues

To distend the vein and make it easier to insert the cannula, place the extremity in a dependent position and gently pat the skin. For very difficult veins, pack the area of the vein with warm packs prior to placing the tourniquet.

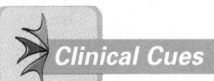

Using a blood pressure cuff rather than a tourniquet sometimes assists in successful venipuncture for the fragile veins of the elderly. Place the cuff about 6 inches above the selected site. Inflate the cuff to about 10 mm Hg above the diastolic pressure to restrict blood flow slightly and dilate the vein. If the patient is fluid depleted, inflate to 20 mm Hg over the diastolic pressure. **If you cannot initiate a patent IV in two attempts, ask another nurse to perform the task.**

In the past, the catheter was secured with tape. For example, a strip of ½-inch tape was placed under the hub, sticky side up; then the ends were crisscrossed to form a "V" over the hub or the ends were folded to form a "U" and then secured to the skin. An antibiotic dressing and a small sterile gauze dressing were then applied at the peripheral IV catheter insertion site. However, gauze dressings obscure the site and transparent dressings are now more commonly used. Antibiotic ointment is not recommended because it can actually contribute to the growth of fungal infections and antimicrobial resistance (Kraemer-Cain & Siegel, 2006). In 2006, the Infusion Nurses Society released new standards and now recommends that catheters should be secured with a manufactured catheter stabilization device, usually with a see-through area, rather than using nonsterile tape.

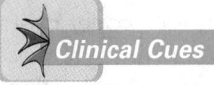

For pediatric patients (or confused elders) who are pulling at the tubing and catheter, a sleeve or roller gauze can be used to cover the site and equipment. Alternatively, a commercial shield shape can be taped over the catheter site (Figure 36-15). Using these devices can prevent accidental dislodgement; however, they do obscure quick visualization of the site.

Selection of the IV Site. Selection of a vein for IV use depends on several factors, including the accessibility of the vein, its general condition, the type of fluid or medication to be given, and the duration of IV therapy. The veins preferred for infusions and intermittent doses of medications are those distal to the antecubital area. The cephalic, basilic, and antebrachial veins of the lower arm and the veins on the back of the hand are the sites of choice for most adult patients (Figure 36-16).

The most distal site is used first so that other sites are available if therapy needs to be continued longer than 48 to 72 hours; a new site cannot be placed distal to an old site.

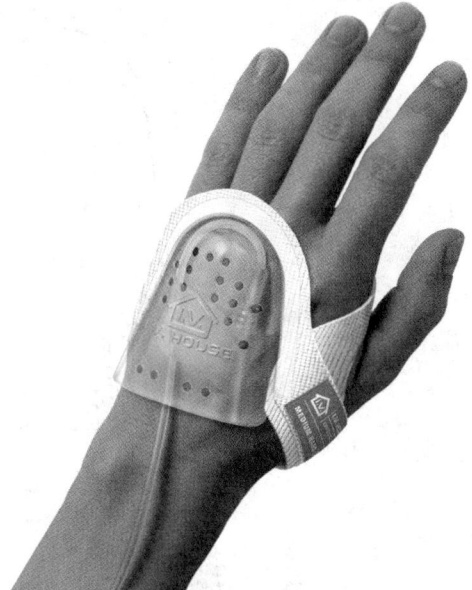

FIGURE **36-15** IV House protective device.

The scalp veins are frequently used in infants because they are easily accessible and the needle is less apt to be dislodged from this site. Veins of the foot are used only when no other site can be used.

Managing Intravenous Therapy

When your patient has an IV, you are responsible for ensuring that the infusion flows at the prescribed rate and that the solution is the one that was ordered. **Movement of the patient can alter the rate.** It is best to check the flow rate after the patient has been ambulating, returns from a test or treatment, is settled after morning care, has been turned in bed, or has been up to the bathroom.

Keeping the IV Solution Running. A primary responsibility is to check the IV each time the patient is observed and to see that it is running properly. Check it every 30 to 60 minutes, and observe each of these points with the eyes traveling from the solution container, down the tubing, and to the catheter site:

- *The IV flow.* The solution should drip into the chamber at regular intervals.
- *The rate of the infusion.* Check the time tape to see if the level of fluid is where it should be for the time elapsed. Count the rate. If it is too fast or too slow, it should be adjusted to the correct infusion rate per minute.
- If a pump is used, check *the programmed rate and volume;* the dripping in the chamber will occur intermittently.
- *The insertion site.* Are there any signs of infiltration or phlebitis?
- *Complaints from the patient.* After the IV has been started, it should not cause any pain or discomfort and there should be no leaking at the site.

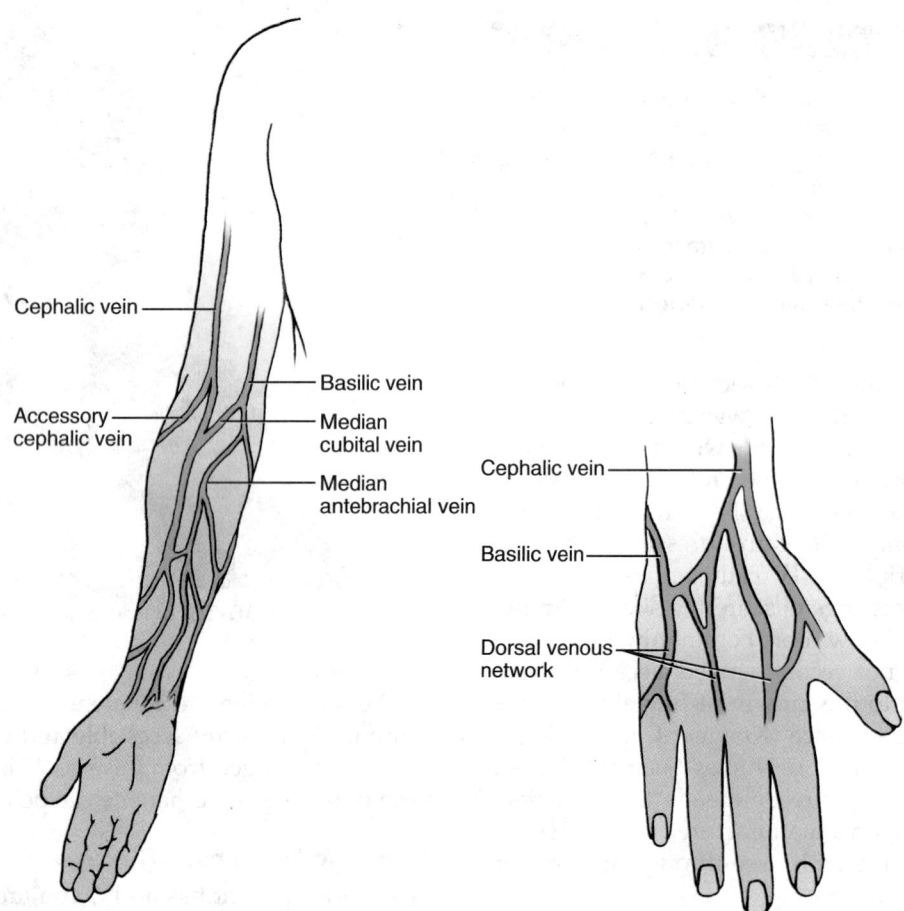

FIGURE **36-16** Sites for insertion of the intravenous cannula.

• *The level of the fluid remaining in the bag.* When there is 50 mL left, a new bag may be added before the current solution is completely infused (Skill 36-2).

The solution container is hung from an IV stand or pole. The tubing should be long enough to provide room for the patient to move about in bed, to turn over, or to carry out necessary activities. Soft restraints are needed for children and confused patients who might pull out the IV or cause it to infiltrate.

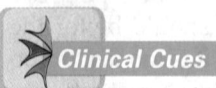

As a courtesy to the oncoming shift and to ensure that the patient's IV continues to flow, check the amount of solution remaining in the bag at the end of your shift and hang a new bag if needed.

Administering Intravenous Medications

Medications can be given by the IV route as one-time (stat) or PRN doses, as multiple doses to be given at regularly scheduled times, or by continuous infusion. Instructions for preparing medications for IV use fre-

quently require diluting the drug in large amounts of fluid (50 to 250 mL or more); this is essential for such drugs as potassium chloride and antibiotics, which, in concentrated form, cause irritation of the vein.

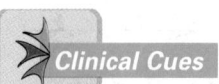

Potassium is always diluted in fluid and is never given as a bolus because it can cause cardiac arrhythmia and arrest.

In coronary or intensive care units, drugs such as lidocaine (Xylocaine) are given very slowly by bolus and by infusion. When the nurse gives the drug in a bolus, the entire amount is injected into the vein over a short period to obtain immediate effects. Therefore, the nurse must be thoroughly familiar with not only the drug's action and side effects but the proper dose parameters and recommended infusion time frames. One of the 2009 National Patient Safety Goals is to "reduce the likelihood of patient harm associated with the use of anticoagulation therapy." Nursing measures to meet this goal would include scrupulous attention

Skill 36-2 | Adding a New Solution to the Intravenous Infusion

When an IV is to remain in place, another container of solution must be hung before the last solution container runs dry. The new solution is hung when the solution that is infusing reaches a level of about 50 mL remaining.

■ Supplies
✓ Ordered IV solution
✓ Alcohol swabs
✓ Medication administration record (MAR)
✓ Time tape

Review and carry out the Standard Steps in Appendix 3.

■ Assessment (Data Collection)

1. ***ACTION*** Determine which solution is required next according to the orders.

   RATIONALE IV solutions are an ordered medication.

2. ***ACTION*** Select the correct solution and inspect it for cloudiness, particles, and other signs of contamination.

   RATIONALE Contaminated solution must not be used.

■ Planning

3. ***ACTION*** Place a time tape label on the container, and mark it appropriately. (Time tapes are not usually used if an infusion pump is being used.)

   RATIONALE A time tape makes it easy to tell at a glance if the IV is flowing on schedule. Infusion pumps will automatically count the volume infused.

■ Implementation

4. ***ACTION*** Go to the patient's bedside, and properly identify the patient. Inspect the IV site for signs of complications.

   RATIONALE Identifying the patient properly helps prevent medication errors. If the IV site shows signs of infection or infiltration, the site should be changed before the new solution is added.

5. ***ACTION*** Hang the IV container on the IV pole. Remove the container that is almost empty, crimp the tubing close to the drip chamber or close the roller clamp, and remove the spike from the used container. Keep the spike from becoming contaminated. Remove the tab from the IV tubing port on the new container, and insert the tubing spike while stabilizing the container with your other hand.

   RATIONALE The tubing must be occluded while you change IV containers to prevent air from entering the tubing. If the spike becomes contaminated, new tubing should be obtained. Stabilizing

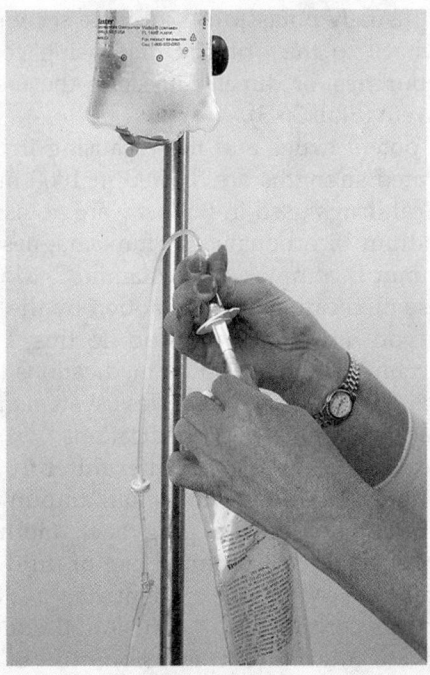

Step **5A**

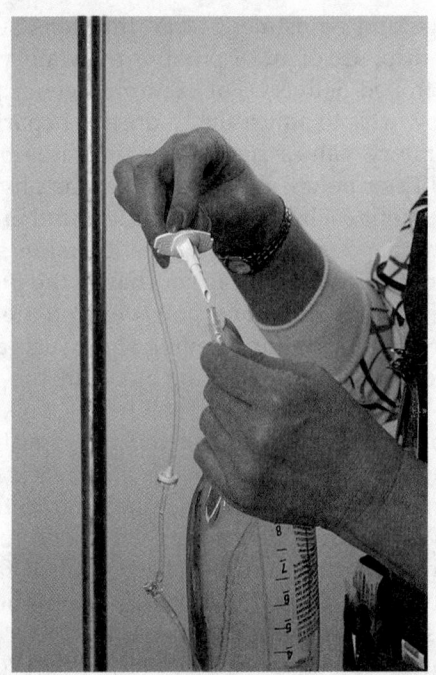

Step **5B**

Continued

Skill 36-2 | Adding a New Solution to the Intravenous Infusion—cont'd

the container helps prevent slipping and contaminating the spike while it is being inserted into the container.

6. **ACTION** Remove any air bubbles that entered the tubing by tapping the tube with your finger or a pencil as you stretch it taut. Squeezing the tubing below the bubbles will sometimes encourage them to move up to the drip chamber.

   RATIONALE Air bubbles can cause an air embolus if sufficient air collects. Patients are disturbed by the sight of air bubbles in the IV tubing. Air will move upward to the drip chamber when dislodged from the side of the tubing.

7. **ACTION** Check the flow rate and readjust it as needed to the prescribed rate.

   RATIONALE The greater quantity of fluid in the new container causes a bigger pressure gradient, and the new solution may flow more rapidly.

8. **ACTION** Dispose of the empty container in the proper receptacle. Remove and destroy any labels that include the patient's name.

   RATIONALE Some agencies require that the container be drained dry before discard. Careful handling of materials with patient's name prevents violations of the Health Insurance Portability and Accountability Act (HIPAA).

■ Evaluation

9. **ACTION** Before leaving the room, check the solution label with the order again, assess the site for signs of infiltration, and make certain that the drop rate is correct.

   RATIONALE Verifies that the solution is the one ordered and that it is running correctly through a patent site.

■ Documentation

10. **ACTION** Record the added fluid on the IV flow sheet.

    RATIONALE The amount and type of fluid added and the infusion rate are charted along with an assessment of the IV site.

?CRITICAL THINKING QUESTIONS

1. You are performing the initial morning assessment for your patient. You find that the bag that is infusing is not the correct solution according to the report that you received at shift change. What would you do?

2. At what point would you switch out the old IV solution for the new solution? (How much is left in the bag?) Why would you choose to change the solution at this point?

---

to dosage and adjustment of IV infusions such as a heparin drip; use of an IV pump is mandatory for safe and controlled delivery. For example, agency protocol may allow RNs to adjust the IV dose of heparin based on laboratory values such as partial thromboplastin time (PTT), or policy may dictate that the physician is notified about each laboratory value and then he will order specific dosage adjustments. **Nursing students should not adjust the dosage or change the pump settings of heparin infusions;** however, you are responsible for monitoring for bleeding signs such as bruising, bleeding of the gums, or blood in the stool or urine.

If a medication is administered too rapidly, speed shock may occur. Speed shock is a systemic reaction that occurs when a substance unfamiliar to the body is infused rapidly. Signs of speed shock are lightheadedness, tightness in the chest, flushed face, and irregular pulse. The patient may lose consciousness, go into shock, and suffer cardiac arrest.

Various methods are used to administer IV medications, such as adding medications to the primary bag

of fluids (usually potassium), adding a secondary line or piggyback to the primary line, using controlled-volume burettes, or directly injecting the medication into the vein (Skill 36-3).

Some potent drugs and those causing irritation in concentrated strengths are diluted in 1000 mL of fluids. Typical drugs used in this way are potassium, insulin, sodium bicarbonate, calcium, magnesium sulfate, vitamin B complex, and vitamin C. Most of the time these medications will be added by the pharmacist, but you must know how to do this. Use strict aseptic technique when adding medications to IV fluids (Steps 36-1, p. 737). Needleless systems are most often used to administer IV medications.

Medications that are given intermittently at timed intervals may be diluted in a small amount of fluid and administered by the piggyback method. The medication is added to a small bag of fluid, usually 50 to 150 mL. When the patient has a PRN lock rather than a continuous IV infusion, the method of hanging an intermittent infusion differs slightly (Skill 36-4, pp. 737-738).

Skill 36-3 | Administering Intravenous Piggyback Medication

Various types of medications are administered intermittently by piggyback or secondary line administration. The drug solution is prepared by the pharmacy. Some drugs in solution must be refrigerated. If this is the case, the medication should be removed from the refrigerator 30 minutes before administration.

■ Supplies
✓ Ordered medication in solution
✓ IV piggyback administration set
✓ Tape (optional)
✓ Alcohol swabs
✓ Medication administration record (MAR)

Review and carry out the Standard Steps in Appendix 3.

■ Assessment (Data Collection)

1. **ACTION** Check the medication with the MAR. Assess for allergies.

   RATIONALE The five rights are used when administering IV medications. Allergy to IV medication can be life threatening.

■ Planning

2. **ACTION** Calculate the flow rate. Check with the pharmacy or consult a drug handbook for the specific drug you will administer.

   RATIONALE Most IV drugs are given over 20 to 90 minutes.

■ Implementation

3. **ACTION** Open the secondary (piggyback) administration set, close the clamp, and insert the spike end of the tubing into the tubing port, using aseptic technique.

   RATIONALE Prepares the solution for infusion.

4. **ACTION** Squeeze the drip chamber while inverting the IV piggyback container, and hang it from an IV hook.

   RATIONALE This maneuver partially fills the drip chamber so that air will not flow into the tubing.

5. **ACTION** Loosen the connector cover; slowly open the clamp, and clear the air by running fluid through the tubing.

   RATIONALE Allows fluid to run through the tubing without allowing more air to bubble into the tubing.

6. **ACTION** Verify the drug and dosage again, and go to the patient's room. Properly identify the patient, checking the identification band. If infusing an antibiotic, reverify any allergies the patient might have.

   RATIONALE Following the five rights helps prevent medication errors. Antibiotic allergies can be life threatening if a drug is infused to which the patient is allergic.

7. **ACTION** Hang the piggyback container on the IV pole. Cleanse the injection port of the primary site with an alcohol swab.

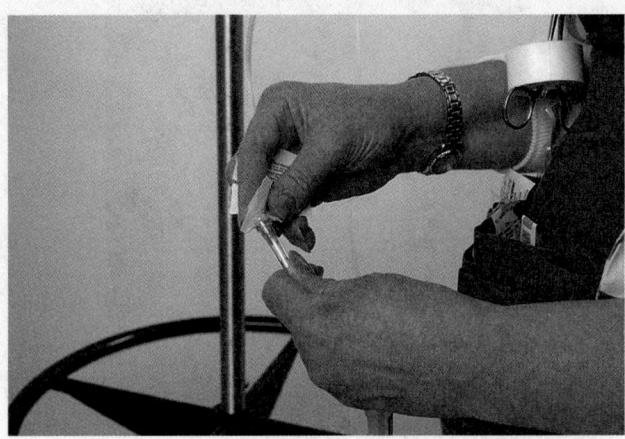

Step **7**

RATIONALE Prevents introduction of microorganism into the bloodstream when the IV piggyback is connected.

8. **ACTION** Attach the IV piggyback tubing to the port with a needleless adaptor or a snap lock device; open the clamp of the secondary set, and adjust the rate of flow. If the piggyback will not flow, lower the primary IV container using an IV hanger.

   RATIONALE The flow rate must be set accurately so as not to cause harm to the patient from too rapid infusion.

■ Evaluation

9. **ACTION** Evaluate whether the medication is effective by assessing for signs of improvement in the problem for which it is being given. Determine that the vein into which the medication is flowing is not becoming irritated.

   RATIONALE Monitoring blood counts and other lab values, as well as vital signs, and assessing the patient's well-being are all part of the evaluation. Some medications are very irritating to the vein.

Continued

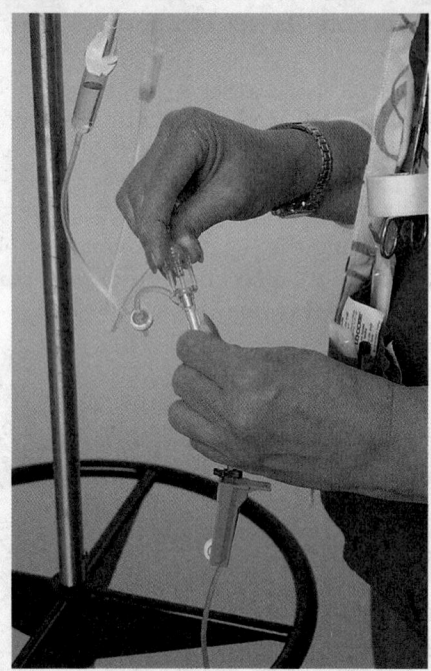

Step **8A**

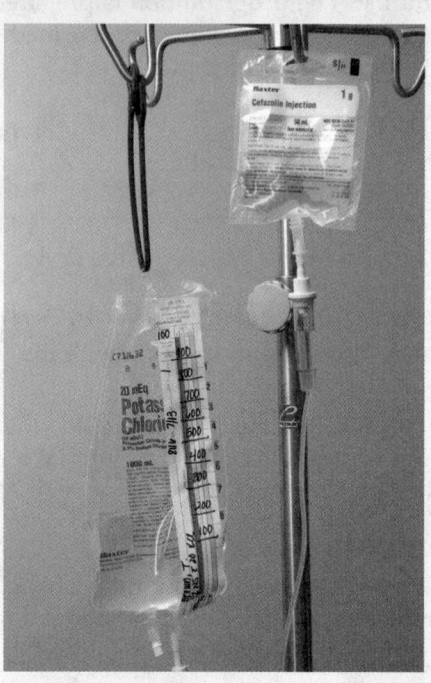

Step **8B**

10. **ACTION** Assess for adverse or side effects to the medication administered.

    RATIONALE If adverse effects occur, the medication needs to be discontinued.

■ Documentation

11. **ACTION** Document the IV medication on the MAR.

    RATIONALE Verifies that the medication has been administered.

■ Special Considerations

✓ Always assess for allergies and adverse effects before infusing *each* dose of medication.

✓ Use a needleless connector with a securing clamp to attach the piggyback to the primary tubing, or tape

the connection so it doesn't pull apart with patient movement.

✓ Always assess the IV site *before* infusing an IV medication to make certain that the IV site is patent.

✓ Note the times IV medications are to be given on your worksheet; for medication drug levels to stay constant, the medication must be started on time.

? CRITICAL THINKING QUESTIONS

1. Can you identify everything you would check before starting to infuse an IV piggyback medication for a patient?

2. What would you need to do if the IV piggyback ordered is incompatible with one of the additives in the main IV solution infusing at the time you are to administer the IV piggyback?

Steps 36-1 | Adding Medication to an Intravenous Solution

The most common medication ordered added to an intravenous infusion is potassium. At times other drugs may be added.

Review and carry out the Standard Steps in Appendix 3.

1. **ACTION** Check the medication and IV solution with the order; calculate the medication dosage if necessary.

   RATIONALE Observing the Five Rights prevents medication errors.

2. **ACTION** Prepare an additive label to be placed on the IV container after the medication is added. The label should include the patient's name, room number, name of the drug, dosage, date, time, and your initials.

   RATIONALE A label indicates what has been added to the solution.

3. **ACTION** Prepare the medication, and draw it up in a syringe using aseptic technique.

RATIONALE Prevents contamination of the medication and the IV solution.

4. **ACTION** Remove the tab from the medication injection port on the IV container, swab it with an antiseptic swab to remove any residue that may have been deposited during manufacture, and inject the medication into the container.

   RATIONALE Deposits the medication into the solution.

5. **ACTION** Place the additive label on the container. Mix the solution with the medication by inverting the container or rotating it several times.

   RATIONALE The medication and solution must be thoroughly mixed to provide the right dilution and distribution of the medication.

Skill 36-4 | Administering Medication via Saline or PRN Lock

When the patient does not need large quantities of IV fluid but does need IV medications intermittently, a capped catheter, or PRN lock, is inserted. If an IV is already infusing, it can be changed to an intermittent IV by removing the tubing and attaching an injection cap to the catheter.

■ Supplies
✓ Gloves
✓ IV cannula and injection cap (or extension set with injection cap)
✓ Normal saline

✓ IV start kit (usually includes: chlorhexidine swabs, alcohol swabs, label, tape, transparent dressing, tourniquet)
✓ Underpad

✓ Syringe and needleless connector or snap connector
✓ Medication administration record (MAR)
✓ Commercial device for securing the site

Review and carry out the Standard Steps listed in Appendix 3.

■ Assessment (Data Collection)

1. **ACTION** Determine need for saline or PRN lock rather than continuous IV; check the orders.

   RATIONALE Intermittent infusion is more comfortable for the patient.

■ Planning

2. **ACTION** Look at the patient's veins and choose the best site for the saline or PRN lock.

   RATIONALE Unless the lock will be used long term, a site near the wrist or on the forearm will be most comfortable for the patient.

■ Implementation
Flushing the Saline or PRN Lock

3. **ACTION** Perform hand hygiene, prepare the skin, don gloves, and insert the IV cannula (see Skill 36-1).

   RATIONALE Provides an IV access.

4. **ACTION** Flush the injection cap (or extension set with cap) with saline and attach it to the catheter; flush with 2 mL of normal saline.

   RATIONALE Places solution in the catheter to help prevent clotting and demonstrates patency of the catheter.

5. **ACTION** Secure the lock with the commercial securement device. Label the site with the date and your initials.

Skill 36-4 | Administering Medication via Saline or PRN Lock—cont'd

RATIONALE Prevents the lock from dislodging. Shows when the lock was started.

Administering Medications via the Saline or PRN Lock

6. **ACTION** Prepare the medication following the Five Rights. The medication may be mixed as an IV piggyback or drawn up in a syringe.

   RATIONALE Helps prevent medication error.

7. **ACTION** Prepare a syringe containing normal saline.

   RATIONALE Saline injection is used to test the patency of the lock. Flushing with saline will clear the lock of medication and leave fluid in the lock to prevent clotting.

8. **ACTION** Cleanse the cap with an alcohol swab. Insert the needleless connector into the bull's eye on the lock or connect the syringe to the lock, and aspirate for blood return to determine the patency of the lock. If you cannot aspirate blood, the lock is not necessarily blocked because the catheter may just be against the side wall of the vein. Slowly inject the saline. If resistance occurs, stop and replace the lock.

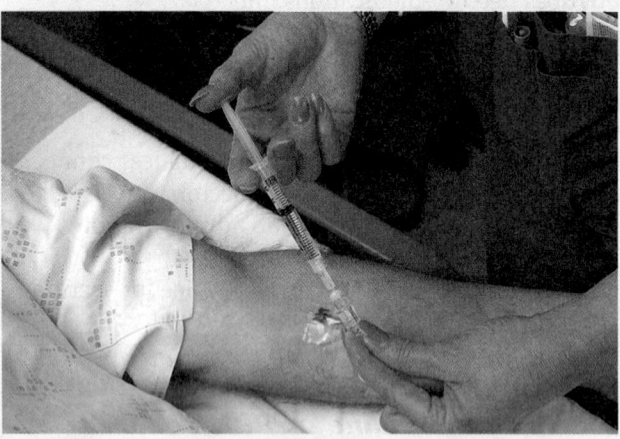

Step **8**

RATIONALE Helps prevent introduction of microorganisms. Verifies that the lock is patent before the medication is injected.

9. **ACTION** Verify the drug, dosage, and patient identification one more time, and then hook up the IV piggyback or inject the medication over the recommended period.

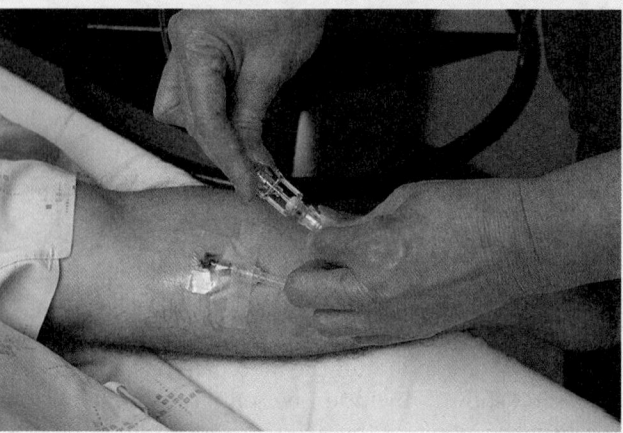

Step **9**

RATIONALE Following the Five Rights helps prevent medication errors.

10. **ACTION** After the medication administration is completed, flush the lock with 2 mL of normal saline. Some agencies follow the flush with a heparin solution; check agency policy.

    RATIONALE Prevents a blood clot from forming and occluding the catheter.

11. **ACTION** Clean up used equipment and make the patient comfortable. Remove the gloves.

    RATIONALE Restores order in the unit. Prevents transfer of microorganisms.

■ Evaluation

12. **ACTION** Observe for blood flow on aspiration of the lock to evaluate patency.

    RATIONALE If no blood flow is seen, injecting 2 mL of saline without pain or swelling at the site indicates that the lock is patent.

■ Documentation

13. **ACTION** Document insertion of the saline or PRN lock on the IV flow sheet. Document each medication administered on the MAR.

    RATIONALE Notes presence of lock and date of insertion.

?CRITICAL THINKING QUESTIONS

1. You can't always obtain a blood return from a PRN or intermittent lock. How would you verify that it is patent before you infuse a medication into the lock?

2. How often should a PRN or intermittent lock be changed to another site?

Another method of administering IV medications is to mix them in a small amount of solution in a controlled-volume burette (Skill 36-5). Medications given by the controlled-volume burette will interrupt the primary infusion of fluids, as does the piggyback setup. The controlled-volume burette is different in two respects that limit its usefulness. First, the medication must be monitored closely, and the clamp must be opened to restart the flow of the primary solution when the medication has infused. Second, the tubing has to be reused for subsequent fluids and additional doses of medication, thus increasing the possibility of contamination. It does enable accurate measurement of the amount of fluid infused at one time. **All medications are administered following the five rights and are documented on the medication administration record (MAR).**

Skill 36-5 | Administration of Medication with a Controlled-Volume Set

A controlled-volume set is still sometimes used when small amounts of fluid are required just to keep a vein open, for pediatric or elderly patients, when infusion pumps are not available, or when backup safety for a pump is needed. They are also sometimes used for diluting doses of medication in place of the IV piggyback container.

■ Supplies
✓ Ordered medication
✓ Alcohol swabs
✓ Medication administration record (MAR)
✓ Medication label
✓ Syringe and needle
✓ In-line burette
✓ IV solution

Review and carry out the Standard Steps listed in Appendix 3.

■ Assessment (Data Collection)
1. **ACTION** Check the medication with the order; calculate the dosage if needed. Verify the compatibility of the drug with primary IV solution.

   RATIONALE Adhering to the Five Rights helps prevent medication errors. Incompatibility may cause the drug to precipitate or may inactivate it.

■ Planning
2. **ACTION** Calculate the drop rate (or the pump setting) to instill the medication in the correct amount of time. Note the ending time on your daily work sheet.

   RATIONALE The medication must be administered over a set period of time. The primary IV must be opened again as soon as the medication finishes.

■ Implementation
3. **ACTION** Prepare the medication, and draw it up in a syringe.

   RATIONALE Provides a way to add the medication to the burette.

4. **ACTION** Take the syringe and the MAR to the patient's bedside. Properly identify the patient, and recheck the medication.

   RATIONALE Helps prevent medication errors.

5. **ACTION** Fill the burette by opening the upper clamp on the tubing to the primary bag and running 50 to 150 mL of fluid, as specified in the order.

Close the clamp on the upper tubing to the solution bag.

   RATIONALE Provides for dilution of the medication.

6. **ACTION** Lower the burette, locate the injection port on the top of it, cleanse the injection port with an alcohol swab, and inject the medication. Mix the medication with the solution by gently tilting the burette back and forth.

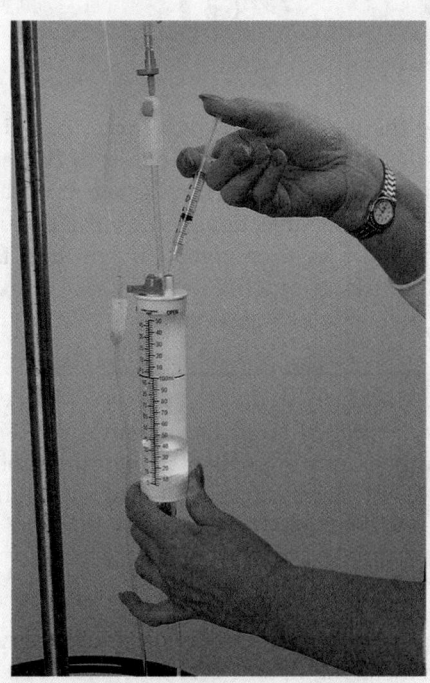

Step **6**

Continued

Skill 36-5 | Administration of Medication with a Controlled-Volume Set—cont'd

RATIONALE Dilutes the medication for the ordered dosage.

7. *ACTION* Open the lower clamp, and adjust the rate of flow from the burette.

   RATIONALE Begins the medication infusion.

8. *ACTION* Label the burette with the name of the drug, dose, time, rate, and your initials.

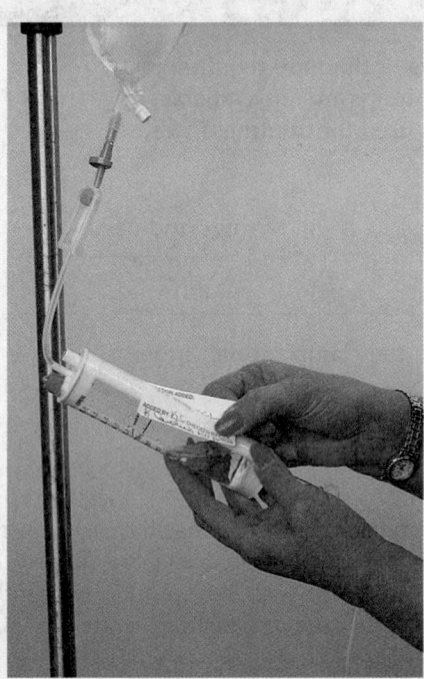

Step **8**

RATIONALE Identifies the contents of the burette.

9. *ACTION* When the burette empties, restart the flow from the primary bag by opening the clamp on the upper tubing. Adjust the flow rate.

   RATIONALE Reinstitutes the primary IV infusion.

■ Evaluation

10. *ACTION* Evaluate the IV site to see if the medication causes irritation of the vein. Evaluate the patient for signs that the medication is effective. Assess for adverse effects.

    RATIONALE Some medications are irritating to the vein. Points to assess for effectiveness of the medication depend on the type of medication and its purpose. Assessment for adverse effects should be accomplished before administering each successive dose.

■ Documentation

11. *ACTION* Document the medication given on the MAR.

    RATIONALE Verifies that the medication dose has been given.

?CRITICAL THINKING QUESTIONS

1. Can you explain what will happen if you forget to clamp off the line from the IV container to the burette when using this controlled-volume device?

Giving the medication directly into the vein over a few minutes is termed giving a bolus, or IV push injection (Steps 36-2, Safety Alert 36-2). The medication can be instilled via the injection port on the IV tubing, or through a PRN lock, or given directly into the vein. Many state nurse practice acts do not allow LPN/LVNs to give a bolus injection.

> ?
> • *Think Critically About* . . . In accordance with *Healthy People 2010*, all health care professionals should be educating patients about their medications. What might cause a nurse to neglect or forget to educate the patient about IV medications?

Administering Antineoplastic Medications

Antineoplastic medications are used to destroy or alter the growth of malignant cells and are very toxic to normal as well as abnormal cells. Many are very irritating to tissue. These drugs are often referred to as *chemotherapy* drugs. Because of their toxicity, special precautions are used in preparing and administering these drugs. Each toxic antineoplastic drug usually has a special label attached with a caution warning (Safety Alert 36-3).

Discontinuing an IV Infusion

When an infusion is to be discontinued, the flow is stopped and the catheter is removed (Steps 36-3). Discontinuation is documented on the IV flow sheet.

Administering Blood and Blood Products

A transfusion is the IV administration of whole blood or one or more of its components. Components frequently transfused include fresh or frozen plasma, packed red blood cells, and platelets. Autologous (from the patient's own body) infusions are common during and after surgery. In this instance, the patient's

Steps 36-2 | Administering an IV Bolus Medication (IV Push)

The physician may order medication to be given by the IV route; although most LPNs/LVNs cannot do this under their state nurse practice act, some locales do allow this with additional training.

Review and carry out the Standard Steps in Appendix 3.

1. **ACTION** Gather equipment and perform hand hygiene.

   RATIONALE Readies equipment for the procedure.

2. **ACTION** Follow the five rights when preparing the medication.

   RATIONALE Prevents medication errors.

3. **ACTION** Check to see that the medication and any IV solution flowing are compatible.

   RATIONALE Prevents precipitation or inactivation of the medication.

4. **ACTION** Perform hand hygiene and don gloves; flush the PRN lock as instructed in Skill 36-4 or cleanse the injection port on the primary tubing closest to the patient (the farthest port should be used for some medications) with an alcohol swab.

   RATIONALE Prevents transfer of microorganisms. Prepares the access for injection of the medication. Some medications, such as promethazine should be given in the most distal port because the medication is very irritating to the veins. Check drug handbooks and consult the pharmacist as needed.

5. **ACTION** Connect the syringe to the port. If using a needleless system, lock the syringe to the port or the PRN lock before injecting.

   RATIONALE Allows the medication to flow into the vein.

6. **ACTION** Occlude the IV tubing above the port while injecting the medication if injecting into a port on the primary tubing.

   RATIONALE Prevents backflow into the tubing.

7. **ACTION** Hold your watch within view as you inject the medication over the recommended time period; inject evenly over the entire time period.

   RATIONALE Prevents injecting the medication too rapidly. No medication should ever be injected in less than 1 minute; some require a 5-minute period or more.

8. **ACTION** Disconnect the syringe from the PRN lock or the IV injection port; slowly open the IV tubing to flush and then reestablish correct rate.

   RATIONALE Ends the medication injection; slowly flushing prevents a rapid bolus of medication that is contained within the section of tubing; reestablishes the correct infusion rate after interruption for bolus delivery.

9. **ACTION** Flush the PRN lock, if used.

   RATIONALE Clears medication from the lock and protects it from clotting.

10. **ACTION** Dispose of equipment in biohazard container; remove gloves and perform hand hygiene.

    RATIONALE Prevents needle sticks and spread of microorganisms.

11. **ACTION** Document the medication administered on the MAR.

    RATIONALE Records the dose administered.

 Safety Alert 36-2

IV Push Promethazine

According to a survey conducted by the *Nurse Advise-ERR* (Institute for Safe Medication Practices, 2006), nurses should use the following measures to reduce the risk of tissue damage from IV push promethazine: dilute the drug, limit the concentration and the initial dose, provide an alert on the MAR, inject the drug into a running IV, use the port that is farthest from the patient's veins, and advise the patient to report discomfort.

 Safety Alert 36-3

Administration of Antineoplastic Medications

Many agencies require special training and certification before a nurse is allowed to administer chemotherapy drugs. Antineoplastic medications can be absorbed through the skin, by inhalation of droplets, or by oral contamination from residue on the hands of the nurse. Frequent or long-term exposure to these drugs can lead to alterations in the cells of ova, sperm, or fetal tissue.

Steps 36-3 Discontinuing an Intravenous Infusion or PRN Lock

When the patient no longer needs IV fluids, IV medications, or access for emergency drugs, the catheter is removed. Standard precautions must be followed when removing an IV catheter because there is almost always a slight amount of bleeding that occurs.

Review and carry out the Standard Steps in Appendix 3.

1. **ACTION** Check the physician's order for discontinuing the IV.

   RATIONALE Prevents inadvertently discontinuing the IV and having to restart it.

2. **ACTION** Identify the patient and remove the IV dressing carefully.

   RATIONALE Patient identification prevents mistakes. Gentle removal of the dressing prevents moving the IV catheter, which might cause tissue irritation.

3. **ACTION** Perform hand hygiene and don gloves; stop the IV flow by clamping the tubing. Hold a sterile gauze pad over the insertion site lightly.

Quickly withdraw the catheter. Examine it to verify it is intact. Immediately apply pressure to the site to stop bleeding.

   RATIONALE Standard Precautions require gloves. If tubing is not clamped, the fluid will continue to drip after the catheter is removed. Sterile gauze will stop the bleeding quicker because it is dry. If the catheter is torn or broken, the patient is at risk for catheter emboli. Applying pressure helps prevent hematoma formation.

4. **ACTION** When the bleeding has stopped, gently clean blood off the skin around the site, and apply an adhesive bandage.

   RATIONALE A bandage protects the insertion site from microorganisms while it heals.

5. **ACTION** Document removal of the catheter.

   RATIONALE Verifies that the catheter was removed.

---

own blood is reinfused. Blood is either collected during surgery (e.g., from chest drainage) or donated by the patient during the weeks prior to surgery for later reinfusion.

A consent to receive blood must be signed by the patient (Legal & Ethical Considerations 36-1). The consent usually must be signed no more than 48 to 72 hours prior to receiving the blood product. If a reaction to the blood occurs, the blood should be instantly shut off. Start the saline (with fresh tubing) to keep the IV access open, in case emergency drugs are needed (Skill 36-6).

Total Parenteral Nutrition

Patients may require IV therapy for long periods. Short-term therapy is usually considered to last up to 2 weeks; long-term therapy is 6 weeks or more (Home Care Considerations 36-1, p. 745). The nutritional status of patients who are NPO and on IV therapy must be assessed every day. Although the IV solution may contain dextrose, the amount of calories supplied is below the total daily requirement; moreover, the patient lacks other essential nutrients and bulk. One thousand milliliters of 5% glucose solution only provides 200 calories. Supplemental calories may be provided by the use of amino acids and fat emulsions. Dextrose in concentrations greater than 10% is best given through central lines because it is irritating to peripheral veins and can lead to thrombophlebitis. TPN is mainly given through a central line. Specially

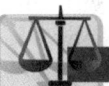

Legal & Ethical Considerations 36-1

Right to Refuse Blood Transfusions

An adult Jehovah's Witness patient may refuse to have a blood transfusion; however, according to U.S. law, if the patient is a minor and the treatment would be lifesaving, a court order can be obtained that allows administration of blood or blood products against the parents' will (Elgindy, 2004). Every effort should be made to understand and treat the family with respect. Blood substitutes or alternative treatments may be used in certain cases.

---

prepared solutions can be given peripherally, but these provide fewer calories because the dextrose content must be less. Information on TPN is found in Chapter 27 and in medical-surgical nursing texts.

Evaluation

Evaluation requires constant assessment of the patient. Evaluation of the effect of intravenous therapy relates to the reason it was given. If fluids are being given to hydrate the patient, check for good skin turgor, adequate urine output, and moist mucous membranes. If TPN is being given, assess the patient's weight gain and monitor the blood glucose level. When IV antibiotics are administered, check the leukocyte count, temperature, and any wound to see if signs of infection are clearing; check for signs or symptoms of al-

Skill 36-6 | Administration of Blood Products

Blood components are administered for a variety of reasons. Packed red cells are commonly given for acute or chronic anemia. Platelets and fresh frozen plasma are transfused to replenish platelets and provide clotting factors. **There is no margin for error when administering blood products because adverse reactions can be life threatening. In accordance with 2009 National Patient Safety Goals, the nurse must use two identifiers for patient identity, and room number or location cannot be used. The patient name and number on the ID bracelet, or the patient verbally stating name and birth date, are suitable identifiers.** Most agencies require that two nurses verify the ordered blood component with the component the blood bank supplies and correctly match up the patient numbers with the blood component unit numbers. In emergency situations, the blood may need to be administered with a pump so that it will flow more quickly. A signed consent is needed before a blood product administration begins. Special tubing with a filter is used for blood components. An extra filter on the bag is required for some blood products. A "Y" tubing set is commonly used for transfusion of packed red cells.

■ Supplies
✓ Blood product administration set
✓ Alcohol swabs
✓ Normal saline 0.9% IV solution
✓ Physician's order
✓ Blood bank slip
✓ Ordered blood component
✓ Tape
✓ Gloves

Review and carry out the Standard Steps listed in Appendix 3.

■ Assessment (Data Collection)
1. *ACTION* See that the patient has a patent IV of at least 19 gauge. Plasma products may be infused via a 22-gauge catheter.

   RATIONALE A catheter with a bore smaller than 19 gauge may break up red cells.

■ Planning
2. *ACTION* Gather the equipment, verify that the patient is ready, and obtain the blood product from the blood bank. (Packed red cells are the component used for this example.)

   RATIONALE Saves time; administration of the blood product must begin within 30 minutes of the time the product leaves the blood bank.

■ Implementation
3. *ACTION* With another nurse, verify the blood component, and compare the donor numbers and the ABO group and Rh type on the request slip with the label and numbers on the blood component bag. One nurse should read the numbers from the blood bank transfusion record slip while the other checks the numbers on the blood component bag. Verify the expiration date on the blood component bag; check the bag for clots.

   RATIONALE For safety, two nurses must verify the order, and match the numbers on the blood component with those on the transfusion record slip. The blood component may not be transfused after the expiration date. If the unit contains clots, it should be returned to the blood bank.

4. *ACTION* Close all clamps on the "Y" administration set. Spike a normal saline container. Prime the filter and tubing with normal saline by opening the slide clamp below the drip chamber of the normal saline and the lower roller clamp. Spike the blood component bag. For packed red cells, invert and lower the packed red cell bag, open the clamp to the bag, and open the slide clamp to the normal saline while keeping the roller clamp closed. Allow about 50 mL of saline to run into the packed red cells. Close the clamps.

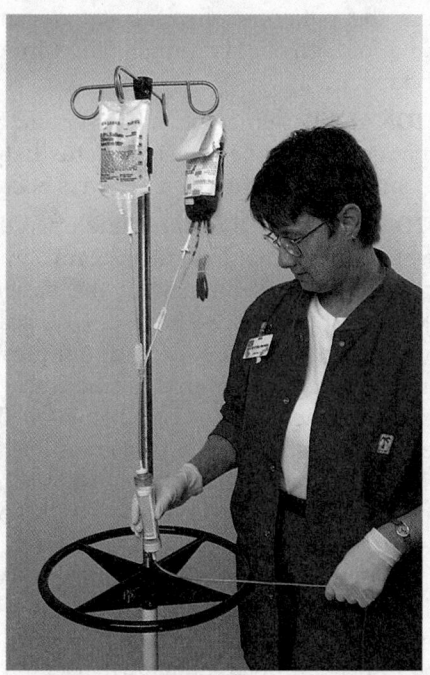

Step **4**

Continued

Skill 36-6 | Administration of Blood Products—cont'd

RATIONALE A "Y" set is always to be used for blood component infusion. Priming the filter and tubing with normal saline removes air and eases the way for blood flow. Combining a small amount of saline with packed red cells, if within agency protocol, decreases the viscosity and helps the blood infuse more easily. Care is taken to close clamps so that none of the blood product is accidentally lost.

5. *ACTION* Take the administration set to the patient's room; properly identify the patient, comparing the full name and hospital identification number on the patient's wristband with the transfusion record information. Compare the blood bracelet identification number with the number on the blood component.

   RATIONALE It is mandatory that all identifying information and numbers match exactly. If discrepancies occur, notify the blood bank. Transfusions are not begun until the discrepancy is resolved.

6. *ACTION* Don gloves, and connect the "Y" administration set to the indwelling catheter. Start the normal saline to clear the catheter, and verify the patency of the site.

   RATIONALE Gloves must be used when contact with blood is likely. The patency of the site must be verified before beginning the transfusion.

7. *ACTION* Obtain baseline vital signs. If the patient's temperature is over 100° F, consult the physician. Assess the patient's physical status, particularly looking for signs or symptoms that mimic a transfusion reaction.

   RATIONALE Baseline data are essential. Knowing the patient's baseline physical status helps determine later if a transfusion reaction is occurring.

8. *ACTION* Clamp off the saline, and open the clamp to the blood. Set the flow rate at 2 mL/min for the first 15 minutes. Remain with the patient for at least the first 5 minutes. Reassess the patient and take vital signs at the end of 15 minutes. If there are no signs of an adverse reaction, the infusion rate may be increased to the calculated flow rate. Take vital signs at the end of 30 minutes and then every 30 minutes until the transfusion is complete. Follow your agency's protocol. Ask the patient to tell you if she feels "funny," or has chills, back pain, itching, or shortness of breath. Watch for flushing. Blood must be infused within 4 hours of release from the blood bank. Monitor the drip rate continuously and use some normal saline to dilute the blood product as needed. Use of an infusion pump is recommended to help control the rate.

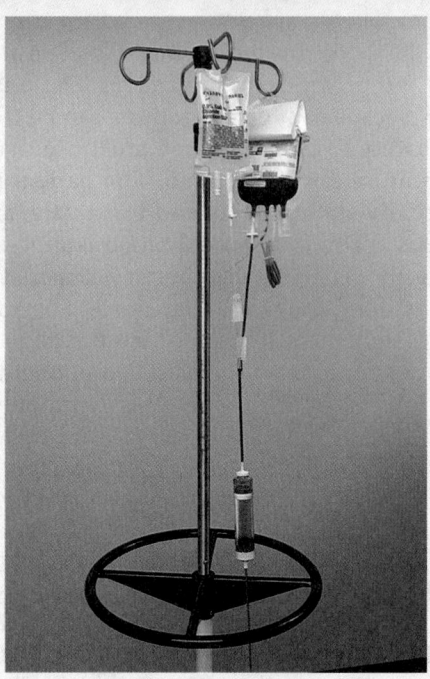

Step **8**

RATIONALE Begins the transfusion. Adverse reactions occur most frequently during the first 5 minutes, although delayed reactions can occur. The patient must be monitored throughout the transfusion for any signs of an adverse reaction. It is essential that the patient understand the importance of reporting any symptoms that differ from normal. Average infusion time is 2 hours per unit. Blood is viscous and the filters will clog and the flow will eventually stop; use of saline dilutes the blood product and decreases viscosity.

9. *ACTION* When the blood component has been infused, flush the line with normal saline. Reinstitute IV fluid orders with a new solution and tubing, or maintain saline at a "keep vein open" rate (30 to 50 mL/hr) until you are certain that the patient is stable and has had no reaction, then convert to a PRN lock, or discontinue the IV site per orders.

   RATIONALE Previously hanging IV solution and tubing are considered contaminated and must be discarded.

■ Evaluation

10. *ACTION* Monitor vital signs and assess for shortness of breath, rash, back pain, apprehension, fever, tachycardia, nausea and vomiting, and other signs of transfusion reaction.

    RATIONALE Evaluates whether a reaction has occurred.

■ Documentation

11. **ACTION** Document the infusion on the IV flow sheet. Add the amount infused to the IV intake record. Attach the label from the blood bag with numbers of the unit and crossmatch identification numbers with the donor type and Rh type; note volume infused, date and time, any reaction signs and symptoms, and your signature. Adverse reactions must be charted in the nurse's notes.

   RATIONALE Documents the transfusion and patient response.

Documentation Example

11/30 1440   Vital signs: T 98.4° F; BP 132/86; P 74; R 16. First unit of packed RBCs via 18 angiocath in rt. forearm. Begun at 2 mL/min. No signs of adverse effects in 15 min. Vital signs: T 98.4° F, BP 136/86; P 76, R 16. Flow rate adjusted to complete unit in 2 hours. Patient voiced no complaints._____
1700 Transfusion complete; line flushed with normal saline. No adverse effects noted _____

_____
(Nurse's signature)

■ Special Considerations

✓ A blood product infusion should begin within 30 minutes of leaving the blood bank.

✓ A blood warmer may be used if the patient is in critical condition or is feeling chilly before infusion.

✓ Blood transfusion should be checked every 15 to 30 minutes to ensure that it is running on time.

✓ Blood components that are still hanging after 4 hours without refrigeration must be discontinued.

✓ In the postinfusion period, the patient's urine is observed for signs of hematuria, indicating a transfusion reaction.

✓ If a transfusion reaction occurs, stop the blood, start saline with fresh tubing (do not merely flush the "Y" tubing with saline because the patient will receive any blood product that remains in the used tubing), stay with the patient, and immediately notify the physician. If shortness of breath occurs, start low-flow oxygen per agency protocol. Return the blood component bag to the blood bank with the transfusion reaction form.

?CRITICAL THINKING QUESTIONS

1. What type of IV fluid is connected to the "Y" tubing when RBCs are given to patients? Why is this IV fluid selected?

2. You are infusing packed red cells and the patient calls you to the room and says that she is feeling short of breath and itchy; what would you do?

Home Care Considerations 36-1

Using Intravenous Medications in the Home

- Intravenous infusions and medications are common in the home care setting. When there is a long-term need for IV therapy, the patient or family may be instructed on how to administer the solutions safely. The solutions and medications are prepared and delivered by a home infusion company. For safety, an infusion pump is often used.

- The patient should be given an emergency telephone number in case a problem arises with the solution or the infusion pump.

- Clearly written instructions in the appropriate language regarding dosage schedules for IV medications, preparation of IV piggyback bags and tubing, PRN lock flushes, changing the primary IV tubing, and so forth must be available for the patient or family member responsible for IV care.

- The patient or family member should give a return demonstration prior to giving unsupervised IV care.

- Coordinate IV teaching with the IV infusion company to avoid conflicting instructions for the patient.

- For home blood transfusion, everything is meticulously checked three times without distractions to prevent error.

---

lergic reaction. When antibiotics are given to prevent infection after surgery, monitor the incision for signs of inflammation and track the body temperature to see if the medication is effective. When a blood product is administered, monitor the blood count to see if values improve. Monitor for signs and symptoms of transfusion reaction.

Documentation

Documentation of IV medication is done on the MAR. Data included in the documentation are similar to those for other types of medications (see Chapter 34 for documentation). In addition, the IV site is assessed every 1 to 2 hours according to agency policy and observations are entered on a flow sheet or in the nurse's notes. IV fluid is counted as intake and recorded on the I & O sheet.

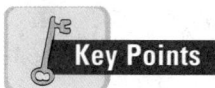
Key Points

- Intravenous solutions supply the body with needed substances or drugs that cannot be supplied as rapidly or efficiently by other means.

- The average adult needs 1500 to 2000 mL of fluid per 24 hours to replace those eliminated by the body.

- Medications may be given as IV solution additives, as piggyback medications, by controlled-volume burette, or by bolus.
- All intravenous solutions must be sterile; interior surfaces of connectors, adaptors, and equipment that comes in contact with the solution must also be kept sterile.
- The three most common infusion tubing sets are the primary, the secondary, and the "Y"-type tubing.
- Regular drop sets deliver 10 to 20 gtt/mL; macrodrip sets deliver 10 gtt/mL, and microdrip sets deliver 60 gtt/mL.
- Infusion pumps deliver fluids more accurately over a set period of time.
- Piggyback (intermittent) IV medications are commonly mixed in 50 to 250 mL of solution.
- The most frequently used peripheral IV sites are the veins of the forearm and hand. Scalp veins may be used in infants.
- PICC and midline catheters are used for IV therapy that requires placement where there is high blood flow; they are also used for long-term IV therapy.
- Central venous catheters are inserted into the subclavian or jugular vein by a physician.
- All IV catheters must be periodically flushed to maintain patency if continuous fluid is not running through them.
- Longer-term intravenous therapy requires a tunneled catheter, PICC line, midline catheter, or implanted infusion port.

- Infiltration is the most common complication of IV therapy; other complications are listed in Table 36-2.
- Assess the site and the patient every 1 to 2 hours when administering intravenous fluids or medications.
- Patients who have a continuous infusion often need more help for activities of daily living.
- A primary nursing responsibility is to correctly calculate the ordered flow rate and regulate the infusion and ensure that the correct fluid is infusing for assigned patients.
- Always clean the port with an alcohol swab prior to flushing or prior to interrupting the system to attach new connectors, adaptors, or IV tubing.
- All intravenous sites and solutions infused are recorded on the IV flow sheet. IV medications are recorded on the MAR.
- Clearly written instructions and demonstrations are given to home care patients who are undergoing intravenous therapy.

 Go to your **Companion CD-ROM** for an Audio Glossary, animations, video clips, and more.

evolve Be sure to visit the companion Evolve site at http://evolve.elsevier.com/deWit/fundamental/ for additional online resources.

NCLEX-PN® EXAMINATION-STYLE REVIEW QUESTIONS

*Choose the **best** answer(s) for each question.*

1. Which solution is the most common vehicle for mixing IV piggyback medications?
   1. 0.45% Saline
   2. 5% Dextrose in water
   3. 10% Dextrose in water
   4. Lactated Ringer's

2. A nurse is assessing the patient who has severe vomiting and diarrhea. The purpose of IV infusion for this patient is to:
   1. provide fluids to reduce elevated temperature.
   2. control the nausea and vomiting.
   3. replenish fluids and correct dehydration.
   4. deliver medication to stabilize blood pressure.

3. An important nursing responsibility when caring for a patient with a central line is to:
   1. use sterile technique during insertion.
   2. flush the line according to agency policy.
   3. verify catheter placement with an x-ray.
   4. rotate the insertion site every 72 hours.

4. A patient is receiving a total of 4000 mL of D_5W over 24 hours. How many calories will this fluid supply?
   1. 800
   2. 600
   3. 500
   4. 250

5. A nurse is adding a secondary piggyback to the patient's existing IV. In order to use the gravity system, the nurse should hang:
   1. the piggyback bag higher than the maintenance IV bag.
   2. the maintenance IV bag at the same height as the piggyback bag.
   3. the piggyback bag and the maintenance IV bag using "Y" tubing.
   4. the maintenance IV bag after the piggyback bag is completed.

6. The nurse needs to establish a peripheral IV access on an adult trauma patient. Which catheter is the best choice?
   1. #24
   2. #22
   3. #20
   4. #18

7. The primary safety advantage of using a burette is that it:
    1. is cost effective because it can be used more than once.
    2. can be used for pediatric and elderly patients.
    3. decreases the likelihood of IV fluid volume overload.
    4. can be used with any type of IV fluid or medication.

8. The nurse must assess for complications of IV therapy. Signs of common complications include: *(Select all that apply.)*
    1. swelling and coolness at the site.
    2. redness along the vein.
    3. pale skin at the insertion site.
    4. fever and fatigue.
    5. erythema and tenderness.
    6. vomiting and diarrhea.

9. The patient is receiving a blood transfusion and begins to have symptoms within 10 minutes after the start of the transfusion. What is the priority action?
    1. Call the physician.
    2. Start low-flow oxygen.
    3. Stop the blood and start normal saline.
    4. Change the IV tubing and solution.

10. A patient returns from physical therapy (PT) and her IV has a very sluggish flow, but it was functioning well before going to PT. What is the priority nursing action?
    1. Call PT and asked if anything happened to the IV during the treatment session.
    2. Discontinue the IV and restart the IV at a new site.
    3. Assess the IV insertion site and tubing and try repositioning the extremity.
    4. Use a heparin flush to clear the line.

11. The doctor orders D_5W (5% dextrose in water) to infuse at 150 mL/hr. The nurse is using macrodrip tubing (10 gtt/mL). What is the drop rate?
    _____ gtt/min

12. The doctor orders 1000 mL of normal saline (0.9% saline) to infuse over 8 hours. What is the pump setting?

CRITICAL THINKING ACTIVITIES *Read each clinical scenario and discuss the questions with your classmates.*

Scenario A
Daris Hostetler has lost a lot of blood from injuries sustained in an automobile accident. The physician orders three units of packed red blood cells (RBCs) for him.

1. Describe the procedure used to prepare to infuse the first unit of packed RBCs.
2. What points are essential to check with another nurse for each unit of packed RBCs?
3. After the second unit is begun, Mr. Hostetler complains of shortness of breath and is very apprehensive. Identify the steps you would take in order of priority.

Scenario B
Sherida Patel, age 82, is receiving IV therapy after surgery for her fractured hip.

1. What areas of assessment (related to the IV therapy) would you pay especially close attention to for this type of elderly patient?
2. Mrs. Patel becomes confused and develops crackles in the bases of the lungs. What would you do?

Scenario C
The patient has a potassium level of 3.2 mEq/L. The physician orders 20 mEq of potassium added to 250 mL of 5% dextrose to infuse over 2 hours.

1. What is the purpose of diluting potassium in the 5% dextrose solution?
2. List at least three nursing actions that you would use to prevent the complications or adverse reactions related to the potassium infusion.

37 Care of the Surgical Patient

evolve http://evolve.elsevier.com/deWit/fundamental/

Objectives

Upon completing this chapter, you should be able to:

Theory

1. Discuss reasons for which surgery might be performed.
2. Assess for potential risk factors for complications of surgery.
3. Explain the nurse's role in the various phases of perioperative nursing.
4. Discuss how robotic surgery has made recovery time shorter.
5. Identify the types of anesthesia used for surgery.
6. State the safety measure now in place to prevent errors regarding the surgical site.
7. Assist the patient with psychological preparation for surgery.
8. Define the nurse's role during the signing of a consent for surgery.
9. Discuss differences in the roles of the scrub person and the circulating nurse.
10. List interventions to prevent each of the potential postoperative complications.

Clinical Practice

1. Implement physical preparation of the patient before surgery.
2. Perform preoperative teaching for the patient and family.
3. Prepare to perform an immediate postoperative assessment when a patient returns to the nursing unit.
4. Promote adequate ventilation of the lungs during recovery from anesthesia.
5. Assess for postoperative pain and provide comfort measures and pain relief.
6. Promote early ambulation and return to independence in activities of daily living.
7. Perform discharge teaching necessary for postoperative home self-care.

Skills

Skills

Skill 37-1 Applying Antiembolism Stockings

Key Terms

Be sure to check out the bonus material on the Companion CD-ROM, including selected audio pronunciations.

anesthesia (ăn-ĕs-THĒ-zē-ă, p. 750)
atelectasis (ă-tĕ-LĔK-tă-sĭs, p. 768)

autotransfusion (p. 755)
conscious (p. 751)
curative surgery (p. 748)
dehiscence (dĕ-HĬS-ĕns, p. 773)
elective (p. 748)
embolus (ĔM-bō-lŭs, p. 771)
evisceration (ĕ-vĭs-ĕr-Ā-shŭn, p. 773)
laser (p. 750)
palliative surgery (PĂL-ē-ă-tĭv, p. 748)
paralytic ileus (păr-ă-LĬT-ĭk ĬL-ē-ŭs, p. 771)
perioperative (pĕr-ē-ŌP-ĕr-ă-tĭv, p. 749)
pneumonia (nū-MŌ-nē-ă, p. 772)
prosthesis (prŏs-THĒ-sĭs, p. 754)
stasis (STĀ-sĭs, p. 755)
thrombophlebitis (thrŏm-bō-flĕ-BĪ-tĭs, p. 755)
thrombosis (thrŏm-BŌ-sĭs, p. 768)
unconscious (p. 751)

REASONS FOR SURGERY

Surgery is performed for a variety of reasons. A procedure may be elective (voluntary), such as when a hernia repair is scheduled a week away. *Emergency surgery* is often necessary in trauma cases in which serious consequences will occur if surgery is not done immediately. Palliative surgery (pain or complication relieving) is performed to make a patient more comfortable. Removing a metastatic tumor that is causing considerable pain from the abdomen is an example. *Diagnostic surgery,* such as a biopsy of a mass, is done to provide data for a diagnosis of the problem. *Reconstructive surgery,* such as mammoplasty after a mastectomy, is done to restore appearance or function. Curative surgery alleviates (cures) a problem, such as when a gallbladder that is full of stones, causing blockage or pain, is removed.

PATIENTS AT HIGHER RISK FOR SURGICAL COMPLICATIONS

The infant and the elderly person are at higher risk for complications of surgery due to either immature body systems or a decline in function of various body systems. Maintaining core body temperature is one concern for these patients. Both age groups are at risk for dehydration or overhydration. Aging causes changes

Table 37-1 | *Surgical Risk Factors*

FACTOR	KEY POINTS
Diabetes mellitus and other chronic diseases	Stress of surgery may cause swings in blood glucose levels that are difficult to control. Patient may receive intravenous insulin during and after surgery. Wound healing tends to be delayed in the diabetic patient, making the risk of dehiscence greater. There is a higher incidence of infection in surgical wounds of diabetic patients. Liver and kidney disease makes it more difficult to metabolize and eliminate anesthesia and waste products.
Advanced age with inactivity	Healing is slower in elderly patients. The risk of disuse syndrome, hypostatic pneumonia, and thrombus formation is higher in an inactive elderly person.
Very young age	Infants have difficulty with temperature control and in maintaining normal circulatory blood volume; they are at risk of dehydration.
Malnutrition	Inadequate nutritional stores lead to poor wound healing and skin breakdown.
Dehydration	Reduced circulating volume reduces kidney perfusion and predisposes to a reduced urine output and thrombus formation. Dehydration also alters electrolyte values. The dehydrated patient is more at risk for problems with pressure areas during surgery.
Obesity	The extremely heavy patient does not breathe as deeply and is at risk of hypostatic pneumonia. Excessive fatty tissue also is a factor in poor wound healing.
Cardiovascular problems	Patients with hypertension, left ventricular hypertrophy, cardiac arrhythmias, or history of congestive heart failure are at a higher risk for myocardial infarction from the stresses of surgery and anesthesia.
Peripheral vascular disease	Poor circulation in the extremities predisposes the patient to possible thrombus formation and pressure sores on the lower legs and feet. Antiembolic stockings or devices are generally prescribed for use during and after surgery.
Substance abuse or alcohol dependence	May alter reaction to anesthetic agents. Alcohol dependence may cause withdrawal symptoms if the use of alcohol is discontinued abruptly.
Smoking	Causes increased lung secretions from anesthesia and predisposes the patient to atelectasis and pneumonia postoperatively. Smokers are more prone to thrombus formation.
Regular use of certain drugs	Aspirin and anticoagulants make the patient more prone to excessive bleeding. Corticosteroids reduce the body's response to infection and delay the healing process.
Excessive fear	Stimulates the sympathetic nervous system and causes the release of hormones, causing swings in the body's chemistry and vital signs. Increased muscle tension makes surgery more difficult. Physical manifestations of fear can interfere with achieving the desired state of anesthesia.

Box 37-1 | *Recommended Measures to Prevent Surgical Site Infections*

- Administer prophylactic antibiotics just before incision time.
- Do not remove hair at surgical site. If removal of hair is essential, remove hair with clippers or a depilatory.
- Hair is to be removed, when essential, immediately before surgery.
- A razor should not be used to remove hair as it causes nicks and abrasions in the skin.
- Glycemic control should be maintained with blood glucose below 200 mg/dL in the first 48 hours postoperatively.
- Body temperature during and after surgery should be maintained at 96.8° to 100.4° F (36° C to 38° C), particularly for those patients having colorectal surgery.

From Daniels, S.M. (2007). Improving hospital care for surgical patients. *Nursing2007, 37*(8), 36-37.

in the cardiovascular, respiratory, renal, integumentary, neurologic, and metabolic systems. Elderly patients must be watched and assessed for complications very closely during and after surgery. Other types of patients who are at higher risk during and after surgery are those with bleeding disorders, cancer, heart disease, chronic respiratory disease, liver disease, immune disorders, chronic pain, upper respiratory infection, or fever, or who abuse street drugs (Table 37-1). These patients are subject to a variety of complications and should be carefully assessed during the postoperative period.

All patients are at risk for surgical site infection. The Institute for Healthcare Improvement launched a campaign to reduce incidents of medical harm. Box 37-1 lists the recommended measures to reduce surgical site infection in patients.

PERIOPERATIVE NURSING

Perioperative nursing refers to the care of the patient from the time of the decision to have surgery through recovery from the procedure. Learning the terminology for surgical procedures will help in identifying what the surgeon is going to do (Box 37-2). Surgery may be performed as a same-day or outpatient procedure or an inpatient procedure in a hospital or surgery center. Minor surgery is often performed in a physician's office. Patients having same-day surgery are admitted early in the morning and discharged in the afternoon. Preparation for surgery is usually begun before admission. The patient has diagnostic tests done in the days just before the scheduled surgery. Teaching for postoperative care must be done effi-

---

Box 37-2 *Terminology for Surgical Procedures*

Suffixes are often attached to a stem word to describe a surgical procedure. For example, *appendectomy* means cutting out the appendix.

Lysis: removal or destruction of (lysis of adhesions—removal of adhesions)

Anastomosis: joining of two parts, ducts, or blood vessels

-ectomy: cutting out or off (colectomy: cutting out a part of the colon)

-oma: tumor (excision of a lipoma: removal of a fat tumor)

-ostomy: to furnish with a mouth or an outlet (colostomy: creating an outlet from the body for the colon)

-otomy: cutting into (thoracotomy: cutting into the chest cavity)

-plasty: revision, molding, or repair of tissue (mammoplasty: revision of the breast)

-pexy: fixation, anchoring in place (orchiopexy: fixation of an undescended testicle in the scrotum)

Home Care Considerations 37-1

Home Care for Discharged Postsurgical Patients

Discharge planning begins at the time of admission. Whether the patient is a same-day surgery patient or an inpatient, the same general points will need to be covered before discharge.

- The patient must know about each medication to be taken and when to take it.
- The diet, any restrictions, and guidelines for fluid intake are discussed. Alcohol must be avoided for 24 hours after surgery.
- Any restrictions on activity are listed and instructions for use of any special equipment such as crutches, splint, walker, and so forth are presented.
- Patients should not drive or make important decisions for 24 hours after anesthesia.
- The type of bath permitted is explained.
- Cleansing and dressing of the wound are discussed along with where to obtain supplies.
- Signs and symptoms to report to the surgeon, such as temperature above 100° F, increasing malaise, severe pain or swelling, bleeding through the bandage, decreased sensation below the surgical site, or severe nausea and vomiting, are listed.
- Instructions as to when to make a follow-up appointment with the doctor are essential.
- Written instructions should be sent home with the patient for all essential points of care.

---

ciently since time of stay is short to reduce hospitalization costs (Home Care Considerations 37-1). Your ability to deliver and reinforce teaching for postoperative and home care is crucial to the well-being and quick recovery of your patients.

ENHANCEMENTS TO SURGICAL TECHNIQUE

LASER SURGERY

Laser (*light amplification by the stimulated emission of radiation*) surgery is common today and is often combined with microscopic, endoscopic, and robotic-enhanced procedures. A laser is a tube that contains a medium such as carbon dioxide or another active gas, which is energized by electricity. Mirrors reflect the energized molecules back and forth and a bright light is generated in the form of a beam. The light beam is converted to heat as tissue absorbs it. There are several varieties of lasers for different uses.

FIBEROPTIC SURGERY

Fiberoptics allows the use of endoscopes with high-resolution video cameras passed through a very small incision for an ever-increasing variety of surgical procedures. Operating microscopes can be combined with an endoscope for microscopic surgery. Small growths and organs can be removed without making a traditional surgical incision. However, two or three other puncture holes are made for the instruments and video camera attachment that provide access and a visual field for the procedure.

ROBOTIC SURGERY

More surgeons are using remote-controlled robots to perform surgeries. Robotics is seen as a key to less invasive, less traumatic surgeries in the future. The robot is operated from a nearby computer while the surgeon views magnified three-dimensional images of the surgical field on the computer's screen. The robot's tiny camera has multiple lenses that allow magnification up to 12 times that of normal vision. There are assistants and a second surgeon next to the patient, but the main surgeon performs the surgery at the computer. For heart surgery, the robot's needle-like "fingers" are introduced through pencil-sized holes in the chest to perform certain heart surgery techniques. Remote-controlled instruments are inserted through small incisions. Various types of robotics that are voice activated by the surgeon are undergoing use. Computer Motion is a firm located in Santa Barbara, California, that is a pioneer in this field. These machines can provide very precise movements for the surgeon.

A big advantage of using the robot is that it has "rock-steady" hands, providing precision that is beyond human dexterity. Because only small incisions are needed, the patient has less pain postoperatively and requires less time to heal. There is less scarring and it seems that fewer infections develop with this new surgical technique.

ANESTHESIA

Anesthesia (the loss of sensory perception) has been in use for surgical procedures since the 1840s. Newer anesthetics and techniques make anesthesia safer than ever, but **there is still a risk any time a patient is anesthetized.** The goals of anesthesia administration are (1) to prevent pain; (2) to achieve adequate muscle relaxation; and (3) to calm fear, ease anxiety, and induce forgetfulness of an unpleasant experience. Anesthetics are administered in a number of ways to achieve these goals. The choice of anesthesia rests with the anesthesiologist. The type of surgery to be performed and the age and physical condition of the patient are the influencing factors.

GENERAL ANESTHESIA

General anesthesia is induced by the administration of an inhalant gas or by medication introduced intravenously. During general anesthesia, the patient is in a deep sleep state with muscle relaxation and is not aware of anything going on in the operating room. There are four stages of general anesthesia (Box 37-3).

When the patient awakens from anesthesia, progression through the stages occurs in reverse. **Quiet must be maintained while the patient is in stage II because noise may cause the patient to become excited, resulting in instability of vital signs.**

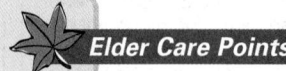
Elder Care Points

- An accurate height and weight of the elderly patient are very important for calculation of anesthetic agents and medication dosages.
- Kidney function is declining in the elderly person, and drugs are not eliminated from the body as quickly. Reduced dosages are often needed.

REGIONAL ANESTHESIA

Regional anesthesia is accomplished by administering a nerve block. It is often more economical than general anesthesia. This may be accomplished by injecting the spinal, epidural, caudal, or peripheral nerve area. The block anesthetizes the local area or the area distal to the block. Spinal or epidural blocks are frequently used for high-risk patients undergoing pelvic or lower extremity surgery; epidural blocks are widely used in obstetric procedures.

PROCEDURAL (MODERATE) SEDATION ANESTHESIA

A local anesthetic agent at the surgical site plus intravenous sedation is used to provide systemic analgesia and conscious (awareness of one's surroundings) sedation as well as depress the autonomic nervous system. The technique can be used for any surgery or procedure that can be done with local anesthesia and is being used more and more frequently. The patient is monitored closely for blood pressure changes, oxygen saturation levels, and heart activity.

Box 37-3 | *The Four Stages of Anesthesia*

- **Stage I:** *The stage of analgesia.* Begins with the administration of the anesthetic agent and ends when the patient becomes unconscious (incapable of responding to sensory stimuli). Hearing is amplified at the end of this stage.
- **Stage II:** *The excitement phase.* Muscles become tense but swallowing and vomiting reflexes are still present. Breathing may become irregular or the breath may be held. The environment should be kept quiet during this period.
- **Stage III:** *Surgical anesthesia state.* Begins with the onset of regular breathing again. Vital functions are depressed, eyes are fixed, and reflexes are lost or temporarily depressed. The surgical procedure is begun during this stage.
- **Stage IV:** *Complete respiratory depression.* Spontaneous respirations are absent. The patient is maintained by the anesthesia machine, which supplies oxygen and a set rate of breaths.

LOCAL ANESTHESIA

Local anesthesia is used for minor procedures such as superficial tissue biopsies, surface cyst excision, insertion of a pacemaker, and insertion of vascular access devices. The patient who has had local anesthesia is transferred directly to the nursing unit and does not need care in the postanesthesia care recovery unit (PACU, also called PAR or PARU).

PREOPERATIVE PROCEDURES

Care of the surgical patient is divided into four phases: preoperative, intraoperative, postanesthesia immediate care, and postoperative care. During the preoperative phase, nonanemic patients may donate their own blood 2 to 4 weeks prior to surgery to be banked in case of postoperative autologous (related to self) transfusion need. This eliminates any possibility of transfusion with blood contaminated with a blood-borne virus, such as human immunodeficiency virus (HIV) or hepatitis B or C.

SURGICAL CONSENT

A surgical consent form must be signed prior to surgery before preoperative medications are given, when the patient's mind is not affected by the medications (Figure 37-1). This is a legal form that must be filled out in ink with the correct spelling of procedures to be done. **The surgeon is responsible for obtaining an informed surgical consent.** The need for the procedure, a description of the procedure to be performed, its risks and benefits, and alternative treatments available and their possible consequences must be explained to the patient in understandable terms, and the explanation (not just the patient's signature) should be witnessed by at least one health care professional. Any questions must be answered. The surgeon often

SPECIAL CONSENT TO OPERATION, POSTOPERATIVE CARE, MEDICAL TREATMENT, ANESTHESIA/SEDATION, OR OTHER PROCEDURE

PATIENT LABEL

1CPROC

Patient _____

Patient No. _____

State law guarantees that you have both the *right* and *obligation* to make decisions concerning your health care. Your physician can provide you with the necessary information and advice, but as a member of the health care team, you must enter into the decision making process. This form has been designed to acknowledge your acceptance of treatment recommended by your physician.

IMPORTANT: HAVE PATIENT SIGN FULL OR LIMITED DISCLOSURE BOX AND SIGNATURE LINE AT BOTTOM.

Full Disclosure

I certify that my physician has informed me of the nature and character of the proposed treatment, of the anticipated results of the proposed treatment, of the possible alternative forms of treatment, and the recognized serious possible risks, complications, and the anticipated benefits involved in the proposed treatment and in the alternative forms of treatment, including nontreatment.

(PATIENT/OTHER LEGALLY RESPONSIBLE PERSON SIGN IF APPLICABLE)

1. I hereby authorize Dr. _____ and/or such associates or assistants as may be selected by said physician to treat the following condition(s) that has (have) been explained to me. (Explain the nature of the condition[s] in professional and lay language.)

_____
_____
_____

2. The procedures planned for treatment of my condition(s) have been explained to me by my physician. I understand them to be as follows. (Describe procedures to be performed in professional and lay language.)

_____
_____
_____
_____

Limited Disclosure

I certify that my physician has explained to me that I have the right to have clearly described to me the nature and character of the proposed treatment, the anticipated results of the proposed treatment, the alternative forms of treatment, and the recognized serious possible risks, complications, and anticipated benefits involved in the proposed treatment, and in the alternative forms of treatment, including nontreatment.
I do not wish to have these risks and facts explained to me.

(PATIENT/OTHER LEGALLY RESPONSIBLE PERSON SIGN IF APPLICABLE)

At: _____
(NAME OF HOSPITAL OR MEDICAL FACILITY)

Any sections below which do not apply to the proposed treatment may be crossed out. All sections crossed out must be initialed by both physician and patient.

3. I recognize that during the course of the operation, postoperative care, medical treatment, anesthesia/sedation, or other procedure unforeseen conditions may necessitate additional or different procedures than those above set forth. I therefore authorize my above named physician, and his or her assistants or designees, to perform such surgical or other procedures as are in the exercise of his, her, or their professional judgment necessary and desirable. The authority granted under this paragraph shall extend to the treatment of all conditions that require treatment and are not known to my physician at the time the medical or surgical procedure is commenced.

4. I have been informed that there are significant risks such as severe loss of blood, infection, and cardiac arrest that can lead to death or permanent or partial disability, that may be attendant to the performance of any procedure. I acknowledge that no warranty or guarantee has been made to me as to result or cure.

5. I consent to the administration of anesthesia/sedation by my attending physician, by an anesthesiologist, or other qualified party under the direction of a physician as may be deemed necessary. I understand that all anesthetics involve risks of complications and serious possible damage to vital organs such as the brain, heart, lung, liver, and kidney and that in some cases may result in paralysis, cardiac arrest, and/or brain death from both known and unknown causes. I understand there is a risk of dental injury during airway management.

6. I consent to the use of transfusion of blood and blood products as deemed necessary, and potential complications associated with this procedure have been explained to me by my physician.

7. Any tissues or parts surgically removed may be disposed of by the hospital or physician in accordance with accustomed practice.

I certify this form has been fully explained to me, that I have read it or have had it read to me, that the blank spaces have been filled in, and that I understand its contents.

DATE _____ TIME _____ A.M. P.M.

_____
PATIENT/OTHER LEGALLY RESPONSIBLE PERSON SIGN

WITNESS _____

_____
RELATIONSHIP OF LEGALLY RESPONSIBLE PERSON TO PATIENT

FIGURE **37-1** Surgical consent form must be signed and witnessed.

explains the procedure with the nurse present, answers questions, and then asks the nurse to obtain the signature of the patient on the form. **If the patient does not understand the procedure, or has further questions for the surgeon, refer the matter back to the surgeon.** If the patient is a minor, is confused, or is mentally incompetent, another responsible party such as a parent, spouse, or guardian must be present for the explanation and may need to be the person to sign the consent form. The signature of the patient or responsible party must be witnessed by another party, usually a staff member. The consent form must show the procedure to be performed and the risks involved, must include the time and date, and must be signed in ink. A witnessed "X" is acceptable if the patient cannot sign with a signature.

If an emergency surgery is needed and the patient is not conscious or able to give consent, an attempt to contact immediate family is made. Telephone permission may be given as long as there are two witnesses on extension lines. If no family can be found, the opinion of a second surgeon regarding the need for surgery is sought and then the surgery may take place. All responsible adults are asked to complete advance directives when admitted to the hospital if they do not already have such a document on file; these are discussed in Chapter 3. Advance directives indicate the patient's desires regarding lifesaving or life-preserving measures in the event of a cardiac arrest or other complication that threatens basic function.

> ? *Think Critically About . . .* You are taking preoperative vital signs and preparing the patient for surgery when he says, "I've changed my mind. I don't want to have this surgery after all." What would you do?

SURGICAL SITE IDENTIFICATION

In 2003, a National Patient Safety Goal was instituted to **"Eliminate wrong-site, wrong-patient, wrong-procedure surgery."** A preoperative checklist verification process is used to ensure that appropriate medical records and imaging studies are available. A process must also be implemented to mark the surgical site and involve the patient in the marking process. This should be done before preoperative medications are given so that the patient is alert to participate in this procedure. Before surgery commences, a "time-out" is called and the correct patient, correct site, and correct body part are verified by the operating team via the chart orders, operative permit, and imaging studies.

PHYSICAL EXAMINATION

The referring physician, surgeon, or surgical resident takes a medical history and performs a physical examination. This may be done in the physician's office.

The dictated report must be in the record before the patient goes to surgery. The patient should be in the best possible physical condition, unless it is an emergency procedure that will be performed.

DIAGNOSTIC TESTS

Diagnostic test data that are usually required before surgery include a complete blood cell count (CBC) and urinalysis. A chest x-ray is performed, and an electrocardiogram (ECG) is often ordered for many patients over 40 years of age. Other tests ordered may be tests to determine pregnancy; tests to determine electrolyte and blood glucose levels; tests indicating blood clotting ability, such as the prothrombin time (PT) and activated partial thromboplastin time (APPT); blood type and crossmatch for transfusion; and a profile that gives data about liver and kidney function. Most surgeons will postpone surgery if the patient's hemoglobin level is below 10 g/dL. The surgeon orders the tests, but you will need to explain to the patient why they are being done. Test values that are outside of normal ranges should be noted on the preoperative checklist as well as brought to the attention of the surgeon.

APPLICATION of the NURSING PROCESS
PREOPERATIVE CARE

During the preoperative period, the patient is prepared physically and psychologically for surgery. As much privacy as possible should be provided. If the patient is very ill, a significant other may join in the interview process. For the best result, focus completely on the patient in an unhurried manner. Ask open-ended questions and avoid judgmental responses.

Assessment (Data Collection)

The nursing history and assessment focus on possible factors that indicate the patient is at higher risk for complications from surgery (see Table 37-1). An important part of your assessment is determining what supplements and herbs a patient is using (Table 37-2). The surgeon and anesthesiologist must be aware of what substances are in the patient's body in addition to their normal medications. Besides checking for drug allergies, it is important to determine whether the patient has a latex allergy.

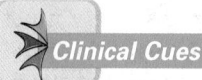 **Clinical Cues**

Indications of latex allergy may be reactions to avocados, kiwifruit, bananas, chestnuts, potatoes, peaches, or apricots.

Psychosocial assessment includes attitudes and concerns about any changes in body image and lifestyle that the surgery may cause (Box 37-4, Communication Cues 37-1).

Table 37-2 *Herbs and Supplements Affecting Surgical Outcomes*

SUBSTANCE	POSSIBLE EFFECT
Echinacea	May cause liver inflammation if used with certain medications
Feverfew	May inhibit platelet aggregation and increase bleeding
Garlic, ginger, ginkgo biloba, ginseng, or valerian	May increase bleeding tendency, particularly if receiving anticoagulants
Goldenseal	May increase blood pressure; may cause increased swelling
Kava	May prolong effects of anesthetics or antiseizure medication; may cause liver damage
Licorice	May alter electrolytes, increase blood pressure, or increase fluid retention
St. John's wort	May prolong the effect of anesthetic agents
Vitamin E or aspirin	May increase bleeding, particularly in conjunction with anticoagulants

Adapted from Lewis, S.L., Heitkemper, M.M., Dirksen, S.R., et al. (2007). *Medical-Surgical Nursing: Assessment and Management of Clinical Problems* (7th ed., p. 347). St. Louis: Elsevier Mosby.

Box 37-4 *Preoperative Psychosocial Data Collection*

Inquire regarding feelings and concerns about the following:
• Body image—scars, loss of body part
• Possible change in role or relationships after surgery
• Specific anxieties or fears about surgery or anesthesia
• Concerns about care after discharge
• Financial concerns
• Effect on lifestyle that surgery may incur
• Past experience of surgery or anesthesia and perceived impressions from others
• Knowledge of surgery, recovery, patient role, and impact on life
• Expectation of result of surgery

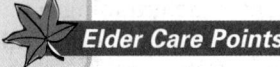 **Elder Care Points**

One of the greatest fears of the elderly person facing surgery is a loss of independence. It is important to stress the measures that will be taken to return the patient to independence after surgery.

Cultural beliefs and values regarding surgery must be taken into consideration (Cultural Cues 37-1). If the patient does not speak the same language as the surgical team, an interpreter should be enlisted to assist with communication. If a female patient's culture has strict rules for female attire, she needs assurance of sufficient privacy and protection of modesty to allay any fears she might have; such issues and interventions must be conveyed to the operating room. If there are certain cultural taboos regarding an aspect of the surgery, the surgical team needs to know about them

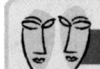 **Communication Cues 37-1**

Preoperative Interaction

Carolyn Silva, age 67, is scheduled for a partial colectomy. She has had several bouts of diverticulitis with considerable pain and malaise. She seems very apprehensive about the surgery.

NURSE: "Mrs. Silva., do you understand what the surgeon is going to do on Wednesday?"

MRS. SILVA: "Yes, but I'm nervous about having this done."

NURSE: "The thought of surgery makes you nervous?"

MRS. SILVA: "Well, it's more than that. I have several family members who have had colon cancer and I can't help thinking that cancer is what will be found."

NURSE: "You are scared you have cancer. As I recall you had a colonoscopy a few weeks ago and it didn't show any lesion suspicious of cancer in the colon."

MRS. SILVA: "That's right, but what if the doctor just didn't see it?"

NURSE: "There are no guarantees until you get a clean pathology report, but the colonoscopy showed that you had severe inflammation in this one part of the colon and that is what is to be taken out."

MRS. SILVA: "Oh, I know. I'm just a worrywart."

NURSE: "Perhaps holding positive thoughts about the outcome of this surgery would help reduce your fears. Try to visualize yourself with a healthy colon with the diseased piece gone and no more episodes of severe pain and illness."

MRS. SILVA: "I'll try it. It does seem foolish to spend energy worrying until I know something more is wrong."

NURSE: "I'll be at the desk charting. If you need me, press the call button."

and plan a way to achieve a good outcome without violating such a taboo. It is especially important to know whether the patient will accept a blood transfusion. Jehovah's Witnesses usually do not wish to have blood administered.

The operating room is notified if the patient is hard of hearing, is essentially blind when glasses are not in place, or has a prosthesis (artificial body part).

Think Critically About . . . The patient has told you during your assessment that she drinks a glass of wine with dinner each night. Later her husband informs you that she tends to drink three to four glasses of wine each evening. What should you do with this information?

Nursing Diagnosis

Nursing diagnoses in the preoperative stage include actual and potential problems identified by your data collection and the RN assessment. Examples of common nursing diagnoses are as follows:
• Anxiety related to the surgical experience and outcome

Prohibition of a Non-Self Blood Transfusion

Jehovah's Witnesses refuse a blood transfusion because it is prohibited by their religion. In years past, many surgeries could not be performed on these individuals because the chance of death was too great. New bloodless medicine strategies have allowed many surgeries to safely occur that were denied before.

- Autotransfusion (transfusion of one's own blood) is one method, using a cell-saver gathering system for blood lost during or in the 2 days after surgery. These cells are washed and then reinfused. This procedure is acceptable to Jehovah's Witnesses as long as there is a continuously closed circuit for collection and reinfusion.
- Hemodilution during surgery may be used, in which up to seven units of the patient's blood are removed and re-placed with crystalloids/colloids. The cells are usually re-infused later, again via a closed system. The replacement fluids decrease blood viscosity and increase blood flow in tissues as well as help maintain oxygen transport and blood pressure.
- The use of lasers, electrocautery, argon beam coagulators, and harmonic scalpels, which cause blood to coagulate after tissue is cut, decreases blood loss.
- If the patient is anemic prior to surgery, epoetin alfa (Epogen, Procrit) is used along with vitamins B_{12} and C to stimulate red blood cell production.

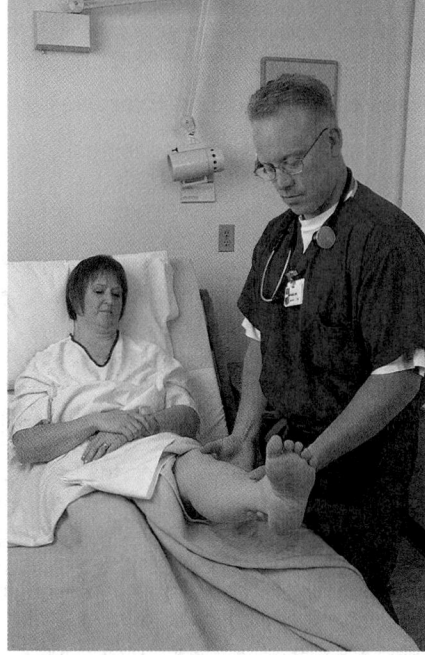

FIGURE **37-2** Teaching postoperative leg exercises.

- Fear related to risk for death, effects of impending surgery, or loss of control due to anesthesia
- Anticipatory grieving related to impending loss of a body function or body part
- Deficient knowledge related to preoperative and postoperative routines
- Sleep deprivation related to stress or unfamiliar environment
- Ineffective coping related to lack of problem-solving skills or adequate support
- Ineffective role performance related to inability to care for children during hospitalization

Planning

Expected outcomes are written for the specific individual nursing diagnoses assigned to each patient. However, *general goals* for all preoperative patients are the same in that the patient will be as follows:

- Prepared for surgery physically and emotionally
- Able to demonstrate deep breathing, coughing, and leg exercises
- Able to verbalize understanding of the procedure and the expectations of him in the postoperative period
- Able to maintain fluid and electrolyte balance throughout the perioperative period

When preoperative patients are assigned, you must plan the work for the shift carefully to have the patients ready without neglecting the needs of other assigned patients. At the beginning of the shift, check to see that any ordered preoperative medications are on hand. Check the surgery schedule and estimate the time that the patient will need to be prepared for surgery.

Implementation

Preoperatively, your time is divided between preparing the patient for surgery and teaching about what will happen and how to assist in the recovery period. The same-day surgery patient receives teaching from the physician's office nurse or a surgical intake nurse. Teaching sessions may be scheduled when the patient comes for diagnostic testing. Sending written instructions home with the patient reinforces what has been taught. The patient should be given a phone number to call for answers to questions that arise before entering the hospital for surgery. Many scheduled surgery patients begin care in the same-day surgery unit rather than spending the night in the hospital before surgery.

Teaching for Postoperative Exercises

Teaching the patient breathing, coughing, turning, and leg exercises is a high priority during the preoperative period. Venous return is often hampered during the surgical procedure due to the position assumed on the operating table and pooling of blood in the lower extremities. The stasis (stoppage of flow) of blood places the patient at risk for thrombophlebitis (blood clot causing inflammation of a vessel). Specific leg exercises help to prevent this complication (Figure 37-2). Explain the importance of doing the exercises and show the patient how to do each one; ask for a return demonstration (Patient Teaching 37-1).

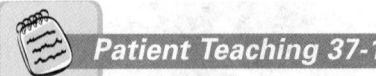

Postoperative Foot and Leg Exercises

- Flex and extend the right foot, moving the toes upward and downward, four or five times.
- Repeat with the left foot.
- Trace circles to the right with the right foot five times; repeat with circles to the left.
- Trace circles to the right with the left foot five times; repeat with circles to the left.
- Bend the right leg at the knee, sliding the foot back toward the buttocks as far as possible; raise the bent leg off the bed, extend the leg and dorsiflex the foot; extend the foot and lower the leg to the bed.
- Bend the left leg at the knee, sliding the foot back toward the buttocks as far as possible; raise the bent leg off the bed, extend the leg and dorsiflex the foot; extend the foot and lower the leg to the bed.
- Tighten the buttocks muscles for a count of 10 and release to exercise the quadriceps muscles.
- Repeat each exercise four more times.

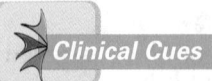

One way for patients to remember to do the exercises is to perform them whenever a commercial comes on TV. The exercises should be done at least 5 to 10 times every hour while awake after surgery until the patient is up and about normally.

For deep breathing and coughing, it is preferable for the patient to sit up with the back away from the mattress or chair. This allows for full lung expansion. The surgical incision should be splinted with a pillow (Figure 37-3).

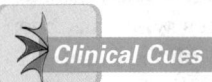

A small, firm, coughing pillow can be made by folding a bath towel and securing it inside a folded pillowcase that is taped together. It is helpful to have a significant other present for these teaching sessions so that coaching and encouragement can later be given to the patient.

Deep breathing and coughing should be performed every 2 hours for 72 hours after general anesthesia. The surgeon may order use of an incentive spirometer. Instruct the patient in its use and supervise until the patient has mastered the technique (Patient Teaching 37-2). Help the same-day surgery patient devise a schedule for doing the exercises.

Show the patient how to turn in bed by flexing the legs to relax the abdominal muscles, grabbing on to the side rail, and slowly turning to the side. This maneuver is also used for getting up out of bed. The pa-

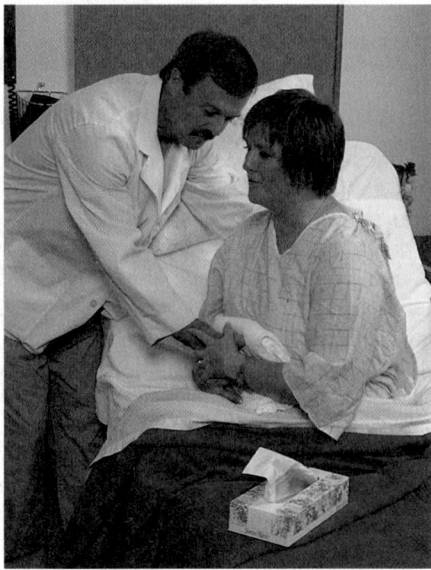

FIGURE **37-3** Teaching deep breathing and coughing.

Lung Exercises

Postoperatively, you will be asked to deep breathe and cough to open the lungs and clear secretions. Sit up away from the mattress when you do these exercises. The exercises should be performed every 2 hours during waking hours.

DEEP BREATHING
- Take a deep breath in through the nose, hold for a few seconds, and slowly exhale.
- Repeat twice more.

FORCED EXHALATION COUGHING
Splint the abdominal or chest incision and:
- Take a deep breath through the nose and cough as you exhale with the mouth open but covered with a tissue.
- If you cannot move secretions with your cough, use a forced exhalation cough.
  - Take a deep breath through the nose and forcibly quickly exhale, producing a huff-cough.
  - Repeat the process.
  - Repeat again, using three short "huffs" as you exhale to bring the secretions to the mouth where they can be expectorated.

USING AN INCENTIVE SPIROMETER
- Insert the mouthpiece, covering it completely with the lips.
- Take a slow deep breath and hold it for at least 3 seconds.
- Exhale slowly, keeping the lips puckered.
- Breathe normally for a few breaths.
- Try to increase the inspired volume by at least 100 mL with each breath on the spirometer.
- Once maximal volume is achieved, attempt to inspire this volume 10 times, resting a few breaths in between each attempt.
- Clean the mouthpiece of the spirometer when finished.

tient is also instructed in what to expect before, during, and after surgery.

NPO Status

Food and fluids will often be restricted before surgery, and the patient is placed on NPO (nothing by mouth) status. A light meal such as toast and clear fluids may be allowed up to 6 hours before surgery and a heavier meal 8 hours prior to surgery. For elective surgery, the American Society of Anesthesiology revised the practice guideline in 1999 for preoperative fasting in healthy patients. Clear liquids such as black coffee, tea, apple juice, or carbonated beverages may be consumed up to 2 hours before surgery in some elective cases. Sometimes the surgeon will allow an oral blood pressure or heart medication to be given with a sip of water the morning of surgery. **Always check the physician's order before giving anything by mouth in the immediate preoperative period.** The purpose of the restriction is to prevent vomiting and aspiration, which can occur with anesthesia, but is rarely seen with modern anesthesia.

Elimination

If the patient is having colon surgery, enemas may be ordered to be given until clear. The patient may be on a special soft or liquid diet for the 3 days prior to surgery to decrease the content of the bowel.

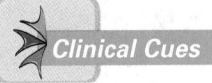
Clinical Cues

Ask the patient to empty the bladder, unless a catheter is in place, as you finish the preoperative checklist. Relaxation induced by medications and anesthesia causes the urge to urinate if the bladder is not empty.

Expected Tubes and Equipment

If a nasogastric tube will be inserted during surgery for postoperative use, explain its purpose, care, and what it will feel like to the patient. Give an estimate of how long the tube will remain in the stomach. Explain the function of other expected tubes such as drains, intravenous (IV) line, oxygen delivery and monitoring devices, chest tube, and urinary catheter, as well as their care and probable duration of use.

Rest and Sedation

It is desirable for the patient to be as well rested as possible prior to surgery so the body is not compromised in meeting the stresses of anesthesia and the procedure. A sedative is usually ordered for the night before surgery, but, if in the hospital, the patient often must ask for it. Same-day surgery patients need to be told how early to take the sedative and retire the night before surgery because it will be necessary to arise early to enter the hospital.

Pain Control

Many surgeons will order a patient-controlled analgesia (PCA) pump for their patients postoperatively. If this is to be the case, patients should receive instruction about the pump and how to operate it prior to surgery. If patients will be receiving injections for pain control, explain that this type of medication is ordered on an as-needed basis every 3 to 4 hours and that they must ask for it.

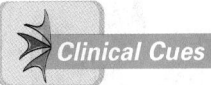
Clinical Cues

Explain that asking for the pain medication before the pain becomes severe makes it easier to control the pain level. The patient will be much more comfortable if pain medication is administered very regularly for the first 48 hours after surgery. Effectiveness of medication delivered by the PCA pump must be assessed and the physician consulted if pain is not being well controlled with the use of the pump.

Skin Preparation

The patient may be asked to shower with a special antibacterial cleanser the night or morning before surgery to remove as many microorganisms from the skin as possible. Removing hair from the operative site may be done just before surgery, but is not generally recommended anymore (see Box 37-1). Explain the process, the area to be prepared, and timing of the prep to the patient (Figure 37-4). Although this is often done in the operating room, it may be part of your job to clip hair or use a depilatory before the patient goes to surgery. (*Refer to Skill 37-2: Performing a Surgical Prep on the* ***Companion CD-ROM.***) If a depilatory is used, a skin test for sensitivity should be performed many hours before its use over the surgical site.

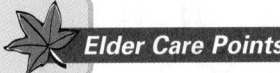
Elder Care Points

- The elderly patient should be taught needed information in short segments to prevent confusion and increase the patient's comprehension.
- Written reminders of the instructions should be given to the patient.

Immediate Preoperative Care

The patient is dressed in a clean hospital gown, without underwear, for the operating room. Hair is covered with a surgical paper cap. Long hair should be dressed so that it will tangle minimally; all hairpins and barrettes must be removed. Jewelry is removed and, along with money and credit cards, is given to a significant other to keep or is secured in a valuables envelope and placed under lock and key. If a wedding band is to be worn to surgery, tape it to the finger without restricting circulation. Dentures are removed, placed in a labeled cup, and kept in a designated place according to hospital policy. Sometimes the anesthesiolo-

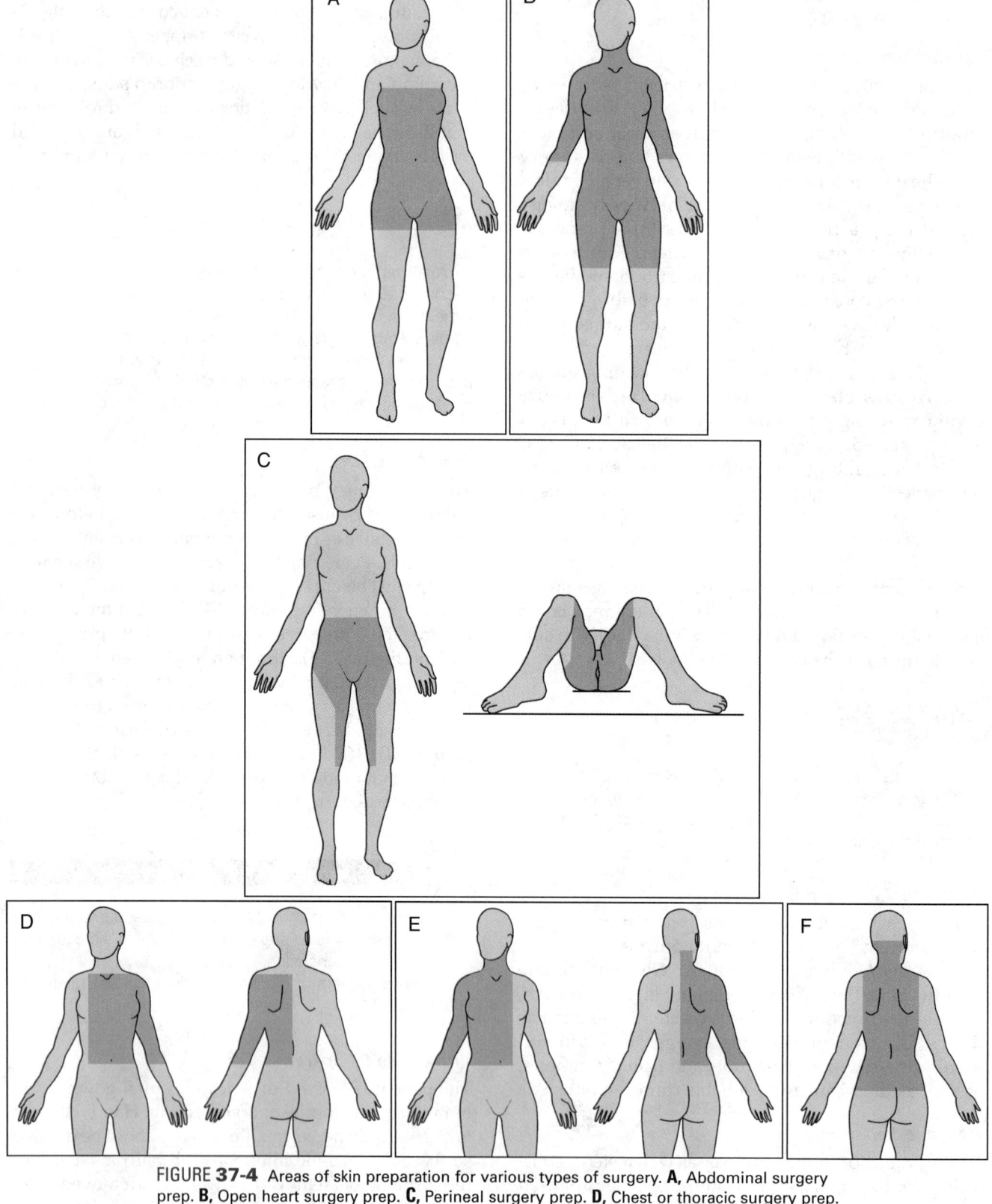

FIGURE **37-4** Areas of skin preparation for various types of surgery. **A,** Abdominal surgery prep. **B,** Open heart surgery prep. **C,** Perineal surgery prep. **D,** Chest or thoracic surgery prep. **E,** Breast surgery prep. **F,** Cervical spine surgery prep.

gist will order the dentures left in place to facilitate the administration of anesthesia by mask.

The patient's identification bracelet is checked with the chart for accuracy to avoid any error or mix-up of patients in the operating room.

Attend to all items on the preoperative checklist that can be handled ahead of time early in the morning (Figure 37-5). This prevents hurrying and mistakes and prevents delaying the departure for the operating room while the list is completed. If the facility wants

PREOP/PREPROCEDURE CHECKLIST/REPORT FORM			PATIENT LABEL

Date		Time	

Surgery/procedure			YES
Correct patient ID band on			☐

	On chart	☐
	Dictated	☐

1SURG

History and Physical
H&P 24 hours to 30 days: update with "No Pertinent Change in History & Physical" stamp
H&P 31-180 days: H&P update form #2396
OB H&P Update for Surgery/Procedures form #2543

	YES	
Initiate Anesthesia Preop order 101.S09. As appropriate initiate OB Anesthesia Order 144.P11	☐	
Include at least one page of patient ID stickers	☐	
Procedural consent: Signed/On Chart	☐	
Procedural site verified with patient/guardian	☐	N/A
Procedural site marked when laterality (including internal laterality), multiple structures (fingers, toes, lesions) or multiple levels (spine). Specify site: _____	☐	☐
Preop antibiotic given	☐	☐
Interpreter if needed	☐	☐
HBOC transfer report on chart (when applicable)	☐	☐
Acuscan MAR-LOS custom report on chart (when applicable)	☐	☐

OB ☐ The Department of Social and Health Services consent for sterilization completed and on chart dated ≥ than 30 days prior to procedure (*unless meets exception criteria, listed in Standards of Care Notebook)

☐ Notify anesthesia provider

Diagnostic ☐ Labs on chart   ☐ X-rays with patient (when appropriate)   ☐ When applicable Glucose: _____/time _____
☐ Type and screen   ☐ ECG (when applicable)   Blood units available: # _____

Medications/IV ☐ MAR on chart   ☐ IV/Saline lock in place   ☐ If TPN running, start second peripheral IV site

Belongings		Labeled	With Patient/Family	To OR
Contacts				
Glasses				
Hearing aids R L Both				
Dentures ☐ Upper ☐ Lower ☐ Partial				

Prep   ☐ Personal clothing removed   ☐ Prep completed
☐ Snap gown   ☐ Voided, time: _____   ☐ Foley
☐ Jewelry/body piercings: ____   ☐ None   ☐ Taped   ☐ Family   ☐ Patient registration safe
☐ Preop teaching done   Last oral/fluid intake: _____   Time: _____

Unit based or bedside procedures: FINAL VERIFICATION
☐ Correct patient   ☐ Correct side/site   ☐ Correct position
☐ Correct procedure   ☐ Correct equipment/trays

REPORT USING SBAR: Provide an opportunity to ask and answer questions. Include significant history/special needs.

INITIALS/OR SIGNATURE IF SIGNATURE PAGE NOT USED

FIGURE **37-5** Preoperative communication record to be filled in as patient is prepared for surgery.

the surgical area marked before the patient leaves the room, confer with the patient and appropriately mark the site according to agency policy. Seek feedback from the patient that the site is marked properly.

Assist in transferring the patient to the stretcher when the transport person comes to take the patient to surgery. Compare the patient's identification bracelet name and numbers with the transport request sheet. Check the chart to make certain that everything ordered has been done and make a final entry in the nurse's notes (Figure 37-6).

Preoperative Medications. Most preoperative medications are given intravenously in the surgical holding area rather than on the nursing unit. Preoperative medications are given for the following reasons:

* To reduce anxiety and promote a restful state
* To decrease secretion of mucus and other body fluids
* To counteract nausea and reduce emesis
* To enhance the effects of the anesthetic

Preparation of the Patient Unit

While patients are in surgery, prepare the patient unit for their return. Make the bed with fresh linen, including a drawsheet placed at shoulder height. Place an underpad at the hip area. Fan-fold the top covers to the far side of the bed or to the bottom of the bed. Have the bed in a raised position at the height of the stretcher that will return the patient and arrange furniture so that the stretcher can be pulled up alongside the bed (Figure 37-7).

Gather an emesis basin, tissues, a frequent vital signs sheet or postoperative record, an intake and output sheet, a small towel and washcloth, and a pencil and place them on the bedside table or console (Figure 37-8). Place an IV pole at the head of the bed. Connect oxygen and suction equipment if their need is anticipated. A thermometer, sphygmomanometer and stethoscope, and pulse oximeter should be close at hand on the patient's return to the unit. If a PCA pump, sequential pneumatic compression devices, or a passive range-of-motion machine will be needed, see that they are obtained and ready.

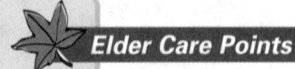
Elder Care Points

* Kidney function is decreased in the elderly, which makes them less tolerant of normal adult dosages of medications. Watch for medication toxicity.
* Meperidine may cause confusion if used continuously.

Evaluation

Evaluation is accomplished by determining if the expected outcomes and goals have been met. If the patient is properly prepared for surgery, is kept NPO, is reasonably calm, and is knowledgeable about the procedure and what is expected of him, then the general goals

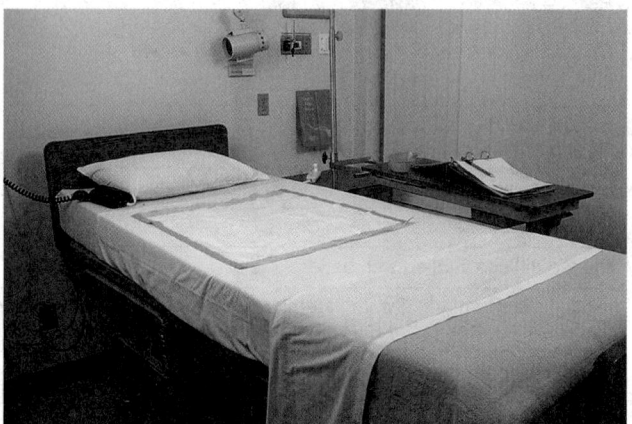

4/10/09 0730 Preop checklist complete. Surgical site & knee verified with patient and marked. - S. Crebs, RN
0800 Took via stretcher. S. Crebs, LPN

FIGURE **37-6** Entry in nurse's notes.

FIGURE **37-7** Postoperative unit prepared for patient.

have been met. If the patient was not ready for transport at the appointed time, then you need to review your steps to see where improvement can occur. Other areas to evaluate are to assess whether the patient's valuables were safely returned after surgery, and dentures, glasses, or hearing aid were found and reinserted. If any of these items were misplaced, then procedures need to be changed. Expected outcomes written for individual nursing diagnoses must also be addressed during evaluation (Nursing Care Plan 37-1).

INTRAOPERATIVE CARE

The patient is transported to a holding room where the circulating nurse will verify the patient's identification and verify that all preoperative orders have been accomplished. The anesthesiologist or nurse anesthetist will start an IV if one is not already in place. Any ordered preoperative medications will be administered. When the operating room (OR) is ready, the patient is transferred to the operating table (Figure 37-9, p. 765). Patient identification is verified again by the circulating nurse. The surgical consent form is checked to ensure that the patient is being prepared for the correct surgery on the correct body part. The surgical site is verified with the patient and marked, if not already done, before medications are given. The patient is positioned with padding to prevent injury to nerves and to minimize pressure over bony prominences. Safety straps are secured around the patient.

All personnel who will be entering the OR wear clean scrub outfits, hair covers, shoe covers, and sterile

POSTOPERATIVE RECORD

Department: _____

Date: _____ Time Received on Unit _____

Type of Surgery: _____

INITIAL POST-OP ASSESSMENT (Circle Appropriate Response)

CONSCIOUSNESS:	Awake	Arousable	Unconscious	Other: _____
AIRWAY:	None	Oral	Nasal	Endotracheal
RESPIRATION:	Deep	Shallow	Regular	Irregular
OXYGEN THERAPY:	_____ liter.	None Cannula mask Vent Tent		Other: _____
COLOR:	WNL	Pale	Cyanotic	Other: _____
PULSES:	Location: _____			
	Strong	Weak	Regular	Irregular
SKIN:	Warm Dry	Cool	Moist Other: _____	
DRESSINGS:	None	Location: _____		
	Dry	Serous	Bloody	Other: _____
DRAINS:	None	Location: _____		Type: _____
		Location: _____		Type: _____
ORTHOPEDIC:	None	Cost: Location: _____		Dry Moist
		Splint: Location: _____		
		Traction: Type: _____ # of weight: _____		
		PAS TEDS		
GI:	Nausea	Emesis		
GU:	Foley	Suprapubic	Other: _____	

RECEIVED BY: _____ R.N.

(See 24 Hours Patient Care Flow Sheet and Nurses Documentation Notes for Ongoing Assessment Date)

	Initial*	15"	30"	1 Hr.	1.5 Hrs.	2.5 Hrs.	3.5 Hrs.			
Actual Time										
Temp.										
B.P.										
Pulse										
Resp. *										
C.M.S.										
TCDB										
Dressing										
Voided/Amt.										
Fluids										
Fundus/Lochia										
Initials										

* Received from PAR

Initials	Signature

Addressograph

H8720-59 (05/02/94) G.e65

FIGURE **37-8** Postoperative record used when patient returns to the unit.

NURSING CARE PLAN 37-1

Care of the Patient Undergoing a Colon Resection

SCENARIO Helen Walters., age 67, has just had a colon resection. She was admitted early this morning, but will stay in the hospital a couple of days. She has a history of diverticulitis (inflammation of pockets in the colon). She is a widow. Her daughter will care for her when she goes home.

PROBLEM/NURSING DIAGNOSIS *Fresh surgical incision*/pain related to surgical incision.
Supporting Assessment Data: Subjective: Moaning and asking for pain medication on return from PACU.
Objective: Abdominal incision for colon resection.

Goals/Expected Outcomes	Nursing Interventions	Selected Rationale	Evaluation
Pain is controlled by analgesia 30 minutes after administration as noted by patient.	Hook up PCA pump immediately after initial assessment and give bolus dose of morphine as ordered if no contraindication is found.	Ability to self-medicate for pain decreases anxiety, and patient usually needs less medication.	*Is pain controlled within 30 minutes?* States is more comfortable.
	Remind patient how to work PCA pump.	Patient must know how to work the pump in order to receive pain medication.	
	Note response to PCA medication and closely monitor respiratory rate.	Morphine can depress the respiratory rate.	Relaxed body posture.
Pain is controlled by oral analgesia by discharge.			*Is pain controlled by oral analgesia?* Not yet.

PROBLEM/NURSING DIAGNOSIS *Skin incision*/Impaired skin integrity related to surgical incision.
Supporting Assessment Data: Objective: Abdominal incision with dressing intact and dry.

Goals/Expected Outcomes	Nursing Interventions	Selected Rationale	Evaluation
Wound will be free of signs of infection.	Keep Hemovac suction functioning properly. Note character and amount of drainage; document.	Hemovac must be compressed to exert suction.	*Are there signs of infection present?* Wound without signs of infection.
	Assess for signs of infection with dressing changes.	Redness, warmth, swelling, and draining pus indicate infection.	
	Monitor temperature and white blood cell (WBC) count.	WBC will rise in presence of infection.	
	Reinforce dressing as needed. Assess for bleeding q hr for 4 hr; then q 2 hr for 24 hr.	Bleeding indicates a complication.	
	Use aseptic technique for dressing changes.	Asepsis prevents wound infection.	
Wound will heal completely.	Assess for signs of proper healing.	Good approximation of wound edges and decreasing redness indicate proper healing.	*Is wound completely healed?* No, but progressing toward outcomes; continue plan.

NURSING CARE PLAN 37-1

Care of the Patient Undergoing a Colon Resection—cont'd

PROBLEM/NURSING DIAGNOSIS *Recovering from anesthesia*/Risk for ineffective airway clearance related to effects of anesthesia, immobility, and incisional pain.
Supporting Assessment Data: Subjective: States had discomfort taking a deep breath or coughing. **Objective:** Under anesthesia for 3 hr; abdominal incision. Resp. 18.

Goals/Expected Outcomes	Nursing Interventions	Selected Rationale	Evaluation
No atelectasis.	Remind how to splint incision to cough.	Splinting when coughing reduces pressure on incision during coughing and helps prevent pain and dehiscence.	*Does patient have atelectasis?* No signs of atelectasis. Splinting adequately.
	Have deep breathe and cough while sitting on side of bed q 2 hr after fully alert.	Sitting to cough aids in lung expansion and expulsion of secretions.	
	Remind to use the incentive spirometer at least q 2 hr.	Sustained inspiration opens alveoli.	
Lung sounds clear.	Auscultate lungs initially and each shift.	Lung sound changes may indicate complications.	*Are lung sounds clear?* Lung sounds clear with decreased sound in bases.
	Encourage ambulation after 8 hr.	Ambulation promotes greater lung expansion and deeper breathing.	
	Monitor temperature and respirations.	Rising temperature and increased respirations may indicate a complication.	Progressing toward outcomes. Continue plan.

PROBLEM/NURSING DIAGNOSIS *NPO status*/Risk for deficient fluid volume related to surgery and nasogastric suction. **Supporting Assessment Data: Objective:** Bowel resection; NPO status.

Goals/Expected Outcomes	Nursing Interventions	Selected Rationale	Evaluation
Fluid balance will be within normal limits.	Maintain low intermittent suction to nasogastric (NG) tube.	Suction must be set as ordered.	*Is fluid balance within normal limits?* Not yet.
	Irrigate with 30 mL normal saline q 2 hr.	Normal saline will not alter electrolyte imbalance.	Suction maintained.
	Monitor character of drainage.	Bleeding in drainage could indicate a complication.	Secretions clear to light brown.
	Check for signs of dehydration. Maintain IV at correct flow rate.	Removing stomach secretions without replacing fluids sufficiently can cause dehydration.	Skin turgor good with moist mucous membranes.
	Monitor for signs of overhydration: auscultate lungs for rales.	Rales or crackles in the lungs indicate moisture, which can be an indication of overhydration.	No signs or symptoms of edema.
	Auscultate for return of bowel sounds each shift.	NG tube cannot be removed until bowel sounds return.	
	Monitor intake and output (I & O).	I & O records help monitor for fluid imbalance.	Intake 660 mL; output 485 mL. Progressing toward outcomes. Continue plan.

Continued

NURSING CARE PLAN 37-1

Care of the Patient Undergoing a Colon Resection—cont'd

PROBLEM/NURSING DIAGNOSIS *Afraid might have cancer*/Anxiety related to outcome of surgery.
Supporting Assessment Data: Subjective: "I hope there wasn't any cancer." **Objective:** Concerned expression on face.

Goals/Expected Outcomes	Nursing Interventions	Selected Rationale	Evaluation
Anxiety will dissipate as evidenced by patient's statements.	Reassure patient that surgeon said there was no sign of a mass in the excised portion of colon.	Reassuring information helps dispel anxiety.	*Do patient's statements indicate anxiety has dissipated?* No signs of anxiety.
	Remind patient that her diagnosis was diverticulitis and not cancer.	Helps patient focus on the positive.	Progressing toward outcomes. Continue plan.

PROBLEM/NURSING DIAGNOSIS *Just had abdominal surgery*/Self-care deficit, bathing/hygiene and grooming related to surgical incision and discomfort.
Supporting Assessment Data: Subjective: States it is difficult to move or bend. **Objective:** Abdominal incision.

Goals/Expected Outcomes	Nursing Interventions	Selected Rationale	Evaluation
Patient will have a daily bath.	Bathing promotes cleanliness and decreases microorganisms on the skin that might lead to a wound infection.	Assist patient with bath, washing feet and back.	*Is patient being bathed daily?* Yes. Meeting outcomes.
Patient will receive assistance with hygiene and grooming.	Assisting with hygiene and grooming conserves energy needed for healing.	Prevent patient from overtiring. Provide dental care equipment and assist as needed with cleansing of the teeth. Apply skin lotion. Assist into a clean gown.	*Is patient assisted with hygiene and grooming?* Yes.

? CRITICAL THINKING QUESTIONS

1. What actions would you take if the patient does not seem to be getting sufficient pain relief when using the PCA pump?

2. Would you expect the intake and output to be essentially balanced for the 24 hours on the day of surgery? What about the day after surgery?

---

gowns and masks, and perform a surgical scrub prior to entering the room. **Strict surgical asepsis is mandatory throughout the surgical area.** The circulating nurse or scrub nurse and OR technician prepare the instruments and sterile supplies (Figure 37-10). As the patient is draped, anesthesia is begun. Further skin preparation is done at this time.

A study found that warming the patient before an operation can reduce the risk of surgical wound infection by 57%. Two different warming systems were used in the study (Melling et al., 2002).

Role of the Scrub Person and Circulating Nurse

A surgical technician or a specially trained nurse (LPN/LVN or RN) may be the scrub person. A licensed nurse usually fulfills the duties of the circulating nurse. Box 37-5 compares the functions of the two.

POSTANESTHESIA IMMEDIATE CARE

Postanesthesia Care Unit

The period immediately following surgery for the patient who had general anesthesia or a major procedure performed with spinal anesthesia is a critical time and requires constant observation by specially trained nurses. The *postanesthesia care recovery unit* (PACU) provides care for all basic needs (Figure 37-11). The patient is positioned to prevent aspiration and promote lung expansion. The patient must be kept warm by covering with warmed blankets and should be reassured that the surgery is over. Vital signs are taken every 5 to 15 minutes until stable. Emergency equipment is on hand. The anesthesia recovery period usually takes 2 to 6 hours. The patient remains in the PACU until the vital signs are stable and the patient is

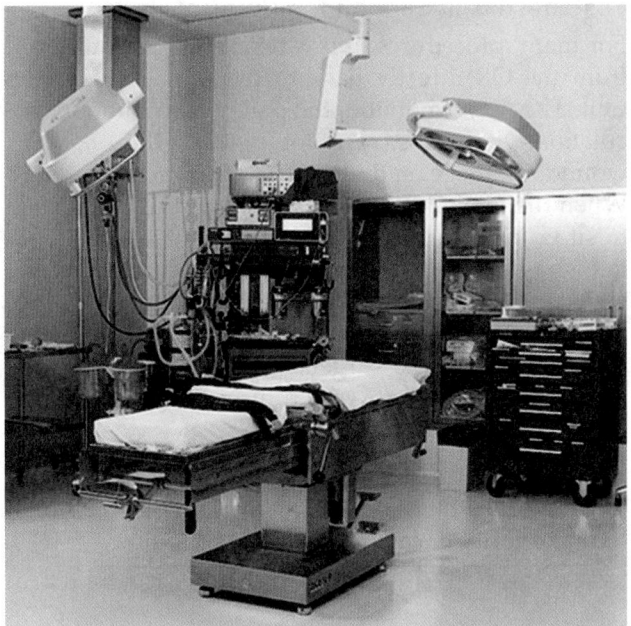

FIGURE **37-9** Traditional operating room.

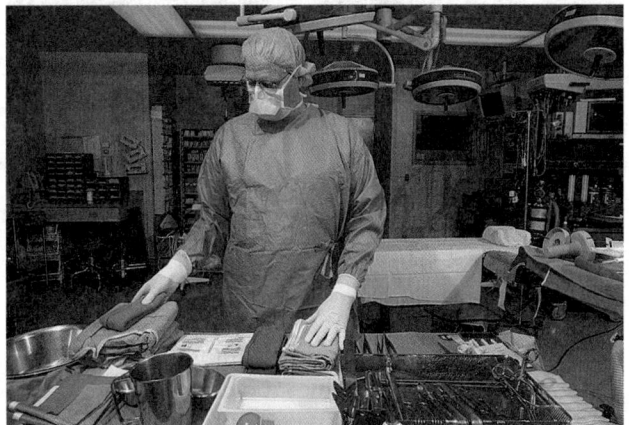

FIGURE **37-10** Preparing the surgical instruments and supplies.

Box 37-5 *Functions of the Circulating Nurse and the Scrub Person*

MAJOR FUNCTIONS OF THE CIRCULATING NURSE
- Coordinates care, oversees the environment, and cares for the patient in the operating room.
- Verifies that consent is signed and accurate and that surgical site is marked.
- Greets patient and performs patient assessment.
- Checks medical record and preoperative forms for completeness.
- Sets up the operating room; adjusts lights, stools, and discard buckets; and ensures supplies and diagnostic support are available.
- Gathers and checks all equipment that is anticipated to be used, ensuring its safe function.
- Opens sterile supplies for scrub nurse.
- Provides needed padding and warming or cooling devices for the operating table.
- Assists with ties of surgical team's gowns.
- Assists with the transfer of the patient to the operating table and positions the patient.
- Places electrocautery ground pad under patient if electrocautery is to be used.
- Assists the anesthesia induction provider with anesthesia.
- May prep the patient's skin before sterile draping occurs.
- Handles labeling and disposition of specimens.
- Coordinates activities with radiology and pathology departments.
- Monitors urine and blood loss during surgery and reports findings to the surgeon.

- Observes for breaks in sterile technique and announces them to the team.
- Monitors traffic and noise within the operating room.
- Communicates information on the surgery's progress to family during long procedures.
- Documents care, events, interventions, and findings.
- Helps transfer patient to gurney and accompanies patient to recovery area, providing report of the surgery and patient condition to the recovery nurse.

MAJOR FUNCTIONS OF THE SCRUB PERSON
- Gathers all equipment for the procedure.
- Prepares all sterile supplies and instruments using sterile technique.
- Gowns and gloves surgeons on entry to operating room.
- Assists with sterile draping of the patient.
- Maintains sterility within the sterile field during surgery.
- Hands instruments and supplies to the operating team during surgery.
- Maintains a neat instrument table.
- Labels and handles surgical specimens correctly.
- Maintains an accurate count of sponges, sharps, and instruments on the sterile field; verifies counts with the circulating nurse before and after surgery.
- Monitors for breaks in sterile technique and points them out.
- Cleans up after the surgery is over.

Adapted from deWit, S.C. (2009). *Medical-Surgical Nursing: Concepts & Practice*. Philadelphia: Elsevier Saunders.

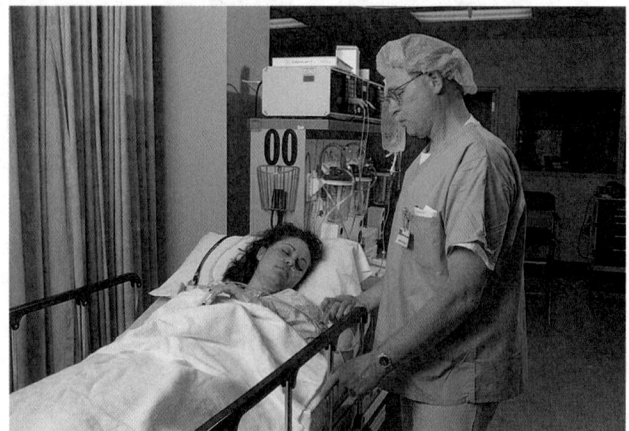

FIGURE **37-11** Postanesthesia recovery unit.

awake and able to respond to stimuli. A form of the Aldrete scoring system may be used to determine readiness for transfer. Activity, respiration, circulation, consciousness, and skin color are each given a score of 1 to 3. A total score of 9 or 10 usually indicates the patient is ready for transfer. Because patients are coming out of anesthesia through the various stages and are unstable, the environment is kept as quiet as possible. Communication among the staff is kept to a minimum and is done in hushed tones. Once the patient is awake, family is sometimes allowed to visit for a few minutes so that they are assured that their loved one is alive and recovering.

Postanesthesia Care on the Surgical Floor

For many procedures, the patient may be transferred from the OR directly back to the same-day surgery unit. The nurse monitors the patient's respiration, circulation, vital signs, neurologic status, fluid balance, wound drainage and dressings, and comfort level. When the vital signs are stable, the patient is allowed to sit up and then is ambulated. When able to ambulate unassisted, the patient may be discharged if vital signs are stable. Recovery time in the same-day surgery unit takes about 1 to 4 hours. Discharge teaching is begun before the surgery and continues once the patient is again alert. Written instructions are always sent home with the patient.

? Think Critically About . . . What is the number one priority of care for the patient in the PACU?

POSTOPERATIVE CARE

Assessment (Data Collection)

Upon receiving the patient from the PACU nurse, checking his identity, and settling him in bed, perform an initial postoperative assessment. This provides a baseline for frequent postoperative assessments performed to prevent or quickly catch signs of complications. Initial postoperative assessment is outlined in Table 37-3. **Vital signs and careful assessment are performed every 15 minutes for 1 hour, every 30 min-**

Table 37-3 *Postoperative Assessment*

AREA	ASSESSMENT	SCHEDULE
Airway	Lung sounds, depth and quality of air movement; respiratory rate.	Auscultate lungs initially; respiratory rate q 15 min until fully aroused from anesthesia, then assess quality of respirations with vital signs assessment.
	Oxygen saturation. Oxygen delivery at rate ordered and patent system.	Note per vital signs schedule and whenever in room. Check oxygen delivery system with initial assessment.
Circulation	Auscultate heart; check peripheral pulses and sensation, especially distal to surgical site. Assess skin color.	Initially, q 4 hr × 2, then with vital signs. If surgery was on an extremity, assess each time vital signs are measured.
Mental status	Level of consciousness and orientation.	Initially and then with full vital signs.
Vital signs	Temperature initially, then q 8 hr once stable. BP, pulse, & respirations.	q 15 min × 1 hr; q 30 min × 4; q 1 hr × 4; q 4 hr × 24–48 hr; or per agency protocol.
Fluid status and hydration	IV site and flow rate; I & O; skin turgor; oral membranes.	Check IV initially and when in room; I & O each shift; skin turgor & oral membranes initially and each shift.
Surgical site	Check for bleeding; mark drainage on dressing; check wound drainage in containers.	Initially and q 1 hr × 4; then with vital signs.
Gastrointestinal	Auscultate bowel sounds; assess abdomen; check NG drainage color, character, amount.	Initially, then q 8 hr. Check drainage whenever in room.
Tubes	Check for patency and function of each.	Initially; then with vital signs after 1 hr.
Kidney function	Assess urine output from Foley catheter; must void within 8 hr if no Foley in place.	Initially and q 1 hr × 4; then if > 30 mL/hr, q 4 hr.
Pain	Use a pain scale and observation of nonverbal behaviors.	Initially and with vital signs; assess at least q 2 hr.
Skin	Pressure areas over bony prominences.	Initially and q 2 hr.

Key: *BP*, Blood pressure; *I & O*, intake and output; *IV*, intravenous; *NG*, nasogastric.

utes for 2 hours, every hour for 4 hours, then every 4 hours until the patient is totally recovered from anesthesia and vital signs have returned to normal. Vital signs are taken more frequently if they are unstable; this is a nursing judgment.

Nursing Diagnosis

Nursing diagnoses commonly used for postoperative patients who had general anesthesia are as follows:
- Pain related to disruption of tissue
- Risk for infection related to surgical wound
- Impaired gas exchange related to the effect of anesthesia on the lungs
- Ineffective airway clearance related to inability to breathe deeply and cough without discomfort
- Self-care deficit, bathing/hygiene related to decreased mobility, tubes, and dressings
- Risk for injury related to sedation, decreased level of consciousness, or excessive blood loss
- Ineffective tissue perfusion related to surgery, anesthesia, and positioning on the operating table
- Ineffective coping related to loss of body part or change in body image

For patients who have undergone spinal anesthesia, include the first two diagnoses on the above list plus the following:
- Impaired physical mobility related to effects of spinal anesthesia
- Risk for injury related to decreased sensation and movement in lower extremities

Planning

The expected outcomes depend on the individual specific nursing diagnoses. General nursing goals are as follows:
- Maintain patent airway and adequate respiratory exchange.
- Maintain adequate tissue perfusion.
- Promote comfort and rest.
- Promote wound healing.
- Promote psychological adjustment to lifestyle or body image changes.
- Prevent complications.

When planning the shift work, you must allow time for frequent postoperative assessments. Careful planning is essential to care for the early postoperative patient properly and not neglect the needs of other assigned patients.

Implementation

Protect the Patient from Injury

Maintaining an open airway is a priority measure. The patient must be positioned on the side or with the head turned to the side to prevent aspiration, if not contraindicated, until fully recovered, alert, and with the swallowing reflex intact.

Side rails are kept raised for safety until patients are fully recovered from anesthesia. Reassure the patient

Table 37-4	*Expected Drainage from Tubes and Catheters Postoperatively*	
TYPE OF DRAINAGE	**AMOUNT OF DRAINAGE IN 24 HOURS**
Urine	500-700 mL for 1-2 days postoperatively, then 1500-2500 mL thereafter depending on intake
Gastric contents	Up to 1500 mL/day
Wound drainage	Variable with procedure and type of drain
T-tube/bile	Up to 500 mL

Adapted from Lewis, S.L., Heitkemper, M.M., Dirksen, S.R., et al. (2007). *Medical-Surgical Nursing: Assessment and Management of Clinical Problems* (7th ed., p. 393). St. Louis: Elsevier Mosby.

who has had spinal anesthesia that it is normal for the legs to feel numb and heavy and that feeling will soon return to normal. Sense of position will return to the legs first, then sensation to deep pressure, then voluntary movement, and finally feeling of superficial pain and temperature. A feeling of "pins and needles" in the legs is common. The patient is prone to hypotension until all effects of the spinal anesthesia are gone. The patient is observed for a spinal headache, but it is not necessary to stay totally flat for the first 12 hours because this has proven to be ineffective. If a headache develops, staying flat reduces the pain.

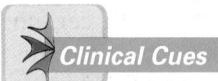
Clinical Cues

Encourage the patient to drink a lot of fluids, including those containing caffeine. The fluids and caffeine raise the vascular pressure at the spinal puncture site and help to seal the hole.

The surgical site is checked when the patient returns to the unit. The dressing should be dry. If it is stained, the area is outlined with pen and the time noted so that further bleeding can be assessed later. If the bleeding has saturated the dressing, reinforce with more dressing supplies; the dressing is not changed without an order to do so. The surgical site should be checked each hour for the first 4 hours, then every 2 hours if bleeding has not been occurring. Excessive bleeding is reported to the surgeon. The bed linens under the patient must be checked as well because sometimes blood runs under the dressing and pools under the patient.

Drains are assessed for patency when the wound is checked, and drainage devices are emptied and recompressed as needed. The amount of drainage is recorded on the intake and output record (Table 37-4). The drainage devices must be positioned so that there is no pulling on the entry sites. During assessment, the tubes are checked for kinking and to ensure that the patient is not lying on them. Common types of drains left in to help remove fluid from the surgical site are Penrose, Hemovac, and Jackson-Pratt (J-P) drains, chest tubes, and a T-tube to the common bile duct.

Promote Respiratory Function

The postoperative patient is at risk for respiratory problems from the effects of anesthesia on the lungs, from being in one position on the OR table for the duration of surgery, and from limited mobility in the immediate postoperative period. The patient may have oxygen per nasal cannula ordered for 24 hours after surgery. Some degree of atelectasis (collapse of alveoli in the lungs) exists after anesthesia. A mild hypoxia is usually present for about 48 hours after surgery. Auscultate the lungs carefully for absence of sound or crackles indicating retained secretions, assess the rate and depth of breathing, and encourage the patient to deep breathe and cough every 2 hours. This is essential to prevent pneumonia and relieve atelectasis. Hypostatic pneumonia occurs when lack of movement or of position change causes stasis of secretions, which become a breeding ground for bacteria. **Coughing may be contraindicated for patients who have had hernia repair or eye, ear, or brain surgery.** Check the physician's orders.

Coughing is for the purpose of moving out secretions. If the patient cannot cough effectively, instruct him to take a deep breath and forcibly exhale with the mouth open; have him repeat the "huff" maneuver again; then ask him to take a deep breath and cough strongly as he exhales to move the secretions out of the airways. Little coughs just clear the throat. Be certain the patient turns every 2 hours as well because this changes the distribution of gas and blood flow in the lungs and helps move secretions.

Signs of complications are complaints of shortness of breath, pain on inspiration, and extreme fatigue, which is related to hypoxemia. The use of an incentive spirometer is especially helpful to prevent atelectasis and hypoventilation. The elderly patient may need extra coaching to master the technique.

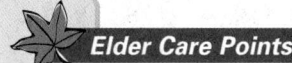
Elder Care Points

The risk of hypoventilation is greater in the elderly because lung expansion may be hampered by calcification of costal cartilage and weakened respiratory muscles.

A pulse oximeter may be utilized to determine blood oxygenation. Monitor the readings periodically and report arterial oxygen saturation (Sao_2) readings below 92% to the physician. Pulse oximetry is covered in Chapter 28.

Promote Circulation

When considerable blood is lost during surgery, transfusion may be ordered. Autologous transfusion may be done if the patient donated blood several weeks prior to surgery or if the patient's blood was collected as it was lost. This blood is filtered and returned to the patient.

When there has been a procedure involving an extremity or the pelvic area, the distal or peripheral pulse is checked during each full assessment. Swelling at the surgical site can compress vessels and decrease blood flow distal to the area. The skin should be warm to the touch and there should be good capillary refill in the fingers or toes.

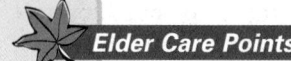
Elder Care Points

- Because skin is fragile and there is less subcutaneous tissue in an elderly person, check bony prominences carefully for signs of breakdown.
- Joint strains can occur from positioning necessary for certain types of surgery; perform position changes slowly and gently.

Blood pressure and pulse should be compared with preoperative values to determine significant changes. An increase in pulse may indicate that internal bleeding is occurring, but it can also signify incomplete pain control. Blood pressure falling below normal baseline level may indicate major bleeding.

The use of antiembolic (elastic) stockings increases venous return from the legs and helps prevent stasis of blood in the lower extremities (Skill 37-1). If the patient is at considerable risk of venous thrombosis (blood clot), the surgeon will order sequential pneumatic compression devices to be applied to the legs. These alternately compress and release, squeezing the vessels and propelling blood along them (Figure 37-12).

Maintain Fluid Balance

The urine output is monitored after surgery. **If the patient has an indwelling catheter, the urine in the bag is observed every hour in the early postoperative period.** There should be a urinometer on the drainage bag for this purpose. If the urine flow is less than 5 mL/kg/hr, it is reported to the charge nurse. If flow is less than 60 mL over a 2-hour period, the surgeon is notified. The catheter is checked to ensure that it is not kinked and that the connecting tubing is not lying beneath the patient. If no catheter is present, the patient must void within 8 hours of surgery. If the patient is unable to empty the bladder spontaneously, an order for catheterization is obtained.

The patient usually has an intravenous infusion running when he returns from surgery. Depending on the type of surgery, IV fluids may be continued for a few days or may be discontinued after the fluid has infused. Check to make certain that the fluid running is the one that the surgeon ordered. **No potassium additive should be given until the urine flow is at least 5 mL/kg/hr.** Potassium may cause hyperkalemia if kidney function is not adequate. The IV site is assessed for patency and lack of complications when vital signs are taken. The IV flow rate is rechecked as well. All IV

Skill 37-1 | Applying Antiembolism Stockings

Many surgeons order some form of antiembolism stockings following major surgery. Patients frequently return from the PACU with the stockings already in place. In such cases, the preoperative orders include fitting the patient for antiembolism stockings, which are then sent with the patient to the operating room.

■ Supplies

✓ Antiembolism stockings
✓ Measuring tape
✓ Powder

Review and carry out the Standard Steps in Appendix 3.

■ Assessment (Data Collection)

1. **ACTION** Check the orders for the type of stocking to be applied.

   RATIONALE Stockings come in three lengths: knee high, thigh high, and full length.

■ Planning

2. **ACTION** Measure the patient's leg length and circumference for the length of stocking ordered. Obtain the correct size stocking.

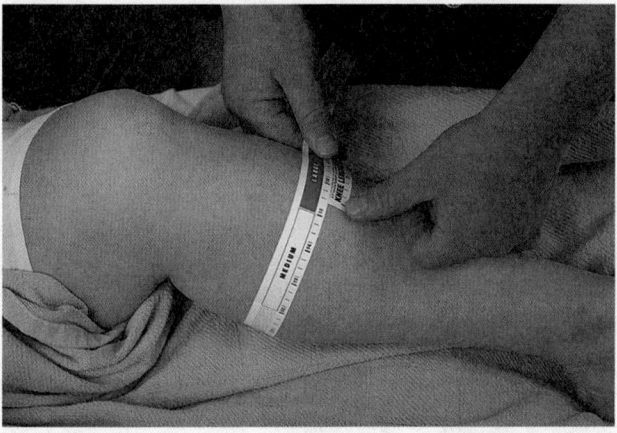
Step **2**

   RATIONALE Ensures that stocking will fit properly.

■ Implementation

3. **ACTION** Be certain the patient's legs are clean and dry; apply a light coating of powder to each leg.

   RATIONALE Powder makes stocking application easier and smoother.

4. **ACTION** Place your hand in one stocking and turn it inside out, down to the heel.

   RATIONALE Makes it easier to slip the stocking onto the foot without discomfort to the patient.

5. **ACTION** Stretch open the stocking at the heel, and fit it over the patient's foot.

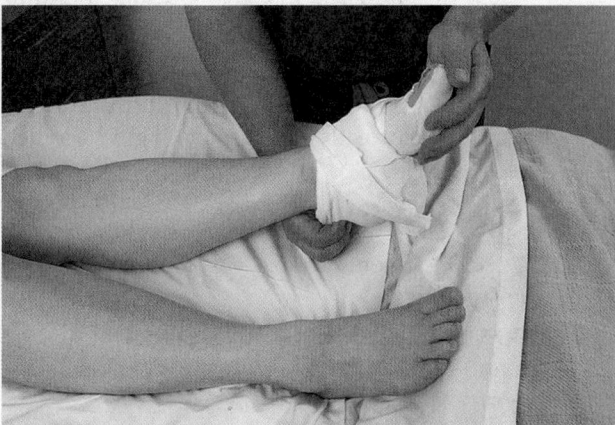
Step **5**

   RATIONALE Stocking must fit smoothly without wrinkles that might damage the skin's surface.

6. **ACTION** Grasp the top of the stocking, and fit it over the ankle and calf.

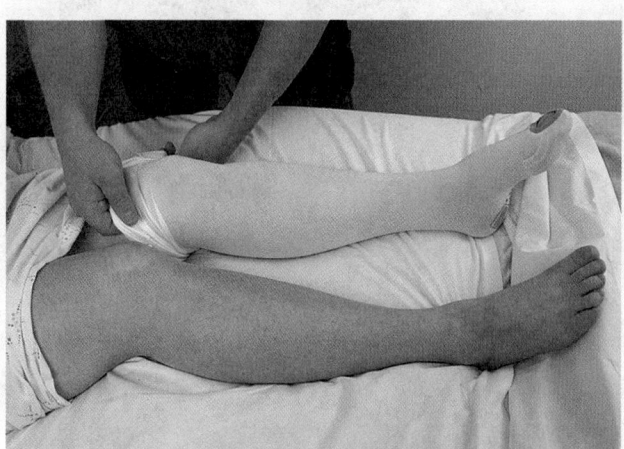
Step **6**

   RATIONALE If knee-high stockings are being used, do not pull over knee or fold the top of the stocking down. The stockings must be the correct length, or they can impair circulation or damage the skin's surface.

7. **ACTION** If thigh high, fit the top of the stocking over the knee and thigh. Smooth the entire surface to eliminate any wrinkles. Repeat steps 4 through 7 for the second stocking. Instruct the patient not

Continued

Skill 37-1 | Applying Antiembolism Stockings—cont'd

to cross the legs or ankles when sitting in a bed or chair.

RATIONALE Crossing the limbs causes pressure points that can hinder circulation.

■ Evaluation

8. **ACTION** Are the stockings at the right height for what was ordered? Are the stockings on smoothly, without any wrinkles? Do the stockings fit properly—not too tight or too loose at any point?

   RATIONALE Answers to these questions indicate whether the correctly fitted stocking is applied properly.

■ Documentation

9. **ACTION** Document the size, type, and application of the stockings.

   RATIONALE Verifies that ordered stockings are in place and supports charges for the stockings.

Documentation Example

2/7 1330 Legs measured and medium regular thigh-high stockings applied.

_____

(Nurse's signature)

■ Special Considerations

✓ Antiembolism stockings should be removed each shift to check the integrity of the skin on the heels and over the bony prominences. Stockings that are too tight may cause skin breakdown.

✓ Stockings should be washed when soiled. Obtain a second pair for use while stockings are drying. To wash, use mild soap and warm, not hot, water. Rinse thoroughly, squeeze out excess water and roll up in a towel to remove further moisture; allow to air dry.

✓ Stockings should not be off the patient for more than 30 minutes at any one time.

?CRITICAL THINKING QUESTIONS

1. What would you do if you measure a patient for thigh-high elastic stockings and the supply room does not have a size available that you need?

2. How does applying dusting powder to the legs make applying elastic stockings easier?

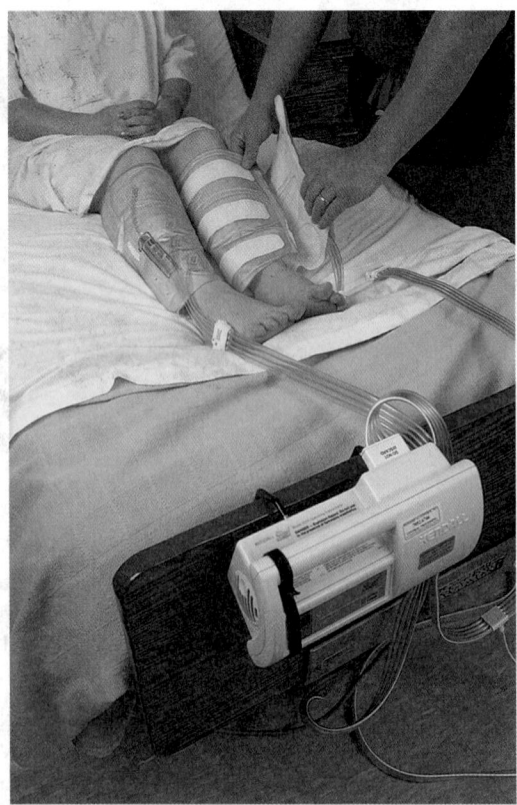

FIGURE **37-12** Applying leg sequential compression devices.

fluid administered is recorded as intake on the intake and output record.

As soon as the patient is conscious and the swallowing reflex has returned, the patient may be offered a few ice chips or sips of water unless there is an order to maintain NPO status. All intake is recorded on the intake and output record. At the end of each shift, the difference between the intake and output is noted. The body will initially retain fluid due to the stress reaction from surgery. Postoperatively, the output will slowly rise until it is more than the intake; after 2 to 3 days, a balance should again occur.

Anesthesia may make the patient nauseated, and vomiting is not uncommon. The emesis basin is kept close at hand, and the patient is positioned on the side to prevent aspiration. The surgeon usually writes an order for medication in the event of excessive nausea or vomiting. It is best to medicate the patient before actual vomiting occurs. After emesis, mouth care should be provided. If vomiting is uncontrolled with medication, a nasogastric tube may have to be inserted to suction stomach contents and prevent further fluid and electrolyte loss.

Surgeons often leave in a nasogastric tube after most abdominal procedures because handling of the gastrointestinal tract, and general anesthesia, causes peristalsis to halt and secretions will not flow through the system properly. When a nasogastric tube is in place, check that the suction is set according to orders, and is working properly. Assess the amount of drainage produced every 1 to 2 hours. **If the tubing is kept above the level of the stomach, drainage will occur more easily.** If the drainage turns dark brown and grainy, it should be checked for blood with a special reagent. The presence of blood should be reported to the surgeon.

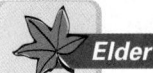

Elder Care Points

- Fluid and electrolyte shifts may cause confusion in the elderly patient after surgery.
- The skin and vessels are more fragile, and the IV site must be assessed frequently for signs of infiltration.
- Adjustment of the body to fluid shifts is more difficult, and the elderly patient is very prone to postural hypotension when changing to a standing position. Be sure to adequately support the patient.

Promote Gastrointestinal Function

Eating is not allowed until bowel sounds have returned after surgery and general anesthesia due to the risk of development of paralytic ileus (failure of forward movement of bowel contents). Listen for bowel sounds at least once per shift. When eating is resumed, the surgeon usually orders clear liquids, followed by full liquids, then a regular diet if the preceding diets have been tolerated. After spinal anesthesia, the patient may be allowed to eat right away.

Once the patient is eating again, he should have a bowel movement within 2 to 3 days. If one does not occur, an order for a suppository may be needed to stimulate a bowel movement. Patients receiving narcotic analgesics may become constipated and require stool softeners or laxatives to produce normal bowel movements.

Promote Comfort

If the patient is complaining of pain upon return to the unit, check through the notes from the PACU and see if any pain medication was given. Note what preoperative medications were administered.

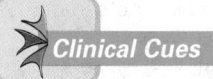

When droperidol plus fentanyl (Innovar) is given as a preoperative medication, narcotic pain medication is reduced by half for the 8 hours after the preoperative medication, or the narcotic analgesic will gravely depress respirations.

If respirations are within normal limits and there is no contraindication to doing so, medicate promptly with the ordered analgesic. If it is too soon to give more analgesia, reposition the patient, be sure the bladder is not distended and causing discomfort, check that the patient is warm enough, and use other comfort measures to relieve the pain, such as distraction and imagery. Note when analgesia is due and have it ready to administer at the appointed time.

The patient may feel cold and should be kept warm with extra blankets or warmed bath blankets applied under the top covers. Placing socks on the feet may help. Some anesthetic agents may cause tremors as they wear off. If uncontrollable shivering occurs, contact the physician for medication orders.

Dressings on extremities should be checked to be certain that they are not so tight that circulation is cut off. Check the distal pulse and skin temperature. Check with the physician or charge nurse before loosening a dressing.

Abdominal distention and considerable flatus may occur after general anesthesia because the gastrointestinal tract action ceases. This may cause discomfort. Ambulating is helpful in moving and evacuating gas. Taking only small amounts of liquid or food at a time, drinking liquids that are neither very hot nor very cold, and refraining from drinking with a straw helps keep flatus to a minimum. If permitted, the patient can try resting in a slight Trendelenburg's position, with the legs and rectum higher than the stomach; this may assist in the evacuation of flatus. Chewing gum, if permitted, may also aid the return of proper gastrointestinal function.

Occasionally continuous hiccups will occur after surgery, making the patient quite uncomfortable. Having the patient breathe into a paper bag will often relieve the hiccups, but persistent hiccups require more vigorous treatment prescribed by the physician.

Rest and Activity

The patient needs to sleep after surgery. The room should be kept quiet and nursing activities grouped to prevent waking the patient more than necessary. Every 2 hours the patient must do the leg exercises and change position. Orders for ambulation may begin 8 hours after surgery. Raise the head of the bed first and let the body adjust to the position change. Then sit the patient on the side of the bed, allowing the legs to dangle over the side with the feet on the floor. After a few minutes, slowly assist the patient to stand. Have the patient walk around the room, or for at least a few steps. Have someone assist you if the patient is very weak. Pain medication can be timed so that it is effective but the patient is not too groggy. Emphasize to the patient that exercise is vital to prevent circulatory problems. **Do not rub the legs to promote circulation. Such an action may disrupt a clot that has formed and cause an** embolus (clot that travels and lodges in a vessel) to the lung, heart, or brain. Praise the patient for any efforts. Continue to ambulate on a set schedule until the patient is up and about independently.

If the patient is on bed rest, range-of-motion exercises must be performed at least four times a day. The patient may do active range of motion on most joints, but passive range of motion on joints the patient is unable to exercise must be done unless physical therapy visits have been ordered. See Chapter 18 for directions for range-of-motion exercises.

Prevent Infection

Aseptic technique must be used when caring for the postoperative patient. Good handwashing is the primary means of preventing infection. Dressing changes are performed with strict aseptic technique while the patient is in the hospital; the patient may use clean technique at home. Encouraging fluids to flush the bladder will help prevent a bladder infection for the patient who was catheterized or has an indwelling catheter. Turning, coughing, and deep breathing, plus ambulation, will assist in preventing pneumonia (inflammation and consolidation of the lung with exudate) from retained secretions and lack of movement.

The surgical wound site should be inspected each shift and assessed for signs of infection: local pain, increased tenderness, warmth, redness, or drainage of pus. The blood count is monitored for increasing leukocytes (WBCs), and the temperature is monitored for unexpected increase.

Complications of Surgery

A major nursing responsibility is continuous monitoring for signs of the various complications that may occur as a result of surgery. Table 37-5 summarizes

---

Table 37-5 *Postoperative Complications*

PROBLEM	SIGNS AND SYMPTOMS	PREVENTIVE INTERVENTIONS
Atelectasis	Decreased breath sounds over areas not aerating; dyspnea	Deep breathing and coughing; use of incentive spirometer; early ambulation; teach to cough properly.
Pneumonia: hypostatic, aspiration, or bacterial	Fever, malaise, increased sputum, purulent sputum, cough, flushed skin, dyspnea, pain on inspiration; abnormal breath sounds, crackles, rhonchi	Deep breathing, coughing, and frequent turning; early ambulation; incentive spirometer use; range-of-motion exercises if unable to ambulate; medication if bacterial.
Paralytic (adynamic) ileus	No bowel sounds 24-36 hr after surgery or fewer than 5 sounds per minute	Monitor bowel sounds; encourage early ambulation; nothing by mouth as ordered. Do not feed until bowel sounds return.
Thrombophlebitis	Pain or warmth in calf of leg, swollen leg, warm area to touch on leg; possible temperature elevation	Encourage leg exercises; keep the patient well hydrated; encourage ambulation; antiembolic stockings or devices.
Urinary retention	Distended bladder; inability to void spontaneously	Palpate bladder; encourage voiding, catheterize if unable to void within 8 hr per order; medicate to increase urinary sphincter tone as ordered.
Urinary tract infection	Dysuria, frequency, foul-smelling urine	Force fluids when allowed; encourage frequent voiding; keep catheter clean and patent; use aseptic technique to empty drainage bag.
Wound infection	Redness, swelling, pain, warmth, drainage, fever, increased leukocytes, rapid pulse and respirations (fever 72 hr after surgery indicates infection in some system or in the wound)	Assess wound characteristics and drainage. Monitor WBC levels and temperature. Use aseptic technique for wound care; encourage adequate nutrition and fluids; encourage activity.
Pulmonary embolus	Shortness of breath, anxiety, chest pain, rapid pulse and respirations, cyanosis, cough, bloody sputum	Antiembolism stockings, adequate fluid intake, frequent turning or ambulation, preventive anticoagulant if ordered.
Hemorrhage and shock	Evidence of copious bleeding; decreased blood pressure, elevated pulse, cold clammy skin, decreased urinary output	Give blood or volume expander; stop bleeding. Place in shock position with feet and legs elevated and head flat; administer ordered medications to raise blood pressure; administer oxygen; frequent vital signs measurement.
Wound dehiscence or evisceration	Discharge of serosanguineous drainage from wound and sensation that "something gave"; separation of wound edges with intestines visible through abdominal incision	Teach to splint properly for coughing. Place patient supine; cover wound with sterile saline-soaked gauze or towels; return to OR for repair; monitor for shock.
Fluid imbalance	*Signs of overhydration:* Crackles in lungs, edema, weight gain *Signs of dehydration:* Weight loss, diminished pulse, dry mucous membranes, decreased tissue turgor	Control IV flow rate. Monitor intake and output; correct imbalances. Output will be less than intake first 72 hr after surgery with general anesthesia. Auscultate lungs each shift. Monitor weight; check for edema.

Key: *IV*, Intravenous; *OR*, operating room; *WBC*, white blood cell.

postoperative complications and nursing actions to prevent them. Dehiscence (separation of the layers of the surgical wound) and evisceration (extrusion of the viscera through the surgical incision) may occur when the patient is coughing, particularly if the abdominal incision is not properly splinted. Research has shown that giving a bolus of IV Plasma-Lyte 148 (20 mL/kg), an isotonic electrolyte solution, prior to surgery can reduce the adverse reactions of drowsiness, headache, nausea, vomiting, and hypotension (Winslow & Jacobson, 1997).

Evaluation

Evaluation is based on whether goals and expected outcomes have been met. Evaluative statements regarding previously stated general goals might be as follows:

- Lungs clear to auscultation; respirations 18
- Pulse 82, BP 136/86, peripheral pulses present
- Pain controlled for 4 hours with analgesia; states pain medication controls pain for about 4 hours
- Incision clean, dry, and without redness
- States is glad he will not have periods of pain and malaise anymore
- No signs of thrombophlebitis or infection

Each nursing care plan is evaluated on whether the individual specific outcomes have been met. Further examples of evaluation are in the nursing care plan for this chapter.

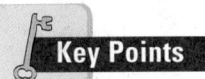

Key Points

- Surgical procedures may be elective, emergency, palliative, diagnostic, curative, or reconstructive.
- The use of lasers, fiberoptic endoscopes with high-resolution video cameras, operating microscopes, and robotic technology has revolutionized surgery.
- Anesthesia is used to prevent pain; achieve adequate muscle relaxation; and calm fear, allay anxiety, and induce forgetfulness of an unpleasant experience.

- Inhalant gases and intravenous medications are used to induce general anesthesia, and the patient progresses through four stages to total anesthesia.
- Regional anesthesia, moderate sedation, or local anesthesia is used for many surgical procedures.
- The surgeon must obtain informed consent from the patient before surgery is performed.
- A variety of preoperative procedures are used to prepare the patient for surgery.
- A thorough assessment is performed by the nurse, and any risk factors for surgery are identified.
- The nursing care plan is amended as the patient progresses through preoperative, intraoperative, and postoperative periods.
- Preoperative teaching of exercises to be performed postoperatively is very important; the patient is taught leg exercises and breathing and coughing exercises.
- The scrub person and the circulating nurse provide care for the patient while in the operating room.
- The PACU monitors patients very closely until they are fully aroused from anesthesia.
- The nurse is vigilant for signs of complications and performs frequent assessments during the postoperative period.
- Nursing interventions are aimed at providing pain control, comfort, and fluid balance; protecting the patient from injury; maintaining vital functions; and preventing infection.
- The nurse tries to prevent or intervene in the many potential complications of surgery.
- Discharge planning begins at admission and covers all areas of basic needs, wound care, and activity restrictions.
- Written instructions regarding all aspects of postoperative care should be sent home with the patient.

 Go to your **Companion CD-ROM** for an Audio Glossary, animations, video clips, and more.

evolve Be sure to visit the companion Evolve site at http://evolve.elsevier.com/deWit/fundamental/ for additional online resources.

NCLEX-PN® EXAMINATION-STYLE REVIEW QUESTION

*Choose the **best** answer(s) for each question.*

1. When signing an informed surgical consent form, the patient is verifying that:
   1. the correct operation is entered on the form.
   2. the risks and alternatives for the surgical procedure have been explained.
   3. all possible consequences of having or not having the procedure are understood.
   4. the surgical procedure and its implications have been explained.

2. Your patient had an appendectomy 2 days ago. To properly auscultate for bowel sounds, you would:
   1. listen in the lower right quadrant for 2 minutes.
   2. listen in both lower quadrants for 2 minutes.
   3. listen in each quadrant for 3 minutes.
   4. listen in all four quadrants for 1 minute each.

3. A similarity of roles for the scrub nurse and the circulating nurse is that they both:
   1. set up initial sterile instruments and supplies.
   2. position lights and step stools.
   3. are communication links with personnel outside the room.
   4. advise the team of breaks in sterile technique.

4. The priority responsibility of the nurse in the PACU when receiving a patient is assessment of:

   1. urine output.
   2. IV line patency.
   3. airway patency.
   4. wound drainage.

5. As part of a patient's immediate care in the PACU, the nurse would: *(Select all that apply.)*

   1. check vital signs every 15 minutes.
   2. assess adequacy of respirations
   3. monitor the dressing.
   4. observe the drainage from the NG tube.
   5. note the amount of urine output.

6. A patient returns to his room after surgery. When he arrives, you notice that he is still groggy from anesthesia and that he has an IV still running in one arm. As you help settle him in bed, you: *(Select all that apply.)*

   1. assess the IV for patency and correct fluid and rate.
   2. position to prevent aspiration while still groggy.
   3. quickly medicate for pain.
   4. take his vital signs every 15 minutes for 1 hour.
   5. reassure him that the surgery is over.

7. If your fresh postoperative patient has not voided within 8 hours of the end of surgery, you would *first:*

   1. seek an order to catheterize the patient.
   2. assist the patient to attempt to void using measures to encourage voiding.
   3. allow another hour in which the patient might spontaneously void.
   4. obtain catheterization equipment and bring it to the bedside.

8. Since your surgery patient returned to her room, you have assisted her to turn and encouraged her to breathe deeply, to cough, and to move her legs at least every 2 hours. By deep breathing and coughing, the patient will be less likely to develop the postoperative complication of _____. *(Fill in the blank.)*

9. The second day after surgery, the nasogastric tube is removed and an order is written for fluids as tolerated and a liquid diet. The patient is eager to try taking fluids. What would you recommend that he do?

   1. Wait until his liquid diet tray arrives at mealtime.
   2. Start with small sips of water at first to see if they are retained.
   3. Take in a variety of fluids totaling 3000 mL/day.
   4. Go ahead and drink all the water he wants.

10. The patient has a PCA pump to be used for pain control. Should her pain not be adequately controlled with use of the pump, you would: *(Select all that apply.)*

    1. administer an oral analgesic in addition to the pump medication.
    2. seek a medication order change from the physician.
    3. straighten the bed and clothing and plump the pillows.
    4. be certain that none of the drainage tubes are kinked.
    5. encourage the use of relaxation techniques.

11. On his third postoperative day, a patient states that he does not feel well and that he has a lot more pain in the incision area. You inspect the incision and notice that the lower end of it is very red. From these symptoms, you suspect that this patient has developed:

    1. an embolus.
    2. an ileus.
    3. a wound infection.
    4. an evisceration.

12. On the sixth postoperative day, a patient complains of malaise and pain in her right lower leg. The lower leg is warm to the touch. She has a positive Homans' sign. You suspect that she may have _____. *(Fill in the blank.)*

CRITICAL THINKING ACTIVITIES *Read each clinical scenario and discuss the questions with your classmates.*

Scenario A

Theresa Hijazi is scheduled for surgery this morning. You are assigned two other patients to care for as well as Theresa. One of these patients is stable and will be going home. The other patient is going for a computed tomography (CT) scan at 11 A.M.

1. Describe in detail how you would plan your morning care for these three patients.
2. Theresa shares with you that she really doesn't understand just what the surgeon is going to do to her. How would you handle the situation?

Scenario B

You have prepared your 16-year-old patient for surgery, given instructions, and left her a clean gown to put on. When you return to assist in transferring him to the stretcher for the trip to the OR, you find he has put on underwear and is wearing a St. Christopher's medal around his neck.

1. What would you do about the underwear?
2. How would you handle the situation with the St. Christopher's medal?

Scenario C

You are told to prepare the unit in 404 for the return of a patient from surgery.

1. What supplies do you need?
2. How would you arrange the unit?
3. How often will you need to take vital signs?
4. How often will you do other assessments?
5. What will you assess?

Theory

1. Describe the physiologic process by which wounds heal.
2. Discuss factors that affect wound healing.
3. Describe four signs and symptoms of wound infection.
4. Discuss actions to be taken if wound dehiscence or evisceration occurs.
5. Identify the advantages of vacuum-assisted wound closure.
6. Explain the major purpose of a wound drain.
7. Compare and contrast the therapeutic effects of heat and cold.

Clinical Practice

1. Perform wound care, including emptying a drainage device and applying a sterile dressing.
2. Provide appropriate care for a pressure ulcer.
3. Perform a wound irrigation.
4. Remove sutures or staples from a wound and apply Steri-Strips.
5. Give a heat or cold treatment to a patient.

Skills & Steps

Skills

Skill 38-1 Sterile Dressing Change
Skill 38-2 Wound Irrigation
Skill 38-3 Applying a Wet-to-Damp or Wet-to-Dry Dressing

Steps

Steps 38-1 Maintaining a Closed Wound Drainage Unit
Steps 38-2 Applying a Hydrocolloid Dressing
Steps 38-3 Removing Sutures or Staples
Steps 38-4 Irrigating the Eye or Adult Ear

Key Terms

Be sure to check out the bonus material on the Companion CD-ROM, including selected audio pronunciations.

abscess (ĂB-sĕs, p. 781)
adhesions (ăd-HĒ-shŭnz, p. 777)
adipose (ĂD-ĭ-pōs, p. 780)
approximate (ă-PRŎX-ĭ-māt, p. 778)
approximation (ă-prŏx-ĭ-MĀ-shŭn, p. 787)
binders (p. 785)
cellulitis (sĕl-ū-LĪ-tĭs, p. 781)
collagen (KŎL-ă-jĕn, p. 777)

débridement (dĕ-BRĒD-măw, p. 782)
erythema (ĕr-ĭ-THĒ-mă, p. 777)
eschar (ĔS-kăr, p. 782)
exudate (ĔKS-ū-dāt, p. 781)
fibrin (p. 776)
first intention (ĭn-TĔN-shŭn, p. 778)
fistula (FĬS-tū-lă, p. 781)
granulation tissue (grăn-ū-LĀ-shŭn, p. 792)
hemostasis (hē-mō-STĀ-sĭs, p. 776)
immunocompromised (ĭm-ū-nō-KŎM-prō-mīzd, p. 780)
integument (ĭn-TĔG-ū-ment, p. 775)
keloid (KĒ-loid, p. 777)
laceration (lăs-ĕr-Ā-shŭn, p. 778)
lysis (LĪ-sĭs, p. 777)
maceration (măs-ĕr- Ā-shŭn, p. 796)
macrophages (MĂK-rō-faj-ĕz, p. 777)
necrosis (nē-KRŌ-sĭs, p. 776)
phagocytosis (făg-ō-sī-TŌ-sĭs, p. 777)
platelet aggregation (PLĀ T-lĕt ăg-rĕ-GĀ-shŭn, p. 776)
purulent (PŪ-rū-lĕnt, p. 780)
sanguineous (săng-GWĬN-ē-ŭs, p. 780)
second intention (p. 778)
serosanguineous (sĕr-ō-săng-GWĬN-ē-ŭs, p. 782)
sinus (SĪ-nŭs, p. 781)
sloughing (SLŬF-ĭng, p. 782)
suppuration (sŭp-ū-RĀ-shŭn, p. 801)
third intention (p. 778)

TYPES OF WOUNDS AND THE HEALING PROCESS

Wounds occur in a variety of ways. Trauma may cause a break in the skin or partial- or full-thickness loss of skin. A surgical incision causes a break in skin integrity. Pressure can cause tissue breakdown and disruption of skin integrity. Burns can partially or completely destroy skin. The skin and mucous membranes are protective barriers for the body against infection. Injury to the integument (skin) brings risk of infection and may cause permanent damage. When the integument is damaged, a complex healing process is initiated. Nurses act to prevent the invasion of microorganisms into wounds and to support and enhance the body's ability to effect wound repair.

Wounds may be *open*, occurring through the skin, or *closed*, without a break in the skin (Table 38-1). Closed wounds are caused by blunt trauma, twisting, pulling, straining, or deceleration force against the body.

Table 38-1 *Wound Types and Characteristics*

TYPE	CHARACTERISTICS	CHARTING DESCRIPTION
CLOSED		
Contusion (bruise)	Tissue injury without breaking of skin	Purple contusion 5 × 7 cm on left thigh.
Hematoma	Tissue injury that disrupts a blood vessel; pooling of blood under the unbroken skin	2-in diameter hematoma on right forearm.
Sprain	Wrenching or twisting of a joint with partial rupture of its ligaments; causes swelling	Swelling of right foot and around malleolus. No bruising noted.
OPEN		
Incision	Surgically made separation of tissues with clean, smooth edges	Approx. 3-in incision on right lower quadrant of abdomen; well approximated; clean and dry with sutures intact.
Laceration	Traumatic separation of tissues with irregular, torn edges	2-in jagged laceration approx. 4 cm deep on lateral aspect of left lower leg.
Abrasion	Traumatic scraping away of surface layers of skin	Raw-appearing abraded area 2½-in diameter beneath left elbow.
Puncture	Wound made by sharp, pointed object through skin or mucous membranes and underlying tissue	Small circular entry wound on bottom of left foot from stepping on nail.
Penetrating	Variable-size open wound through skin and underlying tissues made by a bullet or metal or wood fragment; may extend deeply into body	Jagged deep wound on left chest at third intercostal space, 2 in lateral to sternum.
Avulsion	Tearing away of a structure or a part, such as a fingertip, accidentally or surgically	Avulsion of tip of left little finger from accident with knife. Attached only by skin.
Ulceration	Excavation of skin and/or underlying tissue from injury or necrosis	Ulceration on lateral aspect of left lower leg 4½ cm × 5¾ × 2 cm deep. Yellow drainage present. Wound edges reddened.

Wounds may be partial thickness (superficial) or full thickness. *Partial-thickness* wounds heal more quickly and do so by production of new skin cells by the epithelial cells remaining in the dermal layer of the skin. The fibrin clot that forms acts as the framework, and regrowth occurs across the open area. When a *full-thickness* wound occurs, the dermal layer is no longer present except at the wound margins. In order to heal, all dead (necrotic) tissue must be removed so that granulation tissue can gradually fill in the defect (Figure 38-1). The wound heals by contraction.

Wounds may be *clean* or *dirty*, indicating they are free of microorganisms or contain microorganisms, respectively. A wound is infected when it contains a large number of microorganisms.

When a wound occurs, either regeneration or replacement of cells occurs as it heals. When cells are not damaged beyond recovery, they will restore themselves, and there will be little permanent evidence of injury. If the cellular blood supply has been disrupted and necrosis (fatal injury to cells) has occurred, the affected tissue must heal by *regeneration*. New cells similar in structure and function to the dead ones are produced if the tissue is a type that will regenerate. Skin, mucous membranes, bone marrow, muscle, bone, liver, kidney, and lung tissue can regenerate with tissue that is structurally similar to that which was lost. Heart muscle and nerve cells are generally unable to regenerate. *Replacement* occurs in the form of fibrous connective tissue that does not have the same functional characteristics as the tissue lost when the wound occurred.

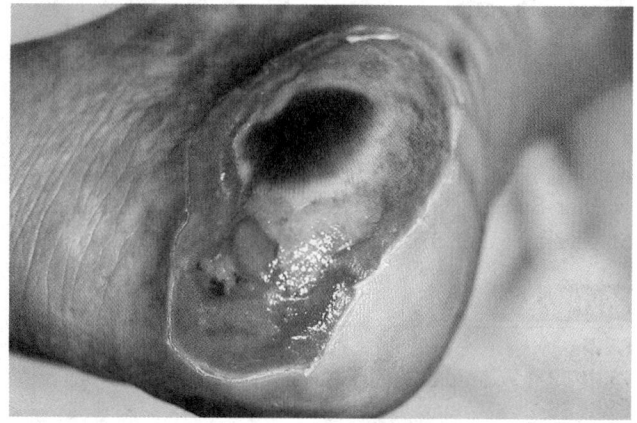

FIGURE **38-1** The brown necrotic tissue must be débrided before healing can take place in this pressure ulcer.

PHASES OF WOUND HEALING

No matter what the cause of the wound, there are three distinct phases of wound healing: the inflammatory phase, the proliferation or reconstruction phase, and the maturation or remodeling phase. **Inflammation** is a localized protective response brought on by injury or destruction of tissues. **The inflammatory phase begins immediately after injury and lasts about 4 days.** It includes constriction of blood vessels, platelet aggregation (clumping), and the formation of fibrin (insoluble protein essential to clotting) from the action of thrombin on fibrinogen and epithelial cell migration. This is the process of hemostasis (arrest of escaping blood by clotting or vessel compression) and clot formation. A scab forms to protect against the invasion of pathogens. Epithelial cells migrate from the margins of the wound toward the base of the scab, and within about 48 hours a thin layer of epithelial tissue forms over the wound. Chemical reactions releasing histamine and prostaglandin occur. Small blood vessels then dilate and become more permeable, causing serous fluid to leak into the traumatized area. The collection of plasma and electrolytes leaking into the interstitial spaces causes edema. The wound becomes reddened, swollen, and tender. More chemical reactions bring phagocytic neutrophils to cleanse the wound. The phagocytic cells remove debris and protect against bacterial invasion by phagocytosis (engulfing of microorganisms or foreign particles). The clinical signs of the inflammatory process are as follows:

- Swelling or edema of the injured part
- Erythema (redness) resulting from the increased blood supply
- Heat or increased temperature at the site
- Pain stemming from pressure on nerve receptors
- A possible loss of function resulting from all these changes

The proliferation stage begins on the third or fourth day after injury and lasts 2 to 3 weeks. Macrophages (monocytes that are phagocytic) continue to clear the wound of debris, stimulating fibroblasts, which synthesize collagen. Collagen (fibrous structural protein of all connective tissue) is the main ingredient of scar tissue. New capillary networks are formed to provide oxygen and nutrients to support the collagen and for further synthesis of granulation tissue. This tissue is deep pink in appearance. A full-thickness wound begins to close by contraction as the new tissue is grown. Scarring is influenced by the degree of stress on the wound. In 15 to 20 days, the risk of wound separation or rupture is less likely (Communication Cues 38-1).

The final stage of healing, maturation, begins about 3 weeks after injury. Scar maturation, or remodeling, is the process of collagen lysis (breakdown) and collagen synthesis by the macrophages to produce the strongest scar tissue possible. Scar tissue slowly thins and becomes paler in color. At the end of this process, the scar is firm and inelastic. The length of each phase is dependent on the type of injury and whether the wound heals by first, second, or third intention. Note that the stages of healing are interwoven rather than linear. Different parts of a wound can be in different stages of healing. The process of wound healing is presented in Concept Map 38-1.

When a wound occurs around a joint, special attention is needed to maintain joint mobility and prevent a **contracture** (abnormal shortening of muscle tissue) that will restrict joint extension. If collagen overgrowth occurs, which is frequent in dark-pigmented skin, a keloid (permanent raised, enlarged scar) occurs (Figure 38-2). In the interior of the body, adhesions (fibrous bands that hold together tissues that are normally sepa-

---

Communication Cues 38-1

Concern About Scarring

Carl Heffner has had open heart surgery and comes to the cardiac rehabilitation center three times a week. The saphenous veins from both legs were used for grafts, so he has three healing incisions from this surgery. He is 64 and divorced.

MR. HEFFNER: "When it gets warm this summer, I will hate wearing shorts to work out with these leg scars. They are so ugly. I feel like I have little red snakes going up my legs."

NURSE: "You are worried about the appearance of your legs?"

MR. HEFFNER: "Yes, people must find these scars repulsive. I've always looked away when I've seen someone in the shower room at the gym with all these scars."

NURSE: "Is it difficult to think of yourself looking different than you did before the surgery?"

MR. HEFFNER: "Yes, I've always taken a great deal of pride in my appearance. There was a time when women told me I was handsome. Now I'm just a wreck."

NURSE: "How are you feeling now, compared with before your surgery?"

MR. HEFFNER: "I feel much better. I'm able to do more and am not fatigued all the time. I'm even thinking of playing tennis again."

NURSE: "So before your surgery, you had fairly constant chest pain, were very fatigued, and had to give up playing tennis. Let's look at what the surgery has meant to your life on the whole."

MR. HEFFNER: "Well, sure, I'm much better after the surgery and I'm grateful to be alive. My stamina is improving daily and it looks like I will be able to play tennis again. I'm really looking forward to that. But, I'm very self-conscious about getting out on the court in shorts. My buddies will probably tease me."

NURSE: "Have any of the other players had heart surgery?"

MR. HEFFNER: "Yes, Charlie has, but he doesn't have these big red scars on his legs."

NURSE: "Did you know him at the time of his surgery?"

MR. HEFFNER: "No, I came to the group a couple of years after that."

NURSE: "I think if you look, you will see that Charlie's leg scar has become white and isn't nearly as noticeable now. Yours will mature in that way also. It just takes time for the scar to mature and the red color to fade."

MR. HEFFNER: "You think they won't be so prominent later on?"

NURSE: "Yes, they will smooth out and fade."

MR. HEFFNER: "I could live with that a lot easier. Plus, players are supposed to keep their eyes on the ball, not on their partner's or opponent's legs!"

NURSE: "That's the spirit, Mr. H.!"

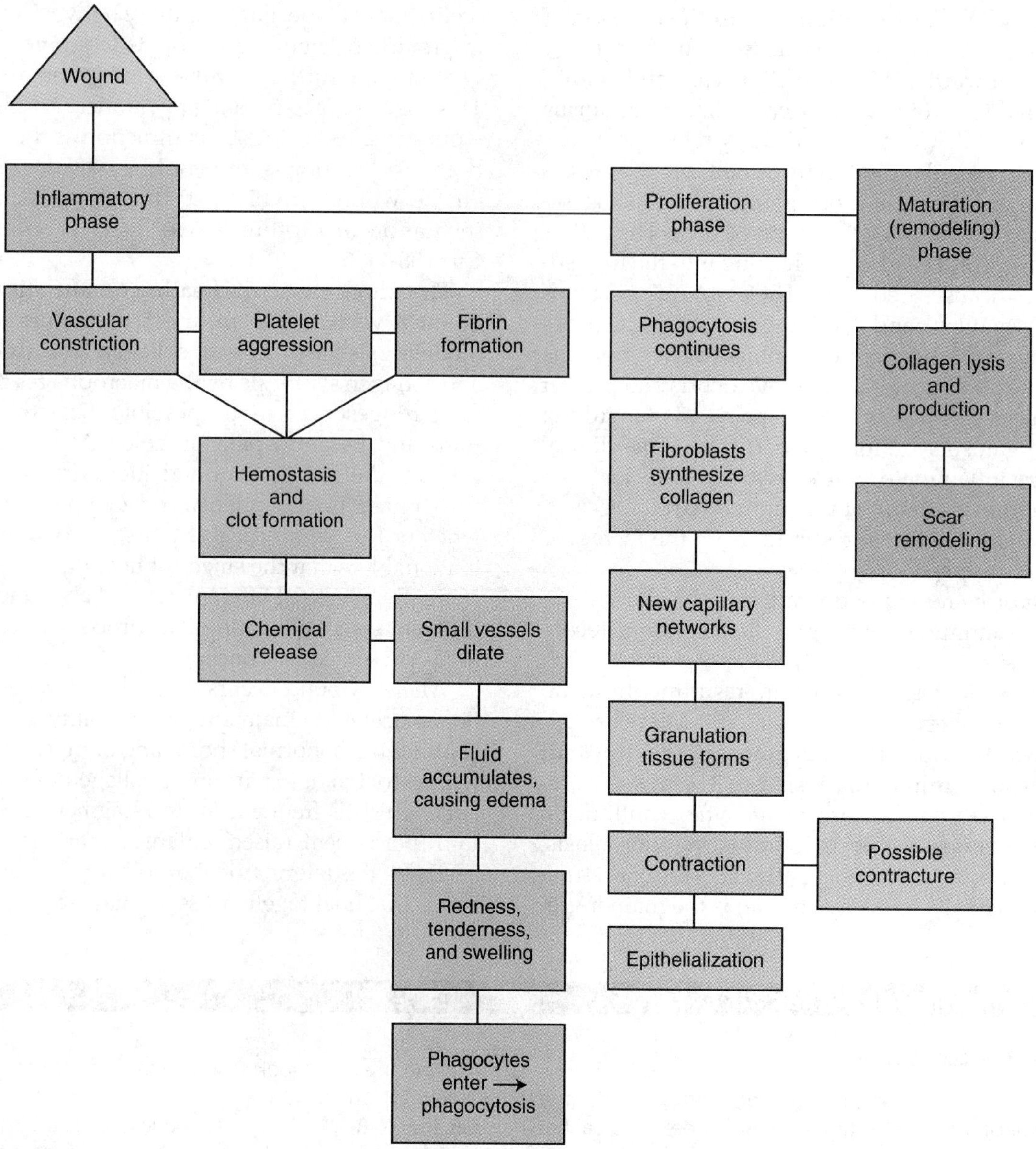

```
                          Wound

        Inflammatory                      Proliferation        Maturation
          phase                              phase              (remodeling)
                                                                  phase

  Vascular        Platelet       Fibrin     Phagocytosis      Collagen lysis
  constriction    aggression   formation     continues            and
                                                                production

            Hemostasis                      Fibroblasts          Scar
            and                             synthesize         remodeling
            clot formation                  collagen

    Chemical          Small vessels         New capillary
    release           dilate                networks

                      Fluid                 Granulation
                      accumulates,          tissue forms
                      causing edema

                                            Contraction     Possible
                      Redness,                              contracture
                      tenderness,
                      and swelling           Epithelialization

                      Phagocytes
                      enter →
                      phagocytosis
```

CONCEPT MAP **38-1** Process of wound healing.

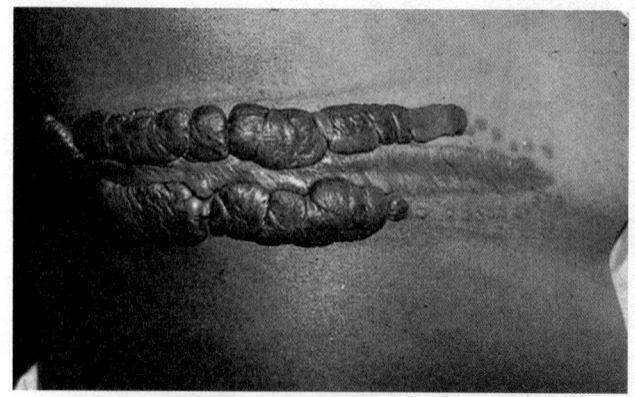

FIGURE **38-2** Keloid along a sutured wound.

rated) may grow and interfere with the normal function of the internal organs around which they form.

A wound with little tissue loss, such as a surgical incision, heals by first intention (closure) (Figure 38-3). The edges of the wound approximate (close together), and there is only a slight chance of infection. A wound with tissue loss, such as a pressure ulcer or severe laceration (a torn, ragged, or mangled wound), heals by second intention. The edges of the wound do not approximate, and the wound is left open and fills with scar tissue. Because of the longer healing period, the chance of infection is higher. Third intention healing, also known as delayed or secondary closure, occurs when there is delayed suturing of a wound. Such wounds are sutured after the granulation tissue has begun to form. An abdominal wound left open for drainage and then later closed is an example of healing by third intention.

Healing
by First
Intention

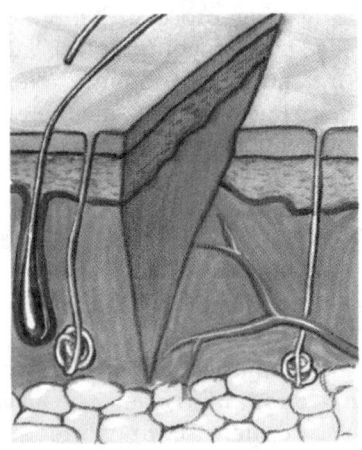 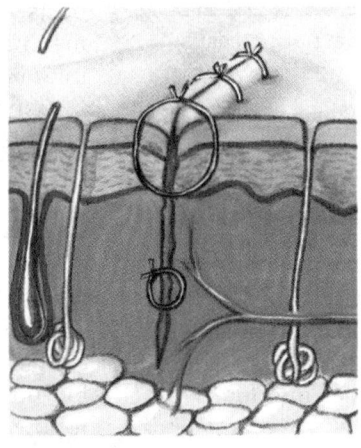 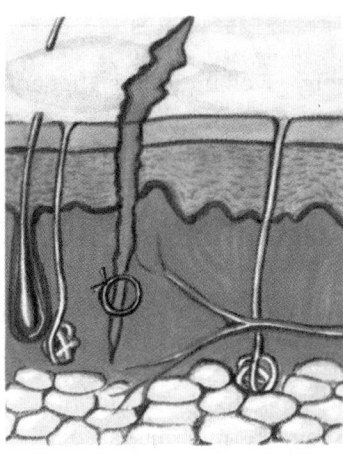

Clean incision Early suture "Hairline" scar

An aseptically made wound with minimal tissue destruction and minimal tissue reaction begins to heal as the edges are approximated by close sutures or staples. No open areas or dead spaces are left to serve as potential sites of infection.

Healing by
Second
Intention
(Granulation)
and
Contraction

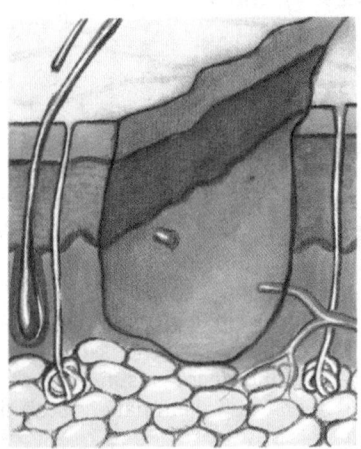 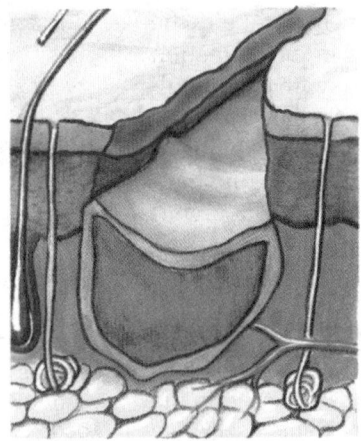 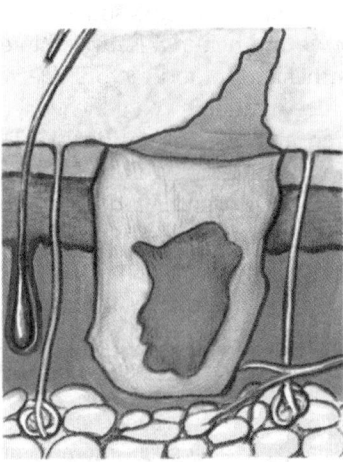

Gaping, irregular wound Granulation and contraction Growth of epithelium over scar

An infected or chronic wound or one with tissue damage so extensive that the edges cannot be smoothly approximated is usually left open and allowed to heal from the inside out. The nurse periodically cleans and assesses the wound for healthy tissue production. Scar tissue is extensive, and healing is prolonged.

Healing by
Third
Intention
(Delayed
Closure)

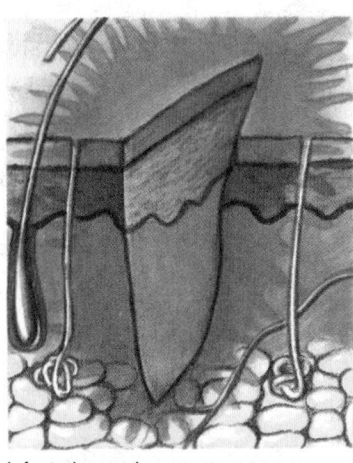 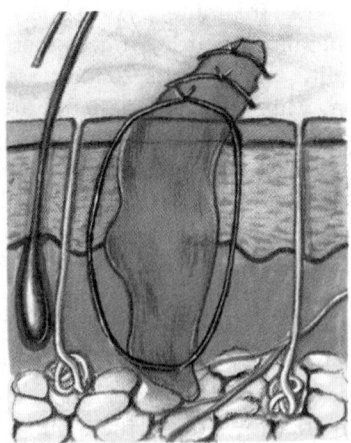

Infected wound Granulation Closure with wide scar

A potentially infected surgical wound may be left open for several days. If no clinical signs of infection occur, the wound is then closed surgically.

FIGURE **38-3** The process of wound healing.

? *Think Critically About . . .* If a patient asks why swelling occurs after an injury, what would you say?

FACTORS AFFECTING WOUND HEALING

AGE

Healthy children and adults heal more quickly than the elderly. Metabolism in the older adult is slower, and regeneration does not occur as quickly. The elderly may have chronic diseases that interfere with healing. Peripheral vascular disease impairs blood flow, which can impede healing. Atherosclerosis and atrophy reduce skin capillaries and impair blood flow to the wound. A decline in immune function reduces the formation of antibodies and monocytes necessary for wound healing. Reduced liver function impairs the synthesis of blood factors. Decreases in lung function reduce available oxygen needed for synthesis of collagen and the formation of new epithelial cells. The skin of the elderly is much thinner and more fragile and is easily damaged; patients' skin should be handled carefully when performing wound care to avoid further wound formation.

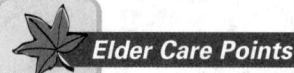

Elder Care Points

Complications of wound healing, such as dehiscence and evisceration, may occur more commonly in the elderly due to the prolonged healing process.

NUTRITION

A diet rich in protein, carbohydrates, lipids, vitamins A and C, thiamine, pyridoxine, and riboflavin, and the minerals zinc, iron, and copper is needed for wound healing. See Chapter 26 for more information on nutrition. Malnourished patients are at risk for delayed wound healing. Added protein and adequate fluid are of great importance when a patient has a chronic wound. Adipose (fatty) tissue has less blood supply and predisposes the obese patient to risk of wound infection and slower healing.

LIFESTYLE

Regular exercise contributes to enhanced blood circulation and promotes healing because blood brings oxygen and nutrients to the wound. Smoking reduces the functional hemoglobin of the blood, which limits oxygen-carrying capacity. Cells need oxygen to function effectively. The person who does not smoke and who exercises regularly will heal more quickly.

MEDICATIONS

Steroids and other anti-inflammatory drugs, heparin, and antineoplastic agents interfere with various aspects of the healing process. Steroids in particular may mask the signs of wound infection because they inhibit the inflammatory response. The fact that infection is occurring would usually be evident due to inflammation, which may not occur when steroids are present.

INFECTION

A wound infection slows the healing process. The acute phase of an infection is characterized by a sudden onset of symptoms as well as by the vascular changes of inflammation, especially swelling caused by fluid collecting in tissue. The acute phase is followed by an increase in white blood cells to overcome the invaders and to clear away the damaged tissues so that healing can occur. A bacterial infection of the skin or mucous membranes frequently causes fluid drainage from the wound or damaged tissue.

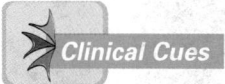

Clinical Cues

Assess drainage for color, consistency, odor, and amount and record the findings. The color may range from creamy yellow to dark green. **Purulent** (containing pus) drainage contains dead phagocytes, bacteria, and tissue and is thick in consistency. As the infection disappears, the drainage has less odor, becomes more serous or watery, and decreases in amount, and the color lightens. All signs of inflammation subside as healing occurs.

CHRONIC ILLNESS

Patients who also have a chronic illness such as diabetes, cardiovascular disease, or a disorder of the immune system may heal more slowly. Slowed wound healing occurs from a decrease of available oxygen and nutrients at the cellular level, disruptions in the normal metabolism of substances in the body, or inability of the body to fight infection adequately.

Patients who are immunocompromised (with poorly functioning immune systems) have delayed wound healing because fibroblast function, collagen synthesis, and phagocytosis are affected. These patients are at high risk for hospital-acquired infection.

COMPLICATIONS OF WOUND HEALING

HEMORRHAGE

Some escape of blood from a wound is normal, but hemorrhage is abnormal. Internal hemorrhage is evidenced by swelling or distention in the area of the wound and, perhaps, sanguineous (bloody) drainage from a surgical drain.

Monitor all patients with fresh surgical wounds for signs of hemorrhage. Be sure to check beneath the patient who had abdominal surgery to be certain blood isn't seeping from the side of the dressing under the patient.

If internal hemorrhage is extensive, hypovolemic shock may occur with a fall in blood pressure, rapid thready pulse, increased rate of respirations, restlessness, diaphoresis, and cold clammy skin. Intervene promptly to prevent a potentially life-threatening situation.

In other cases, a **hematoma** may occur. A hematoma may appear as a swelling that is bluish red. If a hematoma is large, it may place pressure on blood vessels and obstruct blood flow. The risk of hemorrhage is greatest during the first 48 hours after surgery, and when it occurs, it is an emergency. If external hemorrhage occurs, apply extra sterile pressure dressings to the site, closely monitor the patient's vital signs, and report to the surgeon. The patient may need to be immediately returned to the operating room for further intervention.

INFECTION

A wound may be infected with microorganisms at the time of injury, during surgery, or postoperatively. Local signs that a wound is infected include increased pain at the wound site, redness around the wound, warmth in the surrounding tissues, and purulent exudate. Traumatic wounds are more likely to become infected than surgical wounds. A localized infection called an abscess is an accumulation of pus made up of debris from phagocytosis when microorganisms have been present. The liquid may be white, yellow, pink, or green, depending on the infecting microorganisms. Surgical wound infection is often a nosocomial infection, but can be from microorganisms that are present in the colon or on the surface of the skin.

The microorganism most frequently present in wound infections is *Staphylococcus aureus*. Other microorganisms frequently responsible for wound infections include *Escherichia coli*, *Streptococcus pyogenes*, *Proteus vulgaris*, *Aerobacter aerogenes*, and *Pseudomonas aeruginosa*. When wound infection is suspected, a specimen of wound exudate (fluid accumulation containing cellular debris) is obtained and tested. A Culturette tube is used to obtain a specimen for the culture, and a sensitivity test is performed to determine which antibiotic is effective against the offending organism (Figure 38-4). Directions for obtaining a wound culture are found in Chapter 24.

Cellulitis is an inflammation of the tissue surrounding the initial wound, characterized by redness and **induration**. A fistula is an abnormal passage or communication usually formed between two internal organs or

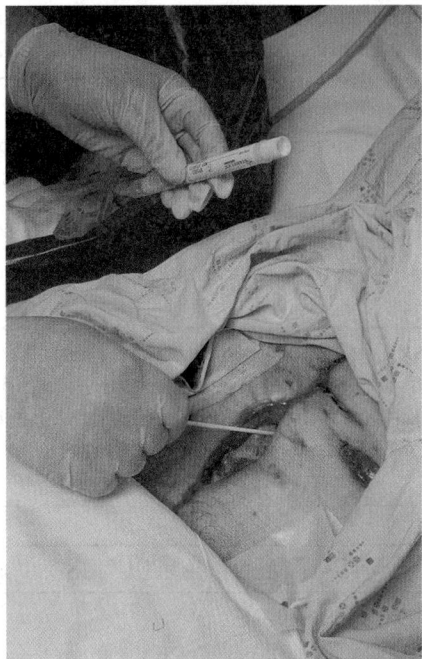

FIGURE **38-4** Take a specimen from the interior of the wound for a culture.

leading from an internal organ to the surface of the body. A fistula may result from an infection, or it may have a congenital origin. Common postoperative fistulas are designated according to the organs or parts with which they communicate, such as a rectovaginal, fecal, anal, or biliary fistula. A sinus is a fistula leading from a pus-filled cavity to the outside of the body.

The best way to prevent wound infection is to maintain strict asepsis when performing wound care. Use sterile equipment, meticulous handwashing, sterile gloves, and sterile dressings. Your hair should be contained so that it is not swinging over the wound during care, and the stethoscope should be removed from around the neck to prevent dropping microorganisms into the wound from it. Refrain from talking while dressing the wound to prevent microorganisms in your mouth or saliva from possibly landing in the wound.

Think Critically About . . . What discharge instructions would you give a patient about assessing for signs of wound infection?

DEHISCENCE AND EVISCERATION

Dehiscence is the spontaneous opening of an incision. Dehiscence of an abdominal wound often involves separation of the layers beneath the skin as well. **Evisceration** is the protrusion of an internal organ through the incision. Risk factors for dehiscence are obesity, poor nutrition, multiple trauma, excessive coughing, vomiting, strong sneezing, suture failure, and dehydration. The greatest risk for wound dehiscence is on the fourth or fifth postoperative day, before extensive collagen has been built up. **A sign of impending de-**

hiscence may be an increase in the flow of serosanguineous (serum and blood mixture) drainage into the wound dressing. When dehiscence occurs, the patient may state that "something has given way." If dehiscence or evisceration occurs, quickly place the patient supine, and place large sterile dressings or towels soaked in normal saline over the incision and viscera. Notify the surgeon immediately and prepare the patient for return to surgery as soon as possible.

> ? *Think Critically About . . .* What would you do if you were ambulating in the hall with a patient who has an abdominal incision and he bends forward suddenly and says "something gave way"?

TREATMENT OF WOUNDS

WOUND CLOSURE

Sutures and staples are used to hold the edges of a surgical wound together until the wound can heal. Traumatic wounds are usually cleaned, trimmed, and sutured. Sutures used to attach tissues beneath the skin are made of absorbable material and are not removed. They disappear within a few days. Skin sutures are made of silk, cotton, linen, wire, nylon, or Dacron. Silver wire clips are also sometimes used. Large retention sutures may be used on a wound when the surgeon believes that there is a danger of dehiscence. These are usually wire, and the portion of the suture outside the skin is covered with rubber. Sometimes the wound is small and Steri-Strips can be used. These are small, reinforced adhesive strips placed over the break in the skin that effectively hold the edges of the wound together while healing takes place.

Dermabond is a synthetic, noninvasive glue that decreases the trauma from removing a dressing, while providing a seal that protects underlying tissue without the need for bandages. This may sometimes be used in place of sutures in small areas. It loosens and comes off in 7 to 10 days. It is not used on mucous membranes.

The recommended method of open-wound classification is based on the color of the wound rather than its cause or dimensions. There are three basic wound types: red, yellow, and black. The type of wound indicates what type of dressing is needed. *Red wounds* are clean and ready to heal. Protection is the best method of treatment. A *yellow wound* has a layer of yellow fibrous debris or exudate. Sloughing (natural shedding of dead tissue) may cause drainage. A yellow wound needs to be continually cleansed and should have a dressing that will absorb the drainage and act to débride the surface mechanically. A yellow wound often becomes infected. *Black wounds* need débridement (removal of all foreign or unhealthy tissue from a wound) of the eschar (sloughing dead tissue, usually caused by a thermal injury or gangrene) to heal. Eschar can be mechanically débrided by a surgeon, softened by soaks or enzyme substances, and gradually removed as it separates.

DRAINS AND DRAINAGE DEVICES

At surgery, one or more drains may be placed to provide an exit for blood and fluids that accumulate during the inflammatory process. The drain may be active or passive. An active drain is attached to a wound suction device. A passive drain has no suction device attachment; it works by gravity and capillary action. The drain is placed within the surgical area and exits through a "stab" wound (a puncture or slit made by the surgeon) at a location different from the incision. A Penrose drain is a flat rubber tube. Often a safety pin is placed at the external end of the drain to prevent it from slipping into the wound (Figure 38-5). Whenever this drain is ordered to be shortened, you would place a new safety pin proximal to where you will cut the drain tubing to the desired length before cutting the tubing. Various sizes of catheters can be used as drains also.

Plastic drainage tubes can be connected to a closed drainage system that is compressed and closed and thus applies slight suction to the drainage tube to help evacuate the fluids within the wound (Figure 38-6). The Hemovac and Jackson-Pratt devices are examples of such a system (Figure 38-7). The drainage device is emptied at the end of each shift, and the fluid is measured and entered on the intake and output record as output (Steps 38-1). Draining excess fluid from a wound area helps prevent the formation of an abscess

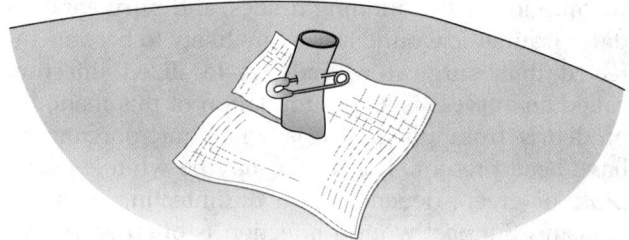

FIGURE **38-5** Penrose drain in a "stab wound" close to an abdominal incision.

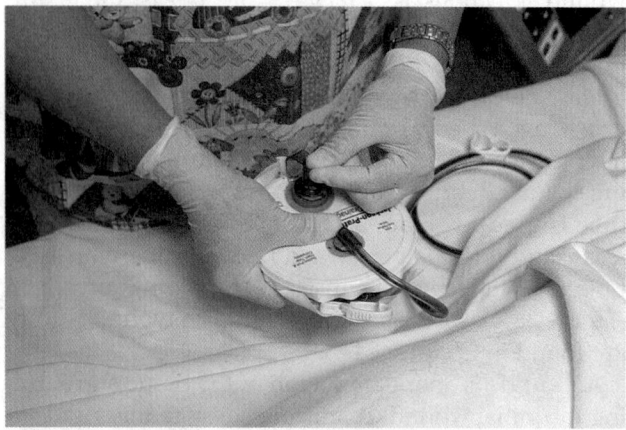

FIGURE **38-6** Compress the Hemovac-type drainage system to activate it.

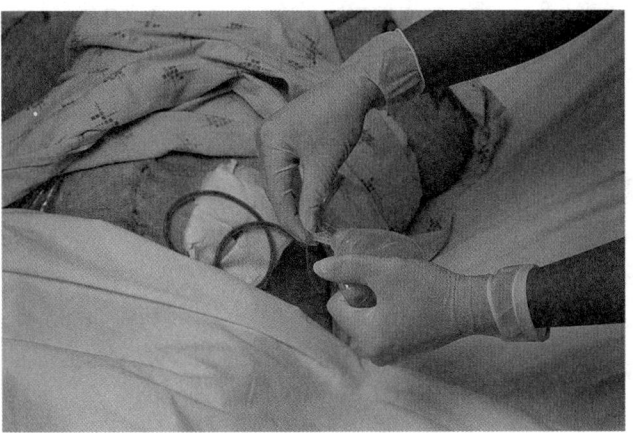

FIGURE **38-7** After emptying drainage, compress the bulb of the Jackson-Pratt–type drainage device to activate it.

or a fistula. Drains are sometimes used when traumatic wounds are sutured as well. The skin around the drain is cleansed during each dressing change.

DÉBRIDEMENT

Necrotic tissue must be removed from the wound before healing can occur. *Sharp débridement* is done at the bedside or in the operating room using sterile scissors, forceps, and a scalpel blade. Sharp débridement is performed when there are signs of cellulitis or sepsis. It is a painful procedure and the wound will bleed afterward. Usually, the surgeon performs this function. Nurses often are directed to perform *enzymatic débridement,* which uses topical substances that break down and liquefy the dead tissue. These substances are placed in the wound and another dressing is placed

---

Steps 38-1   Maintaining a Closed Wound Drainage Unit

A wound drainage unit pulls fluid from a wound to prevent swelling. It promotes healing and helps prevent the formation of an abscess or fistula. Standard Precautions are followed and require the use of gown, mask, protective eyewear, and gloves. Jackson-Pratt drainage system bulbs should be drained and recompressed every 4 hours.

Review and carry out the Standard Steps in Appendix 3.

1. **ACTION** Place a waterproof underpad on the bed under the device. Perform hand hygiene and put on personal protective equipment.

   RATIONALE Protects the bedding if spill occurs. Protects from transfer of microorganisms in splashed fluids.

2. **ACTION** Empty the device when it is two thirds full.

   RATIONALE When overly full, negative pressure needed for suction is diminished.

3. **ACTION** Hold the device with the spout pointing away from you and release the vacuum by removing the plug from the pouring spout.

   RATIONALE Prevents contaminating yourself if fluid splashes out of the spout.

4. **ACTION** Do not touch the drainage spout or plug.

   RATIONALE Touching contaminates these sterile surfaces.

5. **ACTION** Empty the contents into a measuring container. Note the amount and appearance of the drainage.

   RATIONALE Allows accurate output measurement. Provides data for documentation and evaluation.

6. **ACTION** Clean the pouring spout and plug using a separate alcohol sponge for each.

   RATIONALE Prepares for reinitiation of the vacuum and suction.

7. **ACTION** Reactivate the unit by fully compressing it. For a Hemovac, place the unit on a firm surface and compress it equally. For a Jackson-Pratt balloon-shaped device, tightly compress it in your hand. Replace the plug in the spout.

   RATIONALE Compression creates a vacuum and causes negative pressure, which acts to suction drainage into the reservoir.

8. **ACTION** Check to see that the unit remains compressed when you release the manual pressure. Be certain that drainage tubes are not kinked or loose.

   RATIONALE Reinstitutes suction of the wound.

9. **ACTION** Secure the device to the patient's gown below the level of the wound.

   RATIONALE Prevents pulling on the drains and wound if the device is caught on something.

10. **ACTION** Remove and dispose of personal protective equipment (PPE) and wash your hands. Note the amount of drainage on the shift input and output record.

    RATIONALE Prevents the transfer of microorganisms and tracks the amount of drainage.

11. **ACTION** Document amount, color, and odor of drainage and that system is recharged/compressed and drainage tubes are unkinked.

    RATIONALE Provides a record of your actions and findings.

over it to hold them in place. This is very useful for uninfected wounds.

Chemical débridement using Dakin's solution or sterile maggots is occasionally used on a wound with necrotic tissue that isn't responding to other treatments. *Autolytic débridement* is a longer process that uses the body's enzymes to break down nonviable tissue in the wound. It is best used on small, uninfected wounds as the type of dressing provides a warm, moist environment that could encourage growth of bacteria if they are present. The wound must be monitored closely for signs of infection during the autolytic process. *Mechanical débridement* is the physical removal of wound debris by irrigation or hydrotherapy with a whirlpool bath or ultrasound mist. The physical therapist performs the whirlpool procedure. With ultrasound mist therapy, microscopic saline bubbles and sound waves clean and débride the wound bed and remove bacteria while stimulating cell growth. Treatments are usually ordered three times a week. The procedure is painless, but may cause tingling and redness of the site after the treatment. The mist is delivered perpendicular to the wound. The mist is applied in a grid pattern.

Wet-to-dry dressings act to mechanically débride because they stick to the tissue, removing a layer of cells when removed. They are occasionally used but are no longer recommended because they also disrupt newly regenerated tissue.

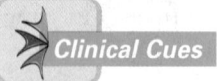
Clinical Cues

The only necrotic wound for which débridement is not recommended is a pressure ulcer on a heel. According to AHCPR guidelines (Bonham, P. [2007]), this type of ulcer is not débrided if edema, erythema, or drainage is not present.

DRESSINGS

Dressings, which are protective coverings placed over wounds, serve a number of different purposes. They prevent microorganisms from entering or escaping freely from the wound, and they absorb drainage. Dressings can be used for applying pressure to control bleeding and for improving the adherence of a skin graft to the grafted site. Finally, dressings help to support and stabilize tissues and reduce the discomfort from the wound.

A wide variety of dressing materials are available for dressing a wound (Figure 38-8). Choices are based on the location, size, and type of wound; whether infection is present or débridement is needed; and the frequency with which the dressing will be changed. Several standard sizes of dry sterile gauze are available: 5 × 5 cm (2 × 2 inch), 10 × 10 cm (4 × 4 inch), and 10 × 20 cm (4 × 8 inch). The size and number of gauze pads needed depend on the size of the wound

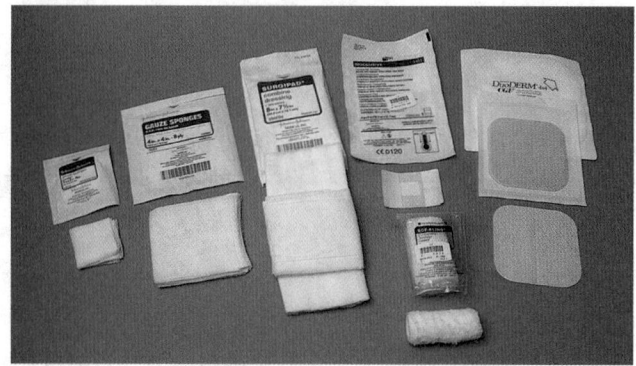
FIGURE **38-8** Various types of dressings.

and the amount of exudate. Dressings may be folded or cut to fit around drains.

Telfa and other nonadherent dressings have a shiny, nonadherent surface on one side that is applied to the wound. Exudate seeps through this surface and collects in the absorbent material on the other side. This dressing causes less trauma to the wound when it is removed.

Surgi-Pads or abdominal pads (ABDs) are used to cover small gauze dressings. They hold the dressings in place and absorb and collect excess drainage. The more absorbent surface of the Surgi-Pad is placed facing the wound; the less absorbent outward side helps protect from external contamination. The outer side is usually indicated by a blue stripe or a seam. Whichever dressings are used, the purpose is to fully cover the wound and supply sufficient absorbent material to contain exudate produced. The outermost dressing should completely cover the inner dressings.

Since the early 1990s, it has been known that superficial wounds heal faster when kept moist than when kept dry. A variety of air or fluid occlusive and semiocclusive wound dressings have been developed, including thin films, hydrocolloids, and foams. These dressings keep the wound moist while insulating and protecting it from external contamination. Foam dressings absorb drainage. These dressings are used more frequently than gauze for chronic or hard-to-heal wounds.

Many combination varieties and other wound dressings are available now. It is important to assess exactly what the desired action for treatment of the wound is before choosing the appropriate dressing. The articles about wound dressings listed in the bibliography for this chapter can provide you with a wealth of specific information. Other types of dressings include hydrogels, foams, calcium alginate, composites, collagens, and enzymatic débriders. The two dressings most commonly used are transparent film and hydrocolloid dressings.

Transparent Film Dressings

Clear film dressings such as OpSite allow you to assess the wound without removing the dressing. The transparent dressing does not require the use of tape and is less bulky than a gauze dressing. These dressings are

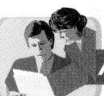

Pressure Ulcer and Wound Observation

Remind UAPs to report any changes such as drainage, increased reddening, or a loose dressing to you. Perform your own assessments of wounds and pressure ulcers. It is not the job of the UAP to assess.

often used to cover intravenous catheter sites and to protect a Stage I or II pressure ulcer. They are useful for superficial, partial-thickness wounds. They do not absorb drainage. A transparent film dressing should be changed when it no longer adheres to the skin properly (Assignment Considerations 38-1). They may remain in place from 3 to 7 days. They are not used over an infected wound.

Hydrocolloid Dressing

Dressings such as DuoDERM keep a wound moist. They are water and air occlusive and self-adhesive. You cannot see through a hydrocolloid dressing. This dressing facilitates autolytic débridement and provides thermal insulation, keeping the wound warm. Once applied, this dressing may stay in place for 3 to 5 days as long as it stays intact with good skin contact on all edges. Hydrocolloids are not recommended for heavily draining wounds.

Securing Dressings

The dressing is secured to the wound using tape, stretch roller gauze (Conform, Kerlix, Kling), mesh netting, an elastic bandage, or Montgomery straps (tie tapes) (Figure 38-9). The correct product must be elected for the purpose. Elastic tape or bandages provide pressure, stretch gauze and mesh netting allow some movement without dislodging the dressing, and Montgomery straps allow changing of the dressing without removing and reapplying tape, which can cause repeated skin irritation (Figure 38-10). Tincture of benzoin may be applied before the tapes are applied to protect sensitive skin (Box 38-1). Strips of hydrocolloid dressing can be placed on either side of the wound edges, the dressing applied, and then tape applied to the hydrocolloid strips for wounds that need frequent dressing changes. Nonallergenic tapes are available for the patient who has an allergy to other types of tape. Ensure that tape adheres to the skin for several inches on both sides of the dressing, and place a length of tape across the middle of the dressing. Do not apply tape over irritated or broken skin. To remove tape, gently loosen the tape ends and gently pull each parallel to the skin surface **toward** the wound while applying light traction to the skin away from the wound as the tape is loosened. If the tape will not loosen, adhesive remover may be used.

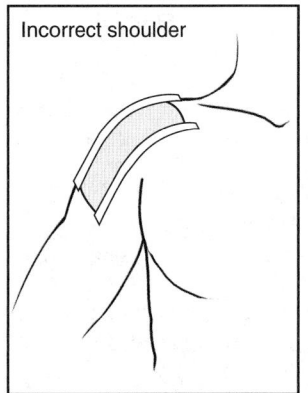
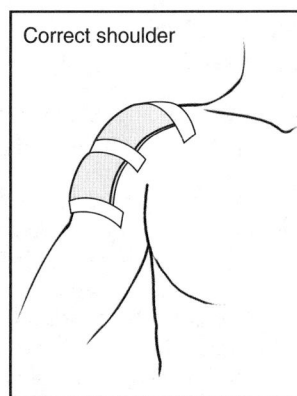
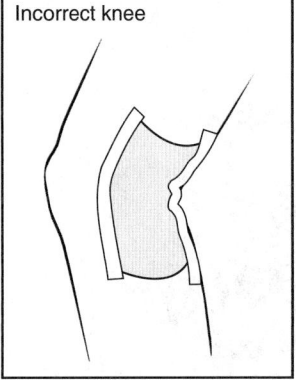
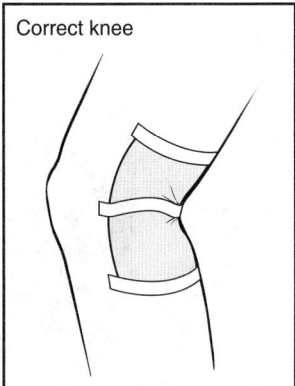

FIGURE **38-9**   Tape across a joint or a crease.

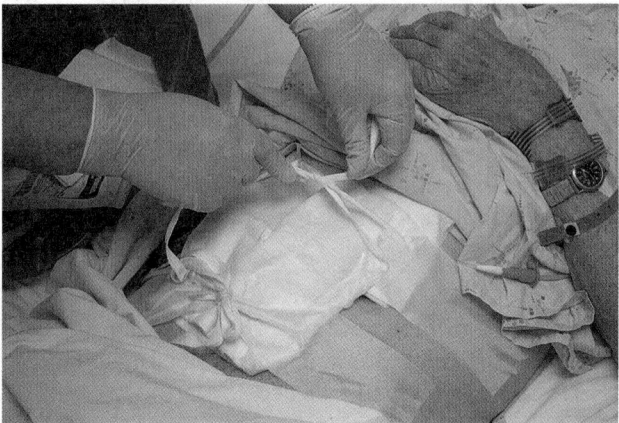

FIGURE **38-10**   Montgomery straps may be used to hold a dressing in place.

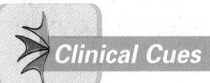

In the home setting, self-adherent plastic wrap can be used to secure dressings on patients who have problems with tape. Use the plastic wrap only for securing dressings over uninfected wounds.

BINDERS

Binders (wide elasticized fabric bands) are used to decrease tension around a wound or suture line, increase patient comfort, decrease lactation after childbirth, or

Box 38-1 *Principles for the Application of Tape on a Dressing*

- Place the tape so that the wound will stay covered by the dressing and the tape will adhere to intact skin. Place strips of tape at the ends of the dressing, and space tape strips evenly across the middle.
- The tape should be long and wide enough to adhere firmly to intact skin on each side of the dressing, but not so long that activity will loosen it.
- Place the tape opposite to body action in the wound location. Tape should go across a joint or crease, not lengthwise along it (see Figure 38-9).
- Turning under the end of the tape leaves a tab, making removal easier.

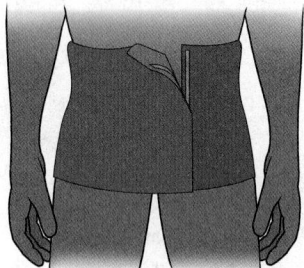

FIGURE **38-11** An abdominal binder provides support.

hold dressings in place. An abdominal binder provides support and comfort for an abdominal incision when the patient must perform deep breathing and coughing exercises and when getting in and out of bed (Figure 38-11). An elastic athletic supporter is used to hold dressings in place on the male scrotum and perineum. Elastic mesh panties or a sanitary belt is used to hold dressings in place for the female perineum.

? *Think Critically About . . .* Why should you assess the number and type of dressings needed for a particular dressing change before taking dressings to the patient's bedside?

NEGATIVE PRESSURE TREATMENT

Wounds that are difficult to heal may respond to negative pressure wound therapy. This treatment can increase healing rate by 40% while minimizing the need for dressing changes. The therapy, known as vacuum-assisted closure (VAC), applies a suction device to a special wound dressing to institute negative pressure at the wound site, drawing the edges together (Figure 38-12). Mechanical stretch of cells occurs, which increases cellular proliferation and tissue growth. The negative pressure and suction remove fluid from the wound, allowing penetration of fresh blood (Box 38-2). After a few days of therapy, bacterial counts in the wound bed drop. The VAC system keeps the wound moist (Figure 38-13). The system may be used on a

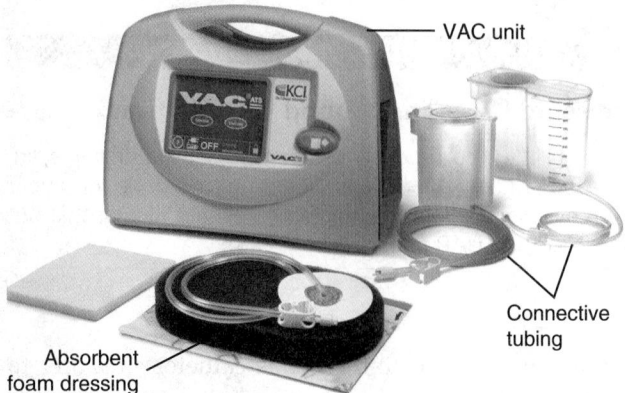

FIGURE **38-12** Wound VAC unit. *Top to bottom:* VAC unit itself, connective tubing to go between VAC unit and VAC absorbent foam dressing.

Box 38-2 *Guidelines for Care of the Vacuum-Assisted Closure (VAC) Dressing*

- Observe the dressing area when assessing vital signs.
- Film covering dressing must remain attached to skin in all areas for negative pressure to be maintained.
- Check the setting on the VAC unit and assess whether it is working properly.
- Assess for proper collapse of the dressing, indicating negative pressure is present. A whistling sound may indicate a leak.
- If a leak is present, press down gently around the drape and/or edges of the foam to better seal the drape. Use excess drape to patch over leaks.
- If the dressing needs to be replaced, check the agency protocol and instructions.
- Assess the patient for any complaints or problems in the wound area.
- Document your findings and that the unit is in place and functioning properly.

wound before a skin graft is performed to close the wound completely. Dressing changes for the system depend on the type of wound being treated. If the wound is infected, the dressing may be changed every 12 to 24 hours. For a clean wound, the dressing is changed three times a week.

TREATMENT OF PRESSURE OR VASCULAR ULCERS

Causes, staging, and prevention of pressure ulcers are presented in Chapter 19. An illustration of an ulcer at each stage is found there also. Treatment is discussed here along with care for all wounds.

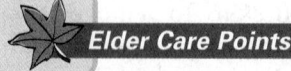

Elder Care Points

Transparent dressing such as OpSite or Tegaderm placed over a reddened area can often prevent skin breakdown in the elderly.

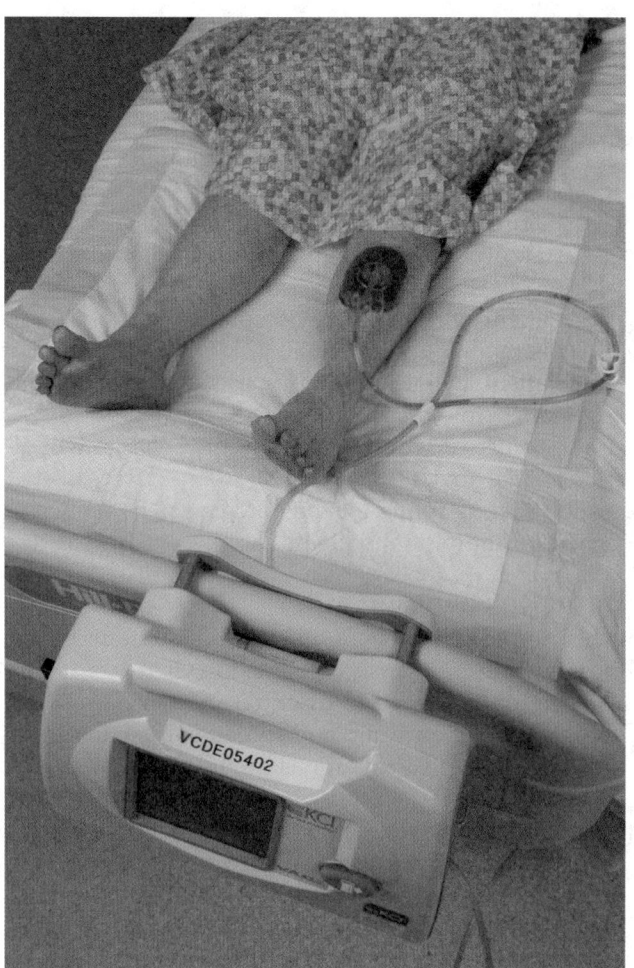

FIGURE **38-13** Wound VAC unit working on a chronic leg wound.

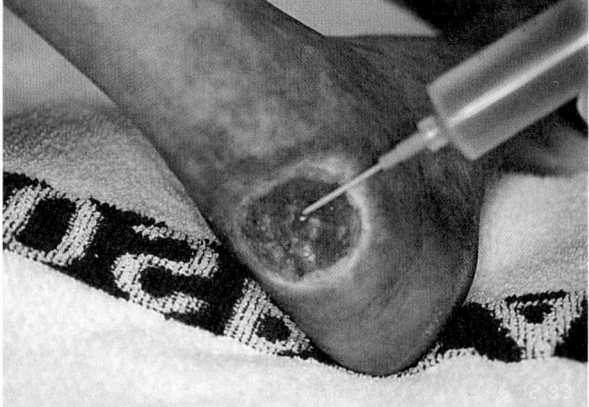

FIGURE **38-14** Wound irrigation using a 35-mL syringe and a 19-gauge plastic intravenous cannula.

APPLICATION of the NURSING PROCESS

Assessment (Data Collection)

Assessment includes a complete inspection of all skin areas. Every abrasion, laceration, contusion, reddened pressure area, **ecchymosis,** and incision should be noted. Be alert for signs of inflammation: redness, swelling, pain, heat, and loss of function. The location and appearance of skin wounds should be documented each day in specific terms because changes can occur quite rapidly.

Wounds are assessed by visual inspection, palpation, and the sense of smell, noting the wound's appearance and any drainage, swelling, odor, separation, and pain. Note the color of the wound and surrounding tissue as well as the approximation (degree of closure) of the wound edges, and determine whether signs of inflammation or infection are present. Assess for signs of systemic infection by checking temperature trend, white blood cell (WBC) count, and feelings of malaise. A temperature greater than 101° F (38.3° C), a WBC count greater than 10,000/dL, and a feeling of malaise may indicate wound infection. Assess acute wounds every 8 hours and chronic wounds once a day. Chronic wounds and pressure ulcers should be measured periodically to determine whether healing is occurring.

In a dark-skinned person, you must rely on localized skin color changes at and around the wound site. The affected skin may be darker than normal skin, or more shiny. Use the back of a gloved hand to detect increased warmth around the wound. Carefully assess the site for surrounding edema. Gently palpate the periphery of the wound for signs of pain.

Assess the progress of healing by checking the decrease in the size of the wound. The size of a nonsurgical wound should be measured and the length, width, and depth recorded. It is especially important to measure chronic wounds such as pressure or vascular ulcers. Moderate postoperative pain is normal for 3 to 5 days, but persistent severe pain or sudden onset of new pain may indicate infection or internal hemorrhage.

Clean ulcers at each dressing change. Use only normal saline and apply light mechanical force with sponges or irrigation fluid to prevent damage to granulation tissue. Use 250 to 500 mL of solution and irrigate using a syringe with a small catheter to reach undermined areas and tunnels (Figure 38-14). Cover the wound with a dressing selected by the characteristics of the wound. Thin film dressings are used on Stage I ulcers to protect them from shearing forces and to keep them moist. For Stage II ulcers that are noninfected, use a hydrocolloid dressing that can be left on for up to a week, which will protect against bacterial contamination. For a Stage III ulcer that is draining, use a dressing that will absorb exudate and maintain a moist environment. **For infected ulcers, a nonocclusive dressing is always used.** Chemical enzyme formulas may be used in the wound to help débride eschar in Stage IV ulcers. Sometimes a wet-to-dry dressing may also be applied to help the sloughing of necrotic tissue by mechanical débridement. Occasionally hyperbaric oxygen chamber treatment is used to treat nonhealing wounds.

If the initial dressing is in place, it is not touched until the physician changes it or leaves orders for the nurse to do so; the dressing is assessed. The appearance of the dressing provides some indirect information about the wound underneath it. The dressing may be dry and intact, or it might be soaked with serous or serosanguineous drainage.

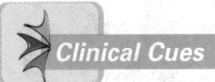
Clinical Cues

Assess for allergy to iodine, medications, cleaning solutions, and tape because many patients are allergic to substances used in wound care.

While changing a dressing, assess the color, consistency, odor, and amount of exudate. Note the number and type of dressings saturated or the diameter of the drainage on the dressing. With a gloved hand, gently palpate around the wound for tautness of tissues and swelling. Assess for drain placement and security, the amount and character of the drainage, and the effectiveness of any suction device. It is important to also assess the patient's reaction to the wound and her readiness to learn to do wound care. Document your findings after the dressing change.

Nursing Diagnosis

Common nursing diagnoses used for patients with wounds are as follows:
- Impaired skin integrity related to surgical incision (or trauma)
- Risk for infection related to nonintact skin or impaired skin integrity
- Acute pain related to infected wound
- Activity intolerance related to pain and malaise from wound infection
- Disturbed body image related to wound appearance
- Deficient knowledge related to care of wound
- Anxiety related to need to perform wound care

Planning

Time for wound assessment and care must be included in the daily work organization plan. Consideration of whether dressings may become damp from bathing dictates whether wound care is provided before or after a shower or bath. Check orders for directives regarding wound care. **Dressing changes require a physician's order, and irrigations may only be done with an order.** Check the chart for the date of wound occurrence or the surgical procedure in order to understand how old the wound is. This information is essential to assess the progress of wound healing. Determine what supplies will be necessary for a dressing change or irrigation.

Sample goals/expected outcome statements related to the nursing diagnoses listed above are as follows:
- Incision will be well approximated without disruption.
- Wound will be clean and dry without redness or swelling.
- Pain will resolve when infection is cleared.
- Activity tolerance will improve when infection resolves.
- Patient will verbalize acceptance of wound appearance.
- Patient will learn to properly perform wound care before discharge.
- Practice of wound care before discharge will alleviate anxiety.

A specific time frame for the outcome to be met is attached for individual patients.

Implementation

When implementing wound care, the nurse must use the principles of asepsis presented in Chapters 16 and 17. Careful technique is essential in preventing contamination of the wound and spread of infection if it is present. Standard Precautions are used for all patient care and are particularly important during wound care, when one comes into direct contact with body fluids. **Sterile gloves or sterile forceps are used whenever an open or fresh surgical wound is touched.** After the wound is sealed, nonsterile disposable gloves may be used. If a dressing becomes wet, it must be changed (Nursing Care Plan 38-1).

Wound Cleansing and Dressing Change

Wounds should be cleaned with warmed isotonic saline or lactated Ringer's solution. Sometimes antibiotic solutions are ordered for wound irrigation. These must be kept refrigerated, and the amount to be used should be allowed to come to room temperature before the irrigation. **Using cold solution lowers the wound temperature, which slows healing.** If antimicrobial solution is used, be sure it is properly diluted. Grossly contaminated or infected wounds are cleaned at each dressing change. Cleaning a healthy wound incorrectly can cause mechanical trauma and delay healing (Safety Alert 38-1). Use gauze squares and avoid using cotton balls to cleanse

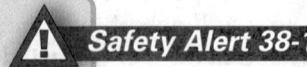
Safety Alert 38-1

Solutions that Damage Granulating Tissue

Certain solutions are toxic to growing and normal cells and should not be used to cleanse granulating wounds. Never use Dakin's solution (sodium hypochlorite), acetic acid, povidone-iodine, or hydrogen peroxide to clean an uninfected, granulating wound.

NURSING CARE PLAN 38-1

Care of the Patient with a Vascular Ulcer

SCENARIO Frank Walters, age 62, has a vascular ulcer on his left lower leg. He had originally bruised the spot when working in the garden. Now he has a stage IV ulcer that is not improving. His physician has admitted him for débridement and whirlpool treatments because he lives 75 miles from the city.

PROBLEM/NURSING DIAGNOSIS *Open wound*/Impaired skin integrity related to injury and decreased peripheral blood supply.

Supporting Assessment Data: *Subjective:* "It's been there for 2 months. It will not heal." *Objective:* 5 × 4½-cm open wound on lower outside aspect of lower left leg with area of black eschar on upper aspect, yellow tissue, and purulent drainage.

Goals/Expected Outcomes	Nursing Interventions	Selected Rationale	Evaluation
Wound will be without infection within 10 days.	Obtain wound culture as ordered.	Culture will determine infecting organism.	*Is infection present?* Culture results pending.
	Administer ciprofloxacin 200 mg IVPB q 12 hr.	Antibiotic will help fight infection.	
	Monitor signs of infection.	Tracking signs of infection will tell whether wound condition is improving.	
	Whirlpool bath to lower leg daily.	Whirlpool flow will help débride and cleanse wound.	
	Débride mechanically with Travase.	Travase enzymatically breaks down necrotic tissue.	
	Maintain sterile wet-to-damp dressing on wound.	Damp wound environment helps break down eschar.	
	Medicate for pain as needed 30 min before whirlpool treatment and dressing change.	Whirlpool and dressing change on a stage IV ulcer may be painful.	
	Measure wound twice a week.	Measurements tell whether wound size is decreasing or increasing.	
	Encourage cessation of smoking to help promote wound healing and prevent further progression of vascular disease.	Smoking contributes to vessel damage that causes vascular disease.	Smoking fewer cigarettes.
	Turn q 2 hr.	Turning prevents formation of new pressure ulcers.	
Wound will close within 1 mo.			*Has wound closed?* Progressing toward expected outcomes; continue plan.

❓ CRITICAL THINKING QUESTIONS

1. Why is smoking particularly contraindicated for this patient? Explain pathophysiology of the effect nicotine and smoking have on the body.

2. Why does eschar need to be removed from the wound? Explain the pathophysiology of how eschar interferes with wound healing.

Key: *IVPB*, Intravenous piggyback.

---

because fibers can become imbedded in the wound. For superficial, noninfected wounds, rinse lightly with normal saline rather than cleansing by using gauze. This reduces mechanical trauma to the wound. Avoid drying a wound after cleaning so that it will stay moist. Surgical wounds are cleansed from the center outward to prevent pulling microorganisms from the skin into the wound. Surgical wound and open wound dressings are changed using sterile technique (Skill 38-1).

Skill 38-1 | Sterile Dressing Change

Sterile dressing changes are performed for surgical wounds, open wounds, and pressure or vascular ulcers. The physician orders the frequency of the dressing change.

■ Supplies

✓ Sterile gloves
✓ Clean gloves
✓ Tape
✓ Plastic discard bag
✓ Scissors

✓ Dressing supplies
  Gauze sponges
  Telfa dressings
  Abdominal combination
    dressings

✓ Sterile normal saline solution
✓ Antiseptic swabs/solution
✓ Transparent film dressings
✓ Cotton-tipped applicators
✓ Bath blanket

Review and carry out the Standard Steps listed in Appendix 3.

■ Assessment (Data Collection)

1. **ACTION** Check the orders for directions for wound care and dressing change.

   RATIONALE A physician's order is required for a dressing change.

2. **ACTION** Determine if the patient is ready for the procedure.

   RATIONALE Saves time if the patient is not involved in another activity.

■ Planning

3. **ACTION** Check the nurse's notes for the types of supplies needed for the dressing change if in doubt as to what is needed, and visually assess the dressing that is in place.

   RATIONALE Ensures that the proper supplies will be on hand during the sterile procedure.

■ Implementation

4. **ACTION** Perform hand hygiene. Loosen the binder or tape; put on clean gloves and remove the old dressing; pull off the tape toward the wound while stabilizing the skin with the other hand. If tape won't loosen, rub over it with an alcohol swab for several seconds or use adhesive remover. Assess the drainage on the dressings and place them in the plastic discard bag. Wet the dressing with normal saline solution if it sticks to the suture line and wait a few minutes before removing it.

   RATIONALE Gloves prevent spread of microorganisms; removing old dressing allows visual assessment of the wound and drainage. Pulling tape toward the wound prevents disruption of the wound. Alcohol helps loosen stubborn adhesive, as does adhesive remover.

5. **ACTION** Inspect the wound, noting degree of healing, presence of pus, and necrosis; check for odor, drainage, and condition of sutures or drain. Remove gloves and discard them. Perform hand hygiene.

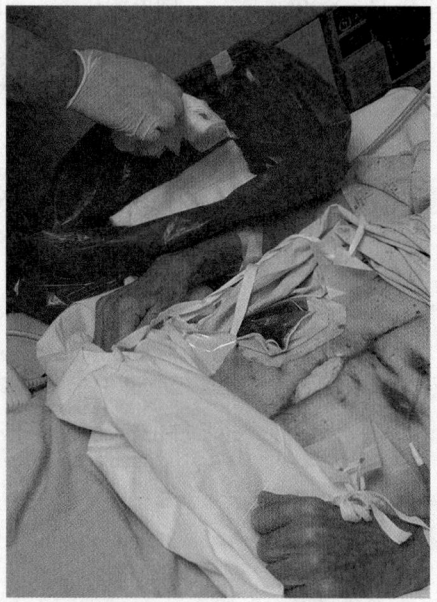

Step **4**

RATIONALE Provides data for determining progress of wound healing or presence of infection.

6. **ACTION** Set up sterile field, placing items in the order in which they will be used. Open the sterile supplies.

   RATIONALE Assists in maintaining a sterile field during the procedure and allows the procedure to be done efficiently. Readies supplies for use.

7. **ACTION** Put on sterile gloves and clean the area around the wound using normal saline or ordered disinfectant. Cleanse by one of the following methods:

   a. Use a separate swab from top to bottom on each side of the incision and continue outward.

   b. Use a separate swab from the wound edge outward on one side and then on the other side from top to bottom. Do not cleanse directly over the wound unless there is excessive drainage and if it is an agency policy. Cleanse the drain sites using a circular motion from the drain outward.

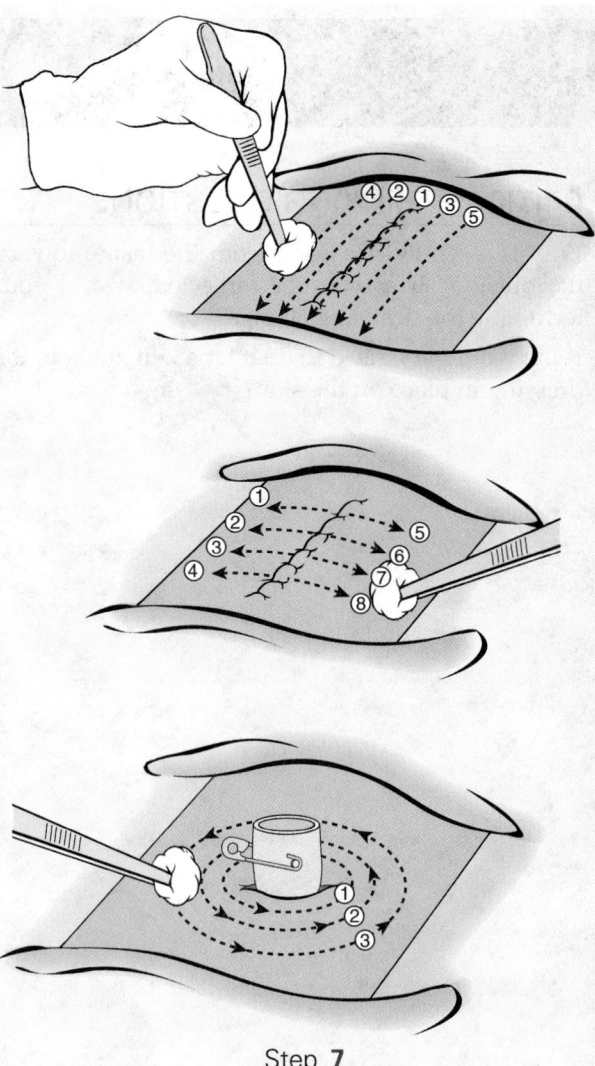

Step 7

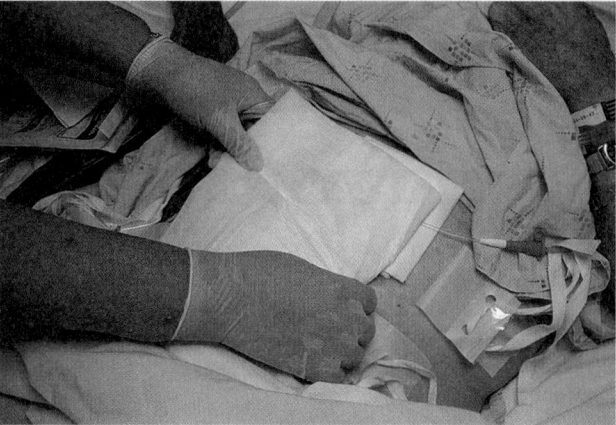

Step 9

c. Use a circular motion from the wound outward in an ever-widening circle.

RATIONALE Sterile technique prevents contamination of the wound. The top of the wound is considered the cleanest area. Cleansing by these methods prevents contaminating the wound. If considerable drainage is present, the wound itself is gently cleansed using a fresh swab for each single stroke.

8. *ACTION* Apply ointment or medication using applicators if ordered.

RATIONALE An order is essential for any medication. Using applicators decreases the chance of contamination of the tube or the medication container.

9. *ACTION* Apply the dressings by positioning them lightly over the wound area; cover the entire wound and do not move dressing once it is placed over the wound. Remove and discard the gloves. Secure the dressing in place. If there is difficulty in getting the tape to stick to the skin, a skin preparation can be used on the skin surface to make the adhesive stick. A binder or Montgomery straps may be used to hold the dressings in place.

RATIONALE Moving the dressing from one area to another may transfer microorganisms; securing the dressing ensures that the wound stays covered.

10. *ACTION* Contain the used dressings in the discard bag and deposit into the biohazard trash container. Perform hand hygiene.

RATIONALE Prevents spread of microorganisms.

■ Evaluation

11. *ACTION* Ask yourself: Are there signs of infection, such as redness and warmth around the wound edges; is thick or colored exudate present? Is the amount of drainage decreasing? Is the wound drain still in place? Had drainage soaked through the dressing? Did the dressing stay intact?

RATIONALE Answers to these questions provide data regarding wound healing and whether the dressing was sufficient to cover the wound and contain the drainage.

■ Documentation

12. *ACTION* Document the condition of the wound, including subjective statements of the patient as well as objective observations. Include health teaching performed for wound care.

RATIONALE Provides data regarding wound healing and patient teaching. Documents use of supplies.

Documentation Example

7/19 1430 Dressing changed with sterile technique using six 4 × 4s and two combined ABDs. Incision clean, dry, and well approximated. Small amount of serous drainage on dressing. Skin cleansed with alcohol swabs. Reinforced teaching re: keeping dressing dry and in place, technique for wound cleansing and dressing change, and signs and symptoms of infection to report immediately.

(Nurse's signature)

Continued

Skill 38-1 | Sterile Dressing Change—cont'd

Home Care Considerations

- Wound care instruments can be cleaned with warm, soapy water and boiled for 10 minutes to sterilize. Allow to air dry and store them in a covered container.
- Remind the patient and family to dispose of soiled dressings in impermeable bags to prevent the spread of infection.
- Montgomery straps can be devised by using wide adhesive tape folded back on itself, making holes in the flap ends, and using a shoelace or rubber bands and safety pins to secure the straps together after they are attached to the skin.
- Provide patients with information on where to obtain dressing materials.
- Provide a wound flow sheet to encourage the patient or family to record the characteristics of the wound when the dressing is changed. Include columns for date and for a description of characteristics of the wound.
- For a child, helping the child change a dressing on a stuffed bear or doll helps decrease anxiety about dressing changes.
- The elderly often have decreased vision and may need more assistance than realized to perform wound care and assess the wound.
- Arthritis in the hands may make it difficult for a person to manage a dressing change independently.

?CRITICAL THINKING QUESTIONS

1. Why is a wound cleansed from the inside toward the outside? If a wound is infected, would your technique for cleansing change?
2. What would you need to do if tape will not hold the dressing in place on the skin?

Think Critically About . . . What interventions would you place on the care plan for a patient with a surgical wound? What interventions might be needed for a patient with an open traumatic wound?

Hydrocolloid Dressings

Hydrocolloid dressings are only applied to uninfected wounds; they keep the wound moist and block entry of microorganisms. A variety of hydrocolloid dressings are available. These are often used on a vascular or pressure ulcer to promote healing after the wound is clean (Steps 38-2).

Wound Irrigation, Débridement, and Packing

An irrigation is the flushing out of an area with a liquid. Wound irrigation is done only with an order from the physician and requires sterile technique. Using a piston syringe instead of a bulb syringe helps prevent the aspiration of drainage and contamination of the syringe. For deep wounds with small openings, a sterile straight catheter may be attached to the syringe. The wound edges may need to be held open so that the solution can reach the depths of the wound. Skill 38-2 presents the steps in irrigating a wound.

A wound may be packed with gauze packing to facilitate formation of granulation tissue (connective tissue with multiple small vessels) and healing by second intention or to débride the wound. Usually moistened or medicated non–cotton-filled gauze is used in the form of fluffed (unfolded and loosely placed) 4 × 4s or strips. Either a wet-to-dry or a wet-to-damp technique is used. In the *wet-to-dry* technique, the dressings are moistened and packed into the wound and allowed to dry between dressing changes, which are done every 4 to 6 hours. As the dressings dry, they trap necrotic material and mechanically débride the wound when the dressing is removed. Removal of the dry packing is painful because it may remove some granulation tissue also. This technique is falling out of favor, but is still occasionally used. The *wet-to-damp* technique for packing is the preferred treatment for *noninfected* wounds (Skill 38-3). Moistened gauze packing is placed in the wound to absorb exudate, but is not allowed to dry before removal and therefore does not damage newly formed tissue.

Steps 38-2 | Applying a Hydrocolloid Dressing

Hydrocolloid dressings are used to provide a moist environment for wound healing in noninfected wounds. They occlude air and promote breakdown of necrotic tissue in wounds, thereby providing an alternative to mechanical débridement. These dressings may be left in place for up to 7 days, with 3- to 5-day adherence being average.

Review and carry out the Standard Steps in Appendix 3.

1. *ACTION* Clip the hair around wound site and cleanse the wound.

   RATIONALE The dressing will adhere better and be less uncomfortable when removed.

2. *ACTION* Choose a large enough dressing to cover a 1¼-inch border of healthy skin around the wound.

   RATIONALE For the dressing to adhere properly and remain in place while absorbing drainage, a 1¼-inch border is necessary.

3. *ACTION* Open the backing paper from the back of the dressing and smooth the dressing in place from the center outward, peeling back the backing as you progress outward. Do not touch adhesive surface.

   RATIONALE Smoothing the dressing prevents pulling and wrinkling of the skin. Adhesive adheres better if not touched.

4. *ACTION* Hold your hand over the dressing for a few minutes until all edges have adhered firmly.

   RATIONALE Warmth helps dressing adhere properly.

5. *ACTION* If dressing does not firmly adhere, cleanse the skin at the edges of the dressing with a skin prep pad and use hypoallergenic tape around the edges. Do not apply skin prep under the dressing.

   RATIONALE Skin prep makes skin tacky so that tape will adhere well. Tape holds the dressing in place. Skin prep over broken skin or wound may cause damage to tissue.

Skill 38-2 | Wound Irrigation

Wound irrigations are ordered by the physician. They are performed when a wound is infected, has large amounts of drainage, or contains necrotic material.

■ Supplies

✓ Sterile gloves
✓ Protective eyewear
✓ Mask
✓ Impermeable gown
✓ Underpad

✓ Sterile solution container
✓ Irrigation set
  Syringe with large-bore blunt needle or sterile angiocath
✓ Normal saline or ordered solution
✓ Basin to catch solution

Review and carry out the Standard Steps listed in Appendix 3.

■ Assessment (Data Collection)

1. *ACTION* Check the orders for wound irrigation to determine solution to be used and whether a sterile or clean irrigation is ordered.

   RATIONALE Solution ordered depends on condition of wound and whether infection is present.

■ Planning

2. *ACTION* Determine if patient is ready for the procedure and if all dressing and irrigation supplies are on hand.

   RATIONALE Saves time and promotes efficiency.

■ Implementation

3. *ACTION* Perform hand hygiene. Put on clean gloves. Using aseptic technique, expose the wound, placing the soiled dressings in the discard bag. Remove gloves and perform hand hygiene.

   RATIONALE Prevents transfer of microorganisms; prepares the wound for irrigation.

4. *ACTION* Aseptically prepare the irrigation set by pouring the solution into the container and checking the action of the syringe plunger. Place an underpad beneath the area to be irrigated. Place a basin to catch drainage against the side of the area being irrigated. Have the patient hold the basin in place if possible.

Continued

Wound Irrigation—cont'd

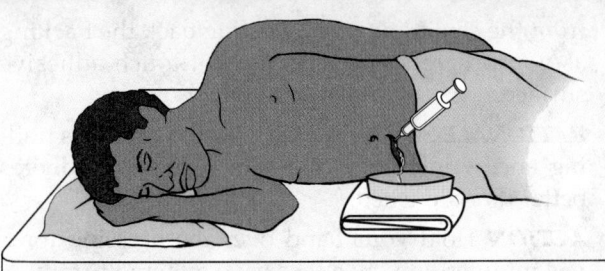

Step **4**

RATIONALE Preparing the irrigation set ensures that the equipment is ready before putting on sterile gloves. An underpad protects linens from moisture. The basin catches most of the irrigation fluid.

5. **ACTION** Don sterile gloves. Draw up solution into the syringe by pulling back on the plunger or squeezing the bulb. Hold the tip of the syringe about 1 inch from the wound surface, and steadily push on the plunger or squeeze the bulb to eject fluid into the wound. Repeat until all debris is washed from the wound or the amount of solution ordered for irrigation has been used. Irrigate all areas of the wound.

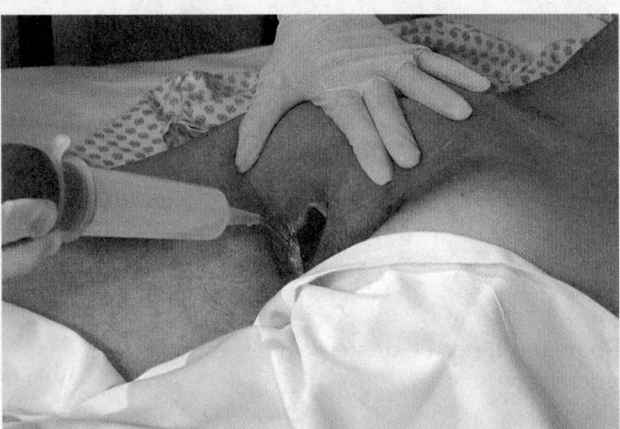

Step **5**

RATIONALE Keeping the syringe tip 1 inch away from the wound surface prevents contamination of the syringe. Using a 20-gauge needle or angiocath on the syringe causes an effective spray to cleanse the wound. Fluid washes out debris and necrotic tissue.

6. **ACTION** Dry the skin with gauze sponges so that tape will stick, and apply a sterile dressing.

RATIONALE Prepares the wound for the dressing; covers the wound.

7. **ACTION** Remove the gloves and discard them. Perform hand hygiene.

RATIONALE Prevents the transfer of microorganisms.

■ Evaluation

8. **ACTION** Was sterile technique maintained if ordered? Was all debris washed from the wound? Were the bed linens kept dry?

RATIONALE Answers to these questions determine whether the procedure was done correctly or if changes need to be made before irrigating the next time.

■ Documentation

9. **ACTION** Document the time of the irrigation and the solution and amount used.

RATIONALE Notes that ordered procedure was performed. Documents use of supplies.

Documentation Example

7/19 1830 Left buttock wound irrigated with 150 mL normal saline using sterile technique. Wound with pink tissue and serous drainage; no odor noted. Sterile dressing applied.

_____
(Nurse's signature)

■ Special Considerations

✓ When the irrigation is not ordered as a sterile procedure, equipment is kept as clean as possible and reused. This is common in the home environment.
✓ All irrigations of deep wounds should be done with sterile technique.
✓ If the patient cannot hold a basin against the area in which it is needed, use pillows covered with plastic and underpads to position the basin firmly against the skin.

 Home Care Considerations

• In the home setting, a plastic trash bag and a towel can be used under the area to be irrigated, or, when wet compress dressings are ordered, to protect the mattress or furniture.

? CRITICAL THINKING QUESTIONS

1. What is a better device for irrigating a wound than a bulb irrigation syringe?

2. If special irrigation solution is ordered and has to be kept refrigerated, why should it be heated? How would you heat it?

Skill 38-3 | Applying a Wet-to-Damp or Wet-to-Dry Dressing

Wet-to-damp dressings are used to keep a wound moist and promote healing; wet-to-dry dressings help débride wounds and encourage cellular growth from the base of the wound up to the surface. Wet-to-dry dressings have been largely replaced by other methods of débridement because they may harm new cell growth when the dressing is removed.

■ Supplies
✓ Gauze sponges
✓ Sterile basin
✓ Tape or binder
✓ Discard bag
✓ Sterile normal saline
✓ Sterile gloves
✓ Clean gloves
✓ Underpad

Review and carry out the Standard Steps listed in Appendix 3.

■ Assessment (Data Collection)

1. *ACTION* Check the order, assess the old dressing if one is in place, and determine if the patient is ready for the procedure.

   RATIONALE Ensures that the proper dressing is applied to the right patient.

■ Planning

2. *ACTION* Plan the appropriate time in your work schedule to perform the dressing change. Determine if all needed supplies are available and on hand at the patient's bedside. Wet-to-damp dressings are changed more frequently than wet-to-dry dressings.

   RATIONALE Assists in performing the procedure smoothly and quickly.

■ Implementation

3. *ACTION* Prepare the work space, and open the dressing packages and sterile container for the wetting solution; perform hand hygiene and don clean gloves.

   RATIONALE Readies the dressings and solution for work. Institutes Standard Precautions.

4. *ACTION For wet-to-damp dressing*, slowly and carefully remove the gauze. If it is stuck to the wound, add a little normal saline to loosen it. *For wet-to-dry dressing*, gently and steadily pull the gauze to remove it, débriding the necrotic tissue. Place used dressings in the discard bag.

   RATIONALE Pulling a stuck dressing loose damages new tissue. A wet-to-dry dressing is not remoistened when removing it.

5. *ACTION* Remove dirty gloves, perform hand hygiene, and pour the sterile wetting solution into the basin.

   RATIONALE Solution should be poured before putting on sterile gloves.

6. *ACTION* Don the sterile gloves.

   RATIONALE Prepares hands for sterile procedure.

7. *ACTION* Place the needed dressings in the wetting solution or moisten by pouring solution on them.

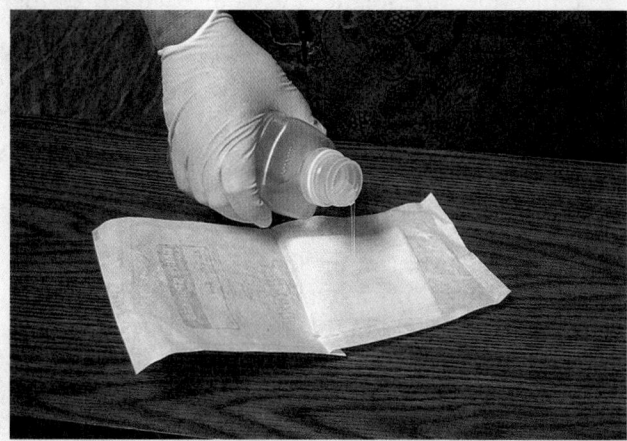

Step **7**

   RATIONALE Dressings should be thoroughly soaked.

8. *ACTION* Wring out dressings one by one and lightly press fluffed gauze into the wound, covering all exposed surface.

   RATIONALE Dressings should be moist without dripping. Moisture encourages healthy tissue growth. Gauze pads must be unfolded and lightly packed to be most effective.

9. *ACTION* Cover with a second moist dressing for a wet-to-damp dressing and then a dry, sterile 4 × 8-inch combined dressing in a single layer on top of the wet dressings. Additional dry dressings may be added as needed to keep the outside dry.

   RATIONALE To promote wound healing, the entire wet-to-damp dressing must be changed at regular intervals before the inner dressing dries out. The physician may order how frequently this is to be done; if not, change the entire dressing at least every 2 hours. If moisture reaches the outside of the sterile dressing, it can provide an avenue for pathogens to enter the wound.

Continued

Skill 38-3   Applying a Wet-to-Damp or Wet-to-Dry Dressing—cont'd

10. ACTION Remove the gloves and discard them; tape the edges of the dressing; perform hand hygiene.

RATIONALE Secures the dressing. A binder may be used in place of tape.

■ Evaluation

11. ACTION Ask yourself: Did the inner dressing stay damp in the wet-to-damp dressing? Did the outer dressing stay dry? Is necrotic tissue being removed from the wound by the wet-to-dry dressing? Is pink granulation tissue appearing in the wound? If the inner dressing for the wet-to-damp dressing is drying, change the dressing more frequently. Add sufficient dressing material to keep the outer dressing dry.

RATIONALE "Yes" answers to these questions determine that the procedure is successful

■ Documentation

12. ACTION Document the times of dressing changes and the procedure as well as the appearance of the wound at the end of the shift.

RATIONALE Verifies that orders were carried out and documents the course of wound healing.

Documentation Example

7/19 1430   Wound packed with fluffed 4 × 4s moistened with normal saline at 0830, 1030, 1230, and 1430. Sterile technique maintained. Wound 2.2 × 3.4-cm area of black eschar at 1500; wound yellow at base. Pink tissue at edges.

_____
(Nurse's signature)

■ Special Considerations

✓ Using a moisture barrier ointment on the skin around the wound protects the skin from maceration (softening of tissue from soaking in moisture). Petroleum jelly protects the skin from moisture.

✓ If a wet-to-dry dressing is ordered, leave out the second moist dressing and cover with only one layer of dry dressing.

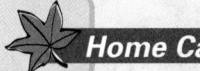
Home Care Considerations

• In the home environment, often clean rather than sterile technique may be used.

Elder Care Points

• Elderly patients have thinner and more fragile skin that is easily damaged. It is preferable to use a stretch gauze wrap or a binder rather than to repeatedly apply and remove adhesive tape during dressing changes.

❓CRITICAL THINKING QUESTIONS

1. Why would a binder be ideal to use to secure a wet-to-damp dressing?

2. Why must black eschar be removed from a wound in order for it to heal?

Clinical Cues

Administer ordered analgesia sufficiently ahead of performing a dressing change on a large or infected wound so that it is effective during the procedure. Wound dressing changes can be very painful, especially when débridement and packing are involved.

Débridement of necrotic tissue may be performed by using enzymatic powder, ointment, or granules that are packed into the wound, or by cutting (sharp débridement) away dead tissue. Enzymes break down the necrotic tissue, and wound packing absorbs the debris. Surgical débridement is performed by a surgeon or an advanced practice nurse. The wound heals slowly from the base upward. In many instances, the body's own healing processes cause sloughing (autolytic débridement) of the necrotic tissue. Petroleum

Elder Care Points

The elder who is discharged home with dressings may have great difficulty performing dressing changes due to poor vision, loss of joint flexibility, and arthritis. Always assess whether the elder can properly perform a dressing change or whether there is someone else available to perform the dressing changes. Teaching regarding the dressing changes must occur before discharge.

jelly may be used on the skin around the wound to prevent maceration from wet dressings.

Patient Teaching for Wound Care

Before the patient is discharged, proper technique for cleaning and dressing the wound must be taught. It is important to send the patient home with sufficient dressings to last until someone in the family can pur-

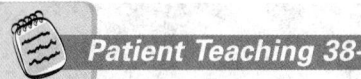

Patient Teaching 38-1

Wound Care

Teaching regarding wound care should begin as soon as possible for the hospitalized patient. Home care patients receive ongoing teaching. Include others in the household who will assist with wound care in all instruction. The following points should be covered in the teaching program:

- Factors that assist with wound healing: exercise, nutrition, rest, not smoking
- Where to obtain needed dressing supplies
- Expected appearance of the wound now and as it heals
- Signs and symptoms of infection to be reported to physician immediately: increased redness, swelling, pain, purulent drainage, persistent increasing fever, increasing malaise
- Importance of keeping the wound and dressing clean and dry
- Limitations on activity related to the wound
- Proper handwashing: the hands should always be washed before and after doing wound care or touching the wound area
- Disposal of used dressing supplies in a sealable plastic bag, following local guidelines for disposal of biohazardous waste

Instruct the patient in dressing change along with demonstration; seek a return demonstration of dressing change. The following points should be covered:

- Removing dressing
- Assessing the wound
- Cleansing the wound; wound irrigation; shower cleansing if allowed
- Caring for a drain
- Caring for wound suction device: emptying, activating suction, positioning to prevent pull on drain
- Applying a new dressing
- Disposing of old dressings

When teaching a patient about wound care in the home:

- Instruct when it is essential to wear gloves.
- If drainage system is in place, explain its purpose.
- Summarize teaching for wound care.
- Provide written instructions.
- Instruct when to call and make an appointment with the physician/surgeon.

---

chase the needed items. By teaching the patient the signs and symptoms of infection, and insisting that they be reported immediately, intervention can be started quickly to treat the infection. Written instructions should be sent home with the patient to reinforce the teaching. Patient Teaching 38-1 reviews points of patient teaching for wound care.

Suture Removal

The physician orders the removal of sutures. Some physicians prefer to remove their own sutures. Some states do not allow LPN/LVNs to remove sutures, but others do. Suture scissors, forceps, and sterile technique are used to remove sutures (Figure 38-15). The suture is clipped so that the exposed part will not be pulled through the skin (Steps 38-3). A special staple remover implement is used to remove staples (Figure 38-16). Inspect the suture after it is pulled out to see that it appears whole. Parts of sutures left under the skin cause inflammation because they are foreign bodies. Steri-Strips are often applied to reinforce the incision as sutures are removed (Figure 38-17).

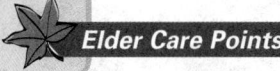

Elder Care Points

Healing time is slower in elderly persons with changes in circulation related to atherosclerosis or arteriosclerosis that can decrease blood flow to the wound area. Sutures may be left in a few days longer than in younger adults.

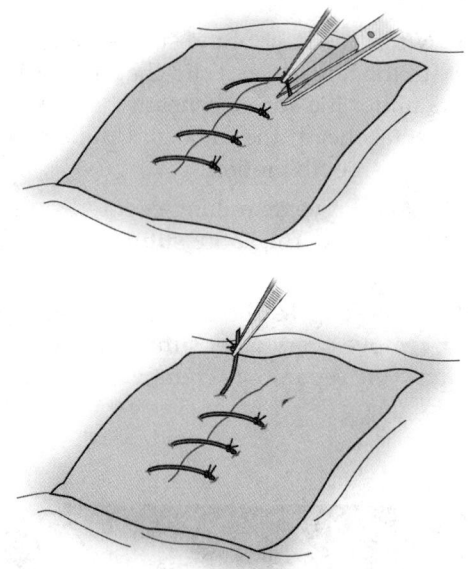

FIGURE 38-15 Clip beneath the knot with the scissors to remove the suture.

Eye, Ear, and Vaginal Irrigations

Irrigations must be performed when the face is involved in an injury and there is a possibility of debris or caustic substance in the eye. Irrigate the affected eye(s) with Standard Precautions and sterile solution or tap water depending on what is available. In the emergency room, special eyecups and a continuous irrigation system are used (Steps 38-4).

Steps 38-3 | Removing Sutures or Staples

Sutures or staples are removed when the wound is well sealed and connective tissue has formed. This occurs in 7 to 10 days, although the time for suture removal may vary. An order is required for removal of sutures or staples.

Review and carry out the Standard Steps in Appendix 3.

1. ***ACTION*** Perform hand hygiene, don clean gloves, and remove the dressing, discarding it in a plastic discard bag. Remove gloves and perform hand hygiene.

   RATIONALE Prevents transfer of microorganisms; exposes the sutures or staples.

2. ***ACTION*** Open the suture removal or staple removal set.

   RATIONALE Prepares the equipment for use.

■ For Sutures

3. ***ACTION*** Pick up the forceps with the nondominant hand and the suture scissors with the dominant hand.

   RATIONALE This allows good control of the instruments.

4. ***ACTION*** Lift the knot of the suture away from the skin with the forceps, and slip the curved tip of the scissors under the suture beneath the knot. The suture is cut beneath the knot and pulled from the skin in one smooth motion.

   RATIONALE Prevents pulling exposed suture back through the skin. The entire suture must be pulled free.

5. ***ACTION*** As long as the skin stays well approximated, remove every other suture. If wound shows no signs of separation, remove the remaining sutures.

RATIONALE Removing every other suture provides a safeguard in case the wound begins to separate.

■ For Staples

3. ***ACTION*** After opening the equipment, place the lower jaw of the staple remover under the staple. Be certain the tip is all the way under the staple.

   RATIONALE Positions the tool to crimp the staple.

4. ***ACTION*** Press the handles of the staple remover together all the way to depress the center of the staple.

   RATIONALE The staple must be firmly pressed between the two parts of the staple remover to allow it to be pulled free of the skin.

5. ***ACTION*** When both ends of the staple are visible, lift it up and away from the skin. Drop the staple into the discard bag.

   RATIONALE Removes the staple; prevents transfer of microorganisms and injury by a sharp object.

■ For Sutures and Staples

6. ***ACTION*** Gently cleanse any dried blood from the suture or staple sites with an antiseptic sponge.

   RATIONALE Suture holes are open to the atmosphere and can admit bacteria. Dried blood may contain microorganisms.

7. ***ACTION*** Place Steri-Strips or a dressing over the incisional area as ordered. Often the incision will simply be left open to the air.

   RATIONALE Secures the wound.

8. ***ACTION*** Place all used supplies in the discard bag. Remove gloves and discard them. Perform hand hygiene.

   RATIONALE Prevents transfer of microorganisms.

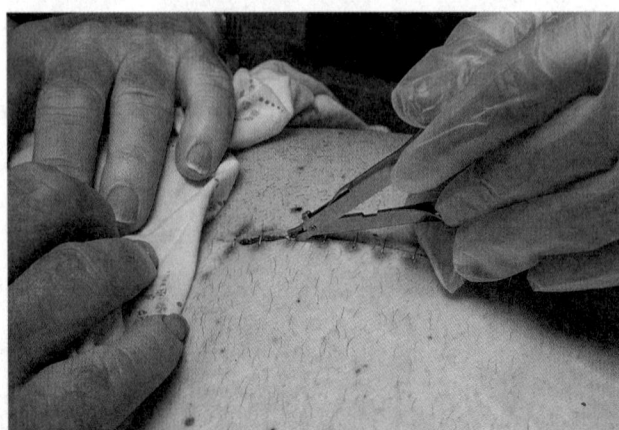

FIGURE **38-16** A special implement is used for staple removal.

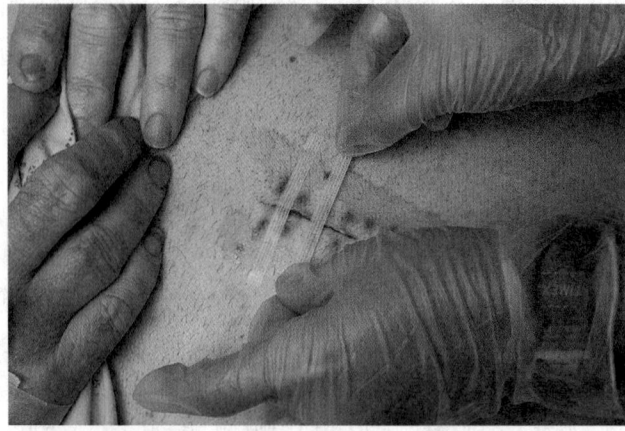

FIGURE **38-17** Apply Steri-Strips to support the incision after suture removal.

Steps 38-4 | Irrigating the Eye or Adult Ear

The eye may need irrigating when it has been injured by debris or chemicals. Irrigation is gently continued until debris is cleared away, or for 10 to 30 minutes after a chemical injury. The ear is irrigated when wax or debris is obstructing the canal and preventing sound from reaching the tympanic membrane.

Review and carry out the Standard Steps in Appendix 3.

■ Eye Irrigation

1. **ACTION** For irrigation with a syringe, place the patient in a supine position and turn the head in the direction of the affected eye. Position the examination light to illuminate the affected eye. Place an underpad and towel on the bed to protect the linens and clothes. Place an irrigation basin close to the face to catch the irrigation solution.

   RATIONALE Irrigation fluid will run away from the eye and not contaminate the other eye. Good light is needed to visualize the area well.

2. **ACTION** Prepare the irrigation set and fluid.

   RATIONALE Fluid should be at room temperature. Sterile normal saline or tap water is used.

3. **ACTION** Don gloves and remove any crusty discharge on the eyelid with a cotton ball moistened with sterile normal saline. Discard the used cotton balls in a discard bag.

   RATIONALE Using a fresh cotton ball for each stroke from the inner canthus to the outer edge maintains aseptic technique.

4. **ACTION** Load the irrigation syringe with fluid. With the nondominant hand, gently but firmly pull the upper eyelid toward the eyebrow and pull the lower lid down toward cheek to expose the conjunctival sac. Ask the patient to look downward.

   RATIONALE Assists in maintaining the eye in an open position to receive the irrigation fluid.

5. **ACTION** Hold the irrigation syringe about ½ to 1 inch above the eye and gently depress the plunger or bulb of the syringe to irrigate the eye, directing the stream from the nasal edge of eye across to the outer edge. Repeat the irrigation until the desired result occurs or the total amount of solution ordered has been used. Allow patient to close eye between washings if large amount of solution is required.

   RATIONALE Solution removes debris or contaminant from eye. Too much pressure of fluid may damage the cornea.

6. **ACTION** Dry the eyelid with a sterile cotton ball.

   RATIONALE Makes the patient comfortable.

7. **ACTION** Record the procedure.

   RATIONALE Documents how procedure was done.

■ Ear Irrigation

1. **ACTION** Place the patient in a sitting position. Drape the shoulder on the side to be irrigated with an underpad and towel, and place the light so that the area is well illuminated.

   RATIONALE The syringe is easier to use with the patient in a sitting position. Underpad and towel help keep the patient dry.

2. **ACTION** Fill the syringe with warm solution (98.6° F, or 37° C). Have the patient hold the basin firmly against the neck under the ear.

   RATIONALE Cool water is very uncomfortable and causes dizziness and nausea through stimulation of the equilibrium sensors in the semicircular canal. Positioning the basin properly prevents water from running down the neck.

3. **ACTION** Straighten the ear canal by grasping the upper portion of the adult pinna and gently pulling upward and backward.

   RATIONALE The canal is straightened so water can penetrate better and debris can be washed out.

4. **ACTION** Place the tip of the syringe just into the entrance of the external meatus, and point the tip upward and inward toward the posterior auditory canal; push the plunger or depress the bulb in slowly and carefully.

   RATIONALE The flow of solution is directed forward to wash out debris.

5. **ACTION** Inspect the ear canal to see that it is clean. Dry the ear and the neck area.

   RATIONALE Cerumen may still be blocking the canal.

6. **ACTION** Repeat until the canal is clean. Be certain solution is still warm.

   RATIONALE Allows visualization of the tympanic membrane and allows sound to reach the membrane.

7. **ACTION** Document the procedure.

   RATIONALE Records how the procedure was done and what result was obtained.

Ear irrigations are used to remove cerumen or foreign bodies that occlude the canal and prevent sound from reaching the tympanic membrane. An ear irrigation is ordered by a physician and should not be performed if there is a possibility that the tympanic membrane is perforated. The irrigation is performed in a fashion similar to the eye irrigation except the solution is directed toward the roof of the auditory canal while holding the pinna of the older adult up and out with the other hand (see Steps 38-4). The pinna for the child is pulled slightly up and back; for the infant, pull the pinna down and back. Sometimes a Water-Pik with a special nozzle is used to irrigate the ear. Only the lowest settings on the device should be used.

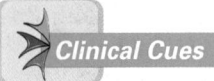

Clinical Cues

Instilling a wax softener such as Cerumenex per agency protocol prior to flushing the ear will make flushing quicker and easier on the patient. Allow the patient to rest for 10 to 20 minutes after instilling the drops before flushing the ear.

A vaginal irrigation may be ordered for infection or surgical preparation of the vagina. Most frequently the patient will administer the irrigation herself. Patient Teaching 38-2 presents the teaching guidelines.

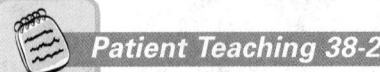

Patient Teaching 38-2

Giving a Vaginal Douche

A douche is most effective when given in the supine position. This may be accomplished by lying down in the bathtub. If a bathtub is not available, you may do the procedure while sitting on the commode.
- Empty the bladder before beginning and perform hand hygiene.
- Prepare the douche solution following the directions for dilution of the medication or antiseptic. The solution should be warm but not too hot.
- Run some of the solution through the tubing and nozzle to clear air from the tubing.
- Hang the bag no more than 18 inches above the hips. A coat hanger over a towel bar may be used to hang the solution container.
- Gently insert the irrigating nozzle, directing it downward and toward the back of the vagina.
- Hold the nozzle in place and open the clamp, allowing the solution to run in slowly and drain out.
- Rotate the nozzle gently during the treatment. Use all of the solution.
- If sitting on the commode, gently hold the labia together to distend the folds of the vagina with solution, then release so the fluid may run out.
- Remove the nozzle when all solution is used.
- Rinse the bag and tubing and wash the nozzle with soap and water and rinse. Allow to dry before storing the equipment.

Hot and Cold Applications

Either dry or moist forms of heat and cold can be applied to the body to promote healing. Usually a physician's order is necessary for a treatment because systemic as well as local effects occur. The order should include the body site to be treated, the type of treatment, and the frequency and duration of the application. Check your agency's policy for various types of heat and cold treatments.

Assessment of the patient and the area to be treated is essential to determine if there are contraindications for the treatment (Box 38-3). Always assess circulation in and around the area to be treated. Be certain that the patient has intact sensation so that damage will not occur from temperature extremes. When cold is applied to a lower extremity, assess for capillary refill, note skin color, and palpate skin temperature and distal pulses so that a baseline of the area can be documented in the chart.

Use of Heat. Heat is applied to the skin surfaces to provide general comfort and to speed the healing process (Table 38-2). Heat is often used for patients with musculoskeletal problems such as joint strains or low back pain. The amount of blood diverted to the skin through vasodilation reduces the blood circulating through internal organs and tissues. The degree of systemic effect is related to the size of the area to which heat is applied. Systemic circulatory changes may cause faintness, a faster pulse, and some degree of dyspnea. If such changes occur, closely monitor the patient's vital signs. The principles for application are the same for each method used when applying heat (Box 38-4). Heat can be applied locally by means of a

Box 38-3 *Contraindications for Heat and Cold Applications*

HEAT
- Heat should not be applied over an area in which active bleeding is occurring as it will increase the bleeding.
- Heat to the abdomen is contraindicated if there is a chance the patient has appendicitis because it may cause the appendix to rupture.
- If a patient has cardiovascular problems, it is unwise to apply heat to a large part of the body, causing massive vasodilation that may divert blood supply from major organs.

COLD
- Cold is not applied to an injury area if it is already edematous because it will slow circulation and prevent absorption of interstitial fluid.
- When neuropathy is present, cold is not applied because the patient is unable to determine if tissue becomes too cold.
- If the patient is shivering, cold is not applied. Shivering raises body temperature.

Adapted from Potter, P.A., & Perry, A.G. (2005). *Fundamentals of Nursing* (6th ed., pp. 554-556). St. Louis: Elsevier Mosby.

Table 38-2 *Therapeutic Effects of Heat and Cold Applications*

PHYSIOLOGIC RESPONSE	THERAPEUTIC BENEFIT
HEAT	
Vasodilation and increased capillary permeability	Increases blood flow to the body part, promotes delivery of nutrients and removal of wastes, and lessens venous congestion in the injured tissues
Reduced blood viscosity	Increases delivery of leukocytes and antibiotics to wound site to fight infection
Reduced muscle tension	Promotes muscle relaxation and reduces pain from spasm or stiffness
COLD	
Vasoconstriction	Reduces blood flow to injured body part preventing edema formation; reduces inflammation
Local anesthesia	Decreases local pain sensation
Reduced cellular metabolism	Reduces oxygen needs of tissues
Increased blood viscosity	Aids blood coagulation at injury site
Decreased muscle tension	Relieves pain

Adapted from Potter, P.A., & Perry, A.G. (2005). *Fundamentals of Nursing* (6th ed., p. 1555). St. Louis: Elsevier Mosby.

Box 38-4 | *Principles of Heat Application*

- Heat causes dilation of blood vessels and increases the supply of blood to the area.
- Heat stimulates metabolism and the growth of new tissues. Heat is effective in clearing away the debris of infection by bringing antibodies and leukocytes to the site and through suppuration (the formation of pus). Hot packs or compresses applied to infected sites promote earlier healing.
- Extreme temperature changes stimulate pain receptors. Heat application may be painful or soothing.
- Applications of heat to portions of the body activate the autonomic nervous system, which produces systemic responses in the body.
- Vasodilation of superficial vessels of the skin decreases the blood supply elsewhere in the body because the blood volume is constant in a closed system. Vasodilation produces skin redness and warmth.
- Water is more effective than air as a conductor of heat.

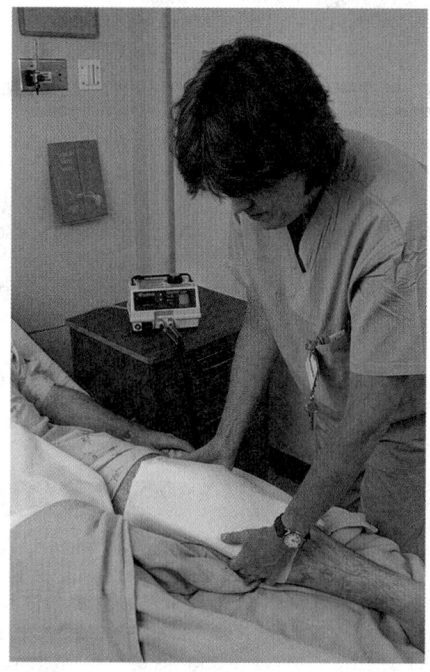

FIGURE **38-18** An aquathermia pad is applied for a heat treatment.

hot water bottle, electric pad, aquathermia pad, or disposable heat pack (Figure 38-18). Moist heat is used in the form of compresses, hot packs, soaks, or a sitz bath. (See Chapter 19 for information about the sitz bath.) Table 38-3 provides general ranges of temperature for heat application, but check the agency procedural manual for recommended temperatures.

To protect patients from burns caused by heat applications, measure the temperature of the liquid if possible. If no thermometer is available, place the prepared pack against the inner aspect of your own arm. If there is any doubt about whether it is too hot, cool it down. Use a flannel or cloth cover for all hot and cold packs. Observe the condition of the skin frequently for signs of burning or blistering and be attentive to complaints. Caution the patient and family not to increase the temperature of heating pads or of water in hot water bottles.

Heat Applications. Hot water bottles are filled two thirds full, the air is expelled, and the plug attached. A heat lamp is a gooseneck lamp with a 60-watt bulb. A heat lamp provides heat by radiation and is placed 18 to 24 inches (45 to 60 cm) from the area of treatment. Heat applications are left in place for 15 to 30 minutes and may be ordered to be repeated each hour or several times a day (Assignment Considerations 38-2).

An aquathermia pad, or K-pad as it is often called, is constructed with tubes containing water (Safety Alert 38-2). An electrically controlled unit pumps warmed water through the tubing network. The reservoir of the K-pad is filled to two thirds full with *distilled* water. The temperature is usually set with a key for 105° F (40.5° C). The pad is covered before application (see Figure 38-18).

When hot compresses are ordered, the solution is heated to the temperature ordered, and gauze or cloth is dipped in the solution and wrung out. When the skin is broken in the area of treatment, sterile technique is required. Sterile gloves and supplies must be

Table 38-3 *Temperature Ranges for Heat and Cold Treatments**

DESCRIPTION	RANGES
HEAT TREATMENTS	
Warm	93°-98° F (34°-37° C)
Hot	98°-105° F (37°-41° C)
Very hot	105°-110° F (41°-46° C) for at-risk adult or child under age 2
	105°-125° F (41°-51° C) for normal adult, dry heat only
COLD TREATMENTS	
Tepid	80°-93° F (26.7°-33.9° C)
Cool	65°-80° F (18.3°-26.7° C)
Cold	55°-65° F (12.3°-18.3° C)
Very cold	Below 55° F (below 12.3° C)

*Discontinue the treatment when numbness occurs.

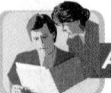

Assignment Considerations 38-2

Applying Heat Treatments

In many states, UAPs are allowed to apply heat treatments or warm moist compresses to wounds under the nurse's supervision. When assigning this task, you should remind the UAP of the proper temperature to maintain for the treatment, the specific time the treatment should be applied, and to notify you when the treatment is complete so that you can assess the wound area and the patient's response to the treatment.

Safety Alert 38-2

Precautions with Heating Pads

When the back is treated with a heating pad, do not let the patient lie on the pad. Heat is not dissipated properly if the patient lies on the pad, and burns can occur. Place the patient prone or on the side to apply the pad.

used. A small amount of solution is heated at a time. Petroleum jelly may be used beneath the compress or pack to protect the skin.

In the home, hot compresses can be made with washcloths dipped in hot water and wrung out. Once the compress is in place, placing a plastic wrap covering on top will help retain the heat longer. A towel may be placed over the plastic wrap. Gel packs are also available that can be heated in a microwave oven. A freshly boiled egg with the shell removed can be placed inside a sock to apply heat to an eye where inflammation is causing discomfort. The egg can be reheated in hot water. Dispose of the egg when treatment is finished.

When a soak is ordered, the part to be treated is submerged in warm water or solution for 15 to 20 minutes. A commercial pack is used to apply heat to a large area of the body.

Whenever heat is used, the safety of the patient must be protected. Some patients are much more likely

Safety Alert 38-3

Safety Factors When Applying Heat

Heat is not usually applied immediately after injury or surgery because it increases bleeding and swelling. Electrical appliances such as heating pads must be checked for defects by the agency engineering department. Check the appliance and the cord before use to prevent shock or sparks. Do not use anything with a frayed cord or loose plug. Avoid using safety pins with a heating pad or K-pad. Use an electric pad with moist packs only when the unit is designed to be used with moisture. When a heating pad is in use on a patient, check the temperature setting frequently.

to suffer burns: those with sensory impairment, impaired mental status with decreased level of consciousness or confusion, and impaired circulation from peripheral vascular disease, diabetes, or congestive heart failure (Safety Alert 38-3). When an appliance is no longer in use, return it to central service immediately so that charges to the patient will cease. Documentation of the use of heat or cold devices each shift is essential for insurance payment to the agency.

? *Think Critically About* . . . What would you do if you had been giving your patient a heat treatment with a heating lamp and, when you return to discontinue the treatment, you find she has lowered the lamp to within 6 inches of the treatment area and now the skin is very red and she says it is more painful?

Use of Cold. Cold is used for two main purposes: (1) to decrease swelling and (2) to decrease pain (see Table 38-2). Cold is often immediately applied to an injury to prevent swelling. When cold is applied to the skin or a part of the body, vasoconstriction causes the skin to become pale and cool. When it interferes with adequate circulation, it can cause damage to body tissues, as in the necrosis caused by frostbite.

Systemic effects of cold are the reverse of those of heat. More blood is sent to the internal organs and the body acts to conserve heat. The autonomic nervous system is activated, and muscle contractions may produce shivering in an effort to produce heat.

The physician will usually indicate the temperature to be used for cold applications (see Table 38-3). Very cold applications are used for 15 to 20 minutes at a time; longer application can damage the skin and underlying tissue.

Cold Applications. Cold is applied in the form of compresses, packs, ice bags, or ice collars, or by hypothermia blanket. Cold compresses consist of gauze or cloth material placed in a basin containing ice chips and a small amount of cold water. The compress is then wrung out and placed on the designated site. The compresses are changed every 15 to 20 minutes.

Cold packs are used for tonsillectomies, perineal wounds, sprains, nosebleeds, fractures of bones, dental extractions, and reduction of postoperative swelling of some parts of the body. Most disposable cold packs are applied directly to the skin, but check the manufacturer's directions. Ice bags or ice collars are reusable. Small ice bags can be made by placing ice chips loosely in a rubber glove and tying it with a knot. This works especially well for applications to the nose or eye. Gel packs are reusable and are placed in the freezer until frozen. When the gel pack becomes warm, it is cleansed and returned to the freezer.

A hypothermia blanket is used to lower body heat for patients who are running a persistently high fever. Because this treatment decreases the rate of metabolic processes, it may be used during surgery to reduce blood flow and oxygen requirements and is often used for patients who have severe brain injuries. The cooling blanket is attached to a machine that supplies the blanket with a cooled solution of distilled water and 20% ethyl alcohol. The blanket is placed in direct contact with the patient's skin. The patient's temperature is continually monitored when the blanket is in use. Chilling to the point of shivering is to be avoided because this activity causes the temperature to rise.

Most cold treatments require a physician's order before application. Care must be taken to assess the skin and circulation in the area of application, and distal to it, before, during, and after the treatment. Prolonged, very cold applications may cause frostbite. Cold therapy is applied for a maximum of 20 minutes at a time. Precautions taken are the same as those for patients who are at risk with heat applications (Home Care Considerations 38-1).

Patient Teaching for Hot and Cold Applications. Assess the caregiver's ability and availability to administer the hot or cold treatment safely. Sterile compresses can be prepared at home in a pressure cooker if one is available. Caution the patient and family not to heat washcloths or other linens in the microwave oven because fire can occur. Check the cords on home lamps to be used for heat treatments and on heating pads. Instruct the patient not to fall asleep on a heating pad and never to use the high setting because burns may occur.

A quick, efficient cold pack may be made by wetting a washcloth, folding it in quarters, and freezing it inside a zipper-locking–type of plastic bag.

Evaluation

Evaluative statements indicating that some previously stated goals/expected outcomes have been met are as follows:

- Wound edges well approximated.
- Wound is clean and dry without redness or swelling.
- Patient states that pain is gone.

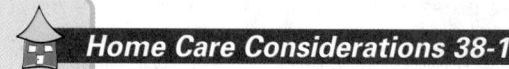

Home Care Considerations 38-1

Use of Cold in the Home Setting

In the home, ice bags can be made with crushed ice in tightly closed plastic bags. These should be wrapped in cloth such as a diaper or dish towel before application to the skin. A bag of frozen peas or corn is very effective when used as a cold pack. The vegetables can be refrozen for repeated treatment, but should be discarded after the end of treatments.

- Patient states that energy has returned and is up walking in the hall.
- Return demonstration of dressing change properly performed.

It is important to evaluate the outcome of the heat or cold treatment. Is it producing the desired effect? If not, it should be discontinued, or another method tried. When the outcome is such that the initial problem is gone, the physician is notified and the treatment is discontinued.

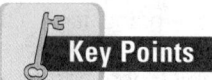

Key Points

- Wounds may be partial-thickness or full-thickness injuries.
- Partial-thickness wounds heal by epithelialization.
- Full-thickness wounds heal by contraction.
- The three phases of wound healing are inflammation, proliferation, and maturation.
- Necrotic tissue interferes with wound healing.
- Surgical wounds heal by first intention because there is little tissue loss at the surface.
- Wounds with tissue loss heal by second intention.
- Wounds are open or closed, clean or "dirty."
- Inflammation is a localized protective response brought on by injury or destruction of tissues.
- The cardinal signs of inflammation are swelling, erythema, heat, pain, and loss of function.
- Signs of inflammation subside as healing occurs.
- The elderly may heal less quickly than children or younger adults.
- A diet rich in protein; carbohydrates; lipids; vitamins A, B, and C; and the minerals zinc, iron, and copper is needed for wound healing.
- Regular exercise enhances blood circulation, bringing oxygen and nutrients to a wound.
- Smoking reduces the oxygen-carrying capacity of the blood and therefore slows healing.
- Steroids, other anti-inflammatory drugs, heparin, and antineoplastic agents interfere with healing.
- Wound infection slows the healing process.
- Chronic illness such as diabetes, cardiovascular disease, or an immune disorder may delay healing.
- Complications of healing are hemorrhage, infection, dehiscence, and evisceration.
- Wounds are closed with sutures or staples; traumatic wounds are trimmed and cleaned, and the edges well approximated when sutured.

- Negative pressure via vacuum-assisted closure may be used for chronic wounds that are not healing.
- The three basic wound types are red, yellow, and black.
- Red wounds are clean and ready to heal.
- A yellow wound contains debris or exudate and often becomes infected.
- A black wound needs débridement before it will heal.
- Wound drains are placed to provide an exit for blood and fluids that accumulate during the inflammatory process.
- To activate a wound suction device, the body of the device is compressed and the outlet is closed.
- The drainage device is emptied at the end of the shift using Standard Precautions; drainage is added to the total output.
- Draining a wound helps prevent the formation of an abscess or fistula.
- Dressings protect the wound and prevent microorganisms from entering or escaping from the wound. Dressings help to support and stabilize tissues and reduce discomfort from the wound.
- Binders are used to provide support as well as to hold dressings in place.
- Clean wounds should only be irrigated with normal saline; antimicrobial solutions damage granulation tissue.
- The dressing placed on an open wound depends on its classification or stage.
- Débridement is accomplished surgically or by enzyme or chemical formulas.
- Wounds must be carefully assessed for appearance, drainage, swelling, odor, approximation of wound edges, and pain; open wounds must be measured.
- Assessment for signs of infection is important; check for purulent drainage, odor, increased redness, pain, and swelling. On an extremity, limitation of movement may indicate infection. Systemic signs include a temperature greater than 101° F (38.3° C), a WBC count greater than 10,000/dL, and a feeling of malaise.
- Progress of healing is determined by decrease in size of the wound as well as appearance.
- Always assess for allergy to cleansing solutions, medications, and tape before beginning wound care.
- Nursing diagnoses always include impaired skin integrity and risk for infection. Other diagnoses are based on individual problems.
- Planning includes checking the physician's specific orders for wound care. Specific goals/expected outcome statements are written for the patient's individualized nursing diagnoses.
- Principles of asepsis are used for wound care; sterile technique is important for all wounds treated in the hospital until the wound is sealed. At home, clean technique may often be used.
- Patient teaching regarding wound care is an important and ongoing nursing intervention.
- Standard Precautions are used for every patient and are especially important during wound care, in which you come into direct contact with body fluids.
- Contaminated or infected wounds are cleaned at each dressing change.

- Hydrocolloid dressings are only applied to uninfected wounds; they keep the wound moist and absorb drainage.
- When irrigating a wound, the solution must reach all undermined areas and tunnels.
- Moist packing and a damp dressing help débride a wound and assist with the formulation of granulation tissue.
- Wet-to-dry dressings débride wounds, are painful when removed, and are not a treatment of choice anymore because they tend to remove new granulation tissue as well.
- Eye irrigation is used to remove debris or chemicals from the eye.
- Ear irrigation is used to remove cerumen or foreign bodies that occlude the auditory canal and prevent sound from reaching the tympanic membrane.
- Vaginal irrigations are ordered for surgical preparation and for medicinal purposes.
- Sutures are usually removed in 7 to 10 days, but may remain longer in elderly patients.
- Heat increases the blood supply, bringing oxygen and nutrients to the tissues and removing waste products and excess fluid, thereby reducing pain by reducing pressure on nerve endings.
- Systemic circulatory effects of applied heat may be faintness, a faster pulse, and some degree of dyspnea; monitor vital signs.
- Local applications of heat are used to relieve congestion and pain, reduce inflammation and swelling, relieve muscle spasm, provide comfort, elevate body temperature, and decrease blood supply in other areas of the body.
- Principles for safety are followed when applying heat. Temperature of the application is closely monitored.
- Heat may be applied by compress, soak, hot pack, hot water bottle, aquathermia pad, heat lamp, heating pad, and hot water bath.
- Cold is used to decrease swelling and pain.
- Care is taken to prevent tissue damage such as frostbite when applying cold.
- When cold is applied, more blood is sent to the internal organs.
- Very cold applications are used for 15 to 20 minutes at a time.
- Cold is applied in the form of compresses, packs, ice bags, or hypothermia blanket.
- Evaluate the outcome of a heat or cold treatment and wound care; determine if goals/expected outcomes are being met.
- Assess the home caregiver's ability to provide wound care or hot and cold treatments. Assess safety factors in the home environment, and check equipment to be used for the patient.

Go to your **Companion CD-ROM** for an Audio Glossary, animations, video clips, and more.

 evolve   Be sure to visit the companion Evolve site at http://evolve.elsevier.com/deWit/fundamental/ for additional online resources.

NCLEX-PN® EXAMINATION-STYLE REVIEW QUESTIONS

*Choose the **best** answer(s) for each question.*

1. Your patient has had abdominal surgery for a ruptured appendix and requires postoperative care and dressing changes. The wound has been left open and irrigations are ordered. When irrigating a wound, it is *most* important to:
   1. irrigate slowly to prevent discomfort.
   2. ensure the solution reaches the depths of the wound.
   3. prevent wetting of the bed and covers.
   4. use vigorous irrigation flow from the syringe.

2. If a wound appears infected, you should:
   1. cleanse it with an antiseptic solution.
   2. obtain an order for a culture to be performed.
   3. apply an antibiotic ointment.
   4. change the dressing every 2 hours.

3. The assessment of the wound indicates healing is occurring when:
   1. the center tissue is white.
   2. bleeding has stopped.
   3. there is no further drainage from the wound.
   4. pink granulation tissue is visible.

4. When assessing for wound infection, you know that signs of wound infection may be: *(Select all that apply.)*
   1. a rise in temperature.
   2. increasingly rapid respirations.
   3. a white blood cell count above 10,000/dL.
   4. restlessness and discomfort.
   5. purulent drainage.
   6. tenderness around the wound.

5. When caring for a pressure ulcer, you know that:
   1. eschar must usually be removed before the wound will heal.
   2. pink granulation tissue should be cleansed with antiseptic solution.
   3. keeping the wound dry and covered will aid healing.
   4. heat treatments hurt new tissue and slow healing.

6. Hydrocolloid dressings are useful for open wound dressings because they:
   1. keep the wound moist while blocking entry of microorganisms.
   2. débride the wound and soften eschar.
   3. supply bacteriostatic action to clean the wound.
   4. contain an antiseptic, allow moisture to evaporate, and protect the wound.

7. If you are assisting a surgical patient to the bathroom and he suddenly says, "It feels like something has given way," you would suspect that _____ has occurred. *(Fill in the blank.)*

8. Proper technique for removal of sutures is to:
   1. clip the suture opposite the knot.
   2. assure the patient that suture removal does not hurt.
   3. refrain from pulling exposed suture through the wound.
   4. apply a Steri-Strip before removing the suture.

9. Cold packs applied during the first 24 hours after injury decrease swelling by:
   1. increasing vasodilation so blood flow will carry away excess fluid.
   2. causing vasoconstriction and decreasing bleeding from damaged blood vessels.
   3. decreasing circulating blood volume so that swelling cannot occur.
   4. dulling pain and thereby reducing cellular enzyme release.

10. Heat is helpful in healing a wound because it:
    1. causes constriction of blood vessels and reduces edema.
    2. soothes nerve endings, lessening pain.
    3. causes vasodilation, bringing oxygen and nutrients to the injury.
    4. causes vasodilation, which moves blood out of the area.

CRITICAL THINKING ACTIVITIES  *Read each clinical scenario and discuss the questions with your classmates.*

Scenario A
Gregory Hansen requires a sterile dressing change for an abdominal incision.

1. How would you determine what is needed in the way of supplies?
2. How would you set up your sterile field? (Be specific.)
3. Because it is best not to talk while doing a sterile procedure, how would you begin to teach Mr. Hansen to do the dressing change himself?
4. Describe the factors you would assess to determine whether Mr. Hansen's wound is infected.

Scenario B
Joshua Weintaub just had surgery on his nose for a deviated septum. Ice packs are ordered. What would you use and how would you perform the ice applications?

Scenario C
Heat lamp treatments are ordered for the donor site from which skin graft material was taken on Bruce Herez's leg.

1. What type of lamp is used for this treatment?
2. How would you set up Mr. Herez and the lamp for the treatment?
3. How often would you check on Mr. Herez during the treatment?

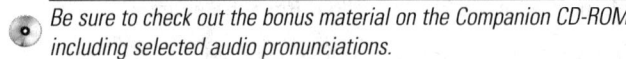

http://evolve.elsevier.com/deWit/fundamental/

Objectives

Upon completing this chapter, you should be able to:

Theory

1. Discuss the effects of inactivity on respiratory exchange and airway clearance.
2. Describe appropriate care of a cast as it dries.
3. Verbalize the differences among an air-fluidized bed, low air-loss bed, and continuous lateral-rotation bed, listing the reasons for their use.
4. Name at least four pressure relief devices that help prevent skin injury in immobile patients.
5. Describe how to perform a neurovascular assessment on an immobilized extremity.
6. Discuss the use of bandages and slings to immobilize a body part.

Clinical Practice

1. Correctly care for the patient undergoing skin or skeletal traction.
2. Teach a patient to properly care for a cast following discharge.
3. Correctly apply an elastic bandage to a stump after an amputation.
4. Use lift sheets and roller or slide devices to move immobilized patients.
5. Transfer a patient using a mechanical lift.
6. Assist a patient with the use of each of the following: walker, crutches, cane, brace, prosthesis, and wheelchair.
7. Devise a plan of care for meeting the psychosocial needs of the alert, immobile patient.

Skills and Steps

Skills

Skill 39-1 Cast Care
Skill 39-2 Care of the Patient in Traction
Skill 39-3 Transferring with a Mechanical Lift

Steps

Steps 39-1 Use of a Continuous Passive Motion Machine
Steps 39-2 Applying an Elastic Bandage
Steps 39-3 Applying a Triangular Bandage Sling

Key Terms

Be sure to check out the bonus material on the Companion CD-ROM, including selected audio pronunciations.

bivalved (BĪ-vălvd, p. 811)
blanch (p. 816)
cast (p. 811)
countertraction force (p. 810)
dorsum (DŌR-sŭm, p. 816)
external fixator (p. 812)
hemiparesis (hĕm-ē-pă-RĒ-sĭs, p. 815)
hemiplegia (hĕm-ē-PLĒ-jă, p. 815)
hydrotherapy (hī-drō-THĔR-ă-pē, p. 824)
hypostatic pneumonia (hī-pō-STĂT-ĭk noo-MŌ-nē-ă, p. 807)
immobilization (ĭ-mō-bĭl-ĭ-ZĀ-shŭn, p. 806)
isometric exercises (ī-sō-MĔT-rĭk, p. 808)
kinetic (p. 813)
moleskin (p. 811)
over-the-bed frame (p. 809)
paraplegics (păr-ă-PLĒ-jĭks, p. 829)
paresthesia (păr-ĕs-THĒ-zē-ă, p. 816)
perfusion (pĕr-FŪ-zhŭn, p. 816)
prosthesis (prŏs-THĒ-sĭs, p. 830)
quadriplegics (kwŏd-rĭ-PLĒ-jĭks, p. 829)
sling (p. 810)
spica casts (SPĪ-kă, p. 811)
splint (p. 809)
traction (p. 806)
trapeze bar (tră-PĒZ, p. 809)

Many conditions require bed rest in order for the patient to heal and recover. Strokes, chronic debilitating illness, trauma, and neuromuscular disorders all can bring periods of immobilization (rendering a part incapable of moving) to the patient. Problems caused by restriction of normal movement include pressure injuries, pneumonia, loss of bone mass, and permanent loss of function in the immobilized part. Many supportive or corrective measures necessary for treatment, such as traction (exertion of a pulling force), casts, or braces, also restrict mobility and may cause the same types of problems (Figure 39-1). Good nursing care is critical in preventing complications for immobilized patients.

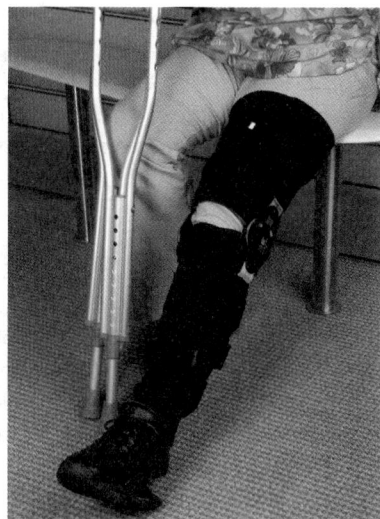

FIGURE **39-1** Patient with a leg brace or splint.

SYSTEMIC EFFECT OF IMMOBILIZATION

Decrease in muscle strength, generalized weakness, easy fatigue, stiff joints, abdominal distention, and diminished coordination begin with just a few days of immobility. Pressure ulcers are a frequent consequence of immobility. Table 39-1 presents the more severe problems that may occur when lack of activity occurs for a longer period of time. Pressure ulcer prevention is presented in Chapter 19.

One of the major concerns when a patient's movement is restricted is the development of respiratory complications. Activity causes people to breathe more deeply, expanding their lungs and encouraging clearing of normal secretions. Without adequate physical activity, these secretions can collect in the lower airways, leading to congestion and, ultimately, to respiratory illness, particularly hypostatic pneumonia (pneumonia caused by stasis of secretions due to inactivity, which provides a medium for bacterial growth) or hospital-acquired pneumonia.

Range-of-motion (ROM) exercises (see Chapter 18), frequent turning, and use of deep-breathing exercises can help prevent pneumonia and increase general oxygenation. Patients who are experiencing pain may be reluctant to move and breathe deeply, and pain control is essential. However, the medications used to control pain may cause sleepiness and further reduce desire to move about. Opioid analgesics such as codeine may depress respirations and further inhibit respiratory clearing (see Chapter 31). Measures to promote respi-

Table 39-1 *Effects and Problems of Immobility*

BODY PART OR SYSTEM	EFFECT OF IMMOBILITY	PROBLEM OR COMPLICATION
Cardiovascular system	Venous stasis	Thrombus formation
	Increased cardiac workload	Thrombophlebitis
	Blood pressure alterations	Pulmonary embolus
		Orthostatic hypotension
		Increased pulse rate
Respiratory system	Stasis of secretions	Hypostatic pneumonia
	Decreased elastic recoil	Bacterial pneumonia
	Decreased vital capacity	Atelectasis
		Decreased gas exchange
Gastrointestinal tract	Anorexia	Weight loss
	Metabolic change to catabolism and negative nitrogen balance	Protein deficiency
	Decreased peristalsis	Abdominal distention
		Constipation
Musculoskeletal system	Decreased muscle mass and muscle tension	Fibrosis of connective tissue
	Shortening of muscle	Atrophy
	Loss of calcium from bone matrix	Weakness
	Decrease in bone weight	Joint contracture
		Osteoporosis
		Bone pain
Urinary system	Stasis of urine	Precipitation of calcium salts
	Urinary tract infection	Frequency
	Renal stones	Dysuria
Skin	Decreased circulation from pressure	Skin breakdown
	Ischemia and necrosis of tissue	Pressure ulcers
Brain/psychological	Decreased mental activity	Disorientation
	Decreased sensory input	Confusion
	Decreased socialization	Boredom
	Decreased independence	Anxiety
		Depression
		Loneliness

ratory function must be included in the plan of care for the immobile patient.

Circulation is also affected by immobilization. Normal movement assists in venous return by compression of the muscles against the venous walls during muscle activity. Healthy, firm muscles provide general support for the venous walls. This is important throughout the body, but especially in the legs, where the force of blood flow is reduced because of the distance from the heart. Various conditions (such as a fracture, trauma, or debilitating illness) and treatments (such as casts, traction, or bed rest) can impair circulation and predispose the patient to pressure injury and permanent loss of function. For these reasons, the general circulatory status of the patient and blood flow to the affected areas of the body must be monitored on a regular basis; this is covered in the "Assessment" section of this chapter, which discusses assessment of color, sensation, and movement.

Increasing fluids to at least 3000 mL/day, encouraging adequate nutritional intake, and increasing fiber in the diet help prevent complications in the gastrointestinal system. The fluid increase also helps prevent urinary complications. Stool softeners and laxatives are ordered as needed for constipation.

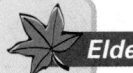 **Elder Care Points**

- Advanced age compromises the respiratory and circulatory systems and places elderly patients at even greater risk for complications of immobility.
- Another problem for the elderly is that inactivity tends to cause anorexia. Interventions for adequate nutritional care should be added to the care plan of the immobile elderly patient. Frequent small feedings and bedtime nourishments may be needed. Having their favorite foods brought in by family and friends can be very helpful.

Performing active or passive range-of-motion exercises helps prevent joint stiffness and muscle atrophy. Encouraging active movement of the unaffected extremities throughout the day assists in maintaining muscle tone. When the patient is on extended periods of bed rest, isometric exercises (exercises performed against resistance) may be appropriate if they are not contraindicated.

Turning the patient every 2 hours, keeping linens smooth and clean, and using pressure relief devices help prevent pressure ulcers. The skin must be kept clean and dry. Skin assessment is performed at least every 8 hours and more frequently for the patient at high risk for skin breakdown.

Children who are immobilized for an extended period may regress to an earlier stage of development. Extensive immobilization of a child often causes developmental delays. Diversionary activities for the child

are a considerable challenge. Access to a computer and computer learning and recreational games is helpful. Scheduled activities of art, story reading, and movies provide distraction. Developing a relationship with a pen pal by e-mail is another recreational possibility.

PSYCHOSOCIAL EFFECTS OF IMMOBILIZATION

Patients faced with movement restriction may experience a variety of emotional responses. Fear can be a major problem for these patients. They may be afraid that they will not be able to return to work and support themselves and those who depend on them. They may fear abandonment by those they love if they cannot function as they did before. Patients who are facing permanent loss may need professional counseling or a support group. This may also be true for significant others affected by the patient's condition. Be supportive, use therapeutic techniques of communication that focus on listening, and allow the patient to verbalize concerns. When signs of fear and stress are observed, take time to listen, and refer these patients to social service as appropriate.

Another frequent problem for the alert immobile patient is boredom. Not all patients like television or enjoy reading, and even those who do will become bored with nothing else to do. Chat with patients about things that interest them while providing their daily care. Some patients may want to do something creative, such as crocheting, crossword puzzles, or crafts. Encourage family and friends to space visits so the patient avoids long periods of loneliness. Family members can also help by contacting friends and relatives and asking them to send notes and cards on a regular basis. In addition to creating bright spots in the day, cards, letters, calls, and visits increase the patient's sense of value to others and feelings of self-worth. Positive feelings are known to play an important role in the healing process.

For the immobile patient being cared for at home, it may be helpful to move the bed into the living room or family room. This move allows the person to participate in family interactions and reduces isolation. It may also save many steps for those providing care, especially if the bedrooms are on a separate floor. Visits by home health aides and friends or respite caregivers can provide a chance for the caregiver to get out of the house and do errands or spend some time with friends or at leisure.

Remember that the nonalert or comatose patient also needs emotional support. Always assume that patients can hear and understand, even when they cannot respond or they respond inappropriately. Talk to the patient in a kind and caring voice. Explain what is being done before and as it is done, and apologize for any unavoidable pain the care may be causing. Talk to the patient about what is going on in the world. If cards or letters arrive, read them to the patient. Patients who have recovered from unconscious states have been known to describe in great detail things that happened while they were unconscious and have expressed thanks to those staff members who continued to treat them as valuable human beings.

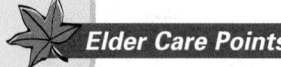

Elder Care Points

Following a stroke, hip fracture, or other condition that causes immobility, elderly patients may worry about becoming a burden to their families. This feeling may be so strong that they feel that it would be better if they died, and they become depressed. Encouragement and praise from the staff, kindness and patience when they attempt self-care or learn a new task, frequent family visits, and expressions of hope for recovery help reestablish their sense of self-worth. Consultation with social services may lead to solutions for financial concerns.

TYPES OF IMMOBILIZATION

SPLINTS

A **splint** is a device that protects an injured part of the body by immobilizing it. A splint may be used as a first aid measure before a cast or traction is applied to an injured part, or it may be used instead of a cast. Box 39-1 presents the guidelines for applying a splint. Several types of commercial splints are available: molded splints, immobilizers, inflatable splints, cervical collars, and traction splints (Figure 39-2). First aid splints are fashioned from materials at hand and require only some rigid material, padding, and something to secure the splint in place. Splints limit movement of the injured part. Inflatable splints help control bleeding as well as immobilize the injured part. The splint should be inflated until fingertips can only indent it 1½ inches (1.3 cm). Immobilizers are made of cloth and foam with Velcro straps. They are often used on an injured knee to prevent movement while an injury heals or during activity to prevent further injury. Molded splints keep the body part in a functional position to prevent contracture. They are used for chronic disorders. Traction splints are applied and hooked to traction ropes, pulleys, and weights to maintain pull on a fracture. An example is the Thomas splint used for a leg fracture.

TRACTION

Traction is the application of a pulling force, and it is used to maintain parts of the body in extension and alignment. It is used to realign bone ends following fracture and to relieve pain and nerve impairment caused by compression or muscle spasm.

The amount of traction is determined by the pull exerted by weights at the end of the traction ropes. The amount of weight must be ordered by the physician

| Box 39-1 | *Applying a First Aid Splint to an Extremity* |

When a serious injury or fracture occurs in the home or outdoor setting, it is advisable to render first aid by splinting the injured part. To apply a splint to an extremity:
- Handle the injured part gently and do not change its position in any way. This decreases the chance of nerve injury and further bleeding.
- Cover any open wounds with material as clean as can be found to help prevent infection.
- Use a rigid splinting material to immobilize the injured part. Flat boards, broom handles, rolled-up newspaper, or similar materials are appropriate. The splint should be long enough to span the joint above and below the injury.
- Pad bony prominences with soft material to prevent pressure wounds.
- Secure the splint with wide bands of material to stabilize the injured limb within the splint.
- Elevate the injured part to decrease edema and swelling.
- Check circulation distal to the injury and loosen the splint ties if tissue becomes pale, cold, or blue.
- Keep the person warm and seek transport to a medical facility.

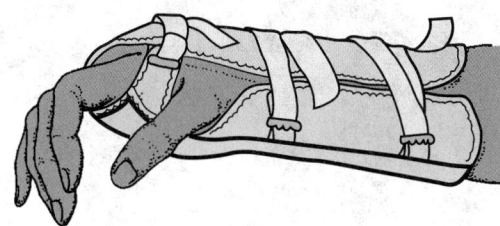

FIGURE **39-2** Wrist and forearm splint.

and often changes over the course of treatment. Initially the muscles tend to be tight and may go into spasm. A heavier weight is required to overcome the muscular pull and allow the body to resume a normal alignment. As time goes on, the muscles tire and relax; the amount of weight is then reduced. The physician will leave orders concerning if and how much the head of the bed may be raised. A slight Trendelenburg position may be ordered to keep the patient from slipping down in the bed. Tape a sign to the head of the bed indicating any restrictions related to bed positioning. **The weights should swing freely without touching the bed or floor.** The ropes must move freely through the pulleys to prevent injury to the patient and alteration in the effects of the traction. Principles to be followed for traction are listed in Table 39-2.

The patient in traction should have an **over-the-bed frame** (rectangular frame to which traction equipment may be attached) with a **trapeze bar** (overhead bar that patient can grab) attached to the bed (see Figure 18-9, *A*). The trapeze bar can be grasped by the patient with the hands to assist in repositioning. Teach the patient how to tell when body alignment is correct in the bed so that as he becomes more active, he can place himself in correct alignment to maintain the traction.

Table 39-2 *Principles of Traction with Nursing Interventions*

PRINCIPLE	NURSING INTERVENTION
Ropes and weights must be free of friction.	Keep ropes free of entanglement in the linens.
Maintain the correct line of pull.	Keep the patient centered in the bed with the body in good alignment.
Weight and pull of the traction must be continuous and as ordered by the physician.	Remove or add weights only by physician's order. Do not interrupt the pull of traction to provide care.
Sufficient countertraction must be maintained.	Keep the patient from sliding down in the bed when in leg or back traction.
	Keep the patient in sidearm traction in the center of the bed.

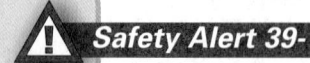

Safety Alert 39-1

Safety with Immobilization

Whenever a patient is in an immobilization device, be sure to check for adequacy of circulation in the affected part by assessing skin temperature and color, capillary refill when appropriate, and sensation.

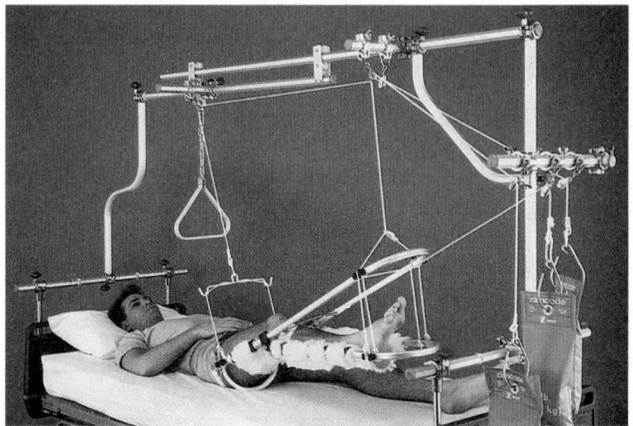

FIGURE **39-4** An example of skeletal traction.

Box 39-2 *Guidelines for Pin Care*

Always follow the physician's orders for cleansing solution and use or nonuse of antibiotic ointment. Some physicians order half-strength hydrogen peroxide in equal parts of normal saline for cleansing.
- Using sterile swabs, cleanse closest to the pin in a circular motion. Use one swab for each circle. Work your way out in succeeding circles until 1½ inches from the pin.
- Apply antibiotic ointment with a sterile swab if ordered.
- Dress with sterile gauze if ordered.
- Secure ends of wires with cork.
- Monitor for infection, assessing for increased pain, redness, edema, tenderness, or purulent drainage.

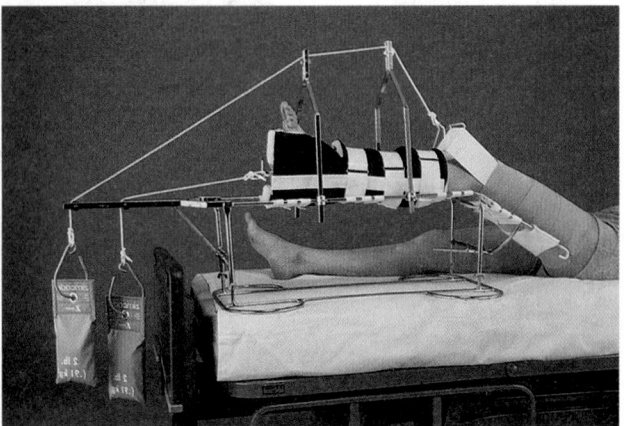

FIGURE **39-3** An example of skin traction.

Skin Traction

In skin traction, a Velcro boot (Buck's traction), belt, halter, or *sling* (bandage for supporting a part) is applied snugly to the skin, and the traction is attached to the appliance (Figure 39-3). Skin traction has the advantage of being noninvasive, and its main purpose is to decrease muscle spasm that accompanies fractures. Damage from skin traction includes blisters, rashes from irritation by adhesives, and skin tears and tissue injuries from the shearing effects of the lateral pull across the skin surface. The amount of weight that can be applied is limited to 5 to 10 lb. The skin must be checked frequently for any indications of injury, and any problems should be reported immediately to the physician or traction technician (Safety Alert 39-1). Any complaints by the patient of skin pain beneath the wrap or appliance must also be reported.

Skeletal Traction

Skeletal traction requires the surgical placement of pins, tongs, screws, or wires that are anchored to or through the bone and, therefore, pierce the skin (Figure 39-4). Traction is thus applied directly to the bone, which can support more weight than the skin. In larger hospitals, an orthopedic technician may set up the traction. The nurse is responsible for maintaining the correct weight and alignment of the traction and for maintaining a balance between traction pull and *countertraction force* (the weight pulling against the weight of the traction). Countertraction is provided by the weight of the patient and the position of the bed. Care of the skin around the openings for the pins, tongs, or wires is done according to the physician's order. Sterile technique is used when performing pin care (Box 39-2). After the sites are healed, they may be left open to the air. Clear fluid drainage is expected initially. Follow the physician's order and the policies of the facility, and report immediately any indication of infection at the wound sites. Circulation checks are performed every hour for the first 24 hours and every 4 hours thereafter.

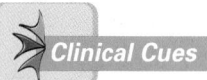

Think Critically About . . . What interventions would you use to prevent skin breakdown on the back and buttocks of the patient in traction?

CASTS

Patients may be placed directly into a cast (a stiff plaster of Paris, fiberglass, or polyester dressing used to immobilize) following a fracture or a variety of orthopedic procedures, or a cast may be applied following a period in traction. The skin is cleansed and inspected and any wounds are treated before a cast is applied. A layer of stockinette is applied first, followed by a thin layer of cotton or synthetic padding and then the cast material. Most casts are made of fiberglass, polyester resin, or thermoplastic material. Plaster of Paris casts are often applied to a lower extremity because they will withstand weight bearing better than the synthetics. Heat may be felt as the casting material is applied, especially with plaster of Paris. Casts made of synthetic material dry rather quickly (7 to 20 minutes), but plaster casts can take from a few hours to a couple of days to dry and be fully hardened. The synthetic cast may be hardened enough to be durable within 30 minutes. **It is critical that the cast be protected from uneven pressure during the drying period because the shape or position can be inadvertently changed.** When handling the cast, use the palm and flat parts of the fingers rather than the fingertips.

Clinical Cues

Dents in the cast can lead to circulatory impairment and pressure injuries, and changes in alignment can alter the position of the healing parts or impede circulation.

Swelling of the tissues is common during the first days after a cast is applied, and if left uncontrolled, this can impair the circulation and cause a pressure injury. A casted extremity should be elevated on pillows. If not padded sufficiently, the edges of the cast may rub or push against bony areas, causing pain and injury. The stockinette may be folded over the outside edge of the cast and taped to protect from chafing, or the cast edge may be "petaled" with waterproof tape. Changing position may relieve the problem, or adding extra padding beneath the edge of the cast may help.

If the cast becomes too tight, it may be bivalved (cut in half lengthwise) to relieve the pressure on the tissues. If there is a wound under the cast that needs

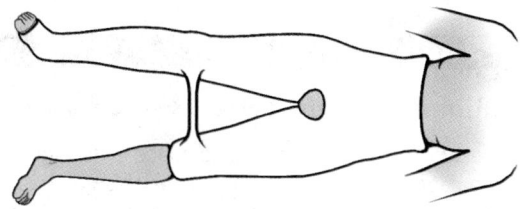

FIGURE **39-5** Hip spica cast.

observation, a window may be cut in the cast over the wound area. When edema has decreased, the cast is secured with outside bandaging or by more casting material. Sometimes after edema subsides, the cast is too loose and must be replaced.

Hip spica (figure-of-8) casts can be particularly challenging for both the patient and caregiver. Hip spica casts encase a portion of the trunk and part or all of both legs (Figure 39-5). A spreader bar is placed between the legs to maintain the desired angle at the hip and incorporated into the cast. **Do not use the spreader bar as a handle for lifting and turning the patient. It may be dislodged, ruining the cast and causing pain and possible injury to the patient.** Grasp the cast over the leg to assist in turning. Because of their size and thickness, hip spica casts often take longer to dry. Frequent turning is necessary, including placing the patient in a prone position to ensure complete and uniform drying.

Clinical Cues

A hair dryer set on low may used to assist in drying the plaster of Paris cast. Just be sure to uniformly dry all areas of the cast and lightly touch the cast frequently to make certain that it isn't becoming so hot that it will burn the patient's skin.

Toileting can be difficult for the patient with a hip spica cast. Ingenuity is needed to protect the cast from soiling. Using disposable plastic wrap around the perineal opening is one method of protection. When elevating a wet cast with pillows, use cloth-covered pillows because plastic-covered ones hamper drying.

Most patients can go home soon after cast placement. If the cast is not yet dry before discharge, instruct the patient and family or caregiver in the proper care of the cast to ensure uniform drying. Show them how to check the cast edges for rough spots or crumbling, how to use pillows to elevate the extremity and prevent swelling, and how to pad the rough edges using tape or moleskin (thick, durable form of adhesive material). Cast condition should be assessed every 8 hours, checking for cracks, crumbling, or rough edges. A damaged cast may need to be replaced (Safety Alert 39-2).

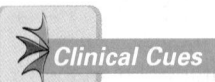

Safety Alert 39-2

Precautions When the Patient Has a Cast

Patients must be cautioned not to place a foreign object under the cast (e.g., wire hanger or stick to scratch an itch). Blowing cool air under the cast with a can of electronic air cleaner may help decrease itching. Discomfort can sometimes be relieved by directing the air of a hair dryer set on "cool" into the cast. Castblast is a commercial product that delivers a soothing layer of talc under the cast.

A major concern for patients with casts is bathing. Plaster casts must be kept dry, or they can disintegrate. Even fiberglass casts are a problem if they become thoroughly wet. The outside material tolerates water, but the padding inside tends to stay wet, causing irritation to the skin. Small casts, such as those that immobilize the forearm or lower leg, can often be covered with a large plastic bag taped in place to allow the patient to shower. Larger casts, however, usually require that the patient take sponge baths until the cast is removed.

When a child is sent home with a cast, it is important to stress the dangers of placing small items inside the cast. These can cause pressure **necrosis** and infection.

Casts are removed using an oscillating saw. The saw is noisy and may frighten the patient. The saw does not cut down to the skin, and the patient needs reassurance about this. After separating the cast material, scissors are used to cut through the stockinette and padding and the cast is removed.

Clinical Cues

It is best to warn the patient that the skin underneath a cast that has just been removed will be dry and dirty in appearance. Otherwise the patient may become quite dismayed at the appearance of the area. Washing with warm soapy water, rinsing, and applying cream or lotion removes dead skin cells and helps the skin return to normal. Vitamin E or other recommended ointment rubbed over the healed incisions may improve appearance also.

EXTERNAL FIXATORS

An external fixator is a metal device, such as a pin, screw, or tong, that is inserted into or through one or more bones to stabilize fragments of a fracture while it heals (Figure 39-6). The metal inserts are attached to a metal frame. This type of immobilization allows the patient to be more active during healing while maintaining immobilization of the fractured area. The pins, screws, or tongs and the frame should be checked for stability every 4 hours. The insertion of the metal device through the skin provides a break in skin integrity

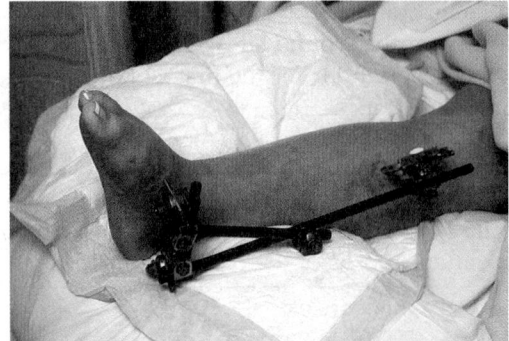

FIGURE **39-6** An external fixator holding fractured bones in place.

that requires regular pin care to prevent infection (see Box 39-2). Pin care is included in Skill 39-2 later in this chapter.

DEVICES USED TO PREVENT PROBLEMS OF IMMOBILITY

SPECIALTY BEDS

On occasion, illness or injury may result in long-term or permanent immobility. Pressure ulcers, complications of immobility, and hospital-acquired infections such as pneumonia are serious concerns. In such instances, patients may benefit from the use of specialty beds or turning frames designed to prevent tissue or structural injury and hospital-acquired infections. A number of manufacturers make such beds and frames, and they serve a variety of purposes. The use of specialty beds is designed to improve patient outcomes and augment nursing care. Because their use is very expensive, thorough ongoing documentation of need is essential.

Air-Fluidized Beds

Air-fluidized beds have tiny silicone beads contained within the bed under a flexible, air-permeable filter sheet (Figure 39-7). Warmed air passes through the small particles, setting them into motion so that they

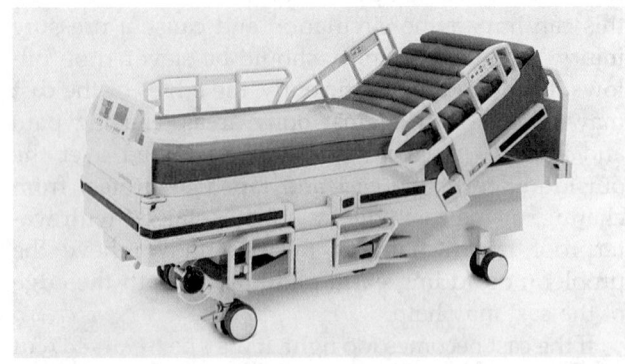

FIGURE **39-7** CLINITRON-Eleixis air-fluidized therapy unit.

act as a fluid that suspends the patient free from contact with any stationary, hard surface. The flotation or buoyancy of the patient on the air-fluidized beads prevents pressure occlusion of blood vessels and shearing of tissues against the mattress during movement, unlike conventional mattresses. The loose filter sheet reduces friction, and the warm air protects the skin from damage by wetness. Air-fluidized therapy is effective in the prevention of pressure injury and helps reduce generalized body pain common among bedridden patients. The indications for use include those patients with full-thickness or multiple pressure ulcers, fresh grafts, or flap repairs of injuries and immobile patients whose general condition puts them at high risk for skin breakdown. Air-fluidized therapy is not recommended for patients with unstable spines or patients who are ambulatory. To maximize the beneficial effects of the therapy, the unit should be in the fluidized mode at all times. Exceptions would be during patient transfer in and out of the bed or during nursing procedures for which the patient needs to be in one stable position for the intervention.

Low Air-Loss Beds

Low air-loss support is achieved by distributing air through multiple cushions connected in a series. The cushions are calibrated to provide maximum pressure relief for the individual patient. Shear and friction are reduced or eliminated because the cushions give with the patient during movement or rest. A low airflow through the cushion controls moisture on the skin. Segments of cushions may be deflated for patient care. The head of the bed can be raised. This bed is contraindicated for the patient with an unstable spine.

Continuous Lateral-Rotation Beds

Lateral-rotation therapy such as that delivered by the Roto-Rest bed is believed to decrease the incidence of lung collapse and hospital-acquired pneumonia, facilitate the normal flow of urine, and reduce the risk for deep vein thrombosis and pulmonary embolism by encouraging venous flow. This intervention may have a significant positive effect on various body systems of the critically ill patient and thereby improve the overall patient outcome. Skin breakdown is reduced by the pressure-reduction foam and gel pack surface. The patient is secured in position on the bed by multiple cushion wedges (Figure 39-8). The bed turns in an arc up to 80 degrees and can be set to pause on either side for up to 30 minutes. The rotation is stopped and the wedge cushions removed as needed for bathing, procedures, or toileting. There is a built-in scale to allow weighing of critically ill patients.

The degree and rate of movement are programmed to meet the individual patient's requirements. The constant side-to-side movement prevents the accu-

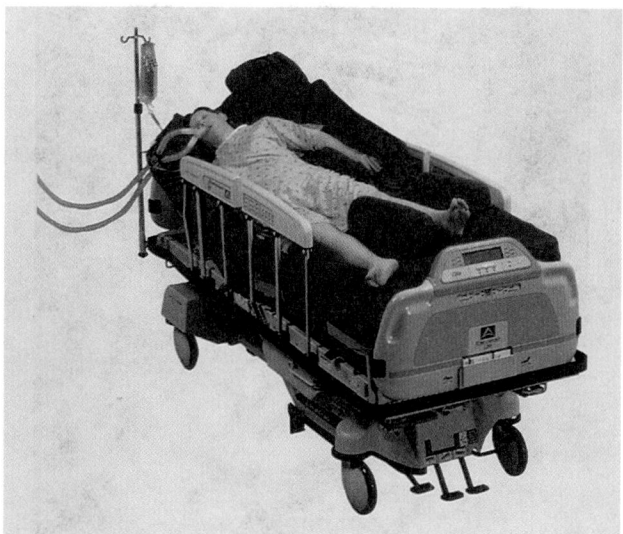

FIGURE **39-8** Roto-Rest Delta continuous lateral-rotation kinetic therapy bed.

mulation of respiratory secretions and promotes respiratory clearing. Other lateral-rotation beds are combined with low air-loss technology to provide relief of tissue pressure.

CircOlectric Bed

The CircOlectric bed is still occasionally used, particularly for the burn patient. It is supported in a large circular frame with the patient secured to a bed frame within the circle. The bed frame can move in a 360-degree arc, allowing a change of position for the patient.

> **?** *Think Critically About . . .* What types of problems, if any, do you think you might encounter when caring for a patient in a kinetic (moving) or air-fluidized bed?

PRESSURE RELIEF DEVICES

There are a variety of accessories that aid in the reduction of skin trauma from pressure for patients in standard hospital beds. These include foam and gel pads, sheepskin pads, heel and elbow protectors, and pulsating air pads and water mattresses that lie on top of the regular mattress (Figures 39-9 and 39-10).

CONTINUOUS PASSIVE MOTION MACHINE

After orthopedic surgery to replace a joint, continuous passive motion is often ordered to restore joint function. A continuous passive motion machine is used to exercise the extremity and joint, thus preventing contracture, muscle atrophy, venous stasis, and thrombus formation. The equipment extends the extremity to a prescribed angle for a specific period of time and then releases the joint, flexing it again. The

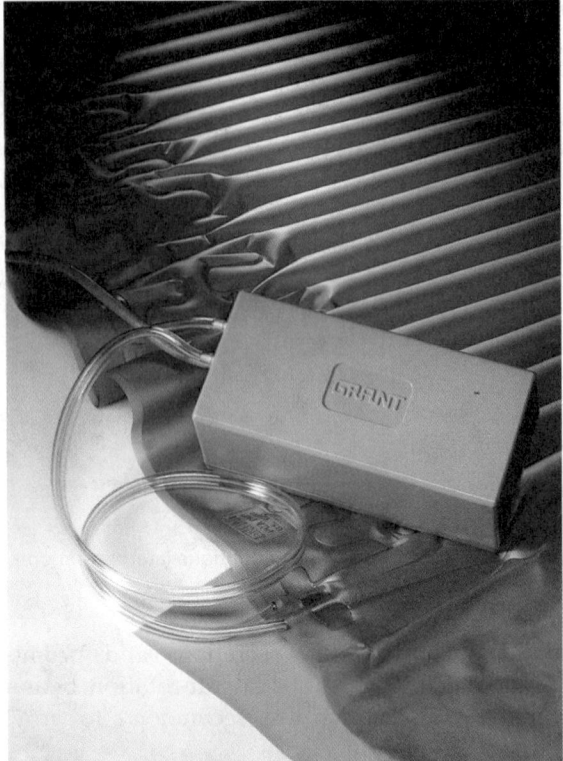

FIGURE **39-9** Alternating air mattress pad.

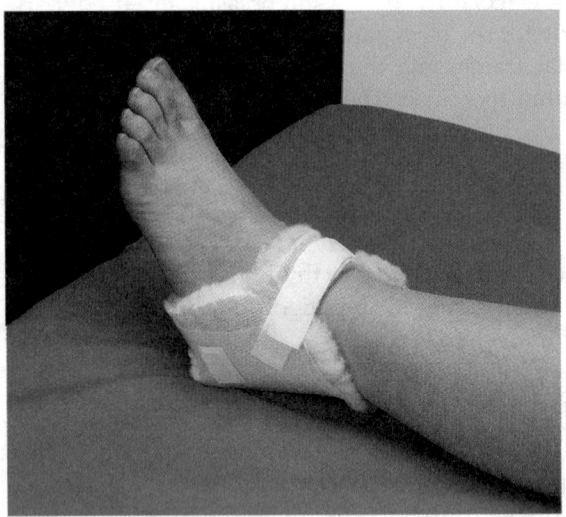

FIGURE **39-10** Heel protector helps prevent skin breakdown.

machine operates continuously as long as it is switched on. As the degree of joint motion is tolerated, the settings are altered to increase the mobility of the joint (Figure 39-11).

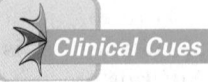

Assess pain level and medicate with ordered analgesia before initiating treatment with this machine. Closely monitor for need of more analgesia throughout exercise. The use of the machine is initially quite painful. **Pain is controlled best when it is treated before it becomes severe.**

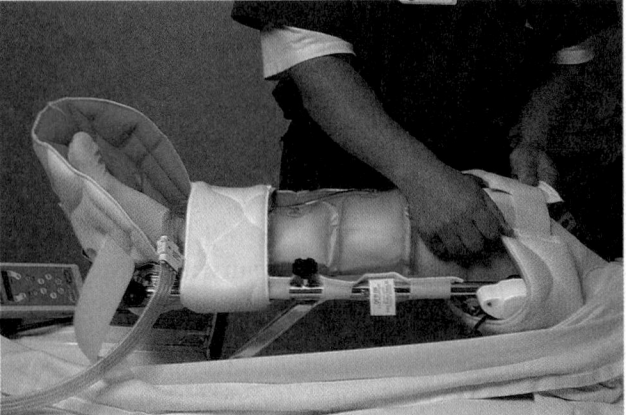

FIGURE **39-11** Continuous passive motion machine for the knee joint.

The dressing is checked for need of reinforcement before attaching the extremity to the machine. The machine is placed in position by two people because it is quite heavy. Checks for function of the machine and electrical safety are performed prior to placing the machine on the bed. Follow Steps 39-1 to initiate therapy.

THERAPEUTIC EXERCISE

Physical therapy is often ordered for the patient who is immobilized for an extended period of time. The physician indicates what the problems are for the patient, and the therapist performs an evaluation and then designs an exercise program to help the patient and to prevent further musculoskeletal problems from occurring. Full ROM exercises should be performed either actively or passively several times a day. (Range-of-motion exercises are presented in Chapter 18.) To prevent joint injury while performing passive ROM exercises, support the limb to be exercised above and below the joint. When the physical therapist is not available, the nurse assists the patient to perform these exercises. A family member or significant other can also be shown how to assist the patient with exercise.

APPLICATION of the NURSING PROCESS
Assessment (Data Collection)

When performing head-to-toe assessment of the immobilized patient, be alert to indicators of circulatory impairment such as reddened areas, pale or blue skin, coldness, or diminished or absent pulses. Look for signs of respiratory impairment such as shallow breathing, rapid or depressed respiratory rate, cough, abnormal lung sounds, use of accessory muscles, retractions or grunting, generalized paleness, duskiness, or cyanosis.

In addition to regular assessment, you should determine which activities of daily living the immobi-

Steps 39-1 Use of a Continuous Passive Motion Machine

The most common use of a continuous passive motion (CPM) machine is for the knee following knee replacement surgery. The nurse is responsible for making certain the machine is attached properly and that the settings are what the surgeon ordered.

Review and carry out the Standard Steps in Appendix 3.

1. **ACTION** Check the order for flexion and extension limits and extremity involved.

   RATIONALE Provides data for setting up the machine.

2. **ACTION** Place machine on bed directly on sheet-covered mattress.

   RATIONALE Provides a stable surface. No extra mattress pad should be under the machine.

3. **ACTION** Connect the control box to the CPM machine and set the limits of flexion and extension.

   RATIONALE Prepares machine for function.

4. **ACTION** Set machine speed control to slow or moderate range.

   RATIONALE Speed is ordered by the physician.

5. **ACTION** Let machine run through one complete cycle.

   RATIONALE Ensures that the CPM is working properly.

6. **ACTION** Stop the machine at end of extension. Center the extremity on machine with sheepskin beneath the extremity and adjust the machine to fit the patient. Align the patient's joint with the machine joint and strap the extremity in place.

   RATIONALE Prepares the machine to work on the joint properly. Avoids pressure on the extremity and protects the skin.

7. **ACTION** Start the machine. When it reaches full flexion, stop the machine and check the degree of flexion.

   RATIONALE Ensures that machine is not flexing the joint more than desired, preventing complications.

8. **ACTION** Set the cycle rate, start the machine, and observe for two full cycles.

   RATIONALE Ensures that machine is functioning correctly. Cycle rate is usually between 2 and 10 cycles per minute.

9. **ACTION** Raise side rails of bed to keep machine in place. Keep bed flat with head raised only 20 degrees if necessary.

   RATIONALE Ensures that machine can function as ordered and patient's body will remain in alignment.

10. **ACTION** Assess patient's comfort level.

    RATIONALE CPM therapy may be initially painful, and patient should be medicated regularly as ordered for pain. When pain is controlled, patient is more able to tolerate increases in speed and flexion.

11. **ACTION** Assess the operative site for bleeding and evaluate alignment of extremity and placement of straps every 2 to 4 hours.

    RATIONALE Prevents complications and promotes patient's compliance with therapy.

12. **ACTION** Assess skin condition over bony prominences and provide skin care every 2 hours.

    RATIONALE Helps prevent pressure ulcers from occurring.

---

lized patient can perform and with which assistance is needed. Incorporate assistance needs into the nursing care plan. Continually assess for pain and discomfort.

Perform a neurovascular assessment for any patient with a cast or traction device (Box 39-3). Assess for cultural beliefs and customs that should be considered in planning care.

When the patient is in traction, assess the pulleys and ropes for proper function and free movement. Ensure that the weights are hanging free and the correct amount of weight is applied. Assess the pin, the wire, or the tong insertion sites for indications of infection.

For the patient in a cast, sniff at the edges of the cast for a foul or musty odor. Other indicators of infection are an elevated temperature, pus-like drainage, and/ or an elevated white blood cell (WBC) count.

Assess any aids to ambulation for structural problems, fit, and safety as well as the patient's ability to use them correctly. Assess the assistive device for correct length or height in relation to the patient's height and posture. Check the foot of the crutch or cane for an intact rubber tip or the walker for properly functioning wheels if they are present. Assess patients' gait with the device to determine their stability (Figure 39-12).

Nursing Diagnosis

Common nursing diagnoses for patients with immobility are as follows:

- Impaired physical mobility related to hemiparesis/hemiplegia (one-sided weakness/one-sided paralysis)

Box 39-3 | **Neurovascular Assessment**

Neurovascular assessment is performed for every patient who has experienced a fracture, whether treated with a cast or traction. It should be performed every hour for the first 24 hours, and if the cast is dry, then every 4 to 8 hours. Check agency protocol for specific time schedule.

Skin: Inspect area distal to the injury. Palpate skin temperature with **dorsum** (back) of the hand; compare with opposite extremity or site.

Movement: Have patient move area distal to the injury, or move it passively. There should be no discomfort.

Sensation: Inquire about feelings of numbness or tingling **(paresthesia).** Check sensation with a paper clip and compare bilaterally. Sensation should be the same.

Pulses: Palpate pulses distal to the injury. Compare bilaterally if possible.

Capillary refill: With thumbnail, press the nail beds distal to the injury to **blanch** (to become pale) and judge time for capillary refill to occur after releasing pressure. Should be within 3 seconds, or within 5 seconds in the elderly.

Pain: Inquire about the degree, location, nature, and frequency of pain, noting any increase in intensity or change in type of pain.

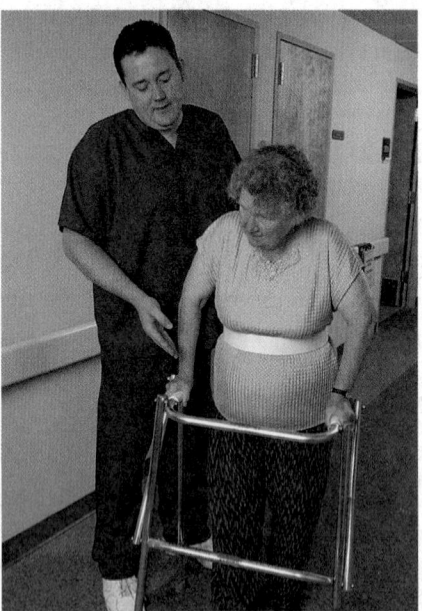

FIGURE **39-12** Assess the gait of the patient learning to use a walker.

- Impaired physical mobility related to fractured extremity in traction or a cast
- Ineffective tissue perfusion (circulation of blood through tissue) related to decreased circulation in the lower extremities
- Impaired tissue integrity related to skin disruption
- Pain related to tissue or bone injury, or muscle spasm

- Ineffective airway clearance related to inactivity and bed rest
- Risk for disuse syndrome
- Risk for peripheral neurovascular dysfunction related to fracture and cast application

Nursing diagnoses related to the psychosocial needs of the immobile person are as follows:

- Social isolation related to immobility
- Disturbed body image related to brace or cast
- Deficient diversional activity related to immobility and bed rest
- Situational low self-esteem related to inability to perform usual roles

Planning

Planning care for the immobile patient requires careful consideration of the time needed to assist the patient with various aspects of activities of daily living, the time needed for treatments, and time to be spent providing diversional activity and socialization. Expected outcomes for some of the above nursing diagnoses might be as follows:

- The patient will demonstrate the ability to cope with physical mobility limitations as evidenced by resumption of as many self-care activities as possible within 10 days.
- The skin will remain intact and free of pressure-related injuries.
- The patient will have pain controlled with medication and alternative techniques.
- The patient will maintain good respiratory status as evidenced by effective airway clearing and normal breath sounds bilaterally.
- The patient will not experience contracture or muscle atrophy from immobilization.
- The patient will show no evidence of peripheral neurovascular dysfunction from swelling and/or cast application.
- The patient will maintain regular contact with significant others, participating in diversional activities.
- The patient will maintain interest in events occurring in the outside world.
- The patient will evidence self-esteem by positive self-statements and voluntary participation in self-care and attention to grooming.

Implementation

Appropriate interventions related to the identified nursing diagnoses would include regular turning and positioning, use of pressure relief devices, coughing and deep-breathing exercises, ROM exercises, assisted ambulation, and visitation or activities addressing the psychosocial needs of the immobile patient. Nursing Care Plan 39-1 presents interventions for a specific patient.

When caring for a patient in a fresh plaster cast, elevate the cast on pillows if possible. This places a soft, yielding surface against the plaster that is less likely to

NURSING CARE PLAN 39-1

Care of the Patient Immobilized by a Stroke

SCENARIO Millie Palmer, age 76, is admitted after suffering an apparent cerebrovascular accident (CVA, stroke). She has left-sided hemiparesis and poor bladder control. She is confused and somewhat groggy. A computed tomography (CT) scan shows that the problem is from a thrombosis (clot), and she is started on heparin to prevent further thrombi from forming.

PROBLEM/NURSING DIAGNOSIS *Stroke with left sided-weakness*/Impaired physical mobility related to weakness of left extremities.
Supporting Assessment Data: *Objective:* Weakness of left arm and left leg; CVA.

Goals/Expected Outcomes	Nursing Interventions	Selected Rationale	Evaluation
Patient will maintain muscle tone in all muscles. Patient will maintain joint mobility in all joints.	Reposition q 2 hr.	Repositioning prevents pressure ulcers and provides comfort for joints.	*Is muscle tone being maintained?* Some tone to muscle.
	Passive ROM to left extremities tid.	Passive ROM will help maintain muscle function and joint mobility.	ROM performed.
	Active ROM to other joints bid. Encourage to perform ADLs as possible.	Active ROM will preserve muscle tone and joint function.	Actively moving other extremities and joints.
	Assess for muscle spasm each shift.	Muscle spasm may occur with hemiparesis and can be painful.	Progressing toward expected outcomes. Continue plan.

PROBLEM/NURSING DIAGNOSIS *Unable to reposition self*/Risk for impaired skin integrity related to decreased mobility and incontinence.
Supporting Assessment Data: *Objective:* Left-sided weakness, confusion; incontinent of urine.

Goals/Expected Outcomes	Nursing Interventions	Selected Rationale	Evaluation
Skin will remain intact.	Assess skin each shift and when turning, with special attention to pressure points.	Frequent inspection of skin reveals reddened areas before pressure ulcers form.	*Is skin intact?* Skin remains intact; area of redness over right ankle; heel protector applied to protect ankle.
	Use cushioning devices under pressure points as needed.	Cushioning reduces pressure over bony prominences.	
	Offer bedpan q 2 hr.	Opportunity to void q 2 hr helps prevent incontinence.	
	Check adult diaper frequently and change quickly when wet; clean and dry the skin.	Moisture contributes to skin breakdown. Keeping skin clean and dry prevents breakdown.	Meeting expected outcomes. Continue plan.

PROBLEM/NURSING DIAGNOSIS *Clot interrupting blood flow in brain*/Ineffective cerebral tissue perfusion related to thrombosis.
Supporting Assessment Data: *Objective:* Cerebral thrombus demonstrated on CT scan.

Goals/Expected Outcomes	Nursing Interventions	Selected Rationale	Evaluation
Neurologic deficits will not increase.	Neuro assessment & vital signs q 2 hr.	Assessment will reveal deteriorating condition in a timely fashion.	*Are there neurologic deficits?* Left-sided weakness present.
	Administer heparin as ordered.	Heparin will help prevent formation of further thrombi.	No change in neurologic status.
	Monitor APTT for therapeutic response to heparin.	APTT levels will demonstrate whether heparin dose is sufficient.	Progressing toward outcomes. Continue plan.

Key: *ADLs,* Activities of daily living; *APPT,* activated partial prothrombin time; *ROM,* range of motion; *tid,* three times daily.

Continued

NURSING CARE PLAN 39-1

Care of the Patient Immobilized by a Stroke—cont'd

PROBLEM/NURSING DIAGNOSIS *Incontinent of urine*/Functional urinary incontinence related to CVA.
Supporting Assessment Data: *Objective:* Left-sided weakness, confusion; incontinent of urine.

Goals/Expected Outcomes	Nursing Interventions	Selected Rationale	Evaluation
Patient will regain continence.	Institute bladder training program in 2 days.	Bladder training regimen can reinstitute urinary continence in many stroke patients.	*Is patient continent?* Not completely; some intermittent uncontrolled voiding.
	Offer bedpan q 2 hr.	Opportunity to void q 2 hr helps prevent incontinence.	Voids in bedpan after meals.
	Obtain order for bedside commode.	With hemiparesis it is easier to transfer to the bedside commode than walk to the bathroom to void.	
	Check diaper frequently; change when wet.		Progressing toward outcomes. Continue plan.

❓ CRITICAL THINKING QUESTIONS

1. How might incontinence affect this patient psychologically?

2. If Mrs. Palmer says that she is too tired to do the exercises and all she feels like doing is sleep, how would you respond?

Key: *ADLs,* Activities of daily living; *APPT,* activated partial prothrombin time; *ROM,* range of motion; *tid,* three times daily.

---

alter the shape of the cast. Elevating the extremity will reduce the likelihood of swelling. Turn the patient hourly so the cast rests on a different area of its surface. This will help the cast to dry evenly, as will a circulating fan. Skill 39-1 presents the points of care for the patient with a cast. For the patient going home with a cast in place, review cast care and assessment of problems with the patient and caregiver (Patient Teaching 39-1).

Care of the patient in traction is time consuming because the patient's mobility is severely limited. Skill 39-2 presents the points of care for the patient in traction.

Bandages Used to Support, Apply Pressure, or Immobilize

Elasticized bandages are applied to immobilize a joint, or to apply pressure to reduce swelling. They may also be used to provide support to a wound and hold dressings in place. Elastic bandages are made in rolls of varying widths; the heavy stretch material conforms to the body part and provides support (Box 39-4, p. 822).

Steps 39-2 on p. 822 show the technique for application of an elastic bandage. The same technique is used for gauze roller bandages. Different bandaging techniques are applied depending on the part to be bandaged.

Circular Turn. Circular turns are used to anchor the bandage and to terminate the wrap. This turn is useful for bandaging the proximal aspect of the finger or wrist. Simply hold the free end of the rolled material in

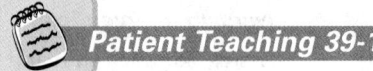

Patient Teaching 39-1

Fracture and Cast Care

To promote healing of your fracture and care for your cast:

- Keep the casted limb elevated above heart level whenever possible to prevent swelling.
- Call the physician if your fingers or toes become numb, tingle, turn blue, or are cold to the touch when the ones on the opposite hand or foot are warm.
- Call the physician if you develop a fever, have unusual pain in the casted extremity, or notice a bad odor coming from the cast. These could be signs of infection.
- Regularly perform the exercises your physician or physical therapist has taught you. These will help you retain your muscle strength while the bone heals.
- If the cast becomes loose or slides, call the physician because it probably will need to be changed.
- Do not get a plaster cast wet. Check with your physician about bathing or swimming with a synthetic cast.
- Do not insert any object inside the cast to relieve an itch. Doing so may damage the skin and result in an infection.
- Do not bear weight on the cast unless your physician has said it is all right to do so.

Skill 39-1 | Cast Care

Casts may be applied to almost any area of the body. The larger and thicker the cast, the longer it takes to dry fully. Hip spica and full-body casts may take 1 to 2 days to dry completely. Synthetic material casts dry much more quickly than plaster casts.

■ Supplies

✓ Tape or moleskin
✓ Pen for marking drainage
✓ Lamb's wool for padding

Review and carry out the Standard Steps in Appendix 3.

■ Assessment (Data Collection)

1. **ACTION** Examine the cast for any dents. Handle the cast gently with the flats of the fingers and the palms, not the fingertips.

   RATIONALE Dents may cause compression on underlying tissues. Fingertip pressure more easily dents the cast because the pressure is on a small area rather than spread over a broader surface.

2. **ACTION** Examine the cast for any areas where blood may have seeped through. Circle any such areas in ink and write the date and time on the cast.

   RATIONALE Bloodstains seeping through the cast are a common occurrence when surgery has preceded the application of a cast. Marking provides a way to judge further bleeding.

3. **ACTION** Assess the cast for rough edges and excessive tightness by running a finger along all cast edges and under the edges next to the skin.

   RATIONALE A finger should slip easily under the edge of the cast. Checking helps to discover problem areas.

■ Planning

4. **ACTION** Plan to reassess a new cast every hour for the first 24 hours and every 2 to 4 hours thereafter or per agency policy.

   RATIONALE Swelling may occur in the period after injury or surgery and may cause pressure on nerves and vessels.

■ Implementation

5. **ACTION** Pad any rough edges by petaling with 1½- to 2-inch pieces of tape or moleskin. Place lamb's wool beneath cast to pad under rough spots.

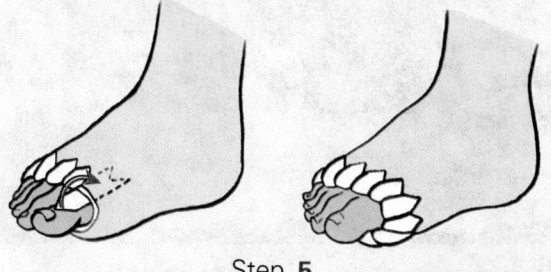

Step **5**

RATIONALE Rough spots will cause skin chafing, abrasion, and breakdown.

6. **ACTION** Notify the orthopedic technician or the physician if any area of the cast is too tight.

   RATIONALE The cast may need to be cut to relieve the pressure.

7. **ACTION** Elevate the casted extremity so that the hand or foot is at the level of the heart.

   RATIONALE Elevation aids in reducing or preventing swelling.

8. **ACTION** For patients in large casts (e.g., hip spica and body), place the bed in a slight Trendelenburg position for the first day or two to help prevent swelling, unless contraindicated by the patient's condition or the physician's orders.

   RATIONALE Patients in large casts may experience swelling in the legs, thighs, perineum, buttocks, and lower abdomen during the first few days. Placing the bed at an approximate 10-degree angle in a Trendelenburg position will help prevent this swelling.

9. **ACTION** Turn the patient at intervals so that all surfaces of the cast are exposed to the air to facilitate even drying and to prevent skin pressure ulcers.

   - When the cast is still wet, turn the patient hourly.
   - As the cast dries, every 2 hours is sufficient unless the patient is uncomfortable.
   - Get adequate help when turning the patient to prevent injury.
   - Use pillows to prop the patient at different angles as the cast dries.

   RATIONALE Air exposure allows moisture to evaporate.

10. **ACTION** Instruct patient not to use sharp, pointed, or rigid items to scratch under the cast.

    RATIONALE The skin under the cast often itches. Using such items to scratch can injure the skin. If itching is severe, ask for an order for medication to control it.

11. **ACTION** Smell the open edges of the cast to assess for infection under the cast.

    RATIONALE Skin injuries may become infected or necrotic and cause a foul or musty odor.

Continued

Skill 39-1 | Cast Care—cont'd

■ Evaluation

12. **ACTION** Evaluate the cast by inspecting for crumbling or cracks. Ask yourself: Is there any discomfort under the cast? Is the cast rubbing the skin anywhere? Are the edges smooth? Is the cast drying evenly? Is swelling in the tissues subsiding?

   RATIONALE Answers to these questions tell whether the interventions are successful in meeting the expected outcomes.

■ Documentation

13. **ACTION** Document assessment findings and interventions on the daily flow sheet or in the nurse's notes.

   RATIONALE Verifies that assessment has been performed and interventions carried out.

Documentation Example

7/29 1015   Received from recovery room alert and stable. Fresh plaster cast encases right leg from mid-thigh to mid-toes. Toes pink, warm, move well; sensation present; capillary refill less than 2 seconds.

Edge of cast easily admits fingertip. Leg elevated on pillows.

_____
(Nurse's signature)

■ Special Considerations

✓ Provide full instructions for cast care for the patient discharged home with a cast.
✓ Instruct to use a hair dryer only on the "cool" setting to help dry the cast or relieve itching.
✓ Demonstrate how to wrap a cast in plastic for showering, if appropriate.
✓ Demonstrate how to handle the extremity when repositioning, supporting the joints.

?CRITICAL THINKING QUESTIONS

1. What would you do if you notice the edge of the cast is crumbling?
2. What would you tell a patient with a long leg cast who keeps slipping a ruler down in the cast to scratch the skin?

Skill 39-2 | Care of the Patient in Traction

Skin traction is mostly used to decrease muscle spasm after a fracture or back muscle injury. Skin traction may be used on small children with a lower extremity fracture. Skeletal traction is used to anchor the traction directly to the bone and is used when significant weight is necessary to maintain bone alignment, such as in the adult with a fractured femur.

■ Supplies

✓ Cleansing agent for pin care
✓ Antibacterial ointment (if ordered)
✓ Small plastic disposal bag
✓ Sterile gloves
✓ Sterile dry swabs
✓ Dressings (if needed)

Review and carry out the Standard Steps in Appendix 3.

■ Assessment (Data Collection)

1. **ACTION** Check the physician's order for the desired amount of weight for traction.

   RATIONALE Ensures that the correct amount of weight is applied.

2. **ACTION** Assess the boot, wrap, or skeletal traction appliance. Check that ropes and pulleys are working smoothly and that weights are hanging free.

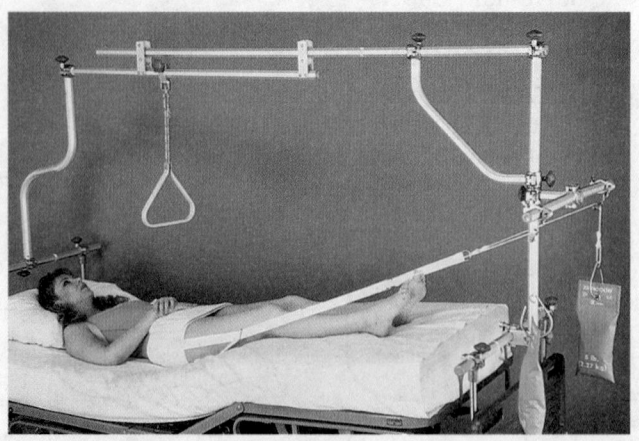

Step **2**

RATIONALE Surface of appliance should be smooth and free of wrinkles or gaps to prevent pressure injury to the skin. Appliance should not be rubbing on any skin surface. Traction will not function properly if ropes are hung up in pulleys or weights are resting on the floor or bed.

3. *ACTION* Assess the skin, distal circulation, and sensation.

   RATIONALE Detects signs of complications.

■ Planning

4. *ACTION* Plan times into work schedule to perform assessments, treatments, and activities of daily living (ADLs).

   RATIONALE Care for the immobile patient in traction takes more time.

■ Implementation

5. *ACTION* Realign the patient in the bed as needed to maintain optimal traction pull.

   RATIONALE A direct straight line is needed for traction to be completely effective. Patients need to be pulled up in the bed periodically.

6. *ACTION* Perform hand hygiene, prepare the supplies, don gloves, and cleanse the skin around pin, wire, or tong insertion sites per agency protocol or physician's orders; maintain sterile technique. Use a different sterile cotton-tipped applicator for each pin site.

   RATIONALE Entry sites into the bone may become infected if sterile technique is not used. Using the same applicator on two different pin sites transfers microorganisms from one site to the other. There is a high risk of osteomyelitis if bone infection occurs.

7. *ACTION* Apply antibacterial ointment if ordered; follow agency protocol.

   RATIONALE Some agencies and physicians do not use antibacterial ointment on insertion sites.

8. *ACTION* Discard used supplies in the plastic discard bag.

   RATIONALE Assists in preventing spread of microorganisms.

9. *ACTION* Remove gloves and perform hand hygiene.

   RATIONALE Reduces transfer of microorganisms.

■ Evaluation

10. *ACTION* Evaluate for signs of complications. Ask yourself: Is there any colored drainage from the insertion sites? Does the patient have a temperature elevation? Is there pain at the insertion sites? Is there a musty or foul odor at the insertion sites? Is the traction apparatus functioning correctly?

    RATIONALE Answers to these questions reveal whether the interventions are successful.

■ Documentation

11. *ACTION* Document interventions performed on the activity flow sheet; note any abnormal assessments in the nurse's notes with action taken.

    RATIONALE Verifies performance of traction care, amount of weight applied, and assessment findings.

Documentation Example

7/30 1300   Pin sites red and swollen; white drainage. Cleansed with normal saline, and Bactroban applied.

_____

(Nurse's signature)

■ Special Considerations

✓ It is important to evaluate and medicate the patient in traction for pain, especially in the first few days when muscle spasm occurs.

✓ Teach family and significant others that they must not tamper with the traction device, ropes, or weights.

✓ A trapeze bar attached to the over-the-bed frame is very helpful so that the patient may assist in repositioning; it also provides opportunity for exercise of the upper extremities.

?CRITICAL THINKING QUESTIONS

1. What would you say to a nurse who is helping a patient move up in the bed if she lifts the weights attached to the leg traction?

2. What activities might be good for a patient who is confined to bed in traction to combat boredom?

one hand and wrap it about the area, bringing it back to the starting point (Figure 39-13, *A*).

Spiral Turn. This turn is used to bandage parts of the body that are uniform in circumference, such as the upper arm or upper leg. The spiral turn partly overlaps the previous turn. The amount of overlap varies from one half to three fourths of the width of the bandage (Figure 39-13, *B*).

Spiral Reverse Turn. Spiral reverse turns are used to bandage body parts that are not uniform in circumference, such as the lower leg or forearm. After securing the bandage with circular turns, the bandage is brought upward at a 30-degree angle. The thumb of the free hand is placed on the upper edge of the bandage to hold it in place while it is reversed on itself. Unroll the bandage about 6 inches (15 cm) and turn the hand so that the bandage falls over itself. Continue the bandage around the extremity, overlapping each previous turn by two thirds the width of the bandage. Make each turn at the same position on the extremity so that the turns of the bandage are all aligned (Figure 39-13, *C*). Care should be taken not to apply undue pressure over a major blood vessel.

Figure-of-8 Turn. Figure-of-8 turns are used to bandage and stabilize an elbow, knee, or ankle, or to immobilize and hold a fractured clavicle in position. Anchor the bandage with two circular turns. Bring the bandage above the joint, around it, and then below it, making a figure-of-8. Continue bandaging above and below the joint, overlapping the previous turn by one third to two thirds the width of the bandage (Figure 39-13, *D*). Secure the bandage above the joint with two circular turns and fasten it.

Box 39-4 *Guidelines for Applying an Elastic or Roller Bandage*

- Elevate the limb and support it while applying the bandage.
- Face the patient and wrap the bandage from the distal to the proximal area.
- Apply even pressure by exerting equal tension throughout the wrapping of the bandage.
- Overlap turns of the bandage equally.
- Smooth the bandage, removing wrinkles, as you wrap it.
- Secure the end of the bandage with self-adherent portion of the bandage, a safety pin, or tape. (Metal clips may come loose and land in the bed, where they can injure the patient.)
- Check the color and sensation of the part distal and proximal to the bandage when finished and at frequent intervals thereafter.
- Remove the bandage for bathing of the body part; assess the skin for irritation or breaks; rewrap the bandage at least twice a day.

Steps 39-2 | **Applying of an Elastic Bandage**

The type and size of the bandage used will depend on the area to be bandaged and the purpose of the bandage. The physician usually orders the type of bandage.

Review and carry out the Standard Steps in Appendix 3.

1. **ACTION** Wash and dry the area to be bandaged.

   RATIONALE Helps prevent infection by removing microorganisms.

2. **ACTION** Elevate the extremity to be bandaged; ask an assistant to help if necessary.

   RATIONALE Elevation encourages venous return and helps prevent swelling. It is easier to wrap the bandage properly if someone else supports the extremity.

3. **ACTION** Stand in front of the patient and unroll the end of the bandage slightly; anchor it in place with the thumb of the nondominant hand on the anterior part of the extremity to be bandaged.

   RATIONALE Secures the bandage while wrapping is occurring.

4. **ACTION** Make two initial circular turns to anchor the bandage in place.

   RATIONALE Securing the bandage end prevents it from becoming loose.

5. **ACTION** Use a circular, spiral, spiral reverse, figure-of-8, recurrent turn, or thumb spica bandaging technique as appropriate for the area to be bandaged.

   RATIONALE The body part to be bandaged will indicate which style of bandaging is best.

6. **ACTION** Apply the bandage smoothly and evenly with light to moderate tension.

   RATIONALE Smoothness helps prevent pressure areas; adequate tension is necessary for the bandage to stay in place.

7. **ACTION** Secure the bandage with self-adherent portion of bandage, tape, or a safety pin.

   RATIONALE The bandage must be secured to remain in place.

8. **ACTION** Assess the bandage for fit and circulation distal to the area bandaged.

   RATIONALE A bandage applied too tightly will impede circulation; a loose bandage will fall off.

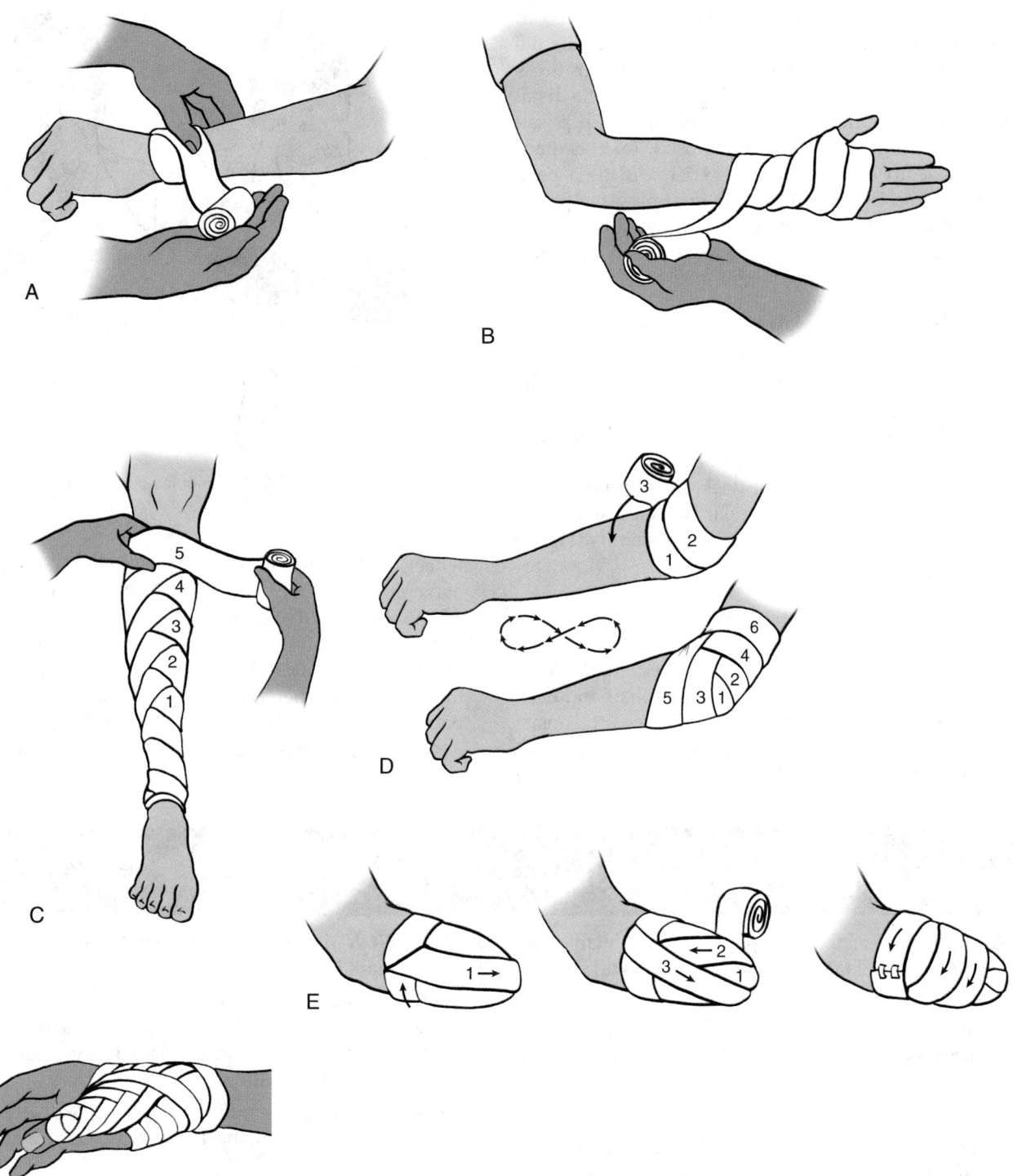

FIGURE **39-13** Applying an elastic bandage: **A,** Starting a bandage with circular turns. **B,** Bandaging with spiral turns. **C,** Bandaging with spiral reverse turns. **D,** Bandaging a joint with figure-of-8 turns. **E,** Recurrent turn bandaging. **F,** Thumb spica bandaging.

Recurrent Turn. This turn is used to cover distal parts of the body, such as the end of a finger, the skull, or the stump left by amputation. The bandage is anchored by two circular turns. It is then folded back on itself and brought centrally over the distal end to be covered. Hold it in place with the other hand and bring the bandage back over the end to the right of the center bandage but overlapping it by two thirds the width of

the bandage. Then bring the bandage back on the left side, overlapping the first turn by two thirds the width of the bandage. Continue alternating bandaging right and left until the area is well covered. Terminate the bandage with two circular turns and secure the end appropriately (Figure 39-13, *E*).

Thumb Spica. This is a variation of the figure-of-8 bandage used to support the thumb in neutral position following a sprain or other injury. The technique can also be used to bandage the hip or shoulder. For the thumb, secure the bandage with two circular turns around the wrist. Bring the bandage down to the distal aspect of the thumb and encircle the thumb. If possible, leave the tip of the thumb exposed. Take the bandage back up and around the wrist, and then back down and around the thumb, overlapping the previous turn by two thirds the width of the bandage. Repeat the above steps, working up the thumb and hand until the thumb is covered (Figure 39-13, *F*).

Immobilizing and Supporting with a Sling

A sling may be used to support and immobilize an injured wrist, elbow, or shoulder. The sling holds the extremity in an elevated position to avoid edema of the hand, pain and discomfort, and fatigue. A commercially made arm sling can be placed about the arm and the straps adjusted about the neck. If this type of support is not available, a triangular bandage sling may be used to support the injured upper extremity (Figure 39-14, Steps 39-3).

Using a Mechanical Lift to Transfer the Immobile Patient

Lifts can be used to move immobile patients from the bed to a stretcher, a chair, or a wheelchair and back again. Mechanical lifts, such as the Hoyer lift, consist of a sturdy metal frame with a wide base of support from which a canvas sling is suspended. The lift is on

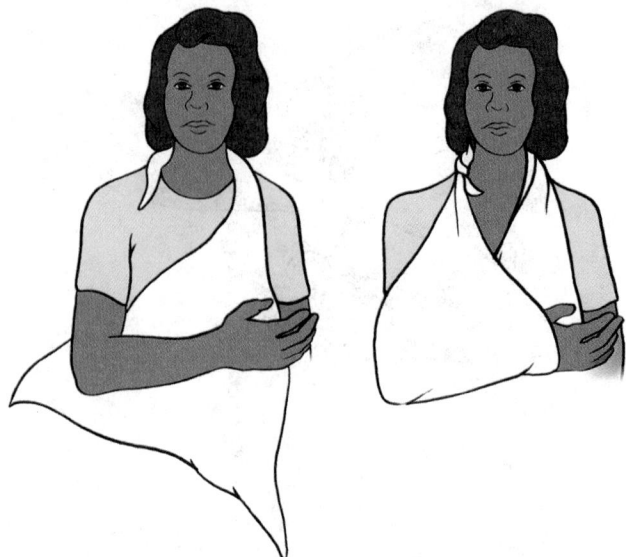

FIGURE **39-14** A triangular sling bandage.

wheels and, when empty, can be easily moved by one person. A hydraulic pump device allows one nurse to lift the weight of the patient, but it takes two people to use a mechanical lift safely—one to raise and move the lift and one to guide the patient into the chair or onto the bed or stretcher. Such lifts are also used to place patients into a tub or whirlpool bath for bathing or hydrotherapy (massage or débridement by moving water).

Steps 39-3 Applying a Triangular Bandage Sling

When a commercial arm support is not available, use a triangular bandage to form a sling. This will support the upper extremity.

Review and carry out the Standard Steps in Appendix 3.

1. **ACTION** Place one end of the triangle over the shoulder on the uninjured side.

   RATIONALE Positions the sling properly.

2. **ACTION** Position the point of the triangle toward the elbow. Ask the patient to bend the injured arm horizontally across the body with the thumb toward the body. Place the bandage under the arm flat against the chest.

   RATIONALE Forms the sling support.

3. **ACTION** Bring the other end over the injured arm and shoulder while the patient keeps the elbow bent at right angles across the lower chest. The hand should be about 4 inches higher than the elbow.

   RATIONALE Finishes forming the sling support. Elevating the hand prevents the fingers from swelling.

4. **ACTION** Tie the two ends at one side of the neck in a square knot.

   RATIONALE Secures the sling; the knot at the side prevents discomfort when the patient lies down and decreased pull on the back of the neck when the arm is in the sling.

5. **ACTION** Fold the point of the triangle neatly over the elbow toward the front and secure it with a safety pin.

   RATIONALE Keeps the elbow and sling from slipping back and forth.

6. **ACTION** Check the circulation in the fingers, comparing color of the nail beds and temperature of the hand with the other hand.

   RATIONALE Fingers should be pink and warm; cold or bluish fingers indicate impaired circulation.

Any patient requiring the use of a lift must never be left unattended in the lift or while in the tub or whirlpool bath. When using a lift, explain to the patient exactly what is being done. Many patients feel somewhat frightened being lifted off the bed or out of a chair by a mechanical device and may need a great deal of reassurance. However, the proper use of a mechanical lift allows the nurse to move weak or helpless patients safely while avoiding self-injury (Skill 39-3).

Before placing a patient on the sling, be sure the skin is clean and dry. Protect the sling as needed with a sheet or bath blanket. If soiled, the sling must be washed with a disinfectant solution before using it again.

Skill 39-3 | Transferring with a Mechanical Lift

Mechanical lifts allow immobile patients to be moved safely between two points some distance apart. A lift may also be used to elevate helpless patients while the bed is changed under them.

■ Supplies
✓ Mechanical lift with sling
✓ Bath blanket or sheet
✓ Chair, wheelchair, stretcher, or clean tub (to receive patient)

Review and carry out the Standard Steps in Appendix 3.

■ Assessment (Data Collection)

1. **ACTION** Determine that lift is functioning correctly and that the sling is clean.

   RATIONALE Promotes smooth, safe use of the lift.

2. **ACTION** Assess patient's readiness to be transferred.

   RATIONALE Patient will suffer less anxiety if prepared for the procedure.

■ Planning

3. **ACTION** Obtain the assistance of a second person.

   RATIONALE Two people are needed to safely transfer a patient using a lift.

■ Implementation

4. **ACTION** Position the chair, wheelchair, or stretcher correctly, clearing away any obstructions; set the brakes if applicable.

   RATIONALE A clear floor is needed to maneuver the lift. Setting the brakes prevents the chair or stretcher from moving while transferring the patient.

5. **ACTION** Raise the far side rail, adjust the bed to working height, and lock the wheels.

   RATIONALE Bed adjustment allows proper use of body mechanics and decreases the risk of injury to the patient and nurse. Locked wheels prevent the bed from moving while transferring.

6. **ACTION** Roll the patient onto the side and place the sling on the bed positioned from back of the head or the shoulders to mid-thigh; roll patient onto the sling.

   RATIONALE Supports entire trunk and positions patient in sling for transfer.

7. **ACTION** Position the lift: Widen the stance of the base of the lift and lock it into place. Position the base under the bed so hooks for the sling are over the patient and in line with the hook openings on the sling.

   RATIONALE Correct positioning prevents the lift from tipping during the transfer. Allows for easy attachment of the hooks to the sling.

8. **ACTION** Lower the sling hooks in a controlled manner, and attach them to the sling. Be certain hooks will not press into the patient's skin when sling is elevated.

   RATIONALE Controlling the hooks prevents them from striking the patient. Checking hook location prevents pressure damage to the patient's skin.

9. **ACTION** Ask the patient to fold the arms over the chest; support the patient's head.

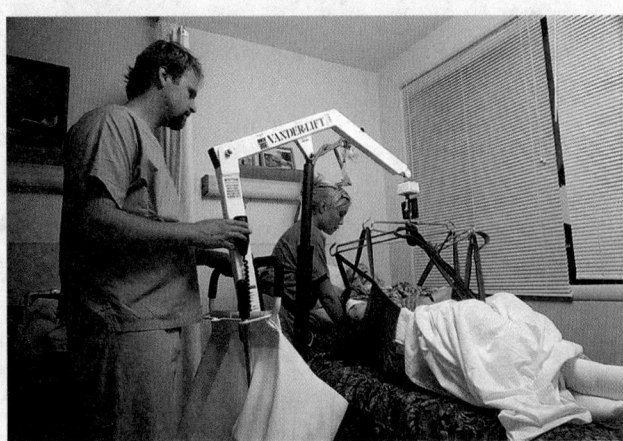

Step **9**

   RATIONALE Head must be supported if sling is not long enough to do so. One person supports the patient's head and guides the sling as the other operates the lift.

Continued

Skill 39-3 **Transferring with a Mechanical Lift**—cont'd

10. **ACTION** Using the lift mechanism, elevate the patient in the sling until it clears the bed by several inches.

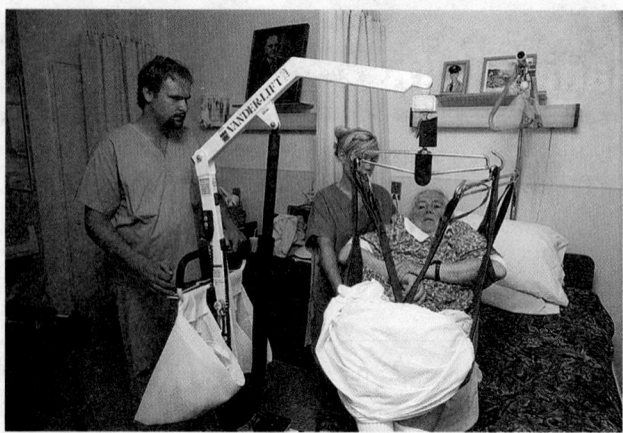

Step **10**

RATIONALE Allows unimpeded transfer of the patient to the chair or stretcher.

11. **ACTION** Roll the lift away from the bed while the second helper safely guides the patient over the chair or stretcher.

RATIONALE Keeps the patient secure and safe. Positions the sling for the transfer.

12. **ACTION** Use the pressure release valve to lower the patient slowly into the chair or onto the stretcher while the helper guides the patient's body. Lower only enough to allow unhooking the sling.

RATIONALE Safely transfers the patient.

13. **ACTION** Unhook the sling, elevate the lift, and roll it away from the patient.

RATIONALE Prevents the hook assembly from striking the patient.

14. **ACTION** Position the patient in good alignment. Smooth the sling or remove it.

RATIONALE The patient is correctly and safely transferred and made comfortable.

15. **ACTION** Cover the patient with a blanket or sheet; place call light and needed items within reach. Secure the patient in the chair with a security vest, or on the stretcher as appropriate.

RATIONALE Promotes safety and comfort for the patient.

16. **ACTION** Monitor at least every 15 minutes for sitting tolerance if the patient is in chair.

RATIONALE If patient is unable to use a call light, place chair where it is visible to a nurse at all times, such as in the hallway near the nurse's station.

17. **ACTION** With the help of an assistant, return the patient to the bed using the lift and following the same steps.

RATIONALE An assistant helps prevent injury to the patient.

■ **Evaluation**

18. **ACTION** Ask yourself: Was the patient transferred smoothly and without injury? Was the patient excessively frightened? Did the lift work correctly?

RATIONALE Answers to these questions provide data to evaluate the effectiveness of the interventions.

■ **Documentation**

19. **ACTION** Document the procedure, noting the use of an assistant. Include the patient's tolerance of the procedure.

RATIONALE Notes transfer of patient and tolerance of procedure.

Documentation Example

7/30 0945   Smooth transfer to wheelchair with lift using an assistant, protective vest in place; chair positioned next to nurse's station. Up in chair × 30 minutes. Returned to bed. Stated it felt good to be out of the bed.

_____
(Nurse's signature)

■ **Special Considerations**

✓ Allow patient to see how the lift works before attempting transfer of patient if at all possible.

✓ In home situation, instruct caregivers thoroughly in use of lift. Use the life to transfer the caregiver to check the function of the lift and to acquaint caregiver with the process.

?CRITICAL THINKING QUESTIONS

1. How would you handle the situation if your patient, who is to be transferred from the bed to a chair with a lift for the first time, is very frightened of this procedure?

2. Why do you think it is essential that the sling for the lift be attached exactly according to the directions that come with it?

Assisting with Aids to Mobilization

Patients require aids to mobility for a variety of reasons, including recent trauma, corrective surgery, and loss of function as a result of stroke or other debilitating conditions. Although the use of ambulatory aids is often taught by a physical therapist or kinesiologist, it is important for you to know the proper techniques so that learning can be reinforced.

Whenever a patient is using an assistive device for mobility, it is important to keep floors clear of clutter and pathways well lighted. The assistive device should be placed within easy reach of the patient when not in use. In the home, the nurse should assess the main pathways the patient will be using and remove hazards.

Walkers. A walker is frequently the first mechanical aid used when training an individual to walk following a loss of function. It is particularly helpful for patients who are weak or tend to lose their balance because it offers a broad base of support.

Walkers are rectangular tubular metal frames that are at least waist high and are open on one side. Most walkers have four rubber-capped tips that rest on the floor, although some have wheels on the front. There are handgrips on the side crossbars. Walkers are adjustable in height. The height is correct if the person's elbow is bent at a 15- to 30-degree angle while standing upright and grasping the handgrips. To use a walker, the individual must have the use of both hands and arms and at least one leg. However, generalized weakness may still allow the patient to use a walker effectively.

Crutches. Depending on the person and the need for assistance with ambulation, the use of crutches may follow the use of a walker or be the first aid to ambulation (Figure 39-15). Although there are a variety of styles of crutches, three basic types are most commonly seen. These are axillary, Lofstrand, and Canadian crutches. Lofstrand and Canadian crutches are shorter and are designed for patients who will permanently need crutches for mobility. Axillary crutches are commonly used for short-term needs. They are adjustable to a variety of heights using wing nuts and are relatively easy to use. They do present one real danger. **Resting the body's weight on the axillary bar puts pressure on vital nerves and can occlude blood vessels in the axilla, causing temporary or permanent damage, including paralysis.** For this reason, it is critical that crutches be adjusted to the proper height and that the patient be instructed to avoid resting the body's weight on the axillary bar.

Crutches need to adjust both in overall length and from the axillary bar to the handgrip. Measure with the patient standing or supine. If standing, be certain the patient's shoes are on the feet. For standing measurement, position the crutches with tips at a point 4 to 6 inches (10 to 15 cm) to the side and 4 to 6 inches in front of the patient's feet. The pads should be ½ to 2 inches (4 to 5 cm) below the axilla. For supine measurement, position the tips 6 inches (15 cm) lateral to the patient's heel. The pad should be 3 or 4 finger breadths under the axilla. Adjust handgrips for both measurements so that the elbow is flexed 15 or 20 degrees when the palms of the hands are resting on the handgrips. When walking, the patient will need to straighten the elbow and the wrist during weight bearing. This should allow the axilla to pass freely over the axillary bar during forward movement (Box 39-5).

Patient Teaching 39-2 provides directions for the most common crutch gaits. Special maneuvers can be taught using Patient Teaching 39-3.

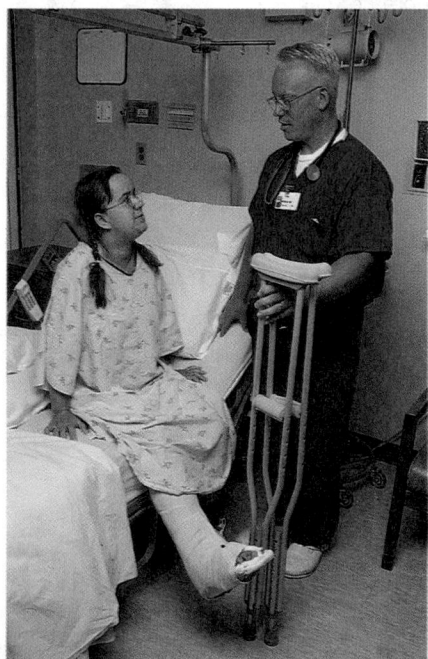

FIGURE **39-15** A patient receiving the beginning of instruction in crutch walking.

Box 39-5 | *Guidelines to Be Considered When Teaching Crutch Walking*

- The head is held up, and the eyes look ahead, as in normal walking.
- The crutches are placed slightly ahead of the patient's feet and to the outside of each foot.
- The hands, not the axillae, are used to support the body's weight.
- The back should be kept straight, and the patient should bend at the hips.
- The crutches and affected foot or leg should be moved forward together (at the same time), except when using a swinging gait.
- A smooth, easy rhythm should be achieved in shifting the weight from the crutches to the unaffected (good) leg and then to the crutches again.
- The crutches should be of the proper length and equipped with heavy rubber suction tips to prevent slipping.
- The gait used will depend on the weight-bearing status of the lower extremities and the patient's abilities.

Patient Teaching 39-2

Common Crutch Gaits

Gait	Description	Pattern
Four-point gait	*Sequence:* 1. Advance left crutch. 2. Advance right foot. 3. Advance right crutch. 4. Advance left foot.	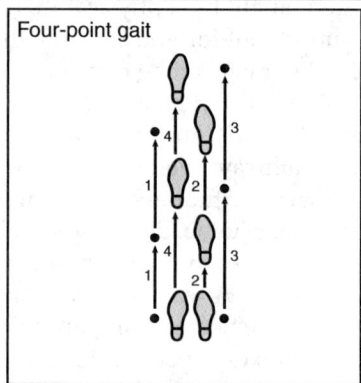
Three-point gait	*Sequence:* 1. Advance both crutches forward with the affected leg and shift weight to crutches. 2. Advance unaffected leg and shift weight onto it. *Advantages:* Allows the affected leg to be partially or completely free of weight bearing. *Requirements:* Full weight bearing on one leg, balance, and upper body strength.	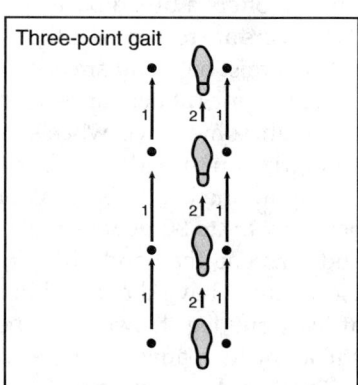
Two-point gait	*Sequence:* 1. Advance left crutch and right foot. 2. Advance right crutch and left foot. *Advantages:* Faster version of the four-point gait, more normal walking pattern (arms and legs moving in opposition). *Requirements:* Partial weight bearing on both legs, balance.	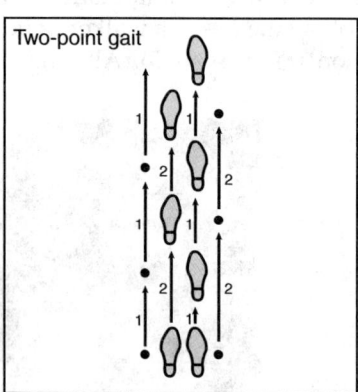
Swing-through gait	*Sequence:* 1. Move both crutches forward. 2. Move both legs forward beyond or even with crutches. Or may keep weight on good foot and move other foot forward and then move good foot forward.	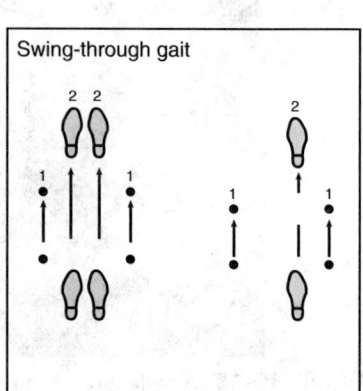

Patient Teaching 39-3

Special Maneuvers on Crutches

Maneuver	Description
Walking upstairs	1. Stand at foot of stairs with weight on good leg and crutch.
	2. Put weight on the crutch handles, and lift the good leg up onto the first step of the stairs.
	3. Put weight on the good leg, and lift other leg and the crutches up to that step.
	4. Repeat for each stair step.
Walking downstairs	1. Stand at top of stairs with weight on good leg and crutches.
	2. Shift weight completely onto the good leg, and put the crutches down on the next step.
	3. Put weight on the crutch handles, and transfer injured leg down on the step with the crutches.
	4. Bring good leg down to that step.
	5. Repeat for each stair step.
Sitting down	1. Crutch walk to the chair.
	2. Turn around slowly so that back is to the chair and the backs of the legs touch the seat of the chair.
	3. Transfer both crutches to the side with the injured leg, and grasp both hand grips with the one hand.
	4. As weight is supported on the crutches and good leg, reach back with free hand and grasp the arm of the chair.
	5. Lower slowly onto the chair seat, using the support of both the crutches and the chair.
	6. Sit back in the chair and elevate the leg, but not to an angle greater than 90 degrees at the hip.
	7. Keep the knee slightly flexed when elevated because too much extension can decrease the circulation.
	8. To get up, bring both crutches along the side of the injured leg, and grasp the hand grip firmly. Make sure the crutch tips are firmly on the floor. Place the other hand on the arm of the chair, and push up.
	9. After becoming upright, transfer one crutch to the other hand for walking.

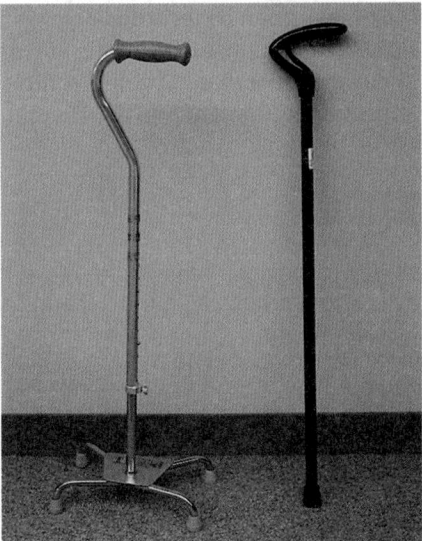

FIGURE **39-16** A regular cane *(right)* provides support, whereas a quad cane *(left)* provides support and stability because of its broad base.

Canes. The most commonly used canes are the standard (one-point) and the quad (four-point) cane (Figure 39-16). An advantage of a quad cane is that it will stand up by itself (Box 39-6).

Wheelchairs. Wheelchairs are used for patients who are not able to ambulate either independently or with aids, such as crutches or a walker. Many paraplegics (those without use of the legs), quadriplegics (those without use of both arms and legs), amputees, and individuals with severe hemiparesis are dependent on

| Box 39-6 | *Guidelines for Using a Cane* |

Instruction for walking with a cane includes ensuring that:
- The cane has an intact rubber tip.
- The patient uses the cane on the unaffected side unless directed by the therapist or physician to use it on the other side for balance reasons.
- The patient does not lean on or bear full weight on the affected leg.
- The caregiver walks beside the patient on the affected side to provide support in case the patient begins to fall.
- The handgrip is at hip level and the person's elbow is bent at a 15- to 30-degree angle when placing weight on the cane.
- The cane's tip is 6 to 10 inches (15 to 25 cm) to the side and 6 inches (15 cm) in front of the near foot.
- The patient looks straight ahead while walking.

wheelchairs for movement from place to place. Patients who are wheelchair dependent over the long term need chairs that are made specifically to their body measurements. When a patient brings a wheelchair to the hospital, see that it is clearly labeled with the owner's name, and never take it for use by someone else.

When moving someone into or out of a wheelchair, always set the brakes. Be sure the person's feet are correctly placed on the footrests and that clothing or lap robes are tucked safely away from the wheels. Shoes, slippers, or bed socks will protect the feet from direct contact with the cold metal footrests. To prevent accidents, keep patients in wheelchairs well away from stairwells, elevators, and doorways if left to sit stationary. **Always have the brakes locked when the chair is not in motion.**

Braces, Splints, and Prostheses for Stabilization. Braces and splints are used to strengthen and support areas of the body affected by weakness or paralysis, such as the legs or back. They may also be used after surgery or trauma to immobilize a part while it heals. Braces and splints are generally made of plastic or metal pieces with padding and straps for attachment. A leg brace may be combined with a shoe. A back brace has metal staves sewn into the fabric; the fabric may be elasticized to provide more support.

A wrist splint is a padded device with an inner metal frame. It is often used to relieve or prevent carpal tunnel syndrome that sometimes occurs with repetitive hand movements and to immobilize a sprained wrist.

Prostheses are used to replace body parts that are missing, either from birth or following amputation. They are specially fashioned to fit the particular patient and assist with lost function. It takes considerable time for a patient to adjust to the use of a prosthesis (artificial substitute for a body part).

All braces, splints, and prostheses have the potential to irritate and injure the tissues and must be monitored closely. The skin should be carefully evaluated during the initial assessment and then reassessed regularly throughout the hospital stay or at home. Any problems must both be noted in the chart and reported promptly to the physician. Handle prosthetic devices carefully as they are made for the specific individual, are expensive, and take many weeks to obtain. Label all the devices with the patient's name and do not allow them out of the room unless in place on the patient.

Rehabilitation

As patients recover from immobilization or from serious illness that restricts usual activity, an exercise prescription may be written to improve muscle tone, joint flexibility, and/or cardiovascular fitness. Parameters for exercise are determined by a target heart rate during activity that is based on age and condition. In a healthy person, the target heart rate for aerobic activity is a minimum of 60% of the age-predicted maximum heart rate (subtract the current age from 220 and multiply by the percentage). The ideal training target is 80% of the age-predicted maximum heart rate.

Patients who have had a joint immobilized are often sent to an outpatient physical therapy facility for an individual exercise program to regain maximum strength and mobility of the joint and extremity.

Evaluation

Evaluation is performed daily by considering whether the specific expected outcomes have been met. Does the skin remain healthy, or are there signs of breakdown? Evaluate the breath sounds, and note any developing cough or signs of dyspnea. Observe the patient's emo-

tional status, including the attitude toward therapy or visitors. Is the patient alert and active in social interactions or withdrawn, hostile, or depressed? If nursing interventions are not achieving the expected outcomes, the plan of care needs to be changed. Evaluation statements indicating that some of the expected outcomes stated earlier are being met might be as follows:

- Performing sponge bath, mouth care, and grooming tasks except for left foot.
- Skin is clean, dry, and without redness or abrasion.
- Respirations normal with clear breath sounds bilaterally.
- Family and friends visiting daily with pleasant interactions.
- Patient is knitting and working on crossword puzzles daily.
- Watching television news show several times a day and discussing events with visitors.
- Asking if a haircut is possible and wants to wear own clothes.

Documentation

Each member of the health care team must maintain a written record of the treatment and its effects. Charting should include any changes in skin integrity, respiratory status, or signs of peripheral circulatory changes. Many aspects of assessment can be recorded on an activity/assessment flow sheet. Because of reimbursement issues, it is vital to document data that indicate a continuing need for use of pieces of equipment and aids to ambulation.

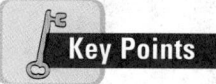 **Key Points**

- It is essential to include measures to prevent the complications of immobility in the nursing care plan (see Table 39-1).
- Particular attention should be paid to respiratory and circulatory function.
- Active or passive exercise is extremely important for the immobilized patient.
- There are special beds and a variety of pressure relief devices available to prevent pressure ulcers and other complications of immobility.
- Attention to psychosocial care as well as physical care is important for the immobile patient.
- Frequent visitors and inclusion of the home patient in family life are important to prevent social isolation.
- The elderly patient is at higher risk for the complications of immobility and may suffer more psychosocial problems.
- Splints are used for immobilization of an injury or for stabilization of an area when paralysis or weakness occurs.
- Traction is used to treat muscle spasm and fractures.
- For traction to be effective, the body must be in correct alignment, the ropes and pulleys must not be impeded, and the weights must hang free without touching anything.

- Skin traction is applied with a Velcro boot, adhesive strips, slings, or wraps; it is noninvasive.
- Skeletal traction requires pins, tongs, or wires attached to the bone; it is invasive.
- External fixators may be used to stabilize a fracture, rather than using a cast, so the patient can be more active during healing.
- Casts are applied to immobilize a particular body part to allow bone healing.
- A cast must be handled gently while drying to prevent altering its shape in any way.
- The cast edges should be smooth and may be "petaled" with tape.
- If a cast becomes too tight, it may be bivalved to relieve pressure on the tissues.
- Nothing small or sharp should be introduced into the cast.
- The air-fluidized, low air-loss, continuous lateral-rotation, and CircOlectric beds are used to prevent complications of immobility.
- The continuous passive motion machine is used to exercise the joint after joint replacement surgery.
- Assessment of neurovascular status, of function of an immobilizing device, and of body systems for signs of complications is performed each shift.
- Nursing diagnoses are related to impaired physical mobility, altered tissue perfusion, the risk of complications, and psychosocial problems.
- Casts are inspected every shift for cracks, crumbling, pressure problems, and signs of infection beneath them.
- Elastic bandages are applied to immobilize a joint or to reduce swelling.
- Neurovascular assessment is performed when an elastic bandage is in place.
- To transfer a patient safely with a mechanical lift, two people should perform the procedure. Always follow the facility's policy.

- A patient is never left alone while suspended in the sling of the lift.
- Aids to mobilization include walkers, crutches, canes, wheelchairs, braces, and prostheses.
- For walkers and canes, the patient's arms should have the elbows placed at a 15- to 30-degree angle when the hands are gripping the device.
- There should be at least two finger breadths of space between the top of the crutch and the axilla when the patient's hands are gripping the crutches.
- Crutches, canes, and walkers should have rubber tips on the feet of the device (unless a wheel is present as on some walkers).
- Wheelchairs are placed in locked position when transferring patients in or out of them, and whenever the patient is placed in a stationary position.
- Braces and prostheses must be handled gently and kept with the patient. Tissue under the device should be assessed before application and when the device is removed.
- Evaluation data are collected to determine whether expected outcomes of the nursing care plan have been met.
- Documentation is vital to obtaining reimbursement for use of immobilization devices and for assistive devices for mobilization. It is essential to document assessment data and interventions instituted for any problems found.

 Go to your **Companion CD-ROM** for an Audio Glossary, animations, video clips, and more.

evolve Be sure to visit the companion Evolve site at http://evolve.elsevier.com/deWit/fundamental/ for additional online resources.

NCLEX-PN® EXAMINATION-STYLE REVIEW QUESTIONS

*Choose the **best** answer(s) for each question.*

1. A 56-year-old woman sustained a fracture of the right femur in an automobile accident. She is in balanced skeletal traction. Immobility causes negative effects on the cardiovascular system. The venous stasis that occurs with immobility can lead to the complication of _____. *(Fill in the blank.)*

2. You are to perform range-of-motion exercises three times a day with your patient who is immobilized. Range-of-motion exercise promotes circulation by:
   1. thinning the blood so that it will move freely.
   2. releasing the one-way valves in the veins and arteries.
   3. contracting the muscles surrounding a vein, forcing blood to move toward the heart.
   4. raising the temperature of the tissues, thereby decreasing blood viscosity so it flows more freely.

3. Passive range-of-motion exercises are performed to prevent the problem of:
   1. formation of a thrombus in the leg.
   2. sluggish circulation in the extremities.
   3. skin breakdown over pressure points.
   4. decreased joint mobility.

4. In addition to good skin care and frequent turning, measures that may help prevent development of pressure ulcers in an immobilized patient are: *(Select all that apply.)*
   1. have family encourage the patient to perform active ROM exercises on unaffected extremities.
   2. restrict calories to reduce weight gain while immobile.
   3. encourage adequate nutritional and fluid intake.
   4. keep the patient's skin clean and dry.

5. When assessing the patient with a new cast on the lower arm, if you find that the cast is tight and almost flush to the skin, you would *first:*

   1. immediately call the orthopedic technician to come and check the cast.
   2. elevate the extremity on two pillows, making certain it is higher than heart level.
   3. report the finding to the charge nurse on the unit.
   4. question the patient as to whether the arm has been kept in an elevated position.

6. A cast that is too tight can directly cause: *(Select all that apply.)*

   1. pressure on nerves and nerve damage.
   2. constriction of blood vessels, decreasing circulation.
   3. blood clot formation.
   4. numbness and tingling in the extremity.

7. The amount of weight exerted by traction is determined by:

   1. the amount of weight placed on traction ropes.
   2. the height of the weight off of the floor.
   3. the ratio of the patient's weight to traction weight.
   4. the position of the patient on the bed.

8. When caring for traction pins and wires, it is most important to:

   1. be very gentle when cleaning around them.
   2. use strict aseptic technique to prevent infection.
   3. rinse the areas cleansed with normal saline.
   4. move them slightly so they do not attach to the bone.

9. You notice that the heel of the foot on your patient who is using a CPM machine is reddened. You should:

   1. pad the portion of the machine that the heel rests on.
   2. stop the machine and notify the physician.
   3. reassess the area in 8 hours.
   4. increase the angle of flexion of the joint to change the pressure on the heel.

10. After applying an elastic bandage to an ankle, you know it is too tight if:

   1. the toes are pink and warm.
   2. the patient complains of pain in the ankle.
   3. there is swelling in the toes and lower foot.
   4. the toes are bluish and cool to the touch.

CRITICAL THINKING ACTIVITIES *Read each clinical scenario and discuss the questions with your classmates.*

Scenario A

Margaret Thies, age 17, received multiple injuries in an automobile accident. She underwent surgery for a lacerated spleen and her right leg is in balanced traction due to two fractures. She will be on bed rest for an extended period.

1. For which complications of immobility do you think Margaret is most at risk?
2. For each complication you identified, list the signs and symptoms that might indicate the complication is occurring.
3. What nursing interventions could you use to help prevent each of the complications listed?

Scenario B

Josh Polaski, age 11, has been treated in the outpatient clinic for a fractured ulna. A short-arm fiberglass cast has been applied.

1. Explain to Josh what he can and cannot do while the cast is in place.
2. Teach Josh's parents how to care for the cast and how to assess for complications.
3. How would teaching differ if the patient were sent home with a plaster cast?

Scenario C

Oscar Nunez, age 38, is in traction for a fractured femur suffered in a motorcycle accident. He has been hospitalized for 4 days and is very bored and restless.

1. What assessments would you make to determine whether his restlessness has a physical cause?
2. If his restlessness seems to be psychological in nature, what activities might you suggest to help him occupy the time and his mind?

40 Common Physical Care Problems of the Elderly

evolve http://evolve.elsevier.com/deWit/fundamental/

Objectives

Upon completing this chapter, you should be able to:

Theory

1. Discuss five age-related common physical care problems of the elderly.
2. Identify three ways to promote mobility in the elderly.
3. List four ways for the elder to prevent falls in the home.
4. Review the physical and psychological consequences of chronic incontinence.
5. Discuss how multiple factors affecting the elderly may lead to an alteration in nutrition.
6. Explain techniques to facilitate communication and safety for the patient with a sensory deficit.
7. Recognize sexual concerns among the elderly population.
8. Identify five reasons why the elder is prone to the problem of polypharmacy.
9. Explain the effect of physical changes on the elderly person's lifestyle.

Clinical Practice

1. Instruct a patient in how to prevent falls.
2. Formulate a plan to assist an elderly patient to decrease or prevent incontinence.
3. Teach an elderly patient specific ways to enhance nutritional status.
4. Assist a patient to develop a self-medication reminder system.

Key Terms

Be sure to check out the bonus material on the Companion CD-ROM, including selected audio pronunciations.

beta-carotene (BĀ-tă KĂR-ō-tēn, p. 840)
cataracts (KĂT-ă-răkts, p. 839)
dyspareunia (dĭs-pă-ROO-nē-ă, p. 841)
glaucoma (glăw-KŌ-mă, p. 839)
macular degeneration (MĂK-ū-lăr dē-jĕn-ĕr-Ā-shŭn, p. 839)
polypharmacy (pŏl-ē-FĂR-mă-sē, p. 841)
postural hypotension (PŌS-chŭr-ăl hĭ-pō-TĔN-shŭn, p. 836)
presbyopia (prĕz-bē-Ō-pē-ă, p. 839)
tinnitus (TĬN-ĭ-tŭs, p. 840)
visual accommodation (p. 839)

GETTING OLDER

With aging, every body system undergoes some change that may not necessarily result in disease or illness, but will cause health problems to be more frequent (Table 40-1). Many of the physical problems, and nursing interventions to help them, are covered in the preceding chapters. This chapter reviews physical problems that are most common to the elderly and nursing interventions to assist the elder to attain an optimal level of function.

Five of the most common physical care problems that plague the elderly population are (1) impaired mobility; (2) alteration in elimination (urinary incontinence, constipation, and fecal impaction); (3) alteration in nutrition; (4) sensory (vision and hearing) deficits; and (5) polypharmacy. Sexuality concerns are also addressed. Table 40-2 presents the causes of and contributing factors that add to these problems. Additional chronic illnesses such as Parkinson's disease, arthritis, emphysema, or cardiac disease may compound these problems. Information on these chronic illnesses may be found in a medical-surgical nursing textbook.

IMMOBILITY

Decreased mobility often leads to numerous complications for the elderly. An acute health condition requiring bed rest may cause further immobility and, consequently, various other problems associated with immobility (see Chapter 39). Diseases that interfere with adequate circulation and oxygenation contribute to activity intolerance and immobility (Concept Map 40-1). For the person with such a problem, personal hygiene, eating, and socializing become too difficult because of exhaustion. Poor nutrition may result from immobility or the lack of energy to obtain or prepare food.

NURSING INTERVENTIONS TO PROMOTE MOBILITY

By immediately addressing mobility needs, you can often quickly get the patient back to her former level of activity, and avoid potential complications. The elderly need to be educated about engaging in activity throughout life that will help maintain optimal mobil-

Table 40-1 *Summary of Common Physiologic Changes with Aging*

SYSTEM AFFECTED	CHANGE NOTED	AGE SPAN (YR)
Height	Average loss 2 in	40-80
Weight		
Men	Peaks in mid-50s, then declines	
Women	Peaks in mid-60s, then declines	
Total body water		
Men	Declines from 60% to 54%	20-80
Women	Declines from 54% to 46%	20-80
Muscle mass	30% decrease	30-70
Taste buds	70% decrease	30-70
Cardiac reserve	Decrease from 4.6 to 3.3 times resting cardiac output	25-70
Maximum heart rate	155-195 beats/min	25-70
Lung vital capacity	17% decrease	30-70
Renal perfusion	Reduced by 50%	30-80
Cerebral blood flow	Reduced by 20%	30-70
Bone mineral content	Reduced by 25%-30% in women; 10%-15% in men	40-80
Brain weight	Reduced by 10%	20-80
Amount of light reaching retina	Diminished by 70%	20-65
Plasma glucocorticoid levels	No change	30-70

Modified from Kenney, P.A. (1982). *Physiology of Aging: A Synopsis.* Chicago: Year Book Medical Publishers; Shock, N.W., et al. (1984). *Normal Human Aging: The Baltimore Study of Aging.* NIH pub. no. 84-2450. Washington, DC: U.S. Government Printing Office; Timiras, P. (2002). *Physiological basis of Aging and Geriatrics,* New York: CBC Press; Beers, M.H., & Berkow, R. (Eds.), (2000). *The Merck Manual of Geriatrics* (3rd ed.). Whitehouse Station, NJ: Merck Research Laboratories.

Table 40-2 *Common Physical Care Problems of the Elderly*

PHYSICAL CARE PROBLEM	EFFECT OF AGING ON SYSTEM	OTHER CONTRIBUTING FACTORS/DISEASES
Impaired mobility	Major loss of calcium, decreased bone density, decreased muscle mass, loss of joint flexibility	Osteoporosis, falls, gout, foot problems, obesity, arthritis, cardiac/respiratory disease, depression, neurologic disorders (e.g., multiple sclerosis)
Urinary incontinence	Altered sphincter control, loss of bladder muscle tone, enlarged prostate, cystocele, rectocele, uterine prolapse, diminished kidney function	Immobility, neurologic disorder (e.g., stroke), urinary tract infection, urinary retention
Constipation	Decreased bowel motility	Immobility, decreased abdominal musculature, insufficient fluid/fiber in diet, hemorrhoids, diverticulosis, depression, nervous system disorders, cognitive impairment, poor dentition, pain medications (e.g., codeine), other medications (e.g., antidepressants and anticholinergics)
Alteration in nutrition	Diseased teeth, poorly fitting dentures, decline in taste buds, decline in sense of smell, dysphagia	Neurologic deficit (e.g., stroke), impaired vision, impaired mobility, anorexia, lack of income/transportation/facilities, dementia, alcohol abuse, depression, taste alterations (e.g., cancer therapy), multiple medications
Vision deficit	Presbyopia, age-related macular degeneration, glaucoma, cataracts	Inadequate income for eye care, diabetes, arteriosclerosis, long-term steroid use
Hearing deficit	Presbycusis, tinnitus, otosclerosis	Long-term exposure to loud noise, heredity, Meniere's disease, labyrinthitis
Polypharmacy	Affects multiple systems	Impaired senses, multiple chronic disorders, impaired cognitive functioning, forgetfulness, multiple physicians prescribing, borrowing drugs from others, use of multiple pharmacies, miscommunication/lack of education, use of over-the-counter medications

ity (Health Promotion Points 40-1). It has been proven that walking 30 minutes a day is very beneficial, but doing this even three times a week is better than not walking at all. Strength training with resistance devices, using free weights or weight machines such as Nautilus, can help prevent muscle wasting, maintain bone density, and improve balance and walking endurance for elders even in their 90s. Dancing, gardening, home maintenance, and swimming can also promote mobility.

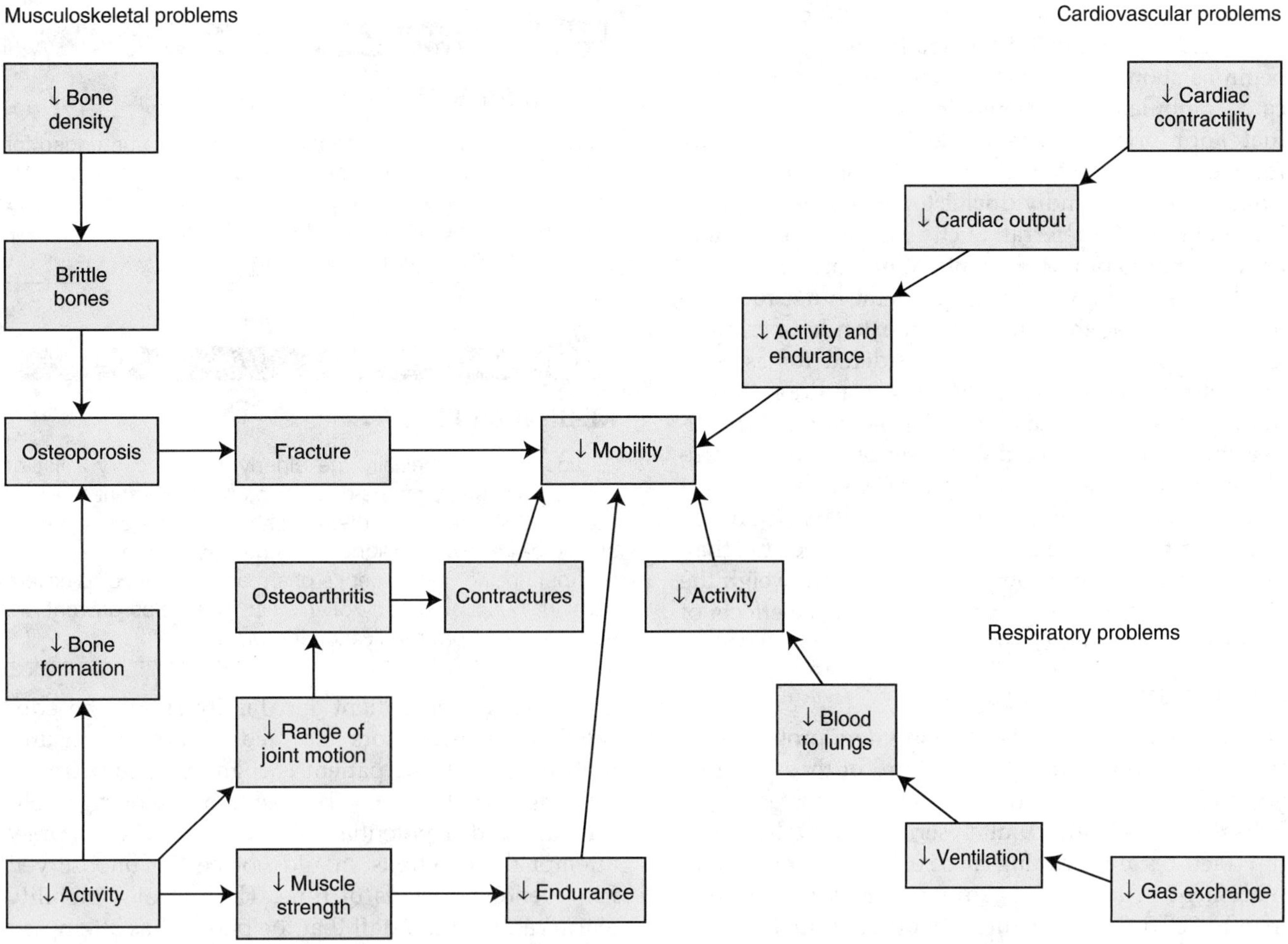

Musculoskeletal problems

Cardiovascular problems

↓ Bone density

↓ Cardiac contractility

↓ Cardiac output

Brittle bones

↓ Activity and endurance

Osteoporosis → Fracture → ↓ Mobility

↓ Bone formation

Osteoarthritis → Contractures

↓ Activity

Respiratory problems

↓ Range of joint motion

↓ Blood to lungs

↓ Activity → ↓ Muscle strength → ↓ Endurance

↓ Ventilation ← ↓ Gas exchange

CONCEPT MAP 40-1 Relationship of physical changes to decreased mobility.

Health Promotion Points 40-1

Healthy People 2010 **Physical Activity**

The Healthy People 2010 *objectives regarding physical activity include:*
- Increase the proportion of adults who engage regularly, preferably daily, in moderate physical activity for at least 30 minutes per day.
- Increase the proportion of adults who perform physical activities that enhance and maintain flexibility.

Participating in craft activities and arthritis programs can assist with preservation of fine motor movement. Proper treatment for arthritis and osteoporosis will help prevent immobility problems. Estrogen replacement therapy (ERT) and adequate dietary or supplemental calcium and vitamin D in combination with weight-bearing exercise are protective against osteoporosis in women. However, ERT's potential side effects make its use controversial. Drugs such as alendronate sodium (Fosamax), risedronate sodium (Actonel), ibandronate sodium (Boniva), calcitonin-salmon (Miacalcin), and raloxifene hydrochloride (Evista) can help rebuild bone or stop its loss. Anti-inflammatory

drugs such as nabumetone (Relafen) or diclofenac sodium (Voltaren) can also help maintain mobility. Etanercept (Enbrel), an immunomodulator, may be used for those patients with rheumatoid arthritis if they have poor response to other treatment.

The period of confined bed rest during illness needs to be as limited as possible. Merely transferring a patient from the bed to a chair has beneficial effects. Teach the bed rest patient active range-of-motion (ROM) activities and isometric exercises (applying pressure against resistance). An example of isometric exercise is instructing the patient to push into the bed with her hands and attempt to lift her hips, while sitting up in bed. If the patient is incapable of performing these exercises, assist with passive ROM exercises to maintain joint flexibility and help prevent muscle wasting. If the elderly patient is noncommunicative, assess for pain using the guidelines in Chapter 31 prior to attempting a ROM program.

Think Critically About . . . ROM exercises may be considered a "chore" for the patient on bed rest. What types of creative exercises/activities can you encourage that would be therapeutic and enjoyable?

With hospital stays so short, every effort to restore the patient to her maximum mobility potential should begin as soon as possible. When it is medically indicated, ambulate the patient with assistance. Make sure that appropriate assistance devices such as sturdy footwear, eyeglasses, walkers, and canes are brought from home. If the individual is too weak, seek a physical therapy (PT) referral. Such rehabilitative services are essential to promote quality of life for the elderly.

The nursing home setting allows the nurse to monitor and promote mobility over an extended period of time. All patients should be considered for assisted ambulation unless an underlying condition/illness (paralysis, severe cardiac disease) prevents it. The elder who is not ambulated will deteriorate and eventually be unable to walk. Although staff may be reluctant to encourage ambulation of a resident with an unsteady gait, many patients would rather risk a fall than be placed in a wheelchair. You may have to weigh the risk of the elder falling versus the negative effects of prolonged immobility.

PREVENTING FALLS

Falls are one of the most common safety problems for the elderly. Approximately one third of those over 65 years old and one half of those over 80 fall each year. Falls may not always result in serious injury; however, hip fractures are a leading cause of hospitalization and placement in long-term care facilities, with approximately 309,500 hip fractures reported annually (Centers for Disease Control and Prevention, 2006). Falls are the most common cause of traumatic brain injuries and accounted for 46% of falls that are fatal among older adults (Centers for Disease Control and Prevention, 2007).

Once an older person has fallen, there is the fear of falling again. This may cause limitation of activities and increased risk for the harmful effects of immobility. Caregivers and family members may also place restrictions on mobility and limit activities to prevent another fall.

Changes in the elder's posture, balance, gait, and vision contribute to the risk of a fall (Health Promotion Points 40-2). Environmental factors such as clutter in walking areas, inadequate lighting or glare, improper footwear, and unsafe furnishings such as scatter rugs predispose to falls.

Medications frequently contribute to falls. With each additional medication consumed, the risk of falls is increased. Sedatives, hypnotics, and tranquilizers can decrease alertness and reaction time. Diuretics, antihypertensives, and antihistamines increase the risk of postural (or orthostatic) hypotension (unusually low blood pressure upon standing), which may cause the patient to become light-headed and fall (Safety Alert 40-1).

Most falls occur in the bedroom or bathroom. The home environment should be assessed to see how the patient navigates in these areas during activities of

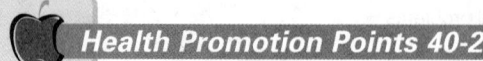

Health Promotion Points 40-2

Tai Chi for Balance

Tai Chi is a form of exercise that is highly recommended for maintaining balance and coordination. It is also good for stimulating the brain. Many community recreation centers and colleges offer classes in Tai Chi. Seniors should be encourage to participate in this activity.

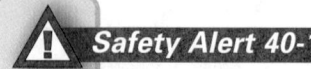

Safety Alert 40-1

Medication Lists

All adults, but especially the elderly, should carry a list of medications and over-the-counter preparations that they are using when they visit their health care provider. The list should be reviewed in light of any new symptom the patient is experiencing. The patient's pharmacist should also have a continually updated copy of this list. This helps prevent adverse events from medication interactions.

daily living. The patient and family should be educated about risk factors and made aware of measures to avoid falls. If the patient is cognitively impaired, a toileting schedule may be used to discourage self-toileting and a potential fall. Patients who unsafely attempt these actions should not be left unobserved for extended periods of time. The use of a mobility alarm can alert the staff that the patient has attempted to move unassisted.

Elderly patients need to be moved slowly out of bed to prevent possible orthostatic hypotension. Elastic support stockings may help prevent or lessen such hypotension. They should use appropriate footwear. A gait belt should be used until independent ambulation is established. Assistance devices, such as a cane or walker that can provide a wider base of support and increase stability, may be needed.

The call bell should be readily available to the patient who is in bed, in a chair, or in the bathroom. Beds should be in the low position with brakes engaged, unless a caregiver is at the bedside. Bells should be answered promptly to avoid unsafe attempts to stand or walk. Health care team members need to remember to keep walking paths clear, adjust lighting, and wipe up spills from the floor as soon as they are noticed.

Protective devices should be used only when there is a documented reason and only after the patient or her guardian has given permission, and they are ordered by the physician. This includes vest or waist devices, safety belts, and geri-chairs. Federal Omnibus Budget Reconciliation Act (OBRA) regulations are very specific about when and what types of devices are permissible. Check the guidelines at your place of employment and follow policy.

Both the patient and significant others need to be taught about hazards in the home and how to prevent

Health Promotion Points 40-3

Preventing Falls

Take the following steps to prevent a fall:
- Use bright, nonglare lighting in each room of the house.
- Keep glasses clean.
- Get up from the bed or a chair slowly and stand before walking.
- Avoid tipping the head backward (extending the neck) to obtain something from a shelf, wash a tall window, or hang clothes as this may cause you to lose your balance.
- Use flat shoes and slippers with nonskid soles. Avoid clothing that is long or loose-fitting that may cause tripping or get caught on furniture or doorknobs.
- Use a night-light in the bedroom and bathroom, or turn on a lamp before arising from the bed at night. Wait for the eyes to adjust to the light before arising.
- If you become dizzy, sit down immediately if possible, or hold on to something solid.
- Avoid using scatter rugs and small bathroom mats that can slide.
- Avoid slick, high polish on floors, and do not walk on wet floor surfaces.
- Use a nonskid mat in the bathtub or shower.
- Install a grab rail in the bath or shower, and also by the toilet, if needed.
- Wipe up spills immediately.
- Watch for pets underfoot.
- Avoid clutter in living spaces.
- Select furniture that provides stability and support, such as chairs with arms.
- Check walking aids routinely for worn rubber tips and replace them as needed.
- Avoid floor coverings with a busy pattern.
- Install handrails on both sides of stairs.

falls in the home. If the individual is being discharged from the hospital and lives alone, a referral may be made for a member of the health care team to assess the home for potential safety hazards. Family members and significant others need to be encouraged to make regular visits to the elder's home to check for unsafe conditions (Health Promotion Points 40-3).

Discourage the elderly from climbing a ladder or standing on a chair to reach high places. If a person needs to reach a high area, a stepstool with a broad base of support should be used. If balance is unsteady, the individual should be instructed not to reach for objects above head level. Devices to assist with reaching can be purchased to avoid the temptation to reach overhead.

ALTERATION IN ELIMINATION

URINARY INCONTINENCE

Incontinence is one of the most common reasons that elder adults are institutionalized. Families who cope with other health problems are often unable to deal

---

Box 40-1 | *Behavioral Approaches to Urinary Incontinence*

- **Bladder retraining:** *Goal:* Restore normal pattern of voiding by inhibiting or stimulating voiding, by lengthening the time between voidings.
- **Prompted voiding:** *Goal:* Teach the patient to be aware of toileting needs and to request assistance from the caregiver.
- **Habit (timed) voiding:** *Goal:* Take confused or cognitively impaired patients to the toilet at regular intervals.

---

with incontinence. Embarrassment, social withdrawal, depression, and low self-esteem are common for the elderly patient who is incontinent.

Urinary incontinence is *not* a normal consequence of aging. Incontinence can be the result of an acute condition or a chronic problem. Approximately 30% of community-dwelling elders and more than 50% of nursing home residents are incontinent of urine (Palmer & Newman, 2004). Causes and treatment of incontinence are presented in Chapter 29. Temporary incontinence may develop as a result of an acute illness. If the patient is assisted to regain continence as soon as the acute episode is over, permanent incontinence can often be avoided. **An underlying cause should always be sought when incontinence occurs.** Bowel incontinence is not as common a problem and is covered in Chapter 30.

Nursing Interventions for Urinary Incontinence

Management of incontinence can be a frustrating problem for both patient and nurse. Incontinence is also costly; annual costs are estimated at $8.6 billion for care within the community and $3.8 billion for nursing home residents (Wilson et al., 2001). Treatment is based on the underlying cause and may include medication, such as oxybutynin chloride (Ditropan) or doxazosin mesylate (Cardura), to relax the smooth muscle of the bladder/prostate. Herbal approaches include the use of saw palmetto and pumpkin seeds, which can reduce prostate swelling (Banschbach, 2002). Treatment may also include surgery or behavioral interventions. Box 40-1 shows behavioral techniques commonly used with elders who experience urinary incontinence. Chapter 29 further describes training procedures, Kegel exercises, and nursing measures to reduce episodes of incontinence.

You can help prevent skin breakdown by keeping the patient who is incontinent clean and dry and by using a product such as Geri-Lav Free as a skin protector. The use of easy-release clothing, protective pads such as the DriStar system for women, and condom catheters such as the Pop-On for men can help hinder skin breakdown, avoid the soiling of bed and clothing, and prevent embarrassment for the patient. Encouraging fluids can decrease the urine concentration so it is less irritating, less predisposing to urinary tract infections, and less odoriferous.

Safety Alert 40-2

Checking for Fecal Impaction

Digital examination should be performed with caution, especially in those patients with cardiac disease. Digital examination can result in an unusually low heart rate due to vagal stimulation. A low heart rate may lead to cardiac arrhythmia and possible cardiac arrest.

Managing urinary incontinence depends not only on effective interventions, but also on a belief by the health care team that improvement is possible. A continence coordinator can be a valuable resource person in providing information and encouraging staff efforts in achieving patient goals.

CONSTIPATION AND FECAL IMPACTION

Constipation is a common problem among the elderly. Many older people believe anything other than a daily bowel movement is abnormal. Before deciding whether constipation is a problem, assess the frequency, amount, and consistency of stools as well as the possible contributing factors addressed in Chapter 30.

Fecal impaction can rapidly develop in the ill elder who, while on bed rest, is receiving pain medication and not eating a normal diet. Signs and symptoms may include abdominal cramping or rectal pain, abdominal distention, the passing of small amounts of liquid stool, and loss of appetite. Digital examination of the rectum often reveals a mass (Safety Alert 40-2). **You need to check whether a physician's order is required at your employing institution before performing this procedure.**

Nursing Interventions for Constipation and Fecal Impaction

Along with the interventions covered in Chapter 30 for constipation, patient teaching should include specific diet remedies such as hot water and lemon juice first thing on arising, prunes, prune juice with carbonated drink, bran cereal or whole-grain breads, and roughage such as raw fruits and vegetables, as well as encouraging fluid intake of at least 2500 mL/day. Encourage an acceptable exercise program and advise the individual to heed the urge to defecate quickly to avoid a potential problem. Impacted stool may require manual removal. An oil-retention enema is ordered to soften stool before impaction removal.

? Think Critically About . . . Beans are an excellent source of fiber for relieving constipation. Your patient complains that beans give her gas. Can you suggest three alternate high-fiber vegetables?

ALTERATION IN NUTRITION

Nutritional needs of the elderly are discussed in Chapter 26. Although there is a decline in energy requirements as a person ages, there are no established recommendations for optimal nutrient intake for the elderly. The present Recommended Dietary Allowances (RDAs) reflect guidelines only for individuals to age 50 and do not consider requirements for additional nutrients as a result of decreased absorption, infection, or chronic illness.

It is recommended that the elderly reduce their sugar and fat intake and increase the roughage in their diet (Health Promotion Points 40-4). Controversy remains as to whether increased nutrients are needed. Some researchers suggest that an increase in whole-grain foods, fruits, and vegetables, as well as additional sources of protein, may help the elderly maintain proper nutrition. Table 40-3 displays dietary recommendations and rationales for the elderly individual. (Refer to MyPyramid for Older Adults in the Supplemental Image Collection on Evolve site http://elsevier.com/deWit/fundamental/.

Obesity contributes to joint problems as well as being a risk factor for hypertension, heart disease, and stroke. Elders should adjust their caloric intake to coincide with their activity to maintain a weight that is within normal limits for their height and body build.

NURSING INTERVENTIONS FOR NUTRITIONAL SUPPORT

Meals can be made more enjoyable for the patient in a long-term care setting by serving the food in an attractive manner and by making the environment as pleasant as possible. Assess for social problems such as annoying table company, and then appropriately address the issue. A nutritionist can assist in determining the nutritional needs of the institutionalized patient. A liquid dietary supplement may be necessary to help the elderly patient meet dietary needs. Tube feedings and parenteral feedings may have to be used if attempts at oral feedings fail. Patients with **dysphagia** (difficulty swallowing) are at high risk for developing a nutritional deficit. These patients need to sit upright or in a high Fowler's position and be fed very small amounts to avoid aspiration. Liquids may need to be thickened. The chin should be tucked when swallowing. The patient should remain in an upright position

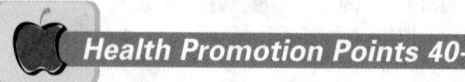

Health Promotion Points 40-4

Dietary Objectives

The Healthy People 2010 *objectives related to nutrition include:*
- Increase the proportion of adults who are at a healthy weight.
- Reduce the proportion of adults who are obese.

Table 40-3 *General Guidelines for Nutrient Needs of the Older Adult*

NUTRIENT	GENERAL GUIDELINE	RATIONALE/EXPLANATION
Calories	Average intake for men = 2000 kcal/day; average intake for women = 1600 kcal/day	Energy requirements tend to decrease with age. Health problems arise when intake totals <1500 kcal/day.
Protein	1-1.25 g/kg, or 63 g/day for average-weight male and 50 g/day for average-weight female	1 g/kg is needed to maintain a positive nitrogen balance.
Carbohydrate	45%-65% of total daily calories from mostly complex carbohydrates	Impaired glucose tolerance may occur in the elderly if too many carbohydrates, especially simple ones such as sugars, are consumed.
Fat	At least 25%-35% of kcal/day	Mostly monounsaturated or polyunsaturated fats should be used. Animal fat intake should be very limited, as should intake of *trans*-fatty acids, because these tend to contribute to cardiovascular disease.
Calcium	1500 mg/day for women and 1200 mg/day for men	Bone demineralization and osteoporosis are common among the elderly.
Vitamin D	10-15 mcg/day (400-600 International Units/day)	Insufficient vitamin D results in bone demineralization. Sunlight provides vitamin D, but not when sunscreen is used.
Other vitamins and minerals	Nutrients should come from foods (i.e., 5-9 servings of fruits and vegetables per day). A multivitamin-mineral tablet per day is recommended.	Vitamins and minerals are needed to maintain optimal nutritional status and health. Most elderly do not consume sufficient fruits and vegetables per day; therefore, a multivitamin-mineral tablet is recommended.
Water	30-35 mL/kg per day; 1500 mL/day minimum intake	Elderly are very susceptible to dehydration. When fluid loss is excessive, water and electrolytes must be replaced.

Adapted from Mahan, L.K., & Escott-Stump, S. (2008). *Krause's Food, Nutrition, and Diet Therapy* (12th ed.). Philadelphia: Elsevier Saunders.

for 45 to 60 minutes after eating. Providing a stress-free environment is essential because stress can make dysphagia more pronounced.

? Think Critically About . . . Your 75-year-old hemiplegic patient with dysphagia is depressed and anxious over her recent stroke. She motions for you to take away her food. What can you do to maintain her nutritional intake?

SENSORY DEFICITS

VISION DEFICITS

Age-related eye changes can be debilitating if they are not recognized and corrected, and may result in a severe limitation of the patient's overall independence. Visual accommodation (the ability to focus on near and far objects) decreases with age as a result of weakening of the muscles that control the lens. Beginning in their 40s, most people need bifocals or reading glasses to correct presbyopia (age-related decreased ability to focus on near objects) and to compensate for loss in accommodation.

The lens of the eye may yellow with age, causing a decline in color perception in the elderly. Because the iris has decreased ability to respond to light changes, the elder may experience difficulty adjusting from light to dark.

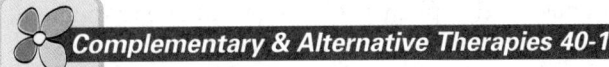

Complementary & Alternative Therapies 40-1

Antioxidant Supplements to Prevent Macular Degeneration

Certain supplements can help stabilize macular degeneration. The vitamins and minerals recommended are vitamin C, vitamin E, carotenoids, selenium, and zinc. Dietary intake of the carotenoids and antioxidants such as anthrocyanidins (e.g., lutein and zeaxanthin) are highly recommended. A diet that contains lots of orange, red, and yellow vegetables and fruits and blue fruits such as bilberries and blueberries is strongly encouraged.

As the blood supply to the retina decreases, depth perception, peripheral vision, and night vision decrease. Any loss of peripheral vision should be further evaluated to rule out glaucoma. Glaucoma, a common disorder of the aging eye, is the accumulation of fluids inside the eye that exert pressure on the optic nerve, eventually causing blindness. It is often asymptomatic and a frequent cause of preventable blindness.

Frequently the elderly develop cataracts, a clouding of the lens. Cataracts occur to some extent in almost all elders, especially those with diabetes. Perhaps the most debilitating eye disorder is age-related macular degeneration, in which the elderly person gradually loses acute, central, and color vision. Unfortunately, there is no proven effective way to halt this disorder (Complementary & Alternative Therapies 40-1). Many medications, especially maintenance drugs such as oral hypoglycemics and thyroid replacement hormones, can affect vision. Thus a careful assessment of the patient's medications, as discussed later in this chapter, is imperative.

Nursing Interventions for the Visually Impaired

Measures to enhance vision include the use of medications, surgery, and prosthetic devices. There are many degrees of vision loss, and interventions are geared to promote the individual's maximum independence.

You must orient the patient to any new environment to avoid potential confusion and anxiety, as well as reduce the risk of accidents. The use of bright lights and bed rails and the removal of hazards in the room are imperative. All members of the health care team should be informed that the patient has a vision deficit. All persons should identify themselves on entering the patient's room, and state when they are leaving to make sure the patient knows of their departure.

Do not rearrange the room or the patient's personal belongings without permission or explanation. Speak before handing an object to her. To promote independence in eating, describe the positions of food on the plate in relation to clock position (e.g., 3 o'clock, 6 o'clock).

When walking with the patient with a visual impairment, offer your arm for guidance. It will be necessary to pause and explain any change in the environment, such as steps, to decrease fear of new surroundings.

For the patient with low vision, devices such as a closed-circuit TV system and the low-vision enhancement system (LVES) are available to magnify and light reading material. Telescopic lenses, TV screen magnifiers, large-print books, talking books, and large-number watches, clocks, and telephones all are examples of aids that can be beneficial. Bright, glare-free light may be necessary for the elderly person to move about safely. Night-lights may also be helpful. During the day, natural light may be preferable.

All interventions to assist with independence need to be explained to family members who may live with the elder at home. Additional teaching or referrals may be necessary for the person who is completely blind. A common concern is the visually impaired elder who continues to drive. This creates a psychosocial issue that involves not only the elder and family, but society as well. In coping with this concern, many states and provinces now require special testing before reissuing licenses to those over a certain age (ranging from 70 to 80 years of age). Individuals may be given limited licenses that restrict driving to specific distances and areas. Older persons who continue to drive must be encouraged to avoid night driving and to wear prescribed hearing aids or glasses to help enhance sensory awareness. The elder should also be advised not to drive under the influence of alcohol or drugs and to avoid driving in inclement weather to avoid a potential accident.

The use of sunglasses when outside and supplementation with vitamin and mineral antioxidants may help protect against macular degeneration. A diet rich in antioxidant foods such as beta-carotene (found in dark green leafy vegetables and deep orange vegetables and fruits), vitamin E (found in seeds, nuts, and wheat germ), and vitamin C (found in citrus fruits and dark green leafy vegetables) should be encouraged as a beneficial food choice.

HEARING DEFICIT

The inability to hear high-frequency sounds usually begins to become noticeable by late middle age. **Presbycusis** is the inability to hear high-pitched sounds and the inability to hear spoken words. This problem is often intensified with the presence of background noise. Tinnitus, or ringing in the ears, may also cause a further loss of hearing.

Presbycusis is commonly exacerbated by cerumen (earwax) accumulation. **Removal of a wax impaction can make a significant difference in the elder's hearing ability.** It is of utmost importance to assess frequently if cerumen is contributing to the hearing loss. Products such as Debrox (carbamide peroxide) are effective in wax removal and can be periodically continued at home.

Hearing loss can lead to ongoing frustration and embarrassment for the individual. The person with a hearing deficit may complain of others mumbling, as well as have a reduced tolerance for loud noises. She may pretend to hear, when she really does not understand what has been communicated. This becomes an important concern when attempting to communicate about health-related issues. Hearing should be checked periodically.

Nursing Interventions for the Hearing Impaired

If the patient has a hearing aid, the nurse should know how to operate it. The hearing aid should be free from earwax and fit properly in the ear canal to function correctly. Chapter 19 describes how to care for the hearing aid. Periodic irrigation of the auditory canal to remove impacted cerumen is a high priority.

Communication with a person with a hearing loss can be difficult for both patient and nurse. Face the patient so she knows you are present, and speak clearly and distinctly in low tones, rephrasing sentences as needed (Figure 40-1). Facial expressions and gestures can be helpful in communicating messages. Conversations should take place in a well-lit area with minimal outside distractions. Speak toward the patient's "good ear" if possible. If the patient wears glasses, they should be worn to aid in seeing facial expressions and to read lips. Environmental noise should be kept to a minimum to avoid confusion and

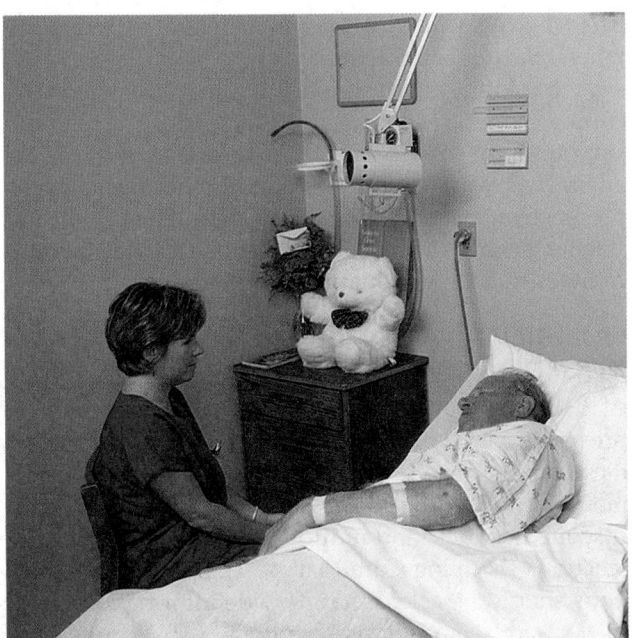

FIGURE **40-1** Communication with the elder with a vision or hearing deficit. Sit in front of the patient where your lips can be seen to communicate. Standing behind the patient causes miscommunication.

improve the clarity of conversation. A pad and pencil can be used if messages are still unclear.

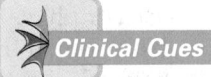
Clinical Cues

When working with a patient with a known hearing deficit, seek feedback regarding instructions given. Do not assume that the patient heard correctly even if a hearing aid is worn.

Family members may become frustrated with an elder who will not get a hearing aid, or who will not wear the hearing aid to communicate. As a result, the individual may gradually stop participating in conversation and become isolated. Work with patients and families to enhance communication techniques. Some patients may benefit from a cochlear implant.

Think Critically About . . . What types of safety measures could you teach the hearing-impaired elder who lives alone?

SEXUALITY

In spite of the general view of the younger generation, the need for sexual expression does not disappear with age. People continue sexual activity into old age. Changing health status, age-related physical changes, and loss of a sex partner do have an effect on the sex-

ual practices of the elderly. Sexual response time slows with age, but the ability to achieve orgasm continues. Sexuality may be difficult for you to discuss with an elderly patient, but it is an area that should be assessed. Try asking questions such as "Are you sexually active?" or "Are you happy with your sex life?" to begin an assessment.

The decreased levels of hormones may result in discomfort or pain (dyspareunia) during intercourse for the female. Thinning and dryness of the vaginal walls predispose to vaginitis. There may be an alteration in the numbers of normal microorganisms in the vagina that leads to a predisposition to vaginal yeast infection. Hormone replacement therapy (HRT) can help alleviate these issues, but because of the potential side effects of those medications, HRT must be closely monitored. Topical vaginal moisteners can be very helpful.

The elderly male may experience a slower sexual arousal. Erection is often less firm than when younger. It takes longer for the elderly male to reach an orgasm and there is less seminal fluid released. Diabetes may contribute to impotence. There are many resources available to help the male achieve erection. Sildenafil citrate (Viagra), vardenafil (Levitra), and tadalafil (Cialis) have been very successful in promoting a satisfying sex life for older men. Vacuum pumps, penile implants, and penile injections are other aids to achieve an erection. An elastic ring can help a man maintain an erection once it is achieved.

Chronic illness or disability may affect one partner or the other's ability to participate in sexual activity. The nurse should explore other ways to help the couple express their sexuality and achieve sexual satisfaction.

A concern is the rise of human immunodeficiency virus (HIV) infection in the older heterosexual population. Elders don't seem to think they need to practice safe sex since pregnancy is no longer an issue. It is imperative to teach about the dangers of unprotected sex and the possibility of the transmission of HIV and other sexually transmitted diseases. It is not uncommon for some elders to strike up a romance within an assisted living facility or a long-term care facility. The incidence of new cases of HIV among heterosexuals in the United States is greatest among the older population.

POLYPHARMACY

The greater the number of medications consumed by an individual, the greater the risk of undesirable reactions, drug interactions, and toxicity. Polypharmacy is the use of multiple medications, often inappropriately and excessively, at the same time. This often occurs when the patient sees multiple physicians and each is unaware of what the other is prescribing. Patients may use a local pharmacy and a mail-order pharmacy as well, so the pharmacist is unaware of all the drugs the

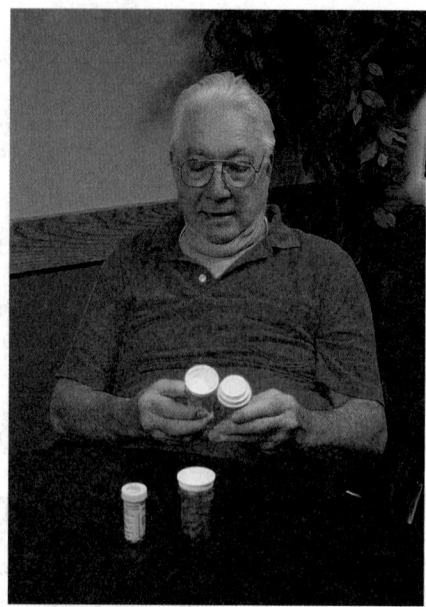

FIGURE **40-2** Elder checking multiple drug bottles.

patient is consuming. Individuals over 65 are the largest users of prescription and over-the-counter (OTC) drugs, and therefore are more likely to experience a polypharmacy situation (Figure 40-2).

In the older person, drug interactions and toxicity can result in behavioral or cognitive changes that may be mistaken for dementia. Unfortunately, when older persons experience adverse drug effects, these problems are often overlooked, inappropriately blamed on the aging process, or treated with yet another medication.

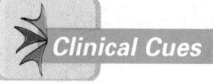

Clinical Cues

Whenever an elderly patient develops confusion or a new symptom, it is wise to first check to see if a new medication or supplement has been taken. A patient may build up a toxic level of a drug after being on it for a few days or weeks and then symptoms of adverse effects appear.

Many factors related to aging alter the rate at which drugs are metabolized and excreted in the elderly person. Absorption, storage, and serum binding factors all affect the way a drug is used within the body. Decreased body water, increased ratio of fat to muscle, and a low serum albumin all predispose the patient to drug toxicity and extended duration of action of drugs (Table 40-4). Alterations in enzyme function, cardiac output, and circulatory function can reduce blood flow to the liver. These changes decrease the liver's effectiveness and speed in metabolizing drugs. As most drugs are metabolized in the liver, the risk of toxicity increases. The risk for toxicity can significantly increase if the elder is malnour-

ished because medications metabolize more slowly when the diet is inadequate.

Aging kidneys are significantly less effective in excreting drugs, resulting in elevated drug levels and symptoms of toxicity. Some medications, such as digoxin (Lanoxin), cause retention of other drugs in the presence of diminished renal function. The use of substances such as alcohol and nicotine can also cause changes in drug elimination in the elderly.

NURSING INTERVENTIONS FOR POLYPHARMACY

A thorough medication history is the initial step in preventing polypharmacy. A comprehensive assessment can help maintain a therapeutic medication regimen, identify educational needs, eliminate unnecessary medications, and reduce the risk of adverse drug reactions (Nursing Care Plan 40-1). Specifically, questions should be asked that provide information about the patient's current prescriptions, OTC drugs, and any vitamins and herbal preparations being taken. Ask the patient to bring a bag with all the drugs she takes at home. Assessment data should also include the patient's current administration schedule, knowledge about her medications, medication-related problems, noncompliance problems, frequency of physician visits, sensory deficits, mental and physical disabilities, ability to purchase and obtain medication, and the use of alcohol and caffeine. Ideally, a pharmacist or physician should address these questions. However, the nurse should be prepared to assess the patient's drug history initially as well as continue to gather information so that a therapeutic medication regimen may be maintained.

In a long-term care facility, it is imperative to assess continually the number of medications, side effects, and the necessity for each being administered to avoid a potentially dangerous situation (Assignment Considerations 40-1).

Think Critically About . . . Your patient mentions to you that she has been using several pharmacies to get the best price for the six prescriptions and four OTC drugs she takes each day. What types of questions might you ask her in your assessment?

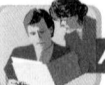

Assignment Considerations 40-1

Medication Administration

If your facility uses nursing assistants who are certified in medication administration, be aware that it is still your responsibility to monitor the patient for correct response and side effects to the medications administered.

Table 40-4 *Age-Related Changes Affecting Drug Therapy in Older Adults*

CHANGE	IMPACT	NURSING MEASURES
Drier mucous membrane of oral cavity	Tablets and capsules may stick to roof or sides of mouth and not be swallowed; can dissolve in and irritate mouth	Offer fluids before drug administration to moisten mouth and ample fluids during administration. Inspect mouth or advise patient to inspect mouth for any tablet or capsule that may not have been swallowed (dentures and reduced sensations may cause patient to be unaware of presence of medication). Unless contraindicated, break large tablets to facilitate swallowing.
Decreased circulation to lower bowel and vagina; lower body temperature	Suppositories require longer time to melt and risk being expelled undissolved	Explore possibility of using alternative route. Allow longer time for suppository to melt. Check/advise patient to check suppository has melted before getting out of bed to resume activities.
Decreased tissue elasticity	Poor seal of tissues after injection, oozing; poor absorption	Use upper, outer quadrant of buttocks for intramuscular injections and rotate sites. Use Z-track injection technique for injections to facilitate sealing. Cleanse any medication that has oozed onto skin.
Decreased pain sensation	Infection or other problem at injection site may not be detected	Check injection sites regularly.
Decreased cardiac efficiency	Greater risk of circulatory overload during intravenous administration of medications	Monitor intravenous drip closely. Observe for signs of circulatory overload (e.g., rise in blood pressure, rapid respirations, coughing, shortness of breath).
Less gastric acid	Slower absorption of drugs that require low gastric pH	Ensure gastric acid is not further reduced by other drugs (e.g., antacids).
Increase in adipose tissue compared to lean body mass; decreased cardiac output	Drugs stored in adipose tissue (lipid-soluble drugs) have increased tissue concentrations and decreased plasma concentrations and accumulate and remain in body for longer duration; plasma levels of drugs can increase while less is deposited in reservoirs (particularly true of water-soluble drugs)	Ensure dosages are age adjusted. Become familiar with adverse effects of drugs administered and observe for these effects.
Reduced serum albumin levels	Administering several protein-bound drugs together can cause drugs to compete for same protein molecules; some drugs may not effectively bind and be less effective	Advise physician of other protein-bound drugs patient is taking when new protein-bound drug is prescribed; highly protein-bound drugs include acetazolamide, amitriptyline, cefazolin, chlordiazepoxide, chlorpromazine, cloxacillin, digitoxin, furosemide, hydralazine, nortriptyline, phenylbutazone, phenytoin, propranolol, rifampin, salicylates, spironolactone, sulfisoxazole, and warfarin. Ensure serum albumin level is evaluated along with blood level of drug (if serum albumin level is low, patient has greater risk for becoming toxic despite normal or low blood levels of drug).
Reduced number of functioning nephrons; decreased glomerular filtration rate; reduced blood flow	Biologic half-life extended; drugs take longer to be filtered from body; increased risk of adverse reactions	Ensure age-adjusted dosages are prescribed for drugs excreted through renal system.

From Eliopoulos, C. *Manual of Gerontologic Nursing* (2nd ed.). St. Louis, 1999, Mosby.

You should attempt to reduce the complexity of the medication regimen by improving self-medication practices. Developing a drug reminder system and a schedule that is appropriate or compatible with the individual's lifestyle can help decrease confusion and increase compliance. A referral to a home health nurse can provide for monitoring of compliance at home. A frequently used medication reminder system is the daily/weekly pill container that is available at pharmacies. A homemade egg

NURSING CARE PLAN 40-1

Care of the Patient at Risk for Polypharmacy

SCENARIO Alice Woo, age 75, who has a history of emphysema, will be discharged on bumetanide (Bumex), digoxin (Lanoxin), and theophylline (Theo-Dur) following treatment for symptoms related to her failure to correctly follow her prescribed medication protocol. When the nurse was reviewing medications during hospitalization, Mrs. Woo consistently confused the medications and exhibited difficulty in remembering when to appropriately take each medication.

PROBLEM/NURSING DIAGNOSIS *Confused about medications*/Ineffective therapeutic regimen management.
Supporting Assessment Data: Subjective: "Sometimes I just can't remember which ones to take in the morning and which ones to take at night." **Objective:** Patient cannot correctly identify three pills by name or use. Hospitalized for symptoms related to improper medication use.

Goals/Expected Outcomes	Nursing Interventions	Selected Rationale	Evaluation
Patient communicates an understanding of need to follow treatment regimen before discharge.	Determine readiness and ability to learn. Reinforce relationship between not following treatment and present hospitalization.	People who are not ready to learn do not learn nearly as well as those who are ready.	*Does patient verbalize an understanding of her treatment regimen?* States she understands the reason for her present hospitalization. Meeting outcome.
Patient correctly identifies all three medications 100% of the time prior to discharge.	Assess patient's ability to read a medication label. If patient cannot see or read labels, use symbol code system on mock medicine bottles marked with large "B," "L," and "T" for easy identification. Review identification method with patient three times a day prior to discharge. Have significant other or pharmacy label patient's medications with letter symbols.	Patient must be able to be read medication labels in order for the medication to be correctly identified.	Despite a vision impairment, patient is now able to easily recognize the coded letters on medication bottles and correctly identify each medication. Meeting outcome.
Patient states the correct dose, frequency, and major side effects of each medication.	Teach patient correct dose, number of pills to take at each dose, and any potential side effects. Reinforce verbal information using large "flash" cards. Ask patient to read each card.	To take medication correctly, patient must know this information.	*Can patient state the correct dose, frequency, and major side effects of each medication?* Patient correctly recites dosage of each medication, number of pills to take at each dose of each medication, and general side effects of each medication. Meeting outcome.
Patient demonstrates ability to monitor effects of medication, by return demonstration of taking pulse correctly and using weight record sheet.	Teach patient to count radial pulse for 1 full minute, noting regularity, and have patient do return demonstration. Teach patient to record weekly weight using a sample calendar form.	Accurately counting the radial pulse allows patient to know when not to take the Lanoxin, or when to report an abnormality to the physician. Tracking daily weight is essential to determine if condition is worsening.	*Is patient monitoring pulse and weight accurately?* Monitoring pulse and weight correctly. Meeting outcome.

NURSING CARE PLAN 40-1

Care of the Patient at Risk for Polypharmacy—cont'd

Goals/Expected Outcomes	Nursing Interventions	Selected Rationale	Evaluation
Patient states intent to call physician if pulse is irregular or below 60; if weight changes by more than 5 lb; if ankle edema develops; or if she experiences gastrointestinal symptoms, neurologic changes, or visual problems.	Instruct patient to promptly call physician if side effects occur or general condition changes. Reinforce instructions; provide clearly printed card with physician's telephone number.	Knowing specific signs and symptoms that indicate a change in condition or side effect will reinforce need to call physician.	*Is patient able to verbalize what to report to the physician?* Able to verbalize when to call physician. Meeting outcome.
Patient states intent to avoid foods/habits that will affect theophylline level, and increase foods that will help prevent potassium loss from Bumex.	Instruct patient to increase fluids, and to limit caffeine products, smoking, and charbroiled foods.	Increasing fluids helps prevent dehydration. Limiting listed items helps maintain a steady theophylline level.	*Can patient identify which foods to avoid and which to increase in diet?*
Patient identifies various types of caffeine products and potassium-rich sources.	Encourage patient to decrease consumption of caffeine and increase consumption of potassium-rich foods.	Intake of potassium-rich foods help prevent hypokalemia.	Patient correctly names several foods to avoid and identifies potassium-rich foods to increase. Meeting outcome.
Patient states intent to avoid taking antacid products within 1 hour of taking Lanoxin.	Give patient list of foods to avoid/increase to promote drug effectiveness. Instruct patient to avoid concurrent use of antacids with Lanoxin to avoid ineffective absorption.	A printed list will aid memory and make it easier for patient to comply.	*Does patient refrain from taking antacid products inappropriately?* Yes; waits for an hour after taking Lanoxin to take her antacid.
Patient demonstrates ability to self-administer prescribed medications.	Give written directions for all medications, doses, and times on a note card in large bold letters.	A reference card helps if patient cannot remember the prescribed dose.	*Is patient able to administer her medications on schedule?* Able to administer medications correctly from 7-day medication planner. Meeting outcome.
	Referring to written instructions, teach method of monitoring self-administration of medication using a pill box system.	Monitoring self-administration of medications is essential to compliance.	
	Allow patient to learn at own rate in a distraction-free environment.	Rushing someone to learn causes anxiety and decreases learning. Learning occurs best in a distraction-free environment, especially for an older adult.	

❓ CRITICAL THINKING QUESTIONS

1. How would you determine Mrs. Woo's readiness to learn?

2. What questions would it be necessary to ask Mrs. Woo to prevent the risk for polypharmacy?

carton container may be substituted for the elder affected with arthritic hands. Other reminder tactics can include the use of check-off systems, calendars, color- or symbol-coded medication bottles, an alarm clock, or a voice-mail system. The use of cueing with daily events such as brushing teeth can also be helpful to promote compliance.

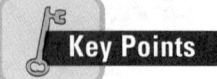

Key Points

- Common health problems that affect mobility include respiratory and cardiovascular diseases, osteoporosis, gout, foot conditions, obesity, and neurologic disorders, as well as psychosocial and emotional disorders.
- Mobility needs that are immediately addressed can allow the patient to quickly resume her former activity level and prevent undesirable consequences.
- Changes in the elder's posture, balance, gait, and vision coupled with chronic conditions and the use of multiple medications greatly increase the risk of a fall.
- Safety may be enhanced in the home by teaching the patient and family about environmental factors that contribute to falls.
- Incontinence is one of the most common reasons for institutionalization of the elderly.
- Incontinence is not a normal consequence of aging, but a condition that is secondary to pathologic, physiologic, and functional contributing factors.
- True constipation can only be identified after assessing the frequency, amount, and consistency of stools as well as possible contributing factors.
- Patient teaching for prevention of constipation includes specific diet remedies as well as a physical exercise plan.
- Physical, social, and psychological factors affect the nutritional status of the elderly.
- The elderly person with a sensory deficit may quickly become confused in a new environment and become subject to safety problems and self-care deficits.
- Socialization may be difficult for the individual with sensory deficits.
- Many people continue sexual activity as they age.
- Individuals over 65 years of age are most likely to experience a polypharmacy situation.
- Changes in body composition as well as in absorption, metabolism, and excretion of drugs in the elderly contribute to the risk of drug toxicity.

 Go to your **Companion CD-ROM** for an Audio Glossary, animations, video clips, and more.

  Be sure to visit the companion Evolve site at http://evolve.elsevier.com/deWit/fundamental/ for additional online resources.

ONLINE RESOURCES

Alzheimer's Association: www.alz.org.

American Dietetic Association: www.eatright.org.

Health Canada, Division of Aging and Seniors: www.hc-sc.gc.ca/seniors-aines.

International Foundation for Functional Gastrointestinal Disorders: www.aboutincontinence.org.

NCLEX-PN® EXAMINATION-STYLE REVIEW QUESTIONS

*Choose the **best** answer(s) for each question.*

1. Prevention of mobility problems in the elderly can be addressed by encouraging: (Select all that apply.)
   1. maintaining a normal weight.
   2. treating arthritis pain adequately.
   3. 30 minutes of walking per day.
   4. strength training exercises.

2. Factors that may contribute to falls in the elderly are: (Select all that apply.)
   1. visual loss.
   2. postural hypotension.
   3. hypertension.
   4. polypharmacy.

3. One of the most common reasons that elder adults are placed in long-term care facilities is:
   1. behavioral problems.
   2. incontinence.
   3. cancer.
   4. delirium.

4. Dietary substances that help prevent constipation include: (Select all that apply.)
   1. hot water and lemon juice in the morning.
   2. eggs.
   3. whole-grain bread.
   4. raw fruits.

5. Dietary recommendations for the elderly include:
   1. between 50 and 63 g/day of protein.
   2. 2000 to 2600 calories per day.
   3. 35% of dietary calories as fat.
   4. 75% of calories from complex carbohydrates.

6. The elder with a sensory impairment as a result of the aging process may:
   1. experience an abrupt awareness of the sensory loss.
   2. be subject to safety problems.
   3. increase socialization patterns.
   4. easily adapt to new environments.

7. Measures to try to prevent the development of macular degeneration include:

    1. wearing sunglasses and a diet of antioxidant foods.
    2. wearing sunglasses and a diet low in calcium oxidate.
    3. artificial tears and a low-roughage diet.
    4. eye exercises and a diet high in vitamin A.

8. Drug toxicity occurs more easily in the elderly due to: *(Select all that apply.)*

    1. decreased kidney function.
    2. slower liver metabolism.
    3. others overdosing them.
    4. diet interaction with drugs.

9. Drug use assessment to identify concerns related to polypharmacy should include:

    1. names of the pharmacies used.
    2. types of insurance coverage.
    3. usual diet consumed.
    4. type of drug reminder system used.

10. The condition most likely to cause a vision loss in the elderly is _____. *(Fill in the blank.)*

CRITICAL THINKING ACTIVITIES *Read each clinical scenario and discuss the questions with your classmates.*

Scenario

Your patient is a 79-year-old widowed woman being discharged from the rehabilitation unit to her home after recovery from a fractured hip secondary to a fall. She states "I'm having trouble swallowing these big 'horse pills' for my osteoporosis."

1. What type of nutritional counseling could you do for this individual?
2. What safety concerns would you have for this individual?
3. What type of community services could be helpful to this individual during her recovery?

Objectives

Upon completing this chapter, you should be able to:

Theory

1. Discuss general principles of care for elderly patients with altered cognitive functioning.
2. Assist with assessment of cognitive changes in the elderly patient.
3. Differentiate characteristics of delirium, dementia, and depression.
4. Identify options for keeping the cognitively impaired senior safe.
5. Implement strategies to decrease agitation, wandering, sundowning, and eating problems in patients.
6. Identify the interrelationship between alcoholism, depression, and suicide in the elder.
7. Identify the four main categories of elder abuse.
8. List five crimes commonly occurring to the elderly.
9. Discuss two future psychosocial issues for the elderly.

Clinical Practice

1. Formulate a plan of care for the cognitively impaired elder.
2. Demonstrate the ability to interact therapeutically with patients with depression and suicidal tendencies.
3. Teach crime prevention suggestions to a group of elders.

Key Terms

 Be sure to check out the bonus material on the Companion CD-ROM, including selected audio pronunciations.

age-associated memory impairment (ĀJ ă-SŌ-sē-ā-tĭd MĔ-mŏ-rē ĭm-PĂR-mĕnt, p. 848)
Alzheimer's disease (ĂWLZ-hī-mĕrz, p. 852)
behavior modification (p. 853)
benign senescent forgetfulness (bē-NĪN sĕ-NĔS-ĕnt, p. 848)
creative behavioral therapies (p. 850)
delirium (dĕ-LĬR-ē-ŭm p. 849)
dementia (dĕ-MĔN-shē-ă, p. 849)
depression (dĕ-PRĔSH-ŭn, p. 854)
electroconvulsive therapy (ECT) (ē-LĔK-trō-kŏn-VŬL-sĭv, p. 856)
nocturnal delirium (nŏk-TŪR-năl, p. 849)
paranoia (păr-ă-NOY-ă, p. 854)
selective serotonin reuptake inhibitors (SSRIs) (p. 856)

Several factors influence the psychosocial status of the elderly, including functional limitations and external forces. Cognitive impairments, such as dementia, and physical care problems, such as altered mobility, are two examples of functional limitations. External forces may include economic and environmental factors such as income, housing, technology, geographic area, community resources, and crime. Individual life circumstances, such as loneliness and depression leading to alcohol abuse or the lack of a support system, can also influence the elder's overall well-being. These factors, individually or in combination, all affect the way elders perceive the health care system and ultimately respond to illness.

CHANGES IN COGNITIVE FUNCTIONING IN THE ELDERLY

There are many misconceptions about the mental functioning of the elderly due to the negative attitudes of our American society toward growing old. People often assume that mental confusion, forgetfulness, and inappropriate behavior are typical of aging. However, very few changes in cognition are attributable to age-related factors alone.

The terms benign senescent forgetfulness and age-associated memory impairment are often used to describe age-related changes in mental processes. These changes include a modest decline in short-term memory and a slight and gradual decline in cognitive skills such as calculation, abstraction, word fluency, verbal comprehension, spatial orientation, and inductive reasoning. **The elderly are as capable of learning new things as younger people, but their speed of processing information is slower.**

Examples of mental changes that are not due to the normal aging process include confusion, disorientation, inappropriate behavior, depression, and the inability to concentrate or follow directions. Any major declines in cognitive functioning typically result from diseases such as dementia and metabolic disorders; stress, such as relocation; alcohol abuse or undesirable medication effects; and vision or hearing impairments. Dispiritedness and depression can occur from becoming withdrawn and detached from social interaction.

?
Think Critically About . . . Can you think of a time you heard someone attribute confusion in an elder to "getting old"?

ASSESSMENT OF COGNITIVE CHANGES IN THE ELDERLY

The older adult with significant changes in mental functioning should be given a comprehensive mental status examination using a tool such as the Mental Status Questionnaire (MSQ). A detailed and accurate medical history and physical examination should also be performed prior to making a judgment about the cause of altered mental functioning.

As a nurse, you need to understand that disorientation and other mental symptoms can have a physiologic basis. You should carefully observe elderly and confused patients and question them and significant others about events preceding admission. Be sure to exercise patience and allow enough time for the elder to respond to questions. Compensate for sensory limitations during all interactions. Assess for factors that may contribute to an altered mental state, such as medication effects, a new environment, disease processes such as pneumonia or a urinary tract infection, fluid and electrolyte imbalance, or psychosocial stressors. All information should be accurately and promptly reported to assist in the appropriate diagnosis and treatment.

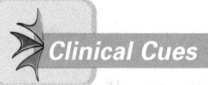
Clinical Cues

An elderly person who is experiencing a situation that makes him very anxious may demonstrate temporary decreased cognitive function. Ask the patient, "Is anything causing you worry at this time?"

COMMON COGNITIVE DISORDERS IN THE ELDERLY

CONFUSION

Patients with confusion have difficulty remembering, learning, following directions, and communicating their needs. Mental confusion can significantly influence a patient's dignity, independence, personality, and support system and may complicate diagnosis and treatment of a patient's illness. It can be caused by delirium, dementia, or numerous other often reversible conditions as listed in Box 41-1.

?
Think Critically About . . . Can you imagine how frustrating it could be to have difficulty remembering your own address? Do you ever have difficulty remembering something?

Box 41-1 | *Conditions Associated with Confusion*

- Vascular insufficiency
- Trauma
- Tumors
- Central nervous system infections
- Hypotension
- Systemic disorders
- Pulmonary/cardiovascular diseases
- Metabolic disorders
- Electrolyte imbalance
- Anemia
- Altered renal function
- Drug toxicity
- Endocrine disorders
- Nutritional deficiencies
- Stress
- Pain
- Anesthesia
- Altered body temperature
- Dehydration
- Anxiety
- Depression/grief
- Fatigue
- Sensory deprivation/overload
- New environment
- Toxic substances

Box 41-2 | *Signs and Symptoms of Sundowning*

Behaviors that occur in the later part of the day indicative of sundowning in the person with dementia are
- Restlessness
- Increased anxiety
- Increased agitation
- Increased confusion
- Uncooperativeness
- More argumentative

DELIRIUM

Delirium is an acute confusional state that can occur suddenly or over a long period as a result of an underlying biologic cause or psychological stressor. Some causes include stroke, tumors, systemic infection, fluid and electrolyte imbalance, acute inflammatory disorders, drug reactions, toxins, and sensory deprivation or overload. If left untreated, delirium can lead to coma or death. Nocturnal delirium, or **sundown syndrome,** is the appearance or increase of symptoms of confusion or agitation associated with the late afternoon or early evening hours and usually continuing into the night (Box 41-2). Little is known about this disorder, which poses a management problem for caregivers. Impaired mental status, dehydration, interruptions in sleep, and recent relocation may contribute to sundowning.

DEMENTIA

Dementia is generally a permanent condition characterized by several cognitive deficits. It is characterized by a slow, insidious onset that affects memory, intel-

Table 41-1 *Differentiation of Delirium, Dementia, and Depression*

	DELIRIUM	DEMENTIA	DEPRESSION
Onset	Sudden	Gradual	Gradual or rapid
Orientation	Disoriented, clouding of consciousness, fluctuating level of awareness	Disoriented	Oriented or disoriented
Affect/Mood	Varies	Labile, inappropriate	Despair, worry
Behavior	Agitation; inability to perform ADLs; changes in sleep-wake cycle	Agitation or apathy, inability to perform ADLs	Apathy, agitation, self-neglect, appetite change
Speech	May be incoherent and inappropriate or coherent and appropriate	Sparse, repetitive, may initially lie to cover deficits; later does not conceal	Coherent, may not want to talk
Memory	Impaired for recent events; memory disturbed	Impaired for recent events, intact remote memory	Impaired; decreased ability to concentrate
Prognosis	Good; resolves with treatment	Poor; no return to predemented state	Resolves with treatment of cause or treatment of depression

Key: *ADLs,* Activities of daily living.

lectual functioning, and the ability to problem-solve. Primarily seen in Alzheimer's disease, it also occurs with brain tumors or with serious medical or surgical disorders. Symptoms of dementia may mask depression. The reverse is also true: The depressed person may present with symptoms similar to dementia, such as confusion and disorientation. Thus careful assessment is essential to determine the cause of the patient's symptoms. Table 41-1 differentiates delirium, dementia, and depression.

The cognitive losses associated with dementia, delirium, and depression are similar; however, each person experiences cognitive changes at different rates, and each responds differently to interventions. Thus interventions must be individualized, with ongoing commitment from both the health care team and family. General principles of care for elders with altered cognitive functioning are summarized in Box 41-3.

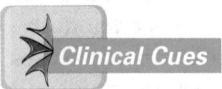
Clinical Cues

Use of a light therapy box in the morning hours may decrease depression as well as alleviate sundown syndrome problems. The patient sits with the light shining on him for 20 to 30 minutes. He can be watching TV, reading, or doing other sedentary tasks while under the light.

Specific Interventions for Confusion and Disorientation

Psychosocial Measures. Because there is little treatment for elders with dementia, a behavioral approach is essential to enhance the elder's quality of life. Two basic types of behavioral management are psychosocial interventions and medication. The plan of care should also include considerations for the patient's family.

The primary goal of psychosocial interventions is to produce a feeling of well-being in the confused

Box 41-3 *Principles of Nursing Care for the Cognitively Impaired Elder*

- Monitor and maintain physical well-being.
- Recognize the underlying meaning of actions/behaviors.
- Adjust the environment accordingly.
- Use concise, direct interactions.
- Maintain and enhance self-esteem and socialization.
- Implement strategies to enhance orientation.
- Maintain adequate nutrition.

and disoriented elder. Although therapy is usually implemented by a social worker or the activity department, you can support therapy during patient care and evaluate changes in the patient's behavior to revise the plan of care as needed.

There are a variety of therapies to help patients who are experiencing confusion and disorientation regain their sense of who they are, and what is happening in the environment around them. It is important to note that once a therapy is initiated, it should be used consistently by everyone in contact with the patient, including the family, to avoid further confusion. Table 41-2 presents several types of psychosocial approaches, their purpose, and related activities.

Other psychosocial interventions include creative behavioral therapies such as art, music, and humor that can allow for self-expression and alleviate anxiety and depression. The goal of creative therapies is to slow the rate of deterioration and prevent institutionalization as long as possible. Having pets available can also meet many needs. They can be someone to talk to, care for, and satisfy the need for touch. Pets may help a person deal with the loneliness caused by the many losses experienced in old age, such as decreased income, death of a spouse, and loss of independence (Figure 41-1).

Table 41-2 | *Psychosocial Approaches for Confusion/Disorientation*

PURPOSE	ACTIVITIES
REALITY ORIENTATION Orient patient to person, place, and time.	Consistent 24-hr/day interaction with staff/family Continual reminders of day, year, time Consistent mealtimes, activities of daily living, treatment Memory aids such as TV, radio, newspaper, clock, calendar
VALIDATION THERAPY Decrease stress, promote self-esteem and communication, reduce chemical/physical restraints, and delay institutionalization.	Group support to encourage respect for the feelings of the individual from his perspective Example activities include singing favorite songs, reminiscing, sharing a memento or family photo
REMINISCENCE Reexamine past to promote socialization and mental stimulation; wrap up unresolved issues.	Individual or group sharing of information about past life/experiences
REMOTIVATION THERAPY Stimulate senses and provide new motivation in life through factual information rather than feelings.	Introduce pictures, plants, animals, or sounds to encourage interaction
RESOCIALIZATION Encourage socialization patterns within a group.	Assign socialization roles in a group, such as serving each other refreshments

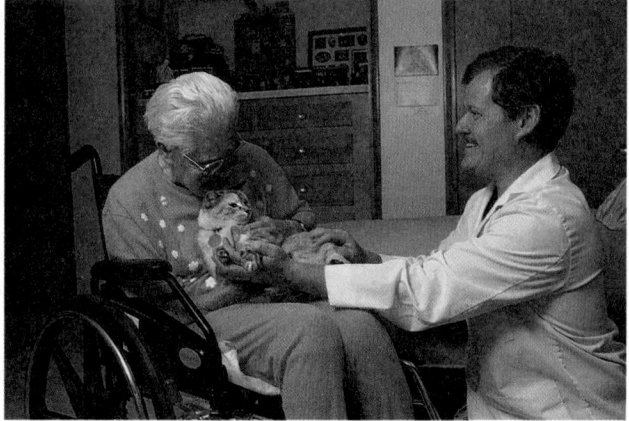

FIGURE **41-1** Pet therapy for the lonely, depressed elderly. A relationship with a pet can provide mutual affection and purposeful activity.

? *Think Critically About . . .* How could you use reminiscence to help an elder adapt to relocating to a nursing home?

Pharmacotherapy. Before any drugs are used to deal with problem behaviors, all other types of nursing interventions must first be used, with documentation of their effectiveness. It is important to use drugs for valid psychological problems, and not just for behaviors that are annoying to others.

Adaptation is necessary when using psychotropic drugs with the elderly. Many psychotropic drugs require an extended period of time to have a therapeutic effect. Toxicity and undesirable side effects such as constipation and orthostatic hypotension are not uncommon. Because of chronic health problems in an individual, some medication may be contraindicated

or require careful administration. Thus patient and family teaching about medications is essential.

Major tranquilizers, such as chlorpromazine (Thorazine) or haloperidol (Haldol), are often prescribed to manage the anxiety, agitation, hostility, and paranoia associated with dementia. Because these drugs can have many side effects, especially in the elderly, patients need to be closely monitored. Minor tranquilizers may also be used to treat symptoms of agitation and anxiety. Antidepressants such as citalopram (Celexa) or duloxetine (Cymbalta) may be used if depression coexists with dementia. These drugs may improve appetite and sleep habits, enhance socialization, and increase energy levels. Hypnotics, antianxiety drugs, and anticonvulsants may also be helpful.

? *Think Critically About . . .* What type of side effects would you assess for in a patient who is receiving major tranquilizers?

Family Support. It is very important to provide emotional and social support to the patient with dementia, as well as to significant others. As caregivers, the entire family often experiences changes in lifestyle, privacy, and socialization. It is not unusual for the caregiver to experience physical and mental exhaustion from providing round-the-clock care.

Adjusting to the reality that dementia is a chronic, nonreversible condition that may result in a lingering death can be very difficult. This places families in a situation of dealing with grief over a long period of time.

Acceptance of a relative with dementia by a loved one depends on personal coping strategies, support, and past experiences. Adjustment can be enhanced by integrating the care of the family into the nursing care plan. Family members will need ongoing support by the entire health care team. They may need an explanation regarding the disease or condition to help them better cope with the days ahead.

Financial problems and multiple role responsibilities add to the burden of caregiving by the spouse or adult children. Caregivers are also subject to loneliness, depression, and social isolation. An assessment of the caregiver's health and functional status, nutrition, and exercise patterns can allow for developing strategies to help families cope more effectively as caregivers. Caregivers may need to be encouraged to take time out and attend to their own well-being.

Nurses can encourage families to consider adult day services or respite care if the elder resides at home. These types of care can provide for much-needed psychological and physical rest for the caregivers. Families may need guidance in locating resources to explore. Referrals may include health care professionals, community mental health centers, area agencies on aging, or support groups for specific diseases such as Alzheimer's disease.

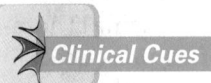

Clinical Cues

Most larger communities have respite care for those with dementia where the family can take the patient while they have a short vacation. Department of Veterans Affairs facilities can often provide this care as well. Often these are special units attached to a hospital or long-term care facility. Families should be encouraged to use this service.

Social implications for the resident in long-term care whose abilities continue to deteriorate relate to maintaining interactions with others for as long as possible. It is important to realize the family will continue to require support from the health care team at this time.

Think Critically About . . . What type of personal stress management strategies could you suggest to a caregiver of an Alzheimer's patient?

ALZHEIMER'S DISEASE

Alzheimer's disease (AD) is the most common form of dementia (70%) in the elderly, and is the fourth leading cause of death in this population. With the graying of America, this disorder may pose a significant public health concern in this new millennium.

The loss of neurons in the frontal and temporal lobes accounts for the AD patient's inability to process and integrate new information as well as retrieve memory. Although there are many diagnostic tools to

---

Box 41-4 *Stages of Alzheimer's Disease and Characteristics and Behaviors*

EARLY
- Mild short-term memory loss
- Difficulty learning new things
- Mild depression

MIDDLE
- Increased short/long-term memory loss
- Suspicion
- Agitation
- Hallucinations
- ADLs affected
- Wanders
- Incontinent

LATE
- Severe memory impairment
- Impaired mobility
- Deteriorating speech
- Bedridden
- Weight loss
- Difficulty swallowing

Key: *ADLs*, Activities of daily living.

rule out some cognitive diseases, few can diagnose AD. Positron emission tomography (PET) has shown reduced lobe activity early in the disease. However, conclusive evidence can be found only at autopsy.

AD has three stages: early, middle, and late. Box 41-4 shows the common behavioral manifestations associated with each stage.

Treatment and Nursing Interventions for Alzheimer's Disease

Treatment is primarily symptomatic. Four cholinesterase inhibitor drugs—tacrine (Cognex), donepezil (Aricept), galantamine (Reminyl), and rivastigmine, (Exelon) produce modest benefits early in the disease by improving memory, alertness, and social engagement. These drugs work by increasing acetylcholine in the cerebral cortex. Cognex is associated with liver toxicity and must be monitored closely. Aricept is administered once a day, and causes less liver toxicity. Memantine (Namenda), a drug developed in Germany and approved in the United States in 2004, is the first treatment option for moderate to severe AD symptoms. Several new drugs are under development for AD, including nerve growth factor drugs.

Other medications found to enhance cognitive functioning, improve behavioral problems, or delay the effects of the disease include estrogen, vitamin E, nonsteroidal anti-inflammatory drugs (NSAIDs), folic acid, and possibly, the cholesterol-lowering statin drugs. General nursing interventions for AD patients depend on the stage of illness. In the early and middle stages, nursing care for a confused patient as previously discussed is necessary. The end of the middle

Box 41-5 | NANDA-I Nursing Diagnoses for the Cognitively Impaired Elder

- Acute confusion
- Anxiety
- Caregiver role strain
- Chronic low self-esteem
- Compromised family coping
- Deficient diversional activity
- Disturbed thought processes
- Fatigue
- Fear
- Functional urinary incontinence
- Imbalanced nutrition: less than body requirements
- Impaired memory
- Impaired physical mobility
- Impaired social interaction
- Impaired verbal communication
- Interrupted family processes
- Risk for injury
- Risk for other-directed violence
- Self-care deficit
- Sleep deprivation

stage, as well as the last stage, requires primarily supportive care measures. Box 41-5 lists some North American Nursing Diagnosis Association–International (NANDA-I) nursing diagnoses that are appropriate for the cognitively impaired older patient.

SAFETY FOR THE COGNITIVELY IMPAIRED

When a senior is cognitively impaired, home safety becomes an issue. When impairment is very mild, the patient may be able to stay in his own home safely. Otherwise, there must be adjustments to the living situation. When a person with dementia goes to live with relatives, there should be alerting systems attached to outside doors to prevent the person from wandering out by himself. Identification should be sewn into clothes and placed in a wallet or purse. An identification bracelet that is not easily removed is helpful if wandering occurs. Measures need to be taken to alert the household if the person leaves the bedroom area at night so that the stove is not used without supervision. Sometimes a residential placement is needed. Options include an assisted-living facility, a board-and-care facility, or a long-term care facility.

If the person still owns a car, driving becomes another safety issue. No one wants to give up independence. Families have great difficulty getting a senior to give up driving. One helpful way is to suggest that a family member take the person wherever he wants to go for a month so that it becomes apparent that giving up the car doesn't mean staying at home. Another option is to research what alternative trans-

portation is available and have a family member accompany the person the first couple of times that transportation is used. If that works well, then it can be pointed out that the person doesn't need to drive anymore to maintain his present lifestyle and independence. Another method is to see if the person will consent to having an outside evaluation by a driver's education firm to determine safe driving capability. Of course, the person should only drive if confusion about direction is not an issue. Helpful information is available in the American Medical Association guide, *Physician's Guide to Assessing and Counseling Older Drivers,* available at www.ama-assn.org/ama/pub/category/10791.html. There are driver rehabilitation specialists that can help sharpen driving skills. Information is available at www.driver-ed.org.

BEHAVIORS ASSOCIATED WITH COGNITIVE DISORDERS

Agitation/Hostility/Paranoia

Violent behavior in the elderly may be the result of a lifelong psychological pattern, an organic condition, or an adverse reaction to multiple medications. Aggressive behavior may also occur as a self-protective response to confusion, fear, or sensory loss. Frequently it is associated with delirium, AD, other dementias, stroke, metabolic disorders, and hypoxia.

Preventing agitation and managing it can be accomplished by watching carefully for signs of this behavior. Some patients will show signs of increasing irritability before a severe problem occurs. Others may have sudden, explosive outbreaks. Notice if patients are talking very loudly, pacing more or faster, or making threats. Before an actual outburst occurs, try to keep the patient engaged in conversation, using some of the therapeutic communication skills discussed in Chapter 8. If seeing reflections in a mirror causes agitation, cover or remove the mirrors.

Matching the tone of the patient's voice may be calming. It may be advisable to step back 4 to 6 feet while conversing. With a disoriented patient or if a sensory deficit is present, you may want to approach more closely to maintain eye contact and touch. This must be done cautiously to protect the safety of everyone. Move other patients or visitors out of the way as necessary.

Behavior modification is also an intervention used to change agitated behavior by giving positive feedback for desired behaviors and negative feedback for undesired behaviors. Distraction may be used for the elder not favorably responding to behavior modification.

If a patient becomes violent, you must remember to protect the patient from his own behavior. You need to call for help and, as a team member, decide what intervention will be most helpful.

Points to consider for intervention are the patient's right to the least restrictive treatment and the federal and state regulations regarding the use of chemical (medication) and physical protective devices. Before giving medications, it is necessary to try behavioral approaches and document their effectiveness. When all else fails and the patient poses a threat to his well-being or others, protective devices may be necessary.

Paranoia can also be caused by dementia as well as psychological conditions such as schizophrenia. Patients with paranoia may misinterpret their environment and believe others are untrustworthy and out to get them. These patients may sound very convincing and logical in their suspicious behaviors.

For the patient with paranoia, developing trust is the most important thing to accomplish. Being consistent and reliable is perhaps the best way to develop trust in the relationship with the paranoid patient. Do not make promises you cannot keep. If you say you will do something, follow up with it. It is of utmost importance not to put any medication in a drink or food without the patient's knowledge so that trust is not broken.

> **?**
> *Think Critically About . . .* Why would it be especially important for you to offer explanations to a hearing-impaired patient experiencing paranoia or thinking that others are talking about him?

Wandering

Wandering may be a problem for the patient affected with a cognitive disorder. Wanderers tend to be individuals who were very active people prior to the onset of disease. For some, wandering may be goal directed, such as looking for the bathroom. For others, it may be a need to combat boredom or restlessness. Nursing interventions might include ensuring the environment is safe for wandering, informing/educating others about this problem, making sure the patient has an identification bracelet, frequently checking the patient, observing for behaviors that trigger the wandering, diverting his attention, and maintaining a regular activity program. Many units are designed for wandering patients and may even include gated outside areas in which to commune with nature.

> **?**
> *Think Critically About . . .* What type of diversional activities could you use for a wandering patient who is trying to go home?

Sundown Syndrome

To alleviate the confusion and fears associated with sundowning, it is important for you to help the patient feel safe in his environment. The use of a night-light, placing the call bell within reach, reducing stimulation in the environment, and moving the patient closer to the nurses' station can help minimize nocturnal confusion (Box 41-6). Protective devices should be used as a

---

Box 41-6 *Strategies and Interventions to Minimize Sundowning*

The following have proven helpful for decreasing sundowning:
- Limit outings and activities to the morning hours.
- For the person with Alzheimer's disease, keep times of sensory stimulation short. Prevent several assaults on the senses from occurring at one time (i.e., television on, noisy children, lots of activity of others in the vicinity, etc.).
- Avoid caffeine drinks and caffeine-containing foods such as chocolate in the afternoon and evening.
- Prevent overnapping during the day, but keep the person well rested.
- Provide soothing music as dusk approaches and through the evening.
- Provide stimulating activities during the day along with exercise, but prevent exhaustion.
- Make certain physical needs are met and that the person isn't hungry, thirsty, wet, soiled, hot, or cold.
- Obtain treatment for arthritis or other discomfort, shortness of breath, urinary tract infection, cold/flu symptoms, etc.
- Provide a private "time-out" place for the person subject to sundowning.
- Keep surroundings as simple as possible with an uncluttered appearance. Remove mirrors and pictures if they seem to cause the person distress. Avoid changing things in the environment around once simplified.

---

last-resort safety measure because they may add to the patient's anxiety.

> **?**
> *Think Critically About . . .* What would it feel like to awaken at night and think that the shadow cast upon the wall is someone leaning over you with a knife?

Eating Problems

Adequate nutrition often becomes a problem for the patient with dementia. Common feeding challenges include lack of appetite, refusal to open the mouth, holding food in the mouth, refusal to swallow food, and choking when swallowing. Nutritional Therapies 41-1 lists strategies to overcome such problems.

DEPRESSION/ALCOHOLISM/SUICIDE

Depression (feelings of sadness, despair, or discouragement) in the elderly is often overlooked and untreated. It is the most common functional mental illness in the elderly. As noted in Table 41-1, it can often be mistaken for delirium or dementia.

Depression is often difficult to recognize because symptoms may be attributed to the aging process. Instead of complaining of a depressed mood, the elderly

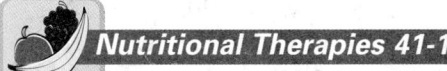

Nutritional Therapies 41-1

Strategies to Improve Nutritional Status of the Cognitively Impaired Elder

- Mealtime companionship in a stress-free environment
- Proper oral hygiene, proper fitting dentures
- Inspection for mouth/gum/dental problems
- Identification of "hungry time" of day
- Meals in same place/same time
- Frequent small meals/snacks
- Serving favorite foods if possible
- Limited food choices served in an attractive manner
- Serving one food at a time to decrease confusion
- Use of liquid thickeners to prevent aspiration
- Reminding patient to open mouth, chew, and swallow
- Avoiding hurrying patient to eat

Box 41-7 | Questionnaire to Determine Presence of Depression

MOOD SCALE (SHORT FORM)

Choose the best answer for how you have felt over the past week:

1. Are you basically satisfied with your life? YES / NO
2. Have you dropped many of your activities and interests? YES / NO
3. Do you feel that your life is empty? YES / NO
4. Do you often get bored? YES / NO
5. Are you in good spirits most of the time? YES / NO
6. Are you afraid that something bad is going to happen to you? YES / NO
7. Do you feel happy most of the time? YES / NO
8. Do you often feel helpless? YES / NO
9. Do you prefer to stay at home, rather than going out and doing new things? YES / NO
10. Do you feel you have more problems with memory than most? YES / NO
11. Do you think it is wonderful to be alive now? YES / NO
12. Do you feel pretty worthless the way you are now? YES / NO
13. Do you feel full of energy? YES / NO
14. Do you feel that your situation is hopeless? YES / NO
15. Do you think that most people are better off than you are? YES / NO

From Original source: Yesavage, J.A., Brink, T.L., Rose, T.L., et al. (1983). Development and validation of a geriatric depression screening scale: A preliminary report. *Journal of Psychiatric Research, 17*(1), 37-49. www.stanford.edu/~yesavage/GDS.html.

may complain of anorexia, sleep disturbances, lack of energy, and loss of interest and enjoyment in life. Depression in the elderly occurs to a great degree as a result of situational factors such as multiple losses. It is helpful to assess the elderly patient's mood periodically (Box 41-7). Undiagnosed and untreated, depression is a major contributor to alcoholism and suicide in the elderly. Focused Assessment 41-1 lists common characteristics of depression to assess in the elderly.

Alcohol abuse, suicide, and depression are interrelated in that they each have similar risk factors associ-

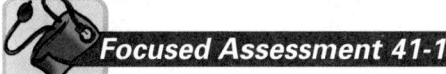

Focused Assessment 41-1

Assessment of Depression in the Elderly

Signs and symptoms to look for include

PHYSICAL ASSESSMENT
- Fatigue
- Headaches
- "Not feeling good"
- Memory impaired
- Vague aches and pains

PSYCHOSOCIAL ASSESSMENT
- Social withdrawal
- Loss of motivation/energy
- Envy/criticism of others
- Increasing demands on others
- Feelings of worthlessness/helplessness
- Appetite changes
- Sleep pattern changes
- Indecisiveness
- Obsessive worrying
- Poor outlook on life

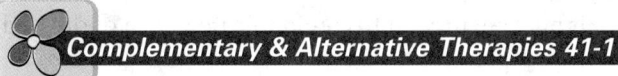

Complementary & Alternative Therapies 41-1

Omega-3 Fatty Acids

New research shows that omega-3 fatty acids may alleviate depression without dangerous side effects. Omega-3 fatty acids also aid impaired cognition. Cod liver oil is rich in omega-3 fatty acids. Eating fish such as salmon, sardines, mackerel, and tuna can increase omega-3 intake. For those who do not like fish, supplement capsules of omega-3 fatty acids are available (Barclay, 2007).

---

ated with multiple loss. Loss of status/power, income, spouse, friends, and health contribute to feelings of despair and hopelessness. The elder's outlook on life is distorted, preventing him from exploring acceptable solutions to his problems.

Alcohol misuse is a serious concern because it can interfere with the management of chronic diseases and heighten the risk of adverse drug reactions due to diminishing liver and kidney function. Alcoholism is often overlooked because so many elder problem drinkers are retired and hidden at home. Clues to alcoholism include depression, insomnia, mental confusion, frequent falls, self-neglect, and uncontrollable hypertension or diabetes, as well as gastritis and anemia.

INTERVENTIONS FOR DEPRESSION, ALCOHOLISM, AND SUICIDE PREVENTION

Patients who are depressed are usually treated with both psychotherapy and antidepressants (Complementary & Alternative Therapies 41-1). Hospitalization may be necessary if the patient is at high risk of suicide.

The three main categories of medications used to treat depression are (1) the tricyclic antidepressants, such as amoxapine (Asendin) and amitriptyline hydrochloride (Elavil); (2) the monoamine oxidase inhibitors (MAOIs), such as phenelzine sulfate (Nardil); and (3) the selective serotonin reuptake inhibitors (SSRIs), such as fluoxetine hydrochloride (Prozac), sertraline hydrochloride (Zoloft), paroxetine hydrochloride (Paxil), citalopram (Celexa), duloxetine (Cymbalta), and venlafaxine hydrochloride (Effexor).

Electroconvulsive therapy (ECT) is a treatment option for those patients who have severe forms of depression and who have failed to respond to several regimens of medication. ECT consists of electric shock to the brain via electrodes attached to the patient's temples, producing tonic-clonic seizures. How this mechanism is effective is not clearly understood. The patient usually receives two or three treatments per week for several weeks.

The primary nursing responsibility for a depressed patient is to protect him from self-injury, especially *after* the patient has initiated antidepressant therapy. Prior to that time, he may not have had the energy to commit suicide.

It may be difficult to communicate with a depressed patient because of his negative thoughts and behaviors. Genuine concern for the patient is essential. You will need to help him set realistic, achievable goals. Start with small goals such as grooming and slowly work toward larger goals. Remember that goal setting and problem solving take concentration and energy that may not be available to the person who is still somewhat depressed. Providing a quiet environment conducive to sleep can help restore energy for individuals who complain of sleep deprivation.

Caregivers need to be alert to signs of potential suicide such as meticulous planning of personal affairs, giving away treasured possessions, sudden euphoria, or statements of death wishes. Assisting the patient to promote self-esteem and meaningful activities may resolve the intent of suicide. It is important for you to build a trusting relationship with the suicidal patient to let him know you care. Spending time with your patient and active listening are very important in showing your concern.

Referrals for outpatient counseling or immediate crisis intervention may be necessary to deter suicidal thoughts or tendencies. However, as with any individual who believes suicide is the only answer, the elder may eventually carry out this act. Thus caregivers and family would need support and possible counseling to resolve their grief.

Think Critically About . . . What type of response would you have for the elder who relates to you he wishes he could go to sleep for the last time?

During patient interviews, health professionals need to assess the use of alcohol by depressed elders. Making the diagnosis of alcohol dependency is not necessarily difficult, but unless there is self-admission of a problem, long-term recovery is unlikely. Initial treatment may consist of detoxification and stabilization of the patient with chlordiazepoxide hydrochloride (Librium). Once the patient is stable, therapy may consist of group or behavioral therapy. Individual therapy may also be instituted for the depressed, alcoholic elder.

Patient and family teaching must include information about the effects of alcohol on medications and on chronic health conditions. Referral to a 12-step program such as Alcoholics Anonymous (AA) for the patient, and Al-Anon for family members, can also be a beneficial part of treatment.

CRIMES AGAINST THE ELDERLY

ELDER ABUSE

Abuse is defined as the intentional infliction of physical or emotional discomfort or the deprivation of basic needs necessary for comfort or survival. It is estimated that only 1 in 14 cases of elder abuse is reported.

Elder abuse is most often inflicted by a spouse or adult children in the home, and is often undetected. It is often related to caregiver stress, unresolved family conflicts, or families with a history of abuse. All forms of abuse are destructive, and at the very least reduce the victim's self-esteem. Box 41-8 identifies the five different categories of abuse.

Think Critically About . . . Can you remember an incident in which perhaps you suspected abuse of an individual or an acquaintance?

Box 41-8 *Categories of Elder Abuse*

- **Physical:** Infliction of physical pain and injury via assault and battery. Using physical restraints or confining persons against their will is also classified as physical abuse. It may also include the inappropriate use of drugs.
- **Sexual:** Infliction of nonconsensual sexual contact of any kind.
- **Psychological:** Verbal harassment, including intimidation, defamation, and isolation. It may also include threats of abandonment or physical violence. Psychological abuse laws vary according to state law.
- **Material:** Theft of elder's money, misuse of funds, or theft or misuse of possessions.
- **Neglect:** Failure to meet the needs of the elder, including leaving the person alone; withholding medication, food, or other necessities; not assisting with activities of daily living or providing inadequate care.

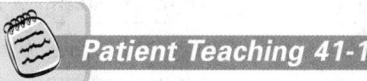

Focused Assessment 41-2

Assessment of Suspected Signs and Symptoms of Abuse in the Elderly

When working with the elderly patient, be observant for:
- Unkempt, inappropriate dress/hygiene
- Malnourished, dehydrated
- Bruises, fractures of undetermined cause; cigarette burns
- Conflicting explanation about elder's condition
- Unusual fear exhibited by the elder
- Confusion, not attributable to other causes
- Abnormal behavior in the caregiver
- Hostility displayed by caregiver in response to questions

Responsibilities of the nurse include identifying those at risk. Assessment of signs and symptoms of suspected elder abuse is described in Focused Assessment 41-2. During assessment of potential abuse, avoid a condescending tone of voice or judgmental expression. The establishment of a confidential, trusting relationship is necessary. Be sure to show a willingness to listen also to the caregiver's perspective. Assess the caregiver's early memories of relationships with the elder to learn of possible long-term conflicts.

You have a legal obligation to report elder abuse and are accorded protection from civil and criminal liability in most states that mandate reporting suspected abuse (Jech, 2002). Evidence of suspected abuse should be reported immediately to the appropriate agency for investigation. **The standard for reporting is usually a reasonable belief that an individual has been or is likely to be abused, neglected, or exploited.**

Be aware that advocacy for the abused may be difficult because you may receive threats from those who resent your involvement. A common frustrating situation is the competent elder with full legal rights who refuses help or desires to remain in an environment that is unsafe or unacceptable. In this case, the health care team must honor the decision after providing counseling about potential dangers. If a person is legally incompetent, steps need to be taken for appropriate guardianship. Testifying in court about an abusive situation can be very stressful for all who are involved.

Individual and/or group psychotherapy is often used to treat both victims and abusers. The victim should be removed from the home before entering treatment to avoid retaliation. Intensive psychotherapy may be necessary for the abuser with psychopathology. Support groups are also available for both victims and abusers. Long-term follow-up is essential to prevent further abuse.

SCAMS/WHITE-COLLAR CRIME

Crime is of particular concern to the elderly because of their sense of vulnerability. Older adults do not suffer any greater physical injury or financial loss than

---

Box 41-9 | *Crimes/Scams Against the Elderly*

- Personal/household theft
- Vehicular theft
- Purse snatching/pickpocketing
- Investment theft
- Mailbox theft
- Rape
- Assault
- Fraudulent schemes through white-collar crime
  - Donations/fundraisers
  - Investments
  - Toll-free numbers
  - Prize offers
  - Funeral planning
  - Home improvements
  - Telemarketing
  - Timesharing
  - Auto repair
  - Medical quackery

Patient Teaching 41-1

Crime Reduction Suggestions for the Elderly

Teach patients and people in the community the following:
- Attend a crime prevention program.
- Identify police/security available in high-risk areas.
- Institute an informal surveillance/buddy system among neighbors.
- Keep doors locked with dead-bolt locks.
- Do not attach ID to key rings.
- If keys are lost, have locks changed.
- Lock windows; draw blinds/curtains at night.
- Keep all hidden entries such as garage/basement door locked.
- Use a peephole. Confirm service person's ID by calling the service agency first before opening the door.
- Do not let strangers at your door or on the telephone know you are alone.
- Beware of phone tricks; do not give information to strangers. Hang up on and report nuisance callers.
- Consider a pet to provide protection.
- Travel in groups.
- Carry/wear a whistle around your neck.
- Carry few valuables on yourself; hide key and other valuables in inside pockets.
- Protect assets; keep money in bank; use direct deposit of Social Security, pension funds.

---

younger people; however, the effects of crime, such as fear, isolation, loneliness, and feelings of powerlessness, may be more detrimental. Location and income are often more significant than age in predicting crime. Some of the various crimes against older adults are listed in Box 41-9.

Nurses can be instrumental in reducing fear of crime and assisting elders in exploring security-conscious behaviors that will decrease vulnerability to victimization (Patient Teaching 41-1).

? *Think Critically About* . . . Can you think of a situation in which an elder you know was subtly scammed by a business?

Nurses also need to learn about referral programs in crime protection, prevention, and victim assistance. Federal programs through the Law Enforcement Assistance Administration, the Office of Community Victim Assistance, the Community Services Administration, and the Department of Housing and Urban Development offer crime prevention and victim counseling. State offices of aging and organizations such as the AARP (formerly the American Association of Retired Persons) have also proved beneficial in enhancing awareness of crime prevention.

FUTURE ISSUES OF CONCERN TO THE ELDERLY

It is not easy to predict what the future will bring, but the best word for the older-aged population may be *increasing*, in both number and age. The elderly will be the fastest growing segment of the population and will have the greatest effect on the delivery of health care. Older adults of the 21st century will be better educated, more involved in community and political activities, and more knowledgeable consumers of health care.

What will be the priorities in the future? How much funding will go toward research of life-threatening diseases of the elderly versus solving environmental problems that affect all populations? With the nation's long list of priorities, what decisions will be made?

? *Think Critically About* . . . What health care issues do you think **you** might face when you become elderly?

PLANNING FOR THE FUTURE

Expanding present services and developing new delivery systems will be challenges for the future. Safe housing and efficient mass transportation to stores and recreational facilities will continue to be needed, as well as one-stop-shopping senior centers. This concept can allow for the arrangement of multiple services such as home-delivered meals and chore services at a nominal cost, which can make a difference as to whether a person can remain at home or must be institutionalized.

Planning for the future will need to include lifelong learning opportunities that assist the elder with maintaining wellness, preparing for retirement and leisure time, financial planning, and advances in technology. Other considerations are job training and retraining for "early retirees" who wish to remain employed.

Health issues to be addressed need to include the rapidly rising rate of acquired immunodeficiency syndrome (AIDS) in the elderly and the health problems specific to the growing proportion of elderly women.

Healthy People 2010 is a federal campaign designed to encourage people to adopt healthy lifestyles to maintain or improve their health. Emphasis is on health promotion, protection, and prevention. State and local governments, the AARP, and business and local industry have been working together since 1990 to achieve the following goal: "Increase the years of healthy life remaining after age 65." New goals have been devised for 2010 that include more objectives that specifically address elders.

Will the programs and services discussed become realities? The answer lies partially with the elderly of today. Individuals over 65 form a powerful political group with real voting power that can effectively make change happen. Combined with the advocacy of nursing power to access necessary resources, the new goals of *Healthy People 2010* can realistically be achieved.

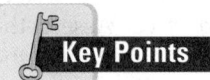 **Key Points**

- Functional limitations and external forces contribute to the psychosocial status of the elder.
- Mental confusion, forgetfulness, and inappropriate behaviors are not solely attributable to the aging process.
- A comprehensive mental status exam, medical history, and physical examination are necessary prior to making a judgment about the cause of altered cognitive functioning.
- The confused or cognitively impaired elderly person must be kept safe.
- Confusion can be caused by delirium, dementia, or numerous other, often reversible, conditions.
- The cognitive changes associated with dementia, delirium, and depression are similar and must be differentiated through careful assessment.
- Behavioral management of the confused patient includes both psychosocial approaches and medication.
- Psychotropic drugs should be used only after psychosocial approaches have been documented as ineffective.
- Drug therapy for cognitive disorders may include major and minor tranquilizers, antidepressants, and hypnotics.
- A significant consideration in managing dementia is to provide emotional and social support to both the patient and significant others.
- Alzheimer's disease is the most common form of dementia and the fourth leading cause of death in the elderly.
- Common behaviors associated with cognitive disorders include agitation, hostility, paranoia, wandering, and sundown syndrome.
- Various strategies can ease the incidence of sundown syndrome.

- Depression is the most common functional mental illness in the elderly.
- Symptoms of depression in the elderly are often attributed to the aging process.
- Alcohol abuse, suicide, and depression are interrelated and have similar risk factors.
- The exact number of abused elders is difficult to determine due to underreporting.
- Protection from civil and criminal liability is accorded to nurses who report abuse in good faith.
- Crimes and scams against the elderly often include white-collar fraudulent schemes by professional people.
- Planning for the future for the elderly should include lifelong learning opportunities that address maintaining wellness; retirement, leisure, and financial planning; job training/retraining; and advances in technology.

 Go to your **Companion CD-ROM** for an Audio Glossary, animations, video clips, and more.

 Be sure to visit the companion Evolve site at http://evolve.elsevier.com/deWit/fundamental/ for additional online resources.

ONLINE RESOURCES

Alzheimer's Association: www.alz.org.

Geriatric Resources, Inc.: www.geriatric-resources.com.

Rush Alzheimer's Disease Center. (2002). *The Rush Manual for Caregivers* (5th ed.). Chicago: Author. Available at: www.rush.edu/cms_docs/rushdoc_26.pdf.

Torres-Stanovik, R. (Ed.). (1990). *Alzheimer's Caregivers Handbook.* San Diego, CA: Caregiver Education and Support Services, San Diego County Mental Health Services. Available at: www.longtermcarelink.net/eldercare/the_caregivers_handbook.htm.

NCLEX-PN® EXAMINATION-STYLE REVIEW QUESTIONS

*Choose the **best** answer(s) for each question.*

1. When it comes to learning, the elderly are:
   1. equally capable as younger persons, but slower to learn.
   2. less able to learn than younger people.
   3. able to learn equally with younger people.
   4. about a third less efficient at learning as a younger person.

2. Confusion is often a reversible condition in patients with:
   1. dementia.
   2. depression.
   3. delirium.
   4. Alzheimer's disease.

3. Measures to keep the cognitively impaired elder safe in a home environment include: (Select all that apply.)
   1. placing alarms on the outside doors.
   2. removing knobs from the stove burners and oven at night.
   3. having the person carry a cell phone at all times.
   4. placing an identification bracelet on the person.
   5. getting the person a guide dog.

4. Which symptoms is the nurse most likely to observe in a depressed, elderly patient? *(Select all that apply.)*
   1. Anger
   2. Poor memory
   3. Insomnia
   4. Loss of motivation

5. Medications that work by increasing acetylcholine in the cerebral cortex may produce:
   1. a calming effect and less hostility.
   2. better ability to organize and carry out tasks.
   3. more ability to concentrate and learn new things.
   4. improved memory, alertness, and more social engagement.

6. Which strategies are the most helpful in managing sundowning? *(Select all that apply.)*
   1. Keeping lights very low after dark.
   2. Keeping a nonstimulating environment in the afternoon and evening.
   3. Diverting the person's attention.
   4. Playing soft music in the late afternoon and evening hours.
   5. Using night-lights in the bedroom and bathroom.

7. When you suspect an elder is considering suicide, the most appropriate intervention is to:
   1. discuss suspicions with a significant other.
   2. ask the patient directly about such plans.
   3. constantly watch the patient.
   4. refer for mental health counseling.

8. The usual standard for reporting elder abuse is one:
   1. of 100% certainty.
   2. of reasonable belief that abuse has occurred/may occur.
   3. that is beyond a shadow of a doubt.
   4. with testimony of one or more eyewitnesses.

9. Long-term recovery from alcohol abuse is most likely to occur when:
   1. the family is supportive.
   2. the patient uses Antabuse.
   3. the patient undergoes detoxification with Librium.
   4. the patient self-admits to a problem.

10. Strategies to help prevent crime include: *(Select all that apply.)*
    1. changing door locks after losing keys.
    2. using direct deposit for pension funds.
    3. using an informal buddy system in the neighborhood.
    4. checking a service person's ID after letting him in.

CRITICAL THINKING ACTIVITIES *Read each clinical scenario and discuss the questions with your classmates.*

Scenario

Your 75-year-old male patient who is being discharged to his daughter's home has just been diagnosed with early-stage Alzheimer's disease. He has a history of alcohol abuse, but has "not had a drink in a couple of years." Aricept has been prescribed in hopes of slowing disease progression.

1. What pharmacologic concerns might you have for this individual?
2. What type of education could you do with his family?
3. What type of community services could you refer the patient's daughter to for help in managing this disorder?

American Nurses Association Standards of Practice

STANDARD 1. ASSESSMENT

The registered nurse collects comprehensive data pertinent to the patient's health or the situation.

Measurement Criteria

The registered nurse:

- Collects data in a systematic and ongoing process.
- Involves the patient, family, other healthcare providers, and environment, as appropriate, in holistic data collection.
- Prioritizes data collection activities based on the patient's immediate condition, or anticipated needs of the patient or situation.
- Uses appropriate evidence-based assessment techniques and instruments in collecting pertinent data.
- Uses analytical models and problem-solving tools.
- Synthesizes available data, information, and knowledge relevant to the situation to identify patterns and variances.
- Documents relevant data in a retrievable format.

STANDARD 2. DIAGNOSIS

The registered nurse analyzes the assessment data to determine the diagnoses or issues.

Measurement Criteria

The registered nurse:

- Derives the diagnoses or issues based on assessment data.
- Validates the diagnoses or issues with the patient, family, and other healthcare providers when possible and appropriate.
- Documents diagnoses or issues in a manner that facilitates the determination of the expected outcomes and plan.

STANDARD 3. OUTCOMES IDENTIFICATION

The registered nurse identifies expected outcomes for a plan individualized to the patient or the situation.

Measurement Criteria

The registered nurse:

- Involves the patient, family, and other healthcare providers in formulating expected outcomes when possible and appropriate.
- Derives culturally appropriate expected outcomes from the diagnoses.
- Considers associated risks, benefits, costs, current scientific evidence, and clinical expertise when formulating expected outcomes.
- Defines expected outcomes in terms of the patient, patient values, ethical considerations, environment, or situation with such consideration as associated risks, benefits and costs, and current scientific evidence.
- Includes a time estimate for attainment of expected outcomes.
- Develops expected outcomes that provide direction for continuity of care.
- Modifies expected outcomes based on changes in the status of the patient or evaluation of the situation.
- Documents expected outcomes as measurable goals.

STANDARD 4. PLANNING

The registered nurse develops a plan that prescribes strategies and alternatives to attain expected outcomes.

Measurement Criteria

The registered nurse:

- Develops an individualized plan considering patient characteristics or the situation (e.g., age and culturally appropriate, environmentally sensitive).
- Develops the plan in conjunction with the patient, family, and others, as appropriate.
- Includes strategies within the plan that address each of the identified nursing diagnoses or

Adapted with permission from American Nurses Association, *Nursing: Scope and Standards of Practice*, © 2004 nursesbooks.org, Silver Spring, MD.

issues, which may include strategies for promotion and restoration of health and prevention of illness, injury, and disease.

- Provides for continuity within the plan.
- Incorporates an implementation pathway or timeline within the plan.
- Establishes the plan priorities with the patient, family, and others as appropriate.
- Utilizes the plan to provide direction to other members of the healthcare team.
- Defines the plan to reflect current statutes, rules and regulations, and standards.
- Integrates current trends and research affecting care in the planning process.
- Considers the economic impact of the plan.
- Uses standardized language or recognized terminology to document the plan.

STANDARD 5. IMPLEMENTATION

The registered nurse implements the identified plan.

Measurement Criteria

The registered nurse:

- Implements the plan in a safe and timely manner.
- Documents implementation and any modifications, including changes or omissions, of the identified plan.
- Utilizes evidence-based interventions and treatments specific to the diagnosis or problem.
- Utilizes community resources and systems to implement the plan.
- Collaborates with nursing colleagues and others to implement the plan.

STANDARD 5A. COORDINATION OF CARE

The registered nurse coordinates care delivery.

Measurement Criteria

The registered nurse:

- Coordinates implementation of the plan.
- Documents the coordination of the care.

STANDARD 5B: HEALTH TEACHING AND HEALTH PROMOTION

The registered nurse employs strategies to promote health and a safe environment.

Measurement Criteria

The registered nurse:

- Provides health teaching that addresses such topics as healthy lifestyles, risk-reducing behaviors, developmental needs, activities of daily living, and preventive self-care.
- Uses health promotion and health teaching methods appropriate to the situation and the patient's developmental level, learning needs, readiness, ability to learn, language preference, and culture.
- Seeks opportunities for feedback and evaluation of the effectiveness of the strategies used.

STANDARD 6. EVALUATION

The registered nurse evaluates progress toward attainment of outcomes.

Measurement Criteria

The registered nurse:

- Conducts a systematic, ongoing, and criterion-based evaluation of the outcomes in relation to the structures and processes prescribed by the plan and the indicated timeline.
- Includes the patient and others involved in the care or situation in the evaluative process.
- Evaluates the effectiveness of the planned strategies in relation to patient responses and the attainment of the expected outcomes.
- Documents the results of the evaluation.
- Uses ongoing assessment data to revise the diagnoses, outcomes, the plan, and the implementation as needed.
- Disseminates the results to the patient and others involved in the care or situation, as appropriate, in accordance with state and federal laws and regulations.

2 American Nurses Association Code of Ethics for Nurses

- The nurse, in all professional relationships, practices with compassion and respect for the inherent dignity, worth, and uniqueness of every individual, unrestricted by considerations of social or economic status, personal attributes, or the nature of health problems.
- The nurse's primary commitment is to the patient, whether an individual, family, group, or community.
- The nurse promotes, advocates for, and strives to protect the health, safety, and rights of the patient.
- The nurse is responsible and accountable for individual nursing practice and determines the appropriate delegation of tasks consistent with the nurse's obligation to provide optimum patient care.
- The nurse owes the same duties to self as to others, including the responsibility to preserve integrity and safety, to maintain competence, and to continue personal and professional growth.
- The nurse participates in establishing, maintaining, and improving health care environments and conditions of employment conducive to the provision of quality health care and consistent with the values of the profession through individual and collective action.
- The nurse participates in the advancement of the profession through contributions to practice, education, administration, and knowledge development.
- The nurse collaborates with other health professionals and the public in promoting community, national, and international efforts to meet health needs.
- The profession of nursing, as represented by associations and their members, is responsible for articulating nursing values, for maintaining the integrity of the profession and its practice, and for shaping social policy.

At the Beginning of the Procedure

Step A. *Perform the task according to protocol.*

Mentally review the steps of the task beforehand. If you are uncertain how to do a task, ask your team leader, resource nurse, instructor, or charge nurse. Plan for efficiency of time and effort while delivering safe care.

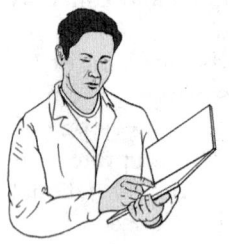 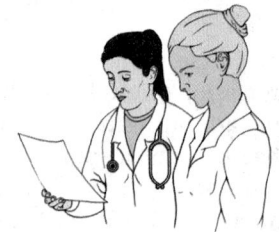

Step B. *Check the order, collect the equipment and supplies, and wash your hands.*

Verify that the procedure is to be done for the patient. Check the agency's policies and procedures manual for the accepted method of performing the procedure. Process equipment and supply charges. Take all equipment and supplies to the patient's room.

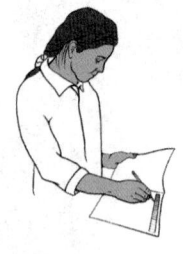 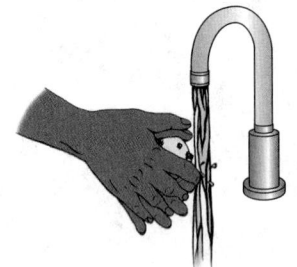

Step C. *Identify and prepare the patient.*

Greet the patient, introduce yourself, and check the patient's identification band. Use two identifiers during the identification process. Explain what you are going to do in terms the patient can understand. Elicit questions and answer clearly. Provide necessary teaching related to the procedure to be performed.

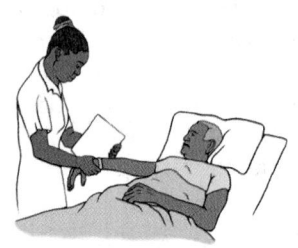 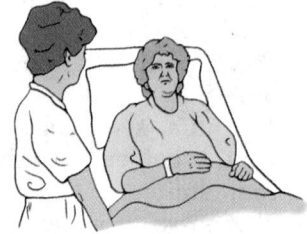

Step D. *Provide privacy and institute safety precautions; arrange the supplies and equipment.*

Close the door or curtains and drape the patient before beginning the procedure or discussing information the person might want kept confidential. Check equipment for breaks or wear and for safety. Set up the equipment and supplies in an orderly, methodical fashion. Raise the bed to an appropriate working height. Raise the side rail before turning the patient and be certain that the wheels are locked. Perform hand hygiene to prevent contaminating the patient with organisms from the chart, the nurses' station, and the supply room.

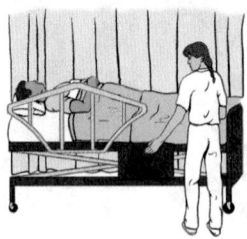 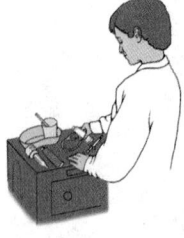

During the Procedure

Step E. *Use Standard Precautions and aseptic technique as appropriate.*

Protect yourself from blood and body fluids by wearing gloves. If there is a danger of splashing blood or body fluids, wear protective glasses or goggles and an impermeable cover gown or apron. Be very careful with sharp instruments and needles so as not to nick your skin. (See Appendix 5: Standard Precautions.)

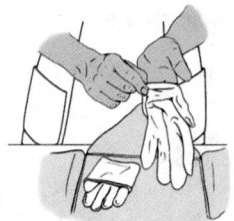 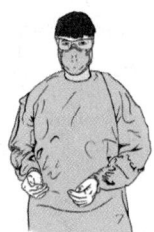

At the End of the Procedure

Step X. *Remove gloves and other protective equipment.*

After making certain the patient is clean and dry, dispose of used supplies, remove goggles and other protective equipment, and discard or store appropriately. To remove gloves without contaminating yourself, begin by pulling one glove off without touching your skin; hold the removed glove in the palm of the remaining gloved hand and then reach to the inside of the other glove and roll it down the hand. Dispose of the gloves in the trash. Perform hand hygiene immediately.

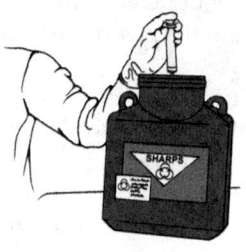 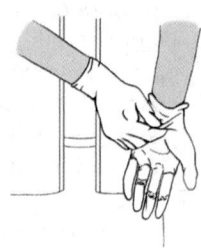

Step Y. *Restore the unit. Collect the used equipment; dispose of, clean, or store items in the proper places.*

Make the person comfortable, tidy the bed and unit, place the call light and personal items within reach, and provide for safety by lowering the bed. Remove used equipment. Soiled linens are placed in a soiled-linen hamper. Reusable items are cleaned and returned to the storage or processing area (central supply). Discontinue use of the equipment on the computer so no further charges will be made. Remove unsightly, odorous, or potentially infectious trash from the room. Inquire if anything else is needed. Perform hand hygiene before leaving the room.

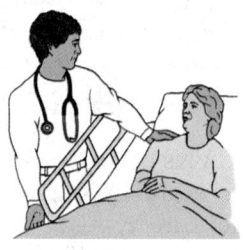 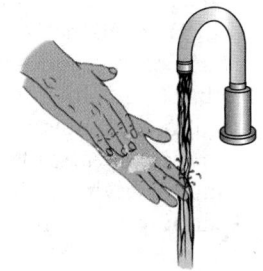

Step Z. *Record and report the procedure.*

Document assessment findings and the details of the procedure performed, or care given, in the chart. Include any problems encountered and the patient's response to the care or treatment. The recording should be accurate, specific, concise, and appropriate and should include the specific time the procedure was performed and how it was done. Report abnormalities encountered to the charge nurse or physician.

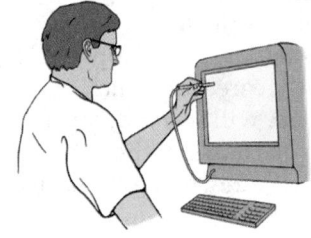 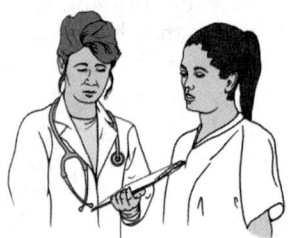

NFLPN Nursing Practice Standards for the Licensed Practical/Vocational Nurse

"Nursing Practice Standards" is one of the ways that NFLPN meets the objective of its bylaws to address principles and ethics and also to meet another Article II objective, "To interpret the standards of practical (vocational) nursing."

In recent years, LPNs and LVNs have practiced in a changing environment. As LPNs and LVNs practice in expanding roles in the health care system, *"Nursing Practice Standards"* is essential reading for LPNs, LVNs, PN, and VN students and their educators, and all who practice with LPNs and LVNs.

NURSING PRACTICE STANDARDS FOR THE LICENSED PRACTICAL/ VOCATIONAL NURSE

PREFACE

The Standards were developed and adopted by NFLPN to provide a basic model whereby the quality of health service and nursing service and nursing care given by LP/VNs may be measured and evaluated.

These nursing practice standards are applicable in any practice setting. The degree to which individual standards are applied will vary according to the individual needs of the patient, the type of health care agency or services and the community resources.

The scope of licensed practical nursing has extended into specialized nursing services. Therefore specialized fields of nursing are included in this document.

THE CODE FOR LICENSED PRACTICAL/VOCATIONAL NURSES

The Code, adopted by NFLPN in 1961 and revised in 1979, provides a motivation for establishing, maintaining, and elevating professional standards. Each LP/VN, upon entering the profession, inherits the respon-

sibility to adhere to the standards of ethical practice and conduct as set forth in this Code.

1. Know the scope of maximum utilization of the LP/VN as specified by the nursing practice act and function within this scope.
2. Safeguard the confidential information acquired from any source about the patient.
3. Provide health care to all patients regardless of race, creed, cultural background, disease, or lifestyle.
4. Uphold the highest standards in personal appearance, language, dress, and demeanor.
5. Stay informed about issues affecting the practice of nursing and delivery of health care and, when appropriate, participate in government and policy decisions.
6. Accept the responsibility for safe nursing by keeping oneself mentally and physically fit and educationally prepared to practice.
7. Accept responsibility for membership in NFLPN and participate in its efforts to maintain the established standards of nursing practice and employment policies that lead to quality patient care.

INTRODUCTORY STATEMENT
Definition

Practical/Vocational nursing means the performance for compensation of authorized acts of nursing that utilize specialized knowledge and skills and that meet the health needs of people in a variety of settings under the direction of qualified health professionals.

Scope

Licensed Practical/Vocational nurses represent the established entry into the nursing profession and include specialized fields of nursing practice.

Opportunities exist for practicing in a milieu where different professions unite their particular skills in a team effort: to preserve or improve an individual patient's functioning and to protect health and safety of patients.

Opportunities also exist for career advancement within the profession through academic education and for lateral expansion of knowledge and expertise through both academic/continuing education and certification.

STANDARDS
Education
The Licensed Practical/Vocational Nurse

1. Shall complete a formal education program in practical nursing approved by the appropriate nursing authority in a state.
2. Shall successfully pass the National Council Licensure Examination for Practical Nurses.
3. Shall participate in initial orientation within the employing institution.

Legal/Ethical Status
The Licensed Practical/Vocational Nurse

1. Shall hold a current license to practice nursing as an LP/VN in accordance with the law of the state wherein employed.
2. Shall know the scope of nursing practice authorized by the Nursing Practice Act in the state wherein employed.
3. Shall have a personal commitment to fulfill the legal responsibilities inherent in good nursing practice.
4. Shall take responsible actions in situations wherein there is unprofessional conduct by a peer or other health care provider.
5. Shall recognize and have a commitment to meet the ethical and moral obligations of the practice of nursing.
6. Shall not accept or perform professional responsibilities that the individual knows he or she is not competent to perform.

Practice
The Licensed Practical/Vocational Nurse

1. Shall accept assigned responsibilities as an accountable member of the health care team.
2. Shall function within the limits of educational preparation and experience as related to the assigned duties.
3. Shall function with other members of the health care team in promoting and maintaining health, preventing disease and disability, caring for and rehabilitating individuals who are experiencing an altered health state, and contributing to the ultimate quality of life until death.
4. Shall know and utilize the nursing process in planning, implementing, and evaluating health services and nursing care for the individual patient or group.
   a. Planning: The planning of nursing includes:
      (1) Assessment/data collection of health status of the individual patient, the family, and community groups

      (2) Reporting information gained from assessment/data collection
      (3) The identification of health goals.
   b. Implementation: The plan for nursing care is put into practice to achieve the stated goals and includes:
      (1) Observing, recording and reporting significant changes that require intervention or different goals
      (2) Applying nursing knowledge and skills to promote and maintain health, to prevent disease and disability and to optimize functional capabilities of an individual patient
      (3) Assisting the patient and family with activities of daily living and encouraging self-care as appropriate
      (4) Carrying out therapeutic regimens and protocols prescribed by personnel pursuant to authorized state law.
   c. Evaluations: The plan for nursing care and its implementations are evaluated to measure the progress toward the stated goals and will include appropriate person and/or groups to determine:
      (1) The relevancy of current goals in relation to the progress of the individual patient
      (2) The involvement of the recipients of care in the evaluation process
      (3) The quality of the nursing action in the implementation of the plan
      (4) A re-ordering of priorities or new goal setting in the care plan.
5. Shall participate in peer review and other evaluation processes.
6. Shall participate in the development of policies concerning the health and nursing needs of society and in the roles and functions of the LP/VN.

Continuing Education
The Licensed Practical/Vocational Nurse

1. Shall be responsible for maintaining the highest possible level of professional competence at all times.
2. Shall periodically reassess career goals and select continuing education activities that will help achieve these goals.
3. Shall take advantage of continuing education and certification opportunities that will lead to personal growth and professional development.
4. Shall seek and participate in continued education activities that are approved for credit by appropriate organizations, such as the NFLPN.

Specialized Nursing Practice
The Licensed Practical/Vocational Nurse

1. Shall have had at least 1 year's experience in nursing at the staff level.

2. Shall present personal qualifications that are indicative of potential abilities for practice in the chosen specialized nursing area.
3. Shall present evidence of completion of a program or course that is approved by an appropriate agency to provide the knowledge and skills necessary for effective nursing services in the specialized field.
4. Shall meet all of the standards of practice as set forth in this document.

GLOSSARY

Authorized (acts of nursing) Those nursing activities made legal through State Nurse Practice Acts.

Lateral Expansion of Knowledge An extension of the basic core of information learned in the school of practical nursing.

Peer Review A formal evaluation of performance on the job by other LP/VNs.

Special Nursing Practice A restricted field of nursing in which a person is particularly skilled and has specific knowledge.

Therapeutic Regimens Regulated plans designed to bring about effective treatment of disease.

Career Advancement A change of career goal.

LP/VN A combined abbreviation for Licensed Practical Nurse and Licensed Vocational Nurse. The LVN is the title used in California and Texas for the nurses who are called LPNs in other states.

Milieu One's environment and surroundings.

Protocols Courses of treatment that include specific steps to be performed in a stated order.

Standard Precautions

RECOMMENDATIONS

IV. STANDARD PRECAUTIONS

Assume that every person is potentially infected or colonized with an organism that could be transmitted in the healthcare setting and apply the following infection control practices during the delivery of health care.

IV.A. Hand Hygiene

IV.A.1. During the delivery of healthcare, avoid unnecessary touching of surfaces in close proximity to the patient to prevent both contamination of clean hands from environmental surfaces and transmission of pathogens from contaminated hands to surfaces.

IV.A.2. When hands are visibly dirty, contaminated with proteinaceous material, or visibly soiled with blood or body fluids, wash hands with either a nonantimicrobial soap and water or an antimicrobial soap and water.

IV.A.3. If hands are not visibly soiled, or after removing visible material with non-antimicrobial soap and water, decontaminate hands in the clinical situations described in IV.A.3.a-f. The preferred method of hand decontamination is with an alcohol-based hand rub. Alternatively, hands may be washed with an antimicrobial soap and water. Frequent use of alcohol-based hand rub immediately following handwashing with nonantimicrobial soap may increase the frequency of dermatitis. Perform hand hygiene:

IV.A.3.a. Before having direct contact with patients.

IV.A.3.b. After contact with blood, body fluids or excretions, mucous membranes, nonintact skin, or wound dressings.

IV.A.3.c. After contact with a patient's intact skin (e.g., when taking a pulse or blood pressure or lifting a patient).

IV.A.3.d. If hands will be moving from a contaminated body site to a clean body site during patient care.

IV.A.3.e. After contact with inanimate objects (including medical equipment) in the immediate vicinity of the patient.

IV.A.3.f. After removing gloves.

IV.A.4. Wash hands with non-antimicrobial soap and water or with antimicrobial soap and water if contact with spores (e.g., *Clostridium difficile* or *Bacillus anthracis*) is likely to have occurred. The physical action of washing and rinsing hands under such circumstances is recommended because alcohols, chlorhexidine, iodophors, and other antiseptic agents have poor activity against spores.

IV.A.5. Do not wear artificial fingernails or extenders if duties include direct contact with patients at high risk for infection and associated adverse outcomes (e.g., those in ICUs or operating rooms).

IV.A.5.a. Develop an organizational policy on the wearing of non-natural nails by healthcare personnel who have direct contact with patients outside of the groups specified above.

IV.B. Personal Protective Equipment (PPE)

IV.B.1. Observe the following principles of use:

IV.B.1.a. Wear PPE, as described in IV.B.2-4,when the nature of the anticipated patient interaction indicates that contact with blood or body fluids may occur.

IV.B.1.b. Prevent contamination of clothing and skin during the process of removing PPE.

IV.B.1.c. Before leaving the patient's room or cubicle, remove and discard PPE.

IV.B.2. Gloves

IV.B.2.a. Wear gloves when it can be reasonably anticipated that contact with blood or other potentially infectious materials, mucous membranes, nonintact skin, or potentially contaminated intact skin (e.g., of a patient incontinent of stool or urine) could occur.

Excerpt from Siegel, J.D., Rhinehart, E., Jackson, M., Chiarello, L., and the Healthcare Infection Control Practices Advisory Committee (2007). *Guideline for Isolation Precautions: Preventing Transmission of Infectious Agents in Healthcare Settings,* June 2007. Available at www.cdc.gov/ncidod/dhqp/pdp/isolation2007.pdf.

IV.B.2.b. Wear gloves with fit and durability appropriate to the task.

IV.B.2.b.i. Wear disposable medical examination gloves for providing direct patient care.

IV.B.2.b.ii. Wear disposable medical examination gloves or reusable utility gloves for cleaning the environment or medical equipment.

IV.B.2.c. Remove gloves after contact with a patient and/or the surrounding environment (including medical equipment) using proper technique to prevent hand contamination. Do not wear the same pair of gloves for the care of more than one patient. Do not wash gloves for the purpose of reuse since this practice has been associated with transmission of pathogens.

IV.B.2.d. Change gloves during patient care if the hands will move from a contaminated body-site (e.g., perineal area) to a clean body-site (e.g., face).

IV.B.3. Gowns

IV.B.3.a. Wear a gown, that is appropriate to the task, to protect skin and prevent soiling or contamination of clothing during procedures and patient-care activities when contact with blood, body fluids, secretions, or excretions is anticipated.

IV.B.3.a.i. Wear a gown for direct patient contact if the patient has uncontained secretions or excretions.

IV.B.3.a.ii. Remove gown and perform hand hygiene before leaving the patient's environment.

IV.B.3.b. Do not reuse gowns, even for repeated contacts with the same patient.

IV.B.3.c. Routine donning of gowns upon entrance into a high-risk unit (e.g., ICU, NICU, HSCT unit) is not indicated.

IV.B.4. Mouth, nose, eye protection

IV.B.4.a. Use PPE to protect the mucous membranes of the eyes, nose, and mouth during procedures and patient-care activities that are likely to generate splashes or sprays of blood, body fluids, secretions and excretions. Select masks, goggles, face shields, and combinations of each according to the need anticipated by the task performed.

IV.B.5. During aerosol-generating procedures (e.g., bronchoscopy, suctioning of the respiratory tract [if not using in-line suction catheters], endotracheal intubation) in patients who are not suspected of being infected with an agent for which respiratory protection is otherwise recommended (e.g., *Mycobacterium tuberculosis,* SARS or hemorrhagic fever viruses), wear one of the following: a face shield that fully covers the front and sides of the face, a mask with attached shield, or a mask and goggles (in addition to gloves and gown).

IV.C. Respiratory Hygiene/Cough Etiquette

IV.C.1. Educate healthcare personnel on the importance of source control measures to contain respiratory secretions to prevent droplet and fomite transmission of respiratory pathogens, especially during seasonal outbreaks of viral respiratory tract infections (e.g., influenza, RSV, adenovirus, parainfluenza virus) in communities.

IV.C.2. Implement the following measures to contain respiratory secretions in patients and accompanying individuals who have signs and symptoms of a respiratory infection, beginning at the point of initial encounter in a healthcare setting (e.g., triage, reception and waiting areas in emergency departments, outpatient clinics and physician offices).

IV.C.2.a. Post signs at entrances and in strategic places (e.g., elevators, cafeterias) within ambulatory and inpatient settings with instructions to patients and other persons with symptoms of a respiratory infection to cover their mouths/noses when coughing or sneezing, use and dispose of tissues, and perform hand hygiene after hands have been in contact with respiratory secretions.

IV.C.2.b. Provide tissues and no-touch receptacles (e.g., foot-pedal–operated lid or open, plastic-lined wastebasket) for disposal of tissues.

IV.C.2.c. Provide resources and instructions for performing hand hygiene in or near waiting areas in ambulatory and inpatient settings; provide conveniently-located dispensers of alcohol-based hand rubs and, where sinks are available, supplies for handwashing.

IV.C.2.d. During periods of increased prevalence of respiratory infections in the community (e.g., as indicated by increased school absenteeism, increased number of patients seeking care for a respiratory infection), offer masks to coughing patients and other symptomatic persons (e.g., persons who accompany ill patients) upon entry into the facility or medical office and encourage them to maintain special separation, ideally a distance of at least 3 feet, from others in common waiting areas.

IV.C.2.d.i. Some facilities may find it logistically easier to institute this recommendation year-round as a standard of practice.

IV.D. Patient Placement

IV.D.1. Include the potential for transmission of infectious agents in patient placement decisions. Place patients who pose a risk for transmission to others (e.g., uncontained secretions, excretions or wound drainage; infants with suspected viral respiratory or gastrointestinal infections) in a single-patient room when available.

IV.D.2. Determine patient placement based on the following principles:

- Route(s) of transmission of the known or suspected infectious agent
- Risk factors for transmission in the infected patient
- Risk factors for adverse outcomes resulting from an HAI in other patients in the area or room being considered for patient placement
- Availability of single-patient rooms
- Patient options for room-sharing (e.g., cohorting patients with the same infection)

IV.E. Patient-Care Equipment and Instruments/Devices

IV.E.1. Establish policies and procedures for containing, transporting, and handling patient-care equipment and instruments/devices that may be contaminated with blood or body fluids.

IV.E.2. Remove organic material from critical and semicritical instrument/devices, using recommended cleaning agents before high level disinfection and sterilization to enable effective disinfection and sterilization processes.

IV.E.3. Wear PPE (e.g., gloves, gown) according to the level of anticipated contamination, when handling patient-care equipment and instruments/devices that is visibly soiled or may have been in contact with blood or body fluids.

IV.F. Care of the Environment

IV.F.1. Establish policies and procedures for routine and targeted cleaning of environmental surfaces as indicated by the level of patient contact and degree of soiling.

IV.F.2. Clean and disinfect surfaces that are likely to be contaminated with pathogens, including those that are in close proximity to the patient (e.g., bed rails, over bed tables) and frequently touched surfaces in the patient care environment (e.g., doorknobs, surfaces in and surrounding toilets in patients' rooms) on a more frequent schedule compared to that for other surfaces (e.g., horizontal surfaces in waiting rooms).

IV.F.3. Use EPA-registered disinfectants that have microbicidal (i.e., killing) activity against the pathogens most likely to contaminate the patient-care environment. Use in accordance with manufacturer's instructions.

IV.F.3.a. Review the efficacy of in-use disinfectants when evidence of continuing transmission of an infectious agent (e.g., rotavirus, *C. difficile*, norovirus) may indicate resistance to the in-use product and change to a more effective disinfectant as indicated.

IV.F.4. In facilities that provide health care to pediatric patients or have waiting areas with child play toys (e.g., obstetric/gynecology offices and clinics), establish policies and procedures for cleaning and disinfecting toys at regular intervals. Category IA

- Use the following principles in developing this policy and procedures:
  - Select play toys that can be easily cleaned and disinfected
  - Do not permit use of stuffed furry toys if they will be shared
  - Clean and disinfect large stationary toys (e.g., climbing equipment) at least weekly and whenever visibly soiled
  - If toys are likely to be mouthed, rinse with water after disinfection; alternatively wash in a dishwasher
  - When a toy requires cleaning and disinfection, do so immediately or store in a designated labeled container separate from toys that are clean and ready for use.

IV.F.5. Include multiuse electronic equipment in policies and procedures for preventing contamination and for cleaning and disinfection, especially those items that are used by patients, those used during delivery of patient care, and mobile devices that are moved in and out of patient rooms frequently (e.g., daily).

IV.F.5.a. No recommendation for use of removable protective covers or washable keyboards. Unresolved issue

IV.G. Textiles and Laundry

IV.G.1. Handle used textiles and fabrics with minimum agitation to avoid contamination of air, surfaces and persons.

IV.G.2. If laundry chutes are used, ensure that they are properly designed, maintained, and used in a manner to minimize dispersion of aerosols from contaminated laundry.

IV.H. Safe Injection Practices

The following recommendations apply to the use of needles, cannulas that replace needles, and, where applicable, intravenous delivery systems

IV.H.1. Use aseptic technique to avoid contamination of sterile injection equipment.

IV.H.2. Do not administer medications from a syringe to multiple patients, even if the needle or cannula on the syringe is changed. Needles, cannulas, and syringes are sterile, single-use items; they should not be reused for another patient or to access a medication or solution that might be used for a subsequent patient.

IV.H.3. Use fluid infusion and administration sets (i.e., intravenous bags, tubing, and connectors) for one patient only, and dispose appropriately after use. Consider a syringe or needle/cannula contaminated once it has been used to enter or connect to a patient's intravenous infusion bag or administration set.

IV.H.4. Use single-dose vials for parenteral medications whenever possible.

IV.H.5. Do not administer medications from single-dose vials or ampules to multiple patients or combine leftover contents for later use.

IV.H.6. If multidose vials must be used, both the needle or cannula and syringe used to access the multidose vial must be sterile.

IV.H.7. Do not keep multidose vials in the immediate patient treatment area and store in accordance with the manufacturer's recommendations; discard if sterility is compromised or questionable.

IV.H.8. Do not use bags or bottles of intravenous solution as a common source of supply for multiple patients.

IV.I. Infection Control Practices for Special Lumbar Puncture Procedures

Wear a surgical mask when placing a catheter or injecting material into the spinal canal or subdural space (i.e., during myelograms, lumbar puncture, and spinal or epidural anesthesia.

IV.J. Worker Safety

Adhere to federal and state requirements for protection of healthcare personnel from exposure to bloodborne pathogens.

Basic Laboratory Test Values

Complete Blood Count

TEST	CONVENTIONAL UNITS	SI UNITS
Erythrocytes (RBCs)		
Males	4.6-6.2 million/mm^3	4.6-6.2 × 10^{12}/L
Females	4.2-5.4 million/mm^3	4.2-5.4 × 10^{12}/L
Children (varies with age)	4.5-5.1 million/mm^3	4.5-5.1 × 10^{12}/L
	4500-11,000/mm^3	4.5-11.0 × 10^9/L
Red cell indices		
Mean corpuscular hemoglobin (MCH)	32-36 g/dL	320-360 g/L
Mean corpuscular volume (MCV)	80-96 mcg/mm^3	80-96 fl L
Mean corpuscular hemoglobin concentration (MCHC)	32-26 g/dL	320-360 g/L
Hemoglobin		
Males	13.0-18.0 g/dL	8.1-11.2 mmol/L
Females	12.0-16.0 g/dL	7.4-9.9 mmol/L
Newborns	16.5-19.5 g/dL	10.2-12.1 mmol/L
Children (varies with age)	11.2-16.5 g/dL	7.0-10.2 mmol/L
Hematocrit		
Males	40-54 mL/dL	0.40-0.54
Females	37-47 mL/dL	0.37-0.47
Newborns	49-54 mL/dL	0.49-0.54
Children (varies with age)	35-49 mL/dL	0.35-0.49
Leukocytes (WBCs)	4500-11,000/mm^3	4.5-11.0 × 10^6/L
Leukocyte differential counts		
Band neutrophils	3%-5%	150-400 × 10^6/L
Segmented neutrophils	54%-62%	3000-5800 × 10^6/L
Lymphocytes	28%-33%	1500-3000 × 10^6/L
Monocytes	3%-7%	300-500 × 10^6/L
Eosinophils	1%-3%	50-250 × 10^6/L
Basophils	0-1%	15-50 × 10^6/L
Platelets	15,000-400,000/mm^3	150-400 × 10^9/L

Urinalysis

TEST	CONVENTIONAL UNITS
Appearance	Clear
Color	Yellow amber
Odor	Aromatic
pH	4.6-8.0
Specific Gravity	1.003-1.030
Protein	Negative
Nitrites	Negative
Ketones	Negative
Bilirubin	Negative
Urobilinogen	0.1-1.0 unit/mL
Glucose	Negative
WBCs	0-4 per low power field
RBCs	= or less than 2
Casts	None
Crystals	None

Blood Chemistry Panel (SMA, Astra-7, Chem-7, Basic Metabolic Panel, Electrolytes)

TEST	CONVENTIONAL UNITS	SI UNITS
Albumin	3.3-5.2 g/dL	33-42 g/L
Alkaline phosphatase	35-150 U/L	35-50 U/L
Aspartate aminotransferase (AST), (SGOT)	1-36 U/L	1-36 U/L
Bilirubin, conjugate	0.1-0.4 mg/dL	1.7-6.8 mcg mol/L
Bilirubin, total	0.3-1.1 mg/dL	5.1-19.0 mcg mol/L
Blood urea nitrogen (BUN)	11-23 mg/dL	8.0-16.4 nmol/L
Calcium	8.4-10.6 mg/dL	2.10-2.65 mmol/L
Carbon dioxide	4-31 mEq/L	24-31 mmol/L
Chloride	96-106 mEq/L	96-106 mmol/L
Creatinine	0.6-1.2 mg/dL	50-110 mcg mol/L
Glucose	70-100 mg/dL	3.9-5.55 nmol/L
Potassium	3.5.0 mEq/L	3.5-5.0 mmol/L
Protein	6.0-8.0 g/dL	60-80 g/L
Sodium	135-145 mEq/L	135-145 mmol/L
Triglycerides	40-150 mg/dL	0.4-1.5 g/L
Uric acid		
Males	2.5-8.0 mg/dL	150-480 mcg mol/L
Females	2.2-7.0 mg/dL	130-420 mcg mol/L

Lipid Panel

TEST	CONVENTIONAL UNITS	SI UNITS
Cholesterol, total	> 200 mg/dL	>5.20 mmol/L
Low-density lipoprotein (LDL)	60-180 mg/dL	1.55-4.65 mmol/L
High-density lipoprotein (HDL)	30-80 mg/dL	0.80-2.05 mmol/L

Thyroid Tests

TEST	CONVENTIONAL UNITS	SI UNITS
Thyrotropin (TSH)	0.4-4/8 mcgIU/mL	0.4-4.8 mIU/L
Thyroxin (T_4)	4.5-12.0 mcg/mL	58-154 nmol/L
Thyroxine, free (FT_4)	0.9-2.1 ng/dL	12-27 pmol/L

Miscellaneous Commonly Performed Tests

TEST	CONVENTIONAL UNITS	SI UNITS
Digoxin level (Lanoxin)	0.8-2.0 ng/mL	>2/4 ng/mL
Prothrombin time (PT)	12.0-14 sec; INR 1.5–2 times control value	85%-100%; INR 20%-30%
Activated partial thromboplastin time (aPPT)	20-25 sec	20-35 sec

7 Therapeutic Diets

Summary of Basic Hospital Diets

FOOD	GENERAL ADEQUATE, OR "HOUSE," DIET	SOFT DIET	FULL LIQUID DIET	CLEAR LIQUID DIET
Milk, cream, buttermilk	Included	Included	Included	Not included
Eggs	Pasteurized or cooked	Included	In beverages (eggnog)	Not included
Cheese	All varieties	Cottage, cream, mildly flavored cheeses	Not included	Not included
Fats	All kinds	Butter, margarine, oil, mayonnaise, and mildly seasoned dressing	Butter, margarine, oil	Not included
Meat, fish, poultry	All included	Tender beef, lamb, veal; liver, bacon, fish and poultry	Not included	Not included
Vegetables	All included	Cooked or canned vegetables of low fiber; tender lettuce; vegetable juices	Vegetable juices, vegetable puree used in soups	
Fruits	All included	Fruit juices, ripe bananas, cooked fruit without skin or seeds	Fruit juices, fruit ades	Strained fruit juices, fruit ades
Breads	All varieties	Refined grain products, rye without seeds, refined crackers	Not included	Not included
Cereals	All varieties	Refined	Cooked, refined cereals	Not included
Cereal products	All varieties	Cooked macaroni, spaghetti, noodles, white rice	Not included	Not included
Soups	All varieties	Clear broth, and consommé; cream and vegetable soups containing allowed items	Clear broth, and consommé; strained vegetable and cream soups	Clear broth and consommé
Beverages	All kinds	All kinds	Tea, decaffeinated or regular coffee, carbonated beverages, eggnog	Tea, decaffeinated coffee, carbonated beverages
Desserts	All kinds	Plain puddings, yogurt, simple cakes and cookies, frozen desserts without nuts, custard, gelatin	Plain gelatin dessert, ice cream or yogurt without nuts and seeds, ices, sherbets, soft custard, pudding	Plain gelatin desserts and ices
Other			Liquid supplements	Elemental liquids

From Mahan, L.K., & Escott-Stump, S. (2003). *Krause's Food, Nutrition, and Diet Therapy* (11th ed.). Philadelphia: Saunders.

Soft Diet

MEAL PLAN	SAMPLE MENU	SERVING SIZE
BREAKFAST		
Fruit	Orange juice	1/2 cup
Cereal	Cooked farina	1/2 cup (cooked weight)
Egg	Poached egg	1
Bread	Toast	1 slice
Butter	Butter or margarine	1 pat
Milk	Milk (2%)	1 cup
Sugar	Sugar	3 tsp
Coffee	Coffee	2 cups
LUNCH		
Soup	Tomato consommé	1/2 cup
Entrée	Baked macaroni and cheese	1 cup
Vegetables	Cooked asparagus tips	1/2 cup
Bread	White bread	1 slice
Butter	Butter or margarine	1 pat
Fruit	Applesauce	1/2 cup
Milk	Milk (2%)	1 cup
DINNER		
Meat	Chicken breast	3 oz
Potato	Mashed potato	1/2 cup
Vegetable	Buttered spinach	1/2 cup
Bread	White bread	1 slice
Butter	Butter or margarine	1/2 pat
Dessert	Chocolate ice cream, ice milk, or frozen yogurt	1/2 cup
Milk	Milk (2%)	1 cup

From Mahan, L.K., & Escott-Stump, S. (2003). *Krause's Food, Nutrition, and Diet Therapy* (11th ed.). Philadelphia: Saunders.

Clear Liquid Diet

MEAL PLAN	SAMPLE MENU	SERVING SIZE
BREAKFAST		
Fruit juice	Apple juice	1/2 cup
Beverage	Coffee (decaffeinated)	2 cups
Sugar	Sugar	2 tsp
AM SNACK		
Fruitade	Lemonade	1 cup
LUNCH		
Soup	Beef broth	1/2 cup
Fruit juice	Grape juice	1/2 cup
Tea	Tea	2 cups
Sugar	Sugar	2 tsp
Fruit ice	Cherry fruit ice	1/2 cup
PM SNACK		
Carbonated beverage	Gingerale	1 cup
DINNER		
Fruit juice	Fruit punch	1/2 cup
Soup	Chicken broth	1/2 cup
Gelatin	Raspberry gelatin	1/4 cup
Tea	Tea	2 cups
Sugar	Sugar	2 tsp
EVENING (h.s.) SNACK		
Fruit juice	Cranberry juice	1 cup

From Mahan, L. K., Escott-Stump, S. (2003). *Krause's Food, Nutrition, and Diet Therapy* (11th ed.). Philadelphia: Saunders.

Full Liquid Diet—Sample Menu

MEAL PLAN	SAMPLE MENU	SERVING SIZE	MEAL PLAN	SAMPLE MENU	SERVING SIZE
BREAKFAST			Coffee or tea	Coffee or tea	1 cup
Fruit	Orange juice	1/2 cup	Sugar	Sugar	2 tsp
Cereal	Cooked farina	1 cup (cooked weight)	**PM SNACK**		
Supplement	Commercial eggnog	1 cup	Supplement	Commercial milkshake (strawberry)	1 cup
Butter	Butter or margarine	2 tsp			
Milk	Milk (2%)	1 cup	**DINNER**		
Sugar	Sugar	2 tsp	Fruit	Apple juice	1/2 cup
Coffee or tea	Coffee or tea	1 cup	Soup	Cream of mushroom (strained) with margarine/butter	1 cup
AM SNACK					
Supplement	Commercial milkshake (chocolate)	1 cup	Supplement	Commercial milkshake	1 cup
			Milk	Ice cream	1/2 cup
LUNCH			Coffee or tea	Coffee or tea	1 cup
Soup	Cream of potato soup (strained) with margarine/butter	1 cup	Sugar	Sugar	2 tsp
			BEDTIME (h.s.) SNACK		
Fruit	Pineapple juice	1/2 cup	Gelatin	Gelatin, strawberry	1/2 cup
Milk	Milk (2%)	1 cup	Supplement	Commercial milkshake (vanilla)	1 cup
	Vanilla pudding	1/2 cup			

From Mahan, L.K., & Escott-Stump, S. (2003). *Krause's Food, Nutrition, and Diet Therapy* (11th ed.). Philadelphia: Saunders.

Low-Fat Diets

FOOD GROUP	CHOOSE	DECREASE
Lean meat, poultry, and fish ≤5-6 oz per day	Beef, pork, lamb—lean cuts, well trimmed before cooking Poultry without skin Fish, shellfish Processed meat—prepared from lean meat (e.g., lean ham, lean frankfurters, lean meat with soy protein or carrageenan)	Beef, pork, lamb—regular ground beef, fatty cuts, spare ribs, organ meats Poultry with skin, fried chicken Fried fish, fried shellfish Regular luncheon meat (e.g., bologna, salami, sausage, frankfurters)
Eggs ≤4 yolks per week (Step I) ≤2 yolks per week (Step II)	Egg whites (two whites can be substituted for one whole egg in recipes), cholesterol-free egg substitute	Egg yolks (if more than 4 per week on Step I or if more than 2 per week on Step II); includes eggs used in cooking and baking
Low-fat dairy products 2-3 servings per day	Milk—skim, ½%, or 1% fat (fluid, powdered, evaporated), buttermilk Yogurt—nonfat or low-fat yogurt or yogurt beverages Cheese—low-fat natural or processed cheese Low-fat or nonfat varieties, such as cottage cheese—low-fat, nonfat, or dry curd (0% to 2% fat) Frozen dairy dessert—ice milk, frozen yogurt (low-fat or nonfat) Low-fat coffee creamer Low-fat or nonfat sour cream	Whole milk (fluid, evaporated, condensed), 2% fat milk (low-fat milk), imitation milk Whole-milk yogurt, whole-milk yogurt beverages Regular cheeses (American, blue, Brie, cheddar, Colby, Edam, Monterey Jack, whole-milk mozzarella, Parmesan, Swiss), cream cheese, Neufchatel cheese Cottage cheese (4% fat) Ice cream Cream, half & half, whipping cream, nondairy creamer, whipped topping, sour cream
Fats and oils ≤6-8 tsp per day	Unsaturated oils—safflower, sunflower, corn, soybean, cottonseed, canola, olive, peanut Margarine—made from unsaturated oils listed above; light or diet margarine, especially soft or liquid forms Salad dressings—made with unsaturated oils listed above; low-fat or fat-free Seeds and nuts—peanut butter, other nut butters Cocoa powder	Coconut oil, palm kernel oil, palm oil Butter, lard, shortening, bacon fat, and hard margarine Dressings made with egg yolk, cheese, sour cream, whole milk Coconut Milk chocolate
Breads and cereals ≥6 servings per day	Breads—whole-grain bread, English muffins, bagels, buns, corn or flour tortilla Cereals—oat, wheat, corn, multigrain Pasta Rice Dried beans and peas Crackers, low-fat—animal type, graham, soda crackers, breadsticks, melba toast Homemade baked goods using unsaturated oil, skim or 1% milk, and egg substitute—quick breads, biscuits, cornbread muffins, bran muffins, pancakes, waffles	Bread in which eggs, fat, and/or butter are a major ingredient; croissants Most granolas High-fat crackers Commercial baked pastries, muffins, biscuits
Soups	Reduced- or low-fat and reduced-sodium varieties (e.g., chicken or beef noodle, minestrone, tomato, vegetable, potato), reduced-fat soups made with skim milk	Soups containing whole milk, cream, meat fat, poultry fat, or poultry skin

From Mahan, L.K., & Escott-Stump, S. (2003). *Krause's Food, Nutrition, and Diet Therapy* (11th ed.). Philadelphia: Saunders.
Data from National Cholesterol Education Program (NCEP) (1993). Second Report of the Expert Panel on Detection, Evaluation, and Treatment of High Blood Cholesterol in Adults (Adult Treatment Panel II). NIH Publication No. 93-3095. Bethesda, MD: National Institutes of Health. National Heart, Lung, and Blood Institute.

Continued

Low-Fat Diets—cont'd

FOOD GROUP	CHOOSE	DECREASE
Vegetables 3-5 servings per day	Fresh, frozen, or canned, without added fat or sauce	Vegetables fried or prepared with butter, cheese, or cream sauce
Fruits 2-4 servings per day	Fruits—fresh, frozen, canned, or dried Fruit juice—fresh, frozen, or canned	Fried fruit or fruit served with butter or cream sauce
Sweets and modified-fat desserts	Beverages—fruit-flavored drinks, lemonade, fruit punch	
	Sweets—sugar, syrup, honey, jam, preserves, candy made without fat (candy corn, gumdrops, hard candy), fruit-flavored gelatin	Candy made with milk chocolate, coconut oil, palm kernel oil, palm oil
	Frozen desserts—low-fat and nonfat yogurt, ice milk, sherbet, sorbet, fruit ice, popsicles	Ice cream and frozen treats made with ice cream
	Cookies, cake, pie, pudding—prepared with egg whites, egg substitute, skim milk or 1% milk, and unsaturated oil or margarine; ginger snaps; fig and other fruit bar cookies; fat-free cookies; angel food cake	Commercial baked pies, cakes, doughnuts, high-fat cookies, cream pies

Sodium-Restricted Diets

FOODS	2-4 g SODIUM	1 g SODIUM
Milk	3 cups milk or yogurt, no processed cheese; natural cheese (1 oz) can replace 1 c milk; free use of low-sodium cheese	2 cups milk or yogurt; up to 1 oz natural cheese can be substituted for 1 c milk; free use of low-sodium cheese
Meat and meat substitutes	Limited use of processed meats; free use of fresh meat	No processed meat; use salt-free canned tuna; limited use of regular peanut butter; free use of low-sodium peanut butter
Breads and cereals	Avoid breads and crackers with salt topping; regular bread may be used in normal amounts; free use of low-sodium bread and cereal products; avoid canned soups and vegetables and cereals with added salt	Up to 2 slices regular bread may be used or 1 serving regular processed cereal; free use of low-sodium breads and cereals
Vegetables and fruits	All fresh, frozen, and dried; all canned fruit but limited use of canned vegetables; free use of low-sodium canned vegetables; no salted products such as potato chips or french fries	Use only low-sodium canned vegetables; limited use of naturally high-sodium vegetables (beets, carrots, celery, spinach); free use of all others
Condiments		
Sweets		
Brown sugar	Free use	Free use
Table sugar	Free use	Free use
Honey	Free use	Free use
Jams and jellies	Free use	Free use
Maple syrup	Free use	Free use
Molasses	Free use	Free use
Sauces		
Catsup	Limited use	Use low-sodium
Mayonnaise	Limited use	Use low-sodium
Mustard	Limited use	Use low-sodium
Soy sauce	Limited use	Use low-sodium
Worcestershire sauce	Limited use	Not allowed
Butter/margarine	Limited use	Use low-sodium
Other		
Cooking oil	Free use	Free use
Vinegar	Free use	Free use
Spices		
Natural	Free use	Free use
Salt-based	Limited use	Not allowed
Lemon	Free use	Free use
Horseradish	Free use	Limited use
Salt	Very limited use (few sprinkles)	Use salt substitute (physician approval)

From Peckenpaugh, N.J., & Poleman, C.M. (2003). *Nutrition Essentials and Diet Therapy* (9th ed.). Philadelphia: Saunders.

High Calorie/Protein Diet

ADDITIONAL FOODS	Kcal	PROTEIN (g)	ADDITIONAL FOODS	Kcal	PROTEIN (g)
PLUS 500 kcal (SERVED BETWEEN MEALS)			**PLUS 1500 kcal (SERVED BETWEEN MEALS)**		
1. 1 cup dry cereal	110	2	1. 2 slices bread	120	4
1 banana	80		2 T peanut butter	172	8
1 cup whole milk	159	8	1 T jam	110	
1 slice toast	60	2	4 graham cracker squares	110	2
1 T peanut butter	86	4	8 oz fruit-flavored yogurt	240	9
	495	16	3/4 cup roasted peanuts	628	28
			1 cup apricot nectar	143	1
2. 8 saltine crackers	99	3		1523	52
1 oz cheese	113	7			
1 cup ice cream	290	6	2. 1 baked custard	285	13
	502	16	Instant Breakfast with whole milk	280	15
			1 cup dry cereal	110	2
3. 6 graham cracker squares	165	3	1 banana	80	
2 T peanut butter	172	8	1 cup whole milk	159	8
1 cup orange juice	122		1 cup orange juice	122	
2 T raisins	52	—	4 T raisins	104	
	511	11	1 bagel	165	6
			2 T cream cheese	99	2
PLUS 1000 kcal (SERVED BETWEEN MEALS)			2 T jam	110	—
1. 8 oz fruit-flavored yogurt	240	9		1514	46
1 slice bread	60	2			
2 oz cheese	226	14			
1 apple	87				
1/4 of 14" cheese pizza	306	16			
1 small banana	81	1			
	1000	42			
2. Instant Breakfast with whole milk	280	15			
1 cup cottage cheese	239	31			
1/2 cup pineapple	95				
1 cup apple juice	117				
6 graham cracker squares	165	3			
1 pear	100	1			
	996	50			

From Mahan, L.K., & Escott-Stump, S. (2003). *Krause's Food, Nutrition, and Diet Therapy* (11th ed.). Philadelphia: Saunders.

Guidelines for High-Fiber Diets*

1. Increase consumption of whole-grain breads, cereals, flours, and other whole-grain products (6-11 servings daily).
2. Increase consumption of vegetables, especially legumes, and fruits, especially those with edible skins, seeds, and hulls (5-8 servings daily).
3. Consume high-fiber cereals, granolas, and legumes as needed to bring fiber intake to at least 25 g daily.
4. Increase consumption of water to at least 2 L (or 2 q) daily.

From Mahan, L.K., & Escott-Stump, S. (2003). *Krause's Food, Nutrition, and Diet Therapy* (11th ed.). Philadelphia: Saunders.
*May increase stool weight, fecal water, and/or gas. The amount that causes clinical symptoms varies among individuals. The age of the individual, the presence of GI disease or malnutrition, any resection of the GI tract, and recent use of the GI tract all impact tolerance.

Medical Terminology

COMBINING FORMS: PREFIXES AND SUFFIXES

Medical terminology is similar to a foreign language. Like a foreign language, it can be analyzed and studied until it becomes a comfortable part of the vocabulary. The main purpose of medical terms is to communicate ideas in such a way that everyone understands exactly what is meant. Many medical terms are derived from Latin and Greek sources. They often consist of two or more simple words or word elements. A word root or *combining form* may be put together with a *prefix* and a *suffix*.

Root—the basis of a word
Example: *nephr*/o/tic (degenerative changes in the kidney)
  Root: nephr- (kidney)

Linking vowel—a vowel that joins the combining form to the suffix or another combining form
Example: nephr/*o*/sis (disease of the kidneys)
  Linking vowel: o
Prefix—the beginning of a word
Example: *hyper*/active (excessively active)
  Prefix: hyper (= excessive)
Suffix — the ending of a word
Example: nephr/*itis* (inflammation of the kidney)
  Suffix — itis (= inflammation)
Combining form — the union of a word root with a linking vowel
Example: *hepato*/megaly (enlargement of the liver)
  Combining form: hepato- (= liver)

Common Prefixes

PREFIX	DEFINITION	PREFIX	DEFINITION
a-	without	ex-	out, away from
ab-	away from	exo-	outside
ad-	toward	extra-	outside
ambi-	both	gastr-	stomach
an-	not	hemi-	one half
ana-	up	hetero-	different
ante-	before, in front of	homo-	same
anti-	against	hyper-	excessive, above normal
auto-	self	hypo-	under, below
bi-	two	im-	not
brady-	slow	in-	in, not
cata-	down	infra-	under, below
circum-	around	inter-	between
co-	with, together	intra-	in, within
con-	with, together	macro-	large
contra-	against	mal-	bad
de-	from, lack of	mesa-	middle
dia-	through, across	meta-	beyond, change
diplo-	double, twofold	micro-	small
dis-	to free or undo	medi-	middle
dys-	bad, painful, difficult, abnormal	mono-	one
ec-	out, out from	multi-	many, much
ecto-	outside	neo-	new
em-	in	osteo-	bone
endo-	in, within	pan-	all
enter-	intestine	para-	near, beside, beyond
epi-	above, upon	per-	through, by
eu-	good, normal	peri-	around

Common Prefixes—cont'd

PREFIX	DEFINITION	PREFIX	DEFINITION
poly-	many, much	sub-	under, below
post-	after, behind	super-	above, excessive
pre-	before, in front of	supra-	above, excessive
primi-	first	sym-	together
pro-	before, in front of	syn-	union, together, joined
pseudo-	false	tachy-	rapid
quadri-	four	therm-	heat
re-	back	trans-	through, across
retro-	backward, behind	tri-	three
scler-	hardening	ultra-	beyond, excess
semi-	one half	uni-	one

Common Suffixes

SUFFIX	DEFINITION	SUFFIX	DEFINITION
-ac	pertaining to	-oma	tumor
-al	pertaining to	-opsy	viewing
-algia	painful condition, pain	-or	one who
-ar	pertaining to	-orrhea	flow, discharge
-ary	pertaining to	-osis	condition, disease
-blast	embryonic	-ous	pertaining to
-cele	hernia, swelling, sac	-para	to bear (offspring)
-centesis	puncture of a cavity	-paresis	partial paralysis
-clasis	break, fracture	-pathy	disease, suffering
-clysis	irrigation, washing	-penia	deficiency, lack of, decrease
-coccus	berry shaped	-pexy	fixation
-crit	to separate	-phagia	eating, swallowing
-cyte	cell	-phasia	speech
-desis	fusion, binding, fixation	-philia	attraction for
-drome	to run	-phobia	fear
-dynia	pain	-physis	to grow
-ectasis	expansion, dilation	-plasia	formation, growth
-ectomy	excision, removal of a body part	-plasm	growth, formation
-emesis	vomiting	-plasty	mold, shape, repair
-emia	blood	-plegia	paralysis
-er	one who	-poiesis	formation, production
-gen	forming, producing, origin	-ptosis	downward displacement, falling
-genesis	forming, producing, origin	-ptysis	spitting
-genic	origin, formation	-rrhage	bursting forth
-grade	to go	-rrhagia	bursting forth
-gram	the record made, mark	-rrhaphy	suture
-graph	instrument for recording, machine	-rrhea	flow, discharge
-graphy	the process, process of recording	-rrhexis	rupture
-ia	condition	-scope	instrument to visually examine
-iasis	morbid condition	-scopy	process of examining, visual examination
-iatry	treatment, medicine	-sis	state of, condition
-ic	pertaining to	-spasm	involuntary spasm
-icle	small, minute	-stalsis	constriction
-ism	condition	-stasis	control, constant level, stop
-ist	one who specializes in, specialist	-stenosis	narrowing, stricture
-itis	inflammation	-stomy	creation of an opening
-lith	stone, calculus	-therapy	treatment
-logist	specialist in the study of	-tic	pertaining to
-logy	process of study	-tome	instrument for cutting
-lysis	dissolution, setting free	-tomy	process of cutting, incision
-malacia	softening, soft	-toxic	poison
-megaly	enlargement	-tresia	opening
-meter	instrument for measuring	-tripsy	surgical crushing
-metry	act of measuring	-trophy	nourishment
-odynia	pain	-ula	small, minute
-oid	form, shape	-ule	small, minute
-ole	small, minute	-y	process
-ology	study or science of		

Continued

ABBREVIATIONS AND ACRONYMS

Health care workers use a vast array of abbreviations and acronyms. It is wise to learn those that are used in the facility and on the units where you work. The first list presents the most common general abbreviations and acronyms encountered in the health care field. These will be encountered in patient charts as well as during the course of conversation and shift report. The following lists organize the abbreviations related to time, to measurements, and to medications.

ABBREVIATION/ ACRONYM	DEFINITION
a	before
aa	of each
AB	abortion
abd	abdomen
ABGs	arterial blood gases
ANCC	American Nurses Credentialing Center
BMR	basal metabolic rate
ACTH	adrenocorticotropic hormone
ADC	aid to dependent children
ADH	antidiuretic hormone
ADL	activities of daily living
ad lib	as desired, at liberty
AFP	alpha-fetoprotein
A/G ratio	albumin-globulin ratio
AHRQ	Agency for Healthcare Research and Quality
AIDS	acquired immunodeficiency syndrome
AKA	above-the-knee amputation
ALL	acute lymphocytic leukemia
ALS	amyotrophic lateral sclerosis
AMA	American Medical Association
AMB	ambulate, ambulatory
AML	acute myelocytic leukemia
ANA	American Nurses' Association; antinuclear antibody
AP	anteroposterior
APTT	activated partial thromboplastin time
ARC	American Red Cross
ARDS	adult respiratory distress syndrome
ARF	acute renal failure
ASHD	arteriosclerotic heart disease
AST	aspartate aminotransferase
ATN	acute tubular necrosis
AV	atrioventricular
AVM	arteriovenous malformation
AVR	aortic valve replacement
BE	barium enema (x-ray)
BKA	below-the-knee amputation
BM	bowel movement
BP, B/P	blood pressure
BPH	benign prostatic hypertrophy
BRP	bathroom privileges
BS	bowel sounds
BUN	blood urea nitrogen
Bx	biopsy
C	Celsius
c̄	with
Ca	cancer; calcium
CABG	coronary artery bypass graft
CAD	coronary artery disease
CAPD	continuous ambulatory peritoneal dialysis
CAL	chronic airflow limitation
cal	calories
CAT	computed axial tomography
CBC	complete blood count
CC	chief complaint

ABBREVIATION/ ACRONYM	DEFINITION
CCPD	continuous-cycle peritoneal dialysis
CCRN	certified critical care registered nurse
CCU	coronary care unit
CDC	Centers for Disease Control and Prevention
CEA	carcinoembryonic antigen
CHF	congestive heart failure
Cl	chloride
CLL	chronic lymphocytic leukemia
CML	chronic myelocytic leukemia
CMV	cytomegalovirus
CNA	certified nursing assistant
CNS	central nervous system
C/O	complains of
CO	cardiac output
COLD	chronic obstructive lung disease
COPD	chronic obstructive pulmonary disease
CP	cerebral palsy
CPK	creatine phosphokinase
CPR	cardiopulmonary resuscitation
CRF	chronic renal failure
crit	hematocrit
CRNA	certified registered nurse anesthetist
CS	central service; central supply
CSF	cerebrospinal fluid
CT scan, CAT scan	computed axial tomography
CVP	central venous pressure
D & C	dilation and curettage
DEA#	Drug Enforcement Administration number
DIC	disseminated intravascular coagulation
Diff	differential white blood cell count
DOB	date of birth
DON	Director of Nurses
DJD	degenerative joint disease
DM	diabetes mellitus
DOA	dead on arrival
DOE	dyspnea on exertion
DPT	diphtheria, pertussis, tetanus toxoid (also DTP)
DRGs	diagnosis-related groups
DVT	deep vein thrombosis
Dx	diagnosis
EBV	Epstein-Barr virus
ECG, EKG	electrocardiogram
ECT	electroconvulsive therapy
EDC	expected date of confinement
EEG	electroencephalogram
EENT	eye, ear, nose, and throat
EMG	electromyogram
ENT	ear, nose, and throat
EOM	extraocular movement
ER	emergency room
ERCP	endoscopic retrograde cholangiopancreatography
ERT	estrogen replacement therapy

ABBREVIATION/ ACRONYM	DEFINITION	ABBREVIATION/ ACRONYM	DEFINITION
ESL	extracorporeal shock-wave lithotripsy	MVA	motor vehicle accident
ESR	erythrocyte sedimentation rate	MVP	mitral valve prolapse
ESRD	end-stage renal disease	MVR	mitral valve replacement
EST	electroshock therapy	Na	sodium
F	Fahrenheit	NANDA-I	North American Nursing Diagnosis Association–International
FBS	fasting blood sugar		
FDA	Food and Drug Administration	NAPNES	National Association for Practical Nurse Education and Service
FH	family history		
FHR	fetal heart rate	NCI	National Cancer Institute
FHT	fetal heart tone	NFLPN	National Federation of Licensed Practical Nurses
FS	frozen section		
FUO	fever of unknown origin	NIH	National Institutes of Health
Fx	fracture	NLN	National League for Nursing
GB	gallbladder	noc	night
GC	gonorrhea	NPH	neutral protamine Hagedorn (insulin)
GI	gastrointestinal	NPO	nothing by mouth (per os)
GTT	glucose tolerance test	NSAID	nonsteroidal anti-inflammatory drug
GU	genitourinary	O	oxygen
gyn	gynecology	OA	osteoarthritis
hct	hematocrit	OB	obstetrics
HDL	high-density lipoprotein	OB-GYN	obstetrics-gynecology
Hgb, HG	hemoglobin	OBS	organic brain syndrome
HIV	human immunodeficiency virus	OOB	out of bed
HMO	health maintenance organization	OR	operating room
HNP	herniated nucleus pulposus	ORIF	open reduction-internal fixation
HPV	human papillomavirus	ORT	orthopedics
H_2O	water	os	mouth
HRC	human rights committee	OSHA	Occupational Safety and Health Administration
HSV	herpes simplex virus		
Ht	height	O.T.	occupational therapy
HTN	hypertension	OV	office visit
HVA	hepatitis A virus	oz	ounce
HVB	hepatitis B virus	P	pulse
hx	history	PA	posteroanterior
IABP	intra-aortic balloon pump	PAC	premature atrial contraction
ICP	intracranial pressure	PACU	postanesthesia care unit
ICS	intercostal space	Pap	Papanicolaou smear
ICU	intensive care unit	PAR	postanesthesia recovery (unit)
I & D	incision and drainage	path	pathology
INR	international normalized ratio	PCA	patient-controlled analgesia
I & O	intake and output	PE	physical exam
IOP	intraocular pressure	PEEP	positive end-expiratory pressure
IUD	intrauterine device	per	through, by
IVP	intravenous pyelogram	PERRLA	pupils equal, round, reactive to light and accommodation
JCAHO	Joint Commission on Accreditation of Healthcare Organizations (now The Joint Commission)		
		PFT	pulmonary function test
		PH	past history
JVD	jugular venous distention	PID	pelvic inflammatory disease
K	potassium	PMH	past medical history
KUB	kidney, ureters, bladder (x-ray)	PMI	point of maximal impulse
lab	laboratory	PMS	premenstrual syndrome
LDL	low-density lipoprotein	PND	paroxysmal nocturnal dyspnea
LLL	left lower lobe	PO	orally
LLQ	left lower quadrant	postop	postoperative
LMP	last menstrual period	PP	postprandial (after meals)
LOC	level of consciousness	preop	preoperative
LP	lumbar puncture	prn	as needed
LPN	licensed practical nurse	pro time	prothrombin time
LRQ	lower right quadrant	PSA	prostate-specific antigen
LUQ	left upper quadrant	pt	patient
LVN	licensed vocational nurse	PT	prothrombin time
lytes	electrolytes	P.T.	physical therapy
MD	medical doctor	PTCA	percutaneous transluminal coronary angioplasty
MI	myocardial infarction		
MRI	magnetic resonance imaging	PTT	partial thromboplastin time
MS	multiple sclerosis	PVC	premature ventricular contraction

Continued

ABBREVIATION/ ACRONYM	DEFINITION
PVD	peripheral vascular disease
R	respirations
RBC	red blood cells, red blood (count)
RBS	random blood sugar
RDA	recommended dietary allowance
REM	rapid eye movement
RLL	right lower lobe
RLQ	right lower quadrant
R/O	rule out
ROM	range of motion
ROS	review of systems, review of symptoms
RN	registered nurse
RR	recovery room
Rx	prescription
s̄	without
SA	sinoatrial
SAH	subarachnoid hemorrhage
SBE	subacute bacterial endocarditis
sed rate	sedimentation rate
SIADH	syndrome of inappropriate secretion of antidiuretic hormone
SLE	systemic lupus erythematosus
SNF	skilled nursing facility
SOB	short of breath
sol	solution
sono	sonogram, sonography
S/P	status post
sp gr	specific gravity
SSE	soapsuds enema
SSRI	serotonin reuptake inhibitor
staph	staphylococcus
stat	immediately
STD	sexually transmitted disease
strep	streptococcus
subcut	subcutaneous

ABBREVIATION/ ACRONYM	DEFINITION
T	temperature
T & A	tonsillectomy and adenoidectomy
TAH	transabdominal hysterectomy
TB	tuberculosis
TENS	transcutaneous electrical nerve stimulation
THA	total hip arthroplasty
THR	total hip replacement
TIA	transient ischemic attack
TJC	The Joint Commission, formerly JCAHO
TKA	total knee arthroplasty
TKR	total knee replacement
TPN	total parenteral nutrition
TPR	temperature, pulse, respiration
TURP	transurethral resection of the prostate
TWE	tap water enema
Tx	treatment, traction
UA	urinalysis
UAP	unlicensed assistive personnel
UGI	upper gatrointestinal
ULQ	upper left quadrant
ung	ointment
URI	upper respiratory infection
US	ultrasound
UTI	urinary tract infection
VA	Veterans Affairs
VD	veneral disease
VDRL	Venereal Disease Research Laboratories test
VLDL	very-low-density lipoprotein
VNA	Visiting Nurse Association
VS	vital signs
WBC	white blood cell (count)
WNL	within normal limits
Wt	weight

Abbreviations Related to Time

ABBREVIATION	DEFINITION
A.M.	before noon
ac, AC	before meals
bid	twice a day
h, H	hour
MN	midnight
pc, PC	after meals
P.M.	after noon, evening
q1h	every hour
q2h	every 2 hours
q3h	every 3 hours
q4h	every 4 hours
q6h	every 6 hours
q8h	every 8 hours
qid	four times a day
tid	three times a day

Abbreviations Related to Medications

ABBREVIATION	DEFINITION	ABBREVIATION	DEFINITION
ac, AC	before meals	ID	intradermal
amp	ampule	IM	intramuscular
cap	capsule	IV	intravenous
comp	compound	pc, PC	after meals
dil	dilute	PP	postprandial
elix	elixir	tab	tablet
ext	extract		
H	hypodermic, hypodermic injection		

Abbreviations Related to Measurements

ABBREVIATION	DEFINITION	ABBREVIATION	DEFINITION
cm	centimeter	mEq	milliequivalent
g, gm	gram		
gr	grain	mg	milligram
kg	kilogram	mL	milliliter
L	liter	tsp	teaspoon
mcg	microgram	tbsp	tablespoon

Chapter 1
1. 1
2. 2
3. 1, 3, 4, 6, and 7
4. 1, 3, 5, and 6
5. 4
6. 4
7. 3
8. 2
9. 2
10. 2

Chapter 2
1. 1
2. 4
3. 4
4. 1
5. 1
6. 2, 4, and 5
7. 5
8. 1
9. 4
10. 3

Chapter 3
1. 1
2. 1, 2, and 5
3. 3 and 5
4. 2
5. 2
6. 3
7. 2
8. 1
9. 2
10. 1, 2, 4, and 5

Chapter 4
1. patient input
2. 3
3. 1, 2, and 3
4. 4
5. 1, 3, 4, 6, and 7
6. 4
7. 2

Chapter 5
1. 4
2. 2
3. 2
4. 2, 4, and 6
5. 2
6. 2, 3, 4, and 5
7. 3
8. 4
9. 3
10. 2

Chapter 6
1. 1, 4, and 5
2. 2, 3, 4, and 5
3. 3
4. 2
5. improvement of nursing care
6. 1
7. 4
8. 1
9. 625 mg

Chapter 7
1. 1
2. 1
3. 2
4. 3
5. 2
6. 1
7. 3
8. 3
9. 4
10. 4

Chapter 8
1. 1
2. 4
3. 3
4. 2
5. 2, 3, 4, and 6
6. 2
7. 1
8. 2

9. 3
10. 4

Chapter 9
1. 4
2. kinesthetic
3. 1
4. 3
5. 2
6. 1
7. 3

Chapter 10
1. democratic
2. autocratic
3. 4 and 5
4. 1, 2, and 5
5. 3
6. 1
7. 4
8. 1, 3, and 4
9. 2
10. 1
11. 3

Chapter 11
1. superego
2. 3
3. 1
4. 1
5. 4
6. 4, 5, 6, and 7
7. 4
8. 1
9. 1
10. 2
11. 1
12. 2
13. 3

Chapter 12
1. blended
2. 3
3. 2
4. 1
5. 4
6. 3

7. 3
8. 1
9. 4
10. 2

Chapter 13
1. 1 and 2
2. 2
3. 4
4. 4
5. 2
6. 2
7. 2
8. 1, 2, and 3
9. 1

Chapter 14
1. 3
2. 2
3. 4
4. 4
5. 2
6. 4
7. 2
8. 2 and 3
9. 2 and 4

Chapter 15
1. 3
2. 4
3. 4
4. 2
5. 1
6. 2
7. 2
8. 3
9. 4
10. 2

Chapter 16
1. 4
2. 2 and 3
3. 2
4. 2, 3, 4, and 5
5. 1, 4, and 5
6. 1, 3, 4, 2
7. 2

8. 4
9. 3

Chapter 17
1. 4
2. 1, 4
3. 1, 2, 3, 5, and 6
4. 3
5. 2 and 3
6. 4
7. 1, 2, and 4
8. 1
9. 3 and 4
10. 1, 2, and 3

Chapter 18
1. 1, 2, and 3
2. 4
3. 1
4. 2
5. 2
6. 4
7. 3
8. 4
9. 2
10. 3

Chapter 19
1. 2
2. 3 and 5
3. 2
4. 4
5. 4
6. 1
7. 3
8. 3
9. 4
10. 1, 3, and 4

Chapter 20
1. 4
2. 2 and 4
3. 3
4. 1 and 4
5. 2
6. 2

7. 4
8. 4
9. pathogenic organisms
10. 3

Chapter 21
1. 3
2. 2
3. 2
4. 2
5. 4
6. orthostatic hypotension
7. 3
8. 2, 3, and 4
9. 4
10. 1 and 3

Chapter 22
1. percussion
2. 2
3. 1
4. 4
5. 2, 3, and 5
6. 2 and 5
7. 1
8. 3 and 4
9. 2
10. 2

Chapter 23
1. 3
2. 2, 3, and 4
3. 3
4. 2
5. 1 and 3
6. 2
7. 1 and 2
8. 2
9. 1, 2, 3, and 4
10. 4
11. 2, 3, and 4

Chapter 24
1. 4
2. 3
3. serology
4. 1, 3, and 4
5. 2
6. 1, 3, and 4
7. 1 and 2
8. aspiration
9. 1
10. 4

Chapter 25
1. 1, 2, 4, and 5
2. 1 and 4
3. 4
4. 610 mL
5. 3
6. 1
7. 2
8. 2
9. 4
10. 1

Chapter 26
1. 1, 4, and 6
2. 2, 5, and 6
3. Cardiac dysrhythmias
4. 3
5. 2
6. 3
7. 2
   (2.2 lb = 1 kg;
   185/2.2 =
   84 kg;
   84 kg × 0.8 =
   67.2 g)
8. 4
9. 2
10. 2

Chapter 27
1. 2, 5, 6, 8
2. 3, 4, 6
3. 4
4. 1
5. 3
6. 2
7. The patient should be positioned with the head of the bed elevated at least 30 degrees to prevent aspiration.
8. 1
9. 4
10. 3

Chapter 28
1. 1 and 2
2. 2
3. 1
4. 2
5. 1, 2, and 4
6. airway obstruction
7. 3
8. 2 and 4
9. 4
10. 1

Chapter 29
1. 3
2. 3
3. 3, 1, 6, 2, 4, 5
4. 1
5. 4
6. 3
7. 4
8. 1

9. 3
10. 2
11. 1
12. 2
13. 3
14. 4
15. 1
16. 4
17. 3

Chapter 30
1. 1, 3, and 4
2. 2
3. 3
4. 2
5. 1
6. 1
7. 4
8. 4
9. 2, 5, 4, 1, 6, 3, 7
10. 4

Chapter 31
1. biofeedback
2. 4
3. 1
4. 2
5. 1 and 3
6. 1
7. 1 and 4
8. 2 and 5
9. 2, 3, 5, 6, and 7
10. 2 and 5

Chapter 32
1. 4
2. mind-body intervention
3. 1
4. 3, 4

5. 2
6. 4
7. 4

Chapter 33
1. 1
2. 3
3. 4
4. 2
5. 4
6. 4
7. 20 kg
8. 7 days

Chapter 34
1. 3
2. 3, 7, 6, 2, 5, 4, 1
3. 2
4. 2
5. 4
6. 1
7. 1
8. 4
9. 2
10. 2

Chapter 35
1. 4
2. 1
3. 2
4. 3
5. 1, 4, 3, 2
6. 2
7. 2
8. 3
9. 2
10. 3

Chapter 36
1. 2
2. 3
3. 2
4. 1
5. 1
6. 4
7. 3
8. 1, 2, 3, 4, and 5
9. 3
10. 3
11. 25 gtt/min
12. 125 mL/hr

Chapter 37
1. 2
2. 4
3. 4
4. 3
5. 1, 2, 3, 4, and 5
6. 1, 2, 4, and 5
7. 2
8. atelectasis
9. 2
10. 2, 3, 4, and 5
11. 3
12. a deep vein thrombosis

Chapter 38
1. 2
2. 2
3. 4
4. 1, 3, 4, 5, and 6
5. 1
6. 1
7. dehiscence
8. 3
9. 2
10. 3

Chapter 39
1. thrombo-phlebitis
2. 3
3. 4
4. 1, 3, and 4
5. 2
6. 1, 2, and 4
7. 1
8. 2
9. 1
10. 4

Chapter 40
1. 1, 2, 3, and 4
2. 1, 2, and 4
3. 2
4. 1, 3, and 4
5. 1
6. 2
7. 1
8. 1 and 2
9. 1
10. macular de-generation

Chapter 41
1. 1
2. 3
3. 1, 2, and 4
4. 2, 3, and 4
5. 4
6. 2, 4, and 5
7. 2
8. 2
9. 4
10. 1, 2, and 3

Bibliography

General References

Ackley, B.J., & Ladwig, G.B. (2006). *Nursing Diagnosis Handbook: A Guide to Planning Care* (7th ed.). St. Louis: Elsevier Mosby.

Adams, M.P., Josephson, D.L., & Holland, L.N. (2005). *Pharmacology for Nurses: A Pathophysiologic Approach.* Upper Saddle River, NJ: Pearson.

Alfaro-LeFevre, R. (2004). *Critical Thinking in Nursing: A Practical Approach* (3rd ed.). Philadelphia: Saunders.

Arnold, E., & Boggs, K.U. (2007). *Interpersonal Relationships: Professional Communication Skills for Nurses* (5th ed.). Philadelphia: Saunders.

Applegate, E. (2006). *The Anatomy and Physiology Learning System* (3rd ed.). Philadelphia: Elsevier Saunders.

Black, J.M., & Hawks, J.H. (2005). *Medical-Surgical Nursing: Clinical Management for Positive Outcomes* (7th ed.). Philadelphia: Elsevier Saunders.

Burke, M.M., & Laramie, J.A. (2004). *Primary Care of the Older Adult: A Multidisciplinary Approach* (2nd ed.). St. Louis: Mosby.

D'Avanzo, C.E., & Geissler, E.M. (2003). *Mosby's Pocket Guide to Cultural Health Assessment.* St. Louis: Mosby.

Dossey, B.M., Keegan, L., & Guzetta, K. (Eds.). (2005). *Holistic Nursing: A Handbook for Practice* (4th ed.). (pp. 91-121). Gaithersburg, MD: Aspen.

Ebersole, P., & Hess, P. (2005). *Geriatric Nursing and Healthy Aging* (2nd ed.). St. Louis: Elsevier Mosby.

Elkin, M.K., Perry, A.G., & Potter, P.A. (2008). *Nursing Interventions and Clinical Skills* (4th ed.). St. Louis: Elsevier Mosby.

Fischbach, F. (2004). *A Manual of Laboratory and Diagnostic Tests* (7th ed.). Philadelphia: Lippincott Williams & Wilkins.

Galanti G.A. (2003). *Caring for Patients from Different Cultures* (3rd ed.). Philadelphia: Penn Press.

Gould, B.E. (2006). *Pathophysiology for the Health-Related Professions* (3rd ed.). Philadelphia: Elsevier Saunders.

Harkreader, H., Hogan, M.A., & Thobaben, M. (2007). *Fundamentals of Nursing: Caring and Clinical Judgment* (2nd ed.). Philadelphia: Saunders.

Healthy People 2010. (2000). *Objectives.* Available at: www.healthypeople.gov/Search/objectives.htm.

Herlihy, B. (2007). *The Human Body in Health and Illness* (3rd ed.). Philadelphia: Elsevier Saunders.

Hill, S.S., & Howlett, H.A. (2009). *Success in Practical/Vocational Nursing: From Student to Leader* (6th ed.). Philadelphia: Saunders.

Hockenberry-Eaton, M., & Wilson, D. (2005). *Wong's Nursing Care of Infants and Children* (8th ed.). St. Louis: Mosby.

Hodgson, B.B., & Kizior, R.J. (2006). *Saunders Nursing Drug Handbook.* Philadelphia: Elsevier Saunders.

Huether, S.E., & McCance, K.L. (2008). *Understanding Pathophysiology* (4th ed.). St. Louis: Elsevier Mosby.

Ignatavicius, D.D., & Workman, M.L. (2006). *Medical-Surgical Nursing: Critical Thinking for Collaborative Care* (5th ed.). Philadelphia: Elsevier Saunders.

Jarvis, C. (2004). *Physical Examination and Health Assessment* (4th ed.). Philadelphia: Saunders.

(The) Joint Commission. (2008). *2008 National patient safety goals.* Available at: www.jointcommission.org/PatientSafety/NationalPatientSafetyGoals.

(The) Joint Commission. (2007). *2007 Hospital/critical access hospital national patient safety goals.* Available at: www.jointcommission.org/PatientSafety/NationalPatientSafetyGoals/07_hap_cah_npsgs.htm.

Kee, J.L., Hayes, E.R., & McCuistion, L.E. (2006). *Pharmacology: A Nursing Process Approach* (5th ed.). Philadelphia: Elsevier Saunders.

Lehne, R.A. (2004). *Pharmacology for Nursing Care* (5th ed.). Philadelphia: Saunders.

Leifer, G. (2007). *Introduction to Maternity and Pediatric Nursing* (5th ed.). Philadelphia: Elsevier Saunders.

Leifer-Hartson, G., & Hartson, H. (2004). *Growth and Development Across the Lifespan: A Health Promotion Focus.* Philadelphia: Saunders.

Lewis, S.L., Heitkemper, M.M., Dirksen, S.R., et al. (2007). *Medical-Surgical Nursing: Assessment and Management of Clinical Problems* (7th ed.). St. Louis: Elsevier Mosby.

Linton, A., & Maebius, N. (2007). *Introduction to Medical-Surgical Nursing* (4th ed.). Philadelphia: Elsevier Saunders.

Macklin, D., & Chernecky, C. (2004). *Real World Nursing Survival Guide: IV Therapy.* Philadelphia: Saunders.

Meiner, S., & Lueckenotte, A. (2005). *Gerontologic Nursing* (3rd ed.). St. Louis: Elsevier Mosby.

Nursing 2008 Drug Handbook (7th ed.). (2008). Philadelphia: Lippincott Williams & Wilkins.

Peckenpaugh, N.J. (2007). *Nutrition Essentials and Diet Therapy* (10th ed.). Philadelphia: Elsevier Saunders.

Pagana K.D., & Pagana, T.J. (2006). *Mosby's Manual of Diagnostic and Laboratory Tests.* St. Louis: Elsevier Mosby.

Pagana, K.D., & Pagana, T.J. (2007). *Mosby's Diagnostic and Laboratory Test Reference* (8th ed.). St. Louis: Elsevier Mosby.

Perry, A.G., & Potter, P.A. (2006). *Clinical Nursing Skills and Techniques* (6th ed.). St. Louis: Elsevier Mosby.

Polan, E., & Taylor, D. (2007). *Journey Across the Life Span* (3rd ed.). Philadelphia: F.A. Davis.

Potter, P.A., & Perry, A.G. (2005). *Fundamentals of Nursing: Concepts, Process and Practice* (6th ed.). St. Louis: Elsevier Mosby.

Purnell, L.D., & Paulanka, B.J. (2003). *Transcultural Health Care: A Culturally Competent Approach.* Philadelphia: F.A. Davis.

Rothrock, J.C. (2003). *Alexander's Care of the Patient in Surgery* (12th ed.). St. Louis: Mosby.

Sorrentino, S.A., & Gorek, B. (2003). *Mosby's Textbook for Long-Term Care Assistants* (4th ed.). St. Louis: Mosby.

Swearingen, P.L. (2004). *All-in-One Care Planning Resource.* St. Louis: Mosby.

Ulrich, S.P., & Canale, S.W. (2005). *Nursing Care Planning Guides for Adults in Acute, Extended and Home Care Settings* (6th ed.). Philadelphia: Elsevier Saunders.

U.S. Department of Health and Human Services. (2000). *Healthy People 2010: With understanding and improving health and objectives for improving health* (2nd ed.). Washington, DC: U.S. Department of Health and Human Services.

Varcarolis, E.M., & Halter, M. (2009). *Foundations of Psychiatric Mental Health Nursing: A Clinical Approach* (6th ed.). Philadelphia: Elsevier Saunders.

White, L. (2005). *Foundations of Basic Nursing* (2nd ed.). Clifton Park, NY: Thompson Delmar Learning.

Wilson, D., & Hockenberry M. J. (2008). *Wong's Clincial Manual of Pediatric Nursing* (7th ed.). St. Louis: Elsevier Mosby.

Zerwekh, J., & Claborn, J.C. (2006). *Nursing Today: Transition and Trends* (5th ed.). Philadelphia: Elsevier Saunders.

Chapter 1

American Nurses Association. (2004). *Nursing: Scope and Standards of Practice.* Silver Spring, MD: American Nurses Publishing.

Armstrong, L. (2006). Healing beyond the bedside. *Nursing2006, 36*(6), 64hn4.

Baier, F. (2006). The Medicare prescription drug benefit. *American Journal of Nursing, 106*(6), 66-72.

Barclay, L. (2006). Licensed practical nurses may be able to fill gap in the nursing shortage. *Medscape Medical News*. Available at: www.medscape.com/viewarticle/541297_print.

Bennett, C. (2007). Evidence-based practice: Taking research to the bedside for optimal patient outcomes. *ADVANCE for Nurses*, 4(5), 15-17.

Buhler-Wilerson, K. (2007). No place like home: A history of nursing and home care in the U.S. *Home Healthcare Nurse*, 25(4), 253-258.

Bullough, V., Bullough, B., & Stanton, M. (Eds.). (1990). *Florence Nightingale and Her Era: A Collection of New Scholarship.* New York: Garland Publishing.

Cowles, L. (2007). On the line: Kaiser Permanente transforms the delivery of healthcare. *ADVANCE for Nurses*, 4(26), 12-14.

DiCenso, A., Guyatt, G., & Ciliska, D. (2005). *Evidence-Based Nursing: A Guide to Clinical Practice.* St. Louis: Elsevier Mosby.

Dolan, J.A., Fitzpatrick, M.L., & Herrmann, E.K. (1983). *Nursing in Society: A Historical Perspective* (15th ed.). Philadelphia: Saunders.

Donahue, M.P. (1985). *Nursing: The Finest Art.* St. Louis: Mosby. (Classic reference).

Gibbs, R.R. (2005). LPNs/LVNs and the changing face of health care. *LPN2005*, 1(6), 4.

Gorski, L.A. (2006). Integrating standards into practice. *Home Healthcare Nurse*, 24, 627-631.

Hartner, K. (2007). Finding evidence: Nurses have an opportunity to effect change through research and action. *ADVANCE for Nurses*, 4(26), 35.

Hill, S.S., & Howlett, H.S. (2005). *Success in Practical/Vocational Nursing: From Student to Leader* (5th ed.). Philadelphia: Saunders.

Nightingale, F. (1859). *Notes on Nursing: What It Is, and What It Is Not.* London: Harrison. (Commemorative edition, 1992. Philadelphia: Lippincott.)

Nolan, S. (2008). Nursing M & M reviews: Learning form our outcomes. *RN*, 71(1), 36-39.

Nursing2008 Eds. (2008). Hit the Web to guide evidence-based practice. *Nursing2008*, 38(1), 59.

O'Toole, M.T. (Ed.). (2005). *Miller-Keane Encyclopedia & Dictionary of Medicine, Nursing, & Allied Health* (7th ed.). Philadelphia: Saunders.

Pravikoff, D.S., Tanner, A.B., & Pierce, S.T. (2005). Readiness of U.S. nurses for evidence-based practice. *American Journal of Nursing*, 105(9), 40-51.

Schorr, T.M., & Kennedy, M.S. (1999). *100 Years of American Nursing.* Philadelphia: Lippincott.

Seago, J.A., Spetz, J., Chapman, S., & Dyer, W. (2006). Can the use of LPNs alleviate the nursing shortage? *American Journal of Nursing*, 106(7), 40-49.

Smith, N. (2007). Supporting evidence: Online tools help nurses find evidence-based practice resources. *NurseWeek*, 20(2), 14.

Waite, R., & Killian, P. (20078). Evidence-based practice: Nurses need to apply all sources of evidence related to their practice area to develop effective nursing practice strategies. *ADVANCE for Nurses*, 5(3), 24-26.

Wood, D.A. (2007). Medicare takes a bold stance. *NurseWeek*, 20(21), 26-27.

Zibell, E. (2006). The many hats of nursing. In *American Journal of Nursing Career Guide 2006*. Philadelphia: Lippincott Williams & Wilkins.

Chapter 2

Adamow, S.M. (2005). Restoring hope. *ADVANCE for Nurses*, 2(20), 113-115.

Benner, P.E., & Wrobel, J. (1989). *The Primacy of Caring: Stress and Coping in Health and Illness.* Menlo Park, CA: Addison-Wesley.

Burggraf, V., & Barry, R.J. (2000). *Healthy People 2010:* Protecting the health of older individuals. *Journal of Gerontological Nursing*, 26(12), 16.

Cannon, W.B. (1967). *The Wisdom of the Body: Revised and Enlarged Edition.* New York: Norton.

Dubos, R. (1965). *Man Adapting.* New Haven, CT: Yale University Press.

Dunn, H.L. (1973). *High Level Wellness.* Arlington, VA: Beatty.

Maslow, A.H. (1970). *Motivation and Personality.* Upper Saddle River, NJ: Prentice Hall.

Nightingale, F. (1859). *Notes on Nursing.* London, Harrison & Sons. (Reprinted, 1969. New York: Dover Publications, Inc.)

O'Toole, M. (Ed.). (2003). *Miller-Keane Encyclopedia and Dictionary of Medicine, Nursing, and Allied Health* (7th ed.). Philadelphia: Saunders.

Perez, M., & Reicherts, M. (1992). *Stress, Coping, and Health.* Seattle: Hogrefe & Huber.

Ringhofer, J. (2008). Treating the "whole" person. *RN*, 71(5), 17.

Selye, H. (1974). *Stress without Distress.* Philadelphia: Lippincott.

Selye, H. (1976). *The Stress of Life* (rev. ed.). New York: McGraw-Hill.

Swinford, P.A., & Webster, J.A. (Eds.). (1989). *Promoting Wellness: A Nurse's Handbook.* Rockville, MD: Aspen.

Chapter 3

Adamski, P. (2007). Implement a handoff communication approach. *Nursing Management*, 38(1), 10-12.

Alford, D.M. (2003). The clinical record: Recognizing its value in litigation. *Geriatric Nursing*, 24(4), 228-229.

American Hospital Association. (1972). *Statement on the Patient's Bill of Rights* (pp. 2-4). Chicago: Author.

American Nurses Association. (2004a). *Code for Nurses* (p. 1). Kansas City, MO: Author.

American Nurses Association. (2004b). *Standards for Clinical Nursing Practice.* Kansas City, MO: Author.

Anderson, F. (2007). Finding HIPAA in your soup: Decoding the privacy rule. *American Journal of Nursing*, 107(2), 66-72.

Austin, S. (2006a). "Ladies and gentlemen of the jury, I present . . . the nursing documentation." *Nursing2006*, 36(1), 56-62.

Austin, S. (2006b). Walk a fine line when your patient wants to leave AMA. *Nursing2006*, 36(12), 49.

Austin, S. (2008). 7 legal tips for safe nursing practice. *Nursing2008*, 38(3), 35-39.

Berry, M. (2004). Saying the right things when things go wrong. *RN*, 67(4), 59-63.

Brooke, P.S. (2005). Understanding HIPAA compliance. *LPN2005*, 1(4), 36-39.

Brooke, P.S. (2006). So you've been named in a lawsuit. *Nursing2006*, 36(7), 44-48.

Brous, E.A. (2008). Malpractice insurance and licensure protection: It's cheap, and you need it. *American Journal of Nursing*, 108(5), 34-36.

Chizek, M. (2006). Litigation in LTC. *ADVANCE for Nurses*, 3(1), 27-28.

Corbo, S.A. (2006). Delegation defined. *ADVANCE for Nurses*, 3(16), 17-19.

Cox, S.S. (2006). How to delegate to UAPs: Follow these guidelines to safe and legal delegation. *Nursing2006*, 36(7), 10-11.

Croke, E.M. (2003). Nurse, negligence, and malpractice. *American Journal of Nursing*, 103(9), 54-63.

Di Luige, K.J. (2004). Giving a deposition? Watch your words! *RN*, 67(1), 63-69.

Ghebrehiwet, T. (2005). The ICN code of ethics for nurses: Helping nurses make ethical decisions. *Reflections on Nursing Leadership*, 31(3), 26-28.

Grace, P.J., & McLaughlin, M. (2005). When consent isn't informed enough. *American Journal of Nursing*, 105(4), 79-84.

Gross, J. (2007). Keeping patients' details private, even from kin. *New York Times*, July 3, 2007.

Haddad, A. (2004). Ethics in action: End-of-life decisions: The family's role. *RN*, 67(1), 25-28.

Haddad, A. (2007). Ethics in action: What the family needs to know. *RN*, 70(11), 23.

Health Privacy Project (n.d.). *Myths and facts about the HIPAA privacy rule.* Available at: www.healthprivacy.org/usr_doc/Myths_and_Facts.pdf (accessed January 22, 2008).

Helm, A., & Kihm, N.C. (2006). Liability insurance: Is it for you? *LPN2006*, 2(3), 14-15.

(The) Joint Commission International Center for Patient Safety. (2007). *National patient safety goals.* Available at: www.jcipatientsafety.org/15148.

Kane, T. (2006). Advance directives. *Nursing2006, 36*(9), 43.

Kentucky Emergency Medical Services. (n.d.) *Do not resuscitate order.* Available at: http://kbems.ky.gov/NR/rdonlyres/09FFFC7BF-C705-4BF1-07BD-76031FF&5215/0/DoNotResuscitateForm.pdf (accessed January 22, 2008).

Levine, C. (2006). HIPAA and talking with family caregivers: What does the law really say? *American Journal of Nursing, 106*(8), 51-53.

Lorenz, J.M. (2007). 2007 Patient safety goals. *ADVANCE for Nurses, 4*(1), 17-19.

Making it clear with an incident report. (2006). *LPN2006, 2*(3), 17-19.

Mason, D.J. (2007). Good nurse—bad nurse: Is it an error or a crime? *American Journal of Nursing, 107*(3), 11.

McCormick-Gendzel, M., & Jurchak, M. (2006). A pathway for moral reasoning in home healthcare. *Home Healthcare Nurse, 24,* 654-661.

Mendler, J. (n.d.) *"Do not resuscitate" bracelets help EMTs honor patient wishes.* Available at: www.ur.umich.edu/9900/April 17_00/12.htm (accessed January 21, 2008).

National Hospice and Palliative Care Organization. (n.d.). *What are advance directives?* Available at: www:caringinfo.org/PlanningAhead/AdvanceDirectives/What are AdvanceDirectives.htm (accessed January 22, 2008).

Olsen, D.P. (2007). Unwanted treatment: What are the ethical implications? *American Journal of Nursing, 107*(9), 51-53.

Otto, S. (2007). Nursing ethics: Request an ethics consult to resolve dilemmas. *Nursing2007 Critical Care, 2*(4), 18-20.

SBAR: *A communication technique for today's healthcare professional.* Available at: www.saferhealthcare.com/index-php>option=com_content+task=view+id=33+itemid=84 (accessed January 22, 2008).

Siewers, M.H. (2008). Legal aspects of restraints. *ADVANCE for Nurses, 5*(9), 29-32.

Sosin, J. (2007). Loose lips: In violation of HIPAA. *Nurseweek, 20*(23) 28.

U.S. Department of Health & Human Services (2008). *General overview of standards for privacy of individually identifiable health information.* Available at: www.hhs.gov/ocr/hipaa/guidelines/overview.pdf.

Vonfrolio, L.G. (2006). Blow the whistle? *RN, 69*(10), 60.

Zonderman, A. (2006). Nursing malpractice insurance. *ADVANCE for Nurses, 3*(17), 33-34.

Chapter 4

Ackley, B.J., & Ladwig, G.B. (2006). *Nursing Diagnosis Handbook: A Guide to Planning Care* (7th ed.). St. Louis: Elsevier Mosby.

Alfaro-LeFevre, R. (2004). *Critical Thinking in Nursing: A Practical Approach* (3rd ed.). Philadelphia: Saunders.

Castillo, S.L.M. (2003). *Strategies, Techniques, and Approaches to Thinking* (2nd ed.). Philadelphia: Saunders.

Covey, S.R. (1990). *The 7 Habits of Highly Effective People.* New York: Simon & Schuster.

Lunney, M. (2001). *Critical Thinking and Nursing Diagnosis: Case Studies and Analyses.* Philadelphia: NANDA-International.

Nicoteri, J. (1998). Critical thinking skills. *American Journal of Nursing, 98*(10), 62-65.

Paul, R., & Binker, A. (Eds.). (1990). *Critical Thinking: How to Prepare Students for a Rapidly Changing World.* Santa Rosa, CA: Foundation for Critical Thinking.

Paul, R.W., & Elder, L. (2001). *Critical Thinking.* Upper Saddle River, NJ: Pearson Education.

Schuster, P.M. (2002). *Concept Mapping: A Critical-Thinking Approach to Care Planning.* Philadelphia: Davis.

Smith-Stoner, M. (1999a). Another 10 tips to think more critically. *Home Healthcare Nurse, 17,* 146-147.

Smith-Stoner, M. (1999b). 10 tips for thinking in a new way: Getting ready for whatever comes next. *Home Healthcare Nurse, 17,* 76-78.

Tucker, S.M., Cannobio, M., Paquette, E., et al. (2000). *Patient Care Standards: Collaborative Planning and Nursing Interventions* (7th ed.). St. Louis: Mosby.

Winningham, M.L., & Preusser, B.A. (2001). *Critical Thinking in Medical-Surgical Settings: A Case Study Approach* (2nd ed.). St. Louis: Mosby.

Chapter 5

Alfaro-LeFevre, R. (2005). *Applying Nursing Process: A Tool for Critical Thinking* (6th ed.). Philadelphia: Lippincott Williams & Wilkins.

American Nurses Association. (1998). *Standards of Clinical Nursing Practice* (2nd ed.). Kansas City, MO: Author.

Bulechek, G.M., & McCloskey, J.C. (2000). *Nursing Interventions: Effective Nursing Treatments* (3rd ed.). Philadelphia: Saunders.

Carpenito, L.J. (2005). *Nursing Diagnosis: Application to Clinical Practice* (11th ed.). Philadelphia: Lippincott Williams & Wilkins.

Doenges, M.E., Moorhouse, M.F., & Geissler-Murr, A.C. (2006a). *Nurse's Pocket Guide: Diagnoses, Interventions and Rationales* (10th ed.). Philadelphia: F.A. Davis.

Doenges, M.E., Moorhouse, M.F., & Geissler-Murr, A.C. (2006b). *Nursing Care Plans: Guidelines for Individualizing Patient Care* (7th ed.). Philadelphia: F.A. Davis.

Huffman, M. (2004). Patient outcomes: What does it all mean? *Home Healthcare Nurse, 22,* 22-27.

Leff, E.W. (2004). Involving patients in care decisions improves satisfaction. *Home Healthcare Nurse, 22,* 297-301.

Moorhead, S., Johnson, M., & Maas, M. (2004). *Nursing Outcomes Classification* (3rd ed.). St. Louis: Mosby.

Ulrich, S.P., & Canale, S.W. (2005). *Nursing Care Planning Guides for Adults in Acute, Extended and Home Care Settings* (6th ed.). Philadelphia: Saunders.

Chapter 6

Durkin, N. (2008). Using record review as a quality improvement process. *Home Healthcare Nurse, 24,* 492-502.

Swearingen, P.L. (2004). *All-in-One Care Planning Resource.* St. Louis: Mosby.

Tucker, S.M., Cannobio, M., Paquette, E., et al. (2000). *Patient Care Standards: Collaborative Planning and Nursing Interventions* (7th ed.). St. Louis: Mosby

Chapter 7

Austin, S. (2006). "Ladies and gentlemen of the jury, I present . . . the nursing documentation." *Nursing2006, 36*(1), 56-62.

Burke, L.J., & Murphy, J. (1998). *Charting by Exception Applications: Making It Work in Clinical Settings* (2nd ed.). Albany, NY: Delmar.

Childers, K.P. (2005). Paying a price for poor documentation. *Nursing2005, 35*(1), 32hn4, 32hn6.

Engram, B.W. (2005). Write this way. *ADVANCE for Nurses, 2*(18), 23-24.

Habel, M. (2003). Document it right. *NurseWeek, 16*(1), 21-22.

Halliday, A. (2005). Creating a reliable time line. *Nursing2005, 35*(2), 27.

Karch, A.M. (2004). What's wrong with U? JCAHO places limits on abbreviations used in practice. *American Journal of Nursing, 104*(6), 65-66.

Lee, T. (2007). *Nursing administrators' experiences in managing PDA use on inpatient units.* Available at: www.medscape.com/viewarticle/550841.

Ligon, K., & Das, E. (2004). The benefits of automated nursing documentation. *Nurse Leader, 2*(5), 29-31.

Lillis, K. (Ed.). (2005). Going paperless. *ADVANCE for Nurses, 2*(12), 36-38.

LPN2005 Eds. (2005). When patients ignore instructions. *LPN2005, 1*(6), 46-47.

LPN2006 Eds. (2006a). Charting tips for long-term care. *LPN2006, 2*(1), 9-11.

LPN2006 Eds. (2006b). Planning your patient's discharge. *LPN2006, 2*(2), 10-12.

LPN2007 Eds. (2007a). Documenting hostile situations. *PLN2007, 3*(6), 9-10.

LPN2007 Eds. (2007b). You're on trial: How to protect yourself. *LPN2007, 3*(2), 16, 18.

LPN2008 Eds. (2008a). Before you say goodbye: Discharge summaries. *LPN2008, 4*(1), 4-5.

LPN2008 Eds. (2008b). Documenting telephone orders. *LPN2008, 4*(4), 4.

Lunney, M., Delaney, C., & Duffy, M. (2005). Advocating for standardized nursing languages in electronic health records. *Journal of Nursing Administration, 35*(1), 1-3.

Martin, R.H. (2006). Incident reports: Documentation of unexpected or unusual events is crucial to promote quality, safety, and risk management. *ADVANCE for Nurses, 3*(21), 23-25.

Moody, L.E., Slocumb, E., Berg, B., et al. (2004). *Electronic health records documentation in nursing: Nurses' perceptions, attitudes, and preferences.* Available at: www.medscape.com/viewarticle/494147.

Nursing2006 Eds. (2006). Documenting general observation. *Nursing2006, 36*(2), 25.

Nursing2007 Eds. (2007). When a patient fails to provide information. *Nursing2007, 37*(11), 29.

Nursing Made Incredibly Easy! Eds. (2004a). Charting challenges: Making an exception in charting. *Nursing Made Incredibly Easy!, 2*(4), 63.

Nursing Made Incredibly Easy! Eds. (2004b). Document now, prevent problems later. *Nursing Made Incredibly Easy!, 2*(3), 59-60.

Nursing Made Incredibly Easy! Eds. (2004c). Making an exception in charting. *Nursing Made Incredibly Easy!, 2*(4), 63.

Olson, C. (2006). Electronic revolution: Electronic documentation lets nurses spend their time providing care instead of doing paperwork. *ADVANCE for Nurses, 3*(23), 27-28.

Poissant, L., Pereira, J., Tamblyn, R., et al. (2005). The impact of electronic health records on time efficiency of physicians and nurses: A systematic review. *Journal of the American Medical Informatics Association, 12*, 505-516.

Smith, K., Smith V., Krugman, M., et al. (2005). Evaluating the impact of computerized clinical documentation. *Computers, Informatics, Nursing: CIN, 23*(3), 132-138.

Smith, L.S. (2004a). Documenting refusal of treatment. *Nursing2004, 34*(4), 79.

Smith, L.S. (2004b). "Erasing" those unavoidable slipups. *Nursing Made Incredibly Easy!, 3*(1), 5.

Smith, L.S. (2005). When a colleague falsifies the record. *Nursing2005, 35*(12), 76.

Smith, L.S. (2006). Documenting discharge planning. *Nursing2006, 36*(5), 18.

World, H. (2004, September 20). Off the charts (to computer). *NurseWeek,* Critical Care Spec Sect, pp. 20-21. Available at www.nurseweek.com/news/Features/04-09/CriticalCareElectronic.asp.

Chapter 8

Adamle, K., & Turkoski, B. (2006). Responding to patient initiated humor: Guidelines for practice. *Home Healthcare Nurse, 24*, 638-644.

Arnold, E., & Underman Boggs, K. (2007). *Interpersonal Relationships: Professional Communication Skills for Nurses* (5th ed.). Philadelphia: Elsevier Saunders.

Bensing, K. (2007). Within boundaries: Professionals walk a thin line to maintain therapeutic relationships with patients. *ADVANCE for Nurses, 4*(15), 14-19.

Burke, M., Boal, J., & Mitchell, R. (2004). Communicating for better care: Improving nurse-physician communication. *American Journal of Nursing, 104*(12), 40-48.

Bylone, M. (2007). Can you hear me now? In the age of wireless communication, healthcare professionals must be careful to ensure patient privacy is not compromised. *ADVANCE for Nurses, 4*(10), 30.

Charting Checkup. (2005). Listen up! How to take verbal and telephone orders. *LPN 2005, 1*(2), 44-45.

Christie, W., & Moore, C. (2005). The impact of humor on patients with cancer. *Clinical Journal of Oncology Nursing, 9*(2), 211-218.

Clayton, M.F. (2006). Communication an important part of nursing. *American Journal of Nursing, 106*(11), 70-72.

Cox, S. (2007). Good communication: Finding the middle ground. *Nursing2007, 37*(1), 57.

Dancer, J. (2006). Message received. *ADVANCE for Nurses, 3*(23), 31.

D'Avanzo, C. (2008). *Mosby's Pocket Guide to Cultural Health Assessment* (4th ed.). St. Louis: Mosby.

Drosey, B. (Ed.). (2007). Safe transport: Concise and confident communication between clinicians is integral to safe patient hand-offs. *ADVANCE for Nurses, 4*(2), 37.

Duda, J.M. (2006). Learning to listen. *NurseWeek, 19*(10), 56-57.

Federwisch, A. (2006). From conflict to collaboration. *NurseWeek, 19*(21), 14-16.

Federwisch, A. (2007). Passing the baton: Bedside shift report ensures quality handoff. *NurseWeek, 20*(20), 14.

Flores, G. (2006). Cases from AHRQ WebM&M: Language barriers are more than an inconvenience. Patient errors range from simple miscommunication to life-threatening. *Medscape Family Medicine.* Available at: www.medscape.com/viewarticle/534045_1.

Hemmila, D. (2006). Talking the talk. *NurseWeek, 19*(17), 16-17.

Kaufman, M.E. (2005). Bridging the English-language gap. *LPN 2005, 1*(5), 10-12.

Lautrette, A., Damon, M., Megarbane, B., et al. (2007). A communication strategy and brochure for relatives of patients dying in the ICU. *New England Journal of Medicine, 356*, 469-478.

LPN2008 Eds. (2008). Documenting telephone orders. *LPN2008, 4*(4), 4.

Maison, D. (2006). Effective communications are more important than ever. *Home Healthcare Nurse, 24*, 178-182.

McPeck, P. (2006). Beyond illegible scrawl: Computerized order entry. *NurseWeek, 19*(10), 48-50.

Miller, C.A. (2008), Communication difficulties in hospitalized older adults with dementia. *American Journal of Nursing, 108*(3), 58-66.

Nahm, E. (2007). Telehealth: Information and communication technologies show potential to improve disease management. *ADVANCE for Nurses, 4*(22), 15-18.

Oliva, N.L. (2008). When language intervenes. *American Journal of Nursing, 108*(3), 73-75.

Pope, B.B., Rodzen, L., & Spross, G. (2008). Raising the SBAR: How better communication improves patient outcomes. *Nursing2008, 38*(3), 41-43.

Pullen, R.L. (2007). Tips for communicating with a patient from another culture. *Nursing2007, 37*(10), 48-49.

Roman, L.M. (2007). Finding the words: How to handle difficult conversations. *RN, 70*(3), 34-38.

Schroeder, S.J. (2006). Picking up the pace: A new template for shift report. *Nursing2006, 36*(10), 22-23.

Schroeder, S.J. (2007). Improving intershift handoff—and patient safety! *LPN2007, 3*(2), 22-23.

Sheldon, L.K., Barrett, R., & Ellington, L. (2006). Difficult communication in nursing. *Journal of Nursing Scholarship, 38*, 141-146.

Shirk, C. & Gianetti, T. (2008). Leave a message: RNs describe solution to phone calls regarding patient care and HIPAA. *ADVANCE for Nurses, 5*(3), 11.

Sirota, T. (2007). Improving the nurse/physician relationship. *LPN2007, 3*(5), 14-17.

Smith, L.S. (2007). Speaking up for medical language interpreters. *Nursing2007, 37*(12), 48-49.

Sosin, J. (2007). Loose lips: In violation of HIPAA. *NurseWeek, 20*(23), 19.

Sullivan, R., & Ferriter, A. (2008). Prevent life-threatening communication breakdowns. *Nursing2008, 38*(2), 17.

Vesterlund, M. (2008). A right to understand: Recognizing the needs of non-English speaking patients. *American Journal of Nursing, 108*(2), 13.

Weber, S. (2007). More effective team interaction. *ADVANCE for Nurses, 4*(11), 11.

Wright, L.D. (2006). Professional boundaries in home care. *Home Healthcare Nurse, 24*, 672-675.

Chapter 9

Canobbio, M.M. (2006). *Mosby's Handbook of Patient Teaching,* (3rd ed.). St. Louis: Mosby.

Haddad, A. (2003). Cutting corners on patient ed? *RN, 66*(7), 23-26.

Health Canada (2002). *Canada Health Act overview.* Available at: www.hc-sc.gc/ca/ahc/media/nr-cp/2002/2002_caresoinsbk4_e.html.

Health Canada (2002).*Canada's health care system at a glance.* Available at: www.hc-sc.gc/ca/ahc/media/nr-cp/2002/2002_caresoinsbk5_e.html.

Hickey, B. (2008). Strategies for educating older adults. *LPN2008, 4*(2), 28-29.

Hindelang, M. (2006). Patient education: Ever so important. *Home Healthcare Nurse, 24*(1), 14-16.

Lillis, K. (2007). Empowering tools: Interactive education and online resources can help foster patient-friendly care. *ADVANCE for Nurses, 4*(19), 25-26.

Lorenz, J.M. (2004). Patient education materials: When preparing written pieces for patients/family members use a reader-friendly format and keep it simple. *Advance for Nurses, 2*(5), 15-18.

Lorig, K.R. (2003). Taking patient ed to the next level. *RN, 66*(12), 35-38.

Neafsey, P.J. (2003). Interactive personal technology education program decreases adverse medication events. *Home Healthcare Nurse, 21*(10), 697-698.

Neder, S. (2003). Individualized education can improve foot care for patients with diabetes. *Home Healthcare Nurse, 21*(12), 837-840.

Polzien, G. (2006). The ABCs of teaching older adults: Implications for home care and hospice. *Home Healthcare Nurse, 24*(8), 487-490.

Ruholl, L. (2003). Tips for teaching the elderly. *RN, 66*(5), 48-52.

Spader, C. (2008). Nurses tap into new teaching tool. *Nurse-Week, 21*(9), 84.

Sutter, P.M., & Sutter, W.N. (2008). Timeless principles of learning. *Home Healthcare Nurse, 26*(2), 82-88.

Weston-Eborn, R. (2004). Home care and the adult learner. *Home Healthcare Nurse, 22*(8), 522-523.

Weston-Eborn, R., & Sitzman, K. (2004). Creating effective learning objectives. *Home Healthcare Nurse, 22*(11), 753.

Weston-Eborn, R., & Sitzman, K. (2005a). Creating teaching plans for the adult learner. *Home Healthcare Nurse, 23*(3), 192-194.

Weston-Eborn, R., & Sitzman, K. (2005b). Selecting effective instructional resources. *Home Healthcare Nurse, 23*(6), 402-403.

Chapter 10

American Association of Critical Care Nurses. (2004). *Delegation handbook.* Available at: www.aacn.org/AACN/practice.nsf/Files/DBEd2/$file/1editedrevisedAACNDelegationHandbook%207-1-2004.pdf.

Ayers, D.M., & Montgomery, M. (2008). Delegating the "right" way. *Nursing2008, 38*(4), 56hn1-56hn2.

Case, B. (2004). Delegation skills. *ADVANCE for Nurses, 6*(16), 17-23.

Hathaway, L.R. (2005). Safely delegating to unlicensed assistive personnel. *LPN2005, 1*(5), 13-14.

(The) Joint Commission International Center for Patient Safety. (2007). *NPSG 2A.* Available at: www.jcipatientsafety.org/22841/.

(The) Joint Commission (2006). Guidelines for accepting and transcribing verbal or telephone orders. *The Source, 4*(7), 6-10.

Lower, J. (2006). Transitioning to charge nurse. *ADVANCE for Nurses, 3*(22), 15-17.

Marriner-Tomey, A. (2004). *Guide to Nursing Management and Leadership* (7th ed.). St. Louis: Mosby.

Orcajada, E., & Rao, L. (2005). The art and science of delegation. *ADVANCE for Nurses, 2*(15), 25-26.

Riley, J.B. (2004). *Communication in Nursing* (5th ed.). St. Louis: Mosby.

Timm, S.E. (2003). Effectively delegating nursing activities in home care. *Home Healthcare Nurse, 21*, 260-262.

Whitman, M.M. (2005). Return and report: Establishing accountability in delegation. *American Journal of Nursing, 105*(3), 97.

Chapter 11

Anderson, S., Schaechter, J., & Brosco, J. (2005). Adolescent patients and their confidentiality: Staying within legal bounds. *Contemporary Pediatrics, 22*(7), 54-59.

Bahr, S.J., Hoffmann, J.P., & Yang, X. (2005). Parental and peer influences on the risk of adolescent drug use. *Journal of Primary Prevention, 26*, 529-549.

Behrman, R., Kliegman, R., & Jenson, H. (2004). *Nelson Textbook of Pediatrics* (17th ed.). Philadelphia: Saunders.

Broderick, M. (2004). Pediatric poisoning. *RN, 67*(9), 37-42.

Cathey, M., & Gaylord, N. (2004). Picky eating: A toddler's approach to mealtime. *Pediatric Nursing, 30*, 101-107.

Condon, M. (2005). Breast is best, but could it be better: What is in breast milk that should not be? *Pediatric Nursing, 31*, 333-338.

Deering, C., & Cody, D. (2002). Communicating with children and adolescents. *American Journal of Nursing, 102*(3), 34-41.

DeRoma, V.M., Lassiter, K.S., & Davis, V.A. (2004). Adolescent involvement in discipline decision making. *Behavior Modification, 28*, 420-437.

Haglund, K. (2006). Recommendations for sexuality education for early adolescents. *Journal of Obstetric, Gynecologic, and Neonatal Nursing, 35*, 369-374.

Henry, L.L. (2005). Childhood obesity: What can be done to help today's youth? *Pediatric Nursing, 31*(1), 13-16.

Ivey, J. (2001). Children's responses to contact with elders. *MCN The American Journal of Maternal/Child Nursing, 26*, 23-27.

Keefe, M., Barbosa, G., Forese-Fretz, A., et al. (2005). An intervention program for families with irritable infants. *MCN The American Journal of Materna/Child Nursing, 30*, 230-236.

Monsen, R. (2001). Children and pets. *Journal of Pediatric Nursing, 16*, 197-198.

Mulryan, K., Cathers, P., & Fagin, A. (2000). Combating abuse: Protecting the child. *Nursing2000, 30*(7), 39-43.

National Coalition for the Protection of Children & Families. *Teen pregnancy.* Available at: www.nationalcoalition.org/resourcesservices/stat.html (accessed June 27, 2007).

O'Dea, J.A. (2005). Improving adolescent eating habits and prevention of childhood obesity: Are we neglecting the crucial role of parents? *Nutrition and Dietetics, 62*(2/3), 66-68.

Polaha, J., Larzelere, R.E., Shapiro, S.K, et al. (2004). Physical discipline and child behavior problems: A study of ethnic group differences. *Parenting, Science and Practice, 4*, 339-360.

Polan, E., & Taylor, D. (2007). *Journey Across the Life Span* (3rd ed., Ch. 5-10). Philadelphia: F.A. Davis.

Ross, J.L. (2005). Near drowning. *RN, 68*(7), 36-41.

Tillett, J. (2005). Adolescence and informed consent: Ethical and legal issues. *Journal of Perinatal & Neonatal Nursing, 19*, 112-119.

U.S. Bureau of the Census. (2007). *Statistical Abstracts of the United States, 2004* (122nd ed.). Washington, DC: U.S. Department of the Treasury.

Chapter 12

Craig, G.J. (1999). *Human Development* (8th ed., Ch. 12-15). Upper Saddle River, NJ: Simon & Schuster.

Davidson, G.J. (2003). *Divorce risk factors.* Available at: www.theologicaleditions.com/Features/TodaysFeature11.htm.

Leifer-Hartson, G., & Hartson, H. (2004). *Growth and Development Across the Lifespan: A Health Promotion Focus.* Philadelphia: Saunders.

Papalia, D., & Olds, S. (2001). *Human Development* (8th ed., Ch. 14, 15). Boston: McGraw-Hill.

PREP, Inc. (2007). What factors are associated with divorce and/or marital unhappiness. Available at: www.prepinc.com/main/docs/what_factors.html.

Rowe, J., & Kahn, R. (1998). *Successful Aging*. New York: Pantheon Books.

Stanley, S.M., & Markman, H. (2007). Predicting divorce. Available at: www.2-in-1.co.uk/articles/preddiv.

Streff, M. B. (2005). Family dynamics. *ADVANCE for Nurses, 2*(23), 19-20.

Taylor, S. (2007). Equal opportunities. *Exchange Magazine*, McCombs School of Business, University of Texas at Austin. Available at: http://mba.mccombs.utexas.edu/mma/info/exchange/2007/equal.asp.

U.S. Bureau of the Census. (2006). *Statistical Abstracts of the United States, 2004* (123rd ed.). Washington, DC: U.S. Department of the Treasury.

Chapter 13

Administration on Aging. (2005). *A Profile of Older Americans: 2005*. Rockville, MD: U.S. Department of Health and Human Services.

Agency for Healthcare Research and Quality (AHRQ) Eds. (2008). Managed care helps the elderly avoid preventable hospitalizations more than traditional Medicare. *AHRQ Bulletin, 330*(Feb), 13.

American Journal of Nursing Eds. (2005). A new look at the old. *American Journal of Nursing, 105*(12), 53-61.

Avidan, A. (2006). Insomnia in elderly. *Advance Newsmagazines for LPNs*. Available at: http://lpn.advanceweb.com/common/editorial/PrintFriendly.aspx?CC=69021.

Bertsch, D.K., & Taylor-Moore, P.C. (2005). Elderly want to 'age in place.' *NurseWeek, 18*(14), 17-18.

Burgess, A.W., & Clements, P.T. (2006). Information processing of sexual abuse in elders. *Journal of Forensic Nursing, 2*, 113-120.

Busko, M., & Lie, D. (2006). *Physical fitness contributes to successful mental aging*. Available at: www.medscape.com/viewarticle/545924.

Butcher, H.K., & McGonigal-Kenney, M. (2005). Depression and dispiritedness in later life: A 'gray drizzle of horror' isn't inevitable. *American Journal of Nursing, 105*(12), 52.

Centers for Disease Control and Prevention. (2007). *Health information for older adults*. Available at: www.cdc.gov/aging/info.htm.

Ebersole, P., Hess, P., & Luggen, A.S. (2004). *Toward Healthy Aging: Human Needs and Nursing Response*. St. Louis: Mosby.

Gray-Vickrey, P. (2005). Elder abuse: Are you prepared to intervene? *LPN2005, 1*(2), 39-41.

Hindelang, M. (2006). Honoring our elders: Hearing their stories, respecting their ways. *Home Healthcare Nurse, 24*, 294-297.

Leff, E., & Sonstegard-Gamm, J. (2006). The home care team approach to self-neglecting elders. *Home Healthcare Nurse, 24*, 249-257.

Lorenz, J.M. (2007). Sex & the older adult. *ADVANCE for Nurses, 4*(13), 14-17.

Mauk, K.L. (2005). Keeping an older adult on her toes with exercise. *Nursing2005, 35*(1), 24.

Mauk, K.L. (2006). Movin' on: Keeping an older adult active with exercise. *LPN2006, 2*(4), 13-14.

Mcreynolds, J.L., & Rossen, E.K. (2004). *Importance of physical activity, nutrition, and social support for optimal aging*. Available at: www.medscape.com/viewarticle/484344.

Meiner, S.E., & Lueckenotte, A. (2006). *Gerontologic Nursing* (3rd ed.). St. Louis: Elsevier Mosby.

Murphy, K. (2007). Is your older patient depressed? *Nursing2007, 37*(6), 22-23.

National Center for Health Statistics. (2004). *Deaths: Final data for 2004*. Available at: www.cdc.gov.nchs/products/pubs/pubd/hestats/finaldeaths04/finaldeaths04.htm.

National Center on Elder Abuse. (2006). *Fact Sheet: Abuse of adults aged 60+ 2004 survey of adult protective services*. Washington, DC: Author.

National Institute of Mental Health. (2007). Older adults: Depression and suicide facts. Available at: www.allaboutdepression.com/gen_20.html.

National Institute on Aging. (2007). Figure 4. U.S. population aging 65 years and older: 1990 to 20 (in millions). Available at: www.nia.nih.gov/ResearchInformation/Conferences And Meetings/WorkshopReport.

National Institute on Aging. (2007). *Growing older in America*. Bethesda, MD: U.S. Deparment of Health and Human Services.

Resnick, B. (2005). Exercise for older adults. *ADVANCE for Nurses, 2*(4), 19-21.

Resnick, B. (2006). Improving care of older adults: You can make a difference. *Geriatric Nursing, 27*, 70-72.

Senior Journal Eds. (2007). Larger number of grandparents taking care of their grandchildren. Available at: www.seniorjournal.com/NEWS/Grandparents/GrndPrntCare.htm.

Senior Journal Eds. (2005). Seniors charging out of poverty while nation sinks. Available at: from www.seniorjournal.com/NEWS/SeniorStats/5-08-31SeniorsLeavePoverty.htm.

U.S. Bureau of the Census. (2002). *Statistical Abstract of the United States, 2002* (122nd ed.). Washington, DC: U.S. Department of the Treasury.

U.S. Bureau of the Census. (2004). *U.S. Interim projections by age, sex, race, and Hispanic origin*. Retrieved from www.census.gov/ipc/www/usinterimproj.

U.S. Bureau of the Census (2004). *Longevity and health characteristics*. Available at: www.census.gov/prod//pop/p.23-190/p.23190/g.pdf.

Weiland, S., & Shellenbarger, T. (2002). Family caregiving at home. *Home Healthcare Nurse, 20*, 113-119.

Wood, D.A. (2006). Elder abuse: Vulnerable seniors need nurses' help. *NurseWeek, 19*(24), 16.

Chapter 14

Bensing, K. (2006a). Prayer and healing: Part 1. *ADVANCE for Nurses, 3*(12), 35.

Bensing, K. (2006b). Prayer and healing: Part 2. *ADVANCE for Nurses, 3*(13), 10.

Boylan, L.N. (2005). Caring for patients of diverse religious traditions: Judaism. *Home Healthcare Nurse, 23*, 794-797.

Brown, I. (2006). Caring for patients of diverse religious traditions: Evangelical "born-again" Christians. *Home Healthcare Nurse, 24*, 677-680.

Crist, J.D. (2005). *Cafecitos* and *telenovelas:* Culturally competent interventions to facilitate Mexican American families' decisions to use home care services. *Geriatric Nursing, 26*, 229-232.

Ellis, G.K. (2005). Taking your patient's spiritual vital signs. *Home Healthcare Nurse, 23*, 634-635.

Galanti, G. (1991). *Caring for Patients from Different Cultures*. Philadelphia: University of Pennsylvania Press.

(The) Joint Commission. (2005). Evaluating your spiritual assessment process. *The Source, Joint Commission on Accreditation of Healthcare Organizations, 3*(2), 6-7.

Killian, P., & Waite, R. (2007). Cultural diversity: Best practices. *ADVANCE for Nurses, 4*(26), 29-31.

Killian, P., & Waite, R. (2008). Weaving culture with care. *ADVANCE for Nurses, 5*(8), 17-18.

Leininger, M.M. (1991). *Culture Care Diversity and Universality: A Theory of Nursing*. New York: National League for Nursing.

Lindberg, D.A. (2005). Integrative review of research related to meditation, spirituality, and the elderly. *Geriatric Nursing, 26*, 372-378.

Lindsay, J., Narayan, M.C., & Rea, K. (1998). The Vietnamese client. *Home Healthcare Nurse, 16*, 693-699.

Lipson, J.G., Dibble, S.L., & Minarik, P.A. (Eds.). (1996). *Culture & Nursing Care: A Pocket Guide*. San Francisco: UCSF Nursing Press.

McCauley, M. (2004). Going the distance for American Indians. *Nursing2004, 34*(12), 46-48.

Miklancie, M.A. (2007). Caring for patients of diverse religious traditions: Islam, a way of life for Muslims. *Home Healthcare Nurse, 25*, 413-417.

Narayan, M.C. (2006). Caring for patients of diverse religious traditions: Catholicism. *Home Healthcare Nurse, 24*, 183-186.

Nardi, D.A., & Siwinski-Hebel, S. (2005). Cultural issues in home care. *ADVANCE for Nurses, 2*(8), 21-25.

Nursing2005 Eds. (2005). Understanding transcultural nursing. *Nursing2005, 35*(Career Directory), 14-23.

Platter, B.K. (2007). Moving past stereotypes with the Roma. *NurseWeek, 20*(23), 14-16.

Purnell, L.D., & Paulanka, B.J. (2003). *Transcultural Health Care: A Culturally Competent Approach* (2nd ed.). Philadelphia: F.A. Davis.

Romero, C. (2007). Caring for culturally diverse patients: One agency's journey toward cultural competence. *Home Healthcare Nurse, 25*, 206-213.

Smith-Stoner, M. (2006). Caring for patients of diverse religious traditions: Considerations for Buddhist clients in home care. *Home Healthcare Nurse, 24*, 459-467.

Spector, R.E. (2000a). *Cultural Care Guides to Heritage Assessment and Health Traditions* (2nd ed.). Upper Saddle River, NJ: Prentice-Hall.

Spector, R.E. (2000b). *Cultural Diversity in Health and Illness* (5th ed.). Upper Saddle River, NJ: Prentice-Hall.

Steefel, L. (2006). On cultural competency. *NurseWeek, 19*(9), 25.

Szabo, L. (2007). *Health system struggles with spiritual care.* Available at: http://usatoday.printhis.clickability.com/pt/cpt?action=cpt&title=Health+system+struggles.

Taylor, E.J. (2008). Promoting spiritual health in home healthcare. *Home Healthcare Nurse, 26*(6), 367-374.

Turkoski, B.B. (2005). Ethical support for culturally sensitive healthcare. *Home Healthcare Nurse, 23*, 355-358.

Ward, J. (2006). Caring for patients of diverse religious traditions: The church of Jesus Christ of Latter-day Saints. *Home Healthcare Nurse, 24*, 396-467.

Weber, D. (2006). Where spirituality and healthcare meet. *RN, 69*(9), 53-54.

Wells, J.N., Spence, C., & Bradley, P.J. (2006). Guiding on Mexican-American cultural values. *Nursing2006, 36*(7), 20-21.

Williams, S. (2006). Beyond belief: Transcultural nurses provide culturally competent care. *NurseWeek, 19*(10), 54-55, 58.

Chapter 15

Allen, C.H. (2008). Providing compassionate end-of-life care. *Made Incredibly Easy!, 6*(4), 46-53.

American Nurses Association. (1987). *Standards and Scope of Hospice Nursing Practice.* Kansas City: Author.

American Nurses Association. (1994). *Position Statement on Euthanasia.* Kansas City: Author.

American Nurses Association. (1995). *Position Statement on Assisted Suicide.* Kansas City: Author.

Bingley, A.F., McDermott, E., Thomas, C., et al. (2006). Making sense of dying: A review of narratives written since 1950 by people facing death from cancer and other diseases. *Palliative Medicine, 20*, 183-195.

Booth, S. (Ed.). (2005). *Palliative Care Consultations in Advanced Breast Cancer.* United Kingdom: Oxford University Press.

Domrose, C. (2007). A time to die: Helping patients fulfill their wishes at the end of life. *NurseWeek, 20*(22), 12-13.

Eilberg, A. (2006). Facing life and death: Spirituality in end-of-life care. *Journal of Jewish Communal Service, Spring*, 157-162.

Ferrell, B.R., & Coyle, N. (2005). *Textbook of Palliative Nursing.* New York: Oxford University Press.

Hester, D. (2006) The quiet man: A dying patient reminded me of why I became a nurse. *Nursing, 36*(4), 64cc5.

Kramer, K. (2005). You cannot die alone (interview of Dr. Elisabeth Kübler-Ross, 1990). *Omega, 50*, 83-101.

Kübler-Ross, E. (1969). *On Death and Dying.* New York: Macmillan.

Kübler-Ross, E. (1975). *Death: The Final Stage of Growth.* Englewood Cliffs, NJ: Prentice-Hall.

Lillis, K. (2008). Compassionate care. *ADVANCE for Nurses, 5*(6), 39.

Louden, K. (2008). End-of-life care provides comfort, dignity. *NurseWeek, 21*(5), 44-45.

LPN2008 Eds. (2008). Managing end-of-life pain. *LPN2008, 4*(4), 45-47.

Lynn, J., Chaudry, E., Simon, L., et al. (2007). *The Common Sense Guide to Improving Palliative Care.* New York: Oxford University Press.

Martinez, J.M. (2005). Hospice and palliative care specialty certification for LPNs and LVNs. *Home Healthcare Nurse, 23*, 121-122.

McCurdy, D. (2008). Ethical spiritual care at the end of life. *American Journal of Nursing, 108*(5), 11.

Mee, C.,(2007). Hospice care. *Nursing2007, 37*(11), 43.

National Center for Health Statistics. (2006). *Trends in health and aging: Death rates by age, sex, rates, and underlying cause. United States 1981—2004 (NMRO4a).*

Nursing2008 Eds. (2008). Documenting a patient's death. *Nursing2008, 38*(7), 19.

Peters, L., & Sellick, K. (2006). Quality of life of cancer patients receiving inpatient and home-based palliative care. *Journal of Advanced Nursing, 53*, 524-533.

Rich, S. (2005). Providing quality end-of-life-care. *Journal of Cardiovascular Nursing, 20*, 141-145.

Ruder, S. (2008a). Incorporating spirituality into home care at the end of life. *Home Healthcare Nurse, 26*(3), 158-163.

Ruder, S. (2008b). The challenges of family member caregiving: How the home health and hospice clinician can help at the end of life. *Home Healthcare Nurse, 26*(2), 131-136.

Stringer, H. (2007). Peaceful passage: Promoting choice in end-of-life care. *NurseWeek, 20*(22), 10-11.

Chapter 16

American Society for Microbiology. (2004). *Guideline for Isolation Precautions: Preventing transmission of infectious agents in healthcare settings.* Available at: www.asm.rg/Policy/index.asp?bid=30034.

Association of Operating Room Nurses. (2006). *Standards, Recommended Practices and Guidelines: Recommended Practices for Sterilization in the Perioperative Practice Setting* (pp. 629-643). Denver: Author.

Barrs, A.W. (2000). *Handwashing: Breaking the chain of infection.* Available at: www.vpico.com/articlemanager/printerfriendly.aspx?article=59659.

Bartlett, J.G., & Perl, T.M. (2005). The new *Clostridium difficile*—what does it mean? *New England Journal of Medicine, 353*, 2503-2505.

Centers for Disease Control and Prevention. (1996). *Guidelines for Isolation Precautions in Hospitals.* Atlanta: Author.

Centers for Disease Control and Prevention. (2002a). *Guidelines for laundry in health care facilities.* Available at: www.cdc.gov/od/ohs/biosfty/laundry.htm.

Centers for Disease Control and Prevention. (2002b). *Hand hygiene guidelines fact sheet.* Available at: www.cdc.gov/od/oc/media/pressrel/fs021025.htm.

Centers for Disease Control and Prevention. (2002c). Overview of CDC Hand Hygiene Guidelines. *MMWR Morbidity and Mortality Weekly Report Recommendations and Reports, 51*(RR-16), 1-4. Available at: www.cdc.gov/handhygiene.

Centers for Disease Control and Prevention. (2006). *Standard precautions.* Available at: www.cdc.gov/ncidod/dhqp/gl_isolation_standard.html.

Centers for Disease Control and Prevention. (2007). *Guidelines for Isolation Precautions: Preventing Transmission of Infectious Agents in Healthcare Settings.* Available at: www.cdc.gov/ncidod/dhgp/pdf/isolation2007/pdf.

Chettle, C.C. (2006). Life-threatening fungal infections on the rise. *NurseWeek, 19*(8), 19-20.

Gagan, M.J. (2003). Probiotics are effective in preventing antibiotic associated diarrhea. *Evidence-Based Nursing, 6*, 2003.

Garner, J.S., for the Hospital Infection Control Practices Advisory Committee. (1996). *Guideline for Isolation Precautions in Hospitals.* Atlanta: Centers for Disease Control and Prevention.

Goldrick, B.A. (2004). MRSA, VRE, and VRSA: How do we control them in nursing homes? *American Journal of Nursing, 104*(6), 50-51.

Johnson, L., & Saravolztz, L. (2005). Community-acquired MRSA: Current epidemiology and management issues. *Infections in Medicine, 22,* 16-20.

Keefe, S. (2007). A good fit: Disposable gloves have become indispensable tools in fighting infection, protecting patients. *ADVANCE for Nurses, 4*(14), 28-29.

McDonald, I.C., Killgore, G.E., Thompson, A., et al. (2005). An epidemic, toxin gene-variant strain of *Clostridium difficile. New England Journal of Medicine, 353,* 2433-2341.

Murray, P.R., Rosenthal, K.S, & Pfaller, M.A. (2006). *Medical Microbiology* (5th ed.). St. Louis: Mosby.

National Institute for Occupational Safety and Health (NIOSH). (1997). *NIOSH Alert: Preventing Allergic Reactions to Natural Rubber Latex in the Workplace.* DHHS (NIOSH) Publication No. 97-135. Cincinnati, OH: U.S. Department of Health and Human Services, Public Health Service.

Oriola, S. (2006). *C. difficile:* A menace in hospitals and homes alike. *Nursing2006, 36*(8), 14-15.

Perry, J., & Jagger, J. (2004). Getting the most from your personal protective gear. *Nursing2004, 34*(12), 72.

Rebmann, T. (2008). Dress up for safety with PPE. *LPN2008, 4*(2), 6-13.

Sebaihia, M., Wren, B.W., Mullany, P., et al. (2006). The multidrug-resistant human pathogen *Clostridium difficile* has a highly mobile, mosaic genome. *Nature Genetics, 38,* 779-786.

Sheff, B. (2005). Mad cow disease and vCJD: Understanding the risks. *Nursing2005, 35*(2), 74-75.

Siegel, J.D., Rhinehart, E., Jackson, M., et al. (2006). *Management of multidrug-resistant organisms in healthcare settings.* Available at: www.cdc.gov/ncidod/dhqp/pdf/ar/mdroGuideline2006.pdf.

Skukla, S. (2005). Community-associated methicillin-resistant *Staphylococcus aureus* and its emerging virulence. *Clinical Medicine & Research, 5,* 57-60.

Todd, B. (2006a). *Clostridium difficile:* Familiar pathogen, changing epidemiology. *American Journal of Nursing, 106*(5), 33-36.

Todd, B. (2006b). The increasing risk of salmonella infections. *American Journal of Nursing, 105*(7), 35-37.

Waknine, Y. (2005). *MRSA outbreak prompts change in prescribing habits.* Available at: www.medscape.com/viewarticl/503059.

Yetman, L. (2006). A new "superbug" leaves the hospital: Community-acquired methicillin-resistant *Staphylococcus aureus. Home Healthcare Nurse, 24,* 213-216.

Chapter 17

Association of Operating Room Nurses. (2006a). Latex guideline. In *Standards, Recommended Practices, and Guidelines.* Denver: Author.

Association of Operating Room Nurses. (2006b). Recommended practices for cleaning and caring for surgical instruments and powered equipment. In *Standards, Recommended Practices, and Guidelines.* Denver: Author.

Association of Operating Room Nurses. (2006c). Recommended practices for maintaining a sterile field. In *Standards, Recommended Practices, and Guidelines.* Denver: Author.

Association of Operating Room Nurses. (2006d). Recommended practices for surgical attire. In *Standards, Recommended Practices, and Guidelines.* Denver: Author.

Association of Operating Room Nurses. (2006e). Recommend practices for traffic patterns in the perioperative practice Setting. In *Standards, Recommended Practices, and Guidelines.* Denver: Author.

Association of Operating Room Nurses. (2006f). Revised statement on patients and health care workers with bloodborne diseases. In *Standards, Recommended Practices, and Guidelines.* Denver: Author.

Association of Operating Room Nurses. (2006g). Sharps injury prevention in the perioperative setting. In *Standards, Recommended Practices, and Guidelines.* Denver: Author.

Berkelman, R.L., & Campos, J.M. (2004). Guideline for Isolation Precautions: Preventing transmission of infectious agents in healthcare settings. *American Society for Microbiology,* 8/04. Available at: www.asm.org/policy/index.asp?bid=30034.

Bobolia, J. (2006). Infection control for the family of the home hospice patient, *Home Healthcare Nurse, 24*(10),624-626.

Centers for Disease Control and Prevention. (2005). *CMS interim final rule regarding placement of alcohol-based hand-rub dispensers,* 3/05. Available at: www.ashe.org/ashe/codes/handrub/index.html.

Centers for Disease Control and Prevention. (2007). *Airborne Precautions, Isolation Precautions in Hospitals.* Available at: www.cdc.gov/ncidod/dhqp/gl_isolation_airborne.html.

Centers for Disease Control and Prevention. (2007). *Contact Precautions, Isolation Precautions in Hospitals.* Available at: www.cdc.gov/ncidod/dhqp/gl_isolation_contact.html.

Centers for Disease Control and Prevention. (2007). *Droplet Precautions, Isolation Precautions in Hospitals.* Available at: www.cdc.gov/ncidod/dhqp/gl_isolation_droplet.html.

Centers for Disease Control and Prevention. (2007). *Standard Precautions, Isolation Precautions in Hospitals.* Available at: www.cdc.gov/ncidod/dhqp/gl_isolation_standard.html.

Cheng, S.M. (2001). Literature review and survey comparing surgical scrub techniques. *AORN Journal, 74*(2), 218, 221-224.

Demmer, R.T., & Desvarleux, M. (2006). Periodontal infections and cardiovascular disease: The heart of the matter. *Journal of the American Dental Association 139*(3), 145-151.

Doody, L. (2004). Bloodborne pathogen exposure. *Nursing2004, 34*(9), 88.

Evans, S. (2006). Personal safeguards. *ADVANCE for Nurses, 8*(25), 33.

Gardner, D., & Anderson-Manz, E. (2001). How to perform surgical hand scrubs. *Infection Control Today.* Available at www.infectioncontroltoday/articles/151bpract.html.

Gilchrist, K. (2006). Infection management: Organized treatment plans bring success and closure of infected wounds. *ADVANCE for Nurses, 8*(21), 34.

Grossman, S., & Mager, D.D. (2008). Managing the threat of methicillin-resistant *Staphylococcus aureus* in home care. *Home Healthcare Nurse, 26*(6), 356-365.

Gruendemann, B., & Bjerke, N. (2001). Is it time for brushless scrubbing with an alcohol-based agent? *AORN Journal, 74*(6), 859-873.

Guinan, M., & McGuckin, M. (2005) Hand hygiene: It does make a difference. *LPN2005, 1*(3), 11-15.

Immunization Action Coalition (2007). *Healthcare personnel vaccination recommendations.* Available at: www.immunize.org, 3/2007. Content CDC reviewed, March, 2007.

Keefe, S. (2005). Inside infection control, *ADVANCE for Nurses, 7*(21), 31.

Keefe, S. (2008). The 'other' bugs. *ADVANCE for Nurses, 5*(8), 15-16.

Lettieri, C. (2007). The emergency and impact of extensively drug-resistant tuberculosis, *Medscape Pulmonary Medicine.* Available at: www.medscape.com/viewarticle/557459.

LPN2008 Eds. (2008). Vanncomycin: Champion against drug-resistant infection. *LPN2008, 4*(1), 6-9.

Martin, S.D. (2006). Infection control matters in home healthcare. *Home Healthcare Nurse, 24*(8), 485-486.

Rebman, T. (2006). The basics of hand hygiene. *LPN2006, 2*(6), 21-23.

Rebman, T. (2007). Protect yourself, protect your patients: The essentials of PPE, *Nursing Made Incredibly Easy!, 5*(1), 30-39.

Rhinehart, E. (2001). Infection control in home care. *Emerging Infectious Diseases, 7*(2), 208-211.

Rothrock, J.C. (2006). What are the current guidelines about wearing artificial nails and nail polish in the healthcare setting? *Medscape Nurses,* 2006; *8*(2). Available at: www.medscape.com/viewarticle/547793.

Rushing, J. (2006). Wearing personal protective gear, *Nursing2006 36*(10), 56-57.

Siegel, J.D., Rhinehart, E., Jackson, M., Chiarello, L., and the Healthcare Infection Control Practices Advisory Committee (2007). *Guideline for Isolation Precautions: Preventing transmission of infectious agents in healthcare settings.* Available at www.cdc.gov/ncidod/dhqp/pdf/guidelines/isolation2007.pdf.

Snow, M. (2006). Preventing *Salmonella* infection, *Nursing2006, 36*(9), 17.

Strelczyk, K., & Wallace, B. (2008). MRSA may be waiting right around the corner. *NurseWeek, 21*(11), 24-29.

Todd, B. (2006). Emerging infections: Beyond MRSA: VISA and VRSA. *American Journal of Nursing, 1006*(4), 28-30.

Todd, B. (2005). Emerging infections: *Legionella* pneumonia. *American Journal of Nursing, 1005*(11), 35-38.

Chapter 18

Ball, S.F. (2008). Ergonomics in healthcare: Keeping a healthy back and body at work: Is a no-life policy in your future? *ADVANCE for Nurses, 5*(10), 27-29.

Baptiste, N.A. (2004). Evidence-based practices for safe patient handling and movement. *Online Journal of Issues in Nursing, 9*(3), Manuscript 3. Available at: www.nursingworld.org/ojin/topic25tpc25_3.htm.

Blocks, M. (2005). Practical solutions for safe patient handling. *Nursing2005, 35*(10), 44-46.

Dunbar, C.N. (2007). Lift smartly, lift safety. *Nursing2007(Spring MED/SURG Specialty Guide)*, 26-27.

Elkin, M.K., Perry, A.G., & Potter, P.A. (2008). *Nursing Interventions and Clinical Skills* (4th ed.). St. Louis: Elsevier Mosby.

Gavin-Dreschnack, D., Nelson, A., Fitzgerald, S., et al. (2005). Wheelchair-related falls: Current evidence and directions for improved quality care. *Journal of Nursing Care Quality, 20,* 119-127.

Gilbey, H., Ackland, T., Wang, A., et al. (2003). Exercise improves early functional recovery after total hip arthroplasty. *Clinical Orthopaedics and Related Research, 408,* 193-200.

Haydon, K.J. (2007). Safe handling saves nurses' backs. *NurseWeek, 20*(9), 12-14.

Hughes, K. (2005). Backing up nurses: Successful strategies to reduce nursing back injuries. *ADVANCE for Nurses, 2*(8), 35-36.

James, E. (2007). Backbreaking work: Minimal lift environments reduce the risk of musculoskeletal injuries. *ADVANCE for Nurses, 4*(1), 20-30.

Lilliss, K. (2007). Safe moves: Successful patient handling programs rely on common factors. *ADVANCE for Nurses, 4*(10), 35-36.

LPN2005 Eds. (2005a). Taking it one step at a time. *LPN2005, 1*(6), 32.

LPN2005 Eds. (2005b). Transfer techniques: Helping your patient move the right way. *LPN2005, 1*(2), 46-47.

LPN2006 Eds. (2006). Bend and stretch: Performing range-of-motion exercises. *LPN2006, 2*(3), 11-13.

McPeck, P. (2006). Watching our backs: RNs get a lift from 'no lift' policies. *NurseWeek, 19*(13), 8-9.

Millsaps, C.C. (2006). Pay attention to patient positioning! *RN, 69*(1), 59-64.

Nursing2006 Eds. (2006). Performing passive range-of-motion exercises. *Nursing2006, 36*(1), 50-51.

Nursing2007 Eds. (2007). Weighing in on lift teams. *Nursing2007, 37*(6), 48hn10-48hn12.

Parsons, K.S., Galinsky, T.L., & Waters, T. (2006). Musculoskeletal disorders in home healthcare workers: Part 2. Life and transfer assistance for non-weight-bearing home care patients. *Home Healthcare Nurse, 24,* 227-233.

Perry, A.G., & Potter, P.A. (2006). *Clinical Nursing Skills and Techniques* (6th ed.). St. Louis: Elsevier Mosby.

Poe, S., Cvach, M.M., Gartrell, D.G., et al. (2005). An evidence-based approach to fall risk assessment, prevention, and management. *Journal of Nursing Care Quality, 20,* 107-116.

Pullen, R.L. (2004). Logrolling a patient. *Nursing2004, 34*(2), 22.

Pullen, R.L. (2008a). Transferring a patient from bed to stretcher. *Nursing2008, 38*(1), 43-45.

Pullen, R.L. (2008b). Transferring a patient from bed to wheelchair. *Nursing2008, 38*(2), 46-47.

Pullen, R.L. (2008c). Smooth patient transfers: Part III: Using a hydraulic lift. *Nursing2008, 38*(3), 54-56.

Quick Tips: Pointers on patient positioning. (2004). *Advances in Skin & Wound Care, 17,* 10.

Todd, J. (2008). Waking up to hospital bed entrapment risks. *Nursing2008, 38*(1), 14-15.

Yauk, S., Hopkins, B.A., Phillips, C.D., et al. (2005). Predicting in-hospital falls. *Journal of Nursing Care Quality, 20,* 128-133.

Chapter 19

Armstrong, G. (2008). Attention nurses! Anticoagulant overdoses prompt Joint Commission to issue new safety requirement. *NurseWeek, 21*(5), 30-33.

Advances in Skin & Wound Care Eds. (2004). The difference between friction and shear. *Advances in Skin & Wound Care, 17,* 222.

Agency for Healthcare Research and Quality (AHRQ). (2007). Clinical informatics and its usefulness for assessing risk and preventing falls and pressure ulcers in nursing home environments. Retrieved from www.ahrq.gov/downloads/pub/advances/vol3/Teigland.pdf.

Bergstrom, N., Allman, R.M., Carlson, C.E., et al. (1992). Pressure Ulcers in Adults: Prediction and Prevention. Clinical Practice Guideline. *Quick Reference Guide for Clinicians,* No. 3. AHCPR Pub. No. 92-0050. Rockville, MD: Agency for Health Care Policy and Research.

Bergstrom, N., Bennett, M.A., Carlson, C.E., et al. (1994). Pressure ulcer treatment. Clinical practice guideline. *Quick Reference Guide for Clinicians,* No. 15. AHCPR Pub. No. 95-0653. Rockville, MD: Agency for Health Care Policy and Research.

Black, J. (2006). Saving the skin during kinetic bed therapy. *Nursing2006, 36*(10), 17.

Catania, K., Huang, C., James, P., et al. (2007). PUPPI: The pressure ulcer prevention protocol interventions. *American Journal of Nursing, 107*(4), 44-52.

Duimel-Peeters, I. (2005). Preventing pressure ulcers with massage? Some say it works, others disagree, Ay, there's the rub. *American Journal of Nursing, 105*(8), 31-32.

Dunleavy, K. (2008). Putting a dent in pressure ulcer rates. *Nursing2008, 38*(1), 20-21.

Elkin, M.K., Perry, A.G., & Potter, P.A. (2008). *Nursing Interventions and Clinical Skills* (4th ed.). St. Louis: Elsevier Mosby.

Harkreader, H., & Hogan, M.A. (2007). *Fundamentals of Nursing: Caring and Clinical Judgment* (2nd ed.). Philadelphia: Elsevier Saunders.

Ignatavicius, D., & Workman, M.L. (2006). *Medical-Surgical Nursing: Critical Thinking for Collaborative Care* (5th ed.). Philadelphia: Elsevier Saunders.

Lorenz, J.M. (2007). Geriatric skin care. *ADVANCE for Nurses, 4*(11), 29-30.

National Pressure Ulcer Advisory Panel. (2007). *Updated staging system.* Available at: www.npuap.org/pr2.htm.

Rasin, J. (2004). Bathing patients with dementia. *American Journal of Nursing, 104*(3), 30-34.

Stokowski, L.A. (2008). *A closer look at pressure ulcers: The name game.* Retrieved from www.medscape.com/viewprogram/12612.

Stotts, N.A., & Gunningberg, L. (2007). Predicting pressure ulcer risk. *American Journal of Nursing, 107*(11), 40-47.

Werkman, H., Simodejka, P., & DeFilippis, J. (2008). Partnering for prevention: A pressure ulcer prevention collaborative project. *Home Healthcare Nurse, 26*(1), 17-22.

Chapter 20

Armstrong, G. (2008). Attention nurses! Anticoagulant overdoses prompt Joint Commission to issue new safety requirement. *NurseWeek, 21*(5), 30-33.

Bolinger, R. (2008). Safety and quality issues for LPNs. *LPN2008, 4*(1), 10-13.

Bucher, G.M., Szczerba, P., & Curtin, P.M. (2007). A comprehensive fall prevention program for assessment, interventions, and referral. *Home Healthcare Nurse, 25,* 174-183.

Center for the Study of Bioterrorism & Emerging Infections. (2001). *Bioterrorism agent fact sheet.* Available at: www.bioterrorism.slu.edu.

Chettle, C., & Habel, M. (2003). Smallpox vaccine: Making an informed decision. *NurseWeek, 16*(5), 29-31.

Duke Center for Nicotine and Smoking Cessation Research. (2007). *Facts about smoking.* Available at: www.duke.edu/web/nicotine/smokingfacts.html.

Eckhart, J. (2006). Ready—or not. *ADVANCE for Nurses, 3*(22), 27-29.

Elkin, M.K., Perry, A.G., & Potter, P.A. (2008). *Nursing Interventions and Clinical Skills* (4th ed.). St. Louis: Elsevier Mosby.

Evans, D., Wood, J., & Lambert, L. (2003). Patient injury and physical restraint devices: A systematic review. *Journal of Advanced Nursing, 41,* 274-282.

Fell-Carson, D. (2003a). Terrorist danger: Part I. *NurseWeek, 16*(2), 19-20.

Fell-Carson, D. (2003b). Terrorist danger: Part II. *NurseWeek, 16*(3), 21-22.

Fischer, R.A. (2007). Prevent fires when using oxygen cylinder regulators. *Nursing2007, 37*(1), 20.

Gallauresi, B.A. (2004). Watch those power connections. *Nursing2004, 34*(2), 27.

Gustafson, S.E. (2007). Assess for fall risk, intervene—and pump up patient safety. *Nursing2007, 37*(12), 24-25.

Hemmila, D. (2007). Banding together for patient safety. *NurseWeek, 20*(1), 24-25.

Hendrich, A. (2007). Predicting patient falls: Using the Hendrich II Fall Risk Model in clinical practice. *American Journal of Nursing, 107*(11), 50-58.

Jasniewski. J. (2006). Help your patient avoid medication-related falls. *LPN2006, 2*(6), 4-7.

Johnson, K., & Maultsby, C.C. (2007). A plan for achieving significant improvement in patient safety. *Journal of Nursing Care Quality, 22*(2), 164-171.

Khadivar, K. (2006). Improving safety. *ADVANCE for Nurses, 2*(20), 38.

Minnick, A.F., Mion, L.C., Johnson, M.E., et al. (2007). Prevalence and variation of physical restraint use in acute care settings in the U.S. *Journal of Nursing Scholarship, 39*(1), 30-36.

Nursing2004 Eds. (2004). No restraints allowed: Legalities and realities. *Nursing2004, 34*(1), 54-55.

Nursing2006 Eds. (2006). Show no restraint. *Nursing2006, 36*(4), 27.

Polzien, G. (2007). Promoting safety and security at home. *Home Healthcare Nurse, 25,* 218-222.

Reed, A.S. (2008). Improving patient safety—everyone's job. *Home Healthcare Nurse, 26*(2), 140.

Resnick, B. (2004). Preventing falls in acute care. *National Guideline Clearing House.* Available at: www.guideline.gov/summary.aspx?doc.

Rosto, L. (2005). Safety plan. *ADVANCE for Nurses, 2*(5), 26-28.

Schlismann, C.A. (2008). Fall risk reduction in home health and hospice. *Home Healthcare Nurse, 26*(5), 301-307.

Sheeran, T., Brown, E.L., Nassisi, P., et al. (2005). Does depression predict falls among home health patients? *Home Healthcare Nurse, 22,* 384-389.

Smith, N. (2007). Preserve independence with fall prevention strategies. *NurseWeek, 20*(3), 12-13.

Swihart, D. (2005). Are we safe yet? *ADVANCE for Nurses, 2*(18), 15-19.

Taschner, M.A. (2008). Responding to a fire. *Nursing2008, 38*(5), 44-47.

Todd, J.F. (2008). Waking up to hospital bed entrapment risks. *Nursing2008, 38*(1), 14-15.

Tullai-McGuinness, S. (2007). Improving patient safety. *Home Healthcare Nurse, 25,* 145-146.

U.S. Consumer Product Safety Commission. (1992). *Home Safety Checklist for Older Consumers.* CPSC Document #4701. Washington, DC: Author.

Weiner, E. (2006). Preparing nurses internationally for emergency planning and response. *Online Journal of Issues in Nursing, 11*(3). Available at: www.medscape.com/viewarticle/546012.

Wilson, P., & Rodgers, B. (2006). Research on falls prevention and physical activity in older adults and a notice of a new web-based quality system by the Agency for Healthcare Research and Quality. *Home Healthcare Nurse, 24,* 632-633.

Yuan, J.R., & Erb, J.K. (2006). Falls prevention, or "I think I can, I think I can." *Home Healthcare Nurse, 24,* 103-110.

Chapter 21

American Heart Association. (2005). Hypertension. Available at: http://hyper.ahajournals.org/cgi/content/full/45/1/42.

Boehringer, S.K. (2004). Hypertension: Review of guidelines and drug therapy management. *NurseWeek, 17*(2), 27-28.

Considine, J. (2005). Consult stat. Taking vitals on a patient with orthostatic hypotension. *RN, 68*(1), 50.

(The) Joint Commission on Accreditation of Healthcare Organizations (JCAHO). (2000). *Pain assessment and management standards.* Available at: www.jcaho.org/standard.

Kestel, F. (2005). The best BP: Eight tips to a more accurate blood pressure. *ADVANCE for Nurses, 2*(22), 32-33.

Khorshid, L., Eser, I., Zaybak, A., et al. (2005). Comparing mercury in-glass, tympanic, and disposable thermometers in measuring body temperature in healthy young people. *Journal of Clinical Nursing, 14*(4), 496-500.

Layne, L. (2008). Discharge planning. *ADVANCE for Nurses, 5*(1), 31-33.

Molony, S.L., Kobayashi, M., Holleran, E.A., et al. (2005). Assessing pain as a fifth vital sign in long-term care facilities: Recommendations from the field. *Journal of Gerontologic Nursing, 31*(3), 16-24.

Nursing2007 Eds. (2007). Take care with tympanic temperature readings. *Nursing2007, 37*(4), 52-53.

Pickering, T.G., Hall, J.E., Appel, L.I., et al. (2005). Hypertension. *Circulation, 45,* 142-161.

Quatrara, B., Coffman, J., Jenkins, T., et al. (2007). The effect of respiratory rate and ingestion of hot and cold beverages on the accuracy of oral temperatures measured by electronic thermometers. *Medsurg Nursing, 16,* 105-108.

Rice, K.L. (1999). Measuring thigh BP. *Nursing99, 29*(8), 58-59.

Schell, K., Bradley, E., Bucher, L., et al. (2005). Clinical comparison of automatic, non-invasive measurements of blood pressure in the forearm and upper arm. *American Journal of Critical Care, 14,* 232-241.

Sclater, A., & Alagiakrishnan, K. (2004). Orthostatic hypotension: A primary care primer for assessment and treatment. *Geriatrics, 59*(8), 22-27.

Thibodeau, G.A., & Patton, K.T. (2007). *Anatomy and Physiology* (6th ed.). St. Louis: Elsevier Mosby.

U.S. Department of Health and Human Services, Joint National Committee on Prevention, Detection, Evaluation, and Treatment of High Blood Pressure. (2003). *Reference card.* Bethesda, MD: National Institutes of Health, National Heart, Lung and Blood Institute.

Williams, M. (2005). *Measuring vital signs in elderly people.* Available at: www.medscape.com/viewprogram/4638.

Yoshikawa, T.T., & Norman D.C. (1998). Fever in the elderly. *Infectious Medicine, 15,* 704-708.

Chapter 22

Carter, K.F. (2003). Identifying primary skin lesions. *Nursing2003, 33*(12), 68-69.

Coviello, J.S. (2004). Cardiac assessment IV. *Home Healthcare Nurse, 22,* 117-123.

Danter, J.H. (2003). Put a realistic spin on geriatric assessment. *Nursing2003, 33*(12), 52-55.

Dulak, S.B. (2004). A practical guide to a thorough history. *RN Supplement, January,* 74 (TNT-19 TNT).

Hathaway, L. (2004). On the right path to deep tendon reflex assessment. *Nursing Made Incredibly Easy!, 2*(2), 54-57.

Katz, M. (2006). Save time! Do a 5-minute initial assessment. *RN, 69*(3), 43-46.

LPN2007 Eds. (2007). Now hear this: How to identify heart sounds. *LPN2007, 3*(1), 4-7.

McCormick, M. (2007). Breathing easy: Interpreting breath sounds. *LPN2007, 3*(6), 27-29.

Nursing Made Incredibly Easy! Eds. (2004). Give me strength! Assessing your patient's motor responses from fingers to toes. *Nursing Made Incredibly Easy!, 2*(1), 58-60.

Nursing Made Incredibly Easy! Eds. (2004). What are normal respiratory signs of aging? *Nursing Made Incredibly Easy!, 2*(3), 64.

Nursing Made Incredibly Easy! Eds. (2004). What's that sound? *Nursing Made Incredibly Easy!, 2*(1), 61.

Chapter 23

Chapman, L. (2007). Discharge planning: A family affair. *Nursing2007, 37*(5), 56hn12, 56hn14.

Davis, M. (2006). Patient Safety Advisory: details, details. *Nursing Spectrum.* Available at: http://community. nursingspectrum.com/MagazineArticles/article. cfm?AID=20104.

Erickson, J. (2002). Making the admission process more efficient. *Home Healthcare Nurse, 20,* 462-465.

Gibbons, J. (2007). A clean exchange: hastily performed patient hand-offs threaten patients' lives. *Advance Online Publications.* Available at: http://nursing.advanceweb.com/ Common/Editorial/PrintFriendly.aspx?CC=97897.

(The) Joint Commission. (2008). *National Patient Safety Goals.* Available at www.jointcommission.org/PatientSafety/ NationalPatientSafetyGoals.

RN Eds. (2004). Communication strategies for smooth patient transfers. *RN, 67*(1), 30hf3.

Walker, C. (2007). Hospital discharge of older adults: how nurses can ease the transition. *American Journal of Nursing, 107*(6), 60-70.

Weber, C., Hogstel, M.O., & Curry, L.C. (2007). Hospital discharge of older adults: How nurses can ease the transition. *American Journal of Nursing, 107*(6), 60-70.

Chapter 24

Adamow, S.M. (2005). On the move: Bringing lab tests to the patient's bedside is both advantageous and challenging for nurses. *ADVANCE for Nurses, 2*(1), 32-33.

Armstrong, M.L., & Elins, L. (2005). Body art and MRI: Tattoos, body piercings, and permanent cosmetics may cause problems. *American Journal of Nursing, 105*(3), 65-67.

Birn, C.S. (2005). Endoscopic ultrasound reveals GI tract secrets. *NurseWeek, 18*(2), 23-25.

Brege, D.J. (2007). Take a look inside the blood vessels with angiography. *Nursing Made Incredibly Easy!, 5*(6), 14-15, 18.

Britt, R.B. (2005). Using EMLA cream before venipuncture. *Nursing2005, 35*(1), 17.

Constantine, L. (2008). C-reactive protein: A marker for cardiovascular disease and stroke. *ADVANCE for Nurses, 5*(2), 29-31.

Crean, C.A. (2007). How can electrophysiology help your patient? *Nursing2007, 37*(7), 60-61.

Dershem, B., Arruss, J., & Schwelnus, E. (2006). Tips to avoid blood redraws. *NurseWeek, 19*(21), 18.

Flasar, C. (2008). What is urine specific gravity? *Nursing2008, 38*(7), 14.

Fox, V.J. (2005). Get the inside story with spiral CT. *Nursing Made Incredibly Easy!, 3*(3), 60-62.

Geiter, H.B. (2006). Contrast-media-induced pulmonary edema. *Nursing2006, 36*(1), 88.

Hathaway, L.R. (2005). Fear factor: Managing a patient with procedural anxiety. *LPN2005, 1*(3), 17-18.

Hutchison, R., & Rodriguez, L. (2008). Capnography and respiratory depression. *American Journal of Nursing, 108*(2), 35-39.

Lange, S., & Malli, S. (2006). Implanted device + MRI = trouble? *Nursing2006, 36*(1), 75.

Lochridge, K. (2005). Do you know where your critical lab values are? *Home Healthcare Nurse, 24*(2), 121-125.

LPN2008 Eds. (2008). Three techniques for collecting wound specimens. *LPN2008, 4*(1), 24-25.

McCarron, K. (2007). Clues in the blood: Know your CBCs. *Nursing Made Incredibly Easy!, 4*(3), 13-17.

Miller, J. (2005). To clot or not to clot . . . *Nursing Made Incredibly Easy!, 3*(6), 4-9.

Minor, J., & George, E.L. (2008). Using mixed venous oxygen saturation to improve patient assessments. *Nursing2008, 38*(1), 56cc1-56cc3.

Nursing2007 Eds. (2007a). Carbon dioxide end-tidal monitoring. *Nursing2007, 37*(5), 49-48.

Nursing2007 Eds. (2007b). Does a high WBC count always signal infection? *Nursing2007, 37*(5), 56hn15-56hn16.

Nursing Made Incredibly Easy! Eds. (2007). Function junction: Testing your patient's liver function. *Nursing Made Incredibly Easy!, 4*(1), 17-19.

Nursing Made Incredibly Easy! Eds. (2008a). A look inside the bowel with colonoscopy. *Nursing Made Incredibly Easy!, 6*(2), 27-28.

Nursing Made Incredibly Easy! Eds. (2008b). Expert infection detection. *Nursing Made Incredibly Easy!, 6*(1), 5.

Nursing Made Incredibly Easy! Eds. (2008c). What you need to know about FOBT. *Made Incredibly Easy!, 6*(4), 32-33.

Ott, L. (2008). Assessing blood flow with CT angiography. *Nursing2008, 38*(1), 26.

Pullen, R.L. (2005a). Performing a modified Allen test. *Nursing2005, 35*(10), 26.

Rushing, J. (2007). Assisting with lumbar puncture. *Nursing2007, 37*(1), 23.

Schoch, L., & Whiteman, K. (2007). Monitoring liver function. *Nursing2007, 37*(11), 22-23.

Shaffer, R. (2006). Groin hematoma following percutaneous coronary intervention. *Nursing2006, 36*(12), 80.

Spader, C. (2006). Diagnostic imaging: Contrast counts. *NurseWeek, 19*(6), 12.

Turka, J. (2006). Deciphering diagnostics: Is this on the level? *Nursing Made Incredibly Easy!, 4*(4), 7-9.

Vertis, M.C. (2008). Is your patient taking the right antimicrobial? *American Journal of Nursing, 108*(6), 49-55.

Wesley, C. (2006). Responding to methemoglobinemia after bronchoscopy. *Nursing2006, 36*(12), 64cc1-64cc2.

Chapter 25

Goertz, S. (2006). Gauging fluid balance with osmolality. *Nursing2006, 36*(10), 70-71.

Holcomb, S.S. (2008). Third-spacing: When body fluid shifts. *Nursing2008, 38*(7), 50-53.

Horne, C., & Derrico, D. (1999). Mastering ABGs: The art of arterial blood gas measurement. *American Journal of Nursing, 99*(8), 26-36.

Karch, A.M. (2004). On the rebound: Maintaining normal fluid intake is critical while on diuretics. *American Journal of Nursing, 105*(10), 73.

Kirksey, K.M., Holt-Ashley, M., & Goodroad, B.K. (2001). An easy method for interpreting the results of arterial blood gas analysis. *Critical Care Nurse, 21*(5), 49-54.

Konivk-McMahan, J. (2008). Calcium imbalances. *ADVANCE for Nurses, 5*(13), 23-25.

McCarron, K. (2008). Recognizing dehydration in patients. *LPN2008, 4*(4), 15-16.

Miller, J. (2006). Potassium in the balance: Understanding hyperkalemia and hypokalemia. *LPN2006, 2*(5), 43-49.

Mills, L.S.E. (2005). Don't forget to drink water. *LPN2005, 1*(4), 10-13.

Nursing Made Incredibly Easy! Eds. (2004a). Balancing: What happens when sodium and water are off-kilter? *Nursing Made Incredibly Easy!, 2*(1), 52-57.

Quillen, R.F. (2005). . . . About hypercalcemia. *Nursing2005, 35*(7), 74.

Sweeney, J. (2005a). What causes hyponatremia? *Nursing2005, 35*(6), 18.

Sweeney, J. (2005b). What causes sudden hypokalemia? *Nursing2005, 35*(4), 12.

Vacca, V. (2008). Hyperkalemia. *Nursing2008, 38*(7), 72.

Woodruff, D.W. (2006). Take these 6 easy steps to ABG analysis. *Nursing Made Incredibly Easy!, 4*(1), 4-7.

Chapter 26

Barclay, L. (2005). Advances in nutritional therapy for attention deficit hyperactivity disorder. *Life Extension, 11*(7), 42-50.

Brugler, L., Stankovic, A.K., & Schlefer, M. (2005). A simplified nutrition screen for hospitalized patients using readily available laboratory and patient information. *Nutrition, 21*, 650-658.

Centers for Disease Control and Prevention. (2007). Prevalence of fruit and vegetable consumption and physical activity by race/ethnicity, United States, 2005. *MMWR Morbidity and Mortality Weekly Report, 56*, 301-304.

Chettle, C. (2008). Food gone bad: What's happening to cause so many outbreaks of foodborne illness in the U.S.? *Nurseweek, 21*(1), 40-44.

Clinical Nutrition Updates. (2008). Soy, isoflavones and bone health. *Arbor Clinical Nutrition Updates 2008, 288*, 1-3.

DiMaria-Ghalili, R.A., & Guenter, P.A. (2008). The mini nutritional assessment. *Amercian Journal of Nursing, 108*(2), 50-55.

Fairfield, K., & Stampfer, M. (2007). Vitamin and mineral supplement for cancer prevention. *American Journal of Clinical Nutrition, 85*(1 Suppl.), 289S-292S.

Fisher, S.G. (2007). Community-based nutrition programs and services are needed to improve the health of older adults. *Journal of the American Dietetic Association, 107*, 272-273.

Fulgoni, V. III, Nicolls, J., Reed, A., et al. (2007). Dietary consumption and related nutrient intake in African-American adults and children in the United States: Continuing survey of food intakes by individuals 1994—1996, 1998, and the National Health and Nutrition Examination Survey 1999–2000. *Journal of the American Dietetic Association, 107*, 256-264.

Georgieff, M.K. (2007). Nutrition and the developing brain: Nutrient priorities and measurement. *American Journal of Clinical Nutrition, 85*(1 Suppl.), 614S-620S.

Gottesman, M.M. (2007). Nursing Resources. HEAT: Healthy eating and activity together. *American Journal of Nursing, 107*(2), 49-50.

Haines, J., & Neumark-Sztainer, D. (2007). Addressing weight-related issues in an elementary school: What do students, parents, and school staff recommend? *Eating Disorders, 15*, 5-21.

Harris, H. (2008). Nursing care of the morbidly obese patient. *Nursing Made Incredibly Easy!, 6*(3), 34-43.

Hathcock, J.N., Shao, A., Vieth, R., et al. (2007). Risk assessment for vitamin D. *American Journal of Clinical Nutrition, 85*, 6-18.

Jacknowitz, A., Novillo, D., & Tiehen, L. (2007). Special Supplemental Nutrition Programs for Women, Infants, Children and infant feeding practices. *Pediatrics, 119*, 281-289.

Lazarides, L. (2005). Nutritional therapy: Not just a load of old bones. *Positive Health, June*(112), 28.

Martin, K.S., & Ferris, A.M. (2007). Food insecurity and gender are risk factors for obesity. *Journal of Nutrition Education and Behavior, 39*, 31-36.

Martinson, W. (2007). Nutrition and fitness—mental health, aging, and the implementation of a healthy diet and physical activity lifestyle. *Journal of Human Nutrition and Dietetics, 20*, 137.

Ojha, R., Amanatidis, S., Petocz, P., et al. (2007). Dieticians and naturopaths require evidence-based nutrition information on organic food. *Journal of Nutrition and Dietetics, 64*, 31-36.

Olendzki, B., Speed, C., & Domino, F.J. (2006). Nutritional assessment and counseling for prevention and treatment of cardiovascular disease. *American Family Physician, 73*, 257-264.

Pitkin, R.M. (2007). Folate and neural tube defects. *American Journal of Clinical Nutrition, 85*(1 Suppl.), 285S-288S.

Rafferty, S. (2007). Nutrition: Are older people eating adequately? *Nursing in the Community, 8*(1), 21-23.

Rasmussen, H.H., Kondrup, J., Staun, M., et al. (2006). A method for implementation of nutritional therapy in hospitals. *Clinical Nutrition, 25*, 515-523.

Rock, C.L. (2007). Multivitamin-multimineral supplements: Who uses them? *American Journal of Clinical Nutrition, 85*(Suppl.), 177S-179S.

Sayer, P. (2007). New nutrition drink boosts vitamin intake at lower cost. *Geriatric Medicine, 37*, 69.

Scott-Smith, J.L., & Greenhouse, P.K. (2007). Transforming care at the bedside: Patient-controlled liberalized diet. *Journal of Interprofessional Care, 21*(2), 179-188.

Sealy, M. (2007). Infant nutrition. *MCN The American Journal of Maternal/Child Nursing, 32*, 125.

Shikora, S.A., Kim, J.J., & Tarnoff, M.E. (2007). Nutrition and gastrointestinal complications of bariatric surgery. *Nutrition in Clinical Practice, 22*, 29-40.

Snyder, L. (2008). Battling obesity at home. *ADVANCE for Nurses, 5*(3), 17-18.

Tanasescu, M., Cho, E., Manson, J.E., et al. (2004). Dietary fat and cholesterol and the risk of cardiovascular disease among women with type 2 diabetes. *American Journal of Clinical Nutrition, 79*, 999-1005.

Tessaro, I., Rye, S., Parker, L., et al. (2007). Effectiveness of a nutrition intervention with rural low-income women. *American Journal of Health Behavior, 31*, 35-43.

Theobald, H. (2007). Childhood nutrition. *Journal of Community Nursing, 21*(2), 25-26, 28.

Vere-Jones, E. (2007). Analysis: Making patient nutrition a top priority. *Nursing Times, 103*(6), 8-9.

Yantis, M.A., & Velander, R. (2007). Get the skinny on *trans* fatty acids. *Nursing2007, 37*(12), 26-27.

Yphantides, N. (2007). For parents: Preventing obesity in your child. *Diabetes Self Management, 24*(1), 62, 64-67.

Chapter 27

Arora, A., Roffe, C., & Crome, P. (2005). An unusual and overlooked complication of nasogastric tube feeding. *Age Ageing, 34*, 84-85.

Bond, W.E. (2005). *Bulimia-nervosa treatment overview.* Available at: www.webmd.com/mental-health/tc.

Breier-Mackie, S.J. (2005). PEGs and ethics revisited: A timely reflection in the wake of the Terri Schiavo case. *Gastroenterology Nursing, 28*(4), 292-297.

Centers for Disease Control and Prevention. (2008). *Overweight and obesity.* Available at: www.cdc.gov/nccdphp/dnpa/obesity.

Coutin, I.B., Kerjriwal, K., Wilde, V.C., et al. (2007). Tube feeding and pneumonia: An unhappy couple. *Long-Term Care Interface, 8*(1), 21-25, 29.

Delegge, M.H. (2007). Parenteral nutrition (PN) use for adult hospitalized patients: A study of usage in a tertiary medical center. *Nutrition in Clinical Practice, 22*, 246-249.

Ellett, M.L.C. (2006). Important facts about intestinal feeding tube placement. *Gastroenterology Nursing, 29*, 112-125.

Enrione, E.B., & Chutkan, S. (2007). Preferences of registered dieticians and nurses recommending artificial nutrition and hydration for elderly patients. *Journal of the American Dietetic Association, 107*, 416-421.

Fairrow, A.M., McCallum, T.J., & Messinger-Rapport, B.J. (2004). Preferences of older African-Americans for long-term tube feeding at the end of life. *Aging Mental Health, 8*, 530-534.

Gorski, L. (2005). Hospital to home care: Discharge planning for the patient requiring home infusion therapy. *Topics in Advanced Practice Nursing, 5*(3), 1-6.

Heller, A.R. (2006). Omega-3 fatty acids improve the diagnosis-related clinical outcomes. *Critical Care Medicine, 34*, 972-979.

Jacobs, B., & Taylor, C. (2005). "Seeing" artificial hydration and nutrition through an ethical lens. *Home Healthcare Nurse, 23*, 739-742.

Kreymann, K.G., Berger, M.M., Deutz, N.E.P., et al. (2006). ESPEN guidelines on enteral nutrition: intensive care. *Clinical Nutrition, 25*, 210-223.

Laino, C. (2005). Home TPN life-sustaining for select patients with incurable cancer. *Oncology Times, 27*(10), 14-15.

Lamondy, A.M. (2006). Hyperemesis gravidarum and the role of the infusion nurse. (2006). *Journal of Infusion Nursing, 29,* 89-100.

LPN2008 Eds. (2008). Caring for a patient with a gastrostomy feeding tube. *LPN2008, 4*(4), 18-21.

Mayo Clinic. (2007). *Weight loss procedures performed at Mayo Clinic.* Available at: www.mayoclinic.org/bariatric-surgery/bariatric-prodedures.html.

Newton, A.F., & Delegge, M.H. (2007). Home initiation of parenteral nutrition. *Nutrition and Clinical Practice, 22,* 57-64.

Nursing2003 Eds. (2003). Clinical rounds. Tube feeding solutions: FDA warns against adding blue dye. *Nursing2003, 33*(12), 33.

Ochoa, J.B., & Caba, D. (2006). Advances in surgical nutrition. *Surgical Clinics of North America, 86,* 1483-1493.

Rader Clinics. (2007). *Anorexia nervosa—it's not your fault.* Available at: www.Raderprograms.com/anorexia.aspx.

Reising, D., & Neal, R. (2005). Enteral tube flushing. *American Journal of Nursing, 105*(3), 58-64.

Rollins, C.J. (2007). Moving initiation of parenteral nutrition to the home. *Nutrition in Clinical Practice, 22,* 55-56.

Rosenthal, K. (2006). Meals to go: Parenteral nutrition. *Nursing Made Incredibly Easy!, 4*(5), 57-63.

Rosenthal, K. (2007). Totally TPN. *Nursing Made Incredibly Easy!, 5*(5), 59-62.

Serna, E., & McCarthy, M. (2006). Heads up to prevent aspiration during enteral feeding. *Nursing2006, 36*(1), 76-77.

Chapter 28

American Heart Association (2005). Highlights of the 2005 American Heart AssociationGuidelines for Cardiopulmonary Resuscitation and Emergency Cardiovascular Care. *Currents in Emergency Cardiovascular Care, 16*(4), 11-16.

Ayers, D.M.M., & Stucky, J. (2004). Act fast when your patient has dyspnea. *Nursing2004, 34*(7), 36-41.

Beattie, S. (2006). Back to basics with O_2 therapy. *RN, 69*(9), 37-40.

Beattie, S. (2007). Respiratory distress. *RN, 70*(7), 34-38.

Coughlin, A.M. (2005a). Clearing the air about suctioning. *Nursing Made Incredibly Easy!, 4*(5), 59-64.

Coughlin, A.M. (2005b). Let's clear the air about suctioning. *LPN2005, 1*(6), 42-45.

Coughlin, A.M., & Parchinsky, C. (2006). Go with the flow of chest tube therapy. *Nursing2006, 36*(3), 36-41.

Hathaway, L. (2006). Breathe easier: A step-by-step guide to MDIs. *Nursing Made Incredibly Easy!, 4*(6), 22-23.

McCarron, K. (2006a). Puzzled about the state of airlessness? *Nursing Made Incredibly Easy!, 4*(1), 60-63.

McCarron, K. (2006b). Take a deep breath: Assessing atelectasis. *LPN2006, 2*(3), 20-25.

McCormick, M. (2007). Every breath you take: Making sense of breath sounds. *Nursing Made Incredibly Easy!, 5*(1), 7-9.

Nursing2005 Eds. (2005). Is your patient's metered-dose inhaler technique up to snuff? *Nursing2005, 35*(8), 50-51.

Nursing Made Incredibly Easy! Eds. (2005). Need to get something off your chest? *Nursing Made Incredibly Easy!, 3*(2), 55-57.

Nursing Made Incredibly Easy! Eds. (2007). Take a look inside the lungs with bronchoscopy. *Nursing Made Incredibly Easy!, 5*(2), 11-12.

Nursing Made Incredibly Easy! Eds. (2008). A close call with carbon monoxide. *Nursing Made Incredibly Easy!, 6*(3), 11-12.

Nursing Made Incredibly Easy! Eds. (2008). Let your patient's fingers do the talking (pulse oximetry). *Nursing Made Incredibly Easy!, 6*(3), 13-15.

Pruitt, B. (2005). Clear the air with closed suctioning. *Nursing2005, 35*(7), 44-46.

Pruitt, B., & Jacobs, M. (2005). Clearing away pulmonary secretions. *Nursing 2005, 35*(7), 37-41.

Pruitt, B., & Jacobs, M. (2006). All clear: How to keep the airways free of pulmonary secretions. *LPN2006, 2*(6), 46-54.

Pruitt, W.C. (2004). The ins and outs of tracheostomy care. *Nursing Made Incredibly Easy!, 3*(6), 58-62.

Pruitt, W.C. (2005a). Teaching your patient to use a peak flowmeter. *Nursing2005, 35*(3), 54-55.

Pruitt, W.C. (2005b). Why is the patient coughing up blood? *Nursing Made Incredibly Easy!, 4*(3), 50-53.

Rokosky, J.M. (2005). Teaching correct use of inhaled medications. *Home Healthcare Nurse, 23,* 766-775.

Rushing, J. (2006a). Assisting with thoracentesis. *Nursing2006, 36*(12), 18.

Rushing, J. (2006b). Using bag-valve-mask ventilation. *Nursing2006, 36*(1), 72.

Salati, D.S. (2008). Responding to foreign-body airway obstruction. *LPN2008, 4*(2), 26-27.

Seckel, M.A. (2005). All about airways. *ADVANCE for Nurses, 2*(1), 23, 28.

Smith, S.K. (2005). Is your patient getting enough oxygen? *LPN2005,* (2), 10-13.

Stiles, S. (2008). *AHA promotes chest-compression-only bystander-initiated CPR.* Available at: www.medscape.com/viewarticle/572238.

Chapter 29

Bray, B., Van Sell, S.L., & Miller-Anderson, M. (2007). Stress incontinence: It's no laughing matter. *RN, 70*(4), 25-29.

Bryan, R.H. (2005). Sanctura an option for treatment of overactive bladder. *ADVANCE for Nurses, 3*(11), 14.

D'Avanzo, C.E. (2008). *Pocket Guide to Cultural Health Assessment* (4th ed.). St. Louis: Elsevier Mosby.

Davis, K. (2004). Need urine from a catheter system? Forget the needle! *Nursing2004, 34*(12), 64.

deWit, S.C. (2009). *Medical-Surgical Nursing: Concepts and Practice.* Philadelphia: Elsevier Saunders.

Ebersole, P., & Hess, P. (2005). *Geriatric Nursing and Healthy Aging* (2nd ed.). St. Louis: Elsevier Mosby.

Elkin, M.K., Perry, A.G., & Potter, P.A. (2005). *Nursing Interventions & Clinical Skills* (3rd ed.). St. Louis: Elsevier Mosby.

Emr, K., & Ryan, R. (2004). Best practice for indwelling catheter in the home setting. *Home Healthcare Nurse, 22,* 820-830.

Gray, M. (2005). Skin care of the incontinent patient. *Advances in Skin & Wound Care, 18,*138-139.

Hairon, N. (2007). Ensuring patient dignity when accessing and using toilets. *Nursing Times, 103*(17), 23-24.

Hathaway, L. (2004). Peritoneal dialysis: Filtering out the bad guys. *Nursing Made Incredibly Easy!, 2*(5), 55-58.

Hathaway, L. (2006). Inserting an indwelling urinary catheter, step by step. *LPN2006, 2*(5), 9-11.

(The) Joint Commission. (2008). *2008 National Patient Safety Goals.* Available at: www.jointcommission.org/PatientSafety/NationalPatientSafetyGoals.

Mauk, K.L. (2005). Conservative therapy for urinary incontinence can help older adults. *Nursing2005, 35*(8), 20-21.

Mennick, F. (2005). Pelvic-floor exercises yield no long-term benefit. *American Journal of Nursing, 105*(5), 22.

Palmer, M.H., & Newman, D.K. (2004). Bladder matters: Urinary incontinence in nursing homes. *American Journal of Nursing, 104*(11), 57-59.

Patraca, K. (2005). Measure bladder volume without catheterization. *Nursing2005, 35*(4), 46-47.

Pullen, R.L. (2004). Inserting an indwelling urinary catheter in a male patient. *Nursing2004, 34*(7), 24.

Pullen, R.J. (2007). Clinical do's & don'ts: Replacing a urostomy drainage pouch. *Nursing2007, 37*(6), 14.

Rushing, J. (2004). Inserting an indwelling urinary catheter in a female patient. *Nursing2004, 34*(8), 22.

Rushing, J. (2006). Caring for your patient's suprapubic catheter. *Nursing2006, 36*(7), 32.

Schultz, J.M. (2004). Urinary incontinence. *Nursing2004, 34*(10), 62-63.

Senese, V., Hendricks, M.B., Morrison, M., et al. (2006). Clinical practice guidelines. Care of the patient with an indwelling catheter. *Urologic Nursing, 26,* 80-81.

Sienkiewicz, J., Wilkinson, G., & Emr, K.D. (2008). The quest for best practice in caring for the home care patient with an indwelling urinary catheter: The New Jersey experience. *Home Healthcare Nurse, 26*(2), 1210-1218.

Specht, J.K. (2005). 9 myths of incontinence in older adults. *American Journal of Nursing, 105*(6), 58-69.

Sterling-Fisher, C. (2004). Is leaking really incontinence? *Home Healthcare Nurse, 22*, 613-623.

Swann, J. (2005). Providing convenient and accessible toilet facilities. *Nursing in Residential Care, 7*, 366-369.

Toughill, E. (2005). Bladder matters: Indwelling urinary catheters. *American Journal of Nursing, 105*(5), 35-37.

Woods, A. (2005). Managing UTIs in older adults. *Nursing2005, 35*(3), 12.

Chapter 30

Amerine, E., & Keirsey, M. (2006a). How should you respond to constipation? *Nursing2006, 36*(10), 64hn1-64hn2.

Amerine, E., & Keirsey, M. (2006b). Managing acute diarrhea. *Nursing2006, 36*(9), 64hn1-64hn4.

Aucoin, M. (2006). Zeroing in. *ADVANCE for Nurses, 4*(5), 19-20.

Brewer, B.W. (2005). United Ostomy Association provides help for ostomy patients and caregivers. *Home Healthcare Nurse, 23*, 353-354.

Centers for Disease Control and Prevention Media Relations. *Hand hygiene guidelines fact sheet.* Available at: www.cdc.gov/od/oc/media/pressrel/fs021025.htm (accessed August 6, 2007).

Clark, J. (2004). *Ileostomy guide.* United Ostomy Association of America Inc. Available at: www.uoaa.org/ostomy_info.

Clark, J., & Dubois, H. (2004). *Urostomy guide.* United Ostomy Association of America Inc. Available at: www.uoaa.org/ostomy_info.

Clark, J., & Grover, P. (2004). *Colostomy guide.* United Ostomy Association of America Inc. Available at: www.uoaa.org/ostomy_info.

Hill, R. (2007). Conquering constipation. *LPN2007, 3*(4), 48-53.

Hurd, L.B., & King, M. (2005). *Dietary guidelines for ileoanal pouch surgery.* The J-Pouch Group. Available at: www.j-pouch.org/diet.html.

Nursing2008 Eds. (2008). Managing opioid-induced constipation. *Nursing2008, 38*(7), 55.

Madsen, D., Sebolt, T., Cullen, L., et al. (2005). Listening to bowel sounds: An evidence-based practice project. *American Journal of Nursing, 105*(12), 40-50.

Mauk, K.L. (2005). Preventing constipation in older adults. *Nursing2005, 35*(6), 22-23.

Medline Plus. *Drugs and supplements: Lubiprostone.* Available at: www.nlm.nih.gov/medlineplus/druginfo/drug_La.html (accessed August 6, 2007).

Pullen, R.L. (2006). Teaching your patient to irrigate a colostomy. *Nursing2006, 36*(4), 22.

Red Flags. (2005). There's trouble down below. *Nursing Made Incredibly Easy!, 3*(1), 60-61.

Ringhofer, J. (2005). Meeting the needs of your ostomy patient. *RN, 68*(8), 37-42.

Scott, B., Curtis, V., Rabie, T., et al. (2007). Health in our hands, but not in our heads: Understanding hygiene motivation in Ghana. *Health Policy and Planning, 22*, 225-233.

Chapter 31

Aguirre, L.L., Nevidjon, B.M., & Clemens, A.E. (2008). Pain diaries. *American Journal of Nursing, 108*(6), 37-39.

Arcidicono, P. (2006). Using a spinal cord stimulator to ease chronic pain. *Nursing2006, 36*(8), 18-19.

Arnstein, P. (2006). Placebo: No relief for Ms. Mahoney's pain. *American Journal of Nursing, 106*(2), 54-65.

Becker, P. (2005). Impact of insomnia on general health and quality of life. *Medscape Psychiatry & Mental Health, 10*(1). Available at: www.medscape.com/viewarticle/505465_print.

Carlock, C. (2007). Ethics and the double bind of palliative sedation. *Nursing Spectrum*, 2007 Spring Med/Surg Specialty Guide, 70-71.

Cohen, M.R. (2007). 10 tips on safe opioid administration. *Nursing2007, 37*(5), 14.

Cole, C., & Richards, K. (2007). Sleep disruption in older adults. *American Journal of Nursing, 107*(5), 40-50.

D'Arcy, Y. (2006a). Phantom limb pain: What it is, how to treat it. *LPN2006, 2*(6), 15-17.

D'Arcy, Y. (2006b). Which analgesic is right for my patient? *Nursing2006, 36*(7), 51-55.

D'Arcy, Y. (2007a). Assessing pain-rating scales. *LPN2007, 3*(6), 13-12.

D'Arcy, Y. (2007b). Climbing the ladder to pain relief success. *Nursing Made Incredibly Easy!, 5*(6), 19-22.

D'Arcy, Y. (2007c). Eyeing capnography to improve PCA safety. *Nursing2007, 37*(9), 18-19.

D'Arcy, Y. (2007d). The fentanyl patch: Convenient, effective pain control. *LPN2007, 3*(3), 4-5.

D'Arcy, Y. (2007e). Managing pain in a patient who's drug dependent. *Nursing2007, 37*(3), 36-41.

D'Arcy, Y. (2007f). New pain management options: Delivery systems and techniques. *Nursing2007, 37*(2), 26-28.

D'Arcy, Y. (2007g). New pain management options: Drugs. *Nursing2007, 37*(1), 26-28.

D'Arcy, Y. (2007h). Safe pain relief at the push of a button. *Nursing Made Incredibly Easy!, 5*(5), 9-12.

D'Arcy, Y. (2007j). Taking a new look at NSAIDs. *LPN 2007, 3*(3), 11-13.

D'Arcy, Y. (2007k). Using adjuvant medications for pain: Antidepressants and anticonvulsants. *LPN2007, 3*(6), 14-19.

D'Arcy, Y. (2007l). Using the WHO analgesic ladder to choose pain medication. *LPN2007, 3*(2), 4-7.

D'Arcy, Y. (2008). How do you spell pain relief? *Made Incredibly Easy!, 6*(4), 12-15, 17.

Dugan, M. (2007). A tale of sleep. *Nursing Made Incredibly Easy!, 5*(3), 28-38.

Flaherty, E. (2008). Using pain-rating scales with older adults. *American Journal of Nursing, 108*(6), 40-47.

Foresman, G. (2007). *Sleep healthy, live healthy.* Available at: www.anaturalbalance.com/Archive/2007/071517.html.

Gervitz, C. (2008a). Bracing and splinting to manage pain. *Nursing2008, 38*(5), 48.

Gevirtz, C. (2008b). How chronic pain affects sexuality. *Nursing2008, 38*(1), 17.

Gevirtz, C. (2007). Treating sleep disturbances in patients with chronic pain. *Nursing2007, 37*(4), 26-27.

Goldberg, R. (2007). Obstructive sleep apnea *ADVANCE for Nurses, 4*(14), 17-19.

Goldsmith, C. (2007). Insomnia: Sleepless in America. *NurseWeek, 20*(5), 16-19.

Hayduk, R. (2002). *Narcolepsy.* Available at: www.medicinenet.com/script/main/art.asp?articlekey=19901&pf=3&page=1.

Hemmila, D. (2007). Sleepless in the USA: Nearly half of women are sleep deprived. *NurseWeek, 20*(15), 24-25.

Horgas, A., & Miller, L. (2008). Pain assessment in people with dementia. *American Journal of Nursing, 108*(7), 62-71.

Karch, A.M. (2007). *Sedative-hypnotic warning.* Available at: www.nursingdrugguide.com/nc_sedativehypnoticwarning.htm.

Kean, M.B. (2007). Assessing complex pain behaviors. *Nursing2007, 37*(12), 18-19.

Keefe, S. (2007). ZZZs & healing. *ADVANCE for Nurses, 9*(1), 37.

Kelly, A.M. (2006). Managing osteoarthritis pain. *Nursing2006, 36*(11), 20-21.

Kozachik, S.L., & Page, G.G. (2008). The skinny on PCAs. *ADVANCE for Nurses, 4*(22), 28-30.

Kwekkeboom, K.L., & Gretarsdottir, E. (2006). Systematic review of relaxation interventions for pain. *Journal of Nursing Scholarship, 38*, 269-277.

LPN2008 Eds. (2008). Oh my aching back! Taking care of low back pain. *LPN2008, 4*(3), 13-18.

Mann, A.R. (2008). Pain management & addiction. *ADVANCE for Nurses, 5*(11), 27-31.

Mauk, K. (2005). Promoting sound sleep habits in older adults. *Nursing2005, 35*(2), 22-25.

McCaffery, M., & Pasero, C. (1989). *Pain Assessment and Pharmacological Management of Pain in Adults.* St. Louis: Mosby.

Metules, T.J. (2007). Hands-on help: Hot and cold packs. *RN, 70*(1), 45-48.

National Cancer Institute. (2005). *Methylnaltrexone relieves constipation caused by pain medication.* Available at: http://cancer.gov/clinicaltrials/results/constipation0605.

Nursing2008 Eds. (2008). Managing opioid-induced constipation. *Nursing2008, 38*(7), 55.

Nursing Made Incredibly Easy! Eds. (2008). Spine-tingling pain relief. *Nursing Made Incredibly Easy!, 6*(2), 17-18.

Pain Pointers. (2007). The path to managing neuropathic pain. *Nursing Made Incredibly Easy!, 5*(1), 26-29.

Pasero, C. (2007). IV opioid range orders for acute pain management. *American Journal of Nursing, 107*(2), 52-60.

Quillen, T.F. (2005). Sounding the alarm for narcolepsy. *Nursing2005, 35*(6), 74-75.

Schaller, J. (2008). . . . About obstructive sleep apnea. *Nursing2008, 38*(1), 27.

Scholz, M. (2007). A way to control breakthrough pain. *RN, 70*(2), 57.

Shields, J. (2008). Sleep apnea: Diganosis and treatment improve quality of life. *Nurseweek, 21*(6), 40-41.

Simon, A.M., & O'Connor, J.P. (2007). Dose and time-dependent effects of cyclooxygenase-2 inhibition on fracture healing. *Journal of Bone and Joint Surgery, 89A*, 500-511.

Smyth, C.A. (2008). Evaluating sleep quality in older adults. *American Journal of Nursing, 1085*, 42-50.

Spader, C. (2008). Depression + pain. *NurseWeek, 21*(12), 22-23.

Springhouse. (2006a). *Nurse's 5 Minute Clinical Consult: Procedures* (pp. 516-517). Philadelphia: Lippincott Williams & Wilkins.

Springhouse. (2006b). PQRST mnemonic. In Cortright, A.B. (Ed.). *LPN Facts Made Incredibly Quick!* Philadelphia: Lippincott Williams & Wilkins.

Teenier, P., & Sender, S. (2007). Assessing pain in the home care environment. *Home Healthcare Nurse, 25*(7), 470-476.

Wheeler, M.S. (2006). Pain assessment and management in the patient with mild to moderate cognitive impairment. *Home Healthcare Nurse, 24*, 354-360.

Willard, R., & Dreher, H.M. (2005). Wake-up call for sleep apnea. *Nursing2005, 35*(3), 46-49.

Wright, D.V. (2008). Non-narcotic options for pain relief with chronic neuropathic conditions. *Journal for Nurse Practitioners, 4*(4), 263-270.

Yemenijian, D. (2007). Honey, you're snoring again. *Advance for LPNs.* Available at: http://lpn.advanceweb.com/common/Editorial/PrintFriendly.aspx?CC+84609.

Chapter 32

Alternatives, Complementary and Alternative Therapies. (2005a). Sweet on peppermint. *Nursing2005, 35*(2), 76.

Alternatives, Complementary and Alternative Therapies. (2005b). Understanding chiropractic practice. *Nursing2005, 35*(1), 73.

Boehringer, S.K. (2003). Herbal medicines: Nurses must help public evaluate pros and cons. *NurseWeek, 16*(4), 15-16.

Cerrato, P.L. (Ed.). (2003a). Complementary therapies update: A "natural" approach to diabetic neuropathy. *RN, 66*(10), 23.

Cerrato, P.L. (Ed.). (2003b). Complementary therapies update: Nerve stimulation relieves the nausea of pregnancy. *RN, 66*(11), 24.

Cerrato, P.L. (2003c). New evidence links fiber to a reduced risk of colon CA. *RN, 66*(10), 20.

Clark, C.C., Eliopoulos, C., Colbath, J.D., et al. (2008). Herbal remedies are often overlooked. *Nurseweek, 21*(9), 78-80.

Cowles, L. (2005). There's no place like "om." *ADVANCE for Nurses, 2*(12), 28-29.

Cowles, L. (2006). Mindful medicine: Nurses use mind over matter with hypnotherapy. *ADVANCE for Nurses, 3*(18), 33-34.

Duffy, K. (2006). *Heaven scent: Clinical aromatherapy can enhance healing process.* Available at: http://lpn.advanceweb.com/common/editorial/PrintFriendly.aspx?CC=66165.

Dunning, T. (2005). Applying a quality use of medicines framework to using essential oils in nursing practice. *Complementary Therapeutic Clinical Practice, 11*, 172-181.

Floyd, J.P., & Fernances, J.H. (2003). Making a place for CAM in the ICU. *RN, 66*(7), 44-47.

Federwisch, A. (2008). Holistic healing. *NurseWeek, 21*(1), 20-23.

Kahn, S. (2006). CoQ$_{10}$'s "other" health benefits. *Life Extension, February*, 51-57.

Learning about tai chi chuan. (2003). *Nursing2002, 32*(12), 86.

Lee, M.S., & Jang, H.S. (2005). Two case reports of the acute effects of Qi therapy (external Qigong) on symptoms of cancer: Short report. *Complementary Therapeutic Clinical Practice, 11*, 211-213.

Lie, D. (2006). *Drinking green tea reduces CVD mortality.* Available at: http://medscape.com/viewarticle/544569_print.

Lillis, K. (2006). Specialty care demands top-level wound care and assessment skills. *ADVANCE for Nurses, 3*(15), 25-26.

McCabe-Maucher, A. (2005). Intro to Reiki. *ADVANCE for Nurses, 7*(26), 38-39.

MD Consult (2005). *Classification of CAM therapies.* Available at: http://home.mdconsult.com/das/news/body/1/ctt/0/94583/1.html?pos=94583.

MedicineNet.com (2004). *Alternative medicine.* Available at: http://medicinenet.com/script/main/art.asp?articlekey=266&pf=3&track=qpa266.

Non-Traditional Choices. (2004a). Herbal remedies: Patient beware. *Nursing2004, 34*(2), 29.

Non-Traditional Choices. (2004b). How herbs can affect your patient's health. *Nursing2004, 34*(7), 70-71.

Non-Traditional Choices. (2004c). More Americans than ever use CAM, says CDC. *Nursing2004, 34*(9), 73.

Non-Traditional Choices. (2004d). The scoop on green tea. *Nursing2004, 34*(4) 73.

Nursing2007 Eds. (2007). How herbal products increase surgical risks. *Nursing2007, 37*(9), 24-25.

Patient Education Series. (2004). Herbal supplements. *Nursing2004, 34*(12), 52.

RN News Watch. (2004). Complementary therapies update. *RN, 67*(1), 27.

Rosick, E.R. (2006). Antioxidants, mitochondrial damage and human aging. *Life Extension, February*, 63-67.

Schmidt, L.M. (2004). Herbal remedies: The other drugs your patients take. *Home Healthcare Nurse, 22*(3), 169-175.

Shields, J. (2007). Probiotics: Bacteria with a healthy slant. *NurseWeek, 20*(23), 22.

Taylor, S. (2006). Research reveals the benefits of meditation. *NurseWeek, 19*(3), 17-18.

Ullman, D. (2003). Ten most frequently asked questions on homeopathic medicine. *Homeopathic Educational Services.* Available at: www.homeopathic.com/articles/view,34.

Vogelzang, J.L. (2004). Alternative and complementary nutrition in chronic cardiac disease. *Home Healthcare Nurse, 22*, 85-87.

Woodruff, D.W. (2004). Herbs and drugs: A bad mix? *Nursing Made Incredibly Easy!, 2*(5), 61-62.

Chapter 33

Aschenbrenner, D.S. (2006). A new format for drug labels. *American Journal of Nursing, 106*(5), 67.

Aschenbrenner, D.S. (2008a). Understanding pharmacokinetics: Part 1: Drug Absorption. *American Journal of Nursing, 108*(5), 55-68.

Aschenbrenner, D.S. (2008b). Understanding pharmacokinetics: Part 2: Drug distribution. *American Journal of Nursing, 108*(6), 68-69.

Aschenbrenner, D.S. (2008c). Understanding pharmacokinetics: Part 3: Drug metabolism. *American Journal of Nursing, 108*(7), 28-29.

Cohen, H. (2008). Be on the alert for high-alert drugs. *Nursing Made Incredibly Easy!, 6*(2), 7-11.

eMedPass (2007). *eMedPass medication administration software introduced to long-term care, assisted living and rehab facilities.* Available at: www.emedpass.com/PR/eMedPassIntroduced.pdf.

Grissinger, M., & Globus, N.J. (2004). How technology affects your risk of medication errors. *Nursing2004, 34*(1), 36-42.

Grissinger, M., & Globus, N.J. (2005). How to make drug delivery safer. *LPN2005, 1*(3), 19-21.

Hamme, M. (2006). Medication management: Educational tools for improving target outcomes. *Home Healthcare Nurse, 24,* 80-86.

Hicks, R.W., & Cousins, D.D. (2004). Preventing drug allergy errors: Nurses are making a difference. *RN, 67*(4), 80.

Hughes, R.G., & Edgerton, E.A. (2005). First do no harm: Reducing pediatric medication errors. *American Journal of Nursing, 105*(5), 79-89.

Institute for Safe Medication Practices. (2004). ISMP issues list of high-alert medications. *Nurse Advise-ERR, 2*(2), 2.

Institute for Safe Medication Practices. (2005a). Inquisitive patients: The last line of defense. *Nurse Advise-ERR, 3*(11), 1.

Institute for Safe Medication Practices. (2005b). Mental slips and lapses: No one is immune. *Nurse Advise-ERR, 3*(10), 1.

Institute for Safe Medication Practices. (2006a). Building a case for medication reconciliation. *Nurse Advise-ERR, 4*(4), 1.

Institute for Safe Medication Practices. (2006b). Safety Wire. Lithium in mg or mEq. *Nurse Advise-ERR, 5*(1), 1.

Institute for Safe Medication Practices. (2006c). Two forms of methylprednisolone: One not for IV use. *Nurse Advise-ERR, 4*(5), 1.

(The) Joint Commission. (2006). Using medication reconciliation to prevent errors. *Sentinel Event Alert, 35.* Available at: www.jointcommission.org/SentinelEvents/SentinelEventAlert.

Karch, A.M. (2004). The grapefruit challenge. *American Journal of Nursing, 104*(12), 33-34.

Ketchum, K., Grass, C.A., & Padwojski, A. (2005). Medication reconciliation. *American Journal of Nursing, 105*(11), 78-85.

Lafleur, K.L. (2004). Tackling med errors with technology. *RN, 67*(5), 29-34.

Luggen, A.S. (2005). Pharmacology update: Inappropriate prescribing in the long-term care setting. *Geriatric Nursing, 26*(4), 233-236.

Manno, M.S. (2006). Preventing adverse drug effects. *Nursing2006, 36*(3), 56-62.

Manno, M.S., & Hayes, D.D. (2006). How medication reconciliation saves lives. *Nursing2006, 36*(3), 63-64.

Mason, D.J. (2005). Making it safer. *American Journal of Nursing, 105*(3), 11.

Math Maze. The dosage calculation two-step. (2004). *Nursing Made Incredibly Easy!, 2*(2), 61-63.

Math Maze. In small doses: Calculating drugs for peds. (2005). *Nursing Made Incredibly Easy!, 3*(3), 57-59.

Meyer, T. (2004). Calculating drug dosages—accurately. *American Journal of Nursing, 104*(11), 13.

Mosocco, D.J. (2006). Using medication reconciliation to prevent errors. *Home Healthcare Nurse, 24,* 483.

Munoz, C., & Hilgenberg, C. (2005). Ethnopharmacology. *American Journal of Nursing, 105*(8), 40-48.

Neafsey, P.J. (2004a). Low-dose aspirin interactions. *Home Healthcare Nurse, 22,* 54.

Neafsey, P.J. (2004b). Practices that alter the efficacy of selected cardiac medications. *Home Healthcare Nurse, 22,* 89-98.

Nursing 2006 Drug Handbook (26th ed.) (2006). Philadelphia: Lippincott.

Paparella, S. (2006). Medication safety. *ADVANCE for Nurses, 3*(5), 18-22.

Phillips, L.D. (2005). *Manual of IV Therapeutics* (4th ed.). Philadelphia: F.A.Davis.

Prows, C.A., & Prows, D.R. (2004). Medication selection by genotype. *American Journal of Nursing, 104*(5), 60-70.

Reading the Label: ISMP, FDA create an educational campaign on error-prone medication abbreviations. (2005). *ADVANCE for Nurses, 2*(21), 38.

RN News Watch Drug Update: As expected, the FDA will begin requiring bar codes. (2005). *RN, 67*(4), 79.

Roark, D.C. (2004). Bar codes & drug administration. *American Journal of Nursing, 104*(1), 63-66.

Santell, J.P., & Camp, S. (2005). How to avoid "wrong patient" errors. *RN, 68*(6), 81.

Santell, J.P., Hicks, R.W., & Protzel, M. (2004). Error watch: Annoyance aside, distractions spell trouble. *RN, 66*(12), 96.

Schull, P.D. (2005). Five rights still resound. *NurseWeek, 18*(2), 21-22.

Vital Signs: Are your patients taking their meds? (2005). *RN, 68*(5), 20.

Wooten, J.M. (2006). New frontiers. *RN, 69*(3), 36-41.

Chapter 34

Adams, M.P., Josephson, D.L., & Holland, L.N. (2005). *Pharmacology for Nurses: A Pathophysiologic Approach.* Upper Saddle River, NJ: Pearson.

Adult Meducation Improving Medication Adherence in Older Adults. (2006). *Dimension 1: social and economic factors.* Available at: www.adultmeducation.com/SocialandEconomicFactors_4.html.

Appel, S.J., & Wright, M.A. (2007). Teach your patient to administer inhaled insulin. *Nursing2007, 37*(1), 49-50.

Drug News. (2006). Birth-control patch: Women warned about clot risks. *Nursing2006, 36*(1), 30.

Ebersole, P., & Hess, P. (2005). *Geriatric Nursing and Healthy Aging* (2nd ed.). St. Louis: Elsevier Mosby.

Exubera. (2007). Available at: www.exubera.com.

Fundamentals of Nursing Made Incredibly Easy! (2007). Philadelphia: Lippincott Williams & Wilkins.

Grissinger, M., & Globus, N.J. (2005). How to make drug delivery safer. *LPN2005, 1*(3), 19-21.

Higgins, D. (2007). Administering a suppository. *Nursing Times, 103*(10), 26-27.

Institute for Safe Medication Practices. (2007a). Getting to the 'route' of the problem: Oral and IV doses differ. *Nurse Advise-ERR, 5*(1), 1.

Institute for Safe Medication Practices. (2007b). Oral syringes: A simple powerful way to prevent patient harm. *Nurse Advise-ERR, 5*(1), 2.

Institute for Safe Medication Practices. (2007c). Pregnancy alert: Can't touch this. *Nurse Advise-ERR, 5*(3), 3.

Institute for Safe Medication Practices. (2007d). Safety Wire. Open packages at bedside. *Nurse Advise-ERR, 5*(1), 2.

Johnson, C.L., DeMass, S.L., & Markle-Elder, S. (2006). Toxic medications. *American Journal of Nursing, 106*(11), 37-38.

Johnson, D. (2006). Prevent soggy patches. *Nursing2006, 36*(7), 8.

Kalemba, J. (2007). Overview of 2007 National Patient Safety Goals and universal protocol. *ADVANCE for Nurses, 5*(2), 33-34.

Krulish, L. H. (2005). MO780: Oral medications. *Home Healthcare Nurse, 23,* 72-76.

LPN2007 Eds. (2007). Administering drugs via the oral mucosa. *LPN2007, 3*(6), 4-7.

Mager, D.R. (2007). Medication errors and the home care patient. *Home Healthcare Nurse, 25,* 151-156.

McErlane, K. (2005). Keeping track of the patch. *American Journal of Nursing, 105*(6), 36-37.

Metules, T.J., & Bauer, J. (2007). JCAHO's patient safety goals: Preventing med errors. *RN, 70*(1), 39-43.

Pullen, R.L. (2008). Administering a transdermal drug. *Nursing2008, 38*(4), 14.

Roark, D.C. (2004). Bar codes and drug administration. *American Journal of Nursing, 104*(1), 63-66.

Rushing, J. (2007). Administering eyedrops. *Nursing2007, 37*(5), 18.

Schulmeister, L. (2007). Stuck on you: Transdermal drug patches. *Nursing Made Incredibly Easy!, 5*(2), 17-19.

Uko-Ekpenyong, G. (2006). Improving medication adherence with orally disintegrating tablets. *Nursing2006, 36*(9), 20-21.

Wolf, Z.R. (2007). Pursuing safe medication use and the promise of technology. *Medsurg Nursing, 16*(2), 92-100.

Wright, M.A., & Appel, S.J. (2007). Inhaled insulin. *Nursing2007, 37*(1), 46-48.

Chapter 35

Barr, D.M., & Thomas, C.M. (2005). IM administration. *ADVANCE for Nurses, 3*(17), 29-30.

Centers for Disease Control and Prevention, Division of Tuberculosis Elimination. (2007). *Mantoux Tuberculosis Skin Test Facilitator Guide.* Available at: www.cdc.gov/tb/pubs/Mantoux/part1.htm.

Diggle, L. (2007). Injection technique for immunisation. *Practice Nurse, 33*(1), 34-37.

Dittman, M. (2005). When health fears hurt health. *Monitor on Psychology, 36*(7). Available at: www.apa.org/monitor/julaug05/fears.html.

Fain, J. A. (2004). Unlock the mysteries of insulin therapy. *Nursing2004, 34*(3), 41-43.

Garnero, T. (2006). More than a shot. *ADVANCE for Nurses, 4*(3), 37-38.

Gillon, H.J., Armstrong, B.G., & Fiese, M.A. (2006). Before you give that vaccination. *Nursing2006, 36*(11), 54-57.

Grace, P. J. (2006). The clinical use of placebos. *American Journal of Nursing, 106*(2), 58-61.

Greenway, K., Merriman, C., & Stratham, D. (2006). Using the ventrogluteal site for intramuscular injections. *Learning Disability Practice, 9*(8), 34-37.

Institute for Safe Medication Practices. (2006). Carpuject syringe mix-ups: It isn't easy being green. *Nurse Advise-ERR, 4*(6), 2.

Institute for Safe Medication Practices. (2007). Pen injectors: Technology not without imPENding risks. *Nurse Advise-ERR, 5*(2), 1.

Kalemba, J. (2007). Overview of 2007 National Patient Safety Goals and universal protocol. *ADVANCE for Nurses, 5*(2), 33-34.

Love, G.H. (2006). Administering an intradermal injection. *Nursing2006, 36*(6), 20.

Nelson, R. (2004). Needlestick injuries: Going but not gone? *American Journal of Nursing, 104*(11), 25-26.

Nursing Made Incredibly Easy! Eds. (2004). Ask an expert. How should I administer an insulin injection? *Nursing Made Incredibly Easy!, 2*(2)64.

Peak Technique. (2005). Are you on track with Z-track injections? *Nursing Made Incredibly Easy!, 3*(1),58-59.

Practice Guide. (2007). Intramuscular injection technique. *Paediatric Nursing, 19*(2), 37.

Pullen, R.L. (2005). Administering medication by the Z-track method. *Nursing2005, 35*(7), 24.

Ridge, R.A. (2007). Boosting insulin safety. *Nursing2007, 37*(2), 14-15.

Rushing, J. (2004). How to administer a subcutaneous injection. *Nursing2004, 34*(6), 32.

Safe Haven. (2005). "Z" is the key to I.M. injections. *LPN2005, 1*(6), 11-12.

Stein, H.G. (2006). Glass ampules and filter needles: An example of implementing the sixth 'R' in medication administration. *Medsurg Nursing, 15*, 290-294.

Wynaden, D., Lansborough, I., McGowan, S., et al. (2006). Best practice guidelines for the administration of intramuscular injections in the mental health setting. *International Journal of Mental Health Nursing, 15*, 195-200.

Zaybak, A., Güneş, Ü.Y., Tamsel, S., et al. (2007). Does obesity prevent the needle from reaching muscle in intramuscular injections? *Journal of Advanced Nursing, 58*, 552-556.

Chapter 36

Adams, M.P., Josephson, D.L., & Holland, L.N. (2005). *Pharmacology for Nurses: A Pathophysiologic Approach.* Upper Saddle River, NJ: Pearson.

Arbique, J., & Arbique, D. (2007). Reducing the risk of nerve injuries. *Nursing2007, 37*(11), 20-21.

Bowe-Geddes, L.A., & Nichols, H. (2005). An overview of peripherally inserted central catheters. *Topics in Advanced Practice Nursing eJournal, 5*(3). Available at: www.medscape.com/viewarticle/508939.

Brosche, T.A. (2005). Signs to watch for when an IV infiltrates. *RN, 68*(4), 69.

Clinical Tips. (2007). Got a tough stick? Here's a formula for success. *RN, 70*(1), 49.

Cohen, M.R. (2007). Medication errors. *Nursing2007, 37*(5), 14.

Consult Stat. (2006). Is it okay to take a shower with a PICC in place? *RN, 69*(7), 48.

Cook, L. S. (2007). Choosing the right intravenous catheter. *Home Healthcare Nurse, 25*(8), 523-531.

Daley, K.A. (2007). Needlestick injuries: How to improve safety in your workplace. *American Nurse Today, 2*(7), 25-26.

David, K. (2007). IV fluids: Do you know what's hanging and why? *RN, 70*(10), 35-40.

Day, M.W. (2006). Tension pneumothorax from a central line placement. *Nursing2006, 36*(11), 80.

Delahanty, K.M., & Myers, F.E. (2007). *Nursing2007* infection control survey report. *Nursing2007, 37*(6), 28-36.

Doellman, D. (2005). Ease a child's anxiety during PICC insertion—without sedation. *Nursing2005, 35*(3), 68.

Dulak, S.B. (2005). Technology today: Smart IV pumps. *RN, 68*(12), 38-44.

Eakle, M., Gallauresi, B.A., & Morrison, A. (2005). Luer-Lok misconnects can be deadly. *Nursing2005, 35*(9), 73.

Eckel, S.F., Anderson, P., Zimmerman, C., et al. (2006). User satisfaction with an intravenous medication safety system. *American Journal of Health-System Pharmacy, 63*, 1419-1423.

Falkowski, A. (2006). Improving the PICC insertion process. *Nursing2006, 36*(2), 26-27.

Federwisch, A. (2005). Learning from smart pumps. *NurseWeek, 18*(15), 14-15.

Frey, A.M. (2006). What's the best way to secure a catheter? *Nursing2006, 36*(9), 30-31.

Gorski, L. A., & Czaplewski, L.M. (2005). Managing complications of midlines and PICCs. *Nursing2005, 35*(6), 68-69.

Hadaway, L.C. (2005a). Administering parental nutrition with other IV drugs. *Nursing2005, 35*(2), 26.

Hadaway, L.C. (2005b). Caring for a nontunneled CVC site. *Nursing2005, 35*(12), 54-56.

Hadaway, L.C. (2005c). Giving medication by retrograde infusion. *Nursing2005, 35*(11), 28.

Hadaway, L.C. (2005d). Reopen the pipeline for IV therapy. *Nursing2005, 35*(8), 54-61.

Hadaway, L.C. (2006a). Five steps to preventing catheter-related bloodstream infections. *LPN2006, 2*(5), 51-55.

Hadaway, L.C. (2006b). Keeping central line infection at bay. *Nursing2006, 36*(4), 58-63.

Hadaway, L.C. (2006c). Tips for using implanted ports safely. *Nursing2006, 36*(8), 66-67.

Hadaway, L.C. (2008). Central venous access devices. *Nursing2008, 38*(6), 34-39.

Hankins, J. (2007). The role of albumin in fluid balance. *Nursing2007, 37*(12), 14-15.

Hathaway, L.R. (2005). Reduce the risk of anaphylaxis. *LPN2005, 1*(3), 37-41.

Hayes, D.D. (2007). How to respond to abnormal serum sodium levels. *Nursing2007, 37*(12), 56hn1-56hn4.

Hayes, D.D. (2007). When potassium takes dangerous detours. *Nursing2007, 37*(11), 56hn1-56hn4.

Hendler, C.B. (2008). A perfect match: Preventing blood incompatibility errors. *NurseWeek, 21*(12), 24-29.

Institute for Safe Medication Practices. (2004). Using FMEA to predict failures with infusion pumps. *Nurse Advise-ERR, 2*(2), 3.

Institute for Safe Medication Practices. (2006a). Double key bounce and double keying errors. *Nurse Advise-ERR, 4*(2), 1.

Institute for Safe Medication Practices. (2006b). Promethazine survey spurs renewed efforts to prevent tissue damage. *Nurse Advise-ERR, 4*(11), 2-3.

Institute for Safe Medication Practices. (2007). Dangerous disconnect when unscrewing syringe from IV port. *Nurse Advise-ERR, 5*(6), 3.

(The) Joint Commission. (2006). Tubing misconnections—a persistent and deadly occurrence. *Sentinel Alert Event, 36.* Available at: www.jointcommission.org/SentinelEvents/SentinelEventAlert.

Kennedy, M. (2005). The state of the science: Focus on IVs and HIV. *American Journal of Nursing, 105*(4), 54.

Kraemer-Cain, J., & Siegel, M. (2006). Venous access devices. *ADVANCE for Nurses, 8*(24), 17.

Krueger, A. (2007). Need help finding a vein? *Nursing2007, 37*(6), 39-41.

LPN2008 Eds. (2008). Calculating I.V. infusion rates. *LPN2008, 4*(3), 21-22.

Ludeman, K. (2008). Which vascular access device is right for your patient? *Nursing Made Incredibly Easy!, 6*(4), 7, 9-11.

Marders, J. (2005). Sounding the alarm for IV infiltration. *Nursing2005, 35*(4), 18-20.

Math Maze. (2004). How fast should the drops drip? *Nursing Made Incredibly Easy!, 2*(4), 60-62.

Moureau, N.L. (2006). Tips for successful IV starts in older patients. *LPN2006, 2*(4), 6-7.

Nursing2008 Eds. (2008). Comparing short peripheral cannula insertion sites. *Nursing 2008, 38*(5), 60.

Nursing2008 Eds. (2008). IV Rounds: What you should know about drug compatibility. *Nursing2008, 38*(3), 15.

Nursing Made Incredibly Easy! Eds. (2008). Complications of peripheral I.V. therapy. *Nursing Made Incredibly Easy!, 6*(1), 14-18.

Palmerchuk, L. (2007). Central command: Making sense of central lines. *NurseWeek, 20.* Available at: http://news.nurse.com/apps/pbcs.dll/article?AID=/20070115/CA09/301150054&SearchID=73301450020626.

Perry, J., & Metules, T. (2004). How to avoid needlesticks. Supplement to *RN, 67*(11), 28ns1-28ns8.

Phillips, L.D. (2005). *Manual of IV Therapeutics* (4th ed.). Philadelphia: F.A. Davis.

Polzien, G. (2006). Home infusion therapy. *Home Healthcare Nurse, 24,* 681-684.

Powers, J., Budgin, C., & Halon, J. (2006). Bad blood: Tips for preventing CR-BSIs. *Nursing Made Incredibly Easy!, 4*(5), 30-39.

Quigley, T. (2004). Smart pumps. *ADVANCE for Nurses, 1*(7), 21.

Randle, J., & Clarke, M. (2007). Maintenance of peripheral intravenous catheters. *Nursing Times, 103*(12), 30-31.

Rosenthal, K. (2004). What you should know about needleless IV system. *Nursing2004, 34*(9), 76.

Rosenthal, K. (2005a). Documenting peripheral IV therapy. *Nursing2005, 35*(7), 28.

Rosenthal, K. (2005b). Initiating intravenous therapy. *LPN2005, 1*(3), 4-10.

Rosenthal, K. (2005c). Kid's stuff: Starting IVs in peds. *Nursing Made Incredibly Easy!, 3*(4), 45-50.

Rosenthal, K. (2005d). Providing safe CVAD site care. *LPN2005, 1*(4), 5-9.

Rosenthal, K. (2005e). Tailor your IV insertion techniques for special populations. *Nursing2005, 35*(5), 37-41.

Rosenthal, K. (2006a). Breaking the link between IV therapy and HIT. *Nursing2006, 36*(5), 22.

Rosenthal, K. (2006b). Navigating safely through a minefield of CVC complications. *Nursing Made Incredibly Easy!, 4*(1), 56-58.

Rosenthal, K. (2006c). One size doesn't fit all...and other perils of IV administration. *Nursing Made Incredibly Easy!, 4*(6), 56-58.

Rosenthal, K. (2006d). What you need to know about ports. *Nursing2006, 36*(1), 20-21.

Rosenthal, K. (2006e). When your patient develops phlebitis. *Nursing2006, 36*(2), 14.

Rosenthal, K. (2006f). The whys and wherefores of IV fluids. *Nursing Made Incredibly Easy!, 4*(3), 8-11.

Rosenthal, K. (2007a). Avoiding common perils of drug administration. *Nursing2007, 37*(4), 20.

Rosenthal, K. (2007b). Bridging the IV access gap with midline catheters. *Nursing Made Incredibly Easy!, 5*(3), 18-20.

Rosenthal, K. (2007c). CVAD site prep with pep. *Nursing Made Incredibly Easy!, 5*(6), 23-24.

Rosenthal, K. (2007d). Reducing the risks of infiltration and extravasation. *Nursing2007, 37*(9), 4-8.

Rosenthal, K. (2007e). What's new in the infusion nursing standards. *Nursing Made Incredibly Easy!, 5*(1),12-13.

Self-Test. (2006). IV challenge, part 1. *Nursing2006, 36*(4), 73-75.

Smith, B. (2006). Updated IV standards. *ADVANCE for Nurses, 3*(13), 23-24.

Smith, B., & Royer, T.I. (2007). New standards for improving peripheral IV catheter securement. *Nursing2007, 37*(3), 72-73.

Tilton, D. (2006). How to fine-tune your PICC care. *RN, 69*(9), 30-36.

Weaver, R., & McDonald, M. (2006). What you need to know about transfusing platelets. *Nursing2006, 36*(6), 26-27.

Chapter 37

Adamow, S.M. (2004). The OR of tomorrow. *ADVANCE for Nurses, 2*(5), 19-20.

Agency for Healthcare Research and Quality (AHRQ) Eds. (2005). Pain management is often inadequate for elderly patients hospitalized for surgery. *AHRQ, 296*(4), 16-17.

Armstrong, M. (2004). Caring for the patient with piercings. *RN, 67*(6), 46-52.

Baldwin, K.M. (2008). FAQs about SSIs. *Made Incredibly Easy!, 6*(4), 36-43.

Barclay, L., & Lie, D. (2004). Electroacupuncture helpful for postoperative nausea and vomiting. *Medscape Medical News.* Available at: www.medscape.com/viewarticle/489936?src=mp.

Barclay, L., & Vega, C. (2006). *Gum chewing may speed recovery from postoperative ileus.* Available at: www.medscape.com/viewarticle/524084.

Barzoloski-O'Connor, B. (2007). Infection control: From scrub to rub: Hand hygiene in the OR. *OR Nurse, 1*(1), 10-12.

Bauer, J. (2004). "Sounds of silence" are as good as music for easing anxiety and pain. *RN, 67*(10), 18.

Baugh, N., Zuelzer, H., & Blandenship, J. (2007). Wounds in surgical patients who are obese. *American Journal of Nursing, 107*(6), 40-50.

Carter-Templeton, H. (2006). Awake to danger: Temperature rising. *Nursing Made Incredibly Easy!, 4*(4), 10-11.

Chettle, C.C. (2008). Shockingly high rates: Surgical site infections remain a constant threat. *Nurseweek, 21*(8), 24-28.

Cofer, M.J. (2005). Unwelcome companion to older patients: Postoperative delirium. *Nursing2005, 35*(1), 32hn1-32hn3.

Daniels, S.M. (2007). Improving hospital care for surgical patients. *Nursing2007, 37*(8), 36-37.

D'Arcy, Y. (2006a). How to care for a surgical patient with chronic pain. *Nursing2006, 36*(3), 17.

D'Arcy, Y. (2006b). Managing postop pain in a patient who's delirious. *Nursing2006, 36*(6), 17.

Day, M.W. (2005). Pulmonary embolism. *Nursing2005, 35*(9), 88.

Dixon, B.A., & O'Donnell, J.M. (2006). Is your patient susceptible to malignant hyperthermia? *Nursing2006, 36*(12), 26-27.

Domrose, C. (2005). Senior surgery: Outcomes improving for elderly patients. *NurseWeek, 13*(22), 10-11.

Doughty, D.B. (2004). Preventing and managing surgical wound dehiscence. *Home Healthcare Nurse, 22,* 365-367.

Dunn, D. (2005). Preventing perioperative complications in special populations. *Nursing2005, 35*(11), 36-43.

Dunn, D. (2006). Age-smart care: Preventing perioperative complications in older adults. *Nursing Made Incredibly Easy!, 4*(3), 30-39.

Evans, S. (2006a). Paging doctor Robot! *ADVANCE for Nurses, 3*(14), 25-26.

Evans, S. (2006b). Robot revolution. *ADVANCE for Nurses, 3*(21), 23-24.

Evans, S. (2006c). Sterile field. *ADVANCE for Nurses, 3*(22), 12-14.

Evans, S. (2006d). Sweet 15: High-tech operating room. *ADVANCE for Nurses, 3*(18), 12-15.

Evans, S. (2007). Perfect harmony: Music therapy eases anxiety and pain in the perioperative setting. *ADVANCE for Nurses, 4*(2), 25-26.

George, J. (2005). Robots finding elbow room in hospital operating suites. *Philadelphia Business Journal.* Available at: http://22.bizjournals.com/industries/health_care/hospitals/2005/04/25/Philadelphia_story8.html.

Goodman, T. (2005). Pressure damage in surgery. *ADVANCE for Nurses, 2*(11), 37-41.

Guajardo, D. (2004). Marks of safety. *NurseWeek, 17*(23), 10-11.

Halliday, A.B. (2006). Shades of sedation: Learning about moderate sedation and analgesia. *Nursing2006, 36*(4), 37-41.

Ho, D. (2005). *Robotic surgical aide 'the first step.'* Available at: www.philly.com/mld/inquirer/living/health.

Hunter, S., Thompson, P., Langermo, D., et al. (2007). Understanding wound dehiscence. *Nursing2007, 37*(9), 28, 30.

(The) Joint Commission. (2003). *Universal Protocol for Preventing Wrong Site, Wrong Procedure, Wrong Person Surgery.* Chicago: Author.

Keefe, S. (2005a). Cell salvaging. *ADVANCE for Nurses, 2*(8), 17-19.

Keefe, S. (2005b). Postoperative ileus. *ADVANCE for Nurses, 2*(14), 26-27.

Litwack, K. (2006). Adjusting postsurgical care for older patients. *Nursing2006, 36*(1), 66-67.

LPN2006 Eds. (2006). You're a witness: Know your role in obtaining informed consent. *LPN2006, 2*(4), 15-16.

Luebbehusen, M. (2005). Bispectral index monitoring. *RN, 68*(9), 50-54.

Mace, S. (2006). Keeping count: "Radio tags" help eliminate retained foreign bodies. *NurseWeek, 19*(22), 14-15.

Mabrey, M.E. (2004). Using insulin to prevent hyperglycemia in surgical patients. *Nursing2004, 34*(10), 22.

Melling, A.C., Ali, B., Scott, E.M., et al. (2002). Effects of preoperative warming on the incidence of wound infection after clean surgery: A randomized controlled trial. *Lancet, 359*(9304), 445-446.

Nursing2006 Eds. (2006). Shades of sedation: Learning about moderate sedation and analgesia. *Nursing2006, 36*(4), 37-41.

Nursing2007 Eds. (2007). How herbal products increase surgical risks. *Nursing2007, 37*(9), 24-25.

Nursing2007 Eds. (2007). Tips for a safe operation. *Nursing2007, 43.*

Nursing Made Incredibly Easy! Eds. (2008). Malignant hyperthermia: Rare by life threatening. *Nursing Made Incredibly Easy!, 6*(3), 56.

Nurseweek Eds. (2008). Massage lessens post-op pain, anxiety. *Nurseweek, 21*(3), 31.

Odom-Forren, J. (2006a). Preventing surgical site infections. *Nursing2006, 36*(6), 59-63.

Odom-Forren, J. (2006b). Winning the battle against surgical site infections. *LPN2006, 2*(3), 44-47.

Perry, K., & Jagger, J. (2005). Pass with care in the OR. *Nursing2005, 35*(2), 70.

Pruitt, B. (2006). Help your patient combat postoperative atelectasis. *Nursing2006, 36*(5), 64hn1-64hn6.

Qaseem, A., Snow, V., Fitterman, N., et al. (2006). *Risk assessment for and strategies to reduce perioperative pulmonary complications for patients undergoing noncardiothoracic surgery: A guideline from the American College of Physicians.* Available at: www.annals.org/cgi/content/full/144/8/575.

Ridge, R.A. (2008). Doing right to prevent wrong-site surgery. *Nursing2008, 38*(3), 24-25.

RN Eds. (2005). Reduce surgical infection: A step-by-step guide. *RN, 68*(5), 32hf1-32hf2.

Schwartz, A.J. (2006). Learning the essentials of epidural anesthesia. *Nursing2006, 36*(1), 44-49.

Schweon, S. (2006). Stamping out surgical site infections. *RN, 69*(8), 36-40.

Smydra, K.E., & Votodian, A.M. (2007). Perioperative management of obese patients. *ADVANCE for Nurses, 4*(2), 21-22.

Stein, R. (2005). *Video robots redefine 'TV doctor.'* Available at: www.washingtonpost.com/wp-dyn/content/article/2005/06/27.

Wilson, J.A., & Clark, J.J. (2004). Obesity: Impediment to postsurgical wound healing. *Advances in Skin & Wound Care, 17*, 426-432.

Winslow, E.H., & Jacobson, A.F. (1997). Preop fluid bolus reduces adverse surgical effects. *American Journal of Nursing, 97*(3), 62.

Chapter 38

Advances in Skin & Wound Care Eds. (2004a). How aging affects wound healing. *Advances in Skin & Wound Care, 18*, 20-21.

Ankrom, M.A., Bennett, R.G., Sprigle, S., et al., for the National Pressure Ulcer Advisory Panel. (2005). Pressure-related deep tissue injury under intact skin and the current pressure ulcer staging systems. *Advances in Skin & Wound Care, 18*, 35-41.

Ayello, E.A. (2005). What does the wound say? Why determining etiology is essential for appropriate wound care. *Advances in Skin & Wound Care, 18*, 98-109.

Ayello, E.A. (2006). New evidence for an enduring wound-healing concept: Moisture control. *Journal of Wound, Ostomy, and Continence Nursing, 33*(65), 51-52.

Bailey, D.L., Jackson, L., & White, D. (2004). HBO therapy: Beyond the bends. *RN, 57*(9), 30-35.

Baldwin, K.M. (2005). How to prevent and treat pressure ulcers. *LPN2005, 1*(2), 18-25.

Baranoski, S. (2005). Wound dressing: A myriad of challenging decisions. *Home Healthcare Nurse, 23*, 307-316.

Baranoski, S. (2008a). Choosing a wound dressing, part 1. *Nursing2008, 38*(1), 60-61.

Baranoski, S. (2008b). Choosing a wound dressing, part 2. *Nursing2008, 38*(2), 14-15.

Baranoski, S., & Ayello, E. (2005). Using a wound assessment form. *Nursing2005, 35*(3), 14-15.

Beattie, S. (2007). Wound dehiscence. *RN, 70*(6), 34-37.

Bergstrom, N., Bennett, M.A., Carlson, C.E., et al. (1994). *Treatment of Pressure Ulcers: Clinical Practice Guideline No. 15* (AHCRP Publication No. 95-0652). Rockville, MD: Agency for Healthcare Research and Policy.

Bonham, P. (2007). Pressure ulcers: A review of successful strategies for risk assessment and staging. *ADVANCE for Nurses, 4*(23), 21-25.

Braden, B.J., & Maklebust, J. (2005). Preventing pressure ulcers with the Braden scale. *American Journal of Nursing, 105*(6), 70-72.

Brett, D.W. (2006). A review of moisture-control dressings in wound care. *Journal of Wound, Ostomy, and Continence Nursing, 33*(65), 53-58.

Brienza, D.M., & Geyer, M.J. (2005). Using support surfaces to manage tissue integrity. *Advances in Skin & Wound Care, 18*, 151-156.

Calianno, C., & Jakubek, P. (2006a). Wound bed preparation: The key to success for chronic wounds, part I. *Nursing2006, 36*(2), 70-71.

Calianno, C., & Jakubek, P. (2006b). Wound bed preparation: The key to success for chronic wounds, part II. *Nursing2006, 36*(3), 76-77.

Calianno, C., & Jakubek, P. (2007). The need to debride. *Nursing Made Incredibly Easy!, 5*(2), 7-10.

Calianno, C., & Martin-Boyan, A. (2005). Snap judgments: Should I photograph my patient's wound? *Nursing2005, 35*(2), 28-29.

Catania, K., Huany, C., James, P., et al. (2007). PUPPI: The pressure ulcer prevention protocol interventions. *American Journal of Nursing, 107*(4), 44-52.

Collins, N. (2004). Adding vitamin C to the wound management mix. *Advances in Skin & Wound Care, 17*, 109-112.

Debelak, S., Estapa, A., Piercey, A., et al. (2004). *Wound V.A.C.—KCI Protocol.* Available at: www.mc.vanderbilt.edu/surgery/trauma/egs/EGSProtocols/WoundVac.pdf.

Duhon, J. (2007). Taking the pressure out of pressure ulcer therapy. *RN, 70*(2), 25-31.

Frantz, R.A. (2005). Identifying infection in chronic wounds. *Nursing2005, 35*(7), 73.

Frantz, R.A. (2006). Uncover the clues to wound infection. *Nursing Made Incredibly Easy!, 4*(5), 10, 12.

Fuller, J. (2007). Help prevent deadly infections when using pulsed lavage. *LPN2007, 4*(5), 9.

Gallagher, S., Langlois, C., Spachy, D.W., et al. (2004). Preplanning with protocols for skin and wound care in obese patients. *Advances in Skin & Wound Care, 17*, 436-441.

Glenn, Y. (2006). When your patient is sensitive to tape. *Nursing2006, 36*(1), 17.

Greer, K.A. (2005). Maggots: Age-old therapy gets new approval. *Home Healthcare Nurse, 23,* 419-420.

Guillett, S.E. (2006). Using a rehabilitation approach to wound care. *Home Healthcare Nurse, 24,* 434-438.

Gupta, S. (2004). Guidelines for managing pressure ulcers with negative pressure wound therapy. *Advances in Skin & Wound Care, 17*(Suppl), 2-15.

Hanson, D., Langemo, D., Anerson, J., et al. (2007). Measuring wounds. *Nursing2007, 37*(2), 18, 21.

Hess, C.T. (2005). The art of skin and wound documentation. *Home Healthcare Nurse, 23,* 502-513.

Hess, C.T., & Trent, J.T. (2004). Incorporating laboratory values in chronic wound management. *Advances in Skin & Wound Care, 17,* 378-386.

Home Healthcare Nurse Eds. (2005). New best practice guidelines for managing pressure ulcers with negative pressure wound therapy published. *Home Healthcare Nurse, 23,* 469.

Kent, D.J. (2007). Getting misty over wound care. *Nursing2007, 37*(9), 36-37.

Lagemo, D., & Hanson, D. (2007). Sizing up your patients' wounds. *LPN2007, 4*(1), 29-30.

Lindsay-Garvey, J. (2005). Long road to wound healing. *NurseWeek, 18*(10), 22-26.

LPN2007 Eds. (2007). Tips for proper wound irrigation. *LPN2007, 4*(4), 27-28.

LPN2008 Eds. (2008a). Assessing the nutritional status of wound-care patients. *LPN2008, 4*(3), 23-26.

LPN2008 Eds. (2008b). Three techniques for collecting wound specimens. *LPN2008, 4*(1), 24-25.

Maklebust, J. (2005). Choosing the right support surface. *Advances in Skin & Wound Care, 18,* 158-161.

Mendez-Eastman, S. (2007). Give stubborn wounds a helping hand. *Nursing Made Incredibly Easy!, 5*(5), 18-20.

Newman, M., Ronel, D.N., Levine, D.S., et al. (2005). Management of a complex Achilles wound. *Advances in Skin & Wound Care, 18,* 83.

Nursing2004 Eds. (2004). Choosing a debridement method. *Nursing2004, 34*(5), 26-27.

Nursing Made Incredibly Easy! Eds. (2007). A fount of wound irrigation tips. *Nursing Made Incredibly Easy!, 4*(1), 14-15.

Nursing Made Incredibly Easy! Eds. (2008). Understanding traumatic wounds. *Nursing Made Incredibly Easy!, 6*(3), 7-10.

Posthauer, M.E. (2005). Hydration: An essential nutrient. *Advances in Skin & Wound Care, 18,* 32-33.

Pullen, R.L. (2005). Tips for using dry heat therapy. *Nursing2005, 35*(12), 18.

Pullen, R.L. (2007). Assessing skin lesions. *Nursing2007, 37*(8), 44-45.

Rushing, J. (2007). Obtaining a wound culture specimen. *Nursing2007, 37*(11), 18.

Salcido, R. (2005). Using our senses in wound care. *Advances in Skin & Wound Care, 18,* 8.

Sardina, D. (2007). Managing and preventing skin tears. *LPN2007, 3*(5), 27-29.

Sarvis, C.M. (2007). Using antiseptics to manage infected wounds. *Nursing2007, 37*(12), 20-21.

Stotts, N.A., & Sparacino, P.S.A. (2005). Assessing the patient with a wound as the basis for home care wound management. *Home Healthcare Nurse, 23,* 83-92.

Wipke-Tevis, D.D., & Sae-sia, W. (2004). Caring for vascular leg ulcers. *Home Healthcare Nurse, 22,* 237-247.

Worley, C.A. (2005). So, what do I put on this wound? Making sense of the wound dressing puzzle: Part II. *Dermatology Nursing, 17,* 204-205.

Zulkowski, K., & Ratliff, C. (2006). Perineal dermatitis or pressure ulcer: How can you tell? *Nursing2006, 36*(12), 22-23.

Chapter 39

Barry, M.E. (2001). Ankle sprains. *American Journal of Nursing, 101*(10), 40-42.

Bennett, P.C. (2007). Foot care: Prevention of problems for optimal health. *Home Healthcare Nurse, 24,* 325-329.

Bonner, S.M. (2007). Fixate on pin site care. *Nursing Made Incredibly Easy!, 5*(4), 22-23.

Bryant, G. (2001). Stump care. *American Journal of Nursing, 101*(2), 67-71.

D'Arcy, Y. (2006). Easing the pain after total joint replacement. *LPN2006, 2*(5), 7-8.

Family Doctor.org. (2005). *Cast care.* Available at: http://familydoctor.org/094.xml?printxml.

Gore, T., & Lacey, S. (2005). Bone up on fat embolism syndrome. *Nursing2005, 35*(8), 32hn1-32hn4.

Habel, M. (2006). Back in action with joint replacements, Part I. *NurseWeek, 19*(20), 15-16.

Hayes, D.D. (2003). How to wrap a below-the-knee amputation stump. *Nursing2003, 33*(2), 28.

LPN2005 Eds. (2005). Getting patients back on their feet. *LPN2005, 2*(5), 15-16.

McConnell, E.A. (2000). Applying a two-piece cervical collar. *Nursing2000, 30*(11), 24.

McConnell, E.A. (2002a). Myths and facts . . . about compartment syndrome. *Nursing2002, 32*(2), 92.

McConnell, E.A. (2002b). Teaching your patient to use a stationary walker. *Nursing2001, 31*(10), 17.

Nursing Made Incredibly Easy! Eds. (2005a). Strains and sprains explained. *Nursing Made Incredibly Easy!, 3*(6), 72.

Nursing Made Incredibly Easy! Eds. (2005b). When the pressure's just too much. *Nursing Made Incredibly Easy!, 3*(2), 53-54.

Olsen, E.V. (1990). The hazards of immobility. *American Journal of Nursing, 90*(3), 43-52. [Classic reference]

Parsons, K.S., Galinsky, T.L., & Waters, T. (2006). Preventing musculoskeletal disorders in home healthcare workers. *Home Healthcare Nurse, 24,* 158-163.

Smith, B. (2005). How to manage that pelvic fracture. *RN, 68*(8), 30-31.

Stewart, K.B. (2000). Open fracture. *Nursing2000, 30*(11), 33.

Tovornik, M., & D'Arcy, Y. {2007). How to control pain and improve functionality after total joint replacement surgery. *Nursing2007, 37*(6 Suppl.), 2-5.

Wollman, S. (2003). Sprains and strains. *Nursing2003, 33*(9), 47.

Chapter 40

Alden, L. (2003). Helping patients and families transition to nursing home care. *Home Healthcare Nurse, 21,* 568.

American Academy of Ophthalmology. (2007). *Antioxidant supplements and age-related macular degeneration.* Available at: http://one.aao.org/printerfriendly.aspx?cid=cb2232ca-253F-4d0d-b136-dda5451-d8e45.

American Dietetic Association. (2000). *Manual of Clinical Dietetics* (6th ed.). Chicago: Author.

Anderson, M.A. (2003). *Caring for Older Adults Holistically* (3rd ed.). Philadelphia: F.A. Davis.

Avidan, A., & Chervin, R.D. (2006). Insomnia in elderly. *ADVANCE Newsmagazines for LPNs.* Available at: http://lpn.advanceweb.com/common/editorial/PrintFriendly.aspx?CC=69021.

Banschbach, M.W. (2002). Nutritional support for the prostate gland. *Townsend Letter for Doctors and Patients.* Available at: www.encyclopedia.com/printable.aspx?id=1G1:86387598.

Brager, R. (2006). Polypharmacy: A hazard to your older patient's health? *LPN2006, 2*(5), 12-15.

Bright, L. (2005). Strategies to improve the patient safety outcome indicator: Preventing or reducing falls. *Home Healthcare Nurse, 23,* 29-36.

Busko, J., & Lie, D. (2006). *Physical fitness contributes to successful mental aging.* Available at: www.medscape.com/viewarticle/545924.

Centers for Disease Control and Prevention. (2007). *Falls among older adults: An overview.* Available at: www.cdc.gov/ncipc/factsheets/adultfalls.htm.

Gallagher, B. (2001). Managing pain in elderly patients at home. *Nursing2001, 31*(8), 18.

Ganz, D.A. (2007). Falls and the elderly: Two simple questions can determine who's at high risk. *Journal of the American Medical Association, 297,* 77-86.

Grogan, T., & Pater, K.S. (2006). Keep our older patients out of medication trouble. *Nursing2006, 36*(9), 44-45.

Jasniewski, J. (2006). Putting a lid on medication-related falls. *Nursing2006, 36*(6), 22-24.

Lorenz, J.M. (2007). Sex & the older adult. *ADVANCE for Nurses, 4*(13), 14-17.

LPN2006 Eds. (2006). Maintaining mobility. *LPN2006, 2*(2), 44.

Mauk, K. (2005). Keeping an older adult on her toes with exercise. *Nursing2005, 35,* 24.

Mcreynolds, J.L., & Rossen, E.K. (2004). Importance of physical activity, nutrition, and social support for optimal aging. *Clinical Nurse Specialist, 18,* 200-206.

Murphy, K. (2007). Is your older patient depressed? *Nursing2007, 37*(6), 22-23.

National Institutes of Health. (2007). *Study sheds new light on intimate lives of older Americans: Older adults are active despite increased sexual problems with age.* Available at: www.niapublications.org/agepages/sexuality.asp.

Neal-Boylan, L. (2007). Health assessment of the very old person at home. *Home Healthcare Nurse, 25,* 388-398.

Palmer, M.H., & Newman, D.K. (2004). Bladder matters: Urinary incontinence in nursing homes. *American Journal Nursing, 104*(11), 57-59.

Podell, R. (1996). Herbal treatments for prostate enlargements. *Nutrition Science News, 1*(9), 12.

Resnick, B. (2005). Exercise for older adults. *ADVANCE for Nurses, 2*(4), 19-21.

Resnick, B. (2006). Improving care of older adults: You can make a difference. *Geriatric Nursing, 27,* 70-72.

Shepler, S.A., Grogan, T.A., & Steinmetz, K. (2007). Helping older patients avoid medication mishaps. *LPN2007, 3*(4), 7-10.

Steffen, K.A. (2003). When your trauma patient is over 65. *Nursing2003, 33*(4), 53-56.

Tanner, E.K. (2003). Assessing home safety in homebound older adults. *Geriatric Nursing, 24,* 250-254.

Truglio-Londrigan, M., & Gallagher, L.P. (2003). Using the seven A's to determine older adults' community resource needs. *Home Healthcare Nurse, 21,* 827-831.

Urinary Incontinence Guideline Panel. (1992). *Urinary Incontinence in Adults: Clinical Practice Guidelines No. 2* (DHHS Publication No. 92-0038). Rockville, MD: Agency for Health Care Policy and Research.

Wallace, M.A. (2008). Assessment of sexual health in older adults. *American Journal of Nursing, 108*(7), 52-60.

Whiteside, M.M., Wallhagen, M.I., & Pettengill, E. (2006). Sensory impairment in older adults: Part 2. Vision loss. *American Journal of Nursing, 106*(11), 52-61.

Wooten, J., & Galavis, J. (2005). Polypharmacy: Keeping the elderly safe. *RN, 68*(8), 44-50.

Zulkowski, K. (2003). Protecting your aging patient's skin. *Nursing2003, 33*(1), 84.

Chapter 41

Alzheimer's Association of Los Angeles. (2007). *Sundowning: Just the facts.* Available at: www.alzla.org/dementia/sundowning.html.

Apply Now Newsletter. (2007). *Sundowning, Alzheimer's disease and dementia.* Available at: http://alzheimers.about.com/od/practicalcare/a/Sundowning.htm.

Arnold, E. (2004). Sorting out the 3 D's: Delirium, dementia, depression. *Nursing2004, 34*(6), 36-42.

Barclay, L. (2007). Fighting depression and improving cognition with omega-3 fatty acids. *Life Extension, 13*(10), 65-70.

Burgess, A.W., & Clements, P.T. (2006). Information processing of sexual abuse in elders. *Journal of Forensic Nursing, 2,* 113-120.

Egan, K.A., & Horvath, G.L. (2006). Family caregiving in the last years of life: Positive experiences in the midst of suffering. *Home Healthcare Nurse, 24,* 554-558.

Evans, L.K., & Cotter, V.T. (2008). Avoiding restraints in patients with dementia. *American Journal of Nursing, 108*(3), 40-49.

Gray-Vickrey, P. (2005). Elder abuse: Are you prepared to intervene? *LPN2005, 1*(2), 39-43.

Greenberg, S. (2007). The geriatric depression scale: Short form. *American Journal of Nursing, 107*(10), 60.

Hajduk, D.B., & Shellenbarger, T. (2004). When dementia complicates care. *RN, 67*(1), 50-55.

Harvath, T.A. (2008). What if Maslow was wrong? *American Journal of Nursing, 108*(4), 11.

Hindelang, M. (2006). Honoring our elders: Hearing their stories, respecting their ways. *Home Healthcare Nurse, 24,* 294-297.

Jech, A.O. (2002). Elder abuse: Mistreatment of older Americans on the rise. *NurseWeek, 15*(23), 23-24.

Keefe, S. (2008). Aging & depression: Geriatric depression calls for long-term follow-up. *ADVANCE for Nurses, 5*(12), 17-18.

Knox, E.A. (2007). *Tips on . . . sundowning.* Available at: www.ec-online.net/Knowledge/articles/sundowntip.html.

Laun, L. (2003). Benefits of pet therapy in dementia. *Home Healthcare Nurse, 21,* 49-52.

Leff, E.W., & Sonstegard-Gamm, J. (2006). The home care team approach to self-neglecting elders. *Home Healthcare Nurse, 24,* 249-257.

Lewis, T.P. (2008). Assessing an older adult for alcohol use disorders. *Nursing2008, 38*(6), 60-61.

Meeks-Sjostrom, D. (2004). A comparison of three measures of elder abuse. *Journal of Nursing Scholarship, 36,* 247-250.

National Institute on Aging. (2007). *Mourning the death of a spouse.* Available at: www.nia.nih.gov/HealthInformation/Publications/spouse.htm.

Rader, J., Barrick, A.L., Hoeffer, B., et al. (2006). The bathing of older adults with dementia. *American Journal of Nursing, 106*(4), 40-48.

Rasin, J. (2004). Bathing patients with dementia. *American Journal of Nursing, 104*(3), 30-33.

Roberson, L. (2003). The importance of touch for the patient with dementia. *Home Healthcare Nurse, 21,* 16-18.

Robinson, K.M. (2003). Understanding hypersexuality: A behavioral disorder of dementia. *Home Healthcare Nurse, 21,* 43-47.

Russo-Meck, P.A. (2004). Nurses can help older drivers steer clear of trouble. *NurseWeek, 17*(22), 31-32.

Schumacher, K., Beck, C.A., & Marren, J.M. (2006). Family caregivers: Caring for older adults, working with their families. *American Journal of Nursing, 106*(8), 40-48.

Stern, S., & O'Boyle, R. (2007). Successful aging: Optimizing life in the second half. Available at: www.ec-online.net/Knowledge/Articles/successfulaging.html.

Turkoski, B.B. (2003). Is this elder abuse? *Home Healthcare Nurse, 21,* 518-521.

Wallace, M., & Shelkey, M. (2008). Monitoring functional status in hospitalized older adults. *American Journal of Nursing, 108*(4), 64-71.

Wood, D.A. (2006). Elder abuse: Vulnerable seniors need nurse's help. *NurseWeek, 19*(24), 16.

Yesavage, J.A., Brink, T.L., Rose, T.L., et al. (1983). Development and validation of a geriatric depression screening scale: A preliminary report. *Journal of Psychiatric Research, 17,* 37-49.

Illustration Credits

Chapter 1

Figures 1-1, 1-2, 1-3, 1-4, Photos courtesy of The American National Red Cross. **Figure 1-5,** Courtesy of the U.S. National Library of Medicine.

Chapter 2

Figure 2-2, Modified from Ignatavicius, D.D., & Workman, M. L. (2002). *Medical-Surgical Nursing: Critical Thinking for Collaborative Care* (4th ed.). Philadelphia: Saunders. **Figure 2-3,** From deWit, S.C. (1998). *Essentials of Medical-Surgical Nursing* (4th ed.). Philadelphia: Saunders.

Chapter 3

Figure 3-1, Courtesy Bassett Healthcare, Cooperstown, New York.

Chapter 5

Figure 5-1, Courtesy Marian Medical Center, Santa Maria, California.

Chapter 6

Figure 6-1, From Ignatavicius, D.D., & Hausman, K.A. (1995). *Clinical Pathways for Collaborative Practice.* Philadelphia: Saunders.

Chapter 7

Figure 7-1, Created by Susan deWit (SCD) RN; Carolyn Sims (CJS) LPN. **Figures 7-6, 7-7,** From Burke, L.J., & Murphy, J. (1995). *Charting by Exception Applications: Making It Work in Clinical Settings.* Albany, New York: Delmar. **Figure 7-11,** Courtesy Solvang Lutheran Home, Solvang, California. **Figure 7-13,** from Potter, P.A., & Perry A.G. (2005). *Fundamentals of Nursing* (6th ed.). St. Louis: Mosby.

Chapter 10

Figure 10-3, From deWit, S.C. (2009). *Clinical Quick Reference for Medical-Surgical Nursing: Concepts and Practice,* Philadelphia: Saunders.

Chapter 11

Figure 11-4, From Bowden, V.R., Dickey, S.B., & Greenberg, C. S. (1998). *Children and Their Families.* Philadelphia: Saunders.

Chapter 16

Figure 16-2, From Kumar, V., Cotran, R.S., & Robbins, S.L. (2003). *Basic Pathology* (7th ed.). Philadelphia: Saunders.

Chapter 17

Figure 17-5, From Phippen, M.L., & Wells, M.P. (2000). *Patient Care During Operative and Invasive Procedures.* Philadelphia: Saunders.

Chapter 19

Figure 19-2, copyright 1998 by Barbara Braden and Nancy Bergstrom. Reprinted with permission. **Figure 19-4,** Modified from Ignatavicius, D.D., & Workman, M.L. (2002). *Medical-Surgical Nursing: Critical Thinking for Collaborative Care* (4th ed.). Philadelphia: Saunders.

Chapter 20

Figure 20-4, Courtesy NOC,• watch, Inc., Crystal Bay, Nevada. Figure 20-5, From deWit, S.C. (2009). *Medical-Surgical Nursing: Concepts and Practice.* Philadelphia: Saunders.

Chapter 21

Figure 21-5, From Elkin, M.K., Perry, A.G., & Potter, P.A. (2008). *Nursing Interventions & Clinical Skills* (4th ed.). St Louis: Mosby. **Figure 21-6,** Courtesy R.G. Medical Diagnostics, Southfield, Michigan. **Figure 21-12,** From Jarvis, C. (2004). *Physical Examination and Health Assessment* (4th ed.). Philadelphia: Saunders. **Figure 21-17,** Courtesy Critikon Inc., Tampa, Florida. **Figure 21-18,** Courtesy Marian Medical Center, Santa Maria, California.

Chapter 22

Figures 22-1, 22-4, 22-5, 22-14, 22-15, From Jarvis, C. (2004). *Physical Examination and Health Assessment* (4th ed.). Philadelphia: Saunders. **Figure 22-6,** Courtesy Welch Allyn, Skaneateles Falls, New York. **Figure 22-10,** From deWit, S.C. (2009). *Medical-Surgical Nursing: Concepts and Practice.* Philadelphia: Saunders. **Figure 22-12,** Adapted from American Cancer Society. (1997). *Breast Self-Examination: A New Approach.* In deWit, S.C. (1998). *Essentials of Medical-Surgical Nursing* (4th ed.). Philadelphia: Saunders. **Unnumbered Figure 22-3 in Skill 22-2, Step 5,** Adapted from Ignatavicius, D.D., & Workman, M.L. (2002). *Medical-Surgical Nursing: Critical Thinking for Collaborative Care* (4th ed.). Philadelphia: Saunders.

Chapter 23

Figure 23-3, Courtesy Marian Medical Center, Santa Maria, California.

Chapter 24

Figure 24-1, From Grainger, R.G., Allison, D.J., Adam, A., & Dixon, A.K. (2002). *Grainger & Allison's Diagnostic Radiology,* (4th ed.). Philadelphia: Churchill Livingstone. **Figures 24-2, 24-6,** From Lewis, S.L., Heitkemper, M.M., Dirksen, S.R. et al. (2007). *Medical-Surgical Nursing: Assessment and Management of Clinical Problems* (7th ed.). St. Louis: Mosby. **Figure 24-3,** From deWit, S.C. (1998). *Essentials of Medical-Surgical Nursing* (4th ed.). Philadelphia: Saunders. **Figure 24-5,** Courtesy Siemans Burdick, Inc., Milton, Wisconsin.

Chapter 25

Figure 25-1, From Copstead, L.C., & Banasik, J.L. (2000). *Pathophysiology* (2nd ed.). Philadelphia: Saunders. **Figure 25-2,** From Leahy, J.M., & Kizilary, P.E. (1998). *Foundations of Nursing Practice: A Nursing Process Approach.* Philadelphia: Saunders. **Figure 25-3,** From Jarvis, C. (2004). *Physical Examination and Health Assessment* (4th ed.). Philadelphia: Saunders. **Figure 25-4,** From Thibodeau, G.A., & Patton, K.T. (2005). *The Human Body in Health & Illness* (4th ed.). St. Louis: Mosby. **Figure 25-5,** From Black, J.M., & Hawks, J.H. (2005). *Medical-Surgical Nursing: Clinical Management for Positive Outcomes* (7th ed.). Philadelphia: Saunders. **Concept Map 25-1,** Redrawn from Black, J.M., & Hawks, J.H. (2005). *Medical-Surgical Nursing: Clinical Management for Positive Outcomes* (7th ed.). Philadelphia: Saunders. From White, B. (1994). Maintaining fluid and electrolyte balance. In Bolander, V.B. (Ed.) (1994). *Sorensen and Luckmann's Basic Nursing: A Physiologic Approach* (3rd ed.). Philadelphia: Saunders.

Chapter 26

Figures 26-2, 26-3, From U.S. Department of Agriculture, Center for Nutrition Policy and Promotion (April, 2005) CNPP-15. **Figure 26-4,** Redrawn from U.S. Food and Drug Administration, Center for Food Safety and Applied Nutrition, November, 2004.

Chapter 28

Figure 28-7, Courtesy AirSep Corporation, Buffalo, New York. **Figure 28-12,** Courtesy Dale Medical Products, Plainville, Maryland. **Figure 28-13,** Courtesy Genzyme Surgical Products, Fall River, Massachusetts. **Figure 28-14,** From Harkreader, H., & Hogan, M.A. (2004). *Fundamentals of Nursing: Caring and Clinical Judgment* (2nd ed.). Philadelphia: Saunders. **Figure 28-15,** From Lewis, S.L., Heitkemper, M.M., Dirksen, S.R., et al. (2007). *Medical-Surgical Nursing; Assessment and Management of Clinical Problems* (7th ed.). Courtesy Atrium Medical Corporation, Hudson, New Hampshire. St. Louis: Mosby. **Figure 28-16,** Courtesy Becton, Dickinson and Company, Franklin Lakes, New Jersey. **Figure 28-20,** From Sorrentino, S., & Gorek, B. (2003). *Mosby's Textbook for Long-Term Care Assistants* (4th ed.). St. Louis: Mosby. **Unnumbered Figure 28-12 in Skill 28-7, Step 9B,** Redrawn from Black, J. M., & Matassarin-Jacobs, E. (1993). *Luckmann and Sorensen's Medical-Surgical Nursing: A Psychopathologic Approach* (4th ed.). Philadelphia: Saunders.

Chapter 29

Figure 29-10, From Elkin, M.K., Perry, A.G., & Potter, P.A. (2004). *Nursing Interventions and Clinical Skills* (3rd ed.). St. Louis: Mosby. **Figure 29-11,** From Black, J.M., & Hawks, J.H. (2005). *Medical-Surgical Nursing: Clinical Management for Positive Outcomes* (7th ed.). Philadelphia: Saunders.

Chapter 30

Figure 30-3, Courtesy C.B. Fleet Company, Lynchburg, Virginia. **Figure 30-8,** Courtesy Hollister, Inc., Libertyville, Indiana.

Chapter 31

Figure 31-4, From Wong D.L., Hockenberry-Eaton M., Wilson D., et al.: *Wong's Essentials of Pediatric Nursing* (6th ed.). St. Louis, 2001, p. 1301. Copyrighted by Mosby, Inc. Reprinted by permission. **Figure 31-5,** From Ignatavicius, D.D., & Workman, M.L. (2002). *Medical-Surgical Nursing: Critical Thinking for Collaborative Care* (4th ed.). Philadelphia: Saunders. **Figure 31-10,** Courtesy of SIMS Deltec, Inc., St. Paul, Minnesota.

Chapter 32

Figure 32-2, From Lindeman, C.A., & McAthie, M. (1999). *Fundamentals of Contemporary Nursing Practice.* Philadelphia: Saunders. **Figure 32-3,** Courtesy Cindy Steury-Lattz, MSN, RN, CS.

Chapter 33

Figure 33-1, Modified from Kee, J.L., & Hayes, E.R. (1997). *Pharmacology: A Nursing Process Approach* (2nd ed.). Philadelphia: Saunders.

Chapter 36

Figure 36-3, Courtesy Beckton Dickinson and Company, Franklin Lakes, New Jersey. **Figure 36-15,** From Potter, P.A., & Perry, A.G. (2005). *Fundamentals of Nursing* (6th ed.). St. Louis: Mosby. Courtesy IV House, St. Louis, Missouri.

Chapter 37

Figures 37-1, 37-5, Courtesy Southwest Washington Medical Center, Vancouver, Washington. **Figure 37-9,** From Lewis, S.L., Heitkemper, M.M., Dirksen, S.R., et al. (2007). *Medical-Surgical Nursing: Assessment and Management of Clinical Problems* (7th ed.). St. Louis: Mosby.

Chapter 38

Figures 38-1, 38-14, From Potter, P.A, & Perry, G.A. (2005). *Fundamentals of Nursing* (6th ed.). St. Louis: Mosby. **Figure 38-2,** From Habif, T.P. (1991). *Clinical Dermatology: A Color Guide to Diagnosis and Therapy* (2nd ed.). St. Louis: Mosby. **Figure 38-3,** From Ignatavicius, D.D., & Workman, M.L. (2002). *Medical-Surgical Nursing: Critical Thinking for Collaborative Care* (4th ed.). Philadelphia: Saunders. **Figure 38-5,** Redrawn from Potter, P.A., & Perry, G.A. (2005). *Fundamentals of Nursing* (6th ed.). St. Louis: Mosby. **Figures 38-12, 38-13,** Courtesy Kinetic Concepts, Inc., San Antonio, Texas. **Unnumbered figure 38-5 in Skill 38-2, Step 5,** From Leahy, J.M., & Kizilay, P.E. (1998). *Foundations of Nursing: A Nursing Process Approach.* Philadelphia: Saunders.

Chapter 39

Figures 39-2, 39-6, From deWit, S.C. (2009). *Medical-Surgical Nursing: Concepts and Practice* (1st ed.) Philadelphia: Saunders. **Figure 39-3, 39-4,** Courtesy Zimmer, Inc., Warsaw, Indiana. **Figure 39-7,** Courtesy Hill-Rom Company, Inc., Batesville, Indiana. **Figure 39-8,** Courtesy Kinetic Concepts, San Antonio, Texas. **Figure 39-9,** Courtesy Grant Dyna-CARE, Grant Airmass Corp., Stamford, Connecticut. **Figure 39-10,** Courtesy J.T. Posey Company, Arcadia, California.

Glossary

A

abduction Moving away from the midline of the body.

abortion Ending a pregnancy before the fetus is viable.

abscess A localized infection consisting of an accumulation of pus made up of debris from phagocytosis when microorganisms have been present.

absorption The uptake of substances into or across tissues (e.g., skin, intestine, and kidney).

acceptance Admission of reality, as in the reality of death; the final stage in the process of dealing with dying and death.

accountability Taking responsibility for one's actions.

achievement stage Life stage dealing with learning and successfully using your abilities.

acidosis An excess of acid or depletion of alkaline substances in the blood and body tissues.

active listening Listening with great concentration and focused energy.

active transport A force that can move molecules into cells regardless of their electrical charge or the concentrations already in the cell.

acupressure A technique that involves applying pressure to various points on the body to relieve pain or other symptoms.

acupuncture A technique that involves the insertion of extremely fine, sterile needles into various points of the body to relieve pain or other symptoms, restoring balance.

acute Sharp, severe; having rapid onset, severe symptoms, and short course.

acute illness An illness that develops suddenly and resolves in a short time.

acute radiation sickness (ARS) Illness that results when most or all of the body is exposed to a high dose of radiation, usually over a short period of time.

adaptation Adjustment in structure or habits.

adduction The act of drawing toward the median plane or toward the axial line of a limb.

adhesion Fibrous band that holds parts together that are normally separated.

adipose Fatty; composed of fat cells.

ADLs Activities of daily living bathing, dressing, grooming, cleansing teeth, shaving, toileting, etc.

advance directive Consent constructed before the need for it arises; it spells out a patient's wishes regarding surgery and diagnostic and therapeutic treatments.

adventitious Acquired; arising sporadically.

adventitious sounds Abnormal lung sounds elicited upon auscultation of the lungs during assessment.

adverse effects Very undesirable side effects with more serious consequences.

aerobic Needing oxygen to live and grow.

afebrile Without a fever.

affective domain Learning domain in which the material is presented in a way that appeals to the learner's beliefs, feelings, and values.

age-associated memory impairment Age-related changes in mental processes, such as a decline in short-term memory and cognitive skills.

ageism Prejudice against aging and aged persons.

aging Continual process of biologic, cognitive, and psychosocial change.

agnostic A person who doubts the existence of God because it can't be proved or disproved.

agonists Drugs that produce a response.

AHRQ Agency for Healthcare Research and Quality, which develops standards of practice based on research.

Airborne Precautions Same as Standard Precautions plus place patient in private room with negative air pressure or in room with a patient with the same infectious organism; wear a respirator when in room with the patient; keep susceptible persons out of patient's room; and limit patient's movement outside room.

alignment Arrangement in a straight line; bringing a line into order.

alkalosis Excess of alkaline or decrease of acid substances in the blood and body fluids.

allergen A substance (antigen drug, foreign protein, or toxin) that produces an anaphylactic (allergic) reaction.

alternative therapies Therapies that are not mainstream or commonly used in medicine in this country.

Alzheimer's disease A progressive, degenerative disease of the brain of unknown origin, resulting in the person's inability to process and integrate new information as well as retrieve memory.

ambulate Walk.

amino acid An organic compound; protein is composed of 20 amino acids.

ampule Small, sterile, all-glass or plastic container used for medication.

anaerobic Able to live and grow only when oxygen is absent.

analgesic Drug that relieves pain without causing loss of consciousness.

anaphylactic shock Serious and profound state of shock brought about by hypersensitivity to an allergen.

From Chabner, D.E. (2004). *The Language of Medicine* (7th ed.). Philadelphia: Saunders.

Pronunciation Guide to Key Terms
The markings ¯ and ˘ above the vowels (a, e, i, o, and u) indicate the proper sounds of the vowels.
When ¯ is above a vowel its sound is long, that is, exactly like its name; for example:

ā as in āpe	ī as in īce	ū as in ūnit
ē as in ēven	ō as in ōpen	

The ˘ marking indicates a short vowel sound, as in the following examples:

ă as in ăpple	ĭ as in ĭnterest	ŭ as in ŭnder
ĕ as in ĕvery	ŏ as in pŏt	

anaphylaxis Severe allergic reaction (hypersensitivity).

anemia Low red blood cell count.

anesthesia The loss of sensory perception.

angiography Method of injecting a dye into an artery and then obtaining an x-ray of blood vessels, tumors, and lesions.

anorexia nervosa Disorder in which the focus is on remaining thin, causing restriction of food intake to the point of danger.

anoxia Condition of being without oxygen.

antagonists Drugs that block a response.

antibiotic An agent that is capable of either killing or inhibiting the growth of microorganisms.

antibody An immunoglobulin molecule that has a specific amino acid sequence that gives it the ability to adhere to and interact only with the antigen that induced its synthesis.

anticipatory grieving Grieving that occurs before the loss actually happens.

antimicrobial A substance capable of either killing or suppressing the multiplication and growth of microorganisms.

antipyretic Relieving or reducing fever.

antiseptic A chemical compound used on skin or tissue to eliminate microorganisms.

anuria Absence of urine.

anus Opening of the rectum at the skin.

aphasia Difficulty expressing or understanding language.

apical pulse Pulse found over the apex of the heart; created as the left ventricle rotates against the chest wall during systole (part of the cardiac cycle).

apnea Absence of breathing.

apothecary system A system used for measuring and weighing drugs and solutions.

appliance Device or apparatus used for therapy or to improve function, including a pouch (bag) that attaches to the skin over an ostomy stoma to collect fecal matter or urine.

apprenticeship Situation where a worker learns a trade or profession by working with a master of the trade or profession.

approximate To close together, as in wound healing.

approximation Degree of closure of a wound.

apprenticeship Learning by doing.

aromatherapy The use of selected fragrances in lotions and inhalants in an effort to affect mood and promote health.

arrhythmia Any variation from the normal rhythm of a heartbeat; also called *dysrhythmia.*

arteriography Radiography of an artery or arterial system after injection of a contrast medium into the bloodstream.

ascites Abnormal accumulation of serous fluid within the peritoneal cavity.

asepsis Destruction and/or containment of infectious agents after they leave the body of a patient with an infectious disease.

aseptic Free of microorganisms.

aseptically Without introducing infectious material.

aspirate Pull back on the plunger of a syringe to see if fluid is obtained.

aspiration Withdrawal of fluid or cells.

assault The threat to harm another, or even to threaten to touch another without that person's permission.

assessment (data collection) Data-gathering activities for the purpose of collecting a complete, relevant database from which a nursing diagnosis can be made.

assignment The asking of ancillary, unlicensed personnel to perform certain duties or tasks.

assimilation The process by which members of a culture change their lifeways to become totally integrated into another culture.

assisted suicide Making available to patients the means to end their lives with knowledge that suicide is their intent.

asymptomatic Without symptoms.

atelectasis Collapsed or airless part of the lung; collapse of alveoli.

atheist A person who does not believe in the existence of God.

atherosclerosis The accumulation of fatty deposits on the walls of blood vessels.

atrophy A decrease in size or a wasting away of a cell, tissue, organ, or part.

auditory learning Learning through what is heard.

auscultation Listening for sounds produced within the body, usually with a stethoscope.

auscultatory gap Period where no sound is heard.

autocratic Leadership style of tight control and unlimited power.

autologous From one's own body.

autonomic Not subject to voluntary control.

autonomy Ability to function independently.

autopsy An examination of the body organs and tissues to determine the cause of death.

autotransfusion Reinfusion of a patient's own blood.

axillary Pertaining to the armpit.

B

baby boomers People born between 1946 and 1964.

bacteria Single-celled microorganisms lacking a nucleus, which reproduce about every 20 minutes.

baptism A religious sacrament marked by the symbolic use of water resulting in admission of the recipient into the community of Christians.

bargaining An attempt to make an arrangement whereby one gives something in order to gain something in return; the third stage in Kübler-Ross' stages of the grieving process.

basal metabolic rate (BMR) The rate at which heat is produced when the body is at rest.

battery Actual physical contact that has been carried out against a person's will.

behavior modification In psychology, a form of treatment used to change behavior by giving positive feedback for desired behavior and negative feedback for undesirable behavior.

behavioral objective Statement of desired change in behavior or addition to current behaviors and attitudes.

belief A conviction or opinion that one considers to be true.

benign senescence Normal physical changes of aging.

benign senescent forgetfulness Term used to describe age-related changes in mental processes, including a slight decline in short-term memory and cognitive skills.

bereavement The state of having suffered a loss by death.

beta-carotene Fat-soluble hydrocarbon found in dark green leafy vegetables and deep orange vegetables and fruits; converts to vitamin A in humans.

bevel Slanted part of a needle tip.

bias A positive or negative attitude or opinion that is unsupported by evidence.

bile Orange or yellow digestive fluid produced by the liver.

binder Support bandage that wraps around the breasts or abdomen and is secured with ties, Velcro, or elastic.

bioavailability The degree to which a drug or other substance becomes available to the target tissue after administration.

biofeedback A specialized relaxation technique using a machine that measures the degree of muscular tension with skin electrodes.

biohazard A biologic agent or condition that can be harmful to a person's health.

biologic theories Theories based on cellular function and body physiology.

biopsy Surgical excision of a small amount of tissue.

bioterrorism The release of pathogenic microorganisms into a community to achieve political and/or military goals.

Biot's respirations Respirations that are shallow for two or three breaths with a period of variable apnea.

bivalve Cut in half lengthwise.

blanch To turn skin white, or on darker skin, to become pale.

bleb A bump, or visible elevation of the epidermis.

body language Nonverbal communication.

body mass index (BMI) Ratio that uses height and weight to estimate fat values at which the risk for disease increases.

bolus Concentrated dose given in short period of time.

bonding Sense of attachment between two people.

bone A dense and hard type of connective tissue.

boomerang children Those who return to the parental home for a period of time.

bore Internal diameter of a needle.

bowel training program A program of timing bowel movements and then scheduling toileting to promote a regular evacuation time.

brachial pulse Pulse found over the brachial artery that can be felt in the upper arm.

bradycardia A slow pulse that is less than 60 beats per minute.

bradypnea Slow and shallow breathing.

brain death The permanent stopping of integrated functioning of the person as a whole; cessation of brain functioning.

bronchoscopy Inspection of the interior of the tracheobronchial tree through a bronchoscope.

bronchovesicular sounds Those lung sounds heard over the central chest or back.

bruit Abnormal sound heard on auscultation of an artery, a kind of swishing sound.

buccal Pertaining to or directed toward the cheek.

buffer A substance that by its presence in solution increases the amount of acid or alkali necessary to produce a unit change in pH.

bulimia An eating disorder characterized by episodic binge eating, followed by behaviors designed to prevent weight gain, including purging, fasting, use of laxatives, and excessive exercise.

burette Tubelike chamber that holds 150 mL of fluid.

bursa A small fluid-filled sac that provides a cushion at friction points in freely movable joints.

C

cachexia A profound and marked state of constitutional disorder; general ill health and malnutrition.

cannula Tube for insertion into a duct or cavity.

capitated cost A set fee is paid for every patient enrolled in the health network each year.

carbohydrate A chemical substance that contains only carbon, oxygen, and hydrogen; category of food.

carcinogen Any cancer-producing substance.

cardiac catheterization Introduction of a catheter into the heart chambers to confirm a diagnosis or to evaluate the extent of the disease process.

cardiac output The pulse rate multiplied by the stroke volume.

career Work that requires specific training; one's occupation or profession.

caries Dental cavities.

carotenoids Antioxidants that protect cells and tissues from damage by free radicals; shown to increase immunity, improve vision, and have a role in cancer prevention.

carotid pulse Pulse found over the carotid artery on the front side of the neck.

carrier An individual who harbors the specific organism of disease without manifesting symptoms and is capable of transmitting the infection.

cartilage A fibrous connective tissue that acts as a cushion.

case management system charting Documentation that tracks variances from the clinical pathway.

cast A rigid dressing, molded to the body while pliable, that hardens as it dries to give firm support.

cataract An opacity (not letting light through) of the lens of the eye, which impairs vision.

cathartics Agents that cause bowel evacuation.

catheter embolus Piece of catheter that travels through a vessel and lodges, obstructing blood flow.

catheterization Insertion of a tube into a body channel or cavity.

cellulitis An acute, spreading inflammation of the deep subcutaneous tissues and sometimes muscle, which may be associated with abscess formation.

centenarians People over 100 years old.

cephalocaudal Proceeding from head to tail.

cerumen A waxy substance secreted by the ceruminous glands; earwax.

chart *n.* Medical record; *v.* to document in the medical record.

charting Documentation of the nursing process, treatment, and associated care.

charting by exception Charting that focuses on deviations from predefined norms, using preset protocols and standards of care.

Cheyne-Stokes respirations Respirations that gradually become more shallow and are followed by periods of apnea (no breathing), with repetition of the pattern.

chi'i Universal life force or energy.

chills Sensations of cold and shaking of the body.

chiropractic A science based on the theory that health and disease are related to the function of the nervous system; chiropractic manipulation involves adjustment and manipulation of the joints and adjacent tissues, particularly the spinal column.

cholesterol A component of fat found only in animal products.

chronic Persisting for a long time.

chronic illness Illness that develops slowly over a long period and lasts throughout life.

chyme Liquefied food and digestive juices

circadian rhythm A biologic rhythmic pattern that is regularly repeated every 24 hours.

circumcision Surgical removal of all or part of the penile foreskin.

circumduction Circular movement of a limb or of an eye.

clinical pathway/care map A collaborative type of plan of care referred to as an interdisciplinary care plan that provides a step-by-step approach to care of the patient.

closure To say goodbye to those people and things that are important.

cognitive The mental process of knowing, remembering, and relating; connected thinking.

cognitive domain Learning domain in which the learner takes in and processes information by listening to or reading the material.

collaborate To work or cooperate with another.

collaboration Working together in a joint intellectual effort.

collagen Fibrous structural protein of all connective tissue.

colon The part of the large intestine extending from the cecum to the rectum.

colonization Development of a bacterial infection; microorganisms take up residence and grow.

colonoscopy The inspection of the entire large intestine for polyps, areas of inflammation, and malignant lesions.

colostomy An artificial opening (stoma) created in the large intestine and brought to the surface of the abdomen for evacuating the bowels.

colostrum The first breast fluid.

colposcopy Gynecologic examination that uses the colposcope to examine the walls of the vagina and the cervix.

comfort care Identifying symptoms that cause the patient distress, and adequately treating those symptoms.

commode chair A chair with a container inserted to catch urine or feces.

communication The exchange of information and ideas by speech, writing, gesture, expression, body posture, intonation, and general appearance.

communion A Christian sacrament in which the bread of the Eucharist is distributed and consumed.

competent Legally fit (mentally and emotionally).

complementary protein Protein from plant sources.

complementary therapies Therapies that are used along with medical therapies to promote health.

complete blood count (CBC) Includes type and number of red blood cells, white blood cells, platelets, and hemoglobin.

complete protein One that contains all nine essential amino acids.

compliance Implementation by the patient of the therapeutic plan that has been established.

compress A pad of gauze or similar dressing, for application of pressure or medication to a restricted area, or for local applications of heat or cold.

computed tomography scan (CT scan) Through use of a computer, cathode ray tubes emit radiation at different depths to show density of tissues and organs, indicating malformations, tumors, and so on; also called computed axial tomography (CAT) scan.

computer-assisted charting Charting in which data are input via the computer.

computerized provider order entry (CPOE) The entering of provider orders into the medical record via computer, eliminating translation error due to poor handwriting or due to human translation error.

concept An idea, thought, or notion derived from experiences and information acquired from one's external environment; an element used in the development of a theory.

conception Union of ovum and sperm.

condom catheter A condom with a tube attached to the distal end that is attached to a drainage bag.

confidential Kept private.

confidentiality The principle of keeping private all information about a patient.

conflict resolution Resolving a conflict.

congestive heart failure Pump failure of the right or left ventricle associated with abnormal retention of fluid.

congruent In agreement.

conization Coring or removal of the mucous lining of the cervical canal and its glands by means of cutting with a high-frequency current; may be performed when a Pap smear indicates abnormal cells.

conscious Having awareness of oneself and one's acts and surroundings.

consent Permission given by the patient or his or her legal representative.

constipation Decreased frequency of bowel movement or passage of hard, dry feces.

constructive criticism Helpful comments to assist the person to improve some plan, action, or interaction.

Contact Precautions Standard Precautions plus never touch with bare hands anything wet that comes from a body surface or cavity; use gloves, impermeable gowns, masks, and protective eyewear when necessary.

contaminate To make unclean.

continuous positive airway pressure (CPAP) Gas (oxygen) delivered at positive pressure to keep open alveoli that would normally close upon expiration.

continuous quality improvement Process of continually evaluating nursing care to identify specific areas that need changes for improvement.

contracture Adaptive shortening of skeletal muscle tissue rendering the muscle highly resistant to stretching; prevents normal joint movement.

contraindications Reasons not to administer (a drug).

convalescence The process of recovering after an illness and regaining health.

convalescent Recovering, getting well.

co-pay The amount an insurance carrier requires the patient to pay for care.

coping Adjusting to or solving challenges.

core Circular piece cut out by the sharp edges of a needle; the center.

core temperature Temperature deep within the body.

coroner A person with legal authority to determine cause of death.

countertraction force The weight pulling against the weight of the traction.

crackles Abnormal, nonmusical sound heard on auscultation of the lungs during inspiration; also called rales.

creative behavioral therapy A psychosocial intervention that includes art, music, and humor, and that can allow for self-expression and alleviate anxiety and depression.

Credé's maneuver Massage from top of bladder to bottom by starting above the pubic bone and rocking the palm of the hand steadily downward.

crisis Abrupt decline in fever.

critical pathway/care map A step-by-step approach to the total care of the patient.

critical thinking Directed, purposeful, mental activity by which ideas are created and evaluated, plans are constructed, and desired outcomes decided.

cross-contamination Transmission of infectious microorganisms from one person or object to another.

cues Pieces of data or information that influence decisions.

cultural awareness Knowledge of a people's history and ancestry and an appreciation for their artistic expressions, foods, and celebrations.

cultural competence Knowing yourself, examining your own values, attitudes, beliefs, and prejudices.

cultural sensitivity Refraining from using offensive language, respecting accepted patterns of communication, and refraining from speaking in ways that are disrespectful of a person's cultural beliefs.

culture (1) The propagation of living organisms or tissue in special media conducive to their growth; (2) values, beliefs, and practices shared by the majority within a group of people.

culture shock Confusion and anxiety confronting a person who is suddenly exposed to a foreign culture.

curandero, -a A Hispanic-American folk healer.

curative surgery Surgery that alleviates or cures a problem.

custom A practice followed by a particular group or region.

cyanosis Bluish discoloration or skin color changes, particularly around the mouth and in the nail beds, due to lack of oxygen.

cystitis Inflammation of the bladder.

cystoscopy The visual inspection of the interior of the bladder for the collection of biopsy specimens, collection of urine separately from each ureter, and treatment of various conditions.

cytology The study of the structure, function, and pathology of cells.

D

dangling The patient position of sitting on the side of the bed with the legs and feet hanging over the side.

data Pieces of information on a specific topic.

database A collection of facts and figure for analysis from which conclusions may be drawn.

death, dying The cessation of all physical and chemical processes that invariably occurs in all living organisms; a stage of life.

débridement Removal of foreign or unhealthy tissue from a wound.

debris Dead tissue or foreign matter.

decision making Choosing the best actions to meet a desired goal.

deductible The amount an insurance carrier requires the patient to pay for care before beginning to pay expenses.

defamation Remarks made by one person about another person that are untrue, and the remarks damage that person's reputation.

defecate Expel feces.

defense mechanisms Strategies used to protect us from increasing anxiety.

defervescence Abatement of fever.

defining characteristics Signs and symptoms that must be present for a particular nursing diagnosis to be appropriate.

degrade Break down.

dehiscence Separation of the layers of the surgical wound; spontaneous opening of an incision.

dehydration Removal of water from a tissue.

delegate Authorize another person to do something; entrust to another.

delegation The assignment of duties to another person.

delirium An acute confusional state that can occur suddenly or over a long period as a result of an underlying biologic cause or psychological stressor.

dementia A neurologic condition characterized by the following cognitive defects: impaired memory, disturbed intellectual function, and inability to problem solve.

democratic Leadership style practicing social equality or majority rule.

demographics Statistics about populations.

denial Defense mechanism in which the existence of intolerable conditions is unconsciously rejected; first stage in the acceptance of death.

dependent nursing action Action requiring a physician's order.

depression A mental state characterized by feelings of sadness, despair, and discouragement, ranging from mild to major symptoms.

dermis The inner, fibrous layer of skin beneath the epidermis

diabetes mellitus A disturbance of the metabolism of carbohydrates and the use of glucose by the body.

diagnosis-related groups (DRGs) Use of a system by which a hospital receives a set amount of money for a patient who is hospitalized with a certain diagnosis.

dialects Regional variations of a language with different pronunciation, grammar, or word meanings.

diaphoresis Excessive sweat production; perspiration.

diarrhea Frequent loose stool.

diastole The phase or part of the cardiac cycle when the ventricles relax and fill with blood.

diastolic pressure the lower pressure exerted on the artery when the heart is at rest between contractions.

Dietary Reference Intakes (DRIs) Guidelines for estimating nutrient intake for planning and evaluating diets of healthy people.

diffusion The process by which substances move back and forth across a membrane until they are evenly distributed throughout the available space.

digestion The process of converting food into chemical substances that can be absorbed into the blood and utilized by the body tissue.

diluent Specified fluid used to dissolve a solute.

diplopia The perception of two images of a single object.

direct contact Contact of the caregiver's hands with a microorganism or with equipment and supplies that have been soiled by body secretions.

discharge planner RN or social worker who implements and organizes the plan for patient discharge.

discrimination To make a decision or treat persons based on a class or group to which they belong, such as race, religion, or sex.

disease A pathologic process with a definite set of signs and symptoms; disease causes illness.

disinfectant An agent that destroys infection-producing organisms.

distention The state of being stretched out or inflated.

distraction Technique of purposeful focusing of attention away from undesirable sensations and/or pain.

diuresis Increased excretion of urine.

do not resuscitate (DNR) Order written by a physician when the patient has indicated a desire to be allowed to die if breathing ceases or the heart stops.

documentation The recording of pertinent data on the clinical record.

dorsalis pedis pulse Pulse found over the dorsalis pedis artery, which is located just lateral to and parallel with the extensor tendon of the big toe in the foot.

dorsiflexion Backward flexion or bending, as of the hand or foot.

dorsum Back.

douche A stream of water or air directed against a part of the body or into a cavity.

Droplet Precautions Same as Standard Precautions plus place patient in private room with negative air pressure or in room with a patient with the same infectious organism; wear mask when in patient's room; and transport patient outside room only when necessary, with patient wearing mask if possible.

drug interaction Process occurring when one drug modifies the action of another drug.

durable power of attorney for health care A legal document that appoints a person chosen by the patient to carry out his or her wishes as expressed in an advance directive.

dysfunctional Not natural or normally functioning.

dyspareunia Abnormal pain during sexual intercourse.

dysphagia Difficulty swallowing.

dyspnea Difficult and labored breathing.

dysrhythmia An abnormal cardiac rhythm.

dysuria Painful urination.

E

ecchymosis Flat, hemorrhagic, blue or purplish patch on the skin or mucous membrane; bruising.

edema Fluid in interstitial spaces.

effluent Discharged fecal matter.

egalitarian A family/household with shared equality between men and women.

ego The problem solver and reality tester portion of the mind that develops with the person's interaction with the environment and the demands of the id. A component of the mind as postulated by Freud.

ego integrity Positive aspect of last psychosocial stage of life in which one reflects on one's achievements and feels self-satisfaction.

egocentric One who perceives everything from his or her own viewpoint and in his or her own way.

elder abuse Any type of abuse of the elderly.

elective Voluntary.

electroconvulsive therapy (ECT) Treatment that consists of electric shock to the brain, for severe depression that fails to respond to medication or psychotherapy.

electroencephalogram (EEG) Tracing of the brain waves.

electrolyte A mineral or a salt that is dissolved in body fluid.

electronic health record (EHR) A health record entered into a computer's software program that is updated via the computer.

embolus Clot that travels and lodges in a vessel.

embryonic Early formation stage of fetal development.

emergency admission Admission for which there is no prior planning.

empathy The ability to understand by seeing the situation from another's perspective.

empty nest syndrome Psychological syndrome occurring when children have left home, causing a sense of loss and sadness.

endorphins Naturally occurring opiate-like peptides that modify the perception of pain.

endoscope An instrument used to view inside a body cavity.

endoscopic retrograde cholangiopancreatography (ERCP) Examination of the biliary system done through a flexible endoscope following instillation of contrast medium into the ampulla of Vater of the pancreas.

endotoxin A heat-stable toxin associated with the outer membranes of certain gram-negative bacteria that is released when the cells are disrupted.

endotracheal Within the trachea.

environment The total of all elements and conditions that surround us and influence our development.

epidemiology Study of the distribution and determinants of health-related states and events in populations, and the application of this study to the control of health problems.

epidermis The outer, thicker layer of skin.

epidural Outside or above the dura mater.

epidural analgesia Analgesia injected into the epidural space outside the dura mater to relieve pain.

erythema Redness of the skin caused by congestion of the capillaries in the lower layers of the skin that occurs with any skin injury, infection, or inflammation.

eschar Slough produced by a thermal burn, corrosive material, or gangrene.

esophagogastroduodenoscopy (EGD) Endoscopic examination of the esophagus, stomach, and duodenum.

essential amino acid Amino acid that must be consumed through food sources.

estrogen replacement therapy (ERT) Hormone medication to replace estrogen levels depleted by menopause.

ethical code Actions and beliefs approved of by a particular group of people.

ethical principles Rules of right and wrong from a moral view.

ethics Actions and beliefs approved of by a particular group of people.

ethics committee A committee that looks at ethical issues of patient care and makes decisions as to whether unethical conduct has occurred, or whether a procedure or treatment would be ethical.

ethnic Referring to a group within a race usually differentiated by geographic, religious, social, or language differences.

ethnocentrism The tendency of human beings to feel that their way of thinking, believing, and doing things is the only way or the only right way.

etiologic factors The causes of a problem.

etiology Study of the cause of disease; origin.

eupnea A normal, relaxed breathing pattern.

euthanasia An easy or painless death; *active euthanasia*, or mercy killing, is the deliberate ending of the life of a person who is incurably and terminally ill; *passive euthanasia* is the withholding of heroic measures and allowing the person to die.

evaluation Judgment of the effectiveness of the intervention or plan.

evidence-based nursing Nursing practice based on validated research.

evisceration Extrusion of the viscera through a surgical incision; protrusion of an internal organ through the incision.

exacerbation Increase in severity of a disease or any of its symptoms.

excoriation Abrasion of the skin.

executive substage Stage of cognitive development of middle adults in which they delegate appropriately, juggle roles, and manage complex situations.

expected outcome A specific statement of the goal the patient is expected to achieve as a result of nursing intervention.

expectorate Cough up and spit out.

expiration Movement of air out of the lungs.

expire To breath out or exhale; to die.

extension posture Arms are stiffly extended, adducted, and hyperpronated with hyperextension of the legs and plantar flexion of the feet; indicates disruption of the motor fibers in the midbrain and brainstem; formerly called decerebrate posture.

external fixator Metal device inserted into or through one or more bones to stabilize fragments of a fracture while it heals.

extracellular Outside of the cell.

exudate Fluid in or on tissue surfaces that has escaped from blood vessels in response to inflammation, and that contains protein and cellular debris.

F

faith A belief that cannot be proven, or for which no material evidence exists.

false imprisonment Preventing a person from leaving a facility or restricting his or her movements within the facility.

fat An essential nutrient made up of fatty acids and glycerol that supplies a concentrated form of energy.

febrile A stage of fever in which the body temperature rises to the new set point established by the hypothalamus and remains there until there is resolution of the cause of the fever.

fecal impaction A collection of hardened feces in the rectum or colon.

fecal incontinence Involuntary passage of feces.

feces Intestinal waste material.

feedback Return of information and how it was interpreted.

feeding pump A pump used in continuous feedings that pumps the liquid formula, drop by drop, into the feeding tube.

femoral pulse Pulse found over the femoral artery in the groin.

fetal Late stage of prenatal development.

fever Elevated temperature.

fiber That portion of carbohydrate that cannot be broken down by intestinal enzymes and juices.

fibrin Insoluble protein essential to clotting.

fibrosis Formation of fibrous tissue.

filtration The movement of water and suspended substances outward through a semipermeable membrane.

first intention A type of wound healing (closure) for wounds with little tissue loss, such as a surgical incision.

fissure A narrow slit.

fistula An abnormal, tubelike passage within body tissue, usually between two internal organs or leading from an internal organ to the body surface.

flatus Intestinal gas released from the anus.

flexion posture Internal rotation and adduction of the arms with flexion of the elbows, wrist, and fingers, resulting from neurologic injury and interruption of voluntary motor tracts; extension of the legs may also be seen; formerly called decorticate posture.

fluoroscopy Examination by means of fluoroscope using x-rays displayed on a fluorescent screen.

focus charting Charging that centers on the patient from a positive perspective and having three components data, action, and response.

fornix/fornices Archlike structure(s).

Fowler's position A position arranged by elevating the head of the bed 60 to 90 degrees.

fructose Fruit sugar.

fungi Tiny, primitive organisms of the plant kingdom containing no chlorophyll that reproduce by means of spores; present in soil, air, and water.

G

gait Style of walking.

gait belt A sturdy belt made of tightly webbed canvas material that is used to ambulate and/or transfer the weak or unsteady patient.

gastrocolic reflex An increase in intestinal and colonic peristaltic activity following the arrive of food into the empty stomach.

gastroscopy The visual inspection of the upper digestive tract and the stomach to obtain specimens of gastric contents, and perform a biopsy on the stomach tissues

gastrostomy tube A feeding tube placed directly into the stomach through the abdominal wall.

gate control theory View of pain transmission as being controlled by a gate mechanism in the central nervous system.

gauge Scale of measurement.

gender The sex of an individual, male or female.

gender roles Behaviors and attitudes a culture expects and approves for males or females.

generalization The formation of a general principle or idea.

generativity Stage of life in which the person guides the lives of younger people.

generic name Drug name not protected by trademark.

genes Segments of DNA that carry the blueprints of development.

germinal Initial stage of prenatal development.

gerontologist A specialist in the study of aging people.

gingiva The part of the oral mucosa covering the tooth-bearing border of the jaw; the gum.

glaucoma The accumulation of fluid inside the eye, which exerts pressure on the optic nerve, eventually causing blindness.

glomerulus A small tuft or cluster of capillaries; it is the integral part of the nephron (the basic unit of the kidney), the function of which is to bring blood to the nephron.

glucometer Small device used to measure glucose content of capillary blood.

glucose The metabolized form of sugar in the body.

gluteal Pertaining to the buttocks.

glycosuria Glucose in the urine.

goal A broad statement describing what is to be accomplished over a specified period.

gram-negative Bacteria that lose the stain in Gram's method of staining.

gram-positive Bacteria that retain the stain in Gram's method of staining.

granulation tissue Connective tissue with multiple small blood vessels.

grief The total emotional response of pain and distress that a person experiences as a reaction to loss.

grieving process A process that occurs over a period of time as a person adapts to and moves through the pain of loss.

guaiac A reagent to test for blood in the stool.

guided imagery Guidance to use the imagination.

gurgles Wet sounds heard when auscultating the lungs; newer term for rhonchi; gurgle sounds also occur in the bowel.

H

half-life The time required for the plasma level of a drug to fall to half of a certain measured level.

halitosis Bad breath.

health The state of functioning well physically and mentally and expressing the full range of one's potentialities.

health care agent Person designated by the patient to make health care decisions when the patient is incapacitated (not able to make those decisions).

health care–associated infections (HAIs) An infection that occurs within a health care facility or because of a treatment or procedure.

health care proxy A person chosen by the patient to carry out the patient's wishes as expressed in an advance directive.

health maintenance organization (HMO) A type of group practice that enrolls patients for a set fee per month and provides a limited network of doctors, hospitals, and other health care providers from which to choose.

helminths Parasitic worms or flukes that belong to the animal kingdom.

hematemesis The vomiting of blood.

hematology Study of blood and its components.

hematoma Localized collection of clotted blood underneath the skin.

hematuria Blood in the urine.

hemiparesis Muscular weakness or partial paralysis affecting one side of the body.

hemiplegia One-sided paralysis.

hemolysis Rupture of erythrocytes with release of hemoglobin into the plasma.

hemoptysis Coughing up and spitting out of blood as a result of bleeding from the respiratory tract.

hemorrhoids Enlarged veins inside or just outside the rectum.

hemostasis Arrest of the escape of blood by either natural (clot formation or vessel spasm) or artificial (compression) means or the interruption of blood flow to a part.

hemothorax Collection of blood in the pleural cavity.

herbals Substances composed of herbs for health promotion.

hernia The abnormal protrusion of part of an organ or tissue through the structures normally containing it.

hierarchy The arrangement of objects, elements, or values in a graduated series.

HIPAA Health Insurance Portability and Accountability Act.

hirsutism Abnormal hairiness, especially in women.

histology Division of anatomy dealing with the structure, composition, and function of tissues.

HMO Health maintenance organization.

holistic Approach to health care that considers the biologic, psychological, sociologic, and spiritual aspects and needs of the person.

homeostasis A tendency of biologic systems to maintain stability in their internal environment while continually adjusting to changes necessary for survival.

hope An inner positive life force, a feeling that what is desired is possible.

hospice A program that provides a continuum of home and inpatient care for terminally ill patients and their families.

host An animal or plant that harbors and provides sustenance for another organism (a parasite).

human immunodeficiency virus (HIV) The causative agent for AIDS (acquired immunodeficiency syndrome).

humidifier A device that supplies moisture to a gas.

humidity The amount of moisture in the air.

hydrostatic pressure Pressure exerted by fluid.

hydrotherapy Massage or débridement by moving water.

hygiene The practice of cleanliness that is conducive to the preservation of health.

hypercalcemia An above-normal level of calcium in the blood.

hypercapnia Excess carbon dioxide in the blood.

hyperchloremia Abnormally high chloride in the blood.

hyperemia An excess of blood in a part.

hyperextension Extension of a limb or a part beyond the normal joint limit.

hyperglycemia Excess of glucose (sugar) in the blood.

hyperkalemia Excessive amount of potassium in the blood.

hypermagnesemia Excess magnesium in the blood.

hypernatremia An excess of sodium in the blood or a loss of body water.

hyperosmolality Increased concentration of solutes within the fluid.

hyperphosphatemia Excess phosphate in the blood.

hypertension Blood pressure elevated above the normal range.

hyperthermia Above-normal body temperature; *malignant hyperthermia:* a syndrome affecting patients undergoing general anesthesia, marked by a rapid rise in body temperature, signs of increased muscle metabolism, and rigidity.

hypertonic Of greater concentration; having a greater tonicity than blood.

hyperventilation A pattern of breathing in which there is an increase in the rate and depth of breaths and carbon dioxide is "blown off," causing the blood level of carbon dioxide to fall.

hypervolemia Abnormal increase in the volume of circulating blood.

hypnosis Therapeutic suggestion, involving inducing a trancelike state using focusing and relaxation techniques and giving the patient suggestions that may be helpful after the return to an alert state of consciousness.

hypocalcemia A below-normal level of calcium in the blood.

hypochloremia Abnormally low chloride in the blood.

hypoglycemia An abnormally low level of glucose (sugar) in the blood.

hypokalemia Abnormally low potassium in the blood.

hypomagnesemia Abnormally low magnesium in the blood.

hyponatremia Abnormally low sodium in the blood.

hypophosphatemia Decreased phosphate in the blood.

hypostatic pneumonia Pneumonia caused by stasis of lung secretions due to inactivity, which provides a medium for bacterial growth.

hypotension Abnormally low blood pressure.

hypothalamus The portion of the diencephalon lying beneath the thalamus at the base of the cerebrum, and forming the floor and part of the lateral wall of the third ventricle of the brain.

hypothermia Subnormal body temperature.

hypotonic Of lesser concentration; containing less solute than extravascular fluid.

hypoventilation Reduction in the amount of air entering the pulmonary alveoli, which causes an increase in the arterial carbon dioxide level.

hypovolemia Decreased volume of circulating blood.

hypoxemia A decreased amount of oxygen in the bloodstream.

hypoxia State of insufficient oxygen in the blood.

I

iatrogenic Referring to any adverse condition in a patient resulting from medical or surgical treatment.

id The body's basic primitive urges as postulated by Freud.

ideology A belief or value system.

idiopathic Of unknown origin.

ileostomy Opening surgically created at the ileum to divert intestinal contents after lower portions of the bowel have been surgically removed.

ileum The distal (farthest) portion of the small intestine, extending from the jejunum to the cecum.

illness Disease of body or mind.

imagery A set of mental pictures or images.

immobilization Rendering a part incapable of moving.

immune response Reaction of the body to substances interpreted as non-self.

immunity Security against a particular disease; nonsusceptibility to the invasive or pathogenic effects of foreign microorganisms or to the toxic effect of antigenic substances.

immunocompromised With poorly functioning immune systems.

impervious Not affording a passage.

implement To put into action.

implementation Performing an intervention and assessing the response.

incident report Documentation of an incident or occurrence that is out of the ordinary, including the facts, who was involved, and who discovered it.

incomplete protein One that does not contain all essential amino acids.

incongruent Verbal and nonverbal messages that do not agree.

incontinence (fecal) Lack of voluntary control over the anal sphincter.

incontinence (urinary) Inability to prevent passing urine.

incubation period The time from invasion of the body by the microorganisms to the onset of symptoms.

independent nursing action An action that does not require a physician's order, but does require critical thinking.

induration An area of the skin that feels hard.

infection Invasion and multiplication of microorganisms (e.g., bacteria and viruses) in body tissues, causing cellular injury.

infection prevention and control The use of medical and surgical asepsis and Standard Precautions to prevent or control the spread of microorganisms.

inferences Conclusions made based on observed data.

infiltrated When solution is deposited in tissue outside the vein.

inflammation Localized protective response brought about by injury or destruction of tissues, which serves to destroy or wall off the injurious agent.

infusion Slow introduction of fluid into a vein.

infusion pump An electronic pump that regulates the flow of an intravenous infusion.

inhaler An apparatus for administering vaporized or volatilized agents by inhalation, or for protecting the lungs from harmful substances in the air.

initiative Willingness to try.

injection The act of forcing a liquid into a part or organ of the body.

input Information put in.

insomnia Difficulty in getting to sleep or staying asleep at night.

inspection Visual examination for detection of abnormal signs or qualities.

inspiration Movement of air into the lungs.

instillation Administration of a liquid drop by drop.

Institute for Safe Medication Practices An institute formed to find ways to prevent medication errors.

insulin pump A programmable pump that delivers insulin directly into the body.

integrated delivery network A set of providers and services organized to deliver coordinated care to promote wellness, care for illness, and promote rehabilitation.

integument The skin covering the body.

integumentary System containing the skin (the largest organ of the body), hair, nails, sweat and sebaceous glands.

intelligence A combination of verbal ability, reasoning, memory, imagination, and judgment.

interdependent action An action that comes from collaborative care planning.

interferon Biologic response modifier that affects cellular growth.

interstitial Placed or lying between.

interstitial fluids Body fluids that are located in the tissue spaces around the cells.

interventions Nursing actions taken to improve, maintain, or restore health or prevent illness.

interview Conversation in which facts are obtained.

intimacy Close, meaningful relationship.

intracellular Within the cell.

intracellular fluid Body fluid that is within the cell walls.

intractable pain Pain that is resistant to treatment.

intradermal (ID) Into the dermis.

intramuscular (IM) Into the muscle.

intrathecal Pertaining to or within the spinal canal.

intrauterine Within the uterus.

intravascular Within a vessel or vessels.

intravenous (IV) Within a vein or veins.

intravenous pyelography (IVP) Injection of a dye into a vein to show urine flow through the renal pelvis, ureters, and bladder on x-ray.

interventions Nursing actions aimed at accomplishing a goal or expected outcome.

invasion of privacy A violation of the confidential and privileged nature of a professional relationship.

invasive procedures Procedures that require entry into the body.

irrigation Washing by a stream of water or other fluid.

ischemia Deficiency of blood in a part, usually due to functional constriction or actual obstruction of a blood vessel.

isolation The separation of infected individuals from those uninfected for the period of communicability of a particular disease; quarantine.

isometric Maintaining the same measurements; of equal dimensions.

isometric exercises Exercises performed against resistance.

isotonic Of equal solute concentration; solutions that have the same concentration, or osmolality, as blood and are used to expand the fluid volume of the body.

J

jaundice Yellowness of the skin, sclera, mucous membranes, and excretions resulting from hyperbilirubinemia and deposition of bile pigments; also called icterus.

jejunostomy or duodenal tube A feeding tube placed directly into the intestines through the abdominal wall.

jejunum That portion of the small intestine that extends from the duodenum to the ileum.

joint The union of two or more bones in the body.

jugular venous distention (JVD) Visible thickening of the jugular veins when the patient is positioned sitting in bed at a 15- to 35-degree angle; assessed as a sign of congestive heart failure or overhydration.

K

keloid Permanent raised, enlarged scar.

ketonuria Acetone bodies in the urine.

kinesiology The study of the movement of body parts, also known as body mechanics.

kinesthetic learning Learning by performing a task or handling items.

kinetic Moving.

Korotkoff sounds Sounds that relate to the effect of arterial wall vibrations during auscultation of blood pressure.

kosher properly prepared in accordance with Jewish dietary laws.

KUB x-ray X-ray of the kidneys, ureters, and bladder.

Kussmaul's respirations Respirations having an increased rate and depth with panting and long, grunting exhalations.

kwashiorkor A condition occurring in infants and young children soon after weaning from breast milk, due to severe protein deficiency.

kyphosis Increased curve in the thoracic spine.

L

laceration A torn, ragged, or mangled wound.

lactation The secretion of milk.

lacto-ovo-vegetarian A diet consisting of dairy products, eggs, and plant foods.

lactose Sugar derived from milk.

lactovegetarian A diet consisting of dairy products and plant foods.

laissez-faire A leadership style that is based on noninterference with what others desire.

laser Acronym for *l*ight *a*mplification by the *s*timulated *e*mission of *r*adiation.

Last Rites A religious rite performed by a clergyman to the individual just prior to death.

lateral position Positioned on the side.

law A rule of conduct established by government.

lesion Damaged tissue.

lethargy Abnormal drowsiness or stupor.

leukocyte White blood cell.

leukocytosis Increase in the number of leukocytes in the blood, due to infection or other causes.

leukoplakia A white patch on a mucous membrane that will not rub off.

liability Responsibility.

liable Responsible.

libel Written defamation.

libido The sex drive.

life span The number of years of a person's life.

ligaments Strong, fibrous connective tissues that support and strengthen the bones of joints.

lipids A group of substances comprising fatty, greasy, oily, and waxy compounds that are insoluble in water and soluble in nonpolar solvents, such as hexane, ether, and chloroform.

living will A document detailing the measures desired for treatment or to prolong life if the person becomes incapacitated; also called advance directives.

logrolling A technique used to turn a patient in bed as a single unit while maintaining straight body alignment at all times.

longevity Length of life.

lordosis Exaggerated lumbar curve.

loss To no longer have or possess an object, person, or situation.

lumbar puncture Insertion of a hollow needle into the subarachnoid space between the third and fourth lumbar vertebrae to withdraw samples of cerebrospinal fluid for analysis and to measure the pressure; also called spinal puncture and spinal tap.

lumen Opening or interior diameter of a needle; channel within a tube.

lymphocyte Any of the mononuclear, nonphagocytic leukocytes, found in the blood, lymph, and lymphoid tissues, that comprise the body's immunologically competent cells and their precursors.

lysis Breakdown, disintegration; also reduction or abatement.

M

maceration The softening of tissue that increases the chance of trauma or infection.

macrobiotic A type of diet consisting mostly of whole grains and beans.

macrodrops 10 gtt/mL of fluid.

macrophage Any of the mononuclear phagocytes found in tissues.

macular degeneration A disorder resulting in a loss of acute, central, and color vision.

magnetic resonance imaging (MRI) Noninvasive diagnostic method based on use of magnetic fields to visualizing soft tissue without the use of contrast media or ionizing radiation.

maladaptation Lack of adjustment.

malaise Discomfort, uneasiness, or indisposition, often indicative of infection.

malnutrition Poor nourishment resulting from improper diet or from some deficit in nutrition that prevents the body from using its food properly.

malpractice Incorrect or negligent treatment of a patient by persons responsible for health care.

managed care plan A health care plan in which all medical care is managed by the insuring group.

marasmus A form of protein-calorie malnutrition occurring chiefly in the first year of life, characterized by growth retardation and wasting of subcutaneous fat and muscle

massage Stimulation of the skin and underlying tissues with varying degrees of hand pressure to decrease pain, produce relaxation, and/or improve circulation.

mastication The act of chewing.

matriarchal A female-dominated family/household.

maturity State of being fully developed physically or emotionally.

meconium Dark-green mucilaginous material in the intestine of the full-term fetus; it constitutes the first stools passed by the newborn infant.

mediate To resolve or settle differences by working with all the conflicting parties.

Medicaid State medical care coverage for individuals and families with reduced or poverty level income.

medical asepsis The practice of reducing the number of organisms present or reducing the risk for transmission of organisms.

medical record (chart) A record that contains all orders, tests, treatments, and care that occurred during the time a person was under the care of a health care provider.

medical social worker (MSW) Individual who provides counseling and information regarding long-term planning, financial assistance, or available community services.

Medicare Health care provided through the Social Security Administration primarily for the elderly retired.

medication administration record (MAR) Patient record of drug orders and administration, on which nurses record the times doses of medication are given.

medication reconciliation A procedure used to compare medications ordered currently with those the patient normally takes at home or during the previous medical facility admission.

meditation Focusing on an image or thought.

melanin The main determinant of skin color.

melena Blood that has changed into a dark, tarry substance as it moves through the stomach or small intestine.

meniscus The curved, upper surface of a liquid being poured for dosage administration.

menopause Cessation of menstruation.

mentor Teacher or coach.

meridian Lines or passageways.

metabolism Cellular chemical reactions in the body.

metered-dose inhaler (MDI) A device that delivers a measured dose of an inhalant medication.

microdrops 60 gtt/mL of fluid.

microorganism Organism only visible with a microscope.

micturition Urination.

mineral An inorganic substance contained in animals and plants.

minister One who is authorized to perform religious functions in a Christian church.

mobility The ability to move in one's environment with ease and without restriction.

moleskin A soft material, often with an adhesive backing, used especially on the feet to protect against chafing.

morals Rules or standards regarding what is right or wrong.

Moro reflex Startle response of the newborn.

murmur A periodic sound of short duration of cardiac or vascular origin.

myocardial infarction (MI) Loss of blood supply to the heart muscle.

MyPyramid The USDA schematic and description of recommended foods and exercise for a healthy diet and lifestyle.

N

NANDA-I North American Nursing Diagnosis Association–International, which identifies, develops, and classifies nursing diagnoses; founded in 1973.

narcolepsy Recurrent, uncontrollable brief episodes of sleep during hours of wakefulness.

narcotic A drug that produces insensibility or stupor; legal definition refers to habit-forming drugs such as opiates and any of many synthetic drugs such as meperidine (Demerol).

nasogastric tube A type of tube that is placed through the nose into the stomach.

nebulizer A device that dispenses liquid in a fine spray, used in inhalation therapy.

necrosis Local death of tissue from disease or injury.

necrotic Of or pertaining to necrosis.

negligence Failing to do something a reasonably prudent person would do or doing something a reasonably prudent person would not do.

neonate Newborn.

nephron The structural and functional unit of the kidney, each nephron being capable of forming urine by itself.

neurotransmitter A substance (e.g., norepinephrine) that is released from the axon terminal of a presynaptic neuron on excitation, and that travels across the synaptic cleft to either excite or inhibit the target cell.

nocturia Voiding during the night.

nocturnal delirium The appearance of or increase of symptoms of confusion or agitation associated with the late afternoon or early evening hours, usually continuing into the night; also known as sundowning or sundown syndrome.

noncompliance When patients do not take the drugs that are prescribed for them on the schedule indicated by the prescription or do not adhere to a prescribed treatment regimen.

nonessential amino acid Amino acid that can be manufactured by the liver.

non–rapid eye movement (NREM) sleep The state of sleep when the body receives the most rest.

nonsteroidal anti-inflammatory drugs (NSAIDs) Drugs with anti-inflammatory properties that do not contain steroids.

nonverbal Without words.

nosocomial Infection acquired during hospitalization.

NPO No food or fluids by mouth.

nurse practice act State law defining the scope of nursing practice and the regulation of the profession by a state board for nursing.

nursing audit Examination of a series of patient records to determine if nursing care for those patients met particular standards.

nursing diagnosis Statement that indicates the patient's actual health status or the risk of a problem developing, the causative or related factors, and specific defining characteristics.

nursing implications Points the nurse needs to remember about a drug or needs to teach patients.

nursing process A goal-directed series of activities whereby the practice of nursing accomplishes its goal of alleviating, minimizing, or preventing real or potential health problems.

nursing theory Statement about relationships among concepts or facts, based on existing information.

nutrient A biochemical substance used by the body that must be supplied in adequate amounts from foods consumed.

nutrition The sum of processes involved in taking in nutrients and absorbing and using them.

nystagmus Involuntary, rapid, rhythmic movement of the eyeball.

O

obesity Excessive accumulation of body fat.

obituary A notice of death published in the newspapers.

objective data Information obtained through the senses or measured by instruments.

observe To see or notice; to watch attentively.

obturator A curved guide that is inserted into the trachea to facilitate placement of a tube.

occult Hidden or concealed.

Occupational Safety and Health (OSH) Act A law passed in 1970 to improve the work environment in areas that affect the worker's health or safety.

olfaction Smelling.

oliguria Diminished amount of urine formation.

one-time (single) order Order written for a drug to be given just one time.

ophthalmic Having to do with the eyes.

ophthalmoscope Lighted instrument used for viewing the interior of the eye.

ordinal position Birth order.

orientation Awareness of one's environment with reference to place, time, and people.

orthopnea The ability to breathe easily only in the upright position.

orthostatic hypotension A fall in blood pressure associated with dizziness, syncope (fainting), and blurred vision, which occurs upon standing; also called postural hypotension.

osmolality The concentration of a solution in terms of osmoles of solute per kilogram of solvent.

osmoreceptors Specialized neurons in the thalamus that are stimulated by increased extracellular fluid osmolality to release antidiuretic hormone (ADH) from the posterior pituitary.

osmosis The movement of pure solvent (liquid) across a membrane.

ostomy Diversion of intestinal contents from their normal path, resulting in an artificial opening into the intestine.

otic Having to do with the ear.

otoscope Lighted instrument used to visualize the tympanic membrane and interior of the ear canal.

ototoxic Having a damaging effect on the eighth cranial nerve (vestibulocochlear) or on the organs of hearing and balance.

outcome-based quality improvement (OBQI) A type of nursing audit that compares actual patient outcomes with desired outcomes so that measures to improve care can be devised.

outcomes Results of actions.

overhydration Excess fluid volume.

over-the-bed frame Rectangular frame to which traction equipment may be attached.

over-the-counter (OTC) Drugs that may be purchased without a prescription.

oximeter Device that measures oxygen in the blood.

oximetry Measurement of oxygen.

P

pain Feeling of distress or suffering, caused by the stimulation of nerve endings.

palliation The act of treating symptoms to relieve pain and provide comfort.

palliative Relieving symptoms when a disease cannot be cured.

palliative surgery Surgery to relieve pain or complications.

pallor Paleness of the skin.

palpate Feel.

palpation Touching with the hands and fingers.

panel Group of tests.

Papanicolaou (Pap) smear A microscopic laboratory examination used to determine the presence of malignant cells using body secretions (from the respiratory, genitourinary, or digestive tract).

paracentesis A needle puncture of the abdomen to remove ascites fluid, perform a lavage, or initiate peritoneal dialysis.

paralytic ileus Obstruction of the intestines from inhibition of bowel motility.

paranoia Behavior characterized by delusions of persecution and/or delusion of grandeur.

paraplegic Person who is paralyzed in the legs and lower part of the body.

parenteral Introduction of a substance into the body by some means other than the gastrointestinal tract.

paresthesia Feeling of numbness or tingling.

pastor A Christian minister.

patent Freely open (e.g., a patent drain).

pathogen Any disease-producing organism.

pathologic fracture Fracture due to weakening of the bone structure brought on by pathologic process, such as cancer and other diseases.

patient advocate One who speaks for, and protects the rights of, the patient.

patient-controlled analgesia (PCA) Analgesia doses controlled by the patient.

patriarchal A male-dominated family/household.

peak action The blood level at which a drug delivers its greatest action.

peers Others of similar age and background.

perception Being aware of something through the senses seeing, hearing, feeling, tasting, and smelling.

percussion Light, quick tapping on the body surface to produce sounds.

percutaneous endoscopic gastrostomy (PEG) tube A feeding tube placed directly into the stomach.

perfusion The act of pouring over or through, especially the passage of a fluid through the vessels of a specific organ; circulation of blood through tissue.

perioperative Period from the time of the decision to have surgery through recovery from the procedure.

periostomal Area around a stoma.

peripheral Situated away from a center or central structure.

peristalsis The action caused by muscle fibers in a tubular organ that propels contents through them in waves.

personal protective equipment (PPE) Items such as gloves, gowns, masks, protective eyewear, and hair covering used to protect the nurse from infectious organisms.

personal space Acceptable or comfortable space between two people when conversing.

petechiae Pinpoint, round, purplish red spots that are not raised; caused by intradermal or submucous hemorrhage; a significant sign for various diseases.

phagocytes Cells capable of ingesting particulate matter (e.g., macrophages).

phagocytosis The engulfing of microorganisms and foreign particles by phagocytes.

pharmacodynamics The study of a drug's effect on cellular physiology and biochemistry and the mechanism of action.

pharmacokinetics The study of how drugs enter the body, are metabolized, reach their site of action, and are excreted.

phimosis Constriction of the foreskin orifice causing inability to push the foreskin back over the end of the penis.

phlebitis Inflammation of a vein.

photophobia Abnormal visual intolerance of light.

phytotherapy Treatment by use of plants.

PIE charting A method of charting in which "P" means problem identification, "I" means interventions, and "E" means evaluation.

pigmentation The deposition of coloring matter in the skin.

pivot Turn or change direction with your feet while remaining in a fixed place.

placebo A medicinal preparation having no specific pharmacologic activity against the patient's illness or complaint, given solely for the psychophysiologic effects of the treatment; a dummy treatment.

planning Determining specific desired outcomes for each nursing diagnosis.

plantar flexion A reflex bending of the toes and foot.

platelet aggregation Clumping of platelets during wound healing.

pleural friction rub Grating or scratchy sound heard on auscultation of the lungs; caused when irritated pleural membranes rub over each other.

pneumonia Inflammation and consolidation of the lung with exudate.

pneumothorax An accumulation of air or gas in the pleural space, which may occur spontaneously or as a result trauma or a pathologic process, or be introduced deliberately.

PO By mouth; orally.

poison A substance that when it is ingested, inhaled, absorbed, applied, injected, or developed within the body, may cause functional or structural disturbances.

polypharmacy The use of multiple medications, often inappropriately and excessively, at the same time.

polyps Growths protruding from a mucous membrane.

polyuria Production of an excessive amount of urine.

popliteal pulse Pulse found over the popliteal artery at the posterior surface of the knee.

posterior tibial pulse Pulse found over the posterior tibial artery between the malleolus and the Achilles tendon in the ankle; also called *pedal pulse.*

postmortem After death.

postoperative After surgery.

postural drainage Removal of lung secretions by changes in the patient's position.

postural hypotension A fall in blood pressure associated with dizziness, syncope (fainting), and blurred vision that occurs upon standing; also called orthostatic hypotension.

practice act Defines activities in which nurses may engage, states the legal requirements and titles for nursing licensure, and establishes the education needed for licensure.

preferred provider organization (PPO) An organization that offers discounted insurance fees in return for a large pool of potential patients who choose a doctor from the list of those associated with the PPO.

prejudice A positive or negative attitude or opinion that is unsupported by evidence.

preoperative Before surgery.

prepuberty Beginning sexual development.

presbycusis Inability to hear high-pitched sounds and some spoken words; occurs in old age.

presbyopia Age-related decreased ability to focus the eye on nearby objects.

prescription A written direction for the preparation and administration of a remedy.

pressure ulcer An ulcer that forms from a local interference with circulation.

priest In many Christian churches, a member of the clergy who may administer the sacraments; in any number of religions, any person having the authority to perform and administer religious rites.

primary illness Illness that develops without being caused by another health problem.

primary intention A type of wound healing (closure) for wounds with little tissue loss, such as a surgical incision.

prions Proteinaceous particles believed to be responsible for transmissible neurodegenerative diseases.

prioritize To put in order of importance.

priority A right of first consideration established on the basis of emergency or need.

privilege Permission to do what is usually not permitted in other circumstances.

PRN Order written to give a medication when the patient requires it.

problem-oriented medical record (POMR) charting Charting that focuses on patient status, emphasizes the problem-solving approach to patient care, and provides a method for communicating what, when, and how things are to be done in order to meet the patient's needs.

proctoscopic examination Examination of the rectum with a lighted instrument.

proctosigmoidoscopy Examination of the rectum and sigmoid colon with a sigmoidoscope.

prodromal period Early or very beginning stage of an illness.

productive cough A cough that produces sputum or mucus.

prolapse The falling down or sinking of a part.

pronation Applied to the hand, the act of turning the palm posteriorly, performed by medial rotation of the forearm; applied to the foot, a combination of eversion and abduction movements.

prone position When the patient is lying face down.

prosthesis Artificial body part.

protective device A mechanical device that prevents a person from getting out of a room, bed or chair (no longer called a restraint); or drugs such as sedatives or tranquilizers used to sedate the patient so that he or she is unable to move about (no longer called chemical restraint).

protein One of a class of complex nitrogenous compounds that occur naturally in plants and animals and yield amino acids when hydrolyzed.

proteinuria An excess of serum proteins in the urine.

protocols Standard procedures.

protozoa One-celled microscopic organisms belonging to the animal kingdom.

proximal Nearest; closer to a point of reference.

prudent Sensible and careful.

psychomotor domain Learning domain in which learner processes the information by doing.

psychosocial Pertaining to both psychological and social aspects.

psychosocial theories Theories related to socialization and life satisfaction.

ptosis Drooping of the upper eyelid from paralysis of the third nerve or from sympathetic innervation.

ptyalin A form of amylase in the saliva of human beings and some animals that catalyzes the hydrolysis of starch into maltose and dextrin.

puberty Sexual maturation.

pulse deficit Deficit between the apical and radial pulse.

pulse pressure The difference between the systolic and the diastolic pressure.

purulent Containing pus.

pyrexia Fever; when a body temperature rises above 100.2° F (38.0° C).

pyrogen A substance that causes fever.

pyuria Pus in the urine.

Q

Qi Gong Type of exercise and stimulation therapy emphasizing breathing, coordination and relaxation.

quadrant Quarter.

quadriceps muscles The large muscles of the thigh.

quadriplegics Individuals who are paralyzed in all four limbs.

R

rabbi Chief religious official of a synagogue (Jewish religious temple).

race A biologic way of categorizing people based on physical characteristics, such as skin color and texture, facial characteristics, and body proportions.

radial pulse Pulse found over the radial artery in the wrist at the base of the thumb.

radiation Energy transmitted by waves through space or through some medium.

radiography The making of film records of internal structures of the body by exposure of film sensitized to x-rays.

radioimmunoassay (RIA) Use of radionuclides, following principles of immunology, to measure materials present in blood in minute amounts.

radionuclides Radioactive substances that disintegrate with the emission of electromagnetic radiation.

radiopharmaceutical A radioactive pharmaceutical substance used for diagnostic or therapeutic purposes.

rapid eye movement (REM) sleep The period of sleep during which the brain waves are fast and of low voltage, and autonomic activities (heart rate and respiration) are irregular; type of sleep associated with dreaming.

rapport A relationship of mutual trust or affinity.

reactive hyperemia A process in which the blood rushes to where there was a decrease in circulation.

reasoning The use of reason to form conclusions, inferences, or judgments; evidence or arguments used in thinking.

reciprocity Recognition of one state's nursing license in another state.

recommended daily allowances (RDAs) Recommended amounts of various nutrients for diet planning.

rectum Distal portion of the large intestine where feces are stored.

reflex An autonomic (automatic) response mediated by the nervous system and not requiring conscious movement.

Reiki Therapy in which a practitioner acts as a conduit for healing energy that is directed into the client's energy field or body.

relaxation Technique for release of tension, which is helpful in reducing pain and in allowing the patient to obtain greater relief from pain medications.

release A legal document that records the patient's permission to perform a treatment or surgery, or to give information to insurance companies or other health care providers; or a legal form to excuse one party from liability.

religion A formalized system of belief and worship.

religious Showing belief in God or a higher power.

reminiscence Reviewing one's life.

remission An abatement of the symptoms of a disease; also, the period during which such an abatement occurs.

residual urine Urine left in the bladder after urination.

residue Remains after digestion or evaporation.

respiration The exchange of oxygen and carbon dioxide in the lungs and tissues, which is initiated by the act of breathing.

respite care Nursing care allowing the caregiver time away from caregiving responsibilities.

responsibility The state of being responsible or accountable.

responsibility stage Stage of middle adulthood concerned with real-life problems and with being in charge of self and others.

retraction Inward movement of respiratory muscles upon inspiration.

return demonstration A review or patient demonstration of what has previously been learned or demonstrated.

rhonchi Continuous dry, rattling sounds heard on auscultation of the lungs; caused by partial obstruction.

Rickettsia A genus of small, rod-shaped to round microorganisms found in tissue cells of lice, fleas, ticks, and mites and transmitted to humans by their bites.

rigor mortis The stiffness that occurs in dead bodies as chemical changes take place.

Rinne test A test to compare bone and air conduction of sound, performed with a tuning fork.

risk management Putting into action policies or procedures that reduce inherent or possible risks.

ritual A ceremonial act.

routine admission Admission that is scheduled in advance.

S

sandwich generation Persons having dependent children at home and dependent elders needing care.

sanguineous Bloody.

saturated fats Fatty acids that come from animal food sources, coconut oil, and palm oil.

SBAR Situation, background, assessment, and recommendation format for accurate communication between health care professionals.

scar A mark remaining after the healing of a wound.

scientific method A step-by-step process used by scientists to solve problems.

scoliosis Pronounced lateral curvature of the spine.

sebaceous A gland that secretes an oily substance called sebum.

sebum An oily substance secreted by the sebaceous glands.

secondary illness Illness that results from or is caused by a primary illness.

second intention A type of wound healing for wounds with tissue loss, as in pressure ulcers; the wound remains open and fills with scar tissue.

selective serotonin reuptake inhibitors (SSRIs) Medications such as fluoxetine, sertraline, paroxetine, and venlafaxine, used to treat depression.

self-actualization Reaching one's full potential.

self-concept The way one views oneself.

semi-Fowler's position A position arranged by elevating the head of the bed 30 to 60 degrees and raising the knees up to 15 degrees.

sensorimotor The first cognitive stage.

sensory deficit A lack or deficiency in one of the senses.

sensory deprivation A condition in which a person receives less than normal sensory input.

sensory overload A condition in which a person receives an excessive or intolerable amount of sensory stimuli.

sentinel event An event of major gravity and importance according to The Joint Commission.

sequential multiple assay (SMA) A chemical analyzer that performs assay tests for a variety of chemical substances on a single blood or serum sample one after another.

serosanguineous Composed of serum and blood.

sexual harassment Unwelcome sexual advances, requests for sexual favors, and other verbal or physical conduct of a sexual nature.

sexual orientation Sexual preference.

sexuality The constitution of an individual in relation to sexual attitudes or activity.

shaman A member of certain tribal societies who acts as a medium between the visible world and an invisible spirit world and who practices for purposes of healing, divination, and control over natural events.

shearing force An applied force that causes a downward and forward pressure on the tissues beneath the skin.

shift report A report on the details of a patient's condition and treatment.

shock Condition of circulatory failure.

shroud A dress or garment for the dead; winding sheet.

sibling Brother or sister.

side effects Results of unintended actions.

side-lying (lateral) position When the patient is resting on his or her side.

sigmoidoscopy An examination of the sigmoid colon using a lighted instrument.

sign Any objective evidence of disease or dysfunction.

Sims' position A side-lying position in which the weight is distributed over the anterior ilium, humerus, and clavicle.

sinus A canal or passageway leading to an abscess.

skeletal muscles Striated muscles that are made of bundles of muscle fibers surrounded by a connective tissue sheath.

slander Oral (spoken) defamation.

sleep apnea Condition in which a person will stop breathing for brief periods during sleep.

sleep disorder A chronic disorder involving sleep.

sling A bandage for supporting a part.

sloughing When a layer of dead tissue separates from living tissue; to shed dead tissue.

smears Specimens for microscopic and cytologic study.

smegma The cheesy secretion of sebaceous glands, especially that found under the penile foreskin.

social competence comfort in public, ability to get along with others.

socialization The process by which society integrates the individual, and the individual learns to behave in socially acceptable ways.

solute Solid material that has been dissolved in a solution.

sore A lesion of the skin or mucous membranes.

source-oriented (narrative) charting Charting that focuses on the problems experienced by the patient as a result of being ill or on the defined nursing diagnoses reflecting those problems.

spansule A medication in the form of tiny time-release pellets within a capsule.

speculum A short, funnel-like tube for examining canals, such as the nasal canal and the vaginal canal.

sphincter Circular muscle that closes an orifice.

sphygmomanometer A device used to indirectly measure blood pressure.

spica cast Figure-of-8 cast.

spiritual distress Feelings of guilt and unworthiness, abandonment, anger, despair, or hopelessness; need to seek forgiveness; conflict between one's religious or spiritual beliefs and medical treatment.

spirituality An intangible element of religion that concerns the spirit or soul.

splint Device that protects an injured body part by immobilizing it.

spores Oval bodies formed within bacteria as a resting stage during the life cycle of the cell; characterized by resistance to environmental changes (humidity or temperature).

sputum Mucous secretions of the lungs ejected through the mouth.

stagnation Inactivity; self-absorption.

Standard Precautions Precautions that protect both the nurse and the patient from infection and are to be used for every patient contact.

standards of care (practice) Rules as defined in nursing procedure books, institutional manuals of procedures or protocols, and nursing journals that outline current skills or techniques.

standing order Order that is carried out until it is canceled by the physician or until the prescribed number of doses have been given.

stasis Stoppage of flow.

stat Immediately.

stat order An order for a single dose of a medication to be given immediately.

statute Legal term for a law.

steatorrhea Stools with an abnormally high fat content.

stereotype A set opinion or belief about a group of people that is applied to an individual.

sterile Without pathologic organisms.

sterilization The process of rendering an article free of microorganisms and their pathogenic products.

stertor Snoring sound produced when patients are unable to cough up secretions from the trachea or bronchi.

stethoscope Device that augments sound.

stoma Opening.

stool Waste eliminated from the colon.

stress The sum of biologic reactions that take place in response to any adverse stimulus.

stressor Adverse stimulus.

stricture Narrowed lumen.

stridor Shrill, harsh sound on inspiration; caused by obstruction of the upper air passages, as occurs in croup or laryngitis.

stroke volume The volume of blood pushed into the aorta per heartbeat.

subculture Smaller group within the culture whose members have similar views and goals in addition to or in place of those of the main culture.

subcutaneous Beneath the skin layers.

subjective data Data obtained orally.

sublingual Under the tongue.

sucrose Table sugar.

superego A further development of the ego that represents the moral component as postulated by Freud.

supination The act of turning the palm of the hand forward or upward.

supine position Resting on the back.

suppuration The formation of pus.

suprapubic Above the pubic bone.

surgical asepsis The practice of preparing and handling materials in a way that prevents the patient's exposure to living microorganisms.

suture A material used in closing a surgical or traumatic wound with stitches.

symmetry Equality in size, form, and arrangement of parts on opposite sides of a plane; a mirror image.

symptom Any indication of disease perceived by the patient; subjective information.

syncope Fainting.

synergistic effect Combined interaction of drugs.

systole The phase or part of the cardiac cycle when blood is pumped from the ventricles and fills the pulmonary and systemic arteries.

systolic pressure The maximum pressure exerted on the artery during left ventricular contraction.

T

tachycardia A heart rate greater than 100 beats per minute.

tachypnea Increased or rapid breathing.

tactile Pertaining to touch.

technique The method of a procedure.

temporal pulse Pulse found over the temporal artery just in front of the ear.

tenacious Adhesive, sticky.

tendons Cords of fibrous connective tissue that connect a muscle to a bone to allow for joint movement.

terminal illness Illness for which no cure is available; it ends in death, usually within a short period of time.

tertiary intention A type of wound healing; delayed or secondary closure, such as a draining abdominal wound.

tetany Continuous tonic spasm of a muscle; characterized by severe muscle cramps, carpopedal spasms, laryngeal spasms, and stridor.

thanatology The medicolegal study of the dying process and death.

theory A belief, policy, or principle proposed or followed as a basis of action.

therapeutic Having medicinal or healing properties.

therapeutic communication Communication that promotes understanding between the sender and the receiver.

therapeutic range Range or level of a drug in the blood that will produce a desired effect without causing toxic effects.

thermoregulation The regulation of heat, such as the body heat of a warm-blooded animal.

third intention A type of wound healing; delayed or secondary closure, such as a draining abdominal wound.

thoracentesis Insertion of a needle through the chest wall to the pleural space to drain fluid or air or to instill medication.

thrombophlebitis Blood clot causing inflammation of a vessel.

thrombosis Formation of a thrombus (blood clot).

time-fixed Tasks that must be done at a set time.

time-flexible Tasks that can be done any time.

time-out Quiet time alone without toys.

tinnitus A noise in the ears such as ringing, buzzing, or roaring.

topical Pertaining to a particular surface area of skin or mucous membrane.

tort A violation of civil law.

total parenteral nutrition (TPN) The technique of providing needed nutrients intravenously.

toxic effects Harmful effects.

toxicity Degree of virulence of a poison.

toxin A poison; a poisonous protein produced by certain bacteria.

tracheostomy Opening into the trachea.

traction The act of drawing or exerting a pulling force, as along the axis of a structure.

trade name Manufacturer's name for a drug or device, protected by trademark.

transcellular Secretions and excretions that move through cell membranes and eventually leave the body.

transcultural nursing Multicultural nursing care that recognizes cultural diversity and is sensitive to the needs of the patient and family.

transcutaneous electrical nerve stimulation (TENS) A form of pain treatment that uses a small electrical stimulator attached to electrodes, which serves to block pain.

transdermal Through the skin.

transducer A wand that emits sound waves.

transfer belt A sturdy belt made of tightly webbed canvas material that is used to ambulate and/or transfer the weak or unsteady patient.

transfusion The introduction of whole blood or a blood component directly into the bloodstream.

Transmission-Based Precautions Those precautions that are based on interrupting the mode of transmission by identifying the specific secretions, body fluids, tissues, or excretions that might be infective.

trapeze bar Overhead bar on a bed, which the patient can grab.

treadmill stress test A test that measures heart rate and blood pressure response to clinically controlled active exercise on a treadmill with a moving belt (a machine on which one walks while staying in one place).

tremors Involuntary fine movement of the body or limbs.

trimester A period of 3 months.

trochanter roll A roll of material used to support the upper legs and hips to prevent external rotation of the legs.

tuberculin syringe Syringe with graduated measurements to 1 mL.

tuning fork A forked metal instrument used to test hearing and the sense of vibration.

turgor Normal tension of a cell; swelling, distention; elastic condition of skin.

tympanic membrane Eardrum.

U

ultrasonography a technique in which deep structures of the body are visualized by recording the reflections (echoes) of ultrasonic waves directed into the tissues.

unconscious Insensible; incapable of responding to sensory stimuli and of having subjective experiences.

unit dose Drugs packaged in single (individual) doses.

unlicensed assistive personnel Unlicensed personnel who, after some training, perform tasks usually performed by nurses.

unsaturated fats Fatty acids that come from vegetables, nuts, or seeds.

urinary incontinence Involuntary emission of urine from the body.

urinary retention Urine retained in the bladder after voiding.

urination Expelling urine.

urinometer An instrument that measures the specific gravity (thinness or thickness) of urine.

urostomy Artificial opening on the abdomen through which urine drains.

urticaria A reaction characterized by reddened, slightly elevated patches known as wheals.

V

vagal response Activation of the vagal nerve.

Valsalva maneuver Closure of glottis and tightening of abdominal muscles after intra-abdominal pressure increases when one holds one's breath; may result in voluntary defecation.

values A measure of worth or efficiency; an ideal, custom, or institution of a society toward which the members of the group have an affective regard (emotional connection).

varicosities Swollen, distended, and knotted veins, usually in the subcutaneous tissues of the leg.

vascular access devices Devices such as needles, cannulas, or catheters that allow direct access to the circulatory system.

vasoconstriction Decrease in the caliber of blood vessels.

vasodilation Dilation of a blood vessel.

vector Carrier that transports an infective agent from one host to another, such as animals, insects, and rodents.

vegan A vegetarian diet in which all animal food sources are excluded.

vegetarian One whose diet is lacto-ovovegetarian, lacto-vegetarian, or vegan.

venesection Phlebotomy.

venipuncture Puncture of the vein with a needle.

ventilation (1) The process or act of supplying a house or room continuously with fresh air; (2) exchange of air between the lungs and atmosphere.

verbal In words; expressed orally.

vernix caseosa A cheesy, waxy substance that protects the skin in fetal life.

vertigo A sensation of rotation or whirling movement; dizziness.

vesicular sounds Soft, rustling sounds heard in the periphery of the lung fields.

viable Capable of living; able to survive outside the womb.

vial A small bottle.

virulence Degree to which a microorganism can cause infection in the host or invade the host.

viruses Extremely small particles of nucleic acids, either DNA or RNA, with a coat of protein, and in some cases a membranous envelope, that can trigger an immune reaction or damage cells in other ways.

viscous Sticky or gummy; having a high degree of viscosity or resistance to flow; thick.

visual accommodation The ability to focus on both near and far objects.

visual learning Learning through what is seen.

vital signs The signs of life, namely pulse, respiration, and temperature.

vitamin An essential nutrient that must be taken in through food sources or supplements.

vocational Related to trade, profession, or occupation.

void Excrete urine.

W

Weber test A test of bone conduction of sound performed with a tuning fork placed in the center of the forehead or the skull.

wellness A dynamic and active movement toward fulfillment of one's potential.

wheeze A high-pitched whistling sound of air forced past a partial obstruction, as found in asthma or emphysema.

whistle-blowing Reporting illegal or unethical actions.

wisdom Having good judgment based on accumulated knowledge.

worldview The perspective a culture takes of the world that is shared by cultural group members, and that influences health and illness beliefs.

wound Bodily injury caused by physical means with disruption of the skin or other structure.

Y

yang A force that is positive, light, warm, or masculine.

yin A force that is negative, dark, cold, or feminine.

yoga A Hindu discipline aimed at training the consciousness for a state of perfect spiritual insight and tranquillity; a system of exercises practiced as part of the discipline to promote control of the mind and body.

Z

Z-track technique Injection technique causing a needle track, or pathway, in the shape of a "Z."

zygote Fertilized egg.

Index

Page numbers followed by a *b* indicate boxes; *f*, figures; *t*, tables.